CORNEAL SURGERY
Theory, Technique, and Tissue

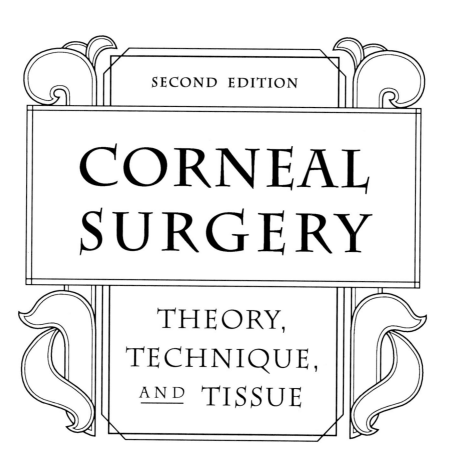

SECOND EDITION

CORNEAL SURGERY

THEORY, TECHNIQUE, AND TISSUE

Edited by

FREDERICK S. BRIGHTBILL, M.D.
Clinical Professor
Department of Ophthalmology
University of Wisconsin
Davis-Duehr Eye Associates
Madison, Wisconsin

*With **928** illustrations
including **215** color illustrations*

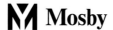 **Mosby**

St. Louis Baltimore Boston Chicago London Philadelphia Sydney Toronto

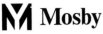 **Mosby**

Dedicated to Publishing Excellence

Editor: Laurel Craven
Managing Editor: Kathryn H. Falk
Assistant Editor: Ellen Baker Geisel
Project Manager: Mark Spann
Production Editor: Carl Masthay
Designer: David Zielinski

SECOND EDITION
Copyright © 1993 Mosby–Year Book, Inc.
A Mosby Imprint of Mosby–Year Book, Inc.

Previous edition copyrighted 1986

Printed in the United States of America

Mosby–Year Book, Inc.
11830 Westline Industrial Drive
St. Louis, Missouri 63146

Library of Congress Cataloging-in-Publication Data
Corneal surgery : theory, technique, and tissue / edited by Frederick
    S. Brightbill. — 2nd ed.
        p.   cm.
        Includes bibliographical references and index.
        ISBN 0-8016-6487-X
        1. Cornea—Surgery. 2. Cornea—Transplantation. 3. Eye banks.
    4. Keratotomy, Radial. I. Brightbill, Frederick S.
        [DNLM: 1. Cornea—surgery. 2. Eye Banks.   WW 220 C8137]
    RE336.C68   1992
    617.7'19—dc20
    DNLM/DLC
    for Library of Congress   92-23630
                                                                                    CIP

93 94 95 96 97 C/WA/WA 9 8 7 6 5 4 3 2 1

Contributors

Richard L. Abbott, M.D.
Director,
Corneal and External Disease Service,
Department of Ophthalmology,
California Pacific Medical Center,
San Francisco, California

Anthony P. Adamis, M.D.
Instructor,
Department of Ophthalmology,
Harvard Medical School,
Massachusetts Eye and Ear Infirmary,
Boston, Massachusetts

Peter J. Agapitos, M.D., F.R.C.S.C.
Assistant Professor of Ophthalmology,
University of Ottawa;
Attending Surgeon,
Ottawa Civic and Ottawa General Hospitals,
Ottawa, Canada

Patricia Aiken-O'Neill, Esq.
President and Chief Executive Officer,
Eye Bank Association of America,
Washington, D.C.

Juan J. Arentsen, M.D.
Professor of Ophthalmology,
Instituto Oftalmológico,
Santiago, Chile

Michael W. Belin, M.D.
Associate Professor of Ophthalmology,
Director, Cornea and External Disease Service,
Department of Ophthalmology,
The Albany Medical College,
Albany, New York

Sandra Belmont, M.D.
Assistant Clinical Professor,
Department of Opthalmology,
Cornell University,
New York Hospital;
Associate Attending Physician,
Manahattan Eye, Ear and Throat Hospital,
New York, New York

Roger W. Beuerman, Ph.D.
Professor,
Departments of Ophthalmology, Anatomy, and
  Psychiatry,
Louisiana State University,
New Orleans, Louisiana

Douglas W. Bond, J.D.
Attorney at Law,
Boca Raton, Florida

S. Arthur Boruchoff, M.D.
Consultant, Cornea and External Diseases;
Professor of Ophthalmology,
Boston University Medical School,
Boston, Massachusetts

William M. Bourne, M.D.
Professor of Ophthalmology,
Department of Ophthalmology,
Mayo Clinic,
Rochester, Minnesota

Frederick S. Brightbill, M.D.
Clinical Professor,
Department of Ophthalmology,
University of Wisconsin;
Davis-Duehr Eye Associates,
Madison, Wisconsin

David G. Buerger, M.D.
Department of Ophthalmology,
Wills Eye Hospital,
Philadelphia, Pennsylvania

Linda L. Burk, M.D., P.A.
Clinical Assistant Professor,
Department of Ophthalmology,
University of Texas–Southwestern,
Dallas, Texas

Douglas F. Buxton, M.D.
Assistant Clinical Director,
New York Eye and Ear Infirmary;
Assistant Attending Surgeon,
Manhattan Eye, Ear and Throat Hospital;
Clinical Assistant Professor,
New York Medical College,
New York, New York

Jorge N. Buxton, M.D.
Chief of Cornea Service,
Surgeon Director,
New York Eye and Ear Infirmary;
Clinical Professor of Ophthalmology,
New York Medical College,
New York, New York

Delmar R. Caldwell, M.D.
Professor and Chairman,
Department of Ophthalmology,
Tulane University Medical Center,
New Orleans, Louisiana

Thomas A. Casey, M.Ch., F.R.C.S., F.C.Oph
Director,
Corneo Plastic Unit and Eye Bank,
Queen Victoria Hospital,
East Grinstead,
Sussex, England

Timothy B. Cavanaugh, M.D.
Department of Ophthalmology,
St. Luke's Hospital;
Clinical Instructor,
Department of Ophthalmolgy,
University of Kansas Medical Center,
Hunkeler Eye Clinic,
Kansas City, Missouri

Mary W. Chaisson, B.A., M.Ed., J.D.
Associate,
Rumberger, Kirk & Caldwell, P.A.,
Tallahassee, Florida

John W. Chandler, M.D.
Professor and Head,
Department of Ophthalmology and Visual Sciences,
The University of Illinois at Chicago,
Chicago, Illinois

Kevin H. Charlton, M.D.
Clinical Assistant Professor,
Department of Ophthalmology,
University of Utah,
Salt Lake City, Utah

Elisabeth J. Cohen, M.D.
Professor,
Department of Ophthalmology,
Thomas Jefferson University School of Medicine;
Attending Physician, Cornea Service,
Wills Eye Hospital,
Philadelphia, Pennsylvania

J. D'Amaro, M.D., Ph.D.
Section Head, Population Genetics and Biostatistics,
Department of Immunohematology,
Leiden University,
Leiden, The Netherlands

Mary Beth Danneffel, R.N., B.S.N.
Executive Director/Manager,
Sierra Regional Eye and Tissue Bank,
University of California, Davis Medical Center,
Sacramento, California

Michael R. Deitz, M.D.
Clinical Associate Professor,
Eye Foundation of Kansas City,
University of Missouri;
Clinical Assistant Professor,
Department of Ophthalmology,
University of Kansas Medical Center,
Kansas City, Kansas

Janet DeMarchi, B.A., C.O.T., N.C.L.E.
Certified Ophthalmic Technician,
Minneapolis, Minnesota

Donald J. Doughman, M.D.
Professor,
Department of Ophthalmology,
University of Minnesota;
Chief,
Department of Ophthalmology,
Veterans Administration Hospital;
Minneapolis, Minnesota

Daniel S. Durrie, M.D.
Children's Mercy Hospital;
St. Luke's Hospital;
Eye Foundation of Kansas City,
University of Missouri;
Hunkeler Eye Clinic,
Kansas City, Missouri

Henry F. Edelhauser, Ph.D.
Ferst Professor of Ophthalmology and Director of Research,
Department of Ophthalmology,
Emory University School of Medicine,
Atlanta, Georgia

Richard A. Eiferman, M.D.
Professor of Ophthalmology and Visual Sciences,
Director, Corneal External Disease Service;
Chief, Ophthalmology,
Veterans Affairs Medical Center,
University of Louisville,
Louisville, Kentucky

Emile J. Farge, Ph.D.
Associate Professor,
Department of Ophthalmology,
Cullen Eye Institute,
Baylor College of Medicine,
Houston, Texas

Robert S. Feder, M.D.
Director, Cornea and External Disease Service,
Department of Ophthalmology,
Northwestern Memorial Hospital;
Assistant Professor of Clinical Ophthalmology,
Department of Ophthalmology,
Northwestern University,
Chicago, Illinois

S. Lance Forstot, M.D.
Clinical Professor,
Department of Ophthalmology,
University of Colorado Medical School,
Denver, Colorado

Gary N. Foulks, M.D.
Professor of Ophthalmology,
Department of Ophthalmology,
Duke University Medical Center,
Durham, North Carolina

George T. Frangieh, M.D.
Associate Professor of Ophthalmology,
Department of Ophthalmology,
Harvard Medical School;
Senior Scientist,
Schepens Eye Research Institute;
Senior Surgeon, Cornea Service,
Massachusetts Eye and Ear Infirmary,
Boston, Massachusetts

Gary E. Friedlaender, M.D.
Professor and Chairman,
Department of Orthopaedics and Rehabilitation,
Yale University School of Medicine;
Chief,
Department of Orthopaedics and Rehabilitation,
Yale–New Haven Hospital,
New Haven, Connecticut

Richard L. Fuller, B.A., M.S.W.
President and Chief Executive Officer,
Tissue Banks International—U.S. Division,
Baltimore , Maryland

Dayle H. Geroski, Ph.D.
Associate Professor,
Department of Ophthalmology,
Emory University,
Atlanta, Georgia

Thomas Gillette, M.D.
Associate Clinical Professor,
Department of Ophthalmology,
University of Washington,
Seattle, Washington

Stephen P. Ginsberg, A.B., M.D.
Ophthalmology, Sub-section chairman
Washington Adventist Hospital
Takoma Park;
Medical Director,
Kensington Eye Center,
Kensington, Maryland

David B. Glasser, M.D.
Director, Cornea/External Disease,
Patuxent Medical Group;
Clinical Associate Professor,
Department of Ophthalmology,
University of Maryland School of Medicine,
Baltimore, Maryland

John D. Gottsch, M.D.
Associate Professor of Ophthalmology,
Department of Ophthalmology,
The Wilmer Ophthalmological Institute,
The Johns Hopkins Hospital,
Baltimore, Maryland

R. Bruce Grene, M.D.
Clinical Assistant Professor,
Department of Surgery,
University of Kansas,
Wichita, Kansas

Frederick N. Griffith
President and Chief Executive Officer,
Tissue Banks International,
Baltimore, Maryland

David H. Haight, M.D.
Attending Surgeon,
Department of Ophthalmology,
Manhatten Eye, Ear and Throat Hospital,
New York, New York

J. Roger Hall, M.D.
Clinical Assistant Professor,
Department of Surgery (Ophthalmology),
University of Kansas School of Medicine at Wichita,
Wichita, Kansas

James C. Hays, M.D.
Private Practice,
Atlanta Eye Surgery Group,
Atlanta, Georgia

Ellen Heck, M.T., A.S.C.P., M.B.A.
Director,
Transplant Services Center,
University of Texas Southwestern Medical Center at Dallas,
Dallas, Texas

Peter S. Hersh, M.D.
Chairman of Ophthalmology,
Department of Ophthalmology,
Bronx-Lebanon Hospital Center;
Associate Professor of Ophthalmology,
Albert Einstein College of Medicine,
New York, New York

Michael E. Hettinger, M.D.
Department of Ophthalmology,
Shawnee Mission Medical Center,
Clinical Assistant Professor,
Department of Ophthalmology,
Kansas University Medical Center,
Kansas City, Kansas

Edward J. Holland, M.D.
Associate Professor,
Department of Ophthalmology,
Director Cornea External Disease Service,
University of Minnesota,
Minneapolis, Minnesota

Gary N. Holland, M.D.
Associate Professor of Ophthalmology,
Department of Ophthalmology,
UCLA School of Medicine,
Los Angeles, California

David S. Hull, M.D.
Professor,
Department of Ophthalmology,
Medical College of Georgia,
Augusta, Georgia

John D. Hunkeler, M.D., F.A.C.S.
Department of Ophthalmology,
St. Lukes Hospital;
Eye Foundation of Kansas City;
Associate Clinical Professor,
Department of Ophthalmology,
University of Kansas Medical Center,
Hunkeler Eye Clinic,
Kansas City, Missouri

Robert A. Hyndiuk, M.D.
Professor, Department of Ophthalmology,
Medical College of Wisconsin;
Director, Cornea–External Disease Unit,
Eye Institute,
Milwaukee County Regional Medical Center,
Milwaukee, Wisconsin

Paul S. Imperia, M.D.
Private Practice,
Rogue Valley Medical Center,
Medford, Oregon;

Michael S. Insler, M.D., J.D.
Associate Professor of Ophthalmology,
Department of Ophthalmology,
Louisiana State University,
New Orleans, Louisiana

Herbert E. Kaufman, M.D.
Boyd Professor of Ophthalmology and Pharmacology and
    Experimental Therapeutics,
Head, Department of Ophthalmology,
Director, Louisiana State University Eye Center,
Louisiana State University,
New Orleans, Louisiana

Margaret C. Kelm
Executive Director,
Wisconsin Eye Bank,
University of Wisconsin Hospital and Clinics,
Madison, Wisconsin

Kenneth R. Kenyon, M.D.
Associate Clinical Professor of Ophthalmology,
Harvard Medical School;
Surgeon in Ophthalmology, Cornea Service,
Massachusetts Eye and Ear Infirmary;
Senior Scientist,
Schepens Eye Research Institute,
Boston, Massachusetts

Natalie C. Kerr, M.D.
Department of Ophthalmology,
University of Florida, Gainesville,
Gainesville, Florida

Shigeru Kinoshita, M.D.
Chairman and Professor,
Department of Ophthalmology,
Kyoto Prefectural University of Medicine,
Kyoto, Japan

†C.C. Kok-van Alphen (Professor Dr.), M.D., Ph.D.
Department of Eurotransplant
University of Leiden
Leiden, The Netherlands

Steven B. Koenig, M.D.
Professor,
Department of Ophthalmology,
Eye Institute,
Medical College of Wisconsin,
Milwaukee, Wisconsin

Jay H. Krachmer, M.D.
Professor and Chairman,
Department of Ophthalmology,
University of Minneapolis,
Minneapolis, Minnesota

Peter R. Laibson, M.D.
Professor of Ophthalmology,
Thomas Jefferson University;
Director, Cornea Service,
Wills Eye Hospital,
Philadelphia, Pennsylvania

Ronald A. Laing, M.D.
Research Professor of Ophthalmology,
Associate Professor of Physiology,
Department of Ophthalmology,
Boston University,
Boston, Massachusetts

Stephen S. Lane, M.D.
Associate Clinical Professor,
Department of Ophthalmology,
University of Minnesota;
Assistant Chief of Ophthalmology,
Veterans Affairs Medical Center,
Minneapolis, Minnesota

Jeffrey Day Lanier, M.D., F.A.C.S.
Clinical Professor,
Department of Ophthalmology,
University of Texas Health Science Center at Houston,
Houston, Texas

Jonathan H. Lass, M.D.
Associate Professor of Ophthalmology,
Department of Ophthalmology,
Case Western Reserve University;
Co-Director, Cornea–External Disease Service,
University Hospitals of Cleveland,
Cleveland, Ohio

David H. Leach, M.D.
Corneal Fellow,
Department of Ophthalmology,
Louisiana State University,
New Orleans, Louisiana

Michael A. Lemp, M.D.
Professor,
Department of Ophthalmology,
Georgetown University Hospital,
Washington, D.C.

Jeremy E. Levenson, M.D.
Clinical Professor,
Department of Ophthalmology,
Jules Stein Eye Institute,
University of California, Los Angeles,
Los Angeles, California

Richard L. Lindstrom, M.D.
Clinical Professor,
Co-Director of the Corneal Fellowship Program,
Department of Ophthalmology,
University of Minnesota,
Minneapolis, Minnesota

Marsha A. Lisitza
Laboratory Director,
Wisconsin Eye Bank,
University of Wisconsin Hospital and Clinics,
Madison, Wisconsin

Michael J. Lynn, Ph.D.
Department of Biometry,
Emory University,
Atlanta, Georgia

Scott M. MacRae, M.D.
Associate Professor of Ophthalmology,
Department of Ophthalmology,
Casey Eye Institute,
Oregon Health Sciences University,
Portland, Oregon

Leo J. Maguire, M.D.
Associate Professor,
Department of Ophthalmology,
Mayo Clinic,
Rochester, Minnesota

†Deceased 1987.

Mark R. Mandel, M.D.
Consultant, Cornea and External Disease,
Medical-Surgical Eye Center,
Hayward, California

Sid Mandelbaum, M.D.
Associate Professor of Clinical Ophthalmology,
Albert Einstein College of Medicine,
Long Island Jewish Medical Center;
Assistant Attending Physician,
Manhattan Eye, Ear and Throat Hospital,
New York, New York

Reizo Manabe, M.D.
Professor and Chairman,
Department of Ophthalmology,
Osaka University Medical School,
Osaka, Japan

Mark J. Mannis, M.D.
Professor,
Department of Ophthalmology,
Director, Cornea–External Disease,
University of California, Davis,
Sacramento, California

Michael M. Marquette, A.F.S.E.
Supervisor,
Lions Eye Bank of Oregon,
Good Samaritan Hospital and Medical Center,
Portland, Oregon

Mamoru Matsuda, M.D.
Department of Ophthalmology,
Osaka University Medical School,
Osaka, Japan

Daniel J. Mayer, M.D.
Private Practice,
Department of Ophthalmology,
Medina General Hospital,
Southwest General Hospital,
Wadsworth-Rittman Hospital,
Medina, Ohio

Lowell H. Mays, A.B., M.Div. D.D.
Vice President and Chief Operating Officer,
The Exutec Group, Inc.
Madison, Wisconsin

Bernard E. McCarey, Ph.D.
Professor,
Department of Ophthalmology,
Emory University School of Medicine,
Atlanta, Georgia

Mark L. McDermott, M.D.
Assistant Professor,
Department of Ophthalmology,
Wayne State University,
Detroit, Michigan

Marguerite B. McDonald, M.D.
Professor of Ophthalmology,
Director, Cornea Service,
Louisiana State University Eye Center,
Louisiana State University,
New Orleans, Louisiana

George N. Meros, Jr., J.D.
Partner,
Rumberger, Kirk & Caldwell, P.A.,
Tallahassee, Florida

Roger F. Meyer, M.D.
Professor of Ophthalmology,
W.K. Kellog Eye Center,
The University of Michigan,
Ann Arbor, Michigan

Elizabeth A. Mindrup, B.S.
Scientist,
Department of Ophthalmology,
University of Minnesota,
Minneapolis, Minnesota

Thomas J. Moore, M.S.
Executive Vice President,
Lions Eye Bank Foundation,
Baylor College of Medicine,
Houston, Texas

Keith S. Morgan, M.D.
Clinical Professor of Ophthalmology,
Louisiana State University Medical Center,
New Orleans, Louisiana

W. Stanley Muenzler, M.D.
Clinical Professor of Ophthalmology,
The University of Oklahoma Health Science Center,
Oklahoma City, Oklahoma

David C. Musch, M.P.H., Ph.D.
Associate Research Scientist,
Departments of Ophthalmology and Epidemiology,
The University of Michigan,
Ann Arbor, Michigan

J. Daniel Nelson, M.D.
Chief,
Department of Ophthalmology,
St. Paul–Ramsey Medical Center and Ramsey Clinic,
St. Paul;
Associate Professor,
Department of Ophthalmology,
University of Minnesota,
Minneapolis, Minnesota

Catherine Newton, M.D.
Assistant Clinical Professor,
Department of Ophthalmology,
University of Louisville,
Louisville, Kentucky

Denis M. O'Day
Michael J. Hogan Professor of Ophthalmology,
Department of Ophthalmology,
Vanderbilt University School of Medicine;
Director,
Corneal and External Disease Service,
Vanderbilt Medical Center,
Vanderbilt University Hospital,
Nashville, Tennessee

Donna M. Oiland
Director, Lions Eye Bank,
University of Washington Medical Center,
Seattle, Washington

Timothy W. Olsen, M.D.
Research Fellow,
Department of Ophthalmology,
University of Minnesota,
Minneapolis, Minnesota

Gregory J. Pamel, M.D.
Corneal Associates of New Jersey,
St. Barnabas Medical Center,
Livingston, New Jersey

Liesbeth Pels, Ph.D.
Section Head, Cornea Bank,
The Netherlands Ophthalmic Research Institute,
Amsterdam, The Netherlands

Jay S. Pepose, M.D., Ph.D.
Associate Professor of Ophthalmology,
Department of Ophthalmology and Visual Sciences,
Washington University School of Medicine,
St. Louis, Missouri

Roswell R. Pfister, M.D., P.C.
Director, Eye Research Laboratory,
Brookwood Medical Center;
Professor of Ophthalmology,
University of Alabama, School of Medicine,
Birmingham, Alabama

Frank M. Polack, M.D.
Private Practice,
Gainesville, Florida

John T. Purcell, Jr., M.D.
Director,
Department of Ophthalmology,
St. Mary's Health Center;
Associate Clinical Professor,
Department of Ophthalmology,
St. Louis University,
St. Louis, Missouri

Peter A. Rapoza, M.D.
Cornea Consultants,
Boston;
Andover Eye Associates,
Andover;
Surgeon,
Massachusetts Eye and Ear Infirmary,
Boston, Massachusetts

William J. Reinhart, M.D.
Assistant Professor,
Department of Ophthalmology,
Case Western Reserve University,
University Hospitals, Metro Health Hospital,
Cleveland, Ohio

Jeffrey D. Robinson, M.D.
Senior Resident,
Department of Ophthalmology,
Medical College of Wisconsin–Eye Institute,
Milwaukee, Wisconsin

Caroline Bunker Rosdahl, R.N., B.S.N., M.A.
Executive Director,
Minnesota Lions Eye Bank,
Department of Ophthalmology,
University of Minnesota;
Assistant Professor,
St. Mary's Campus, College of St. Catherine,
Minneapolis, Minnesota

I. Nelson Rose, J.D.
Professor of Law,
Whittier College School of Law,
Los Angeles, California

J. James Rowsey, M.D.
Professor and Chairman,
Department of Ophthalmology,
College of Medicine,
University of South Florida,
Tampa, Florida

Fred Sanfilippo, M.D.
Director, Immunopathology,
Department of Pathology,
Duke University Hospital;
Professor,
Department of Pathology, Microbiology and
    Immunology, and Experimental Surgery,
Duke University Medical Center,
Durham, North Carolina

Mark R. Sawusch, M.D.
Clinical Assistant Professor of Ophthalmology,
Department of Ophthalmology,
University of Southern California School of Medicine,
Los Angeles, California

Bernd H. Schimmelpfennig, M.D.
Private Practice,
Zürich, Switzerland

Yvonne Schuchard, M.D.
Department of Morphology,
Cornea Bank,
The Netherlands Ophthalmic Research Institute,
Amsterdam, The Netherlands

Gregory S. Schultz, Ph.D.
Professor,
Department of Obstetrics and Gynecology,
Department of Ophthalmology,
University of Florida,
Gainesville, Florida

Ann E. Schwartz, M.D.
Assistant Professor,
Department of Ophthalmology,
University of Wisconsin,
Madison, Wisconsin

Theo W. Seiler, M.D., Ph.D.
Professor of Ophthalmology,
Universitäts-Augenklinik Charlottenburg,
Freie Universität Berlin,
Berlin, Germany

Michael B. Shapiro, M.D.
Assistant Clinical Professor,
Department of Ophthalmology,
University of Wisconsin;
Davis-Duehr Eye Associates,
Madison, Wisconsin

Edward L. Shaw, M.D.
Chairman,
Department of Ophthalmology,
St. Luke's Hospital,
Phoenix, Arizona

Neal A. Sher, M.D., F.A.C.S.
Attending Surgeon,
Phillips Eye Institute;
Clinical Associate Professor,
Department of Ophthalmology,
University of Minnesota,
Minneapolis, Minnesota

Debra L. Skelnick, B.S.
President,
Insight Biomed, Inc.,
Minneapolis, Minnesota

Ronald E. Smith, M.D.
Professor and Vice Chairman,
Department of Ophthalmology,
University of Southern California,
Los Angeles, California

Mark G. Speaker, M.D., Ph.D.
Cornea Service,
Department of Ophthalmology,
The New York Eye and Ear Infirmary;
Associate Professor,
Department of Ophthalmology,
New York Medical College,
New York, New York

Tomy Starck, M.D.
Fellow,
Department of Ophthalmology,
Massachusetts Eye and Ear Infirmary,
Harvard Medical School,
Boston, Massachusetts;
Department of Ophthalmology,
University of Texas Health Science Center,
San Antonio, Texas

Walter J. Stark, M.D.
Professor of Ophthalmology,
Director, Cornea Service,
The Wilmer Eye Institute,
Johns Hopkins Hospital,
Baltimore, Maryland

Thomas L. Steinemann, M.D.
Assistant Professor,
Department of Ophthalmology,
University of Arkansas for Medical Sciences,
Little Rock, Arkansas

Roger F. Steinert, M.D.
Associate Surgeon,
Department of Ophthalmology,
Massachusetts Eye and Ear Infirmary;
Assistant Clinical Professor,
Department of Ophthalmology,
Harvard Medical School,
Boston, Massachusetts

Kenneth D. Sterner, B.A., M.A.S.
Senior Vice President,
Tissue Distribution and Information Center,
Tissue Banks International,
Baltimore, Maryland

Mary Jayne Stevens
Executive Director,
Utah Lions Eye Bank,
University of Utah Health Sciences Center,
Department of Ophthalmology,
University of Utah,
Salt Lake City, Utah

R. Doyle Stulting, M.D.
Assistant Professor,
Department of Ophthalmology,
Emory University,
Atlanta, Georgia

Alan Sugar, M.D.
Professor of Ophthalmology,
W.K. Kellogg Eye Center,
The University of Michigan,
Ann Arbor, Michigan

Michael E. Sulewski, M.D.
Assistant Professor,
Scheie Eye Institute,
University of Pennsylvania;
Chief, Department of Ophthalmology,
Philadelphia Veterans Administration,
Philadelphia, Pennsylvania

William R. Sullivan, M.D., P.C.
Clinical Instructor,
Department of Surgery,
University of Tennessee,
Knoxville Unit,
Knoxville, Tennessee

Casimir A. Swinger, M.D.
Assistant Clinical Professor,
Department of Ophthalmology,
Mount Sinai School of Medicine of CUNY;
Park West Eye Center,
New York, New York

Emanuel Tanne, M.D.
Clinical Assistant Professor,
Department of Ophthalmology,
Oregon Health Science University;
Adjunct Associate Professor,
Department of Applied Physics and Electrical
Engineering,
Oregon Graduate Institute of Science and Technology,
Portland, Oregon

Daniel M. Taylor, M.D.
Frances E. Solomon Professor and Chairman,
Department of Ophthalmology,
University of Connecticut Health Center,
Farmington;
Grove Hill Clinic,
New Britain, Connecticut

Richard A. Thoft, M.D.
Professor and Chairman,
Department of Ophthalmology,
Montefiore University Hospital,
University of Pittsburgh,
Pittsburgh, Pennsylvania

Vance M. Thompson, M.D.
Ophthalmology Ltd.,
Sioux Falls, South Dakota

Richard C. Troutman, M.D.
Clinical Professor,
Department of Ophthalmology,
Cornell Medical Center;
Professor Emeritus,
State University of New York Downstate Medical Center;
Chief, Corneal and Refractive Surgery,
Manhattan Eye, Ear and Throat Hospital,
New York, New York

Audrey W. Tuberville, M.D.
Associate Professor,
Department of Ophthalmology,
University of Tennessee,
Center for the Health Sciences,
Memphis, Tennessee

Charles T. Valmadrid, M.D., M.P.H.
Department of Epidemiology,
Johns Hopkins University,
School of Hygiene and Public Health;
Tissue Banks International,
Baltimore, Maryland

Emily D. Varnell, B.S.
Assistant Professor,
Department of Ophthalmology,
Louisiana State University,
New Orleans, Louisiana

Margaret S. Verble, Ed.D.
President,
Verble, Worth & Verble, Instructional Consultants,
Lexington, Kentucky

Richard A. Villaseñor, M.D.
Associate Clinical Professor,
Department of Ophthalmology,
University of Southern California,
Los Angeles, California

H.J. Völker-Dieben, M.D., Ph.D.
Senior Ophthalmic Surgeon,
Department of Ophthalmology,
Diaconessenhuis-Leiden;
Honorary Member,
Netherlands Ophthalmic Research Institute,
University of Amsterdam,
Leiden, The Netherlands

George O. Waring III, M.D., F.A.C.S.
Professor,
Director of Refractive Surgery,
Department of Ophthalmology,
Emory University,
Atlanta, Georgia

Mark J. Weiner, M.D.
Chief, Department of Ophthalmology,
R.T. Jones Regional Hospital;
Weiner Eye Center,
Canton, Georgia

Theodore P. Werblin, M.D., P.C.
Department of Ophthalmology/Surgery,
Princeton Community Hospital,
Princeton, West Virginia;
Clinical Associate Professor,
Department of Ophthalmology,
University of Virginia,
Charlottesville, Virginia

José A. Westphalen, M.D.
Cornea and External Disease Fellow,
New York Eye and Ear Infirmary,
New York, New York;
Attending Surgeon,
Department of Ophthalmology,
Hospital São Vicente de Paulo,
Rio de Janeiro, RJ, Brazil

Peter Y. Windt, Ph.D.
Associate Professor,
Department of Philosophy,
University of Utah,
Salt Lake City, Utah

Thomas O. Wood, M.D.
Professor,
Department of Ophthalmology,
University of Tennessee;
Baptist Memorial Hospital Central;
Memphis, Tennessee

Judy K. Worth, M.A.
Partner,
Verble, Worth & Verble, Instructional Consultants,
Lexington, Kentucky

TO
CALVIN C. COVERT
Chairman of the Board and Chief Executive Officer
Woodward Governor Company
Rockford, Illinois
Corneal transplant recipient and
dedicated friend of Eye Banking
and
To the eye bank professionals and
volunteers throughout the world who
serve to bring the gift of sight to others

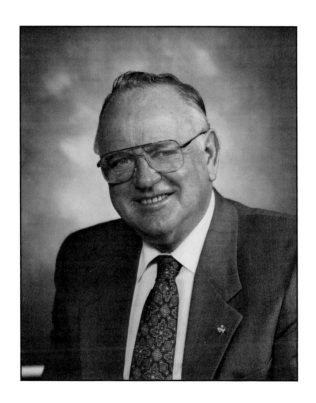

Preface

The first edition of *Corneal Surgery: Theory, Technique, and Tissue* evolved from the first International Cornea and Eye Banking Symposium held in San Diego, California, in 1985 and quickly became a standard reference for corneal surgeons and eye banks throughout the world.

This second edition, in my opinion, represents a significant step up. Although nearly all retained chapters and subchapters have been revised by their authors, 16 chapters and subchapters from the first edition have been omitted and replaced with 35 entirely new chapters. The book features 33 new contributing first authors and three entirely new subsections including (1) concepts of corneal function applicable to surgery, (2) non–laser refractive keratoplasty, and (3) refractive surgery with lasers.

The research section in the first edition has been deleted and those topics of most interest integrated into the main text. The sections on medical and administrative aspects of eye banking have been consolidated and include the completely updated 1992 Medical Standards of the Eye Bank Association of America (EBAA).

In an effort to allow for expansion of the textbook, limit its purchase price, and include 215 colored illustrations, The Woodward Governor Company Charitable Trust of Rockford, Illinois, has again donated a large sum of money to defray costs. For this generosity I believe we owe an unending debt of gratitude. All proceeds from this book will again be donated to the Eye Bank Association of America.

I wish to express my thanks to the EBAA, its officers, and members for their work and confidence in me. The primary force behind this effort has been The Wisconsin Eye Bank and the cooperation I have received from Margaret Kelm, Executive Director. Jan Hyland provided outstanding secretarial assistance over the 2-year period of this project. Others who assisted in the project whom I wish to thank include Marsha Lisitza, Dr. Courtney W. Moffatt, Linda Taylor, Gundega Korsts, and Kim Thomas.

Kathy Falk, Ellen Baker Geisel, and others at Mosby–Year Book provided the professional support and personal encouragement that allowed me to persevere during this project. Indeed, I would be remiss if I failed to recognize my unending respect for Carl Masthay, whose linguistic ability and attention to detail once again brightens these pages.

Finally, I wish to express my sincere appreciation to the book's many contributors whose chapters speak for themselves. The ophthalmologic community will certainly be more informed through your efforts. Congratulations and thanks!

Frederick S. Brightbill, M.D.
Editor
Madison, Wisconsin

Contents

Part I

CONCEPTS OF CORNEAL FUNCTION APPLICABLE TO SURGERY

Chapter 1

The Preocular Tear Film in Corneal Grafting

MICHAEL A. LEMP

The production, distribution, and maintenance of adequate tear film is essential for the establishment and renewal of a normal corneal and conjunctival surface. The intimate relationship between the preocular tear film and the corneal surface is well recognized. The successful healing of a corneal graft requires epithelial resurfacing, in addition to stromal and endothelial healing. The role of the preocular tear film in facilitating epithelial renewal and healing is further complicated by innervational and topographic variations after penetrating keratoplasty. A review of factors important in the formation and maintenance of tear film, a discussion of tear film abnormalities, and the factors important in the renewal of the ocular surface (a more detailed description of ocular surface physiology is contained in another chapter) are presented. Finally, special considerations in the corneal grafting circumstance are discussed in detail.

STRUCTURE, FORMATION, AND MAINTENANCE OF THE TEAR FILM

The preocular tear film provides an environment essential for the normal structure and function of the corneal and conjunctival epithelium.[14] The tear film fills in and smoothes out spaces caused by reticulations on the epithelial surface 0.5 μm high and 0.3 μm wide.[18] The tear film then acts as the anterior refracting surface of the eye, preventing image degradation that would otherwise occur as a result of these reticulations. The tear film is approximately 7 μm in thickness. The structure of the tear film is three layered: the outermost lipid layer of secretion of the meibomian glands of the lid, the intermediate aqueous layer, which is produced by secretion of the main and accessory lacrimal glands, and the innermost mucin layer.[39] The mucin layer is believed to consist of two parts, that is, the inner glycocalyx produced by the epithelial cells and the outer, more loosely bound mucin blanket produced by the goblet cells of the conjunctiva.[30]

Aqueous tears are secreted at a rate of approximately 1.2 μl/min.[29] The secretion from the main accessory and lacrimal glands appears to be identical. The number of accessory lacrimal glands varies considerably from one individual to another. All aqueous tear secretion appears to be reflex driven.[15] The aqueous component of tears provides over 90% of the thickness of the tear film.[3] Aqueous tears are secreted as an isotonic or slightly hypotonic solution. The flow of aqueous tears originates in ductular openings of the main and accessory lacrimal glands. The fluid flows through the forniceal spaces into the lacrimal rivers and over the exposed portions of the corneal and conjunctival surface. The flow of aqueous fluid is from temporal to medial and is driven by the action of the orbicularis oculi muscle. The fluid is drawn into the two punctal openings in a relaxation phase immediately subsequent to a blink. Some aqueous fluid is lost through evaporation and reabsorption through the conjunctival surface, but the majority of fluid flows out through the punctal openings into the canaliculi, the lacrimal sac, the nasolacrimal duct, and then into the inferior meatus in the nasal cavity.[6,25] There is, however, considerable reabsorption of fluid across the mucosa of the nasolacrimal duct.

The lipid layer of the tear film consists of the material secreted by the meibomian glands of the lids. There are approximately 20 meibomian glands in each upper and lower lid. The factors controlling secretion rates from meibomian glands are poorly understood. The lipids of the meibomian glands, however, are made up of a variety of lipid entities, including primarily nonpolar sterol and waxy esters. The lipid excreta as a liquid flows onto the aqueous preocular tear film and spreads quickly to form a "duplex" film. During blinking, this lipid layer undergoes considerable compression and decompression. This layer is characterized by a high degree of stability. The lipid layer serves to retard evaporation from the tear film, prevent contamination of the tear film by the more polar liquids secreted by the sebaceous glands of the eyelids, and lowers the surface tension of tears, which, in turn, draws water into the tear film and thickens the aqueous phase.[12]

The mucin layer consists mostly of mucous (hydrated) glycoproteins associated with a mixture of protein, electrolytes, and cellular material. The innermost component of the mucin layer is tightly bound to the epithelial surface and is believed to constitute a glycocalyx secreted by subsurface epithelial vesicles.[10,30] Above this is a much looser "mucus blanket," believed to be the product of the goblet cells of the conjunctiva. The difference in the physical chemical properties of these two components of the mucin layer has not been well studied. The outer mucin layer, however, does form a tenuous covering over epithelial cells, which is important in enabling the overlying aqueous layer to provide a continuous covering. It is believed that a tenuous hydrophilic surface is produced by the mucin component though the exact nature of the epithelial surface and its relationship to the overlying mucin layer remains an area of controversy.

Key to the formation and maintenance of preocular tear film is the action of the lids. The upper lid moves over an area covering approximately three fourths of the surface of the cornea. The lower lid does not move much and has considerably less force than the upper lid. The upper lid serves to distribute the tear film and provides a shearing force against the corneal surface. The action of the lid by periodic blinking is necessary to reestablish tear film, which tends to disruption between blinks secondary to evaporation and thinning of the tear film. If blinking is prevented or is incomplete, dry spots develop within the tear film because of contamination of the mucin layer by overlying lipid. The aqueous layer then retracts from these areas, causing large areas of discontinuity in the tear film and subse-

quent drying of the epithelium.[13] It is essential for all elements of tear production and distribution in the ocular surface to be intact to maintain a normal preocular tear film and provide the environment essential for a normal ocular surface.

TEAR-FILM ABNORMALITIES

The term "dry eye" is a rubric to describe a variety of ocular conditions characterized by a disturbance in the preocular tear film and sharing signs of ocular surface abnormalities. These conditions are of diverse pathogenesis and include decreased aqueous tear secretion, abnormalities of conjunctival mucin secretion, dysfunction of the meibomian glands of the lids, lid surfacing abnormalities, and primary ocular surface epithelial abnormalities. Based on the considerations discussed earlier, I have devised a classification of tear abnormalities.[14] Although there is some overlap between these categories, each of the deficiency states is characterized by a breakdown in one of the essential mechanisms described earlier.

Aqueous Tear Deficiency (Keratoconjunctivitis Sicca, KCS). Aqueous tear deficiency is probably the most common cause of tear film abnormalities in the developed world. Although there are rare forms of aqueous tear deficiencies such as familial dysautonomia (Riley-Day syndrome) and congenital alacrima, the most common form of aqueous tear deficiency occurs with increasing frequency with advancing age. Tear secretion diminishes with age, and in some individuals there is an exaggeration of this process. This condition occurs most commonly in the fifth decade of life and later. The most common symptoms are ocular irritation, burning, or foreign-body sensation. This condition occurs with particularly high prevalence in women. The most commonly observed clinical signs include increased debris in the tear film, a scanty marginal tear strip, increased mucus threads within the tear film, particularly in the inferior fornix, decreased wetting of Schirmer test strips, and staining of the exposed portions of the corneal and conjunctival surfaces with Rose Bengal stain. More severe cases can progress to a debilitating filamentary keratitis. Eyes with KCS are particularly susceptible to infection. There is a breakdown in several aspects of the normal ocular surface defense mechanisms, including a decrease in enzymes within the tears, that is, lysozyme, betalysine, and lactoferrin, and the flushing action of the tears is impaired. There is a high prevalence of concomitant lid infections of patients with KCS, and this can lead to more serious infections of the ocular surface, including conjunctivitis and keratitis.

Although most cases of KCS occur in the absence of any other overt systemic abnormality, there is a frequent association of KCS with systemic disease. The prevalence of KCS in women, particularly in the menopausal and postmenopausal age groups, is suggestive of a relationship to hormonal changes. Recent studies have identified hormonal receptors in the lacrimal glands[13] and changes in the morphology of conjunctival surface cells in association with the menstrual cycle.[19]

The most common association of KCS with systemic disease has been with collagen vascular disorders. A variety of systemic autoimmune diseases has been associated with the development of dry eye. Approximately 14% to 15% of patients with rheumatoid arthritis have KCS. When KCS occurs as part of a larger systemic abnormality, it is referred to as "Sjögren's syndrome." Primary Sjögren's syndrome is the association of dry eye, dry mouth, and other systemic inflammatory abnormalities in the absence of a defined systemic disease. When a specific systemic disease is present, the condition is referred to as "secondary Sjögren's syndrome." In these patients, there is a tendency for more severe aqueous tear deficiency, and there is evidence that there is a primary inflammatory abnormality of the ocular surface that is immunogenic in origin. This subset of patients with Sjögren's syndrome represents a more severe type of dry eye, and these patients are prone to more severe complications of the disease process, including associations with scleritis, rheumatoid nodules of the sclera, and peripheral corneal ulceration, which can sometimes lead to perforation. KCS is usually a bilateral disease.

Mucin Deficiency. In contrast to the previously described aqueous-deficient dry-eye states, there exists a group of conditions that are characterized primarily by changes in the conjunctival morphology, leading to a decrease in conjunctival goblet cells and, in turn, an instability of the tear film. Several conditions adversely affect the goblet cell population of the conjunctiva. These include hypovitaminosis A, cicatricial ocular pemphigoid, erythema multiforme, chemical burns, and other severe inflammatory conditions affecting the conjunctiva, such as trachoma.

Vitamin A deficiency represents the prototype of the mucin-deficient process. It is characterized by a dropout of goblet cells and the appearance of areas of nonwettability on the conjunctival and corneal surface. Further development of this condition leads to keratinization of both the cornea and conjunctiva. There is a rapid breakup of the tear film, even in the absence of adequate aqueous tear production. In more severe cases, the scarring that occurs occludes the opening of the main and accessory lacrimal gland ductules, giving rise to a secondary aqueous tear deficiency.[20,23]

Lipid Abnormalities. The problems associated with this condition are those of glandular dysfunction rather than glandular absence. Congenital anhidrotic ectodermal dysplasia is a rare condition associated with the absence of the meibomian gland openings. More commonly, however, meibomian gland dysfunction is associated with abnormalities of excreta thickness and volume of meibomian glands. In more pronounced cases, an obstructive meibomian gland dysfunction occurs with a decreased volume of excreta, which results in an increase in tear film osmolarity, probably associated with accelerated evaporation from the ocular surface. This can in turn give rise to a type of "pseudo–dry eye state."[22] Secondary infection of the meibomian glands, usually with staphylococci, further complicates this problem, leading to tear film instability and punctate epitheliopathy of the cornea and conjunctiva.

Lid Surfacing Abnormalities. The tear film must be continually reformed by blinking, since it is inherently unstable. When normal lid movement is compromised, the area of the cornea and conjunctiva not covered by the excursion of the upper lid represents a well-defined area of nonwetting, resulting in local desiccation. Eventually, secondary changes (keratinization) will occur in the desiccated epithelium, making the area even less wettable.

Localized drying is seen in lesions of the seventh cranial nerve and is referred to as "exposure keratitis." Lid movement can also be restricted by the presence of symblepharons, which are particularly prominent in cicatrizing ocular pemphigoid, erythema multiforme, and chemical burns. Successful maintenance of the preocular tear film also presupposes a reasonable congruity between the lids and the ocular surface in order to produce sufficient and uniform shear. In the absence of proper apposition between the lid and the ocular surface, the shear diminishes, and the tear layer is not surfaced properly.

Epitheliopathy. Because of the intimate relationship between the corneal surface and the tear film, alterations in the normal morphology of the epithelium can affect the stability of the tear film. The corneal epithelium is normally thrown into multiple microvillous projections, allowing for more adsorptive sites for tear mucin. Abnormalities in the morphology of the corneal surface give rise to problems in tear surfacing that lead to desiccation, epithelial breakdown, and frank ulceration. Nervous innerva-

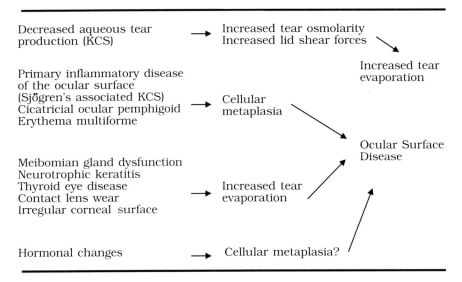

Fig. 1-1. Factors causing dry eye symptoms. (From Lemp MA: *The dry eye: a comprehensive guide*, New York, 1992, Springer-Verlag.)

tion of the cornea is essential in maintaining corneal integrity. Corneal anesthesia frequently results in corneal epithelial abnormalities ranging from superficial punctate erosions and coarse mucus plaques to corneal ulceration, melting, and even perforation.

There are multiple factors in the production of ocular surface disease in dry eye states. These include desiccation secondary to decreased aqueous tear production, increased evaporation from the tear film, decreased lubricity between the upper lid and the ocular surface, resulting in an increased shearing force and abrasive effect, cellular metaplasia of the conjunctival surface, particularly in patients with Sjögren's syndrome, hormonal changes in menopausal and postmenopausal women, primary inflammatory disease of the ocular surface, particularly in patients with Sjögren's syndrome, and, finally, associated conditions such as meibomian gland dysfunction.

It is probable that the origin of ocular surface disease differs in different dry eye states and is, in many of them, multifactorial. Fig. 1-1 displays a schema listing the factors resulting in ocular surface disease giving rise to dry eye symptoms.[22]

RENEWAL OF THE OCULAR SURFACE

Corneal epithelial cells (and, by implication, conjunctival epithelial cells, though less is known about their life cycle) are in a continual state of renewal. There is a gradual upward and outward movement of new cells starting in the basal cell layer until the cells reach the surface; this movement ultimately culminates in sloughing (exfoliation) of dead cells from the surface. The average life cycle of a new epithelial cell is from 3½ to 7 days.[11] The mitotic activity in the central corneal area is insufficient, however, to keep up with the loss of cells from the ocular surface. Over the past two decades, attention has focused on the limbal area of the cornea as a major regenerative site for epithelial cells.[5] The limbal area, an annular band of tissue approximately 1 mm in width and surrounding the cornea proper, is characterized by deep subepithelial outpouchings of richly vascularized papillae, the palisades of Vogt.[9] Between the papillae are numerous invaginations of goblet cell–free epithelial cells. There are a variety of clinical conditions in which a streaming of epithelial cells from the periphery to the surface becomes evident when the epithelial cells become visible by an accumulation of pigment, iron, or metabolic products. Bron has postulated that this represents a sliding of cells reflective of a general radial centripetal movement from the limbus to the corneal center.[2]

More recent studies employing a variety of methodologies, including intracellular markers, chemical studies, morphologic studies, in vitro growth studies, and monoclonally produced keratin-specific antibodies have all pointed to the limbal area as a critical area for epithelial cell regeneration.[4,7,33,34,37] It is believed that epithelial cells undergo intensive cell division in the limbal area and migrate centrally forming swirling, radiating lines, which give rise to vortex patterns. These are usually not visible because of the transparency of corneal tissue, but given an accumulation of substances within epithelial cells in a variety of clinical conditions such as Fabry's disease, toxic keratopathies such as those occurring with chloroquine and amiodarone therapy, striate melanokeratosis, healing corneal abrasions, band keratopathy, and corneal edema, this vortex pattern can be evident by slitlamp examination.[2]

Recent studies employing specular microscopy have indicated that at least one of the driving forces in the centripetal movement of epithelial cells may be a preferential exfoliative loss of cells from the central cornea driven by the shearing force of the upper lid.[21,24] The upper lid is capable of considerable posterior force on the corneal surface; presumably this is greatest near the corneal apex, giving rise to a preferential loss of cells in the central cornea. In conditions such as keratoconjunctivitis sicca, this process appears to be accentuated.

SPECIAL CONSIDERATIONS IN CORNEAL GRAFTING

The healing of the grafted cornea is dependent not only on stromal and endothelial healing, but also on healing of the epithelial surface of the graft. The fate of donor epithelium is somewhat unclear. There is some evidence of early sloughing and replacement by the recipient epithelium, at least in moist chamber-stored whole donor eyes.[38] On the other hand, tests with animal models indicate that donor epithelium can be retained for long periods, and slitlamp observations of donor epithelial rejection support the notion that donor epithelium can remain on the graft surface for many months.[1,16,17]

The movement of epithelial cells from the limbal area to the center of the newly grafted cornea presents a special set of circumstances that may well deviate from the normal significantly. Indeed, a variety of epithelial abnormalities are noted clinically in the corneal graft. These changes can range from mild superficial punctate erosions, epithelial dots, microcysts and filaments, to pronounced vortex keratopathy and frank epithelial defects.[26,28,32] Many of these changes disappear with time, particularly after suture removal.

Epithelial surfacing problems may occur even in recipient diseases, such as keratoconus, under special circumstances. Topographic irregularities in the corneal surface and annular depressions just central to the placement of long or tight sutures may interfere with shearing forces of the lid on the surface of the eye and limit epithelial cell renewal and centripetal movement of cells. Kaye [16] has reported the frequent occurrence of multiple intraepithelial white dots within annular depressions, which may persist until suture removal. Subsequently, they move over a period of weeks toward the center of the eye before disappearing.

The grafted cornea remains in a state of denervation for some time after surgery.[35] When corneal sensitivity does return, it is slow and may occur centrally in a graft as early as 18 months after surgery.[27] Other grafts, however, show no central return of sensation, even up to 32 years after keratoplasty.[31] This persistent lack of corneal sensitivity may give rise to epithelial abnormalities. The tear film itself may reflect surfacing abnormalities associated with topographic differences and epithelial abnormalities associated with denervation.

The prognosis for a successful corneal graft decreases in those conditions associated with significant abnormalities of the tear film and ocular surface, such as keratoconjunctivitis sicca, ocular pemphigoid, Stevens-Johnson syndrome (erythema multiforme), chemical burns, and severe ocular inflammatory states, particularly those that have destroyed a significant percentage of tissue in the limbal area.

Complete corneal denervation is generally considered, in itself, an absolute contraindication to penetrating keratoplasty. Partial degrees of denervation resulting in decreased but still present corneal sensation can be associated with successful keratoplasty, as after corneal scarring from zoster ophthalmicus. Each of these conditions must be approached carefully and individually. Several strategies have been designed to increase the likelihood of success in dealing with these problems. After chemical burns in which most of the regenerative area of the limbus has been destroyed, transplantation of normal limbal tissue from a contralateral normal eye or even from cadavers has been advocated and tried with some success.[36] Preoperative treatment of active problems such as meibomian gland dysfunction with lid hygiene and systemic broad-spectrum antibiotics, such as tetracycline or doxycycline, can be very helpful. In some recipient conditions in which there is a problem with the ocular surface or tear film, the use of a partial tarsorrhaphy at the time of surgery may be very helpful in protecting the corneal graft surface. Presumably the tarsorrhaphy works by (1) decreasing the exposed surface of the eye and thereby decreasing evaporation, (2) providing a steady proximity of the conjunctival blood vessels to the ocular surface (though decreased oxygenation can be a problem, and there are those who argue against complete tarsorrhaphies for this reason), and (3) an immobilization of the lid neutralizing the shearing force of the upper lid against the ocular surface.

A careful assessment of the condition of the tear film and the ocular surface is essential before a decision is made to perform a keratoplasty. Careful evaluation and planning of strategies to create the most favorable environment for the healing of the ocular surface to occur will greatly increase the likelihood of success in corneal grafting.

REFERENCES

1. Alldredge OC, Krachmer JH: Clinical types of corneal transplant rejection, *Arch Ophthalmol* 99:599-604, 1981.
2. Bron AJ: Vortex patterns of the corneal epithelium, *Trans Ophthalmol Soc UK* 93:455-472, 1973.
3. Bron AJ: Prospects for the dry eye, *Trans Ophthalmol Soc UK* 104:801-826, 1985.
4. Buck RC: Hemidesmosomes of normal and regenerating mouse corneal epithelium, *Virchows Arch Cell Pathol* 41:1-16, 1982.
5. Davenger M, Evensen A: Role of pericorneal papillary structure in renewal of the corneal epithelium, *Nature* 229:560-561, 1971.
6. Doane MG: Blinking and the mechanics of the lacrimal drainage system, *Ophthalmology* 88:844-851, 1982.
7. Ebato B, Friend J, Thoft RA: Comparison of central and peripheral human corneal epithelium in tissue culture, *Invest Ophthalmol Vis Sci* 28:1450-1456, 1987.
8. Frey WH, Nelson JD, Frink ML, Elde RP: Prolactin immunoreactivity in human tears and lacrimal gland: possible implications for tear production in the preocular tear film. In Holly FJ, editor: *The preocular tear film in health, disease and contact lens wear*, Lubbock, Texas, 1986, The Dry Eye Institute.
9. Goldberg MF, Bron AJ: Limbal palisades of Vogt, *Trans Am Ophthalmol Soc* 80:155-169, 1982.
10. Greiner JV, Weidman TA, Korb DR, Allansmith MR: Histochemical analysis of secretory vesicles in non-goblet conjunctival cells, *Acta Ophthalmol* 63:89-92, 1985.
11. Hanna C, O'Brien JE: Cell production and migration in the epithelial layer of the cornea, *Arch Ophthalmol* 64:536-539, 1960.
12. Holly FJ: Formation and rupture of the tear film, *Exp Eye Res* 15:515-524, 1973.
13. Holly FJ, Lemp MA: Wettability and wetting of the corneal epithelium, *Exp Eye Res* 11:239-250, 1971.
14. Holly FJ, Lemp MA: Tear physiology and dry eyes, *Surv Ophthalmol* 22:69-87, 1977.
15. Jordan A, Baum JL: Basic tear flow, does it exist? *Ophthalmology* 87:920-930, 1980.
16. Kaye DB: Epithelial response in penetrating keratoplasty, *Am J Ophthalmol* 89:381-387, 1980.
17. Kinoshita S, Friend J, Thoft RA: Sex chromatin of donor corneal epithelium in rabbits, *Invest Ophthalmol Vis Sci* 21:434-441, 1981.
18. Klyce SD, Beuerman RW: Structure and function of the cornea. In Kaufman HE et al, editors: *The cornea*, New York, 1988, Churchill Livingstone.
19. Kramer P, Lubkin V, Potter W, et al: Cyclic changes in conjunctival smears from menstruating females, *Ophthalmology* 97:303-307, 1990.
20. Lemp MA: The mucin-deficient dry eye. In Holly FJ, Lemp

MA, editors: *The preocular tear film and dry eye syndrome*, International Ophthalmology Clinics 13:185-189, Boston, 1973, Little, Brown.
21. Lemp MA: The surface of the corneal graft: in vivo color specular microscopic study in the human, *Trans Am Ophthalmol Soc* 87:619-657, 1989.
22. Lemp MA: Basic principles and classification of dry eye disorders. In *The dry eye—a practical guide to the diagnosis and treatment of the dry eye*, New York, Springer-Verlag. (In press.)
23. Lemp MA, Dohlman CH, Holly FJ: Corneal desiccation despite normal tear volume, *Ann Ophthalmol* 2:258-261, 1970.
24. Lemp MA, Mathers WD: Corneal epithelial cell movement in humans, *Eye* 3:438-445, 1989.
25. Lemp MA, Weiler HH: How do tears exist? *Invest Ophthalmol Vis Sci* 24:619-622, 1983.
26. Mackman GS, Polack FM, Sychys L: Hurricane keratitis in penetrating keratoplasty, *Cornea* 2:31-34, 1983.
27. Mathers WD, Jester JV, Lemp MA: Return of human corneal sensitivity in grafts following penetrating keratoplasty, *Ophthalmology* 92:1408-1411, 1988.
28. Mathers WD, Lemp MA: Vortex keratopathy of the corneal graft, *Cornea* 10:93-99, 1991.
29. Mishima S: Some physiological aspects of the precorneal tear film, *Arch Ophthalmol* 73:233-241, 1965.
30. Nichols BA, Chiappino ML, Dawson CL: Demonstration of mucus layer of the tear film by electron microscopy, *Invest Ophthalmol Vis Sci* 26:464-473, 1985.
31. Rao GN, John T, Ishida N, et al: Recovery of corneal sensitivity in grafts following penetrating keratoplasty, *Ophthalmology* 92:1408-1411, 1985.
32. Rotkis WM, Chandler JW, Forstot SL: Filamentary keratitis following penetrating keratoplasty, *Ophthalmology* 89:946-949, 1982.
33. Schirmer A, Galvin S, Sun T-T: Differentiation-related expression of a major 64K corneal keratin in vivo and in culture suggests limbal location of corneal epithelium stem cells, *J Cell Biol* 103:49-62, 1986.
34. Shapiro MS, Friend J, Thoft RA: Corneal re-epithelialization from the conjunctiva, *Invest Ophthalmol* 21:135-142, 1981.
35. Skriver K: Reinnervation of the corneal graft, *Acta Ophthalmol* 56:1013-1015, 1978.
36. Thoft RA: Conjunctival transplantation, *Arch Ophthalmol* 95:1425-1427, 1977.
37. Thoft RA, Friend J: Biochemical transformation of regenerating ocular surface epithelium, *Invest Ophthalmol* 16:14-20, 1977.
38. Thoft RA, Friend J, Freedman H, et al: Corneal epithelial preservation, *Arch Ophthalmol* 93:357-361, 1975.
39. Wolff E: Anatomy of the eye and orbit, ed 4, New York, 1954, Blakiston & Co, pp. 207-209.

Chapter 2

Ocular Surface Maintenance

RICHARD A. THOFT

The concept of the ocular surface and its diseases and therapy were introduced by Thoft and Friend, nearly 14 years ago.[13] At that time, there were ample histologic and biochemical data to distinguish the conjunctival epithelium from the corneal epithelium but little reason to be suggestive of a consolidation of these two areas into a single biologic continuum. The term "ocular surface" emphasized the emerging realization that these two portions of the ocular covering are not entirely independent but that the cornea, at least, depends on the health of the conjunctiva for its own well-being.

The current definition of the "ocular surface" refers to the epithelial and subepithelial tissues that cover the globe and adnexae, beginning at the gray line at the lid margin, extending over the back of the lids into the fornices, reflecting back up over the globe to the limbus, and extending to and covering the cornea. Included are the subjacent connective tissue of the conjunctiva, since the subepithelial regions are the locus of many of the important pathologic processes that affect the surface.

As originally defined, disease as well as trauma of the ocular surface is present when there is concurrent involvement of both the conjunctival and corneal surfaces. This definition excludes conditions that are localized to only one of the regions. Examples of this are the recurrent erosion syndrome, which, as far as is known, only affects the cornea, and bacterial conjunctivitis, which seems to have no primary effect on the cornea. For simplicity, the term "ocular surface disease" has been restricted to those conditions that are noninfectious. Therefore epidemic keratoconjunctivitis involving both the cornea and conjunctiva has not been grouped into the class of ocular surface diseases, even though such inclusion would be entirely plausible.

The following box lists those conditions that fall easily into the category of ocular surface disease.

CHARACTERISTICS OF OCULAR SURFACE DISORDERS

Characteristic of the ocular surface disorders is a tendency for vascularization of the cornea with accompanying scarring. The autoimmune phenomena and trauma manifest significant scarring in the fornices, which is the forerunner of lid distortion, trichiasis, and, in the late stages, decrease in tear secretion.

A detailed description of the histologic changes that accompany the autoimmune phenomena is beyond the scope of this article. Such descriptions are available in the work of Foster[3] and Mondino and Brown,[8] who amplified earlier descriptions of

---

OCULAR SURFACE DISORDERS

Probable autoimmune diseases
    Ocular cicatricial pemphigoid
    Stevens-Johnson syndrome
    Atopic keratoconjunctivitis
Chemical or thermal trauma
Radiation keratoconjunctivitis
Aniridia
Contact lens–induced keratopathy
Superior limbic keratoconjunctivitis (SLK)

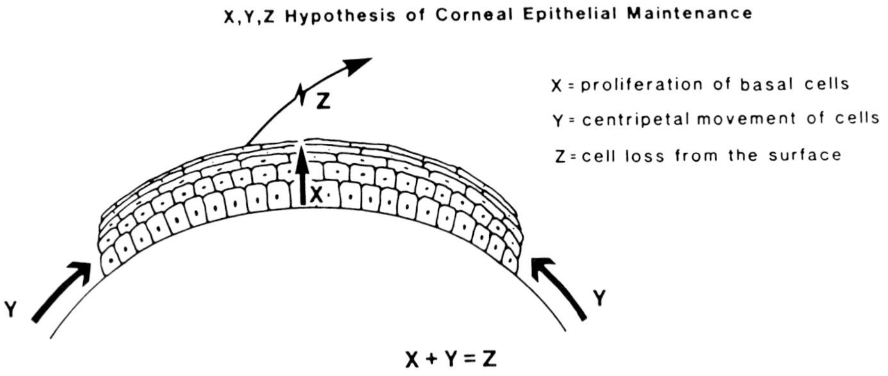

X,Y,Z Hypothesis of Corneal Epithelial Maintenance

X = proliferation of basal cells

Y = centripetal movement of cells

Z = cell loss from the surface

X + Y = Z

Fig. 2-1. The X, Y, Z hypothesis of corneal epithelial maintenance.

Andersen and co-workers.[2] One of the characteristics, the thickening of the epithelial cells, has been related to a hyperproliferation of the epithelial cells.[19]

Another feature of the autoimmune and atopic diseases is the presence of squamous metaplasia. This abnormality has been emphasized by Tseng and co-workers and has been used as a measure of the well-being of those cells.[20] The measurement of squamous metaplasia has been achieved by evaluation of impression cytology of superficial cells removed with a variety of porous surfaces, the most common one being that of a Millipore filter.[9] This method has not received wide application because of the difficulty in obtaining consistent values. Nevertheless the technique has highlighted the abnormality of surface differentiation in the ocular surface disorders.

Another important feature of the ocular surface disorders is their propensity for corneal persistent epithelial defect (PED) formation. These defects can be acute, as in the case of traumatic events, or can be chronic, as in the case of radiation keratitis, aniridia, and autoimmune phenomena, or contact lens–induced keratopathy. PED presents the most compelling need for therapeutic intervention in most of these disorders, though the defect formation may not ultimately be as serious as the scarring and loss of tears.

THE X, Y, Z HYPOTHESIS OF CORNEAL EPITHELIAL MAINTENANCE

One of the hypotheses that has served an important role in the formulation of an understanding of ocular surface disease is the X, Y, Z hypothesis published by Thoft and Friend in 1983.[18] As diagrammed in Fig. 2-1, maintenance of the corneal epithelial cell mass is believed to represent the balance of three separate variables.

In this diagram, X represents basal cell prolifera-tion, Y represents centripetal movement, and Z represents the loss of cells from the corneal surface. Although there is considerable experimental and clinical evidence to support this hypothesis, some of the most important depend on the concept that there are "stem cells" at the limbus that act as an ongoing source of cells to contribute to corneal epithelial renewal.[11]

TRANSDIFFERENTIATION OF THE OCULAR SURFACE

Because reepithelialization from the conjunctiva is a process that follows all acute corneal epithelial loss, further investigation of this process was undertaken. Experiments done in rabbits by Shapiro[12] made it possible to stage the reepithelialization on the basis of its histologic appearance. The initial epithelial covering of the denuded cornea is nondescript, with a prominent "bloom" of goblet cells at about 3 weeks. Thereafter, there is an abrupt transformation of the phenotype to normal corneal epithelium. This observation led to the development of the procedure of conjunctival transplantation.

EPITHELIAL ABNORMALITIES IN OCULAR SURFACE DISORDERS

Epithelial changes associated with ocular surface disorders included superficial punctate keratitis, vortex epitheliopathy, and persistent epithelial defect. These three phenomena are likely variations on a common theme, that of inadequate epithelial cell maintenance. For example, the superficial keratitis seen in the presence of trichiasis is secondary to a mechanical loss of cells, leaving pits and microdefects in the surface that are filled in by either local cell proliferation or sliding of cells from adjacent regions. The persistence of a defect after chemical trauma appears to be an exaggeration of the inability of the epithelial cells to fill in the defect.

TREATMENT FOR EPITHELIAL DEFECTS

Medical
  Artificial tear substitutes
  Lubricants
  Hypertonic drops and ointments
  Anti-inflammatory agents
    Topical corticosteroids
    Nonsteroidal anti-inflammatory agents
    Mitogens
Epithelial growth factor, other growth factors
Adhesion enhancers
    Fibronectin
    Mollusk tissue glue
    Laminin, other basement membrane components
    Antibiotic—tetracycline
    Therapeutic contact lenses
Surgical
    Conjunctival flap
    Tarsorrhaphy
    Keratoplasty
      Lamellar
      Penetrating

THERAPY OF PERSISTENT CORNEAL EPITHELIAL DEFECTS

In this discussion the healing epithelial defects are confined to the ocular surface diseases. Nevertheless, the methods and medications employed have been used for all types of epithelial defects, and there is nothing specific about these methods that limit their application to the defects found in ocular surface disease. The methods that have been used for treatment of epithelial defects are shown in the Box.

It is not the intention of this work to detail any of the therapies listed in the box or to comment on their usefulness in any particular clinical situation. It is to the point, however, to indicate that any one or a combination of all of these treatments is used in most recalcitrant persistent epithelial defects and that the defect occasionally does not respond to therapy. This is the case particularly in chemical trauma, the autoimmune ocular surface diseases, radiation keratitis, and contact lens keratopathies. This particular group of problems is more likely to lead to stromal ulceration, infection, and subsequent vascularization and scarring when healing does eventually occur. It is the frustration with these therapeutic alternatives that led to exploration of epithelial replacement.

CONJUNCTIVAL TRANSPLANTATION

In 1977, a procedure to replace the ocular surface was developed.[13] The intention of conjunctival transplantation is to provide a new, healthy epithelial source for resurfacing of the cornea. It thus differs fundamentally from a conjunctival flap, where the goal of the surgery is to bring a vascularized curtain of tissue over the area of thinning, defect, or ulceration, by the application of the raw, vascularized underside of the flap to the affected area. Although conjunctival flaps have long been recognized as effective treatment of severe corneal problems,[4] their nature is to obscure the visual axis with vessels and not to provide a stable surface capable of nonvascularized repair. Another important difference in the two procedures is that conjunctival transplantation requires the presence of a healthy, noninvolved donor eye, a condition of no relevance in doing a conjunctival flap.

The procedure of conjunctival transplantation has changed very little since the original method was described. In an effort to free the cornea of all its scarring and to give the transplanted tissue an opportunity to "colonize" the periphery, a keratectomy is done beginning 5 mm posterior to the limbus. Having done a 360-degree peritomy down to the sclera, one continues the excision of tissue toward the cornea, across the limbal area (being aware that Schlemm's canal lies not too deep at that point) and up onto the dome of the cornea. It should be emphasized that the earlier procedures were done entirely with sharp dissection in the limbal and corneal regions. This fact serves to lay to rest the suggestion that limbal epithelium might have remained behind to repopulate the cornea.[7]

After the surface of the cornea is cleared of its superficial scar, the eye is then ready to receive the new surface. Initially, there were some misgivings on the part of the patients about using tissue from their only good eye, but experience in conjunctival surgery and biopsies in particular indicate that no harm is caused by even generous excision of tissue from the donor eye.

The original conjunctival transplants were characterized by too generous an extension of the donor tissue onto the cornea. This resulted undoubtedly from the fear that leaving a broad expanse of cornea raw would lead to ulceration, an event that did not occur. The result of this placing of the explants well onto the cornea was that there is a less striking cosmetic result for the patient, though there were no other adverse consequences.

The explants are secured to the host eye at the limbus, and their apices are drawn onto the peripheral cornea with a 10-0 nylon suture that is gently

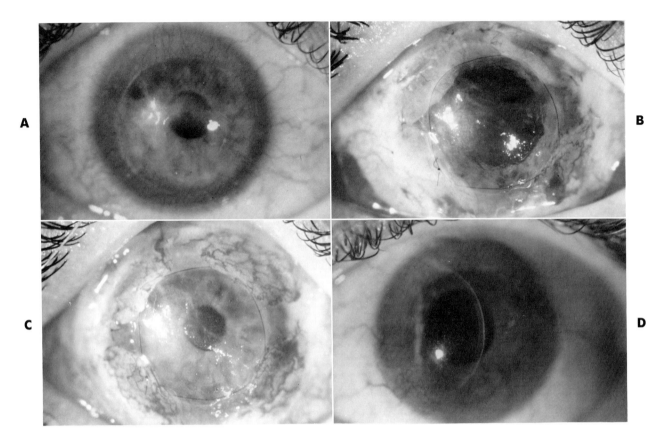

Fig. 2-2. A, Surface scarring and vascularization of a graft 3 years after the keratoplasty. **B,** After a superficial keratectomy, the conjunctival grafts are in place, anchored
with 10-0 nylon sutures. **C,** Four days postoperatively, the transplants are recanalized.
D, At 1 year, graft is still compact, and there is very little central scarring.

tightened to keep the whole explant in apposition to
the raw stroma. A soft contact lens is put into place
to keep the lid movements and globe movement
from disturbing the position of the grafts. Routine
topical antibiotic therapy is continued until the surface has healed.

One of the surprises in the procedure is the rapid
recanalization of the vessels in the transplants.
Within 2 to 3 days there appears a violaceous hue
that is followed in a day or two by blood flow in the
vessels in the transplanted conjunctiva. This phase is
accompanied by swelling and edema of the grafts.
Over the next 2 months the vessels regress, leaving a
reasonably clear central axis, and a less prominently
vascularized peripheral cornea (Fig. 2-2).

Because of the rarity of patients who have chemical injury that is unilateral, conjunctival transplants
are done infrequently. A follow-up study of the original patients was published in 1979,[14] and a paper
discussing the indications for the procedure ap-

peared in 1982.[15] There was prompt acceptance of
this procedure in the corneal surgery community,
and other applications soon appeared.

One of the first applications devised was that published by Vasteen and co-workers,[22] who reported
several cases of fornix reconstruction using conjunctival tissue from the opposite, uninjured eye. They
were able to release symblepharons and to restore
adequate motion and lid coverage in eyes that had
received severe damage. Such a use of tissue from
the opposite eye encouraged others to view the good
eye as a source of tissue for other ocular surface procedures.

The procedure that received the greatest attention
was conjunctival transplantation for pterygium. In
this procedure, the pterygium is excised in the usual
bare-sclera technique that had been devised by Ombrain.[10] The change in the technique is to use conjunctiva from the uninvolved eye to cover the defect
caused by the excision. This procedure was refined

and applied to several patients by Kenyon, and publication of the procedure led to its wide acceptance, even in the treatment of primary pterygium.[5] In Fig. 2-3, *A*, a patient who had had two prior excisions of a pterygium shows the dense scarring that is frequently associated with diplopia and limitation of motion.

Conjunctival transplantation can be particularly useful in these cases, where removal of the superficial scarring and vascularization soon reveals the depth of the fibrous tissue formation, frequently involving the rectus muscle. With careful dissection and identification of the rectus muscle, the scarred tissue can be removed. There remains such a broad area of exposed subepithelial tissue, however, that scarring is sure to recur unless new, noninflamed tissue is put in place to prevent scarring. Fig. 2-3, *B*, shows the result 6 months after a conjunctival transplant in the same patient. This result was accompanied by a considerable reduction in the limitation of gaze and consequent diplopia.

KERATOEPITHELIOPLASTY

To overcome some of the limitations of conjunctival transplantation, a variation on the technique was introduced in 1984.[16] This procedure uses thin lenticules of donor cornea, covered by epithelium, to serve as the source of new cells for surface renewal. The procedure has two significant differences from the conjunctival procedure: use of donor tissue and the use of cells that are already corneal in phenotype. The advantages of the procedure therefore include an available source of donor material for patients who have bilateral disease or injury and no need for transdifferentiation of cells to create a normal corneal surface.

The procedure was first devised for a very small subgroup of patients who were one eyed and who had had penetrating keratoplasty for chemical injury. In this group of patients the development of persistent epithelial defects is to be expected within 1 or 2 years after the keratoplasty, despite vigorous prophylactic treatment with ocular lubricants and the use of topical corticosteroids to prevent immune graft reaction. An example of such a case is shown in Fig. 2-4. In this case the keratoplasty was done 2 years before, with the formation of the persistent defect occurring about 1 year thereafter.

Characteristic of the defect in this case, as is true in the defects after keratoplasty in most chemical injuries, the configuration changes slowly, seemingly unrelated to treatment. The other important feature of this sort of defect is the relative lack of inflammation that accompanies it. It would be reasonable to

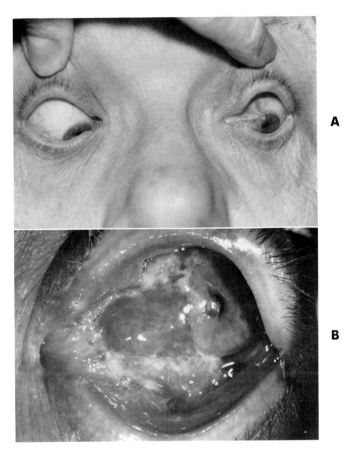

Fig. 2-3. A, Preoperative appearance of an eye that has failed two prior simple excisions of symblepharons. **B,** Appearance 6 months after excision of scar and application of a conjunctival transplant from opposite eye.

assume that there would not be high levels of inflammatory mediators in the tear film and that the environments into which the transplanted epithelium is placed should be benign.

Conjunctival transplantation has demonstrated that it is safe to undertake the same surgical preparation on the host eye for keratoepithelioplasty, with an extensive peritomy, excision of conjunctiva and limbus, and clearing of the corneal surface with a superficial keratectomy. Up to this point the procedure is identical to that employing conjunctiva as the source of epithelial cells.

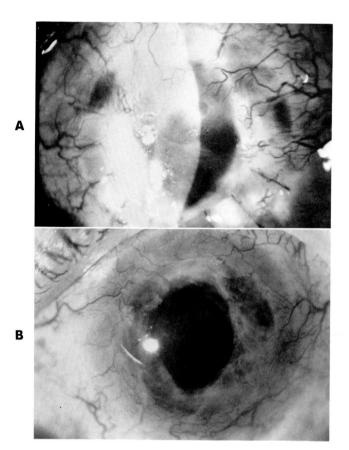

Fig. 2-4. A, Two years after a penetrating keratoplasty for a severe alkali injury, a recalcitrant epithelial defect developed, unresponsive to conventional therapy. **B,** Keratoepithelioplasty on eye healed the surface and produced a relatively smooth surface without significant vascularization at 6 months after procedure. Cornea has remained stable for 4 years.

In keratoepithelioplasty, however, a fresh donor cornea serves as the source of the cells for surface renewal. As described in the original publication, thin stromal lenticules are "carved" from the intact globe. This maneuver requires elevating the pressure in the donor eye to retain the normal curvature of the cornea, so that the disposable cataract knife can be used to remove the stromal tissue with its overlying epithelium.

It is apparent that the epithelium must be in the very best condition possible to enhance the likelihood of its surviving the operative procedure. In contrast to using the patient's own conjunctiva, the corneal epithelium on the donor globe is subject to the adverse conditions inherent in eye retrieval, processing, and transport. Maintaining the epithelium in best condition requires prompt removal of donor tissue, prompt refrigeration, and prompt transfer to

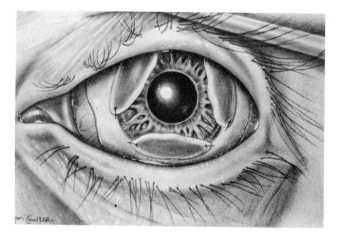

Fig. 2-5. This illustration shows the lenticules on recipient eye. Edge of lenticule closest to center of cornea is seen to be reversed from that on donor. Opacity comes from scleral tissue that supports that portion of lenticule. In addition, two 10-0 monofilament nylon sutures used to anchor lenticule at limbus are shown. In this case, three lenticules were created, rather than four.

the surgeon. These steps are increasingly difficult as eye banking becomes more complicated.

The second feature of the donor material is the need for a whole donor globe. There is difficulty in preparing the lenticules in a uniform fashion without the support of the globe as they are cut. This need for a whole globe and the necessity for the freshest possible tissue make getting donor material a very significant limitation in the application of keratoepithelioplasty.

The limbal cells are oriented so that they are closest to the corneal portion of the host eye. This means, therefore, that the lenticules are reversed from the position they occupied in the donor eye. This is illustrated in Fig. 2-5, where the reversed location of the lenticules is apparent because of the white appearance of the sclera that underlies the limbal portion of the lenticules.

As in the case of conjunctival transplantation, the lenticules are sutured to the host eye at the limbus. Because of the rigidity of the stromal carriers, however, it is not necessary to secure the edges of the grafts with suture. A soft contact lens in put in place to protect the epithelium in the postoperative period.

The results of keratoepithelioplasty have been described recently in a small group of patients.[21] The procedure has been most useful in those patients who have persistent epithelial defects after keratoplasty for chemical injury. Other useful results have been achieved in patients with the pannus and defect formation found in aniridia and for elimination of the superficial scarring and vascularization found in contact lens—induced keratopathy. The follow-up period has ranged as long as 6 years in some of these patients, and there is no evidence up to now that the positive results are only temporary.

In addition to the need for very fresh donor tissue, keratoepithelioplasty has at least one other important disadvantage that is not shared by conjunctival transplant, that being the high likelihood of immunologic rejection of the donor epithelium. Although epithelial graft rejection is not as frequent in keratoplasty as endothelial rejection is (or at least is not recognized so frequently), its occurrence after surface renewal would obviously eliminate any positive benefits from the procedure. As described by Khodadoust[6] and Alldredge and Krachmer,[1] the epithelial rejection can take the form of scattered subepithelial opacities which resemble those seen in epidemic keratoconjunctivitis, or can take the form of an elevated epithelial line, thought to be similar in its cellular makeup to the endothelial line described by Khodadoust.

In all the cases we have treated, topical steroids have been an integral part of the postoperative long-term therapy, and so one would not expect that an epithelial rejection would occur in these patients.

SUMMARY

When conventional measures do not halt the ulceration and vascularization secondary to chronic persistent epithelial defects in ocular surface disease and injury, surgical intervention may be useful. Both conjunctival transplantation and keratoepithelioplasty provide a healthy population of cells at the periphery of the cornea. These are good results in terms of stabilizing the surface, with enhancement of vision in most cases.

REFERENCES

1. Alldredge OC, Krachmer JH: Clinical types of corneal transplant rejection, *Arch Ophthalmol* 99:599-604, 1981.
2. Andersen SR, Jensen OA, Kristensen EB, et al: Benign mucous membrane pemphigoid: III. Biopsy, *Acta Ophthalmol* (Copenh) 52:455, 1974.
3. Foster CS: Cicatricial pemphigoid, *Trans Am Ophthalmol Soc* 84:527-663, 1986.
4. Gundersen T: Conjunctival flaps in the treatment of corneal disease with reference to a new technique of application, *Arch Ophthalmol* 60:880-888, 1958.
5. Kenyon KR, Wagoner MD, Hettinger ME: Conjunctival autograft transplantation for advanced and recurrent pterygium, *Ophthalmology* 92:1461-1470, 1985.
6. Khodadoust AA, Silverstein AM: Studies on the nature of the privilege enjoyed by corneal allografts, *Invest Ophthalmol* 11:137-148, 1972.
7. Kruse FE, Chen JJY, Tsai RJF, Tseng SCG: Conjunctival transdifferentiation is due to the incomplete removal of limbal basal epithelium, *Invest Ophthalmol Vis Sci* 31:1903-1913, 1990.
8. Mondino BJ, Brown SI: Ocular cicatricial pemphigoid, *Ophthalmology* 88:95, 1981.
9. Nelson JD, Havener VR, Cameron JD: Cellulose acetate impressions of the ocular surface: dry eye states, *Arch Ophthalmol* 101:1869-1872, 1983.
10. Ombrain A: The surgical treatment of pterygium, *Br J Ophthalmol* 32:65-71, 1948.
11. Schermer A, Galvin S, Sun T-T: Differentiation-related expression of a major 64K corneal keratin in vivo and in culture suggests limbal location of corneal epithelial stem cells, *J Cell Biol* 103:49-62, 1986.
12. Shapiro MS, Friend J, Thoft RA: Corneal re-epithelialization from the conjunctiva, *Invest Ophthalmol Vis Sci* 21:135-142, 1981.
13. Thoft RA: Conjunctival transplantation, *Arch Ophthalmol* 95:1425-1427, 1977.
14. Thoft RA: Conjunctival transplantation as an alternative to keratoplasty, *Ophthalmology* 86:1084-1091, 1979.
15. Thoft RA: Indications for conjunctival transplantation, *Ophthalmology* 89:335-339, 1982.
16. Thoft RA: Keratoepithelioplasty, *Am J Ophthalmol* 97:1-6, 1984.
17. Thoft RA, Friend J: Biochemical transformation of regenerating ocular surface epithelium, *Invest Ophthalmol Vis Sci* 16:14-20, 1977.
18. Thoft RA, Friend J: The X, Y, Z hypothesis of corneal epithelial maintenance, *Invest Ophthalmol Vis Sci* 24:1442-1443, 1983.
19. Thoft RA, Friend J, Kinoshita S, et al: Ocular cicatricial pemphigoid associated with hyperproliferation of the conjunctival epithelium, *Am J Ophthalmol* 98:37-42, 1984.
20. Tseng SCG: Staging of conjunctival squamous metaplasia by impression cytology, *Ophthalmology* 92:728-733, 1985.
21. Turgeon P, Nauheim R, Stopak S, et al: Indications for keratoepithelioplasty, *Arch Ophthalmol* 108:233-236, 1990.
22. Vasteen DW, Stewart WB, Schwab IR: Reconstruction of the periocular mucous membrane by autologous conjunctival transplantation, *Ophthalmology* 89:1072-1081, 1982.

Chapter 3

Biology of Persistent Epithelial Defects

ROSWELL R. PFISTER

Closure of an epithelial defect of the cornea usually proceeds in an orderly and timely fashion. Cells move toward the center over the denuded basement membrane until the surface is confluent and the normal thickness is restored. In a variety of either temporary or permanent conditions, this normal process is abrogated, delaying or preventing the restoration of epithelial integrity. The persistence of an epithelial defect may initiate a cascade of events that might result in corneal scarring, vascularization, ulceration, perforation, infection, and ultimately loss of the eye. Prevention of these disastrous consequences lies in an understanding of the biology of cell locomotion, cell regeneration, and cell-to-cell and cell-to-substratum interactions in those diseases and conditions that interfere with normal repair.

NORMAL EPITHELIAL REPAIR

Epithelial cells at the edge of an abrasion immediately separate from one another, begin to swell, and subsequently become enmeshed in fibrin. Polymorphonuclear leukocytes (PMN) aggregate along this interface (Fig. 3-1). Motility of adjacent epithelial cells into the defect begins within minutes if the defect is very small but can be delayed up to 6 hours after a 6 mm abrasion.[4,34] A variety of membrane elaborations develop in basal cells at the leading edge of the defect, including ruffles, filopodia, and lamellopodia (Fig. 3-2). These membrane perturbations signal the beginning of cellular locomotion and cease only when the defect is closed.

The driving force behind the movement of corneal epithelium is under some debate. One theory is that the migration of epithelium appears to be medi-

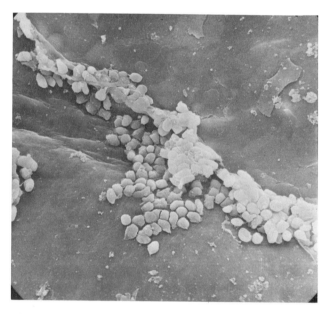

Fig. 3-1. Six hours after corneal abrasion, variable numbers of polymorphonucleocytes are found at wound edge and on adjacent basement membrane. (From Pfister RR: *Invest Ophthalmol* 14:648, 1975.)

ated by the contraction of the intracytoplasmic proteins actin and myosin. These proteins are the same type of fibers found in skeletal muscles, effecting movement by longitudinal shortening. Actin composes 10% of the protein in nonmuscle cells and has been identified in the cytoplasm of human corneal epithelial cells in two coexisting patterns, as follows: (1) within numerous parallel and convergent linear bundles known as "stress fibers" and (2) diffusely in the cytoplasm, with a increased density in the corti-

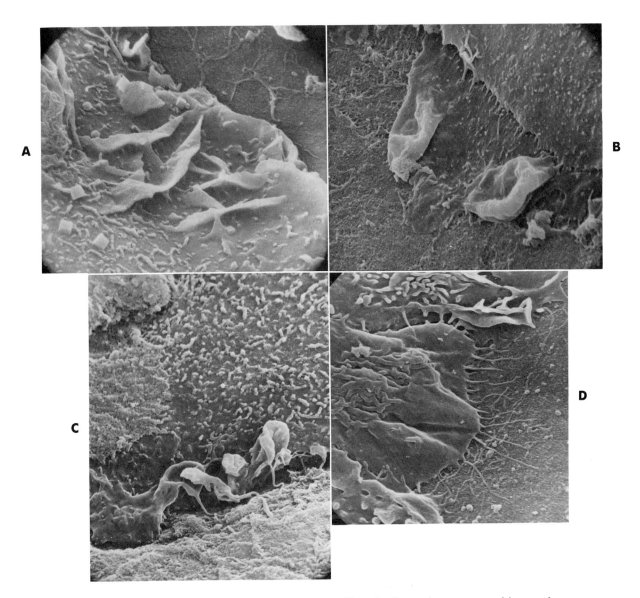

Fig. 3-2. Fifteen hours after abrasion. **A,** Ruffles of cell margin present as thin membranous leaves giving evidence of impending motion. **B,** Broad, thick ruffles appear to develop from circumscribed elevations near cell edge. **C,** Broad lamellipodia extend out over basal lamina combined with filopodia. **D,** Filopodial extensions of cell spread out ahead of cell. Intermediate and distal portions of filopodia are in tight contact with basement membrane. (From Pfister RR: *Invest Ophthalmol* 14:648, 1975.)

cal region under the cell membrane.[47] Several techniques have demonstrated these fibers in filopodia of cells in the leading front.[15,46] The epithelial cell sheet might be drawn forward by the actions of these actinomycin fibers on adhesion plaques. These focal contacts possess the protein components vinculin integrins, talin, and alpha-actinin. Adhesion plaques are localized regions of filopodia where there is interaction between actin microfilaments, the plasmalemma, and the substrate. To support this

concept, it has been demonstrated that migrating rat corneal epithelial cells show actin fibers located in basal regions of cells. Furthermore, cell movement is inhibited in rat epithelium by cytochalasin, a potent inhibitor of stress fiber formation.[16,17,22] Some investigators do not believe that stress fibers are required for cell motility. In fact, motile rabbit corneal epithelium shows only a diffuse distribution of actin fibers, not arranged into stress fibers. In the rabbit, there is evidence indicating that the leading edge may be important for adherence but that the collective pressure of cells behind the edge is responsible for its advancement.[3]

The thickness of the epithelium becomes attenuated as the defect is covered. This is especially true at the leading edge where only a single layer of cells may cover the basement membrane. During this active phase of cell movement, mitotic activity is inhibited for 96 to 120 hours, whereupon cell division begins to restore the normal compliment of cells in the corneal epithelium. During this time the appearance of the surface cells returns to normal.

CLINICAL SETTING OF A PERSISTENT EPITHELIAL DEFECT

A persistent corneal epithelial defect may be defined as a full-thickness loss of cells that fails to show the expected rate of healing for the time course.

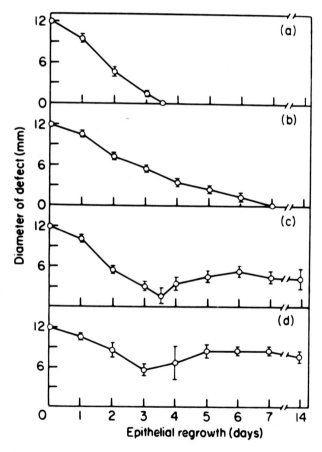

Fig. 3-3. Initial epithelial regrowths of 12 mm corneal injuries are compared. **a,** Abrasion. **b,** Keratectomy. **c,** 1 N NaOH burn. **d,** Keratectomy burn. Notice rate of epithelial regrowth of abrasions is double that of keratectomy. Reversal of epithelial regrowth at 84 hours occurs in each alkali burn regardless of size of defect. *Circle,* Mean; *brackets,* standard deviation. (From Pfister RR: *Exp Eye Res* 23:519, 1976.)

The normal rate of healing of an epithelial defect in the rabbit is a representative model for the anticipated time in the human (Fig. 3-3). For this reason, it is possible to monitor the rate of healing with respect to this model and consider intervention if more than 2 to 4 days pass without progress. The conditions potentially giving rise to a persistent epithelial defect are as follows:

Tear film abnormalities
Intrinsic epithelial disorders
Basement membrane disorders
Lid abnormalities—exposure
Metabolic disturbances
Iatrogenic
Trauma
Neurogenic
Infectious
Inflammation
Nutrition
Immune disease

A detailed expostulation on each of the conditions causing this failure is beyond the purview of this discussion.[6]

BASEMENT MEMBRANE

The attachment of the epithelium to its underlying basement membrane is crucially important to its epithelial integrity. Basement membrane is a secretion product of the basal corneal epithelial cells, requiring about 6 weeks to reform after its destruction.[26] During this interval the epithelium adheres poorly to the underlying stroma except at its leading edge. In contrast, epithelium that has migrated over preformed basement membrane tightly adheres over its entirety in 6 days. In either case strong adherence is correlated with the presence of many electron densities (hemidesmosomes) along the basal cell membrane. These hemidesmosomes radiate osmophilic fibers bridging the narrow space under the cell and penetrate basement membrane, ending in Bowman's layer. These anchoring fibrils are believed to represent the major adhesive strength between the epithelium and substratum.

Damage to the basement membrane and its disappearance or failure to regenerate appears to constitute the major reason for poor adherence of the epithelium in many diseases. In a biopsy specimen examined by electron microscopy, traumatic recurrent corneal erosion syndrome showed the absence or discontinuity of basement membrane in the affected area.[18] In addition, metaherpetic erosions are frequently correlated with therapeutic caustic scrubs of the cornea that damage basement membrane.[23] Dystrophic processes, characterized by corneal erosions, such as anterior membrane dystrophy and Reis-Bücklers' dystrophy, represent multilamination or absence of the basement membrane. The shield lesion of vernal catarrh also represents an erosive phenomenon consequent to the abrasive effect of upper lid vegetations and severe mast cell degranulation. Diabetics are subject to epithelial erosions, especially after surgery, though evidence to implicate an abnormally thickened basement membrane is not convincing.[48] Substantial damage to the basement membrane has also been demonstrated in patients with keratoconus who had been treated by thermokeratoplasty.[11] Only in the epithelial recovery after an alkali burn does this correlation between basement membrane injury and recurrent erosion break down. Disappearance of the basement membrane after the burn is correlated with loss of progression of epithelial migration, but this reversal in epithelial movement occurs even after an alkali burn in a cornea previously subjected to a lamellar keratectomy.[26]

PROBLEM OF ALKALI BURNS

Severe alkali burns present a classic example of an epithelial defect that will not heal.[41] For the first 72 hours the rate of epithelial migration for alkali burns is identical to that of corneal abrasion.[35] By 84 hours migration stops, and by 96 hours the front recedes by peeling back (Fig. 3-3). Disappearance of the basement membrane at 72 hours is not the cause for this phenomenon, since a keratectomy preceding the burn is still characterized by epithelial reversal (Fig. 3-3). Loss of motility is concurrent with cessation of membrane activity at the leading edge of the cell layer. Specifically, cells at the leading edge cease ruffling, and their filopodia and lamellopodia lose their firm attachments to the underlying stroma, resulting in cell retraction. Once this line of attachment is broken, the epithelial sheet loses it polarity and healing progress ceases.

MECHANICAL PROTECTION OF THE CORNEAL EPITHELIUM

It is important not to overlook some simple and direct mechanical approaches to assist epithelial healing. Temporary closure of the eyelid with patch or tape is occasionally useful if excessive ocular exposure is brief and self-limited. Temporary or permanent tarsorraphy is indicated when corneal exposure is prolonged, as in lagophthalmos from seventh nerve palsy or the neurotrophic problems associated with herpes zoster ophthalmicus. A variety of other trophic and devitalized ulcers are also likely to respond to a one- or two-pillar tarsorrhaphy.

The mainstay of treatment of persistent epithelial defects, not of an exposure type, is the therapeutic soft contact lens. In a series of 22 persistent epithelial defects occurring after penetrating keratoplasty, 16 healed with the continuous use of a Bausch & Lomb O4 therapeutic soft contact lens.[19] In the same study, collagen shields derived from sclera did not heal any of 7 eyes with persistent epithelial defects; 5 of 6 subsequently healed under a soft contact lens. Collagen shields may protect epithelium and encourage healing of short-term defects but appear to have little place in the treatment of defects of a persistent character.

FIBRONECTIN AS AN ENHANCER OF EPITHELIAL HEALING

Fibronectin has been implicated as a key element in wound healing for its involvement in cell-to-cell and cell-to-matrix adhesion and cell spreading.[28] Fibronectin is a large glycoprotein that may originate from blood or from cells bordering the injury. Corneal abrasion probably results in leakage of serum components from conjunctival blood vessels into the precorneal tear film. By this mechanism large proteins such as fibrinogen may reach the bare basement membrane where polymerization and deposition take place. Immunofluorescent techniques have shown a carpet of fibronectin ahead of as well as under the advancing epithelial layer, which gradually disappears over a period of several weeks.[13] In vitro studies of rabbit corneas show accelerated epithelial healing in the presence of fibronectin.[38]

Fibronectin eye drops have been used to treat a variety of conditions with persistent epithelial defects. Epithelial defects occurring in herpetic keratitis, trophic corneal ulcers, and defects after cataract surgery consistently responded to fibronectin drops when used in an open-labeled study.[30-32] An alternative explanation is suggested by an animal study conducted by Boisjoly who found that albumin eye drops were as effective as fibronectin in the treatment of persistent epithelial defects.[2] This indicates that whatever favorable effect is noted it might be a nonspecific response. The determination of the value of fibronectin in epithelial disease is currently under investigation in two prospective, randomized clinical trials using fibronectin derived from recombinant technology or isolated from serum.

A severe alkali burn of the eye causes the epithelium to become trapped in a phase of proteolytic débridement. The secretion of plasminogen activator, putatively produced by the basal epithelial cells, is capable of degrading both fibrin and fibronectin. The fact that fibronectin disappears much more rapidly from under the regenerated epithelial cells after an alkali burn indicates that its premature degradation might trigger a loss of adhesions before hemidesmosome formation.[1] Despite this, the simple addition of fibronectin eye drops to the regimen of treatment of the alkali-injured eye has failed to show any more than a 1-day advancement in epithelial healing before recurrence of a persistent epithelial defect.[13]

INFLUENCE OF TEAR LAYER

The quantity of the tear film layer is also critically important to the health and integrity of the epithelial layer. The intermediate aqueous layer composes the bulk of the thickness of the precorneal tear film (about 7 μm). Between blinks this film thins because of its evaporation as well as flow into the nasolacrimal passages. As the aqueous portion disappears, the superficial lipid layer approaches the deepest mucin layer. If the aqueous component of the tear film is not replenished by blinking, lipid contamination of the mucin coacervate adjacent to the surface cells creates a localized hydrophobic epithelium. If such a dry area persists, partial or full-thickness epithelial breakdown may occur. The effects of aqueous tear deficiency, as occurs in keratoconjunctivitis sicca, include surface drying, punctate epithelial staining, mucus plaques, and nonhealing epithelial defects, especially after corneal or cataract surgery.

The influence of the quality of the tear film on epithelial integrity is more difficult to assess. Lipid deficiencies are rare, except when extensive loss or scarring of the lid margins has occurred. Vitamin A deficiency reduces mucin production through the loss of conjunctival goblet cells. When weaning guinea pigs are fed vitamin A–deficient diets, goblet cells disappear from the conjunctiva in 7 weeks[37]

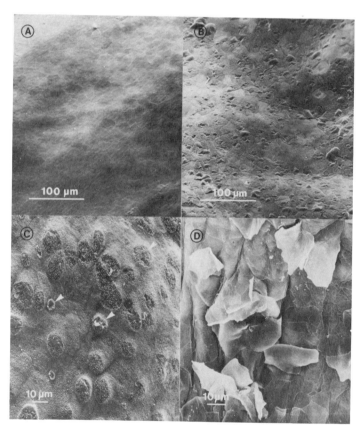

Fig. 3-4. Control cornea. **A,** Smooth, continuous sheet of flat polygonal epithelial cells is found. **B,** Seven-week vitamin A–deficient cornea. Entire surface layer of cells shows extensive separation and desquamation from epithelial sheet. **C,** Control conjunctiva. Numerous goblet cells, *arrowheads,* in various stages of maturation, stud the surfaces of palpebral and cul-de-sac conjunctiva. **D,** Six-week vitamin A–deficient conjunctiva. Keratinized epithelial cells show extensive separations and desquamation from surface epithelial sheet. Total absence of goblet cells is a striking finding. (From Pfister RR, Renner ME: *Invest Ophthalmol* 17:874, 1978.)

(Fig. 3-4). Keratinization of the ocular surface, loss of surface microprojections, epithelial defects, corneal ulceration, and keratomalacia are common in the case of chronic vitamin A deficiency (Fig. 3-4). Goblet cell deficiencies occur in a variety of unrelated conditions including erythema multiforme, pemphigoid, alkali burns, and even keratoconjunctivitis sicca. In many people this condition leads to a lifetime of ocular irritation caused by nonwetting of the ocular surface. As a consequence, recurrent corneal epithelial defects, ulceration, and vascularization are frequent.

The lids distribute the tear film over the ocular surface in an even and efficient manner. Congruity of the lids to the globe may be disturbed by lid scarring, malposition, or neurogenic malfunction. Large irregularities on the surface of the globe interfere with smooth resurfacing of the mucin coacervate by the lids, thus creating hydrophobic areas. In rabbit experiments a retinal implant sponge placed subconjunctivally at the nasal limbus creates an S-shaped deformity of the upper lid causing dry spots to appear on the adjacent cornea.[36] (Fig. 3-5). Fluid disturbances over the surfaces of living cells accelerate death and desquamation. The remaining cells at the base of the dry spot are relatively hydrophobic. As a consequence, evaporation from this area continues without replenishment from the tear film. In this area the epithelium thins and the stroma becomes compacted producing saucerized excavations known as "dellen." Although a true persistent epithelial defect does not usually result from these classical circumstances, the same pathophysiologic changes can induce persistent epithelial defects in a variety of conditions, including alkali-injured eyes or those eyes after cataract or corneal transplant surgery.

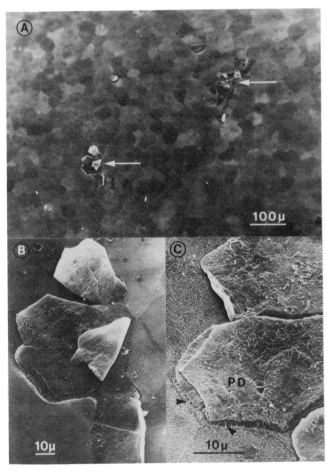

Fig. 3-5. A, Epithelial irregularity of two dry spot areas, *arrows,* is evident on an otherwise smooth corneal surface. **B,** This dry spot consisted of a cluster of five corneal epithelial cells separating from contiguous surface. **C,** Separating epithelial cells in a dry spot show loss of surface microprojections and irregularity and disruption of plasma membrane. Retraction fibrils, *arrowheads,* and discrete anterior cellular edges mark disrupted attachments with adjacent cells. *PD,* Pachymetry depth. (From Pfister RR, Renner ME: *Invest Ophthalmol* 16:1025, 1977.)

INFLUENCE OF DRUGS ON SURFACE EPITHELIUM

The use of eye drops is a time-honored approach to the treatment of many ocular diseases. Included in these formulations are a variety of additional compounds to stabilize and maintain the active compound or preserve the preparation from microbial contamination. A single instillation may produce significant abnormalities in the surface and deeper layers of epithelial cells.[40] When these solutions are used frequently or for a prolonged period, the damage may be profound, with secondary changes of scarring and vascularization.

Scanning electron microscopy of the surface of corneal epithelium showed that most antibiotics had little effect on the plasma cell membrane. Antiglaucoma drugs caused only mildly to moderately disruptive effects in the membrane, but severe damage occurred when preservatives such as benzalkonium chloride were employed[40] (Fig. 3-6). When benzalkonium chloride is used in the presence of regenerating epithelium, there is loss of tight adherence of the leading edge, loss of membrane activity, and peeling back of the advancing layer (Fig. 3-7). Idiosyncratic reactions or chronic use of drugs, particularly topical anesthetics, has been repeatedly documented to cause and maintain epithelial defects. The reason for this effect is that topical anesthetics probably disrupt actin assembly in the epithelium, which is essential for normal wound healing.[20]

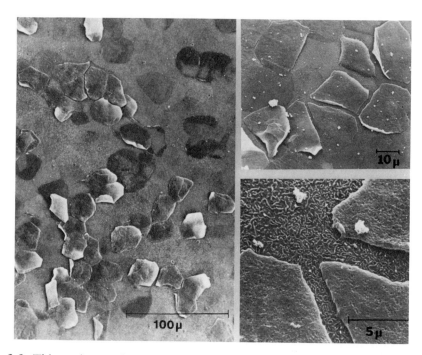

Fig. 3-6. Thirty minutes after two drops of a 0.01% benzalkonium chloride solution applied to the eye, most of the top layer of cells are desquamating. *Insets,* Severe degenerative membrane changes are notable in these dying cells. (From Pfister RR, Burstein N: *Invest Ophthalmol* 15:246, 1976.)

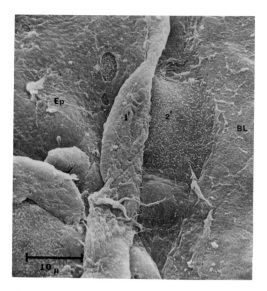

Fig. 3-7. Thirty minutes after 0.01% benzalkonium chloride was applied to actively migrating corneal epithelial cells, *Ep.* Advancing layer of cells lose their locomotory activity (ruffles and filopodia) showing extensive membrane degeneration. This cell, *1',* peeled back, exposing the underlying cell, *2',* which also shows some separation of leading edge. *BL,* Basal lamina. (From Pfister RR, Burstein N: *Invest Ophthalmol* 15:246, 1976.)

Chronic topical treatment of a cornea with or without an epithelial defect may cause a persistent defect induced or perpetuated by medication alone. For this reason the first step in the treatment of some persistent defects is to remove all medications from topical use.

ROLE OF INFLAMMATION

The influx of inflammatory cells into the cornea after injury prepares the tissue for the repair process but may also interfere with healing. Inflammatory mediators released from injured local tissues appear to trigger the initial wave of polymorphonuclear (PMN) leukocytes. Successive waves are probably stimulated to enter the cornea by other mediators including leukotrienes, C5a, C3a, and superoxide-lipid-serum albumin complexes. Corneas with epithelial defects cultured in vitro showed significant inhibition of epithelial healing when the perfusate contained either viable stimulated PMN or a PMN lysate.[51] It appears that large numbers of polymorphonuclear leukocytes in corneal tissues, especially anteriorly, are likely to encourage the development or persistence of epithelial defects as well as ulceration.

The use of topical steroids in eyes with persistent epithelial defects is controversial. Neutrophils inhibit epithelial migration, tending to prolong the healing of epithelial defects. Steroids limit the inflammatory response by stabilizing lysosomal and other membranes required for inflammatory mediator release. Reducing the recruitment of polymorphonuclear leukocytes diminishes the inflammatory response. Steroids do not, however, affect phagocytosis or the respiratory burst and superoxide radical production.[42] Excessive use of steroid drops for prolonged periods also inhibits epithelial migration as well as wound healing. When combined with the excessive elaboration of collagenase from polymorphonuclear leukocytes, the chance for corneal ulceration is enhanced. For these reasons the use of steroids must be monitored carefully.

A new and clinically untried idea is the inhibition of polymorphonuclear leukocytes in situ by topical citrate. Sodium citrate prevents the accumulation, phagocytosis, and subsequent release of degradative enzymes and free oxygen radicals from polymorphonuclear leukocytes. Animal and laboratory studies with citrate have shown it to be a chelator of extracellular Ca^{2+}. Calcium is probably necessary for the activation of the polymorphonuclear leukocytes, acting as an important intracellular second messenger. Inhibition of the polymorphonuclear leukocytes through calcium depletion may be caused by interference with calcium-calmodulin modulated microfilament or microtubule interfaces in the polymorphonuclear leukocyte plasma membrane.[39] Hence topical treatment with citrate may bring the entire set of polymorphonuclear leukocyte activities to a halt.

The ulceration associated with persistent epithelial defects may lead to corneal perforation. In these circumstances ocular integrity and anatomic restoration of tissues must be reestablished before healing will take place. If the hole is less than 0.5 mm in size, tissue adhesive (isobutylcyanoacrylate) may be applied to the cornea to seal the perforation. With or without a hard contact lens, the adhesive inhibits chemotaxis, respiratory burst, enzyme release, and phagocytosis of polymorphonuclear leukocytes into the cornea and their degradation.[24] This inhibition is probably caused by the diffusion of a breakdown product of the adhesive, most likely formaldehyde, into the tissues.[42] Bonding of the adhesive to the collagen surrounding the perforation site excludes epithelium that will return only after the adhesive has fallen off.

Exogenous ascorbate improves the substratum of the cornea of the alkali-injured eye by encouraging collagen synthesis from scorbutic fibroblasts in the tissue.[38] Calcium chelators and tissue adhesives have also been shown to decrease corneal ulceration in al-

kali burns of the eye. Despite this fact, there is no evidence to show that the epithelium grows over this improved substrate any better. This indicates that there are additional factors involved.

Persistent epithelial defects are especially common in Sjögren's syndrome where the progression to ulceration and perforation may occur rapidly. Most of the eyes with this disease do not show a significant inflammatory component. If the epithelial defect can be encouraged to close by soft lens application or by immunosuppressive therapy, ulceration stops, and active disease abates.[43] The presence of an epithelial defect in this disease process appears to be secondary to degradative changes in the corneal stroma and an abnormal tear film.

GROWTH FACTORS

Epidermal growth factor (EGF) is a polypeptide originally isolated from mouse submaxillary gland that has been shown to enhance the rate of healing and induce hyperplasia in corneal epithelium.[7,12,21] It exercises its effect by binding to the cell membrane at glycoprotein-receptor sites and by subsequent internalization.[5] In the rabbit its effect on the cornea is nontoxic, but cell-mediated immunity is stimulated by all routes of administration.[10] The replacement of mouse EGF with recombinant human EGF eliminates these potential problems. EGF stimulated complete epithelial healing after alkali injury in two studies,[9,45] but in each instance recurrent erosions reestablished the defect. In another study only marginal acceleration of epithelial healing occurred shortly after the injury.[14]

Although no beneficial effect on epithelial migration could be shown by topical administration of mouse EGF after penetrating keratoplasty in the human, epithelial defects healed in half the time over epikeratophakia lenticules using human EGF.[8] The latter study is of special importance, since persistent epithelial defects do occur after epikeratophakia, sometimes leading to ulceration and requiring replacement of the lenticule. EGF clearly stimulates epithelial proliferation but its utility in corneal diseases is unknown. Its use may be limited in persistent epithelial defects where adhesion problems are most severe. Growth factors may find a more favored place in the acceleration of wound strength[52] by the mechanism of enhancement of macromolecular synthesis.[44]

INFLUENCE OF TOTAL EPITHELIAL LOSS

The initial size of the epithelial defect influences the speed and possibly the permanence of epithelial recovery. In the absence of basement membrane or stromal injury, epithelial defects that do not exceed the limits of the cornea usually heal without incident. When epithelial defects destroy the limbal palisades of Vogt, movement of conjunctival epithelium significantly slows corneal reepithelialization and substantially increases the incidence of persistent corneal epithelial defects. This process of transdifferentiation of conjunctival epithelium to corneal epithelium requires substantial anatomic and biochemical changes.[49] The conjunctival epithelium must change from a two- to a four-layer structure with few desmosomes and many goblet cells to a five- or six-layer structure both devoid of goblet cells and firmly attached by desmosomes and hemidesmosomes, the latter to the basement membrane. This process involves a biochemical shift from the conjunctiva, which has high activities of the glycolytic, tricarboxylic acid cycle, and respiratory chain enzymes to the hexose monophosphate shunt in the cornea where glycogen is accumulated intracellularly.

The transplantation of healthy conjunctiva into the alkali-injured eye is reported to improve the vision and stability of the ocular surface.[27,50] Superficial lamellar keratectomy to remove scar tissue, followed by surgical onlay of conjunctival epithelium at the limbus, obtained from the other eye, allows new epithelium to grow out onto the bare stroma. In these studies, 7 of 10 eyes had improved sight, but all showed an improved and more stable ocular surface.

The discovery of a discrete group of stem cells in the depths of the perilimbal conjunctival epithelium has led to newer surgical approaches to corneal reepithelialization. Evidence that these cells are unique includes reaction to a specific monoclonal antibody,[53] the presence of a specific 64,000-dalton keratin, and an enhanced growth curve compared to corneal or conjunctival epithelium. Excision of limbal epithelium leads to poor epithelialization and corneal vascularization, a sign that a critical element has been removed from the generative source of corneal epithelial cells. This basic data give substance to current recommendations of limbal conjunctival autograft from the uninjured eye to the injured eye for those patients who have sustained unilateral stem cell injury.[25] This works well in conditions such as chemical injury or after pterygium excision but relies on homografts in bilateral chemical injuries or in systemic conditions.

REFERENCES

1. Berman M, Manseau E, Law M, Aiken D: Ulceration is correlated with degradation of fibrin and fibronectin at the corneal surface, *Invest Ophthalmol Vis Sci* 24:1358, 1983.
2. Boisjoly HM, Beaulieu A, Giasson M, Menard, C.: The effect of fibronectin compared to albumin on rabbit epithelial wound healing, *Invest Ophthalmol Vis Sci* 28(suppl):52, 1987.
3. Buck RC: Cell migration in repair of mouse corneal epithelium, *Invest Ophthalmol Vis Sci* 18:767, 1979.
4. Busche W: Morphologic changes in cells of corneal epithelium in wound healing, *Arch Ophthalmol* 41:306, 1949.
5. Carpenter G, Cohen S: Epidermal growth factor, *Annu Rev Biochem* 48:193, 1979.
6. Cavanagh HD, Pihlaja D, Thoft RA, Dohlman CH: The pathogenesis and treatment of persistent epithelial defects, *Trans Am Acad Ophthalmol Otolaryngol* 81:754, 1976.
7. Cohen, S.: Isolation of a mouse submaxillary gland protein accelerating incisor eruption and eyelid opening in the newborn animal, *Am J Ophthalmol* 98:411, 1984.
8. Eiferman R, Brightwell J, Rowsey J, et al: Acceleration of corneal epithelial resurfacing and keratocyte migration in primate epikeratophakia by biosynthetic human EGF, *Invest Ophthalmol Vis Sci* 26(suppl):204, 1985.
9. Eiferman R, Schultz GS: Treatment of alkali burns in rabbits with epidermal growth factor, *Invest Ophthalmol Vis Sci* 28(suppl):52, 1987.
10. Elliott J: Epidermal growth factor: in vivo ocular studies, *Trans Am Ophthalmol Soc* 78:629, 1980.
11. Fogle JA, Kenyon KR, Stark WJ: Damage to epithelial basement membrane by thermokeratoplasty, *Am J Ophthalmol* 83:392, 1977.
12. Frati L, Daniele S, Delogue A, Covelli I: Selective binding of EFG and its specific effects on the epithelial cells of the cornea, *Exp Eye Res* 14:135, 1972.
13. Fujikawa LS, Foster CS, Harrist TJ, et al: Fibronectin in healing rabbit corneal wounds, *Lab Invest* 45:120, 1981.
14. Fujisawa K, Ketakami C, and Yamamoto M: Effect of epidermal growth factor on epithelial cells and keratocytes during wound healing of alkali-burned cornea, *Invest Ophthalmol Vis Sci* 31(suppl):225, 1990.
15. Gipson IK, Anderson RA: Actin filaments in normal and migrating corneal epithelial cells, *Invest Ophthalmol Vis Sci* 16:161, 1977.
16. Gipson IK, Keezer L: Effects of cytochalasins and colchicine on the ultrastructure of migrating corneal epithelium, *Invest Ophthalmol Vis Sci* 22:643, 1982.
17. Gipson IK, Westcott MJ, Brooksby MG: Effects of cytochalasins B and D and colchicine on migration of the corneal epithelium, *Invest Ophthalmol Vis Sci* 22:633, 1982.
18. Goldman JN, Dohlman CH, Kravitt BA: The basement membrane of the human cornea in recurrent epithelial erosion syndrome, *Trans Am Acad Ophthalmol Otolaryngol* 73:471, 1969.
19. Groden LT, White W, Updegraff S: Porcine collagen corneal shield treatment of persistent epithelial defects following penetrating keratoplasty, *Invest Ophthalmol Vis Sci* 30(suppl):340, 1989.
20. Higbee RG, Hazlett LD: Topical ocular anesthetics: effect on corneal cytoskeleton, *Invest Ophthalmol Vis Sci* 25(suppl):321, 1984.
21. Ho PC, Davis WH, Elliott JH, Cohen SP: Kinetics of corneal epithelial regeneration and epidermal growth factor, *Invest Ophthalmol Vis Sci* 13:804, 1974.
22. Jester JV, Rodrigues MM: Actin filament localization in normal and migrating rabbit corneal epithelium, *Curr Eye Res* 3:955, 1984.
23. Kaufman HE: Epithelial erosion syndrome: metaherpetic keratitis, *Am J Ophthalmol* 57:983, 1964.
24. Kenyon KR, Berman M, Rose J, and Gage J: Prevention of stromal ulceration in the alkali-burned rabbit cornea by glued-on contact lens: evidence for the role of polymorpho-

nuclear leukocytes in collagen degradation, *Invest Ophthalmol Vis Sci* 18:570, 1979.

25. Kenyon KR, Tseng SC: Limbal autograft transplantation for ocular surface disorders, *Ophthalmology* 96:709, 1989.
26. Khodadoust AA, Silverstein AM, Kenyon KR, Dowling JE: Adhesion of regenerating corneal epithelium: the role of basement membrane, *Am J Ophthalmol* 65:339, 1968.
27. Kinoshita S, Friend J, Thoft RA: Ocular surface epithelial regeneration and disease, *Int Ophthalmol Clin* 24:169, 1984.
28. Mosher DF: Cross-linking of cold-insoluble globulin by fibrin-stabilizing factor, *J Biol Chem* 250:6614, 1975.
29. Nishida T, Nakagawa S, Awata T, et al: Fibronectin promotes epithelial migration of cultured rabbit cornea in situ, *J Cell Biol* 97:1653, 1983.
30. Nishida T, Nakagawa S, Manabe R: Clinical evaluation of fibronectin eyedrops on epithelial disorders after herpetic keratitis, *Ophthalmology* 92:213, 1985.
31. Nishida T, Ohashi Y, Awata T, Manabe R: Fibronectin, *Arch Ophthalmol* 101:1046, 1983.
32. Nishida T, Yagi J, Fukuda M, et al: Spontaneous persistent epithelial defects after cataract surgery, *Cornea* 6:32, 1987.
33. Nishida T, Ohashi Y, Awata T, Manabe R: Fibronectin, *Arch Ophthalmol* 101:1046, 1983.
34. Pfister RR: The healing of corneal epithelial abrasions in the rabbit: a scanning electron microscope study, *Invest Ophthalmol Vis Sci* 14:648, 1975.
35. Pfister RR: The alkali burned cornea. I. Epithelial and stromal repair, *Exp Eye Res* 23:519, 1976.
36. Pfister RR: The histopathology of experimental dry spots and dellen in the rabbit cornea: a light microscopy and scanning and transmission electron microscopy study, *Invest Ophthalmol Vis Sci* 16:1025, 1977.
37. Pfister RR: The corneal and conjunctival surface in vitamin A deficiency: a scanning electron microscope study, *Invest Ophthalmol Vis Sci* 17:874, 1978.
38. Pfister RR: Ascorbic acid in the treatment of alkali burns of the eye, *Ophthalmology* 87:1050, 1980.
39. Pfister RR, Haddox JD, Dodson RW, Deshazo WJ: Polymorphonuclear leukocytic inhibition by citrate, other metal chelators, and trifluoperazine, *Invest Ophthalmol Vis Sci* 25:955, 1984.
40. Pfister RR, Burstein N: The effects of ophthalmic drugs, vehicles, and preservatives on corneal epithelium: a scanning electron microscope study, *Invest Ophthalmol Vis Sci* 15:246, 1976.
41. Pfister RR: Diseases of the external eye: alkali burns, *Clin Signs in Ophthalmol* (Alcon) 8(2):1-12, 1986.
42. Pfister RR, Haddox JL, Dodson RW, Germann VP: The effect of citrate and other compounds on PMN incubated *in vitro:* further studies on the site and mechanism of action of citrate, *Cornea* 3:240-249, 1985.
43. Pfister RR, Murphy GE: Corneal ulceration and perforation associated with Sjögren's syndrome, *Arch Ophthalmol* 98:89, 1980.
44. Serdarevic O, Menasche M, Ben-Rayana N, et al: Stimulation of stromal macromolecular biosynthesis after penetrating keratoplasty by human epidermal growth factor, *Invest Ophthalmol Vis Sci* 31:226, 1990.
45. Singh G, Foster CS: Epidermal growth factor in alkali-burned corneal epithelial wound healing, *Am J Ophthalmol* 103:802-807, 1987.
46. Soong HK, Cintron C: Calmodulin inhibitors and F-actin formation in corneal epithelium, *Invest Ophthalmol Vis Sci* 25:322, 1984.
47. Soong HK, Fairley JA: Actin in human corneal epithelium, *Arch Ophthalmol* 103:565, 1985.
48. Taylor HR, Kimsey RA: Corneal epithelial basement membrane changes in diabetes, *Invest Ophthalmol Vis Sci* 20:548, 1981.
49. Thoft RA: Biochemical transformation of regenerating ocular surface epithelium, *Invest Ophthalmol Vis Sci* 16:14, 1977.
50. Thoft RA: Conjunctival transplantation, *Ophthalmology* 86:1084, 1979.
51. Wagoner MD, Kenyon KR, Gipson IK, et al: Polymorphonuclear neutrophils delay corneal epithelial wound healing in vitro, *Invest Ophthalmol Vis Sci* 25:1217, 1984.
52. Woost PG, Brightwell J, Eiferman TA, Schultz GS: Effect of growth factors with dexamethasone of healing of rabbit corneal stromal incisions, *Exp Eye Res* 40:47-60, 1985.
53. Zieske JD, Bukusoglu H: Numbers of limbal basal cells expressing a 50-kD antigen increase after wounding, *Invest Ophthalmol Vis Sci* 31(suppl):538, 1990.

Chapter 4

Corneal Topography

Principles

J. JAMES ROWSEY
JAMES C. HAYS

Keratorefractive surgery continues to be one of the most exciting and rapidly changing fields in ophthalmology.[1-9] The key to understanding how each surgical procedure works lies in understanding the shifts in corneal topography caused by the surgery. The major refracting surface of the eye is the air-to-tear film interface. It is here that small changes in shape can have great effects on refraction.

We have suggested the "ten caveats in keratorefractive surgery," nine of which are reviewed for clinical complications in this chapter. Basic rules of refractive surgery are as follows:

1. The normal cornea flattens over any incision.
2. Radial corneal incisions flatten the adjacent cornea and the cornea 90 degrees away.
3. The cornea flattening effect increases as incisions approach the visual axis.
4. The cornea flattens directly over any sutured incision.
5. The limbal cornea flattens adjacent to loose sutures.
6. The limbal cornea steepens adjacent to tight sutures.
7. The cornea flattens over a wedge resection or tuck.
8. The cornea steepens anterior to wedge resections or tucks.
9. Tissue removal produces corneal flattening over the site of tissue removal, whether traumatic or surgically induced.
10. Full-thickness corneal tissue addition produces corneal steepening over the site of the

tissue addition and flattens the adjacent cornea.

Most keratorefractive operations consist in one or more of the following four components: (1) corneal incision, (2) corneal suturing, (3) tissue addition, and (4) tissue removal. The purpose of this chapter is to describe how each of these components alters corneal astigmatism.

Corneal astigmatism is affected by the incision length, location, and angulation. When the incision is being closed, the type of suture material, number of suture bites, length of bites, and suture tension help determine the final refractive result.

By breaking each procedure into components and considering the effect of each component, one can understand the overall effect of the operation.

INCISIONS

The normal cornea flattens over any incision. This effect is attributable to gaping of the wound. A corneal incision slices through the corneal lamellae and intraocular pressure spreads the edges apart. This increases the radius of curvature of the cornea across the incision and flattens the cornea (Fig. 4-1). The incision heals with a greater surface area, essentially a microwedge addition.

Perpendicular Versus Shelved Corneal Incisions. Eisner[5] has observed that a perpendicular wound gapes more than a shelved wound. In a perpendicular wound, intraocular pressure spreads the edges of the wound. In a shelved wound, intraocular pressure forces the inside lip to oppose the outside lip like a valve and help seal the wound. The no-stitch technique of a shelved phacoemulsification incision utilizes this valve insight for success. Not until a higher intraocular pressure is reached will the lips slip apart and gape. Likewise, a low pressure may allow the wound to gape open and cause endophthalmitis with no-stitch surgery.

Incision Depth. Deeper corneal incisions leave fewer intact lamellae and therefore gape more than shallower corneal incisions. The increased wound gaping causes increased corneal flattening. Deeper incisions in radial keratotomy surgery are believed to give more effect than shallow incisions.[4,14,15] This depth of incision increases corneal flattening according to Laplace's law.

$$\text{Stress (grams/mm}^2) = \frac{\substack{\text{Pressure} \\ \text{(grams/mm}^2)} \times \substack{\text{Radius} \\ \text{(mm)}}}{2 \times \text{Thickness (mm)}}$$

Note that as the thickness (T in Fig. 4-1) decreases, the stress of the incision increases tremendously, forcing the tissue forward and bending it.

Length. The length of an incision also helps determine how much wound gaping will occur. Since the lamellae are intact at each end of the wound, the wound gaping will be maximal in the center of the wound if the wound is a consistent depth. A longer wound will allow more gaping than a shorter wound.

The corneal flattening effect of an incision increases as the incision approaches the center of the cornea.[9] A smaller optical zone is consequently associated with greater effect in radial keratotomy surgery.[1,4,8,10,14,15]

Radial and Circumferential Incisions. The location and direction of corneal incisions also help determine what their refractive effect will be. Incisions may be placed radially in the cornea. Radial incisions, if carried across the cornea, bisect the cornea into two equal parts (Fig. 4-2). Circumferential, or tangential, incisions do not bisect the cornea into two equal parts.

Both circumferential and radial incisions flatten the cornea across their length because of wound gaping. However, radial incisions flatten the cornea 90 degrees away from their location, whereas circumferential incisions steepen the cornea 90 degrees away.[6,7,9]

It is very important to understand the difference in the effect of radial and circumferential incisions 90 degrees to their axis. Consider the limbus as a ring with a constant circumference. Any force that stretches the ring in one direction (flattening) tends to narrow the ring (steepening) in the meridian 90 degrees away. To visualize this concept, take a rubber band and compress and reshape it without stretching it.

A circumferential incision flattens the cornea (increased radius of curvature) across the width of the incision because of wound gape (Fig. 4-2). It will steepen the cornea 90 degrees away by causing a slight constriction of the diameter of the cornea, since the perpendicular meridian has enlarged a bit. Consider any of the four nonradial incisions in Fig. 4-2. The cornea flattens vertically with these incisions. The shaded strip of cornea serves as a constricting band, not allowing stretching of the central cornea. Therefore the shaded strip of cornea will steepen as the vertical meridian flattens.

Now consider an incision made radially. The longer incision in the shaded bank in Fig. 4-2 is ra-

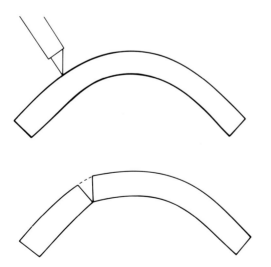

Fig. 4-1. Corneal incision allows wound gaping and increase in radius of curvature of cornea.

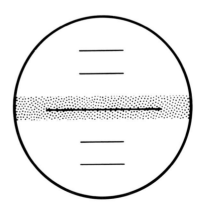

Fig. 4-2. Comparison of radial incision, *shaded area*, with nonradial incisions, *above and below.*

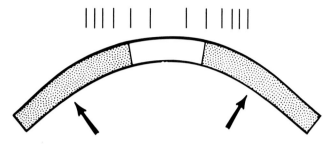

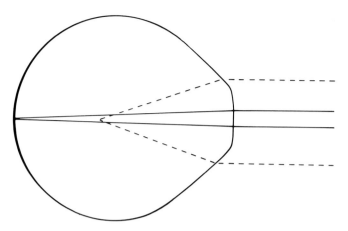

Fig. 4-3. Effect of radial keratotomy. Radial incisions allow bulging of midperipheral cornea, *shaded*, and subsequent central corneal flattening, *white*. Relative positions of corneoscope rings are demonstrated above cornea. Wide central rings document central corneal flattening.

Fig. 4-5. Midperipheral light rays are refracted more than central rays after radial keratotomy.

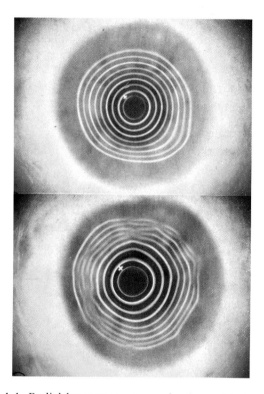

Fig. 4-4. Radial keratotomy on eye-bank eye. Notice central corneal flattening with wider spaced rings with relative midperipheral steepening.

dial. This causes flattening in the vertical meridian because of wound gape, just as any of the other parallel incisions do. Because this central constricting band has been cut, it is allowed to relax and assume a new shape. The cornea will flatten along a radial incision. Consider what happens in radial keratotomy surgery. Fig. 4-3 shows that there will be bulging of the cornea along the incision, flattening the central cornea and causing relative steepening of the periphery. This explains the topographic picture seen in radial keratotomy (Fig. 4-4). The central cor-

nea will be quite flat, and the midperiphery will be relatively steep. This midperipheral knee partly explains why patients who have undergone radial keratotomy complain of decreased night vision.[10]

In Fig. 4-4 (a 16-incision radial keratotomy with a 4.0 mm optical zone in an eye-bank eye), notice the pronounced widening of the central corneal rings and relative steepening of rings five, six, and seven. As seen in Fig. 4-5, light entering the eye through a small pupil will be refracted less than light entering through a widely dilated pupil. The postoperative radial keratotomy patient will experience a return of some of his original myopia when the pupil dilates. Our radial keratotomy patients who have trouble seeing at night tend to request 0.75 diopter more minus in their spectacles than they need during the day. Postoperative radial keratotomy patients overcorrected by at least 0.50 dioper have fewer complaints of decreased night vision.

Ruiz Incision. The Ruiz procedure for the correction of astigmatism takes advantage of the fact that circumferential and radial incisions have opposite effects on the cornea 90 degrees from their axis. By making stepladder incisions, with both radial and circumferential incisions in the same axis, one can greatly steepen the cornea in one axis with relatively little effect 90 degrees away. The final refractive state of the healed procedure is exceedingly difficult to quantitate. However, the topographic insights are useful for prescribing astigmatism surgery. Fig. 4-6, *A*, show a freshly enucleated eye-bank eye. Fig. 4-6, *B*, shows the topographic effect of putting in only the steps of the ladder. Notice that in the axis of the steps the cornea flattens greatly but 90 degrees away it actually steepens. When the radial cuts are added

University of Oklahoma
Department of Ophthalmology

Dean McGee Institute
Research Division

Patient name: Eye bank eye   *Eye:* E.B.

File: EBU13S3.PRE

TX MX: Preop. for Ruiz incisions

Cycloplegic Ref.: None   *Photo date:* 9/13/83   *Printed:* 9/16/83

Control value: 7.96   *Photo Mag.:* 4.81   *I.R.:* 1.3375

M.D. location: Rowsey/MEI   *PERK #:* EBank   *Med. Rec. #:* None

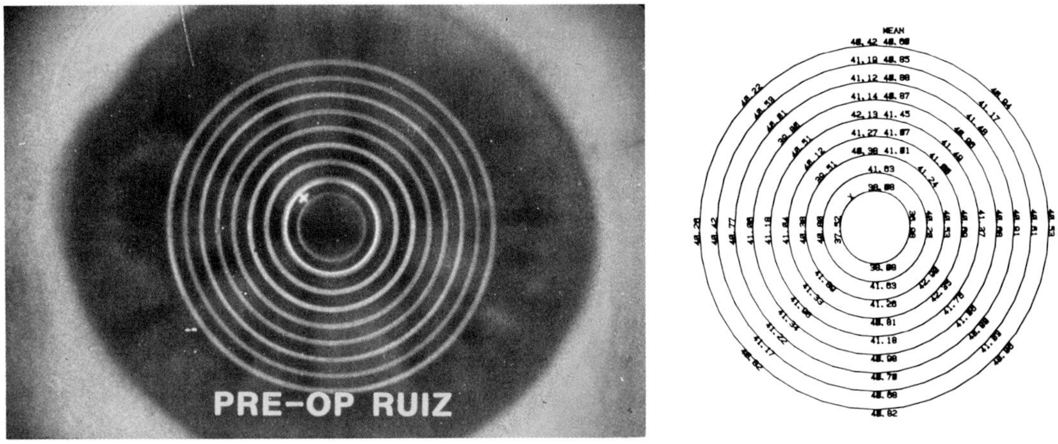

Fig. 4-6. Ruiz procedure on eye bank eye. **A,** Preoperative.
Continued.

(Fig. 4-6, *C*), notice that the axis of the incisions flatten even further whereas the cornea 90 degrees away flattens almost to the preoperative readings (Fig. 4-6, *A*). This procedure could also be combined with additional radial incisions to flatten the uninvolved axis. The Ruiz procedure has the potential to correct large amounts of astigmatism. The exact surgical parameters to predictably correct astigmatism with this procedure are still under investigation. Our experience suggests that placement of only two tangential incisions 2 mm in length (essentially two steps of the Ruiz procedure) are adequate to correct most astigmatism.

Our current nomogram for astigmatism surgery is as follows:

10 minus astigmatism in diopters =
    Optical zone in millimeters

Two (2 mm) tangential incisions are placed with a forward-cutting diamond knife to 90% of the ultrasonic corneal thickness at the desired optical zone in the steep axis of the cornea. No smaller than a 5.0 mm optical zone is utilized. Fig. 4-7 demonstrates the efficacy of this technique with a patient with 9 diopters of astigmatism, in pellucid marginal degeneration.

Scarred corneal tissue does not react as described to incisions. We have attempted, unsuccessfully, to place relaxing incisions in corneas scarred by herpes simplex keratitis. The results in these cases have been quite variable. In addition, scars extending through Descemet's membrane tether the cornea, precluding adequate bowing forward after relaxing incisions. We have not been able to achieve satisfactory flattening of the scarred cornea, prompting us to discontinue placing relaxing incisions in scarred tissue.

SUTURES

The usual purpose of sutures is to hold wound edges in apposition so that healing can proceed. The surgeon attempting to reduce corneal astigmatism may utilize sutures to alter corneal topography. Sutures are placed very tightly in an attempt to steepen the cornea.[3,9] Anterior to the suture (caveat 6), they may also be placed in quadrants 90 degrees away from relaxing incisions to increase the flattening effect of the relaxing incision.

Suture tension is important when one is determining the initial postoperative astigmatism effect of corneal surgery. However, the effect of suture tension decreases as a contributor to the determination of long-term corneal astigmatism.

Sutures vary in their contributions to corneal shape over time. They can be tied tightly, either intentionally or unintentionally producing tissue com-

CORNEASCOPE READING CENTER

University of Oklahoma
Department of Ophthalmology

Dean McGee Institute
Research Division

Patient name: Eye bank eye   *Eye:* E.B.   *File:* EBU13S3.ROL

TX MX: Ruiz procedure   Rings on ladder

Cycloplegic Ref.: None   Photo date: 9/13/83   *Printed:* 9/16/83

Control value: 7.96   Photo Mag.: 4.81   *I.R.:* 1.3375

                   PERK #: EBank   *Med. Rec. #:* None

M.D. location: Rowsey/MEI   Chord one is 102 degrees.

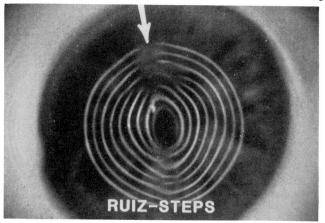 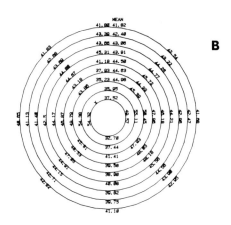

CORNEASCOPE READING.CENTER

University of Oklahoma
Department of Ophthalmology

Dean McGee Institute
Research Division

Patient name: Eye bank eye   *Eye:* E.B.   *File:* EBU13S3.FIN

TX MX: Compled Ruiz procedure   Diamond knife at .85 mm.

Cycloplegic Ref.: None   Photo date: 9/13/83   *Printed:* 9/16/83

Control value: 7.96   Photo Mag.: 4.81   *I.R.:* 1.3375

                   PERK #: EBank   *Med. Rec. #:* None

M.D. location: Rowsey/MEI   Chord one is 103 degrees.

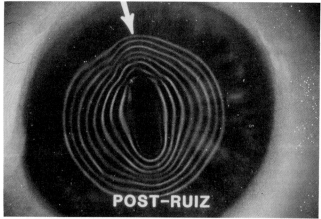 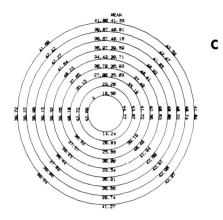

Fig. 4-6, cont'd. Ruiz procedure on eye bank eye. **B,** After step incisions are added. **C,** After radial incisions are added.

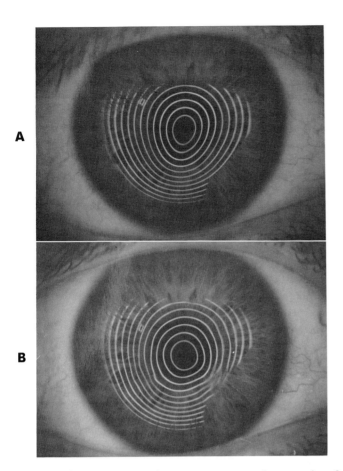

A

B

Fig. 4-7. A, Preoperative corneoscope photograph of right eye of 33-year-old man with pellucid marginal degeneration at 6 o'clock position. Manifest refraction (MR): $-6.75 + 5.50 \times 165$. **B,** Postoperative corneoscope photograph of same eye with 4.00 mm optical zone, 2.5 mm length, and tangential incisions to 90% of corneal thickness at 165 degrees with four semiradial incisions at 165 degrees to the 4.00 mm optical zone. MR: $-150 + 0.75 \times 25$.

pression, or essentially a microwedge resection. Sutures can be tied loosely providing tissue relaxation or essentially a microwedge addition. Sutures "cheesewire" through their suture canals and loosen. Sutures may loosen as edematous, traumatized tissue deturgesces and thins. In addition, sutures may cause epithelial defects that may lead to corneal melting or transplant rejection.

Sutures may break or may be removed when necessary to decrease astigmatism. As long as a corneal suture is intact and demonstrating a compressive topographic vector, however, it does play a major role in astigmatism.

Tight Sutures. Tight corneal sutures have the effect of flattening the cornea over the sutures but

steepening the cornea central to the tight sutures (caveat 6). This insight is helpful in the modification of astigmatism. Fig. 4-8, *A*, shows a postoperative corneoscope photograph of an eye that underwent a wound revision and resuturing for 4.50 diopters of against-the-rule astigmatism. An area of wound gaping could be seen at the 100-degree axis at the old cataract incision. A flat, beveled incision was placed with a diamond knife through the area of wound gape, and the incision was tightly closed with long bites of 10-0 nylon sutures. Approximately 4.00 diopters of plus axis astigmatism was induced postoperatively, based on the corneoscope appearance. In this sequence of photographs, the tight suture at the 11 o'clock position is seen to be compressing the wound. Refraction is $-2.50 +1.50 \times 123$ degrees. The appearance in the corneoscope photograph of a tight suture is similar to a finger pressing into a rubber ball or balloon at the point of the tight suture. The suture itself may be observed when one changes the focal plane of the camera anteriorly (Fig. 4-8, *B*). By using a corneoscope photograph, one can easily identify the precise suture causing the astigmatism (Fig. 4-8, *B*). As the suture is cut, this excessive tension is relieved and the central corneoscope rings round out (Fig. 4-8, *C*). This is more accurate than trying to determine which suture is tight based on keratometry alone.[12,13]

Tight sutures in transplants or cataract surgery may be recognized by corneoscopy, retinoscopy, or slitlamp appearance.

The most important observation for the presence of tight sutures on corneoscopy include Placido disc ring information (Fig. 4-8, *D*). The greatest vector of indentation is observed closest to the suture. More importantly, in refractive surgery, the corneal apex is decentered away from tight sutures and toward loose sutures (Fig. 4-9).

Fig. 4-10, *A*, shows an eye-bank eye with an incision placed from the limbus to the central cornea. Notice that the cornea is flattened by the incision (caveat 1). If this incision were closed with equally spaced and equally tight sutures along the length of the incision, the sutures would further flatten the cornea at the 6 o'clock position[9] (caveat 6). Instead, this incision was closed with only two sutures. The second epicenter of the Placido disc image on the corneoscope photograph, seen between the sutures inferiorly in the cornea, indicates extreme corneal flattening. These two peripheral sutures were tied extremely tight because tight sutures cause the central corneal topography to steepen. Notice that the central cornea anterior to the sutures is desirably round, not flat (Fig. 4-9, *B*).

We recommend that attention be paid to the antic-

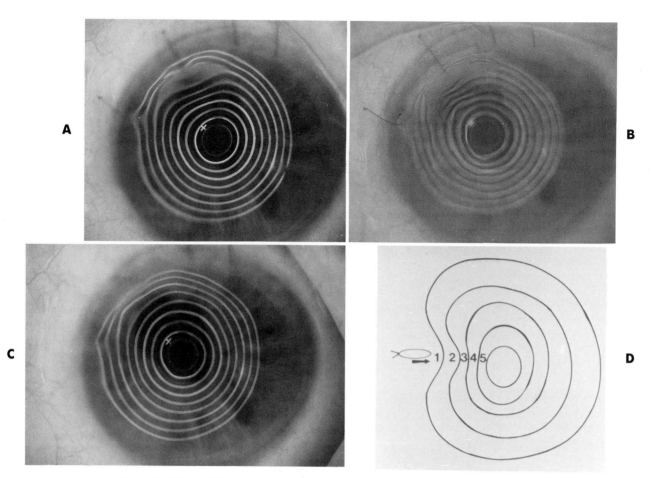

Fig. 4-8. Effect of tight suture. **A,** Tight suture at 11 o'clock position. Note V vector of indented corneal tissue under suture. Wide seventh ring is also a sign of tabletop-like flattening of cornea in this area. Ninth ring of corneoscope photograph remains closer to limbus at 9 o'clock to 12 o'clock position indicating presence of higher or flatter cornea in this quadrant, compared to 2 o'clock ring position. Original wound dehiscence is manifested as a microwedge tissue addition, which therefore persists at 10 o'clock position. **B,** Corneoscope photograph focused anteriorly on sutures demonstrates flattening between the 10 o'clock suture and adjacent tissue indentation. **C,** Effect of suture removal is to increase corneal sphericity. **D,** Indentation vector of single peripheral corneal sutures. Compressive effect of peripheral suture decreases as central corneal rings are approached.

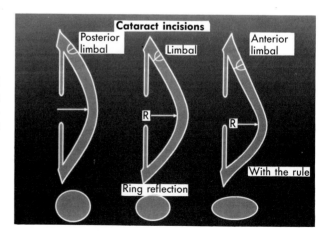

Fig. 4-9. Tight limbal sutures steepen central cornea and move corneal apex *away* from the tight sutures. Patient views environment through side of corneal mountain. Astigmatism surgery should be designed both to reduce astigmatism and to center corneal apex over visual axis.

ipated astigmatic result at the time of the initial repair of ocular trauma.[12] Vertical incisions should be closed first to allow for inflation of the anterior chamber. Shelving incisions should be closed secondarily with longer limbal sutures (flattening the peripheral cornea and steepening the center) and shorter central corneal sutures observing for central sphericity. Even well-apposed corneal wounds will flatten excessively unless compressive sutures are used to steepen the central cornea. Application of these principles at the time of initial corneal wound repair may help lessen postoperative astigmatism and aid in rehabilitating the eye without further reconstructive surgery.

Loose Sutures. Loose or broken limbal sutures cause flattening of the cornea in the meridian of the loose sutures (caveat 5). This is accompanied by steepening of the cornea 90 degrees away. This effect is reminiscent of the effect of a relaxing incision.

If we consider a wound dehiscence from broken or loose sutures as a relaxing incision, the effect is much easier to understand.

Loose sutures in a corneal transplant closure cause wound-edge disparity with elevation of the donor cornea. This pattern may be detected with a corneoscope photograph, even when it is so subtle as to be imperceptible on slitlamp examination.

Fig. 4-11, *A*, shows the appearance of an eye with running 10-0 nylon suture in place. When the running suture was removed, wound dehiscence occurred at the 3 o'clock meridian. The pattern of wound dehiscence is seen in Fig. 4-11, *B* and *C*. The wound was resutured with interrupted sutures. The corneoscopic appearance of the eye 24 hours after wound resuturing is seen in Fig. 4-11, *D*.

Fig. 4-12, *A*, shows the appearance of an eye after penetrating keratoplasty. The running suture was removed immediately after corneoscope photogra-

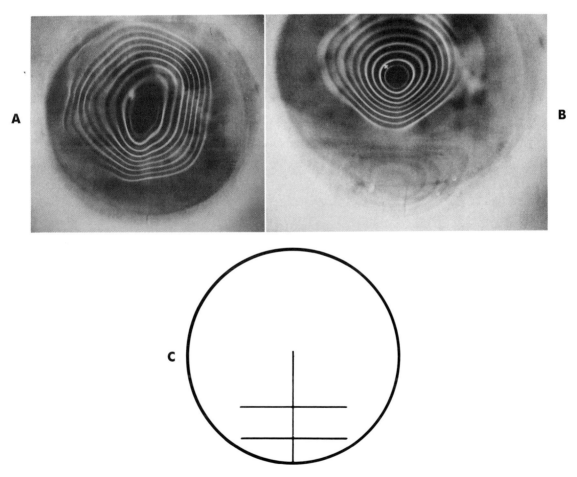

Fig. 4-10. Repair of corneal laceration. **A,** Laceration from 6 o'clock to center of cornea. Noticeable flattening of cornea vertically (caveat 1). **B,** Closure with two large compressive sutures in periphery. Notice round central topography and second epicenter of rings over sutures (caveats 4 and 6). **C,** Suture pattern.

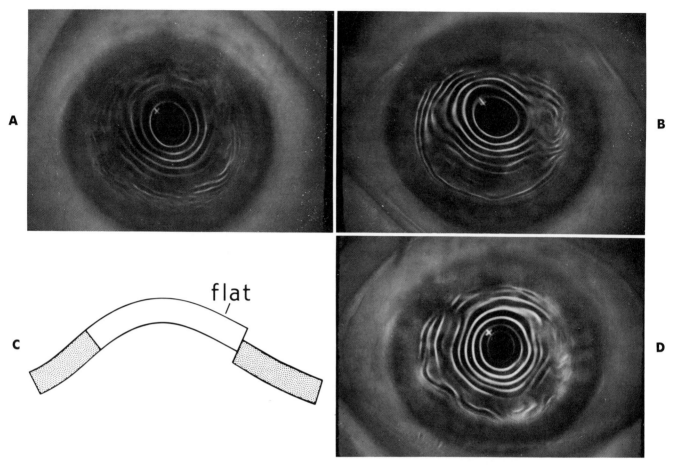

Fig. 4-11. Wound dehiscence on removal of corneal transplant sutures. **A,** Presuture removal. **B,** Immediately after wound dehiscence. **C,** Diagram of corneal flattening. **D,** After resuturing, 3 o'clock cornea astigmatism is reduced.

phy. Fig. 4-12, *B,* shows the appearance 1 month later with the intraocular pressure increased to 35, causing a subtle wound dehiscence at the 1 o'clock position. Lowering the pressure to 14 caused a regression of the bulging of the wound, as seen in Fig. 4-12, *C.*

When the occult patterns of wound dehiscence are observed after corneal transplantation, the appropriate astigmatism surgery is resuturing of the wound in the area of the dehiscence. It may be necessary to reincise the donor-recipient interface if some healing has taken place. This advice is important for the surgeon planning to correct posttransplant astigmatism with relaxing incisions based on keratometry readings. It is impossible to tell by keratometry readings if there is a subtle wound dehiscence, which should be repaired. Instead, the information from keratometry readings might lead the surgeon to perform relaxing incisions in the steeper (normal) part of the incision. Whenever a surgical approach is de-

signed to correct astigmatism, the surgeon should try to correct the effect that is responsible for the astigmatism. This is a better approach than trying to make the healthy cornea match up with the defect.

TISSUE ADDITION

Tissue addition is becoming an increasingly popular method of changing the refractive power of the cornea. Tissue may be added as intrastromal inlays, epikeratophakia onlays, or wedge additions.

Stromal Implants. Intrastromal inlays may be made of either donor human corneal material or synthetic material. The major indication for intrastromal inlays has been for the correcting of large spherical refractive errors, as in aphakia. Intrastromal inlays have not yet been used for the correction of astigmatism. Astigmatism can be introduced with this surgery if the lenticule is not precisely centered.[15]

Epikeratophakia. Epikeratophakia lenticules are

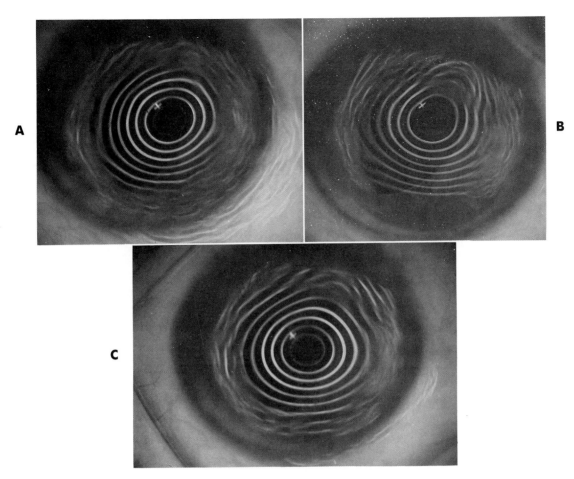

Fig. 4-12. Impending wound dehiscence from high intraocular pressure (IOP). **A,** Postoperative corneal transplant with sutures removed. **B,** Wound dehiscence at 1 o'clock; IOP, 35 mm Hg. **C,** IOP returned to normal. Wound dehiscence pattern has returned almost to normal.

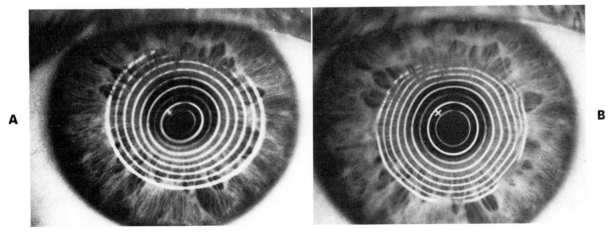

Fig. 4-13. Epikeratophakia for keratoconus. **A,** Preoperative. **B,** Six months postoperatively there is pronounced flattening and sphericity of central cornea.

also primarily used to correct large spherical refractive errors. However, some work has been done to investigate the possibility of correcting astigmatism with epikeratophakia. Schanzlin and Villaseñor[17] reported early experience in toric lathing of the cornea to correct astigmatism. Werblin, Blaydes, and Kaufman[20] have reported early experience with the results of using elliptical epikeratophakia lenticules for correction of astigmatism.

Compressive epikeratophakia lenticules may correct the astigmatism associated with keratoconus. Fig. 4-13 shows the preoperative and 6-month postoperative appearance of the corneal topography change that occurred with epikeratophakia performed by Daniel Durrie (M.D., Kansas City, Missouri). The advantageous flattening effect is readily appreciated in Fig. 4-13, *B*. Although long-term follow-up study is not yet available, this procedure seems to hold promise for the correction of keratoconus.

Traumatic Avulsion. Wedge additions of corneal tissue can correct astigmatism after corneal trauma. If corneal trauma is associated with tissue loss, tight sutures will be necessary to close the gaping wound. If the wound is in the central cornea, penetrating keratoplasty will probably be necessary to remove the scar and restore normal topography. If the

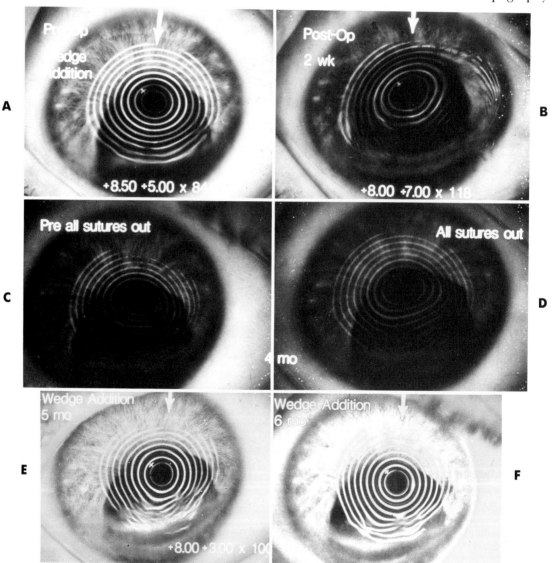

Fig. 4-14. Wedge addition for corneal laceration. **A,** Corneoscope photograph. **B,** Two weeks postoperatively. **C** and **D,** Four weeks postoperatively before and after suture removal. **E,** Five months postoperatively. **F,** Six months postoperatively improved corneal sphericity allows contact lens refitting.

wound is outside the visual axis, it is possible to reincise the scar and a wedge of corneal tissue to replace the lost tissue.

The effect of tissue loss in a corneal laceration in the peripheral or midperipheral cornea is similar to a wedge resection. Fig. 4-14 shows the appearance of a patient who suffered a knife injury to the inferior cornea. The lens was also damaged and was removed. The patient was unable to tolerate a contact lens to correct his aphakia because of his distorted corneal topography. A 0.55 mm wedge of crescent-shaped glycerin-preserved cornea was placed into his original, reincised wound. His 6-month follow-up corneoscope photograph (Fig. 4-14, *F*) shows significant rounding of his central cornea. He is now able to tolerate a contact lens to correct his aphakia.

TISSUE REMOVAL

Loss of corneal tissue can have a profound effect on corneal topography. The actual loss flattens the cornea over the site of the loss. If tight sutures are needed to correct the wound gaping, further flattening over the tissue loss will occur (caveat 9). If the tissue loss is in the midperipheral or peripheral cornea, these tight sutures will cause steepening of the central cornea (caveat 8).

Wedge Resection. This pattern of altered topography occurs after accidental trauma to the cornea. The same principles can be applied to the planned surgical removal of corneal tissue. Troutman[3,17,18] has developed the concept of wedge corneal resection for the correction of astigmatism. His initial work was performed to correct high levels of post-transplant astigmatism.

After identifying the flat corneal meridian, Dr. Troutman excises a wedge of tissue 90 degrees wide and 90% depth from the donor-recipient scar. The width of the crescent is determined by the amount of the refractive error he wishes to correct. After removing the tissue, he closes the incision to achieve a 50% overcorrection. Dr. Troutman's results show that a 1.0 mm wedge gives about 10 diopters of astigmatic correction. He notes that the flatter meridian will steepen and that the steeper meridian will flatten with a ratio of steepening to flattening of 2:1. A 1.0 mm wedge should therefore steepen the flatter meridian approximately 6.6 diopters and flatten the steeper meridian approximately 3.3 diopters.

Keratomileusis. Keratomileusis is a procedure developed by Dr. José Barraquer in which the patient's cornea is resected with a microkeratome and frozen.[2] The cornea is then lathed to a different shape and resutured onto the corneal bed.

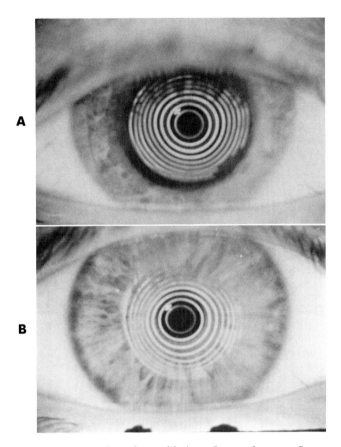

Fig. 4-15. Excimer laser ablation of central cornea for myopia of 5 diopters. **A,** Preoperative photograph. **B,** Postoperative photography demonstrating round central rings and flattened cornea.

Keratomileusis holds the promise of being able to correct both hyperopia and myopia.

Barraquer has reported the average induction of less than 1 diopter of astigmatism in performing keratomileusis.[2] His experience is extensive, however, and in less experienced hands there is the potential for lathing errors and suturing problems.

Excimer Laser. Excimer laser sculpting of the corneal provides an excellent method of flattening the cornea over the visual axis without providing excessive corneal scarring. Fig. 4-15 demonstrates the preoperative and postoperative topography of a myopic postepikeratophakia eye demonstrating stable corneal flattening of 7 diopters after excimer ablation. The wide central rings indicate the ablation site. It is important to enter the ablation zone over the visual axis, or induced astigmatism may occur with the patient seeing through the side of the mountain of the cornea. The excimer laser has the potential for removing corneal tissue at 0.22 μm per pulse or a submicrometer level of refinement of our surgical technique.

REFERENCES

1. Arrowsmith PN, Sanders DR, Marks RG: Visual refractive and keratometric results of radial keratotomy, *Arch Ophthalmol* 101:873, 1983.
2. Binder PS, editor: Refractive corneal surgery: the correction of aphakia, hyperopia, and myopia, Boston, 1983, Little, Brown.
3. Binder PS, editor: Refractive corneal surgery: the correction of astigmatism, Boston, 1983, Little, Brown.
4. Deitz MR, Sanders DR, Marks RG: Radial keratotomy: an overview of the Kansas City Study, *Ophthalmology* 91:467, 1984.
5. Eisner, G: *Eye surgery: an introduction to operative technique*, New York, 1980, Springer.
6. Fyodorov SN, Durnev VV: Operation of dosaged dissection of corneal circular ligament in cases of myopia of mild degree, *Ann Ophthalmol* 11:1885, 1979.
7. Krachmer JH, Fenzl RE: Surgical correction of high post-keratoplasty astigmatism, *Arch Ophthalmol* 98:1400, 1980.
8. Lavery GW, Lindstrom RL, Hofer LA, Doughman DJ: The surgical management of corneal astigmatism after penetrating keratoplasty, *Ophthalmic Surg* 16:165, 1985.
9. Rowsey JJ: Ten caveats in keratorefractive surgery, *Ophthalmology* 90:148, 1983.
10. Holladay JT, Lynn MJ, Waring GO III, et al: The relationship of visual acuity, refractive error, and pupil size after radial keratotomy, *Arch Ophthalmol* 109:70, 1991.
11. Rowsey JJ, Balyeat HD, Rabinovitch B, et al: Predicting the results of radial keratotomy, *Ophthalmology* 90:642, 1983.
12. Rowsey JJ, Hays JD: Refractive reconstruction for acute eye injuries, *Ophthalmic Surg* 15:569, 1984.
13. Rowsey JJ, Isaac MS: Corneoscopy in keratorefractive surgery, *Cornea* 2:133, 1983.
14. Rowsey JJ, Reynolds AE, Brown R: Corneal topography: corneoscope, *Arch Ophthalmol* 99:1093, 1981.
15. Rowsey JJ, Fowler WC, Terry M, Scoper SV: Use of keratoscopy, slit-lamp biomicroscopy and retinoscopy in the management of astigmatism after penetrating keratoplasty, *Refract Corneal Surg* 7:33-41, 1991.
16. Sanders D, editor: *Radial keratotomy*, Thorofare, NJ, 1984, Slack.
17. Sanders DR, Hofmann RF, editors: *Refractive surgery: a text of radial keratotomy*, Thorofare, NJ, 1985, Slack.
18. Schanzlin D, Villaseñor RA: *Toric lathing of the cornea for the correction of astigmatism*, Presented at the Estelle Doheny Eye Foundation Residents' Day, Los Angeles, June 11, 1982.
19. Troutman R: Microsurgical control of corneal astigmatism in cataract and keratoplasty, *Trans Am Acad Ophthalmol Otolaryngol* 77:563, 1973.
20. Troutman RC, editor: *Microsurgery of the anterior segment of the eye. II. The cornea: optics and surgery*, St. Louis, 1977, Mosby–Year Book.
21. Werblin TP, Blaydes JE, Kaufman HE: Epikeratophakia: the surgical correction of astigmatism: preliminary experimental results, *CLAO J* 9:61, 1983.

Lessons from corneal topography

LEO J. MAGUIRE

Keratorefractive surgery caused two revolutions in eye care. The first revolution was the birth of modern keratorefractive surgery itself. The second and much more silent revolution was a renewal of activity in a very old field of study: analysis of the topography of the cornea. Recently these two fields of science, keratorefractive surgery and topography analysis of the cornea, began to nurture each other in a wonderfully symbiotic way that should speed the day when we can offer patients a keratorefractive operation with superb optical performance and excellent refractive stability.

Topography studies are important to anyone interested in corneal surgery because these studies show the strange and highly individualistic ways corneas change shape after such surgery. When one understands the results of topography studies of radial keratotomy,[1] epikeratoplasty,[4,6] excimer laser photorefractive surgery,[9,14] and penetrating keratoplasty,[3] one understands how inadequate and insensitive our previous measures of surgical success were.

Topography studies have shed light on the topography of the normal cornea and the cornea with noninflammatory ectatic degeneration as well. Since the interested reader can find recent exhaustive reviews describing the theory behind keratoscope-based topography systems[11] and reviews showing how topographers applied these systems to clinical practice,[5,13] I need not repeat those discussions here. Instead the chapter is a review of the keratorefractive studies that identified a need for improved analysis of corneal curvature, then a description the topography systems that evolved, and finally a discussion of the lessons corneal specialists learned from topography studies.

IDENTIFYING THE NEED FOR IMPROVED TOPOGRAPHY ANALYSIS

At the beginning of the twentieth century, Helmholtz and others interested in the physiologic optics of the normal eye suggested that the central portion of the cornea approximated a spherocylindrical optical system. This simplified notion approximates reality well enough to be useful for most clinical conditions found in normal eyes. We must understand that the keratometer, the instrument used most commonly in clinical practice to measure the curve of the

Supported in part by an unrestricted grant from Research to Prevent Blindness, Inc., New York, and the Mayo Foundation, Rochester, Minnesota.

central cornea, operates under the assumption that the cornea enclosed by the keratometer mire is spherocylindrical. When this assumption is not correct, keratometry measurements cannot represent corneal surface power accurately.

Most early studies of radial keratotomy, epikeratoplasty, and excimer laser ablation showed that changes in keratometry correlated inexactly with changes in refractive error after surgery.[12] Since the keratometric results did not correlate well with the refractive results, investigators began to suspect that at least some patients undergoing keratorefractive surgery had a postoperative cornea with an optical composition that differed from a spherocylindrical optical system.

Other studies that corroborated that hypothesis followed. In 1987 Santos, Waring, and associates wrote a classic paper that suggested indirectly that the amount of corneal irregularity induced by radial keratotomy differed among individual patients.[10] PERK (Prospective Evaluation of Radial Keratotomy) Study patients with cycloplegic refractions showing significant residual myopia showed on average a two-line better uncorrected Snellen acuity when compared to patients with the same cycloplegic refraction who had no surgery. This finding indicated that the cornea altered by radial keratotomy could have an optical surface that could produce a degraded image that could nonetheless be resolved over a wider refractive range than a normal cornea that gives superior resolution over a restricted refractive range. Investigators looked at these results and reasoned that the change in corneal curvature caused the change in the resolving power of these patients, but they had no effective way of measuring these corneas to understand the relationship between corneal topography and optical performance. They did not know what happened to the cornea when refractive instability or poor visual results were observed.

In short, keratorefractive surgeons were confused about their clinical results and knew they would stay confused until somebody made a machine that could show them the patterns of corneal power caused by their surgery.

KERATOSCOPE-BASED TOPOGRAPHY SYSTEMS

Once scientists understood they needed a system that would allow them to study the changes in power distribution on the cornea caused by keratorefractive surgery, they had to ask what they would require of an ideal system. The ideal system would simultaneously measure with accuracy the location and re-

fractive power of thousands of points evenly distributed over the entire corneal surface. The system would also have to translate these thousands of pieces of information into a form clinicians could understand without a crash course in topography analysis.

Since keratoscopes cover a large portion of the corneal surface, why not measure power at many points around the circumference of each keratoscope ring and use that information to interpolate surface power between these points? In 1985 Klyce introduced a prototype system that performed such analysis.[8] The system digitized keratoscope photos from a flat target keratoscope. Algorithms were used to calculate the location and corneal power of individual points around the circumference of each keratoscope ring. Almost 2000 measurements were made altogether. Since so many points in proximity were measured, algorithms that could infer power between the keratoscope rings could be developed. Klyce's greatest innovation was the introduction of color-coded maps to show patterns of corneal power distribution. Each color defines a range of corneal power, and the scale is set so that colors in the blue spectrum represent low power and red colors represent the highest power (Fig. 4-16).

Commercial systems soon followed. Computed Anatomy (New York City) introduced the Corneal Modeling System, which has more keratoscope rings and covers a larger portion of the surface of the cornea. The map format remained the same, but the ar-

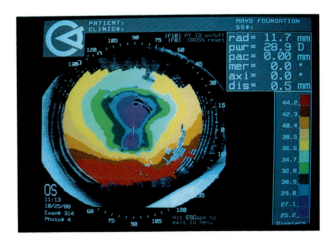

Fig. 4-16. Topography map of a patient complaining of visual disability despite a best corrected vision of 20/20 after radial keratotomy. Power ranges from 25.2 diopters to greater than 44.2 diopters. Each color represents a 1.9-diopter range of surface power. (Adapted from Maguire LJ, Bourne WM: *Refract Corneal Surg* 5:394, 1989.)

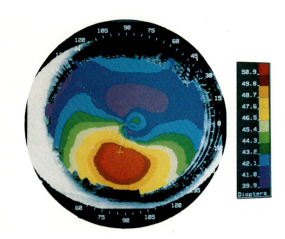

Fig. 4-17. Color-coded topographic map of a patient with early keratoconus generated by Corneal Modeling System. Each color represents a defined range of surface power (in this case 1.1 diopters). Blue areas are lowest power and colors closer to red spectrum represent areas of higher power. Red area identifies location of inferiorly displaced cone. Despite corneal irregularity, this patient could see 20/20 with a spectacle correction of −2.50. This map emphasizes that visual acuity and refractive results are an insensitive measure of corneal irregularity. (Adapted from Camp JJ, Maguire LJ, Cameron BM, et al: *Am J Ophthalmol* 109:379, 1990.)

eas of the cornea that could be analyzed increased. Most of the topography studies of the late 1980s used this system. Others systems like the EyeSys system and Computed Anatomy's TMS system followed in the early 1990s.

LESSONS FROM TOPOGRAPHY STUDIES

Rather than describe all topography studies in detail, let's review the lessons corneal specialists learned once they used topography analysis in their practice.

LESSON 1. Visual acuity and refractive error are inadequate and insensitive measures of corneal irregularity.

An airplane pilot complains of debilitating visual aberration after radial keratotomy even when a spectacle correction with moderate hyperopia and astigmatism improves vision to 20/20. Why should he complain when he sees 20/20 with spectacle correction? The topography map from the patient (Fig. 4-17) explains. Corneal power varies from 27.0 diopters to greater than 48 diopters. Each color represents a 2.1-diopter range. No one would argue that this is severe corneal distortion even though the patient sees 20/20. This example reminds us that clinical assessment of visual performance (visual acuity charts) and clinical assessment of ametropia (refractive er-

ror) are based on the assumption that the physiologic optics of the eye remain constant regardless of the method of correction of refractive error. This assumption is so basic it is rarely discussed in clinical texts on refraction. It is mentioned here because keratorefractive procedures and other corneal procedures do disturb the eye's optical system. In cases like our unfortunate airline pilot it may produce an optical system that makes an image capable of resolution but with much poorer image quality than the normal cornea. Snellen vision and residual refractive error are not good ways to measure corneal irregularity after corneal surgery. They are too insensitive. We must realize that an object like a high-contrast visual acuity letter can undergo tremendous image degradation and still be perceived. Topography analysis provides a more sensitive measure of surgical success.

LESSON 2. Not all corneas that look normal are normal.

Topography studies are helpful in identifying important abnormalities in corneas that would be considered normal using standard methods of measurement such as keratometry and slitlamp biomicroscopy. Let's illustrate with an example. A patient walks into the office wishing to have radial keratotomy. The slitlamp examination is normal. Vision is

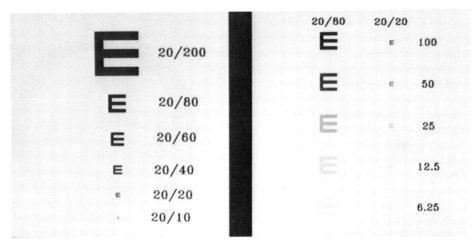

Fig. 4-18. These 20/20 and 20/80 letters of variable contrast (100%, 50%, 25%, 12.5%, 6.25%) are used as objects in a raytracing method that models optical performance of cornea. (Adapted from Camp JJ, Maguire LJ, Cameron BM, et al: *Am J Ophthalmol* 109:379, 1990.)

20/20 with a refraction of −2.50. Keratometry readings are 43.12 × 43.87. A perfect case for RK? Fig. 4-16 shows the patient's topography map. Each color represents 1.5 diopters of refractive power. Surface power ranges between 39.9 and 52 diopters. Power is distributed in a way characteristic of early keratoconus. Without topography analysis, this patient would have been an RK patient. How many of the so-called "outlyers"—patients with bad results after RK—were such "normals" who weren't normal?

LESSON 3. Topography analysis identifies design problems and surgeon errors that were not appreciated previously.

This fact was understood during the first clinical application of Klyce's topography system—the study of the topography of epikeratoplasty for myopia.[4] Klyce's epikeratoplasty design predicted that the zone of uniform power in the epikeratoplasty graft would be 6 mm. Topography analysis showed it was rarely larger than 4 mm. The study also showed that surgeons had inadvertently decentered the grafts in half the cases. Topography studies showed similar problems in the earliest reports of excimer laser photorefractive keratectomy for myopia.[9,14] Ablation zone sizes were often smaller than predicted, and decentration was common.

LESSON 4. Serial analysis of corneal topography can document corneal instability.

Serial studies shed important information on nonsurgical causes of corneal instability such as keratoconus[7] and contact lens–induced corneal warp.[15]

Wilson's study showed that contact lens decentration is a risk factor for developing warpage. Superior riding lenses produced a superior flattening and an inferior corneal steepening that mimicked the appearance of early keratoconus, but unlike keratoconus the pattern regressed over time. Topography returned to normal in 16 of 21 patients. Five patients showed some residual irregularity.[2] The Louisiana State University group was the first to use serial topography analysis to study refractive instability after keratorefractive surgery when they reported on their first 17 normally sighted patients who had excimer laser photorefractive keratectomy for myopia.[14] They showed that only 12 of 17 patients stabilized their topography during the first 7 postoperative months.

LESSON 5. Topography systems can help us to understand the optical consequences of corneal irregularity.

Topography analysis has improved our knowledge of the patterns of power distribution that can occur after surgical procedures. But what are we to make of the patient with a moderately irregular surface, 20/20 vision, and vague complaints of visual aberration? A need exists for methods that allow a more sensitive and direct measurement of the optical performance of the cornea. One method advocated is the electronic optical bench—a computer program that uses topography analysis as a component part of software that simulates the function of an optical bench.[2] The computer simulates objects in space such as visual acuity letters of varying contrast (Fig.

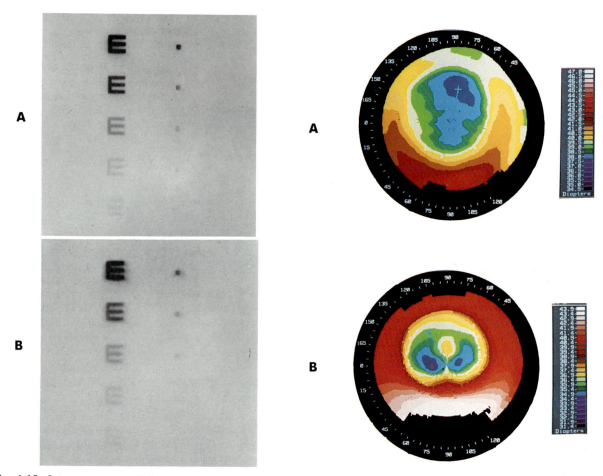

Fig. 4-19. Images generated from two patients after excimer laser photorefractive keratectomy for myopia. **A,** Image generated from topography map shown in Fig. 4-20, *A*. Letters are well resolved with even the lower contrast letters being visible. There is a slight loss of contrast and edge definition when compared to Fig. 4-18. This patient saw 20/20. **B,** Image generated from topography map shown in Figure 4-20, *B*. There is more loss of contrast, and 20/20 letters are not resolved. This patient sees 20/25, but analysis indicates that high-contrast 20/25 letter must be severely degraded. (Adapted from Maguire LJ, Zabel RW, Parker P, Lindstrom RL: *Refract Corneal Surg* 7:122-128, 1991.)

Fig. 4-20. Topography maps after excimer laser photorefractive keratectomy. In both maps each color represents a 0.5-diopter range of power. **A,** The map shows a well-centered ablation zone with minimal corneal irregularity. **B,** Map used to generate image in Fig. 4-19, *B*. The ablation zone is decentered and more irregular than that in Fig. 4-20, *A*. (Adapted from Maguire LJ, Zabel RW, Parker P, Lindstrom RL: *Refract Corneal Surg* 7:122-128, 1991.)

4-18). The lens is the cornea as represented by the topography system. Raytracing analysis produces an image at a defined vergence and presents the image on a video screen for analysis (Fig. 4-19). Fig. 4-19 shows how raytracing analysis may help clinicians understand the optical consequences of corneal irregularity. The images were generated by raytracing analysis of two patients after excimer photorefractive keratectomy for myopia. Fig. 4-19, *A*, is derived from a topography map that showed fairly good centration and a relatively uniform power centrally (Fig. 4-20, *A*), whereas Fig. 4-19, *B*, is derived from a patient who showed more decentration and more irregularity (Fig. 4-20, *B*). The first figure shows good resolution of the letters even at low contrast, whereas the second shows loss of contrast, poor edge definition, and poorly resolved low-contrast letters. These are the types of clinically important information that cannot be obtained from refractive and visual acuity results, keratometry, or even inspection of topography maps.

I hope that this chapter helps convince the reader of the important role topography studies play in the study of both medical and surgical causes of corneal irregularity. They are particularly important in studies of keratorefractive surgery where surgeons are making optical systems of a type different from those we usually associate with the cornea.

Investigators who learn the lessons topography studies have to teach will identify deficiencies early, correct them, and speed the day when we can guarantee keratorefractive patients a stable surface with superior optical performance.

REFERENCES

1. Bogan SJ, Maloney RK, Drews CD, Waring GO: Computer-assisted videokeratography of corneal topography after radial keratotomy, *Arch Ophthalmol* 109:834, 1991.
2. Camp JJ, Maguire LJ, Cameron BM, Robb RA: A computer model for the evaluation of the effect of corneal topography on optical performance, *Am J Ophthalmol* 109:379-386, 1991.
3. Frangieh GT, Kwitko S, McDonnell PJ: Prospective corneal topographic analysis in surgery for postkeratoplasty astigmatism, *Arch Ophthalmol* 109:506, 1991.
4. Maguire LJ: Corneal topography of patients with excellent Snellen visual acuity after epikeratoplasty for aphakia, *Am J Ophthalmol* 109:162, 1990.
5. Maguire LJ: Topography analysis and corneal disease, *Ophthalmol Clin North Am* 3:651-663, 1990.
6. Maguire LJ, Lowry JC: Identifying progression of subclinical keratoconus by serial topography analysis, *Am J Ophthalmol* 112:41-45, 1991.
7. Maguire LJ, Singer DE, Klyce SD: Graphic presentation of computer analyzed keratoscope photographs, *Arch Ophthalmol* 105:223, 1987.
8. Maguire LJ, Klyce SD, Singer DE, et al: Corneal topography in myopic patients undergoing epikeratophakia, *Am J Ophthalmol* 103:404, 1987.
9. Maguire LJ, Zabel RW, Parker P, Lindstrom RL: Topography and raytracing analysis of patients with excellent visual acuity 3 months after excimer photorefractive keratectomy for myopia, *Refract Corneal Surg* 7:122-128, 1991.
10. Santos VR, Waring GO III, Lynn MJ, et al: Relationship between refractive error and visual acuity in the Prospective Evaluation of Radial Keratotomy (PERK) study, *Arch Ophthalmol* 105:86, 1989.
11. Wang J, Rice DA, Klyce SD: A new reconstruction algorithm for improvement of corneal topographical analysis, *Refract Corneal Surg* 5:397, 1989.
12. Waring GO, Lynn MJ, Strahlman ER, et al: Stability of refraction during four years after radial keratotomy in the prospective evaluation of radial keratotomy in the prospective evaluation of radial keratotomy study, *Am J Ophthalmol* 111:133-144, 1991.
13. Wilson SD, Klyce SD: Advances in the analysis of corneal topography, *Surv Ophthalmol* 35:269, 1991.
14. Wilson SE, Klyce SD, McDonald MB, et al: Changes in corneal topography after excimer laser photorefractive keratectomy for myopia, *Ophthalmology* 98:1338, 1991.
15. Wilson SE, Lin DTC, Klyce SD, et al: Topographic changes in contact lens–induced corneal warpage, *Ophthalmology* 97:734-744, 1990.

Chapter 5

Stromal Wound Healing

MARK L. McDERMOTT

Understanding corneal wound healing is essential for the corneal surgeon. Corneal wound healing influences preoperative evaluation, operative procedure selection, and postoperative care for all reconstructive and refractive corneal procedures. In this chapter the central emphasis is on describing the events that occur in the human corneal stroma during wound healing after a full-thickness, central, circular, sutured incision. During the course of this discussion other wound types including partial-thickness, unsutured, linear, and ablative are mentioned but only as a source of comparison to highlight differences in wound healing. The effects of sutures, topical drugs, host factors, and technique on wound healing are presented. Common clinical problems in keratoplasty wounds are reviewed. Several summaries on the subject exist for additional review.[5,7,19,38,41]

CORNEAL STROMAL ANATOMY

The corneal stroma represents 80% of the corneal thickness. Its three principle constituents are collagen fibrils, proteoglycans (PGs), and keratocytes. The collagen fibrils consist mainly of collagen type I.[47] The principle role for the collagen is to provide tensile strength to the corneal matrix. The proteoglycan content is approximately 60% keratan sulfate proteoglycan and 40% dermatan sulfate proteoglycan. Proteoglycans consist of a protein chain to which multiple polyanionic carbohydrate polymers are covalently bound.[51] The protein chains that form the core proteins are heterogeneous with significant variation in amino acid sequence. They vary in size from 11,000 to 220,000 daltons. The glycosaminoglycan component consists of multiple chains made up of polymerized disaccharides. The physical properties of the glycosaminoglycan determine the behavior of the proteoglycan.[51] All glycosaminoglycans are polyanions with increasing charge density in the more highly sulfated types. In aqueous solutions proteoglycans have large bound water compartments, and their tertiary structure is one of a large hydrated sphere. Proteoglycans are large hydrophilic molecules that act as space maintainers. This role is essential in maintaining a regular spatial arrangement of the collagen fibrils to promote corneal transparency. The keratocyte serves to continually renew the other two stromal elements. It has the capacity to phagocytose collagen and glycosaminoglycans, to resynthesize new collagen and glycosaminoglycans, and to deposit them in an orderly array.

CORNEAL WOUND HEALING

Incision. Corneal wounding produces zones of tissue death, injury, and distortion. Depending on the wounding implement, the zones can be very narrow or relatively broad. Techniques using scissors to excise donor buttons and prepare recipient beds produces the widest zones of trauma. Such zones are produced because of the substantial crush injury to the areas adjacent to the incision. The thicker the tissue that is attempted to be divided, the greater is the crush effect. In addition to the crush effect, scissors incisions have the potential to create scrolls of both Descemet's membrane and Bowman's membrane. These scrolls are often incarcerated into the incision and may adversely affect wound healing.[35,42,45,46] It appears that Descemet's membrane may act as a barrier to ingrowth of fibroblastic cells creating a focal area of weakness where stroma and Descemet's membrane abut.[46] This weakness has also been seen in human full-thickness lamellar keratoplasties where a weakened total graft-host bond was observed in the area where donor Descemet's membrane is adjacent to recipient stroma.[44]

Use of corneal trephines to punch the donor button and to cut to the level of Descemet's membrane in the recipient bed reduces this crush effect. The findings after use of a disposable trephine include disruption and distortion of the corneal epithelium.[52] Such damage is attributable to a combination of compressive and shear forces created as the trephine is placed on the recipient bed and rotated.[32] It is also related to the construction of the trephine blade itself. All trephines have a tapering bevel on the outside surface of the barrel. It is this bevel that creates the shear effect. The magnitude of this effect increases as the downward pressure is increased.[32] As the trephine enters Bowman's membrane and deeper stromal layers, it may wander axially as well as anteroposteriorly. This results in noticeable variation in the surface contour of the "walls" of the incision.[32] On an ultrastructural level stromal lamellae are irregularly frayed and torn with jagged transitions from one lamella to the next deeper one.[52] Keratocytes are torn, stretched, and exposed.[32] Insertion of the corneal scissors to complete the incision through Descemet's membrane during suturing causes additional trauma through crushing both by the scissors itself and by focal application of the tissue-fixation forceps. This crush effect also damages the peripheral recipient endothelium. Focal application of the forceps and stretching of the recipient Descemet's membrane also results in endothelial loss.[2]

The nature of the other half of the wound, the incision in the donor button, is similar but with less trauma, since scissors are not used in its preparation. Full-thickness punching out of the corneal button with the endothelial side up results in a 1% to 2% endothelial cell loss adjacent to the trephine incision.[2] What is different, however, is the fact that the donor cornea has been incubated in a storage medium for a period of time of up to 1 week. During this time there is uptake of colloids such as dextran or chondroitin sulfate from the medium into the stroma. At the same time stromal glycosaminoglycans have been shown to be eluted from the stroma into the storage medium.[30,54] Moreover, the degree of loss is dependent on the medium, with dextran-

free media showing the greatest loss of glycosaminoglycans.[54]

With this background the nature of the keratoplasty wound can be summarized. It is full thickness with an annular surface epithelial wound created by scissors, forceps, and the trephine; a grossly vertical stromal wound created by scissors, forceps, and trephines; and an annular endothelial wound created by scissors. When the wound is sutured, the stored, edematous, and traumatized corneal stroma of the donor is abutted against a similarly traumatized recipient stroma, which retains a preexisting pathologic condition. There is an epithelial defect overlying the stromal incision and an endothelial defect lying below.

Early Noncellular Events. The immediate events surrounding a corneal wound have been determined almost exclusively through animal model experiments. In the majority of studies the animal model is a rabbit. There are several important differences between these studies and the in vivo event as practiced by corneal surgeons. Species differences include absence of Bowman's membrane in the rabbit; the tendency for rabbit wounds to gape open; the proliferative ability of the rabbit endothelium, which allows rabbit wounds an additional posterior source of fibroblastic cells in healing; the relatively young age of the rabbit tissue; the presence of a nictitating membrane; and the greater iris vascularity and greater anterior chamber inflammatory response of the rabbit. There are also significant differences in the types of wounds made. In most rabbit studies one produces the wounds by performing a full-thickness, central, 2 mm trephination and removing the button, thus creating a 2 mm diameter full-thickness corneal defect that is left unsutured with the defect to be plugged by a fibrin clot. Although this wound is substantially different from a human keratoplasty incision, it may provide an indicator of the sequence of events but not necessarily the magnitude of the events involved in wound healing.

The earliest soluble event in both human and rabbit wounds appears to be the deposition of fibrin, fibronectin, and other elements of the clotting cascade in the wound. In the rabbit the source of the fibrin is a protein-rich exudate from the iris and vascular arcade that literally forms a clot in the anterior chamber and extends to form a fibrin-rich plug in the defect.[9] In humans this degree of fibrinous anterior chamber response is rare, usually seen in diabetic patients with iris neovascularization who undergo prolonged retinal procedures.

In humans the source of fibrin is probably from a combination of anterior chamber exudation, limbal vessels, and conjunctival vasculature. In the rabbit the deposition of the fibrin clot is important, since it acts as a scaffold for migrating corneal epithelium to guide the cells to close the epithelial defect.[15] It also serves as a matrix for proliferating fibroblasts to move through.[15] In humans the size of the epithelial defect at the wound margins is smaller, but fibrin and fibronectin have been shown to be important in assisting with epithelial migration thus facilitating closure. The contribution of fibrin to human stromal wound healing is unclear. A well-opposed wound leaves little space for large amounts of fibrin, but even the small amount present may provide important chemotactic functions. Larger amounts of fibrin may be counterproductive, since an epithelial plug may subsequently form within the anterior incision and such a formation alters wound healing.

Large amounts of fibronectin are synthesized by stromal keratocytes as well.[61] This fibronectin plays a role in the adhesion and migration of both fibroblasts and epithelial cells.

Besides ingress of factors from the clotting cascade, there is tissue necrosis. Keratocytes within a few hundred micrometers of the wound edge die[8,45] and at 1 to 2 hours the cells adjacent to the wound appear pyknotic.[9,33] These cells rapidly decrease in number creating a narrow (200 μm) hypocellular band adjacent to the walls of the incision.[9,33] There is also edema of the wound margins,[33] which may in part be attributable to loss of corneal proteoglycans[30] as well as fluid accumulation. The elastic Bowman's membrane and Descemet's membrane retract from the incision.

Cellular Response. The cellular changes occurring after wounding center on the death, alteration, and proliferation of keratocytes and epithelial cells as well as the influx of leukocytes. In a penetrating keratoplasty with viable keratocytes and structural matrix in the donor button, the cellular constituents come from both donor and recipient tissues. This is in contrast to epikeratophakia where the cellular response is totally from the recipient.[31] In the zone beyond keratolysis, that is, a zone 200 to 500 μm from the wound, keratocytes show morphologic changes within hours of wounding.[33] The alterations include hypertrophy of cytosolic granules, extension of cytoplasmic limbs, and the appearance of multiple nucleoli.[33] The appearance of nucleoli indicates increased protein synthesis, which corresponds well to autoradiographic experiments indicating increased uptake of ^{3}H-thymidine and ^{3}H-leucine in a zone 500 to 900 μm from the wound edge within hours of the incision.[9] This progressive keratocyte hypertrophy, migration, and transformation continues for about 1

week, with a peak between the third and sixth day.[9,15,33] Other studies have confirmed the role of transformed keratocytes in supplying fibroblasts to the healing wound.[58,59]

In rabbit-wound healing the early cell density along the wound margin from anterior to posterior is not uniform. There is greater cell density in the anterior portion of the wound than posteriorly.[15] This relative anterior stromal hypercellularity may reflect an interaction between the overlying epithelium and stromal fibroblasts.[15,19,20] In human keratoplasty wounds this cellular disparity is probably less because of differences in wound type.

It is important to understand that the keratocyte is not the sole source of a fibroblastic type of cell. Circulating monocytes may enter the wound[15] through tears, aqueous humor, neovascularization, or stromal migration and be transformed into fibroblasts. In partial-thickness incisions from the endothelial surface, aqueous humor was shown to be a significant source of fibroblastic cells.[3]

An important early role for keratocytes and fibroblasts is phagocytosis. Human keratocytes have been shown to possess phagocytic abilities in cell culture, and this ability is probably contributory in the degradation of damaged proteoglycans and collagen lamellae at the wound edge.[34] Moreover, the local deposition of fibronectin in the wound[61] may enhance this phagocytic activity by opsonic effects.[43] Fibroblastic cells as well possess phagocytic activity. There appears to be concomitant secretion of collagenase with fibroblast phagocytic activity.[4] Other enzyme systems have also been shown to be present at the wound margin. In rabbit keratectomy wounds urokinase type of plasminogen activator has been found localized to the margins.[56] The plasminogen activator–plasmin system appears also to play a degradative role either directly through plasmin or as a result of plasmin-catalyzed conversion of precollagenases to collagenases.[56]

In addition to keratocyte and fibroblast activity, the early wound is characterized by the influx of polymorphonuclear leukocytes. Although entry to the area can occur through migration within the stroma, it appears that a significant portal of entry for polymorphonuclear leukocytes is into the wound itself from tears.[1,28] Neutrophils have been seen as soon as 1.5 hours after wounding, peaking at 12 hours and slowly declining over 72 hours.[9,28] In the keratoplasty incision there is little gaping, which may make neutrophil entry into the incision more difficult, but there is also the presence of sutures, which penetrate into deep stroma thus providing an easy portal of entry for tear neutrophils. In patients with preexisting ocular inflammatory disease and vascularized corneas, neutrophil ingress probably occurs to a greater degree. The presence of neutrophils is important in the phagocytosis of dead keratocytes and damaged stromal collagen and matrix. In studies attempting to quantify stromal destruction from inflammation it appeared that stromal loss was the result of neutrophil activity and that stromal collagen synthesis was not decreased.[50] In addition, this loss of stromal collagen was preventable by corticosteroids, which reduced the entry of neutrophils into the area.[50]

Epithelial cells appear to play a major role in stromal wound strength. In rabbits, sutured central partial-thickness wounds of which the epithelium was debrided daily had a 66% reduction in tensile strength compared to similarly wounded corneas of which the epithelium was allowed to heal.[25] In primates who underwent central, full-thickness, unsutured incisions in octanol-debrided corneas showed a 66% reduction in burst strength compared to corneas with an intact epithelium.[11] To a degree, presence of epithelial cells in a corneal wound is beneficial in maximizing tensile strength. Excessive accumulation and persistence of epithelium within a human corneal incision to form an epithelial plug, however, weakens the incision. In unsutured, deep, partial-thickness, radial incisions in humans (radial keratotomy) persistence of the epithelial plug is of long term (years) and is presumed to be contributory to the incomplete healing of such wounds.[7,18] The presence of epithelium within the wound in human radial keratotomy specimens was associated with reduction in fibroblastic activity in the surrounding stroma.[18]

This conflicting role of the epithelium in wound healing can be rationalized in the following manner. The production of a small epithelial defect during wounding and its attendant healing may result in cellular and soluble mediators that stimulate stromal fibroblastic activity as well. In this respect the epithelium assists in augmenting stromal tensile strength. If, however, there is wound gaping or malapposition of the wound, epithelium enters the wound forming a plug and by contact inhibition prevents stromal fibroblasts from crossing the area. In rabbits this epithelial plug is expelled and fibroblasts do cross the area, but in humans the epithelial plug is not readily expelled and may persist for years.[18]

Matrix Changes. Rabbit corneal wound healing studies have shown time-dependent, distinct alterations in proteoglycan type and concentration in both the corneal scar as well as in the adjacent stroma.[13,17,24] During the first week a presumed elution from adjacent stroma of native, previously synthesized proteoglycans into the wound itself occurs.[13] Dermatan sulfate proteoglycan (DSPG) appears to be closely associated with the fibrin clot.[13] Native, highly sulfated keratan sulfate proteoglycan (KSPG) also enters the wound from the cut stromal edge.[13] There is a nonuniform distribution of these native proteoglycans within the wound scar. They are concentrated in the anterior and middle portions of the scar with little deposition posteriorly.[13] Adjacent areas of stroma show relative depletion of these same proteoglycans compared to more remote areas of normal stroma. By the second week there is evidence of de novo synthesis within the scar of sparsely sulfated keratan sulfate proteoglycan and greatly sulfated dermatan sulfate proteoglycan.[17,24] The sparsely sulfated KSPG is antigenically distinct from native greatly sulfated KSPG.[24] The cause for this difference is presumed attributable to alterations in the keratan sulfate glycosaminoglycan (less sulfation), since the core proteins of sparsely sulfated KSPG and greatly sulfated KSPG appears immunologically similar.[24] The DSPG from scar tissue is also different from native DSPG. It consists of two populations: one of higher and the other of lower size than that of native DSPG.[17] Besides being opposite to normal corneal proteoglycans in the degree of sulfation, the rate of KSPG to DSPG is altered in the scar. There appears to be a preponderance of DSPG within the scar.[13] In normal corneal stroma the ratio of KSPG/DSPG is 2.3, in the scar it is 0.6, and in adjacent stroma 1.5.[17] In addition, the proteoglycans in the adjacent stroma show a higher charge density than that in either normal stroma or the scar.[17]

As additional time elapses, the rate of proteoglycan synthesis decreases but the quantity of proteoglycan in the scar and adjacent stroma increases.[17] After several years proteoglycan content tends to revert toward normal stromal composition.

In addition to proteoglycan synthesis, the corneal wound must synthesize new collagen to provide tensile strength for the tissue. During the first 4 weeks of experimental full-thickness keratoplasty wounds in rabbits there is both a small increase in collagenolysis and a larger increase in collagen synthesis.[37] In other studies using rabbit models, collagen of types I, III, V, and VI are synthesized and deposited within the wound.[12,14,15] The predominant quantity is of collagen type I trimer with lesser amounts of collagen types V and VI.[12,14] Small quantities of collagen type III are present, restricted to the most posterior aspect of the wound.[16] The amount of type III collagen disappears with increasing wound age.[16]

The organization of this collagen deposition changes with time as well. In rabbit wounds in the first week after wounding the area contains multiple flat fibroblasts that lie tangentially to the wound surface.[15] Collagen deposition is in the form of single filaments or bundles that run along the surface of the fibroblasts.[15] By three weeks after wounding a dense network of fibrils is present. Some are in the form of tight parallel bundles, whereas others are randomly oriented.[15] At 4 months after wounding no discernible pattern of collagen deposition is seen. The matrix appears granular and a random meshwork of fibrils is seen. In rabbit tissue followed for 2 years after wounding the lamellar collagen pattern is reapproximated, but the area of scar may be identified by the shorter and narrower lamellae present.

Course. There are few human or primate data on the course of healing in keratoplasty wounds. Most studies are histopathologic examinations obtained post mortem.[35] Nevertheless, it is improbable that human corneal wounds heal by reanastamosing of the cut ends of stromal lamellae.[41] More likely there is a deposition of a tangle of new fibrils within the wound that then intercalate with adjacent stromal lamellae.[41]

The architecture of the keratoplasty wound in humans may play some role in healing. Penetrating keratoplasty wounds are seldom perpendicular. The interface at the graft-host junction often assumes an S or V configuration.[35,42] Incarcerated epithelium, Bowman's membrane, or Descemet's membrane within the wound are not uncommon findings in the postkeratoplasty wound.[35,42,45,46] The presence of this tissue invariably weakens the wound and may be associated with excessive keratometric astigmatism.[35] In lamellar keratoplasty using full-thickness donor tissue the apposition of donor Descemet's membrane with deep recipient stroma resulted in poor healing.[44] Poor wound alignment may result in anterior stromal outgrowth if significant anterior override is present.[27] Actual wound gaping is quickly filled with epithelium to form an epithelial plug. The presence of epithelium, however, mimics the healing of a radial keratotomy incision resulting in a weaker wound.[8,18] Posterior gaping of the wound is contributory to retrocorneal membrane formation and iridocorneal adhesions.[35]

Even with "complete" healing the tensile strength of the corneal wound is less than intact corneal tissue. In rabbits the tensile strength of full-thickness central sutured corneal wounds was determined over time for up to 100 days.[25] For up to the first week after wounding there was essentially no tensile strength. From day 10 through day 40 tensile strength increased from 8% to 36% of intact tissue. From day 40 to day 100 the rate at which tensile strength increased slowed, rising from 36% to 50% that of intact tissue. Although no animals were followed by later observation, the decline in the rate of tensile strength gain is suggestive that noticeable gains greater than 50% are unlikely. The location of the wound also affects ultimate tensile strength. In rabbits the same sutured incisions placed paralimbally in the cornea showed greater tensile strength than central wounds at the same period of time after wounding.[25] This time-dependent increase in wound strength has also been observed in human time. Corneas obtained post mortem at various times after a clear corneal section showed a slow increase in the breaking load with time.[53] The difference between this study and the rabbit study was that the 50% tensile strength level did not occur until 2 to 3 years postoperatively in humans.[53]

This relatively long period until tensile strength is regained may account for the incidence of keratoplasty wound separations occurring shortly after suture removal.[6] In that study interrupted suture removal during the first 3 months postoperatively was associated with focal wound separations, usually in the inferotemporal quadrants.[6] Even with adequate healing the graft-host junction is a source of weakness.[23] After blunt trauma the rupture always occurs at the graft-host junction[21,23,49,57] often with loss of the lens and uveal prolapse. The prognosis is often guarded because of posterior segment trauma.[49,21]

MODIFIERS OF HEALING

Sutures. Sutures provide several functions in the healing corneal wound. They precisely align tissue edges to minimize override or underride, which in turn reduce the incidence of stromal outgrowth and retrocorneal membrane formation. They eliminate wound dead space thereby minimizing the migration distance that fibroblasts must travel and limit epithelial ingrowth. During the early lytic phase of wound healing they provide tensile strength. They serve as a nidus of inflammation to stimulate the production of tear leukocytes and macrophages, which in turn assist in lytic and synthetic phases of healing. They also provide a portal of entry for the same cells into the deep stroma for more complete healing. Characteristics of sutures that affect the inflammatory response of those sutures include (1) the material, (2) their gauge, and (3) the pattern of suturing.

From studies in cutaneous incisions stainless steel and nylon materials incite the least inflammatory response, with organic materials such as silk or gut inciting the most response. The larger the suture gage, the greater is the mass of foreign body and subsequent inflammatory response. Primate studies have characterized the inflammatory response to indwelling interrupted 10-0 nylon sutures as predominantly lymphocytic surrounding the sutures.[42] Intimately associated with the sutures was an extensive fibroblastic proliferation.[42]

In general, the inflammatory response is variable depending on the manner of suturing. A running 10-0 nylon with 4 or 5 bites per quadrant probably has a greater mass of suture within the wound compared to 16 interrupted sutures, but the interrupted sutures have a focal area of greater bulk in the vicinity of the knot.

In comparing a sutured deep partial-thickness radial keratotomy wound with similar deep unsutured wounds one can gain an idea as to the effect of sutures on wound healing. In a primate model identical corneal wounds were prepared, with the only difference being the presence of one or more buried 10-0 nylon sutures in one eye compared to its unsutured paired mate.[42] The presence of the sutures resulted in several notable differences histopathologically in tissues examined 2.5 to 8 months postoperatively. Sutured wounds (1) lacked epithelial plugs, (2) showed complete healing, (3) showed significant subepithelial fibroplasia with a hypertrophic scar, and (4) showed fibroblasts and lamellae that spanned the wound. In comparison, unsutured wounds (1) showed a prominent and chronic epithelial plug, (2) had less complete healing, (3) lacked subepithelial fibroplasia, and (4) showed fibroblasts and lamellae that ran parallel to the wound edges rather than spanning across the wound. Similar findings were present when human sutured keratoplasty wounds examined post mortem were compared to postmortem radial keratotomy wounds.[42]

Before suture removal, one of the most indeterminant areas is estimation of the completeness of wound healing. Because of the irregular collagen lamellae within the wound, light is scattered resulting in a visible scar. In general, the amount of scarring optically present increases with time.[40] A dense scar is often a good indicator of sufficient healing, especially if it is associated with loosening of previously tight sutures. The loosening of sutures is associated with wound contraction, probably attributable to fibroblast activity as well as some contractibility of the scar itself.[39] Heavy scar, however, is not always foolproof as an indicator of wound healing. A dense-appearing scar may be just superficial stromal outgrowth from wound-edge mismatch, and the wound could be really quite immature.[27] In addition, incarcerated Descemet's membrane or Bowman's membrane may focally weaken an otherwise dense-appearing scar.[45,46]

Besides scarring, the presence of a blood vessel within the wound or crossing it proper is usually very good evidence that sufficient healing in that area has occurred. Also if the recipient bed is vascularized, rapid healing is the usual course. Another important host factor is age. Keratoplasty incisions in children heal over a period of weeks compared to their adult counterparts, which take months to years.

Corticosteroids. Topical corticosteroids have been shown to reduce the strength of the fresh corneal wound. This effect appears to be dose related. In rabbits receiving a full-thickness central linear incision with the placement of interrupted 7-0 silk sutures a 50% reduction in tensile strength was seen in the animals receiving 0.1% dexamethasone topically 12 times a day.[26] Animals wounded in an identical fashion showed no reduction in tensile strength when treated with either 0.01% dexamethasone 12 times a day or 0.1% dexamethasone 4 times a day.[26] A later study using rabbits receiving a central full-thickness, linear incision was able to show a modest (20%) reduction in burst strength in animals treated with 1% prednisolone acetate four times a day.[48] It is likely that the level of corticosteroids commonly used clinically (that is, prednisolone acetate 1% four times a day) in the postoperative period after keratoplasty does not cause enough wound strength reduction to be clinically significant. If, however, more frequent daily dosing is used, their effect on wound healing may become clinically important.

Similarly, if a keratoplasty wound is subjected to higher than normal distending forces as in poorly controlled glaucoma, the modest reduction in wound strength from 1% prednisolone acetate 4 times a day may be significant enough to cause a wound dehiscence.

Other. Besides corticosteroids, the keratoplasty wound is exposed to a variety of antibiotic, antiviral, and antihypertensive drops and ointments. Their effect on wound healing may be mediated through several routes. One way is a direct effect of the drug on stromal wound healing. Antivirals are often cited as having this effect on wound healing. In one study either idoxuridine (IDU) or vidarabine (adenine arabinoside, ara-A) ointment applied 4 times a day after a full-thickness central trephination in rabbits caused an approximate 40% reduction in burst strength 21 days after wounding.[36] A later study showed differing results. In that study 0.1% IDU drops given 8 times a day or 1% trifluorothymidine drops given 8 times a day to eyes after a full-thickness central trephination in rabbits resulted in no significant reduction in burst strength compared to vehicle-treated controls 21 days after wounding. 3% ara-A drops at the same frequency actually resulted in an increase in burst strength.[22] These results indicate that the direct effect of antivirals on stromal wound healing is unclear.

Another important way any topical medication including antivirals may affect stromal wound healing is by inhibition of epithelial closure over the wound. Any reduction in the rate of epithelial closure will significantly retard stromal wound strength.[11,25]

In this regard, all three antiviral drops 0.1% IDU, 3% ara-A, and 1% trifluorothymidine cause clinically and histopathologically apparent toxic changes in regenerating corneal epithelium.[22] Topical antibiotic solutions also affect corneal epithelial healing rates. Five percent cefazolin and the commercial mixture of neomycin, polymixin B, and gramicidin had the smallest reduction in healing rates, whereas the aminoglycosides and 0.5% chloramphenicol had the greatest reductions in healing rate.[55]

Besides the parent compund contained within any medication, the effect of the vehicle on epithelial healing must also be considered. The most important component of the vehicle is the preservative used. Benzalkonium chloride 0.01% is probably the most toxic preservative to the healing corneal epithelium. Other vehicle components such as purified mineral oil and white petrolatum have been shown to have no effect on epithelial healing.[29]

In distinction to all other classes of drugs, growth factors may actually strengthen corneal wounds. Full-thickness central corneal wounds in rabbits showed a highly significant increase in tensile strength over vehicle-treated controls 5 days after wounding when treated topically with 0.5 mg/ml mouse epidermal growth factor (mEGF) 3 times daily.[60] Human epidermal growth factor (hEGF) 0.5 mg/ml given 4 times a day resulted in a doubling of burst strength in full-thickness central corneal incisions in primates.[11] Human EGF in the same dose has also been shown to accelerate the rate of epithelial closure in both epithelial débridement and anterior keratectomy wounds.[10]

REFERENCES

1. Anderson JA, Murphy JA, Gaster RN: Inflammatory cell responses to radial keratotomy, *Refract Corneal Surg* 5:21-26, 1989.
2. Bahn CF et al: Effect of 1% sodium hyaluronate (Healon®) on a nonregenerating (Feline) corneal endothelium, *Invest Ophthalmol Vis Sci* 27(10):1485-1494, 1986.
3. Baum JL: Source of the fibroblast in central corneal wound healing, *Arch Ophthalmol* 85:473-477, 1971.
4. Berman M, Leary R, Gage J: Collagenase from corneal cell cultures and its modulation by phagocytosis, *Invest Ophthalmol Vis Sci* 18(6):588-601, 1979.
5. Binder PS: What we have learned about corneal wound healing from refractive surgery, *Refract Corneal Surg* 5:98-119, 1989.
6. Binder PS et al: Keratoplasty wound separations, *Am J Ophthalmol* 80(1):109-115, 1975.
7. Binder PS et al: *Symposium on medical surgical diseases of the cornea*, St. Louis, 1980, Mosby—Year Book.
8. Binder PS et al: An ultrastructural and histochemical study of long-term wound healing after radial keratotomy, *Am J Ophthalmol* 103:432-440, 1987.
9. Bracher R: Radioautographic analysis of the synthesis of protein, RNA, DNA, and sulfated mucopolysaccharides in the early stages of corneal wound healing, *Invest Ophthalmol Vis Sci* 6(6):565-573, 1967.
10. Brazzell RK et al: Human recombinant epidermal growth factor experimental corneal wound healing, *Invest Ophthalmol Vis Sci* 32(2):336-340, 1991.
11. Brightwell JR et al: Biosynthetic human EGF accelerates healing of neodecadron-treated primate corneas, *Invest Ophthalmol Vis Sci* 26(1):105-110, 1985.
12. Cho H, Covington HI, Cintron C: Immunolocalization of type VI collagen in developing and healing rabbit cornea, *Invest Ophthalmol Vis Sci* 31(6):1096-1102, 1990.
13. Cintron C, Covington HI, Kublin CL: Morphologic analyses of proteoglycans in rabbit cornea scars, *Invest Ophthalmol Vis Sci* 31(9):1789-1798, 1990.
14. Cintron C, Hong B: Heterogeneity of collagens in rabbit cornea: type VI collagen, *Invest Ophthalmol Vis Sci* 29(5):760-766, 1988.
15. Cintron C et al: Scanning electron microscopy of rabbit corneal scars, *Invest Ophthalmol Vis Sci* 23(1):550-563, 1982.
16. Cintron C et al: Heterogeneity of collagens in rabbit cornea: type III collagen, *Invest Ophthalmol Vis Sci* 29(5):767-775, 1988.
17. Cintron C et al: Biochemical analyses of proteoglycans in rabbit corneal scars, *Invest Ophthalmol Vis Sci* 31(10):1975-1981, 1990.
18. Deg JK, Zavala EY, Binder PS: Delayed corneal wound healing following radial keratotomy, *Ophthalmology* 92(6):734-740, 1985.
19. Duke-Elder S, editor: *Diseases of the outer eye, part II*, Vol. VIII, *The healing and regeneration of the corneal stroma*, St. Louis, 1965, Mosby—Year Book.
20. Eiferman RA: Corneal wound healing and the future of refractive surgery, *Refract Corneal Surg* 5:73-74, 1989.
21. Farley MK, Pettit TH: Traumatic wound dehiscence after penetrating keratoplasty, *Am J Ophthalmol* 104:44-49, 1987.
22. Foster CS, Pavan-Langston D: Corneal wound healing and antiviral medication, *Arch Ophthalmol* 95:2062-2067, 1977.
23. Friedman AH: Late traumatic wound rupture following successful partial penetrating keratoplasty, *Am J Ophthalmol* 75(1):117-120, 1973.
24. Funderburgh JL et al: Immunoanalysis of keratan sulfate proteoglycan from corneal scars, *Invest Ophthalmol Vis Sci* 29(7):1116-1124, 1988.
25. Gasset AR, Dohlman CH: The tensile strength of corneal wounds, *Arch Ophthalmol* 79:595-602, 1968.
26. Gasset AR et al: Quantitative corticosteroid effect on corneal wound healing, *Arch Ophthalmol* 81:589-591, 1969.
27. Girard LJ et al: Corneal stromal outgrowth, *Am J Ophthalmol* 76(4):445-450, 1973.
28. Haik BG, Zimny ML: Scanning electron microscopy of corneal wound healing in the rabbit, *Invest Ophthalmol Vis Sci* 16(9):787-796, 1977.
29. Hanna C et al: The effect of ophthalmic ointments on corneal wound healing, *Am J Ophthalmol* 76(2):193-200, 1973.

30. Kangas TA et al: Loss of stromal glycosaminoglycans during corneal edema, *Invest Ophthalmol Vis Sci* 31(10):1994-2002, 1990.

31. Katakami C et al: Keratocyte activity in wound healing after epikeratophakia in rabbits, *Invest Ophthalmol Vis Sci* 32(6):1837-1845, 1991.

32. Kerr-Muir MG et al: Ultrastructural comparison of conventional surgical and argon fluoride excimer laser keratectomy, *Am J Ophthalmol* 103:448-453, 1987.

33. Kitano S, Goldman JN: Cytologic and histochemical changes in corneal wound repair, *Arch Ophthalmol* 76:345-354, 1966.

34. Lande MA et al: Phagocytic properties of human keratocyte cultures, *Invest Ophthalmol Vis Sci* 20(4):481-489, 1981.

35. Lang GK, Green WR, Maumenee AE: Clinicopathologic studies of keratoplasty eyes obtained post mortem, *Am J Ophthalmol* 101:28-40, 1986.

36. Langston RHS, Pavan-Langston D, Dohlman CH: Antiviral medication and corneal wound healing, *Arch Ophthalmol* 92:509-513, 1974.

37. Lass JH et al: Collagen degradation and synthesis in experimental corneal grafts, *Exp Eye Res* 42:201-210, 1986.

38. Lemp MA: Cornea and sclera, *Arch Ophthalmol* 94:473-490, 1976.

39. Luttrull JK, Smith RE, Jester JV: In vitro contractility of avascular corneal wounds in rabbit eyes, *Invest Ophthalmol Vis Sci* 26(10):1449-1452, 1985.

40. Mathers WD, Lemp MA: In Cavanaugh WD, editor: *The cornea: Transactions of the World Congress on the Cornea III,* New York, 1988, Raven Press.

41. Maurice DM: The biology of wound healing in the corneal stroma, *Cornea* 6(3):162-168, 1987.

42. Melles GRJ, Binder PS: A comparison of wound healing in sutured and unsutured corneal wounds, *Arch Ophthalmol* 108:1460-1469, 1990.

43. Mishima H et al: Fibronectin enhances the phagocytic activity of cultured rabbit keratocytes, *Invest Ophthalmol Vis Sci* 28(9):1521-1526, 1987.

44. Morrison JC, Swan KC: Full-thickness lamellar keratoplasty, *Ophthalmology* 89(6):715-719, 1982.

45. Morrison JC, Swan KC: Bowman's layer in penetrating keratoplasties of the human eye, *Arch Ophthalmol* 100:1835-1838, 1982.

46. Morrison JC, Swan KC: Descemet's membrane in penetrating keratoplasties, *Arch Ophthalmol* 101:1927-1929, 1983.

47. Newsome DA, Gross J, Hassell JR: Human corneal stroma contains three distinct collagens, *Invest Ophthalmol Vis Sci* 22(3):376-381, 1982.

48. Phillips K et al: Effects of prednisolone and medroxyprogesterone on corneal wound healing, ulceration and neovascularization, *Arch Ophthalmol* 101:640-643, 1983.

49. Raber IM, Arentsen JJ, Laibson PR: Traumatic wound dehiscence after penetrating keratoplasty, *Arch Ophthalmol* 98:1407-1409, 1980.

50. Trinkaus-Randall V et al: Quantification of stromal destruction in the inflamed cornea, *Invest Ophthalmol Vis Sci* 32(3):603-609, 1991.

51. Ruoslahti E: Structure and biology of proteoglycans, *Annu Rev Cell Biol* 4:229-255, 1988.

52. Serdarevic ON et al: Excimer laser trephination in penetrating keratoplasty: morphologic features and wound healing, *Ophthalmology* 94(4):493-505, 1988.

53. Simonsen AH, Andreassen TT, Bendix K: The healing strength of corneal wound in the human eye, *Exp Eye Res* 35:287-292, 1982.

54. Slack JW, Kangas TA, Edelhauser HF: Loss of stromal proteoglycans during corneal preservation, *Invest Ophthalmol Vis Sci* 30(3)(suppl):342, 1989.

55. Stern GA et al: Effect of topical antibiotic solutions on corneal epithelial wound healing, *Arch Ophthalmol* 101:644-647, 1983.

56. Tervo T et al: Plasminogen activator and its inhibitor in the experimental corneal wound, *Exp Eye Res* 48:445-449, 1989.

57. Topping TM et al: Traumatic wound dehiscence following penetrating keratoplasty, *Br J Ophthalmol* 66:174-178, 1982.

58. Weimar VL: The transformation of corneal stroma cells to fibroblasts in corneal wound healing, *Am J Ophthalmol* 44:173-180, 1957.

59. Weimar VL: The sources of fibroblasts in corneal wound repair: a quantitative analysis, *Arch Ophthalmol* 60:93-109, 1958.

60. Woost PG et al: Effect of growth factors with dexamethasone on healing of rabbit corneal stromal incisions, *Exp Eye Res* 40:47-60, 1985.

61. Zieske JD et al: Biosynthetic responses of the rabbit cornea to a keratectomy wound, *Invest Ophthalmol Vis Sci* 28(10):1668-1677, 1987.

Chapter 6

Endothelium: Development, Morphology, Disease, and Repair

NATALIE C. KERR

GREGORY S. SCHULTZ

RICHARD A. EIFERMAN

The corneal endothelium performs the essential function of maintaining corneal transparency by actively pumping ions from the corneal stroma. Maintenance of stromal dehydration requires a critical number of functioning endothelial cells, without which the cornea becomes edematous and cloudy. Aging, disease, and surgical trauma reduce the number of endothelial cells. This creates a severe problem in the human adult eye because human corneal endothelial cells (HCEC) rarely mitose in vivo to compensate for cell death or loss. At present, the only way to replenish the endothelial cell population and corneal clarity is by penetrating keratoplasty.

A substantial amount of research has been directed at understanding and modulating the endothelial cell's response to damage in hopes of developing a better way to replace damaged or lost endothelial cells than to use penetrating keratoplasty. Current studies of endothelial development, morphology, aging, disease, surgical trauma, and peptide growth factors are creating a body of knowledge about the corneal endothelium that may lead to improved endothelial preservation and wound healing. The following is a review of current theories and research in each of these areas as they relate to the mechanism of maintenance, loss, or restoration of the corneal endothelial cell population.

EMBRYOLOGY AND DEVELOPMENT

The corneal endothelium is formed from neural crest cells that separate from the neural plate and are present at the optic cup rim at 40 days after ovulation in the primate.[56,61,84] At this stage, the primary cornea is a loose fibrillar structure between the lens vesicle and surface ectoderm. Neural crest cells migrate over a layer of fibronectin in the developing cornea to form the endothelium. By the eighth week of human gestation, the multilayer sheet of migrated neural crest cells thins to form a monolayer of endothelial cells and starts to deposit Descemet's membrane. Between the eighth and sixteenth week, gap junctions and the apical band develop and Descemet's membrane forms a complete layer. This maturation to the adult configuration parallels the beginning of aqueous secretion in the eye.

The endothelium shares its origin with the cells of the anterior part of the iris, trabecular meshwork, and the ocular periendothelial vascular tissues.[52] Congenital diseases of the endothelium often involve these related structures in the anterior chamber. Corneal endothelial cells do not share a common origin with vascular endothelium. Differentiation of neural crest cells into the different anterior chamber structures is determined in part by the locus of origin on the neural crest, as well as glycoproteins in the environment.[56] The formation of the endothelial monolayer is mediated by contact inhibition with its adjacent structures and cells, and persistent multilayering may occur if the lens vesicle is removed.[23,55] Ultimate maturation of endothelial pump function and dehydration of the corneal stroma have been related to thyroid function in the chick.[13,47] Thyroid function may also play a role in mammalian systems, since transthyretin (prealbumin), a transport protein for thyroxine (T_4) and retinol, has been immunohistochemically localized to the corneal endothelium of the rat.[18]

AGING AND MORPHOLOGY

Corneal endothelial cell density is highest at birth, as high as 7500 cells/mm^2.[4,78,84] The rapid decline in density during the first year of life is compatible with a fixed population spreading over an enlarging cornea. Specular microscopy of normal children from 5 to 14 years of age shows that cell density is variable among individuals, with a range of 3591 ± 399 cells/mm^2 at 5 years to 2697 ± 246 cells/mm^2 in older subjects.[57] Decreases in cell density of 13% between 5 and 7 years of age and 12% between 7 and 10 years have been recorded. The rate of loss slows into the midtwenties, and even lower rates of approximately 0.52% loss per year continue into old age.[53] The critical endothelial cell density below which the human cornea decompensates is approximately 300 to 500 cells/mm^2.[50]

In childhood, normal endothelial cells have a uniform size and hexagonal shape.[57] As cell density decreases with age, individual cells enlarge and lose their hexagonal shape.[50,84] Computer-assisted morphometric analysis can determine the frequency of large or irregular cells in a given population and can generate a coefficient of variation for cell size and cell shape. As cells enlarge, they tend to lose their hexagonal pattern. Hexagonality can be measured and expressed as a percentage of total cells. Polymegethism, the irregularity in the normally regular mosaic pattern, may be quantified as a coefficient of variation in cell size.

Changes of cell shape with age are similarly observed in nonprimates.[5,78,84] Increased polymegethism or coefficient of variation of cell size correlate with the endothelium's susceptibility to traumatic cell loss, presumably reflecting a "weakened" state. However, cell morphology and function have not been clearly linked, and thus this coefficient remains most useful as a tool for comparing intraocular surgical techniques with regard to endothelial damage and not as a measure of the endothelium's ability to dehydrate the cornea.[84]

Little is known about mechanisms involved in aging of HCEC, but it is clear from studies of organ cultures, HCEC cultures, and graft survival that the younger the donor, the better is their survival and response to mitogens.[79] Metabolic injuries that accumulate with aging, such as the effect of oxidants, may play a role in this observed phenomenon. Catalase has been shown to protect the tissues of the anterior chamber from the toxic effects of hydrogen peroxide and has been observed to decline in activity with age in the iris and endothelium of rabbits.[68] Lipid-soluble antioxidants such as vitamin E have been studied in the preservation of rabbit corneal endothelial cells. Vitamin E–treated corneas survived twice as long as nontreated corneas in perfusion studies.[43] The nontreated cells showed damage largely in the endoplasmic reticulum and mitochondria, whereas the plasma and nuclear membranes remained normal.[59] Interestingly, mitochondrial dysfunction and accelerated corneal endothelial aging has been reported in a patient with Kearns-Sayre disease (mitochondrial encephalomyopathy secondary to an enzyme deficiency). The endothelial cells of this patient showed early signs of aging, with decreased cell density, severe polymegethism, and pleomorphism in both eyes.[60]

Normal endothelial cell cytoplasm contains large numbers of mitochondria, rough and smooth endoplasmic reticulum, and a well-developed Golgi apparatus, indicative of high levels of active transport and protein synthesis. HCEC are 5 μm in height and 18 to 20 μm wide. The posterior surface (anterior chamber side) is covered by microvilli, which project into the aqueous. The anterior surface abuts Descemet's membrane but has no anchoring structures. This may explain its susceptibility to surgical touch injury.[84] There are interdigitations of the cell membranes on the anterior surface but no desmosomal attachments.[74] The ionic-pump systems responsible for corneal deturgescence are located in the cell membranes. One theoretical model places the active sodium-potassium ATPase pump at the basolateral membrane and an enzymatically activated sodium bicarbonate exchange occurs at the anterior cell membrane.[84] The gap junctions, which are believed to compose the terminal bar, show dye and electrical coupling properties. With the aid of electron microscopy, apical tight junctions have also been found in this area. These tight junctions are believed to perform the barrier function that helps maintain corneal dehydration.[87] Also forming the apical band are actin filaments, which may participate in cell-migration response to injury.[84]

DISEASE STATES

Anterior Chamber Cleavage Syndromes. Endothelial dysgenesis, or abnormal migration of the neural crest cells, results in anterior chamber cleavage syndromes.[56,84,86] Eponyms for these entities include Axenfeld's anomaly, Axenfeld's syndrome, Rieger's anomaly, Rieger's syndrome, Axenfeld-Rieger syndrome, and Peter's anomaly. Clinical differentiation between these anomalies is based on the presence or absence of glaucoma or mesenchymal/neural crest anomalies involving the teeth, facial bones, and melanocytes. The corneal abnormalities associated with the Axenfeld-Rieger syndromes are pleomorphism of endothelial cells, attenuated Descemet's membrane, and posterior embryotoxin (anteriorly displaced Schwalbe's line, made prominent by an abnormal layer of collagen, Figs. 6-1 and 6-2). These are referred to clinically as peripheral developmental defects because the only clinically visible anomalies are in the peripheral area of the cornea. However, Peter's anomaly is a central defect, which has clinically detectable thinning of the central posterior cornea with overlying opacity of the cornea. The central endothelium is attenuated or absent, as is Descemet's layer. The basement membrane may contain giant collagen fibrils, which have also been demonstrated in congenital hereditary endothelial dystrophy.[38]

Congenital Hereditary Endothelial Dystrophy, Posterior Polymorphous Dystrophy, and Iridocorneal Endothelial Syndrome. Congenital hereditary endothelial dystrophy (CHED) is a rare disease that presents as bilateral, diffuse corneal edema in children and young adults.[84,86] It can be inherited as an autosomal dominant or recessive disorder and has a range of histologic findings. As in Peter's anomaly, the central corneal endothelium may be absent, or the endothelial cells may demonstrate fibroblast type of changes (Fig. 6-3). Also like Peter's anomaly, this entity probably represents a failure of neural crest migration to the central cornea but has the added feature of secondary endothelial metaplasia and abnormal secretion of collagen (hence the designation as a dysplasia or dystrophy). When this disease occurs during the amblyogenic period, penetrating keratoplasty is indicated, though grafts in this age range have high failure rates (Fig. 6-4). Reports of similar pathosis in posterior amorphous and polymorphous corneal dystrophies indicate a probable similar process with CHED, and it has been suggested that CHED may represent the earlier and more severe spectrum of these posterior dystrophies.[11]

The iridocorneal endothelial syndrome (ICE) falls somewhere in between a dystrophy and a dysplasia

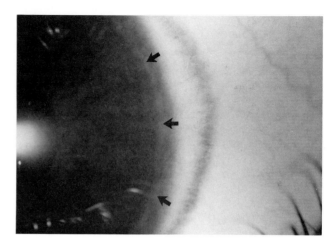

Fig. 6-1. Axenfeld's anomaly demonstrating a prominent Schwalbe's line *(arrows)*.

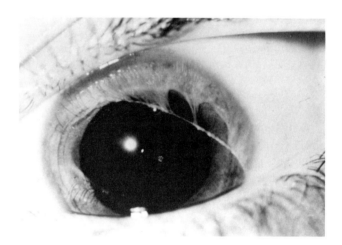

Fig. 6-2. Rieger's anomaly with anteriorly displaced Schwalbe's line and iris processes.

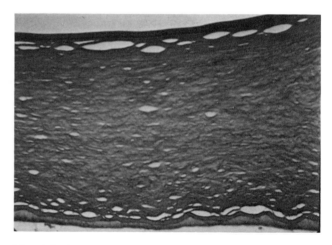

Fig. 6-3. Corneal button from a patient with congenital hereditary endothelial dystrophy demonstrating atrophic corneal endothelium. (H&E, 400×.)

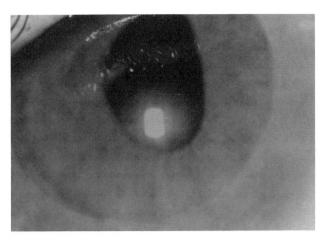

Fig. 6-4. Clear corneal graft in a child with congenital hereditary endothelial dystrophy.

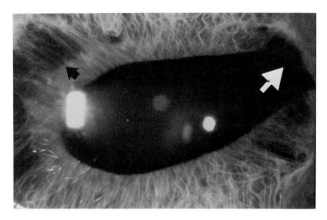

Fig. 6-5. Iridocorneal endothelial syndrome with thinning of the iris *(black arrow)*, corectopia, and peripheral anterior synechiae with ectropion uveae *(white arrow)*.

(Fig. 6-5).[70,84] There are three subdivisions of the ICE syndrome: essential iris atrophy, Chandler's syndrome, and the Cogan-Reese syndrome. All are unilateral diseases that have the appearance on specular reflection of a hammered-silver endothelium. Also present is the so-called ICE cell, which has an irregular shape and altered density. Early in the disease process, these cells are interspersed with groups of normal cells. However, the dystrophic cells gradually replace the normal cells, and it is at this stage that the intraocular pressure starts to rise. As normal endothelial cells undergo necrosis on the posterior surface of the cornea, there is proliferation of endothelial cells onto the iris. This occurs in the absence of mitosis.[1,2] These endothelial cells on the iris, along with a collagenous layer, form the "glass membrane" that is seen in ICE. The rise in pressure results from the blockage of outflow caused by these proliferating cells on the trabecular meshwork. ICE has been attributed to abnormal crest cell migration[70] as well as delayed expression of abnormal neural crest cell development or an inflammatory disease.[84] The presence of a normal Descemet's layer under the posterior collagenous layer does indicate a postnatal onset of the cause.[1] ICE syndrome has been linked to posterior polymorphous s dystrophy (PPMD) because of the increased expression of cytokeratins and epithelioid hyperplasia, which are features common to both of these diseases.[71]

The occurrence of CHED, ICE, and PPMD in the same families, as well as their association with other forms of mesenchymal dysgenesis, also indicates a common cause for these neurocristopathies.[11,29] PPMD is clinically recognizable as clusters of vesicular lesions at the level of Descemet's membrane (Fig.

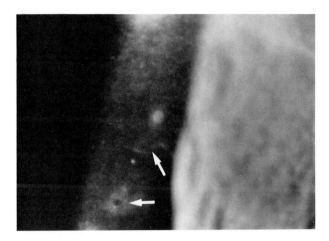

Fig. 6-6. Posterior polymorphous dystrophy with vesicles *(arrows)* and endothelial striae.

6-6). Histologically, PPMD is characterized by epithelioid cells forming multiple layers and overgrowing normal cells. Unlike normal endothelium, these cells have desmosomal junctions, but expression of keratin cytoskeleton indicates that they derive from endothelial cells, not surface ectoderm.[51] The clinical appearance of vesicles is produced by a thick collagenous layer, deposited by the epithelioid cells, which project into the anterior chamber or fill in folds in Descemet's membrane.[66]

Fuchs' Dystrophy. The most common endothelial dystrophy is Fuchs', which manifests in adulthood as central guttae, corneal edema, and reduced vision (Figs. 6-7 and 6-8).[84,90] It is more common and more severely expressed in women, though it is an autosomal dominant disease. The primary histologic fea-

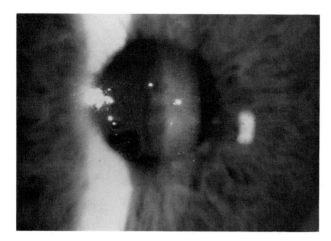

Fig. 6-7. Large bullae, central stromal edema, and epithelial edema in Fuchs' dystrophy.

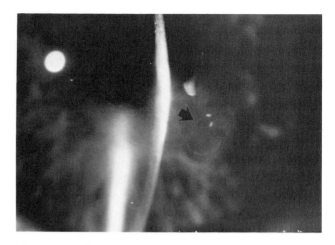

Fig. 6-8. Fuchs' dystrophy with large bullae and stromal and epithelial edema.

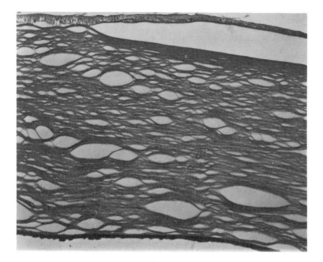

Fig. 6-9. Prominent corneal guttae with epithelial and stromal edema in Fuchs' dystrophy (H&E, ×400).

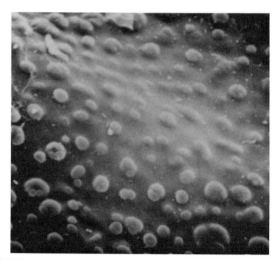

Fig. 6-10. Scanning electron microscopic view of corneal guttae in Fuchs' dystrophy.

ture of Fuchs' dystrophy is multiple excrescences of posterior Descemet's membrane with decreased endothelial cell density and increased cell size (Figs. 6-8 to 6-11). Endothelial pump function is significantly increased in the earlier stages of disease, delaying the onset of corneal edema.[9,24] Eventually, the total endothelial pump function falls below a level sufficient to maintain corneal clarity. The cause of Fuchs' remains unknown. One theory implicated a faulty fibrinolytic system in the aqueous humor with fibrin and fibrinogen deposition,[84] but a recent study found no statistical difference between levels of aqueous humor total fibrinogen–related antigen, small molecular weight fibrinogen–derived metabolites, ascorbate, glucose, carbon dioxide, bicarbonate, and pH in normals and patients with Fuchs'.[89] They

concluded that Fuchs' dystrophy is a primary disease of the corneal endothelium.

Diabetes. Patients with diabetes have altered endothelial cell morphology and function.[72] Two findings implicate a process for this corneal endotheliopathy different from that for the vasculopathy seen in diabetic patients. First, there is no increase in the thickness of Descemet's membrane as in the other basement membranes of diabetics.[75] Secondly, the degree of endothelial morphometric abnormality does not correlate with duration of disease or glycemic control.[48] Abnormal aldose reductase activity in the corneal endothelium has been implicated in the decreased cell density and increased cell size seen in the diabetic endothelium,[15] though the decreased ability of the diabetic corneal endothelium to main-

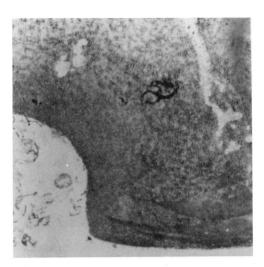

Fig. 6-11. Transmission electron microscopic view of cornea guttata. Notice thickened Descemet's membrane.

tain stromal dehydration appears to be related to endothelial pump dysfunction and not to an abnormal osmotic substance in the stroma.[31] This altered function would explain the observation that diabetics are slow to recover from postoperative corneal edema,[62] despite findings of normal endothelial cell density, coefficient of variation of cell size, or cell loss in pseudophakic diabetics when compared to age-matched nondiabetics.[22]

Surgical Trauma. Trauma from intraocular surgery results in endothelial cell loss, which, if it progresses beyond the critical level required for deturgescence, results in bullous keratopathy. Factors that culminate in corneal decompensation can be divided into preoperative disease, intraoperative damage from touch or pharmacologic insult, and postoperative cell loss caused by inflammation or chronic contact injury.

One recent study indicates that fellow eyes in pseudophakic or aphakic bullous keratopathy may have, on average, a lower cell count and increased thickness when compared to age-matched controls.[35] The recognition of a nonguttate dystrophy explains why some eyes with normal preoperative appearance and atraumatic surgical course experience postoperative bullous keratopathy.[8] It has been suggested that longitudinal observation of endothelial cell loss may be the best prognosticator for postoperative corneal edema.[42]

Intraocular surgery causes both an acute and chronic endothelial cell loss in addition to that normally attributed to aging.[10,19,42] A review of the large body of literature that addresses the causes and prevention of endothelial cell loss during in-

traocular surgery is beyond the scope of this chapter. However, a brief discussion of the factors known to accelerate cell loss during and after surgery will provide background information for the following discussion on wound-healing experiments.

Mechanical trauma from endothelial touch contributes more to endothelial cell loss during uncomplicated cataract extractions than any other single factor.[10,84] The superior area of the cornea is where the incision is made and where instruments, the natural lens, and the lens implant enter and exit the eye, and most cells lost are in the region of the superior area of the cornea.[73] One month after surgery, morphologic changes have been observed in the central cornea. The appearance of the central endothelial cells becomes stable within 3 months, with or without a posterior chamber lens.

Viscoelastic substances have allowed anterior segment surgery to be performed with greater ease than the techniques employing an air bubble to maintain the anterior chamber and protect the endothelium from touch. Exposure of the endothelium to air is, in itself, mildly traumatic.[20,82] Protection of the endothelium from air bubbles during phacoemulsification has become one criterion for choosing a particular viscoelastic agent.[14] There is now evidence that the viscoelastic substance sodium hyaluronate not only protects the endothelium by its viscous properties, but also actually has receptors on the endothelium that bind with it to form a continuous layer over the endothelium.[44]

The pharmacologic agents used during intraocular surgery can also play a significant role in endothelial cell loss.[19] Balanced salt solutions for irrigation during intraocular surgery lessen trauma to the endothelium better than normal saline solution does.[82] The irrigating solution should contain calcium to maintain endothelial junctional complexes, glucose for aerobic metabolism, glutathione for the protection of sulfhydryls in the endothelial membrane, and a bicarbonate buffer.[19] The use of miotic agents can promote endothelial cell damage. One group has reported a 37.2% increase in endothelial cell size after cataract extraction with the use of the miotic acetylcholine in the anterior chamber.[49] This is compared to a 7.08% increase in the operated group receiving no acetylcholine. Another study has demonstrated a pronounced toxic reaction to 1% acetylcholine by HCEC in organ culture as compared to 0.01% carbachol or the irrigating balanced salt solution BSS Plus.[91] Higher concentrations of commercially available epinephrine (1:1000) can cause irreversible corneal edema from damage to endothelial cells, and current recommendations are to use a 1:5000 solution of commercially available epinephrine.[19,91] Significant postoperative edema can also be caused by detergents left in irrigating cannulas after cleaning.[58]

Intraocular lenses have, over the history of their use, been a leading cause of corneal demise after cataract surgery. Advancements in fixation and loop design have remedied many of the problems experienced with anterior chamber lenses, and posterior chamber lenses appear to have little effect on the postoperative cell count in uneventful surgery.[73] However, if the intraocular poly(methyl methacrylate), or PMMA, lens touches the endothelium during or after insertion, the endothelium is basically denuded in that area of touch. One proposal to decrease the abrasive effect of PMMA lenses is to coat them with a permanent, chemically bound, hydrophilic, polymer surface.[32]

WOUND REPAIR

From the previous discussion on corneal disease and decompensation, it is clear that HCEC have a limited capacity to regenerate in vivo. This is puzzling in the face of early reports from animal-model studies of endothelial wound healing that demonstrated that large central transcorneal freeze injuries to the endothelium of rabbits healed exclusively by mitosis of endothelial cells adjacent to the injury and migration of the daughter cells to cover the wound.[65] These tritiated thymidine-labeled cells persisted in the wound area for up to 4 years after the injury, indicating that they returned to their amitotic state once the monolayer was reestablished. Rabbit endothelial cells readily mitose in vitro and form pure cultures, which are capable of repeated passaging[63] and can synthesize basement membrane.[64] Bovine corneal endothelial cells also readily mitose in vitro.[28] Although it is not known why mitosis in endothelial wound healing is limited in certain species and not others, this information points out the need for an animal model tissue in which to study HCEC wound healing different from rabbit or bovine tissue.

Cats and primates have proved to be more suitable models for HCEC wound healing than rabbits. Van Horn and Hyndiuk reported on transcorneal freeze injuries to primate and cat corneas healed in vivo by enlargement and migration of the marginal endothelial cells with no clear evidence of endothelial cell mitosis.[85] This report closely parallels reports by Doughman and co-workers,[17] who studied HCEC repair in organ culture after freeze injury. They reported that HCEC responded to cell loss by enlargement and migration of uninjured endothelial cells at the wound margin with no evidence of mitosis. One

study has found mitosis to play a role in cat corneal endothelial healing, though it was a relatively small contributor to the overall cellular response to injury (148.5 ± 74.5 and 206.8 ± 40.1 mitotic figures at 3 and 4 days after injury versus 3999 ± 746 and 3129 ± 877 multinuclear, amitotic cells for the same time periods).[40] Morphologic studies of cat endothelial cells after injury have confirmed that they share a similar response to chronic stress as human endothelium.[83]

Does this mean that adult HCEC, cat, and primate endothelial cells have lost the cellular mechanisms required for large-scale mitotic regeneration, or do they just lack the proper environmental stimulus to replenish their population? The latter appears to be the more likely culprit. Two areas of study have confirmed this hypothesis. First, HCEC can be cultured. Second, mitotic activity has been demonstrated in human organ culture after injury.

Baum and co-workers[6] cultured fragments of Descemet's membrane with endothelium to obtain outgrowths of endothelial cells. Thirteen of 19 corneas from donors less than 20 years of age produced cultures that grew to confluency. These cells had the typical morphologic characteristics of endothelial cells, and one cell line was passaged six times in 6 months. Nayak and Binder reported the successful outgrowth and passaging of HCEC from 12 of 31 corneoscleral rims, again finding the best results from donors less than 20 years of age.[54]

Simonsen, Sørensen, and Sperling used tritiated thymidine to document HCEC mitotic activity in organ culture.[77] Donors ranged in age from 19 to 89 years, and corneal buttons were incubated in Eagle's medium with 8% dextran and 10% fetal calf serum at 37° C for 6 days. All five wounded corneas contained labeled nuclei, predominantly in the central cornea. Few nuclei were labeled in the uninjured controls. Zagorski reported mitotic figures and nuclei labeled with tritiated thymidine in human corneas injured by freezing and then placed in organ culture with medium containing 20% fetal calf serum.[92] Treffers found similar results in 85 organ-cultured human corneas and two corneas injured in vivo and cultured in vitro in medium containing 10% fetal calf serum.[80] No labeling was observed at 24 hours after injury in the organ-cultured corneas, but extensive labeling was observed at 48 and 72 hours. Pulse labeling after 72 hours revealed very little labeling, indicating that mitotic activity occurred in the period from 24 to 72 hours. The two in vivo cases were taken from scheduled enucleations for malignant melanoma of the choroid. Transcorneal freeze injuries were made 48 or 72 hours before scheduled surgery. Immediately after enucleation, the corneas were removed and incubated with tritiated thymidine for 1 hour. Thirty labeled cells were found in the 48-hour-old injury, and 76 labeled cells in the 72-hour-old cornea. Finally, evidence that HCEC can, though rarely does, mitose in vivo was presented by Laing and co-workers who observed mitotic figures by specular microscopy in a patient who had undergone penetrating keratoplasty.[39]

GROWTH FACTORS IN WOUND HEALING

Growth factors are substances that act at nanomolar concentrations at specific high-affinity receptor sites to control development, proliferation, and wound healing of the target cell.[81] Peptide growth factors, such as fibroblast growth factor (FGF) and epidermal growth factor (EGF), have been studied in the context of corneal endothelial wound healing. Both of these factors are known to accelerate the regeneration of bovine corneal endothelial cells in organ culture.[26] They have therefore been targeted for study in the relatively amitotic endothelium of cats, primates, and humans.

One of the first growth factor–human organ culture studies used a partially purified component present in mouse submandibular glands, mesodermal growth factor (MGF).[88] In four wounded corneal buttons from donors less than 60 years of age, MGF produced a mean increase of 100 more mitotic figures per whole mount than paired controls. However, in the four corneas from donors more than 60 years of age, there was no statistically significant increase in mitosis with MGF. Subsequent purification and separation of MGF into its components revealed that MGF is a protease of the kallikrein family and has four times the peptidase activity on a molar basis than pure trypsin.[30] The mechanism of MGF stimulation of HCEC is not known, but it may act directly, as has been reported for proteases such as thrombin,[30] or indirectly by the proteolytic release of the active form of an inactive membrane bound precursor for growth factors such as EGF of TGF-alpha.

Using the more potent purified growth factor EGF, Fabricant and colleagues conducted an experiment in primates to study the in vivo effect of this growth factor on endothelial wound healing.[21] They removed a 6 mm autograft and wiped away all the endothelium with a cotton-tipped swab before suturing it back into its bed. EGF in buffered solution was injected into the test eyes at the time of surgery and 3 weeks later. Ten weeks after the initial autotransplantation, the grafts were removed and flat mounts of the endothelium prepared. Cell densities were significantly higher in the EGF-treated corneas than the controls. However, separating the effects of migration versus mitosis in the endothelial regeneration could not be ascertained with this technique. This is an important determination to make in the study of primate endothelial regeneration because large wounds (two thirds of the endothelium) still demonstrate total closure within 7 to 9 days.[85] However, the dehydrating capacity of the endothelial tissue does not return to normal because the overall cell number is not restored (such as migration without mitosis).

Not all studies have found a positive effect of EGF on wound healing. Brogdon and co-workers made 8 mm diameter transcorneal freeze injuries to cats and injected EGF in water into the anterior chamber.[7] Pachymetry and endothelial specular microscopy of the corneas was able to show no difference between eyes injected with EGF or vehicle. The authors speculated that the vehicle used did not retain EGF in the anterior chamber for a period sufficient to stimulate endothelial cells.

The mitotic effect of EGF on HCEC has been demonstrated in organ culture of fetal and adult donor tissue. Hyldahl found that EGF stimulated mitosis in human fetal organ culture, as well as in primary cell cultures from human embryonic corneas.[33] Couch and co-workers studied 25 adult human corneas that were transected, and one half were placed in McCarey-Kaufman (MK) storage media alone and the other half were placed in MK media with EGF.[12] After incubation for 96 hours, an endothelial flat mount was stained and mitotic figures were counted. Endothelial cell mitosis was significantly increased in MK media by the addition of EGF. The use of paired corneas divided into halves verified the increase in mitotic activity in each donor with the addition of EGF to each of the test media.

Landshman and colleagues studied FGF in cats after a large in vivo endothelial injury produced by a 180-degree corneal incision and crush injury to the cornea with a modified chalazion clamp.[41] They found that cell density in the wound was significantly increased in FGF-treated eyes and that the most noticeable difference was 2 weeks after injury, though a difference persisted up to 12 weeks after injury. The presence of significant iritis in several eyes raises the issue of how intraocular inflammation may alter the results of in vivo endothelial wound healing studies. Protein factors released by polymorphonuclear leukocytes have been reported to modulate cell shape and collagen gene expression in corneal endothelial cells.[36] Other studies have indicated a possible role for prostaglandins in mediating corneal endothelial wound healing.[25,36] Therefore, in addition to the clinical observation that intraocular inflammation compromises endothelial cells,[10] laboratory investigations at the molecular level show that endothelial wound healing might be altered by inflammation.

To study the influence of EGF on corneal endothelial wound healing so as to distinguish migration versus mitosis and reduce the effects of rapid egress of EGF from the anterior chamber and altered wound healing from excessive inflammation, an experimental model was utilized in which an endothelial touch injury was made through a small incision and EGF was mixed with the viscoelastic sodium hyaluronate as the test solution.[67] A single injection of EGF in the viscoelastic increased endothelial cell density 38% over control corneas, and the number of endothelial cell nuclei labeled with tritiated thymidine by 75% compared to control corneas. This demonstrates that increased endothelial cell density in EGF-treated eyes is at least partially attributable to mitosis, not just migration. Also, treatment with EGF increased the percentage of hexagonal cells by 13% and decreased the coefficient of variation of cell size (polymegethism) by 30%. The effect of EGF to normalize the parameters of endothelial cell morphology after touch injury indicates that intraocular growth factors may be clinically useful.

Relatively little is known about endogenous growth factors in the anterior chamber and their role in the natural course of endothelial wound healing. We recently analyzed cat anterior chamber fluid after touch injury for transforming growth factor-alpha (TGF-alpha).[69] TGF-alpha is structurally related to EGF and interacts with EGF receptors in a similar fashion as EGF.[45] Two hours after the injury the level of TGF-alpha increased fourteenfold and the general level of mitogenic activity increased tenfold when compared to the preinjury levels.[69] The level of TGF-alpha in the anterior chamber decreased to preinjury levels by 24 hours after injury. Mitogenic activity of the anterior chamber fluid was decreased 20% by the addition of neutralizing antibody to TGF-alpha. The source of the TGF-alpha that was detected in the anterior chamber fluid after injury may be the endothelial cells themselves, since immunoreactive TGF-alpha was measured in extracts of bovine corneal endothelial cells. Anterior chamber fluid obtained from six humans just before cataract surgery also had detectable levels of TGF-alpha. This information, coupled with other studies of TGF-alpha, indicates that TGF-alpha may be involved in corneal endothelial healing by an autocrine mechanism.[16,46]

ENDOTHELIAL GRAFTING

The ability of HCEC to mitose in cell culture and organ culture raises the possibility of grafting cells to injured or diseased corneas, rather than performing a penetrating keratoplasty. Skelnick and colleagues established HCEC cultures in 20% fetal calf serum-containing medium and seeded cat corneas with these HCEC cultures over 9 days.[76] Endothelial cell density was approximately twice as high as companion (nonseeded) corneas at 6 weeks after keratoplasty. Other researchers have cultured bovine corneal endothelial cells onto cat or rabbit corneas denuded of their endothelium with varying results. Denuded rabbit corneas seeded with multipassaged bovine corneal endothelial cells were transplanted back to the same or a different rabbit.[26] All nine rabbits had clear corneas for many months. Similar techniques were used to repopulate denuded cat corneas with 8 of 9 remaining totally clear.[27]

In contrast, Bahn and colleagues found that cat corneas repopulated with bovine corneal endothelial cells remained clear for 2 weeks and then became opacified and edematous secondary to a host response directed at the bovine corneal endothelial cells.[3] Controls remained clear. They postulated that the difference in results may be attributable to the greater cell surface antigenicity of early passage cells used in their study as compared to the multipassaged cells of Gospodarowicz and colleagues.

Insler and Lopez studied eight human corneal buttons that were denuded of endothelium, incubated with infant HCEC cultures for 144 hours, and transplanted into African green monkeys.[34] Six corneas cleared after transplantation and remained so for the 12-month follow-up period. All control eyes showed advanced edema and neovascularization. Studies such as this raise hopes that corneal tissue for transplantation may one day be more readily available to the hundreds of thousands of patients worldwide who would benefit from a corneal transplant.

THE FUTURE

The studies and experiments discussed in this chapter illustrate where our knowledge of corneal endothelial cell loss and regeneration both originates and leads. Better understanding of the mechanisms of cell death in disease, aging, and trauma will generate better techniques of preserving corneal clarity. By identification of the factors that promote HCEC mitosis in vivo, it may be possible to stimulate regeneration of one's own diseased endothelium and avoid the morbidity associated with penetrating keratoplasty.

REFERENCES

1. Alvarado JA et al: Pathogenesis of Chandler's syndrome, essential iris atrophy and the Cogan-Reese syndrome I, *Invest Ophthalmol Vis Sci* 27:853-872, 1986.
2. Alvarado JA et al: Pathogenesis of Chandler's syndrome, essential iris atrophy and the Cogan-Reese syndrome II, *Invest Ophthalmol Vis Sci* 27:873-882, 1986.
3. Bahn CF et al: Complications associated with bovine corneal endothelial cell–lined homografts in the cat, *Invest Ophthalmol Vis Sci* 22:73-90, 1982.
4. Bahn CF et al: Postnatal development of corneal endothelium, *Invest Ophthalmol Vis Sci* 27:44-51, 1986.
5. Baroody RA et al: Ocular development of aging I. Corneal endothelial changes in cats and free-ranging and caged rhesus monkeys, *Exp Eye Res* 45:607-622, 1987.
6. Baum JL et al: Mass culturing of human corneal endothelial cells, *Arch Ophthalmol* 97:1136-1140, 1979.
7. Brogdon JD et al: Effect of epidermal growth factor on healing of corneal endothelial cells in cats, *Am J Vet Res* 50:1237-1243, 1989.
8. Brooks AM, Grant GB, Gillies WE: Bullous keratopathy due to nonguttate corneal endothelial dystrophy, *Aust NZ J Ophthalmol* 18(3):335-341, 1990.
9. Burns RR, Bourne WM, Brubaker RE: Endothelial function in patients with guttata, *Invest Ophthalmol Vis Sci* 20:77-85, 1981.
10. Cameron JD: Surgical and nonsurgical trauma. In Tasman W, Jaeger EA, editors: *Biomedical foundations of ophthalmology*, vol 3, Philadelphia, 1989, Lippincott.
11. Chan CC et al: Similarities between posterior polymorphous and congenital endothelial dystrophies, *Cornea* 1:155-172, 1982.
12. Couch JM et al: Mitotic activity of corneal endothelial cells in organ culture with recombinant human epidermal growth factor, *Ophthalmology* 94(1):1-6, 1987.
13. Coulombre AJ, Coulombre JL: Corneal development III. The role of the thyroid in dehydration and transparency, *Exp Eye Res* 3:105-114, 1975.
14. Craig MT et al: Air bubble endothelial damage during phacoemulsification in human eye bank eyes: the positive effects of Healon and Viscoat, *J Cataract Refract Surg* 16(5):597-602, 1990.
15. Datiles MB et al: The effects of sorbinil, an aldose reductase inhibitor, on the corneal endothelium in galactosemic dogs, *Invest Ophthalmol Vis Sci* 31(11):2201-2204, 1990.
16. Derynck R: Transforming growth factor α, *Cell* 54:593-595, 1988.
17. Doughman DJ et al: Human corneal endothelial layer repair during organ culture, *Arch Ophthalmol* 94:1791-1796, 1976.
18. Dwork AJ et al: Distribution of transthyretin in the rat eye, *Invest Ophthalmol Vis Sci* 31(3):489-496, 1990.
19. Edelhauser HF, Van Horn DL, Records RE: Cornea and sclera. In Tasman W, Jaeger EA, editors: *Biomedical foundations of ophthalmology*, vol 2, Philadelphia, 1989, Lippincott.
20. Eiferman RA, Wilkins EL: The effect of air on human corneal endothelium, *Am J Ophthalmol* 92(3):328-331, 1981.
21. Fabricant R et al: Regenerative effects of epidermal growth factor after penetrating keratoplasty in primates, *Arch Ophthalmol* 100:994-995, 1982.
22. Furuse N et al: Corneal endothelial changes after posterior chamber intraocular lens implantation with or without diabetes mellitus, *Br J Ophthalmol* 74(5):258-260, 1990.
23. Genis-Galves JM: Role of the lens in the morphogenesis of the iris and cornea, *Nature* 210:209-210, 1966.
24. Geroski DH et al: Pump function of the human corneal endothelium, *Ophthalmology* 92:759-763, 1985.
25. Gerritsen ME et al: Arachidonic acid metabolism by cultured bovine corneal endothelial cells, *Invest Ophthalmol Vis Sci* 30(4):698-705, 1989.
26. Gospodarowicz D, Greenburg G: The effects of epidermal and fibroblast growth factors on the repair of corneal endothelial wounds in bovine corneas maintained in organ culture, *Exp Eye Res* 28:147-157, 1979.
27. Gospodarowicz D, Greenburg G, Alvarado J: Transplantation of cultured bovine corneal endothelial cells to rabbit cornea: clinical implications for human studies, *Proc Nat Acad Sci USA* 76:464-468, 1979.
28. Gospodarowicz D, Mescher ML, Birdwell CR: Stimulation of corneal endothelial cell proliferation in vitro by fibroblast and epidermal growth factors, *Exp Eye Res* 25:75-89, 1977.
29. Grayson M: The nature of hereditary deep polymorphous dystrophy of the cornea: its association with iris and anterior chamber dysgenesis, *Trans Am Ophthalmol Soc* 72:516-559, 1974.
30. Haraguchi KH et al: Synergistic growth stimulation of corneal fibroblasts by components of mesodermal growth factor from murine submaxillary glands, *J Cell Physiol* 111:1117-1132, 1982.
31. Herse PR: Corneal hydration control in normal and alloxan-induced diabetic rabbits, *Invest Ophthalmol Vis Sci* 31(11):2205-2213, 1990.
32. Hofmeister FM et al: In vitro evaluation of iris chafe protection afforded by hydrophilic surface modification of polymethylmethacrylate intraocular lenses, *J Cataract Refract Surg* 14(5):514-519, 1988.
33. Hyldahl L: Control of cell proliferation in the human embryonic cornea, *J Cell Sci* 83:1-21, 1986.
34. Insler MS, Lopez JG: Extended incubation times improve corneal endothelial cell transplantation success, *Invest Ophthalmol Vis Sci* 32(6):1828-1836, 1991.
35. Insler MS, Robbins RG: Fellow eyes in aphakic and pseudophakic bullous keratopathy, *J Cataract Refract Surg* 16(1):92-95, 1990.
36. Jumblatt MM, Paterson CA: Prostaglandin E$_2$ effects on corneal endothelial cyclic adenosine monophosphate synthesis and cell shape are mediated by a receptor of the EP$_2$ subtype, *Invest Ophthalmol Vis Sci* 32(2):360-365, 1991.
37. Kay EP, Rivela A, He YG: Corneal endothelium modulation factor released by polymorphonuclear leukocytes: partial purification and initial characterization, *Invest Ophthalmol Vis Sci* 31(2):313-322, 1990.
38. Kenyon KR, Maumenee AE: Further studies of congenital hereditary dystrophy of the cornea, *Am J Ophthalmol* 76:419-439, 1973.
39. Laing RA et al: Evidence for mitosis in the adult corneal endothelium, *Ophthalmology* 91:1129-1134, 1984.
40. Landshman N, Solomon A, Belkin M: Cell division in the healing of the corneal endothelium of cats, *Arch Ophthalmol* 107(12):1804-1808, 1989.
41. Landshman N et al: Regeneration of cat endothelium induced in vitro by fibroblast growth factor, *Exp Eye Res* 45:805-811, 1987.
42. Liesegang TJ: The response of the corneal endothelium to intraocular surgery, *Refract Corneal Surg* 7:81-86, 1991.
43. Lux NO, Millar TJ: Lipid soluble antioxidants preserve rabbit corneal cell function, *Curr Eye Res* 9(2):103-109.
44. Madsen K et al: Hyaluronate binding to intact corneas and cultured endothelial cells, *Invest Ophthalmol Vis Sci* 30(10):2132-2137, 1989.
45. Marquadt H et al: Rat transforming growth factor type 1: Structure and relationship to epidermal growth factor, *Science* 223:1073-1082, 1984.

46. Massague J: Transforming growth factor α, *J Biol Chem* 35:21393-21396, 1990.

47. Masterson E, Edelhauser HF, Van Horn DL: Role of thyroid hormone in the development of the chick corneal endothelium and epithelium, *Invest Ophthalmol Vis Sci* 16:105-115, 1977.

48. Matsuda M et al: Relationship of corneal endothelial morphology to diabetic retinopathy, duration of disease and glycemic disease, *Jpn J Ophthalmol* 34(1):53-56, 1990.

49. Menchini U et al: Clinical evaluation of the effect of acetylcholine on the corneal endothelium, *J Cataract Refract Surg* 15(4):421-424, 1989.

50. Mishima S: Clinical investigations of the corneal endothelium, *Am J Ophthalmol* 93:1-29, 1982.

51. Morgan G, Patterson A: Pathology of polymorphous degeneration of the cornea, *Br J Ophthalmol* 51:433-437, 1967.

52. Mooy CM, Clark BJ, Lee WR: Posterior axial corneal malformation and uveoretinal angiodysgenesis—a neurocristopathy? *Graefes Arch Clin Exp Ophthalmol* 228(1):9-18, 1990.

53. Murphy C et al: Prenatal and postnatal cellularity of the human corneal endothelium, *Invest Ophthalmol Vis Sci* 25:312-322, 1984.

54. Nayak S, Binder PS: The growth of endothelium from human corneal rims in tissue culture, *Invest Ophthalmol Vis Sci* 25:1213-1216, 1984.

55. Nelson GA, Revel JP: Scanning electron microscopic study of cell movements in the corneal endothelium of the avian embryo, *Dev Biol* 42:315-337, 1975.

56. Noden DM: Periocular mesenchyme: neural crest and mesodermal interactions. In Tasman W, Jaeger EA, editors: *Biomedical foundations of ophthalmology*, vol 1, Philadelphia, 1989, Lippincott.

57. Nucci P et al: Normal endothelial cell density range in childhood, *Arch Ophthalmol* 108(2):247-248, 1990.

58. Nuyts RMMA et al: Toxic effects of detergents on the corneal endothelium, *Arch Ophthalmol* 108:1158-1162, 1990.

59. Ogita Y et al: Histochemical studies of mitochondrial activities of cultured corneal endothelial cells of cat during wound-healing, *Jpn J Ophthalmol* 34(2):200-215, 1990.

60. Ohkoshi K et al: Corneal endothelium in a case of mitochondrial encephalomyopathy (Kearns-Sayre syndrome), *Cornea* 8(3):210-214, 1989.

61. Ozanics V, Jakobiec FA: Prenatal development of the eye and its adnexa. In Tasman W, Jaeger EA: *Biomedical foundations of ophthalmology*, vol 1, Philadelphia, 1989, Lippincott.

62. Pardos GJ, Kratchmer JH: Comparison of endothelial cell density in diabetes and a control population, *Am J Ophthalmol* 90:172-174, 1980.

63. Perlman M, Baum JL: The mass culture of rabbit corneal endothelial cells, *Arch Ophthalmol* 92:235-237, 1974.

64. Perlman M, Baum JL: Synthesis of a collagenous basal membrane by rabbit corneal endothelial cells in vitro, *Arch Ophthalmol* 92:237-239, 1974.

65. Polack FM: Four year retention of ^{3}H-thymidine by corneal endothelium, *Arch Ophthalmol* 75:659-660, 1966.

66. Polack FM et al: Scanning electron microscopy of posterior polymorphous corneal dystrophy, *Am J Ophthalmol* 89:575-584, 1980.

67. Raphael B et al: Effect of epidermal growth factor in a viscoelastic on corneal endothelial wound healing in cats. (Submitted for publication.)

68. Riley MV: Physiologic neutralization mechanisms and the response of the corneal endothelium to hydrogen peroxide, *CLAO J* 16(1 suppl):S16-21, 1990.

69. Rotatori DS et al: Detection of TGF-α in cat anterior chamber fluid after endothelial injury. (Submitted for publication.)

70. Sassani JW: Glaucoma. In Tasman W, Jaeger EA, editors: *Biomedical foundations of ophthalmology*, vol 3, Philadelphia, 1989, Lippincott.

71. Scheie HG, Yanoff M: Iris nevus (Cogan-Reese) syndrome: a cause of unilateral glaucoma, *Arch Ophthalmol* 93:963-970, 1975.

72. Schultz RO et al: Corneal endothelial changes in type I and II diabetes mellitus, *Am J Ophthalmol* 98:401-410, 1984.

73. Schultz RO et al: Response of corneal endothelium to cataract surgery, *Arch Ophthalmol* 104(8):1164-1169, 1986.

74. Sherrard ES, Ng YL: The other side of the corneal endothelium, *Cornea* 9(1):48-54, 1990.

75. Shetlar DJ, Bourne WM, Campbell J: Morphological evaluation of Descemet's membrane and corneal endothelium in diabetes mellitus, *Ophthalmology* 96:247-250, 1989.

76. Skelnik DL et al: Culturing and application of HCE in human corneal endothelial enhancement, *Invest Ophthalmol Vis Sci* 26:247A, 1985.

77. Simonsen AH, Sørenson KE, Sperling S: Thymidine incorporation by human corneal endothelium during organ culture, *Acta Ophthalmol* (Copenh) 59:110-118, 1981.

78. Speedwell L et al: The infant corneal endothelium, *Arch Ophthalmol* 106:771-775, 1988.

79. Squires EL, Weimar VL: Stimulation of repair of human corneal endothelium in organ culture by mesodermal growth factor, *Arch Ophthalmol* 98:1462-1466, 1980.

80. Treffers WF: Human corneal endothelial wound repair, *Ophthalmology* 89:605-613, 1982.

81. Tripathi BJ, Kwait PS, Tripathi RC: Corneal growth factors: a new generation of ophthalmic pharmaceuticals, *Cornea* 9(1):2-9, 1990.

82. Tsubota K et al: Effects of air and irrigating solutions on the corneal endothelium, *Cornea* 7(2):115-121, 1988.

83. Tuberville AW et al: A correlative electron microscopic and freeze-fracture examination of cat corneal endothelial wound repair, *Curr Eye Res* 8(4):365-377, 1989.

84. Tuft SJ, Coster DJ: The corneal endothelium, *Eye* 4:389-424, 1990.

85. Van Horn DL, Hyndiuk RA: Endothelial wound repair in primate cornea, *Exp Eye Res* 21:113-124, 1975.

86. Waring GO, Rodrigues MM: Congenital and neonatal corneal abnormalities. In Tasman W, Jaeger EA, editors: *Biomedical foundations of ophthalmology*, vol 1, Philadelphia, 1989, Lippincott.

87. Watsky MA et al: Corneal endothelial junctions and the effect of ouabain, *Invest Ophthalmol Vis Sci* 31(5):933-941, 1990.

88. Weimar VL, Haraguchi KH: A potent new mesodermal growth factor from mouse submaxillary gland: a quantitive, comparative study with previously described submaxillary gland growth factors, *Physiol Chem Phys* 7:7-21, 1975.

89. Wilson SE et al: Aqueous humor composition in Fuchs' dystrophy, *Invest Ophthalmol Vis Sci* 30(3):449-453, 1989.

90. Yanoff M, Fine BS: Cornea and sclera. In Tasman W, Jaeger EA, editors, *Biomedical foundations of ophthalmology*, vol 3, Philadelphia, 1989, Lippincott.

91. Yee RW, Edelhauser HF: Comparison of intraocular acetylcholine and carbachol, *J Cataract Refract Surg* 12:18-22, 1986.

92. Zagorski Z: Replication capacity of the regenerating human corneal endothelium in organ culture. In Naumann GOH, Gloor B, editors: *Wundheilung des Auges und ihre Komplikationen*, München, 1980, JF Bergmann Verlag.

Chapter 7

Techniques for Evaluating Endothelial Cell Function

HENRY F. EDELHAUSER

DAYLE H. GEROSKI

DAVID B. GLASSER

MAMORU MATSUDA

Methods available for the laboratory evaluation of eye bank tissue have expanded considerably from those employed in the original studies that utilized dye exclusion[57] to allow assessment of endothelial cellular viability. Techniques currently being applied to the quantitation of the functional capacity of donor-stored corneas include measurement of endothelial pump sites, using patch-clamp procedures to define the status of ion channels in individual endothelial cells[49] and using more sensitive probes, such as carboxyfluorescein, to measure endothelial barrier function in donor corneas.[66] These newer techniques will provide new data on the functional changes that occur during donor corneal storage and thus be quite useful in the evaluation of any new preservative media.

The early physiologic evaluations of eye bank tissue and endothelium were established by the use of trypan blue, a vital and supravital stain, which stained damaged endothelial cells.[13,55] Later Robbins and co-workers[51] used the nitro-blue tetrazolium stain as the primary method of evaluating corneal

cryopreservation. Endothelial ultrastructure was the next procedure used to evaluate alterations in endothelial cells that occurred during moist-chamber storage, after cryopreservation, and after storage in McCarey-Kaufman storage (MK) medium.[46,48,62,63]

The classical temperature-reversal studies were the first laboratory physiologic tests performed on eye bank tissue after moist-chamber storage.[22] Subsequent studies coupled temperature reversal and in vitro specular microscopy for evaluation of moist-chamber storage eyes[23] and MK medium−stored corneas.[44,45]

Further laboratory evaluation of moist-chamber storage and cryopreserved corneal tissue included measurements of corneal water, sodium, potassium, and the measurement of corneal uptake and removal of dimethyl sulfoxide (DMSO).[11,12] Measurements of corneal oxygen consumption[61] and corneal glucose metabolism[15] were also used to evaluate the stored and preserved tissue.

Ultimately the analysis of whether a corneal preservation procedure has successfully maintained the endothelium is the graft's ability to maintain transparency after keratoplasty. Once the graft is in place, the endothelial cells can be followed by specular microscopy, endothelial function can be assessed

Supported in part by NIH grants EY00933, EY05609, P30 EY06360 (a Departmental Core Grant), and Research to Prevent Blindness, Inc.

by measurement of corneal thickness, and endothelial barrier function can be monitored by fluorophotometry.[5]

This chapter is a description of some of the newer physiologic methods currently being used to evaluate eye bank tissue stored in different media.

WILD-FIELD SPECULAR MICROSCOPY

Wide-field specular microscopic evaluation of donor corneal endothelium has valuable clinical and research applications. Clinically the integrity of the corneal endothelium is vital to the success of penetrating keratoplasty. Donor corneas with large numbers of healthy endothelial cells that can participate in endothelial wound healing after transplantation can be assumed to be of superior quality compared with corneas with low cell densities. Bourne's[5] demonstration of progressive endothelial cell loss during the first 2 years after keratoplasty indicates that a cell density of at least 2000 cells/mm^2 may be desirable in donor tissue.

Although the traditional criteria for donor selection (donor age, cause of death, associated systemic or ocular conditions, time from death to enucleation, preservation time, and slitlamp assessment of corneal thickness and endothelial and epithelial status) have succeeded in maintaining a low incidence of primary graft failure, they may not be accurate indicators of endothelial cell density and viability. For example, many surgeons prefer to use corneas from younger donors[3] because younger tissue is believed to have a higher number of endothelial cells and greater functional integrity than older tissue.[5,6,33,35,41,48] However, donor age has no effect on clinical results,[14,31,52] and correlation between donor age and the cell density of the graft endothelium is poor.[10,36,40]

One can observe the donor endothelium with the slitlamp using specular reflection, but the field of view is so narrow that any estimate of cell density or viability is subject to unacceptably large sampling errors. At least 100 adjacent cells in a large single field should be evaluated to minimize sampling error.[5,32] Wide-field specular microscopy provides the capability for several hundred cells to be photographed in one field and allows the examiner to rapidly scan the entire central cornea in search of localized abnormalities (Fig. 7-1). Morphologic analysis of endothelial cells may provide even more information regarding donor viability. Several studies indicate that endothelial morphology (degree of polymegethism and pleomorphism) is more closely related to the functional reserve of the corneal endothelium than cell density is.[50,54,55,58]

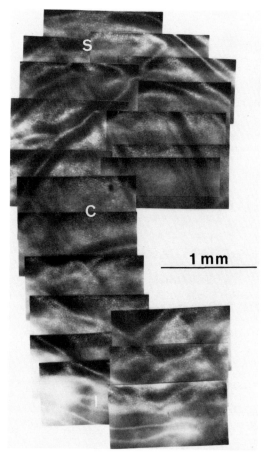

Fig. 7-1. Montage of donor cornea demonstrating capability of scanning large areas of endothelium. *S,* Superior cornea; *C,* central cornea; *I,* inferior cornea.

We performed wide-field specular microscopy and pachymetry on 92 donor corneas to evaluate the nature and degree of changes that occur in the endothelium during moist-chamber storage at 4° C. The endothelial changes were evaluated by computer-assisted morphometry. The donor corneas were divided into two groups: younger (38 eyes, mean age of 34 years) and older (54 eyes, mean age of 72 years).

No significant differences in endothelial cell density, coefficient of variation in cell area (polymegethism), percentage of hexagonal cells (pleomorphism), or central corneal thickness were noted between the younger and older donors after any of the storage intervals studied (0-12, 13-24, 25-48 hours). In both groups, although cell density remained constant, a great increase in the extent of polymegethism and pleomorphism developed when storage was prolonged beyond 12 hours. These changes may, in part, be attributable to buildup of toxic products in the stagnant aqueous humor.[4] During this period,

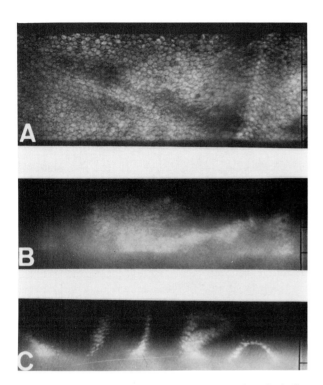

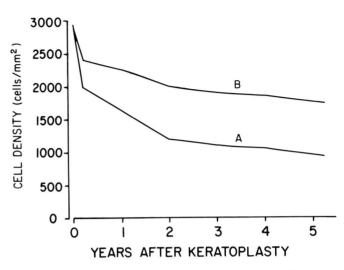

Fig. 7-3. Endothelial cell density (central) as a function of time after keratoplasty. *A,* McCarey-Kaufman medium storage (data adapted from Matsuda M, Bourne WM: *Arch Ophthalmol* 103:1343, 1985). *B,* Hypothetical performance using an improved storage medium or technique.

Fig. 7-2. A, Good-quality wide-field view of endothelium obtained from donor eye stored for 10 hours in a moist chamber at 4° C. **B,** Fair view of endothelium, adequate for cell density and morphologic analysis, obtained from a donor eye stored for 20 hours. **C,** Poor view of endothelium obtained after 30 hours of storage.

corneal thickness also increased significantly, but there was no correlation between thickness and the extent of the endothelial changes. These results indicate that evaluation of endothelial morphology by specular microscopy may be a more reliable method of screening donor tissue than donor age or corneal thickness. A significant number of corneas that may have been rejected on the basis of donor age or corneal thickness demonstrated morphologically normal endothelia with cell densities. Although some or all of these corneas may be useful for penetrating keratoplasty, their functional status is currently unknown.

Specular microscopy employing Polaroid film and commercially available matching grids can be used by eye bank personnel to evaluate donor corneas for endothelial cell density and polymegethism (coefficient of variation).[70] Whole globes and corneas stored in MK medium can be photographed. A limitation of this technique is that the quality of the photographs begins to deteriorate when tissue storage is prolonged beyond 12 hours (Fig. 7-2), particularly when the corneoscleral rim has been removed from the globe.

Research applications of wide-field specular microscopy in eye banking are equally promising. The fate of the transplanted endothelium is the ultimate test of the effectiveness of a corneal preservation medium or technique. Bourne's[5] prospective, longitudinal evaluation of MK medium–stored corneas before and after transplantation has provided a valuable groundwork for comparison with new methods of corneal preservation such as organ culture and media containing chondroitin sulfate. In addition to prolonging usable storage time, an improved medium might also be able to reduce the initial cell loss after keratoplasty (Fig. 7-3).

Morphology and cell-density measurements also may be used to investigate the effects of different donor disease processes on the quality of the donor endothelium. For example, polymegethism and pleomorphism have been observed in corneas from donors maintained on mechanical ventilators for periods of 3 days or longer.[69]

MEASUREMENT OF ENDOTHELIAL BARRIER FUNCTION IN DONOR CORNEAS

A sensitive and accurate technique for the in vitro measurement of endothelial permeability in the isolated rabbit cornea has been described by Araie.[1] This technique involves endothelial perfusion of the isolated cornea mounted in the specular microscope and the use of 5(6)-carboxyfluorescein to determine endothelial permeability. We have adapted this technique to measure endothelial permeability in human

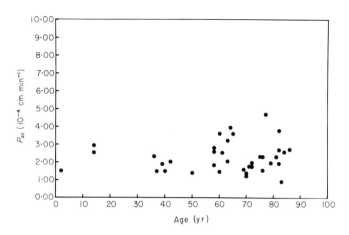

Fig. 7-4. Endothelial permeability (P_{ac}) versus donor age for human donor corneas ($n = 39$). No correlation was found between donor age and endothelial permeability. (From Watsky MA, McDermott ML, Edelhauser HF: *Exp Eye Res* 49:751, 1989.)

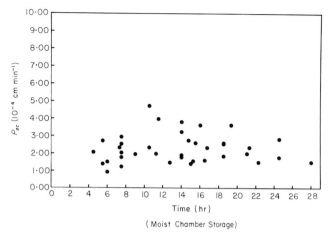

(Moist Chamber Storage)

Fig. 7-5. Endothelial permeability (P_{ac}) versus moist chamber storage time for human donor corneas ($n = 39$). No correlation was found between storage time and endothelial permeability. (From Watsky MA, McDermott ML, Edelhauser HF: *Exp Eye Res* 49:151, 1989.)

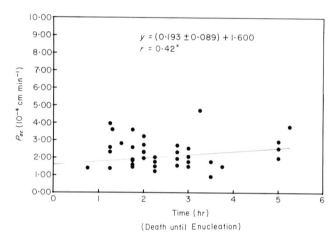

(Death until Enucleation)

Fig. 7-6. Endothelial permeability (P_{ac}) versus time between death and enucleation for human donor corneas ($n = 39$). A significant correlation ($p < 0.05$) was found between permeability and time between death and enucleation. Equation represents slope ($\pm$SE) of its shown regression line. (From Watsky MA, McDermott ML, Edelhauser HF: *Exp Eye Res* 49:751, 1989.)

donor corneas and have investigated factors that might influence endothelial barrier function in donor tissue.[66] Factors examined include donor age, time between death and enucleation, tissue storage time, diabetes, and cataract surgery before the death of the donor.

In human donor corneas, no significant correlation was found between donor age (Fig. 7-4) or moist chamber storage time (Fig. 7-5) and endothelial permeability to carboxyfluorescein. A significant and positive correlation was found, however, between endothelial permeability and the time period between death and enucleation (Fig. 7-6). Endothelial permeability was found to increase as this time period increased.

Endothelial permeability data for control human corneas compared to the donor operative and diabetic donor (types I and II) groups are shown in Table 7-1. Permeability values for aphakic (3.88×10^{-4} cm/min), pseudophakic posterior chamber (PC) implant (3.30×10^{-4} cm/min), and anterior chamber (AC) implant donor corneas (3.53×10^{-4} cm/min), as well as pooled pseudophakic corneas (3.48×10^{-4} cm/min), were all significantly greater ($p < 0.05$) than values for control corneas (2.26×10^{-4} cm/min). Central corneal thickness for aphakic and pooled corneas was also significantly greater than the central corneal thickness of control corneas. Diabetic donor corneas, both type I and type II, were found to have endothelial permeabilities entirely comparable to control donor corneas.

These data indicate that, with prolonged donor death to enucleation times, hypoxic metabolites may accumulate within the anterior chamber, stroma,

and endothelial cells resulting in a progressive breakdown of the endothelial barrier. Furthermore, donor eyes having undergone previous cataract surgery, regardless of the procedure, were shown to have an increased endothelial permeability when compared to control donor corneas. This elevated permeability did not approach the value for corneas completely denuded of endothelium (12.85×10^{-4} cm/min), illustrating that the endothelial barrier was not completely abolished. The decreased endothelial cell density observed in donor eyes that had under-

Table 7-1. Permeability ($\times$ 10^{-4} cm/min) and corneal thickness data for human donor corneas

	Control	Pooled	Aphakic	PC	AC	Diabetic Humans Type I	Diabetic Humans Type II
Number	39	22	3	10	9	6	10
Age*	62 ± 21	80 ± 10	78 ± 13	78 ± 7	80 ± 10	67 ± 10	65 ± 9
CCT	589 ± 43	629 ± 58†	625 ± 61	622 ± 54	639 ± 67‡	634 ± 89	621 ± 41
P_{ac}	2.26 ± 0.84	3.48 ± 1.30†	3.88 ± 1.78‡	3.30 ± 1.37‡	3.54 ± 1.20‡	2.25 ± 0.72	1.98 ± 0.50

AC, Anterior chamber; *CCT*, central corneal thickness; P_{ac}, endothelial permeability of AC; *PC*, posterior chamber.
*Age indicates the mean (±S.D.) age of the donor (years).
†Significantly different from control (p <0.01, Student's *t*-test).
‡Significantly different from control (p <0.05, least-significance difference multiple comparison).

gone cataract surgery in the present study (data not shown) and in previous studies[42] implies surgical trauma to the endothelium. This trauma, whether physical, chemical, or attributable to the inflammatory process, appears to damage the endothelial cell junctions such that endothelial permeability is increased. The full-thickness stromal incision performed during the cataract procedure may also contribute to the increase in permeability.

MEASUREMENT OF ENDOTHELIAL PUMP FUNCTION IN DONOR CORNEAS

Corneal transparency is mediated by the well-established barrier and pump functions of the endothelium. As long as the leak rate is exactly matched by the rate of the metabolic pump, stromal hydration is maintained at 78% and corneal transparency is maintained. Clinically, corneal edema will develop when the rate of fluid leak exceeds endothelial pump capacity.

An essential component of the endothelial fluid pump is Na/K ATPase,[8,18,37,59] an enzyme located in the lateral endothelial cell membranes.[34,38] The cardiac glycoside ouabain is a specific inhibitor of this enzyme to which it is bound quantitatively.[20] By utilization of the specific and high binding affinity of tritiated ouabain to endothelial Na/K ATPase, it has been possible to quantitate the density of these Na/K "pump sites" in the rabbit[16] and human[19] corneal endothelia. These studies have demonstrated that the density of Na/K pump sites is relatively high and comparable to that seen in other tissues having a high transport function.

Pump function of the human corneal endothelium is of particular interest, since failure of the pump to adapt to increased endothelial leak is a presumptive mechanism for the development of corneal edema. Na/K pump-site density has been studied in a group of 26 pairs of human donor corneas with donor eyes ranging from 11 through 91 years. In this group of

corneas, pump-site density was found to remain constant and independent of donor age (Fig. 7-7). Since the permeability of the corneal endothelium to fluorescein has also been shown to remain constant with age,[7,65,66] these data document that, in the normal aging cornea, barrier and pump functions remain balanced despite a constant gradual loss of endothelial cells. On the other hand, when the endothelium becomes leaky as occurs in Fuchs' dystrophy,[9,65] pump-site density was found to be significantly increased, a change demonstrating that, before decompensation, barrier and pump remain matched and corneal transparency is preserved. The human corneal endothelium thus has reserve adaptive pump capacity, which is manifest by the appearance of additional pump sites in Fuchs' dystrophy. When this physiologic reserve is exceeded, pump and leak

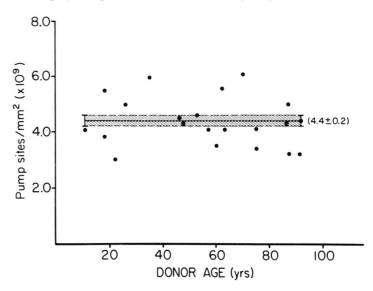

Fig. 7-7. Endothelial Na/K pump-site density versus donor age for human corneas. Pump-site density remains constant (4.4 ± 0.2 × 10^9 sites/mm²) and independent of donor age in normal human cornea. *Shaded region*, Mean ± standard-error density.

can no longer be matched and decompensation will occur. Recent cytochemical data indicate that in decompensated Fuchs' dystrophy Na/K pump activity becomes severely reduced,[53] a finding indicating that the pump has literally burned itself out.

Recent data thus demonstrate that although the corneal endothelium does possess considerable adaptive pump capacity the tissue's physiologic reserve is limited. It is quite reasonable to assume that successful keratoplasty depends to a large extent on utilization of donor tissue having a minimally compromised reserve. The preservation of endothelial pump capacity is therefore of major importance in donor-tissue storage. The newer tritiated ouabain-binding methods enable specific, quantitative measurements of endothelial pump-site density. Utilizing these techniques to evaluate methods of donor tissue storage will thus provide quantitative data on the ability of the various storage methods to preserve endothelial pump function and reserve.

We have recently compared the effects of corneal storage in two commonly used preservation media—modified McCarey-Kaufman (mMK) and K-Sol—on endothelial Na/K pump site density and carboxyfluorescein permeability in human donor corneas.[47]

For the permeability measurements, one member of a matched pair of donor corneas underwent immediate permeability determination, whereas its mate was stored (4 or 7 days) in either mMK medium or K-Sol. Endothelial permeability (P_{ac}) was then determined after 4 or 7 days of storage.

Endothelial Na/K pump-site density was measured after storage in another group of paired corneas. For this group of corneas, one member of each matched pair was placed in mMK medium, whereas its mate was placed into K-Sol. Both corneas were stored at 4° C, and after 7 days of storage, endothelial Na/K pump-site density was measured with use of the tritiated ouabain-binding method.

Table 7-2 shows endothelial permeability after 4 and 7 days of storage in mMK and K-Sol media. These data indicate that after 4 days of storage no significant change in P_{ac} was seen between fresh and stored mate corneas in either storage medium. Normal endothelial permeability was preserved through 7 days of storage in mMK medium as well. Seven days of storage in K-Sol, however, resulted in a significant ($p < 0.05$) increase in P_{ac}. Endothelial permeability of the K-Sol–stored corneas increased to 1.5 times that of their unstored mate corneas.

Fig. 7-8 shows the results of the ouabain-binding studies for paired corneas stored for 7 days in K-Sol and in mMK media. Also shown are data obtained from seven pairs of control (unstored) corneas. These

Table 7-2. Permeability Data for Human Corneas after Storage in mMK or K-Sol*

| Storage | P_{ac} ($\times 10^{-4}$ cm/min) | |
	Unstored Mate	Stored Mate
4 days		
mMK	2.42 ± 0.68	2.31 ± 0.31
K-Sol	2.58 ± 0.93	2.44 ± 0.60
7 days		
mMK	2.46 ± 0.42	2.82 ± 0.80
K-Sol	2.18 ± 0.54	3.33 ± 0.90†

*$n = 5$ pairs of corneas for each medium at each time; values are mean ±SD.
†$p < 0.05$ compared to unstored mate.

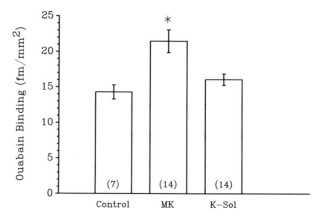

Fig. 7-8. Ouabain binding by endothelia of corneas stored 7 days in modified McCarey-Kaufman (mMK) or K-Sol medium compared to ouabain binding by endothelia of fresh, unstored tissue. Bars represent mean (±SE). Values in parentheses represent its number of corneas studied. $p < 0.01$ compared to fresh controls or K-Sol–stored tissue. *$p < 0.01$ compared to fresh controls or K-Sol–stored tissue. (From McDermott ML et al: *Cornea* 10:44, 1991.)

data indicate that after 7 days of storage endothelial pump-site density in the mMK-stored corneas (21.5 fm/mm^2) was significantly ($p < 0.001$) greater than either unstored control tissue (14.3 fm/mm^2) or the paired K-Sol–stored tissue (16.8 fm/mm^2).

These results show that endothelial permeability and Na/K pump-site density of human corneas stored in mMK or K-Sol media under eye bank conditions change with storage time. Both storage media studied maintained endothelial barrier function through 4 days of storage; however, after 7 days of storage changes in endothelial function were measured in each solution. Endothelial permeability to carboxyfluorescein, after 7 days of storage, was preserved by mMK medium but not by K-Sol. Hull and co-workers[25] also found mMK medium to better preserve endothelial barrier function in stored rabbit corneas. The ouabain-binding data also indicate that significant alterations in endothelial Na/K ATPase pump-site density can occur during donor corneal storage. After 7 days of storage, a significant increase in Na/K site density was measured in mMK-stored corneas compared to either K-Sol–stored mates or control, unstored tissue. This elevation of pump-site density may be indicative of stressed tissue. On the other hand, the increased ouabain binding seen in the mMK-stored tissue may, indeed, reflect an increased endothelial transport capacity. The functional significance of these findings is presently uncertain. Although additional studies are necessary to define the functional significance of these changes, it is clear that changes in endothelial barrier and pump functions do occur during donor tissue storage. An understanding of these functional alterations will be essential to one optimizing storage medium.

STROMAL PROTEOGLYCAN LOSS DURING DONOR CORNEAL STORAGE

Corneal transparency is derived from the parallel arrangement and regular spacing of the stromal collagen fibrils.[42] Proteoglycans (PGs), which consist of a protein core with covalently bound polyanionic glycosaminoglycans (GAGS), are interspersed between and interact with the stromal collagen fibers. Stromal PGs through their interactions with the collagen fibrils affect the regularity in fibril spacing and therefore assume a principal role in determining corneal transparency.[2]

Kangas and co-workers[30] have described the loss of stromal PGs during corneal edema. Proteoglycan loss can result in collagen fibril aggregation, disruption of the regular arrangement of collagen fibrils, and a decrease in corneal transparency. The fate of stromal PGs during corneal storage is unknown. Since alterations in stromal PGs that might occur during corneal storage could affect corneal transparency, we initiated studies aimed at determining the fate of stromal PGs during corneal storage.[56]

For these experiments, stromal PGs of New Zealand White rabbits were labeled in vivo using anterior chamber injections of a 50:50 mixture of ^{35}S-sulfate and D-[6-^{3}H]-glucosamine hydrochloride. The animals were euthanatized, their corneas were excised and stored at 4° C for up to 14 days in mMK, K-Sol, CSM (chondroitin sulfate medium), or Dexsol medium. PG loss was measured by collection of 200 µl aliquots of storage media daily and deter-

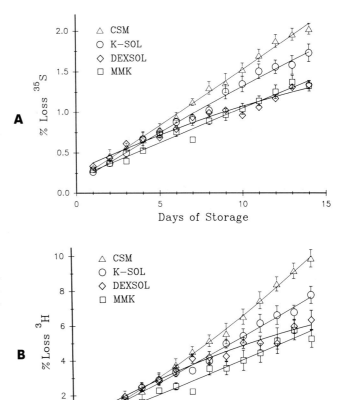

Fig. 7-9. A, Percent of total ^{3}H radioisotope loss from labeled corneas into the preservation media over 14 days of storage. Each point represents the mean (±SE) of six measurements. **B,** Percent of total ^{35}S radioisotope loss from labeled corneas into the preservation media over 14 days of storage. Each point represents the mean (±SE) of six measurements.

mining isotope loss using scintillation spectroscopy. After storage, corneas were digested, and stromal isotope content was measured. DEAE chromatography was also performed on each medium sample to confirm that isotope loss corresponded to PG and GAG loss (data not shown).

Fig. 7-9 depicts the progressive, nearly linear, time-dependent loss of incorporated ^{3}H and ^{35}S from stored corneas. Fig. 7-9, *A,* shows that the greatest loss of incorporated ^{3}H occurred in corneas stored for 14 days in CSM medium. Corneas stored in K-Sol showed intermediate levels of loss, whereas corneas stored in mMK or Dexsol lost the least incorporated ^{3}H. The loss of incorporated ^{35}S-sulfate, which more closely represents proteoglycan loss, is shown in Fig. 7-9, *B.* Again, the greatest loss of incorporated label occurred with CSM storage, followed by K-Sol.

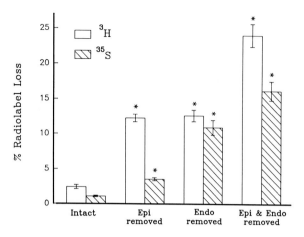

Fig. 7-10. Comparison of the percentage of radiolabeled corneal components lost during 4 days of storage in mMK medium with an intact or selectively removed epithelium or endothelium, or both. Each histobar represents the mean (±SE) of six measurements. *$p < 0.05$ statistical comparisons are to the corresponding value for the intact group.

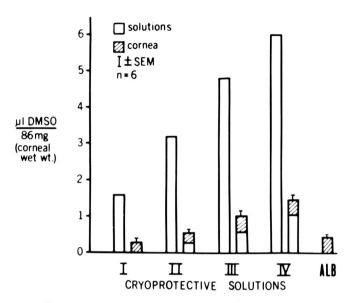

Fig. 7-11. Uptake of DMSO (dimethyl sulfoxide) by rabbit corneal tissue in each of four cryoprotective solutions *(I-IV)* and residual DMSO remaining in cornea after freezing, thawing, and 10 minutes of postthaw incubation in 25% human serum albumin (ALB). *Matched lines,* Amount of DMSO taken up during 10-minute incubation in each solution. *Open bars,* Amount of DMSO present in each of four cryoprotective solutions. (From Edelhauser HF et al: *Cryobiology* 8:104, 1971.)

In an additional group of corneas, the epithelium, the endothelium, or both, were removed before the tissue was stored for 4 days in mMK medium. Fig. 7-10 shows the results of these experiments. Removal of the epithelium or endothelium effected a significantly greater loss of incorporated isotope. Epithelial removal resulted in a fivefold greater loss of ^{3}H and a threefold greater loss of ^{35}S compared to the epithelium intact group. Endothelial removal resulted in a fivefold increase in ^{3}H loss and a tenfold increase in ^{35}S loss. Removal of both the epithelium and endothelium resulted in a 24% loss in ^{3}H and a 16% loss in [35]S.

These results demonstrate a progressive loss of proteoglycans during corneal storage. Furthermore, after long-term storage, the loss of PGs was reduced in corneas stored in mMK and Dexsol compared to corneas stored in CSM and K-Sol media, suggestive of a protective effect of dextran. Dextran may be dehydrating the epithelial and endothelial layers, making it more difficult for the labeled PGs to diffuse from the stroma into the storage medium.

The percentage of PGs lost during storage is relatively small (<2.0%) as long as the epithelium and endothelium remain intact, but the degree of PG loss increases dramatically with either epithelial or endothelial removal. These data emphasize the importance of maintaining intact epithelium and endothelium in the storage media.

IN VITRO LABORATORY EVALUATION OF EYE BANK TISSUE

With any new or modified storage medium such as MK or organ culture media with chondroitin sulfate, it is most important to determine the corneal uptake and removal of the various chemicals that compose the storage medium. The first such studies were performed on the uptake and removal of DMSO (dimethyl sulfoxide) in rabbit and human corneas.[12] The results of this study showed that the DMSO in the cornea did not reach equilibrium during the 40 minutes of incubation in the cryoprotective solutions that preceded the controlled-rate freezing of the tissue (Fig. 7-11). The post-thaw incubation in 25% albumin for 10 minutes at 4° C removed 56% of the DMSO. The residual DMSO within the cornea then diffused into the aqueous humor after transplantation. The half-time, for removal of the residual DMSO from the corneal button to the aqueous humor was 14.6 minutes (Fig. 7-12). Similar studies were performed by Hull and co-workers[26] for dextran, the osmotic agent in MK medium. These authors reported that the dextran in the cornea and MK medium reached equilibrium in 24 hours and that the postkeratoplasty dextran afflux is rapid,

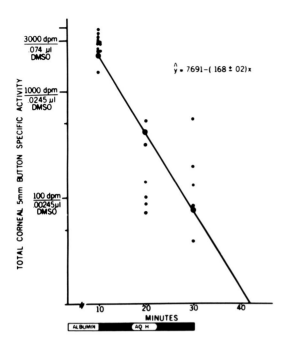

Fig. 7-12. In vitro removal of residual DMSO from a 5 mm cryopreserved rabbit corneal button. The half-time was 14.6 minutes. (From Edelhauser HF et al: *Cryobiology* 8:104, 1971.)

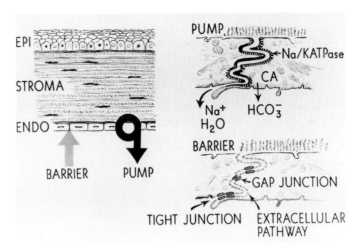

Fig. 7-13. Drawing illustrating location of corneal endothelial metabolic pump and barrier. *EPI*, Epithelium; *ENDO*, endothelium. (From Waring GO III et al: *Ophthalmology* 89:531, 1982.)

with 70% to 75% being lost by 1 to 3 hours and 98% being lost in 12 hours.

In a more recent report by Yau and colleagues[68] it has been found that corneas stored in MK medium containing 100 μg/ml of gentamicin for 3 days before surgery take up sufficient amounts of gentamicin. However, the concentration of gentamicin 1 hour after keratoplasty in the donor tissue was 8.9 μg/ml and in the aqueous humor 2.8 μg/ml. These levels were sufficient to inhibit bacterial growth; by 6 hours there were only trace amounts of gentamicin found in the tissue and aqueous humor.

With the addition of chondroitin sulfate (CDS) to storage media, it will be most important to determine the tissue uptake and removal of the CDS. One report[64] states that corneas stored in unpurified CDS showed more corneal edema after keratoplasty than those stored in purified CDS. It was suggested that the corneas in the unpurified CDS may take up the low-molecular-weight CDS by diffusion, which causes swelling of the donor corneal tissue when placed within the eye. Removal of the low-molecular-weight CDS in the purification procedure prevented the corneal uptake. With any slight modification of a new corneal storage medium, it is essential to determine the corneal uptake and release of the various components of the medium.

Since the corneal endothelium acts as both a bar-

rier and a pump, any new storage medium should protect both of these functions (Fig. 7-13). The endothelial barrier function can be assessed in vitro by use of tracers such as inulin and dextran or carboxyfluorescein.[27,28] Similarly, in vitro studies on endothelial pump function may employ flux studies for $Na^{+ \, 2,7,24}$ and $HCO_3^{- \, 21}$ and ouabain binding. In the formulation of a new storage medium, it will be of importance to determine the ability of the medium to preserve the endothelial barrier and pump.

Metabolic studies are also necessary to establish the effect of a storage medium on the endothelium. Intracellular potentials[67] can be used to determine the ability of the storage media to protect endothelial cells, to assess the cell's ability to regulate volume, and to maintain their membrane potential. Similarly, intracellular pH, glutathione,[29] and endothelial glucose utilization[16] can be measured for assessment of the ability of the storage medium to maintain each of these. Studies with the newer techniques such as patch clamping the endothelial cell membrane[49] will be able to provide specific information on the ability of storage media to maintain membrane ionic channels.

All these techniques are currently being used to evaluate corneal endothelial function and should permit the development of new storage media that will preserve maximal endothelial function and thereby reduce the continual loss of endothelial cells that occurs after keratoplasty.

REFERENCES

1. Araie M: Barrier function of the corneal endothelium and its intraocular irrigation solutions, *Arch Ophthalmol* 104:475, 1986.

2. Balazs EA: Glycosaminoglycans and glycoproteins of the cornea. In Balazs EA, Jeandoz RW, editors: *The amino sugars,* vol 2A, London, 1965, Academic Press, p 444.
3. Binder PS: Eye banking and corneal preservation. In *Symposium on medical and surgical diseases of the cornea,* Trans New Orleans Acad Ophthalmol, St. Louis, 1980, Mosby–Year Book.
4. Bito LZ, Salvador EV: Intraocular fluid dynamics. II. Postmortem changes in solute concentrations, *Exp Eye Res* 10:273, 1970.
5. Bourne WM: Morphologic and functional evaluation of the endothelium of transplanted human corneas, *Trans Am Ophthalmol Soc* 81:403, 1983.
6. Bourne WM, Kaufman HE: Specular microscopy of human corneal endothelium in vivo, *Am J Ophthalmol* 82:319, 1976.
7. Bourne WM, Nagataki S, Brubaker RF: The permeability of the corneal endothelium to fluorescein in the normal human eye, *Curr Eye Res* 3:509, 1984.
8. Brown SI, Hedbys BO: The effect of ouabain on the hydration of the cornea, *Invest Ophthalmol* 4:216, 1976.
9. Burns RR, Bourne WM, Brubaker RF: Endothelial function in patients with cornea guttata, *Invest Ophthalmol Vis Sci* 20:77, 1981.
10. Culbertson WM, Abbott RL, Foster DK: Endothelial cell loss in penetrating keratoplasty, *Ophthalmology* 89:600, 1982.
11. Edelhauser HF et al: Experimental rehydration of cryopreserved corneal tissue, *Invest Ophthalmol* 10:100, 1971.
12. Edelhauser HF et al: Uptake and removal of dimethylsulfoxide in rabbit and human corneas during cryopreservation, *Cryobiology* 8:104, 1971.
13. Evans HM, Schulemann W: The action of vital stains belonging to the benzidine group, *Science* 39:443, 1944.
14. Foster RK, Fine M: Relation of donor age to success in penetrating keratoplasty, *Arch Ophthalmol* 85:42, 1971.
15. Geroski DH, Edelhauser HF: Metabolic evaluation of cryopreserved corneal tissue, *Arch Ophthalmol* 91:130, 1974.
16. Geroski DH, Edelhauser HF: Quantitation of Na/K ATPase pump sites in the rabbit corneal endothelium, *Invest Ophthalmol Vis Sci* 25:2056, 1984.
17. Geroski DH, Edelhauser HF, O'Brien WJ: Hexose monophosphate shunt response to diamide in the component layers of the cornea, *Exp Eye Res* 26:611, 1978.
18. Geroski DH, Kies JC, Edelhauser HF: The effects of ouabain on endothelial function in human and rabbit corneas, *Curr Eye Res* 3:331, 1984.
19. Geroski DH et al: Pump function of the human corneal endothelium, *Ophthalmology* 92:759, 1985.
20. Glenn I, Karlish S: The sodium pump, *Annu Rev Physiol* 37:13, 1975.
21. Green K, Buyer JG, Hull DS: Cornea endothelial bicarbonate fluxes following preservation in solutions of varying composition, *Invest Ophthalmol Vis Sci* 17:1117, 1978.
22. Harris JE, Byrnes P: Reversal of induced hydration of human corneas stored in a moist chamber at refrigeration temperatures for various periods of time. In Capella JA, Edelhauser HF, Van Horn DL, editors: *Corneal preservation,* Springfield, Ill, 1973, Charles C Thomas, Publisher.
23. Hoefle FB, Maurice DM, Sibley RC: Methods of evaluating corneal donor material. In Capella JA, Edelhauser HF, Van Horn DL, editors: *Corneal preservation,* Springfield, Ill, 1973, Charles C Thomas, Publisher.
24. Huff J, Green K: Demonstration of active sodium transport across the isolated rabbit corneal endothelium, *Curr Eye Res* 1:113, 1981.
25. Hull DS, Berdecia R, Green K: Corneal storage in MK medium and K-Sol: effect on ionic and non-ionic fluxes, *Invest Ophthalmol Vis Sci* 28:2088, 1987.
26. Hull DS, Green K, Bowman K: Dextran uptake into and loss from corneas stored in intermediate-term preservative, *Invest Ophthalmol Vis Sci* 15:663, 1976.
27. Hull DS, Green D, Bowman K: Corneal endothelial permeability following storage in moist chamber and MK medium, *Acta Ophthalmol* 57:999, 1979.
28. Hull DS, Green K, Buyer M: Corneal endothelial bicarbonate fluxes following storage in moist chamber, MK medium, and MK medium with added hydrocortisone, *Invest Ophthalmol Vis Sci* 18:484, 1979.
29. Hull DS et al: Intracellular pH and glutathione levels in rabbit corneal endothelium following storage in moist chamber and MK medium, *Invest Ophthalmol Vis Sci* 24:214, 1983.
30. Kangas TA: Loss of stromal proteoglycans in corneal edema, *Invest Ophthalmol Vis Sci* 31:1994, 1990.
31. Jenkins MS, Lempert SL, Brown SI: Significance of donor age in penetrating keratoplasty, *Ann Ophthalmol* 11:974, 1979.
32. Karaki T: Establishing a standard method of studying the corneal endothelium using a digitizer, *Folia Ophthalmol Jpn* 32:2241, 1981.
33. Kaufman HE, Capella JA, Robbins JE: The human corneal endothelium, *Am J Ophthalmol* 61:835, 1966.
34. Kaye G, Tice L: Studies on the cornea. V. Electron microscopic localization of adenosine triphosphatase activity in the rabbit cornea in relation to transport, *Invest Ophthalmol Vis Sci* 5:22, 1966.
35. Laing RA et al: Changes in the corneal endothelium as a function of age, *Exp Eye Res* 22:585, 1976.
36. Laing RA et al: Morphologic changes in corneal endothelial cells after penetrating keratoplasty, *Am J Ophthalmol* 82:459, 1976.
37. Langham M, Kostelnik M: The effect of ouabain on the hydration and adenosine triphosphatase activity of the cornea, *J Pharm Exp Ther* 150:298, 1965.
38. Leuenberger P, Novikoff A: Localization of transport adenosine triphosphatase in rat cornea, *J Cell Biol* 60:721, 1974.
39. Lim J: Na^+ transport across the rabbit corneal endothelium, *Curr Eye Res* 1:255, 1981.
40. Linn JG et al: Endothelial morphology in long-term keratoconus corneal transplants, *Ophthalmology* 88:761, 1980.
41. Lorenzetti DWC et al: Central cornea guttata, *Am J Ophthalmol* 64:1155, 1967.
42. Matsuda M et al: Specular microscopic evaluation of donor corneal endothelium, *Arch Ophthalmol* 104:259, 1986.
43. Maurice DM: The structure and transparency of the cornea, *J Physiol* 136:263, 1957.
44. McCarey BE: In vitro specular microscope perfusion of M-K and moist chamber-stored human corneas, *Invest Ophthalmol Vis Sci* 16:743, 1977.
45. McCarey BE, Kaufman HE: Improved corneal storage, *Invest Ophthalmol Vis Sci* 13:165, 1974.
46. McCarey BE, Sakimoto T, Bigar F: Ultrastructure of M-K and refrigerated moist chamber-stored corneas, *Invest Ophthalmol Vis Sci* 13:859, 1974.
47. McDermott ML: Human corneal storage in modified McCarey-Kaufman and K-Sol media: effect on endothelial Na^+/K^+ ATPase pump site density and permeability, *Cornea* 10:44, 1991.
48. Mishima S: Clinical investigations on the corneal endothelium, *Am J Ophthalmol* 93:1, 1982.
49. Rae JL et al: Potassium channel in rabbit corneal endothelium activated by external anions, *J Membr Biol* 114:29, 1990.
50. Rao GN et al: Pseudophakic bullous keratopathy: relation to

preoperative corneal endothelial status, *Ophthalmology* 91:1135, 1984.

51. Robbins JE et al: Study of endothelium in keratoplasty and corneal preservation, *Arch Ophthalmol* 73:242, 1965.

52. Salleby SS: Keratoplasty: results using donor tissue beyond 48 hours, *Arch Ophthalmol* 87:538, 1972.

53. Sasaki Y et al: Em localization of the Na/K ATPase activity in Fuchs' corneal dystrophy, *Invest Ophthalmol Vis Sci* 26(suppl):53, 1985.

54. Schultz RO et al: Corneal endothelial changes in type I and type II diabetes mellitus, *Am J Ophthalmol* 98:401, 1984.

55. Shaw EL et al: The functional reserve of the corneal endothelium, *Trans Am Acad Ophthalmol Otolaryngol* 85:640, 1978.

56. Slack JW, Kangas TA, Edelhauser HF: Loss of stromal proteoglycans during corneal storage, *Invest Ophthalmol Vis Sci* 30(suppl):342, 1989.

57. Stocker FW et al: Comparison of two different staining methods for evaluating corneal endothelial viability, *Arch Ophthalmol* 76:833, 1966.

58. Sweeney DF et al: The clinical significance of corneal endothelial polymegethism, *Invest Ophthalmol Vis Sci* 26(suppl):58, 1985.

59. Trenberth A, Mishima S: The effects of ouabain on the rabbit corneal endothelium, *Invest Ophthalmol* 7:44, 1968.

60. Van Horn DL: Evaluation of trypan blue staining of human corneal endothelium. In Caspella JA, Edelhauser HF, Van Horn DL, editors: *Corneal preservation*, Springfield, Ill, 1973, Charles C Thomas, Publisher.

61. Van Horn DL, Edelhauser HF, DeBruin J: Functional and ultrastructural changes in cryopreserved corneas, *Arch Ophthalmol* 90:312, 1973.

62. Van Horn DL, Schultz RO: Ultrastructural changes in cryopreserved and experimentally rehydrated corneal tissue. In Capella JA, Edelhauser HF, Van Horn DL, editors: *Corneal preservation*, Springfield, Ill, 1973, Charles C Thomas, Publisher.

63. Van Horn DL, Schultz RO: Ultrastructural changes in the endothelium of human corneas stored under eye bank conditions. In Capella JA, Edelhauser HF, Van Horn DL, editors: *Corneal preservation*, Springfield, Ill, 1973, Charles C Thomas, Publisher.

64. Varnell ED, Kaufman HE, Beuerman RW: A new preserving medium for 14 day storage of donor corneas, *Invest Ophthalmol Vis Sci* 26(suppl):238, 1985.

65. Waltman SR, Kaufman HE: In vivo studies of human corneal endothelial permeability, *Am J Ophthalmol* 70:45, 1970.

66. Watsky MA, McDermott ML, Edelhauser HF: In vitro corneal endothelial permeability in rabbit and human: the effects of age, cataract surgery and diabetes, *Exp Eye Res* 49:751, 1989.

67. Wiederholt M, Koch M: Effect of intraocular irrigating solutions on intracellular membrane potentials and swelling rate of isolated human and rabbit cornea, *Invest Ophthalmol Vis Sci* 18:313, 1979.

68. Yau CW, Busin M, Kaufman HE: Distribution of gentamicin from preservative medium to ocular tissues after penetrating keratoplasty, *Invest Ophthalmol Vis Sci* 26(suppl):148, 1985.

69. Yee RW: Unpublished data, Milwaukee, 1985.

70. Yee RW, Matsuda M, Edelhauser HF: Wide-field endothelial counting panels, *Am J Ophthalmol* 99:596, 1985.

Part II

PENETRATING KERATOPLASTY

Chapter 8

Indications and Contraindications

JORGE N. BUXTON

DOUGLAS F. BUXTON

JOSÉ A. WESTPHALEN

DEFINITION OF TERMS

Penetrating keratoplasty (penetrating corneal transplant, penetrating corneal graft) is the surgical procedure in which abnormal full-thickness corneal tissue is removed from a host and substituted with full-thickness donor corneal tissue. The term "penetrating" is used to connote full thickness, in contrast to "lamellar," or partial, thickness.

Presently, only *homografts* (tissue or organs from the same species) or *autografts* (donor material from same individual) are employed in human penetrating keratoplasty. Autografts may be *contralateral* (OD to OS, or OS to OD) or *rotating ipsilateral* (autograft rotated in the same eye). *Isografts* are transplants between homozygotic twins, and *xenografts (heterografts)* are transplants between different species.

HISTORICAL CONSIDERATIONS AND EVOLUTION

During the nineteenth and early twentieth centuries various types of tissue substitutions were attempted, including glass, xenografts, and homografts without much success. The first human, full-thickness, successful corneal transplant was performed in 1905 by Dr. Edward Zirm in a severe bilateral lye burn.[56]

Over the past 3 to 4 decades there has been a remarkable turnabout in the success of penetrating keratoplasty attributable in great measure to the work of many pioneering surgeons. This success is vividly demonstrated by the fact that penetrating keratoplasty was still an uncommon, even rare procedure 30 years ago, whereas in 1990, according to the Eye Bank Association of America (EBAA), over 40,631 grafts were performed in the United States. Additionally, that same year the EBAA collected 38,364 tissues for research and training.

Many factors are responsible for this dramatic increase in corneal transplants, not the least of which are major scientific and technological innovations. The advent of the surgical microscope, coupled with advances in microsurgical instrumentation, nonreactive 10-0 suture material, microsurgical techniques, and improved preoperative and postoperative management, including the introduction of corticosteroids and other immunosuppressive agents, such as topical cyclosporin A[5,27] have contributed to the development of penetrating keratoplasty as the most frequently performed transplantation procedure in the United States. More sophisticated methods of donor-cornea processing, including acquisition, evaluation, matching, storage, and handling, have played a role in this greater success. The ever-increasing number of elderly recipients with greater life expectancy has also expanded the indications for corneal grafting.

GENERAL INDICATIONS

Optical Prime purpose being improvement in vision

Tectonic Restoration of altered corneal structure (thinning, perforation, and so on)

Therapeutic Tissue substitution for refractory corneal disease

Cosmetic Replacement without hope of visual improvement[16]

These categories are far from absolute. Frequently, several purposes are addressed when a transplant is performed. For example, if a patient with aphakic bullous keratopathy is grafted for optical reasons, one may achieve improved vision, decreased pain, and a more regular thickness. Similarly, if a patient with uncontrolled bacterial keratitis is grafted for therapeutic indications, one may achieve not only control of the infection, but also an increase in structural integrity and perhaps an increase in visual acuity.

In bilateral disease, especially if progressive, the indication for surgery is unequivocal. In unilateral cases there is some controversy, but with a vastly improved prognosis, corrective surgery should be attempted, especially in older patients to avoid dangerous falls with possible fractures. If successful, it will maintain binocular vision and decrease the anxiety of the monocular patient, even if only improvement in peripheral vision is anticipated because of a preexisting macular disorder. A properly informed patient will obtain enhanced peripheral fusion with increased visual function and safety. Certain unilateral conditions, including impending perforations or refractory corneal ulcerations, are mandatory indications for penetrating keratoplasty.

Semitransparent scars and postlaceration leukomas may cause a sharp decrease in vision because of glare and irregular astigmatism. Therefore a trial with contact lenses should be attempted (PMMA, rigid gas permeable, or, rarely, soft contact lenses including "piggy-back"[4] or tandem). Furthermore, a semitransparent scar may fade or the induced astigmatism may decrease over a period of a year, obviating corneal surgery.

CHANGING INDICATIONS

The diagnostic indications have also changed dramatically over the past 25 to 30 years. In the 1950s, when only a small number of transplants were being performed, the most common indications for corneal grafting were herpetic scarring, regrafts, and keratoconus.[2,45] Transplants for bullous keratopathy were almost nonexistent because of the high failure rate. In 1952, Dr. Frederick Stocker reported the first successful graft for aphakic bullous keratopathy.[49] However, it was Dr. Max Fine who first popularized penetrating keratoplasty for this indication by presenting a successful series of 49 eyes at the

Cornea World Congress held in Washington, D.C., in 1964.[26]

As recently as, say, 1975 the main indication for transplants remained regrafts followed by keratoconus while aphakic bullous keratopathy was rapidly emerging as an important indication for corneal transplantation.[2,49] The advent of intraocular lenses[31,48] made pseudophakic bullous keratopathy (PBK) an important complication of cataract surgery and a leading indication for penetrating keratoplasty.[9,30,32,44,47] Herpes, after the introduction of antiviral drugs, has fallen as a leading indication.[25]

Recent data tabulated from 1983 through 1988 from the Wills Eye Hospital (U.S.A.) indicate that pseudophakic bullous keratopathy (22.9%), Fuchs' dystrophy (16.3%), and keratoconus (15.1%) were the leading indications for corneal transplants.[9] However, in a study at Moorfields Eye Hospital (U.K.) for the period from 1985 through 1987, the most common indications for penetrating keratoplasty were keratoconus (34.2%), regrafts (17.2%), and bullous keratopathy (12.6%).[37] Similar results were reported by Brooks and Weiner from Australia.[10]

Table 8-1 lists indications for penetrating keratoplasty of 543 cases performed by one of the authors (J.N.B.), from 1984 to 1989. It is important to note that the frequency of each indication reflects the average over a 6-year period. Column 4 represents the percentage of indications solely for 1989.

In 1984 our personal experience revealed that pseudophakic bullous keratopathy was the primary indication for penetrating keratoplasty representing 21.3% of the total, followed by aphakic bullous keratopathy (18.1%) and keratoconus (11.7%). Paralleling the recent increase in IOL implantation, pseudophakic bullous keratopathy has increased from 4.39% in 1984 to 29.0% in 1988 but in 1989 fell behind to pseudophakic graft decompensation (21.9%), which was only 5.3% of our indication in 1984.

The surprisingly high percentage of pseudophakic graft decompensation is probably attributable to the referral nature of our practice, as well as to our proclivity of retaining certain "benign" anterior chamber and iris-fixated intraocular lenses at the time of initial keratoplasty in the late 1970s and early 1980s, especially in individuals over 70 years of age. In fact, if all regrafts are taken as a separate indication, regardless of the original diagnosis (keratoconus, herpetic keratitis, chemical burns, and so on), PBK represents the most frequent preoperative diagnosis (28.3%) in all years except one (1986) during the study period of 1984 through 1989. This is consis-

Table 8-1. Indications for Penetrating Keratoplasty—1984 to 1989

Recipient Population: 543 Eyes

Follow-up Study at 6 Years: Indications	Patients	01/1984 to 12/1989 %	1989 %
Pseudophakic bullous keratopathy	114	21.0%	14.0%
Keratoconus	70	12.9%	7.8%
Aphakic bullous keratopathy	70	12.9%	7.8%
Pseudophakic graft decompensation	60	11.1%	21.9%
Fuchs' dystrophy	59	10.8%	12.5%
Graft failure	42	7.7%	6.3%
Aphakic graft decompensation	39	7.2%	4.7%
Corneal scars	33	6.1%	4.7%
Herpes keratitis	18	3.3%	6.3%
Corneal ulcers	15	2.7%	4.7%
Corneal dystrophies	11	2.0%	4.7%
Miscellaneous	12	2.2%	1.5%

tent with other series in the literature, which range from 10% to 30%.[2,7,42,47]

PREOPERATIVE EVALUATION

General Considerations. The decision for surgery in cases of optical penetrating keratoplasty should be a joint one between the surgeon and an informed consenting patient. There are no strict visual acuity criteria for performing corneal transplants, just as there are none for performing cataract surgery. Surgical intervention is generally indicated when the patient's vision is no longer sufficient for his needs, be they social, economic, or related to the patient's personal autonomy.[53]

Visual Evaluation. Preoperative visual testing is directed toward predicting postoperative visual outcome. A history of strabismus, amblyopia, or poor vision secondary to other ocular conditions arising before corneal clouding should be elicited. Visual evaluation should, of course, include a measurement of visual acuity in both the proposed surgical eye and the fellow eye.

It is essential to evaluate the best potential visual acuity of the affected eye. If only peripheral vision is expected, the understanding of the value of peripheral function and binocularity should be explained and emphasized to the patient. In semitransparent scars, vision should be tested with a trial contact lens and a trial lens with a pinhole, followed by a dilated pupil with a trial lens and pinhole. Depending on these findings a potential acuity meter (Mentor O &

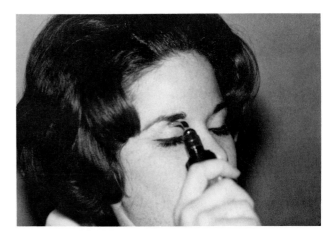

Fig. 8-1. Auto-ophthalmoscopy technique. Muscle light is applied to closed lids and patient is asked to describe intensity and extent of visual field including scotomas.

O, Inc., Norwell, Massachusetts) or laser interferometer should be employed. In opaque corneas, functional tests including evaluation of light projection (with variable intensities of light), two-light discrimination, and auto-ophthalmoscopy should not be underestimated in their predictive value.

Auto-ophthalmoscopy is a transillumination technique that one can perform with a muscle light through closed lids to diagnose and evaluate macular disease or glaucomatous field defects by way of entoptic phenomena, using when possible the contralateral eye as a normal control (Fig. 8-1). Visual evoked response tests and electroretinograms have also been effective in predicting peripheral visual outcome.[54] Additionally, ruling out media and fundus lesions with A and B scan ultrasonography should be routinely performed but is not helpful in determining postoperative central visual acuity.

Lids and Adnexa. Abnormalities of the lids and ocular adnexa must be corrected before corneal surgery. Trichiasis, entropion, ectropion, other lid defects, and symblepharon interfere with adequate lubrication of the graft and may interfere with epithelial healing. Dacryocystitis and blepharitis should be medically or surgically controlled before penetrating keratoplasty is attempted.

Conjunctiva. The conjunctiva should be free of infection. More importantly, tear function must be satisfactory. Moderate and severe forms of dry eye are considered contraindications to penetrating keratoplasty. A decreased number of goblet cells (Stevens-Johnson syndrome, ocular pemphigoid, chemical burns, and so on) will decrease tear-film mucin and create inefficient lubrication. This will invariably lead to poor postoperative results.

Intraocular Pressure. Determining intraocular pressure is frequently difficult, requiring measurements at different corneal sites to avoid scars and false readings. This is best accomplished by employment of different types of instruments including Goldmann applanation, pneumotonometry, and Schiøtz tonometry with two weights.

A past history of glaucoma will necessitate close investigation for the presence of clinically significant peripheral field cuts and central scotomas. In opaque corneas, auto-ophthalmoscopy should be performed, as previously described. If surgery is postponed, careful frequent monitoring of the affected eye is mandatory because of possible progressive glaucomatous damage, especially in children.

Intraocular pressure may be increased by partial loss of the filtration angle, which is occasionally aggravated by penetrating keratoplasty. Postoperative management generally includes corticosteroids, which may also increase preexisting elevated intraocular pressure.[8] Intraocular pressure must be well controlled before transplantation; otherwise endothelial decompensation is more likely to occur. As a general rule, if intraocular pressure is not adequately and consistently controlled with no more than two topical medications without dependence on carbonic anhydrase inhibitors (CAI), an initial glaucoma procedure should be seriously contemplated. Medical management should be accomplished without chronic use of CAI because this measure should not be continued for prolonged periods of time, especially in elderly patients. If moderate medical management fails preoperatively, a filtering procedure or Molteno implant must be performed initially. Cyclocryotherapy is our last preference. Glaucoma surgery performed after a successful corneal graft may adversely affect graft clarity.

Intraocular Inflammation. Active uveitis must be controlled before surgery and may even require systemic corticosteroids or nonsteroidal anti-inflammatory agents, as well as postponement of surgery for several months. Postoperatively, a decreased endothelial population can be expected in the face of chronic, active inflammation.

Cornea. An examination of the cornea preoperatively should include evaluation of the following:

Regularity or variation of corneal thickness and structural integrity, especially if ectasia extends near or to the limbus.[16,33] It may be difficult to obtain proper wound coaptation, and sutures may "cheesewire" through the recipient.

Degree and level of neovascularization. Diffuse, segmental, and particularly deeper vessels have a much higher association with endothelial rejection.

Superficial vascularization tends to complicate future contact lens wear. The presence of significant neovascularization indicates the necessity for variation in suturing technique (for example, a combination of interrupted and continuous suturing versus continuous suturing alone; the former permits segmental removal when necessary).

Status of ocular surface. Dry eye, surface disease, or chemical or radiation burns may hinder repopulation of the central epithelium and wound healing.

Morphologic features of the corneal disorder. The size of the graft necessary to eliminate the disorder in question should be estimated. Smaller transplants, less than 6.5 mm, create higher degrees of astigmatism, whereas larger grafts, greater than 8.5 mm, closer to the vascular limbus, have a higher incidence of rejection.

For localized, central scars with good peripheral endothelial morphology and function, one should

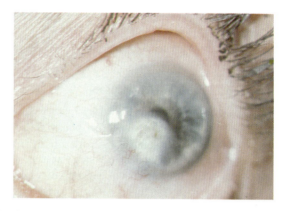

Fig. 8-2. Corneal scar of unknown origin involving visual axis. K: 40.00/48.75 × 55; acuity with +4.00 × 65, 20/60+2, pinhole 20/50.

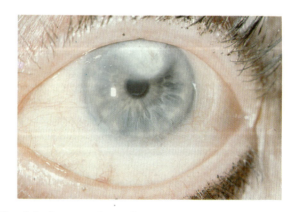

Fig. 8-3. Same patient after rotational autograft. Size of rotated graft 9 mm. K: 43.62/48.87 × 120, 5 years postoperatively; acuity with +0.50 −1.25 × 30, 20/30+2.

consider an ipsilateral rotating autograft (Figs. 8-2 and 8-3) that would rotate the scar out of the visual axis with no chance of graft reaction.[28] In rotating autokeratoplasty, larger grafts (8.5 mm or greater) should be performed so that apposition of thicker peripheral cornea with thinner central cornea, creating both scarring near the visual axis and high astigmatism, does not occur.

Systemic Evaluation. Before surgery the patient should be evaluated systemically, just as for any intraocular procedure. General anesthesia may be indicated for the younger, more apprehensive patients; in cases of difficult previous local anesthesia; or in patients who may be undergoing lengthier, more complicated procedures (triple procedure,

penetrating keratoplasty with posterior intraocular lens exchange with scleral fixation, and so forth).

Psychosocial Considerations. Preoperatively, the patient should have a complete understanding of the necessity for long-term follow-up examination and strict therapeutic compliance. The patient should be capable of either self-administering medications or have someone close at hand to assist. Geographic proximity to either the corneal surgeon or another ophthalmologist who is able to recognize an early graft reaction may be critical to the success of the graft. Typewritten instructions are routinely given to patients 8 to 12 weeks after surgery.

The patient should be aware that complete visual rehabilitation may not be possible within the first few

Table 8-2. Prognosis for Graft Clarity

Group 1 Excellent prognosis 90% or more	Diagnosis:	1. Keratoconus 2. Central or paracentral inactive scars 3. Granular dystrophy 4. Central Fuchs' dystrophy (early) 5. Rotating grafts or autografts
	Morphology:	Avascular central corneal thinning, scarring, or edema surrounded by healthy corneal tissue
Group 2 Very good prognosis 80%-90%	Diagnosis:	1. Advanced Fuchs' dystrophy 2. Pseudophakic bullous keratopathy 3. Aphakic bullous keratopathy 4. Inactive herpes simplex keratitis 5. Iridocorneal endothelial syndromes 6. Interstitial keratitis 7. Macular dystrophy
	Morphology:	Lesion that extends partially or totally to periphery with an adequate surface and mild-to-moderate vascularity
Group 3 Fair prognosis 50%-80%	Diagnosis:	1. Active bacterial keratitis 2. Active herpes simplex keratitis 3. Congenital hereditary endothelial dystrophy and breaks in Descemet's membrane associated with birth trauma 4. Active fungal keratitis 5. Mild chemical burns 6. Moderate keratitis sicca 7. Lattice dystrophy 8. Congenital glaucoma
	Morphology:	Extremes of corneal thickness, perforations, peripheral descemetoceles, active disease, recurrent disease
Group 4 Poor prognosis 0-50%	Diagnosis:	1. Severe chemical burns 2. Radiation burns 3. Ocular pemphigoid 4. Stevens-Johnson syndrome 5. Neuroparalytic disease 6. Epithelial downgrowth 7. Anterior chamber cleavage syndromes 8. Multiple graft failures
	Morphology:	Severe fibrovascular replacement of cornea and conjunctival ischemia, partial anterior chamber obliteration

This table is meant to be a guideline and is certainly not absolute. The prognosis for each group is worsened by the presence of elevated intraocular pressure, intraocular inflammation, lid and conjunctival defects, and other ocular surface disorders as well. Failed grafts are generally considered to possess the prognosis for the group of their primary diagnosis, or slightly less.

postoperative months and that it may take a year or more before some form of correction can be provided, though a large proportion of patients can be fitted with glasses or contact lenses after 2 to 3 months. Patients should also be aware that graft reaction or opacification is a lifelong possibility and that they must be cognizant of the earliest symptoms.

A lack of awareness by the patient may lead to poor compliance and a poor outcome with severe disappointment.

An informed patient with a good result but who suffered from poor and distorted vision can be a source of enormous gratification to the ophthalmologist.

PROGNOSIS

The prognosis for a successful visual result is based on multiple factors. Patient selection is determined by an exhaustive preoperative evaluation, including the general ocular, systemic, and psychosocial considerations previously discussed. Technical ability and experience in handling complications are important intraoperatively. Postoperatively, early recognition of complications, especially those potentially leading to graft rejection, is vital. The timing and refractive effect of postoperative suture removal must be considered. Visual rehabilitation may require meticulous refraction, and at times the fitting of rigid gas permeable contact lenses. Secondary procedures such as relaxing incisions and wedge resections,[6,22,52] may be necessary to correct eyes with high postoperative astigmatism. It is clear that the ophthalmologist's experience and expertise with both corneal surgery and postoperative management is crucial to a successful outcome.

Today, with strict patient selection, excluding those with severe dry eyes, active inflammation, increased intraocular pressure, and other pathologic conditions, one can obtain a clear graft more than 90% of the time, but grafts frequently must be performed on eyes in less than optimal health. Table 8-2 presents a prognostic classification for graft clarity based on several surgeons' results.[1,18,23,36,38-41,51,55]

The prognostic percentage for maintaining corneal graft clarity depends on the initial pathologic condition under consideration.

Group 1. Excellent, 90%+; diagnosis: (1) keratoconus (Fig. 8-4), (2) central or paracentral inactive scars, (3) granular or macular dystrophies, (4) central Fuchs' dystrophy, (5) rotating grafts or autografts.

The quiescent, avascular, and centralized nature of these conditions places them in an excellent prog-

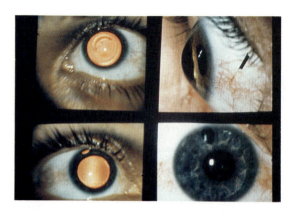

Fig. 8-4. Red reflex highlights round cone, and same eye from side demonstrates pronounced corneal steepening, *above.* Postoperatively clear graft with peripheral iridectomy, *below.*

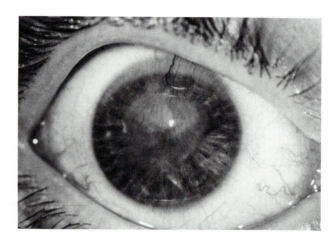

Fig. 8-5. Postherpetic scarring, vascularized.

nostic group. Inactive, traumatic, central or paracentral scars have a good prognosis unless the opacity is postherpetic (Fig. 8-5). Granular and macular dystrophies as well as central Fuchs' dystrophy are all in this good prognostic category.

Group 2. Very good, 80%-90%; diagnosis: (1) advanced Fuchs' dystrophy, (2) pseudophakic bullous keratopathy, (3) aphakic bullous keratopathy, (4) inactive herpes simplex keratitis, (5) iridocorneal endothelial syndromes, (6) inactive interstitial keratitis, (7) lattice dystrophy.

These are relatively avascular corneal disorders extending partially or totally to the periphery with a relatively stable ocular surface. These features are most commonly encountered in advanced Fuchs' dystrophy and pseudophakic and aphakic bullous keratopathy. Despite peripheral extension to the limbus, there appears to be a positive influence from the transplanted endothelial cells onto the edema-

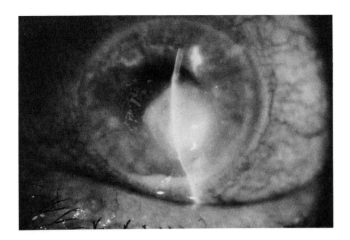

Fig. 8-6. Corneal *Pseudomonas* infection in a soft contact lens wearer, pathologic condition does not reach limbus, which is a better prognosis for corneal grafting.

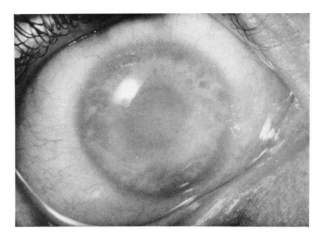

Fig. 8-7. Congenital hereditary endothelial dystrophy.

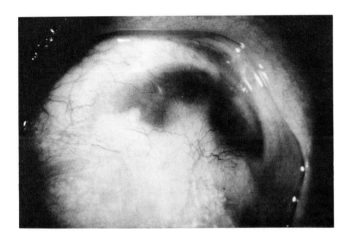

Fig. 8-8. Preoperative view of severe chemical burn from hot aluminum; acuity 6/200, pinhole 20/80.

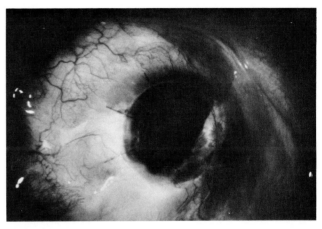

Fig. 8-9. Same eye as in Fig. 8-7 6 years postoperatively; acuity 20/50.

tous periphery. It is possible, however, that these grafts are of shorter longevity than those that do not have this peripheral involvement.

Corneal sensitivity in cases of inactive herpes simplex keratitis is a crucial feature in the outcome of penetrating keratoplasty. The retention of peripheral corneal sensitivity usually indicates a better prognosis. The best evaluation of sensitivity is performed just within the limbus with a Cochet-Bonnet anesthesiometer (Luneau, Paris). If this instrument is not available, a fine wisp of cotton may be employed. Care must be taken that the patient's responses are not related to perceived movements of the hand holding of the instrument near the eye. There is always the risk of reinfection of the graft by herpesvirus, especially if there is a dependence on steroid therapy. Initially, herpetic grafts should be protected with antiviral drugs. Preliminary results with the iridocorneal endothelial syndromes have been satisfactory; however, long-term prognosis is dubious because of frequent development of intractable glaucoma.[21,50]

Group 3. Fair, 50%-80%; diagnosis: (1) active bacterial keratitis (Fig. 8-6), (2) active herpes simplex keratitis, (3) active fungal keratitis, (4) congenital hereditary endothelial dystrophy (Fig. 8-7), (5) mild chemical burns of the acidic type, (6) moderate keratitis sicca.

Group 4. Poor, 0-50%; generally these conditions are contraindications to penetrating keratoplasty though there may be rare exceptions (Figs 8-8 and 8-9). Lower success rates are associated with eyes demonstrating anesthesia, neurotrophic disturbances, or moderate-to-severe dryness.

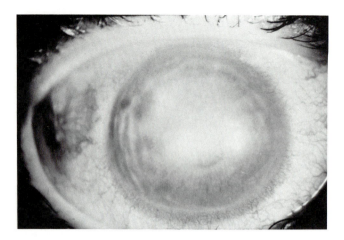

Fig. 8-10. Neuroparalytic keratitis with poor healing with fifth cranial nerve dysfunction not responding to multiple therapies including contact lenses.

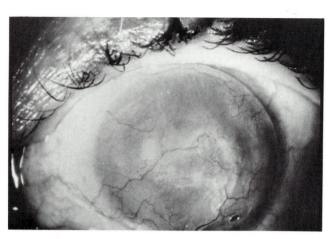

Fig. 8-11. Total thin conjunctival flap for this disorder with rigid gas-permeable contact lens, 2 years, 2 months postoperatively.

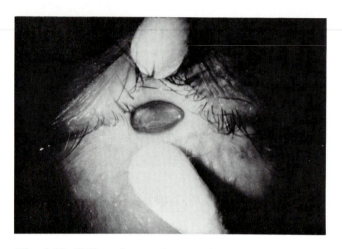

Fig. 8-12. Fifth and seventh nerve involvement with extensive nasal and temporal tarsorrhaphies.

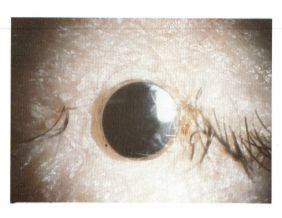

Fig. 8-13. Keratoprosthesis with tarsorrhaphy for advanced ocular pemphigoid has extremely guarded prognosis. This therapy should be avoided if at all possible, especially if other eye has useful vision.

CONTRAINDICATIONS

The only absolute contraindication to penetrating keratoplasty is when the anticipated surgical stress and anesthesia risk creates a situation of significantly increased morbidity and mortality. However, a blind, elderly patient in poor general health may tolerate the procedure well and obtain a good visual outcome without systemic complications if proper anesthesia and medical precautions are taken.

The following diagnostic considerations are considered relative contraindications, each with significant clinical exceptions.

Ocular

Corneal anesthesia. Secondary to neuroparalytic keratitis with poor healing secondary to corneal hypoesthesia or anesthesia (fifth cranial nerve dysfunc-

tion). An alternative management option is a total, thin, conjunctival flap. Subsequently, a rigid gas-permeable contact lens is fitted. This frequently produces adequate visual rehabilitation in these difficult neurotrophic conditions (Figs. 8-10 and 8-11).

Exposure keratitis. Seventh cranial nerve dysfunction (that is, after removal of an acoustic neuroma), uncorrected lid deformities resulting in inadequate lid closure with epithelial healing problems. If corneal grafting becomes necessary, permanent nasal and temporal tarsorrhaphies should be performed at the time of surgery. Alternatively, upper lid gold weights and wire springs as well as lower lid auricular implants may be employed.[34,35,46] In cases of both fifth and seventh cranial nerve involvement, the only possibility of preserving the eye is with ex-

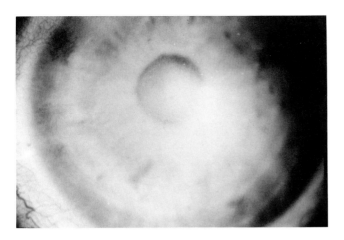

Fig. 8-14. Fuchs' dystrophy and cataract.

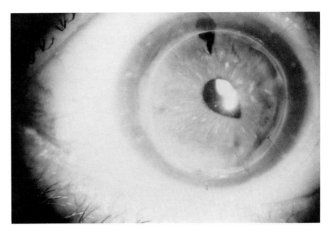

Fig. 8-15. Postoperative results in eye in Fig. 8-13. Successful triple operation, but with symptomatic edema outside graft resistant to all therapies.

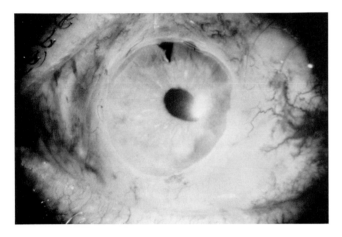

Fig. 8-16. Annular conjunctival flap for symptomatic corneal edema outside graft.

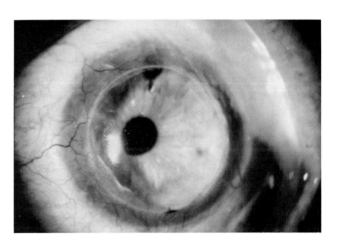

Fig. 8-17. Annular conjunctival flap, 4½ years postoperatively; acuity with −7.00 −2.25 × 30, 20/25−.

tensive permanent nasal and temporal tarsorrhaphies (Fig. 8-12).

Severe Dry Eye. Ocular pemphigoid, Stevens-Johnson syndrome, severe keratitis sicca. In these conditions, if one eye is still functional, surgery should be deferred. If surgery becomes mandatory, a keratoprosthesis (Fig. 8-13) with guarded prognosis should be considered in one eye only. Other modalities may involve contralateral conjunctival transplantation, buccal mucosa grafting, rigid gas-permeable contact lenses, etc.

Systemic. Patients who are malnourished, diabetic, or alcoholic are likely to have healing difficulties and higher susceptibility to infection. Compliance may certainly be a problem in patients with senility, mental retardation, alcoholism, and drug addiction.

GENERAL APPROACH IN SPECIAL CORNEAL PROBLEMS

Peripheral Edema. After successful penetrating keratoplasty for corneal edema (advanced Fuchs', aphakic and pseudophakic bullous, and so on), if the patient becomes symptomatic because of peripheral host edema (outside the graft), a thin annular conjunctival flap is the procedure of choice[14] (Figs. 8-14 to 8-17) when conservative management is ineffective.

This same technique is useful in the unlikely central progression of a Brown-McClean syndrome (idiopathic peripheral corneal edema after intracapsular cataract extraction).[11-13]

The use of a total thin conjunctival flap for symptomatic, diffuse corneal edema is a well-known option when corneal grafting is contraindicated and

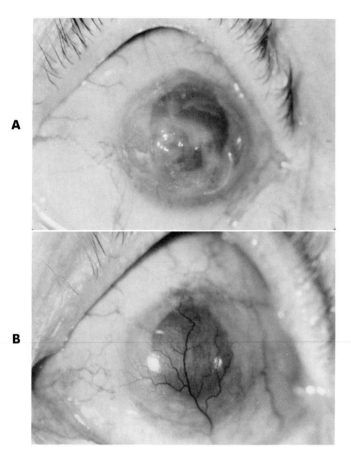

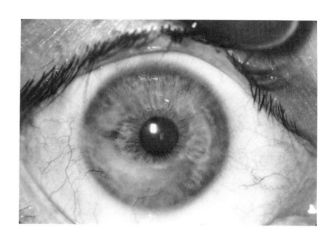

Fig. 8-20. Terrien's dystrophy with increasing thinning and astigmatism, K: 41.40/51.00 × 75; acuity with −8.50 +6.50 × 75, 20/30.

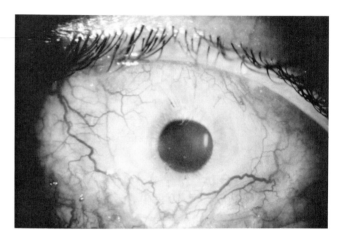

Fig. 8-18. Bullous keratopathy noticeably symptomatic refusing corneal grafting and contact lenses, **A,** preoperative and, **B,** total therapeutic conjunctival flap.

Fig. 8-21. Terrien's dystrophy, annular conjunctival flap, 1 month postoperatively; acuity 20/300, pinhole 20/25.

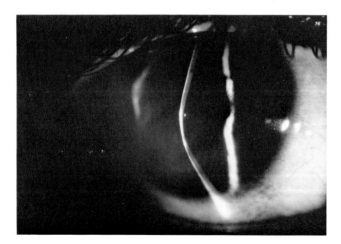

Fig. 8-19. Keratoconus with thinning reaching limbus below and temporally in oval or sagging cone.

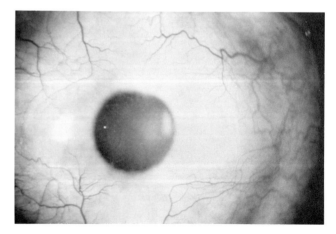

Fig. 8-22. Terrien's dystrophy, annular conjunctival flap, 7 years postoperatively, K: 41.50/54.50 × 75; acuity with contact lens and −4.00 −0.50 × 18, 20/20.

therapeutic contact lenses are poorly tolerated[15,17,29] (Fig. 8-18).

Corneal Thinning. The classic example of noninflammatory thinning is keratoconus, especially in the oval or sagging variety in which the ectatic process reaches the inferotemporal limbus.[33] Fitting of contact lenses in this situation is problematic. Frequently decentered grafts are necessary with an increased risk of immune reactions[19,20,24] (Fig. 8-19).

Terrien's margin dystrophy usually progresses slowly. Exceptionally, pinpoint perforations may occur.[3,43] The best follow-up examination is with serial keratometry or computerized corneal imaging. If thinning or irregular astigmatism progresses, we find that partial or annular therapeutic conjunctival flaps tend to arrest the process (Figs. 8-20 to 8-22). In extremely thin Terrien's an adequate partial lamellar graft is indicated covered by a partial therapeutic conjunctival flap.

In very dry eyes, especially in rheumatoid arthritis, localized areas of extreme thinning, descemetocele formation, or perforations are encountered. In this situation the best therapy is a small lamellar graft covered by a partial conjunctival flap and a small temporal tarsorrhaphy over the area of disorder. If the small lamellar graft is not covered by the conjunctival flap, there is an increased risk of graft necrosis or dehiscence.[15,17]

REFERENCES

1. Arentsen JJ, Laibson PR: Surgical management of pseudophakic corneal edema: complications and visual results following penetrating keratoplasty, *Ophthalmic Surg* 13:371, 1982.
2. Arentsen JJ, Morgan B, Green WR: Changing indications for keratoplasty, *Am J Ophthalmol* 81:313, 1976.
3. Austin P, Brown SI: Inflammatory Terrien's marginal corneal disease, *Am J Ophthalmol* 92:189, 1981.
4. Baldone JA, Clark WB: Contact lenses in the aphakic child, *Contact Lens Med Bull* 3:25, 1970.
5. Belin MW et al: Topical cyclosporine in high-risk corneal transplants, *Ophthalmology* 96:1144, 1989.
6. Belmont SC, Troutman RC: Compensating compression sutures in wedge resection, *J Refract Surg* 1:104, 1985.
7. Bigar F, Witmer R: Corneal regrafts, *Dev Ophthalmol* 14:117, 1987.
8. Boruchoff SA: Therapeutic keratoplasty. In Smolin G, Thoft RA, editors: *The cornea: scientific foundations and clinical practice*, Boston, 1983, Little, Brown.
9. Brady SE et al: Clinical indication for and procedures associated with penetrating keratoplasty 1983-1988, *Am J Ophthalmol* 108:118-122, 1989.
10. Brooks AM, Weiner JM: Indications for penetrating keratoplasty: a clinicopathological review of 511 corneal specimens, *Aust NZ J Ophthalmol* 15(4):277, 1987.
11. Brown SI: Peripheral corneal edema after cataract extraction, *Am J Ophthalmol* 70:326, 1970.
12. Brown SI, McLean JM: Peripheral corneal edema after cataract extraction: a new clinical entity, *Trans Am Acad Ophthalmol Otolaryngol* 73:465, 1969.
13. Brown SI, McLean JM: Peripheral corneal edema after cataract extraction: a new clinical entity. In Hughes WF, editor: *The year book of ophthalmology 1970*, Chicago, 1970, Mosby–Year Book.
14. Buxton DF, Buxton JN: Treatment of unusual complications following penetrating keratoplasty, *Ocular Surg News* 8(7):12, 1990.
15. Buxton JN: Therapeutic conjunctival flaps and tarsorrhaphy, *Contact and Intraocular Lens Med J* 7:150, 1981.
16. Buxton JN: Corneal surgery. In Collins JF: *Handbook of clinical ophthalmology*, New York, 1982, Masson.
17. Buxton JN, Buxton DF, Andrade COR: Colgajos conjuntivales totales y parciales. In Arentsen JJ, editor: *Cirugía del segmento anterior del ojo*, Buenos Aires, Arg, 1990, Editora Médica Panamericana SA.
18. Buxton JN, Chambers CE: Indications for surgery. In Bronson NR II, Paton RT, editors: *Advances in keratoplasty*, Boston, 1970, Little, Brown.
19. Buxton JN, Hoefle F, Koverman J: Contact lenses in keratoplasty, *Contact Lens Med Bull* 2:3, 1969.
20. Buxton JN, Keates RH, Hoefle FB: The contact lens correction of keratoconus. In Dabezies OH, editor: *The CLAO guide to basic science and clinical practice*, Boston, 1988, Little, Brown, pp 55.1-55.14.
21. Buxton JN, Lash RS: Results of penetrating keratoplasty in the iridocorneal endothelial syndrome, *Am J Ophthalmol* 98:297, 1984.
22. Buzard KA, Haight D, Troutman, RC: Ruiz procedure for postkeratoplasty astigmatism, *J Refract Surg* 3:40, 1987.
23. Castroviejo R: *Atlas of keratectomy and keratoplasty*, Philadelphia, 1966, Saunders.
24. Cohen EJ, Adams CP: Postkeratoplasty fitting for visual rehabilitation. In Dabezies OH, editor: *The CLAO guide to basic science and clinical practice*, Boston, 1988, Little, Brown, pp 52.1-52.7.
25. Ficker LA et al: Longterm prognosis for corneal grafting in herpes simplex keratitis, *Eye* 2:400, 1988.
26. Fine M: Keratoplasty in aphakia. In King JG Jr, McTigue JW, editor: *The Cornea World Congress*, Washington, DC, 1965, Butterworth.
27. Goichot-Bonnat EL, Pouliquen YJM: Topical cyclosporin A in high-risk keratoplasty. In Cavanagh HD, editor: The cornea, Transactions of the World Congress on the Cornea III, New York, 1988, Raven Press.
28. Groden LR, Arentsen JJ: Ipsilateral rotating autokeratoplasty, *Ann Ophthalmol* 15:899, 1983.
29. Gundersen T, Pearlson HR: Conjunctival flaps for corneal disease: their usefulness and complications, *Trans Am Acad Ophthalmol* 67:78, 1969.
30. Hyman L, Susel R, Lance B: *The keratoplasty evaluation project.* Presented at May 1985 meeting of Association for Research in Vision and Ophthalmology, Sarasota, Florida (New Rochelle, New York, headquarters).
31. Jaffe NS: The outlook for intraocular lenses through 1990, *J Cataract Refract Surg* 12:267, 1986.
32. Kozarsky AM et al: Results of penetrating keratoplasty for pseudophakic corneal edema with retention of intraocular lens, *Ophthalmology* 91:1141, 1984.
33. Kretzer F: Possible ultrastructural and biochemical mechanisms of stromal thinning in keratoconus, *Invest Ophthalmol* 19:202, 1980.
34. May M: Gold weight and wire spring implants as alternatives to tarsorrhaphy, *Arch Otolaryngol Head Neck Surg* 113:656, 1987.
35. May M et al: Management of the paralyzed lower eyelid by

implanting auricular cartilage, *Arch Otolaryngol Head Neck Surg* 116:786, 1990.

36. Moore TE Jr: Keratoplasty. In Leibowitz HM: *Corneal disorders: clinical diagnosis and management*, Philadelphia, 1984, Saunders.

37. Morris RJ, Bates AK: Changing indications for keratoplasty, *Eye* 3:455, 1989.

38. Paton D, Jones DB: *Penetrating keratoplasty*, Alcon Monogram Series 1, No. 1, Oct 1976, Fort Worth, Texas.

39. Polack FM: *Corneal transplantation*, New York, 1977, Grune & Stratton.

40. Price FW, Whitson WE, Marks RG: Graft survival in four common groups of patients undergoing penetrating keratoplasty, *Ophthalmology* 98:322, 1991.

41. Raju VK: Corneal surgery. In Duane TD, Jaeger EA, editors: *Clinical ophthalmology*, New York, 1984, Harper & Row, vol 5, Chapt 6.

42. Rapuano CJ et al: Indications for and outcomes of repeat penetrating keratoplasty, *Am J Ophthalmol* 109:689, 1990.

43. Richards WW: Marginal degeneration of the cornea with perforation, *Arch Ophthalmol* 70:610, 1963.

44. Robin JB et al: An update of the indications for penetrating keratoplasty, *Arch Ophthalmol* 104:87, 1986.

45. Smith RE et al: Penetrating keratoplasty, changing indications, 1947 to 1978, *Arch Ophthalmol* 98:1226, 1980.

46. Soll DB: New surgical approaches to the management of ocular exposure secondary to facial paralysis, *Ophthalmic Plast Reconstr Surg* 4:215, 1988.

47. Stanley JA: Indications for corneal transplant surgery, *Int Ophthalmol Clin* 28:5-13, 1988.

48. Stark WJ et al: Trends in intraocular lens implantation in the United States, *Arch Ophthalmol* 104:1769, 1986.

49. Stocker FW: Successful corneal graft in a case of endothelial and epithelial dystrophy, *Am J Ophthalmol* 35:349, 1952.

50. Stulting RD, Cavanagh HD, Crawford G: *Penetrating keratoplasty in the management of iridocorneal endothelial syndrome*, Presented at the Castroviejo Society Meeting, Nov 1984, Atlanta, Georgia.

51. Sugar A: An analysis of corneal endothelial and graft survival in pseudophakic bullous keratopathy, *Trans Am Ophthalmol Soc* 87:762, 1990.

52. Troutman RC: Corneal wedge resections and relaxing incisions for post keratoplasty astigmatism, *Int Ophthalmol Clin* 23(4):161, 1983.

53. Waring GO 3d: Selecting patients for penetrating keratoplasty, *South Med J* 74:1243, 1981.

54. Wendel RT, Mannis MJ, Keltner JL: Role of electrophysiologic testing in the preoperative evaluation of corneal transplant patients, *Ann Ophthalmol* 16:788, 1984.

55. Wilson SE, Kaufman HE: Graft failure after penetrating keratoplasty, *Surv Ophthalmol* 34:325, 1990.

56. Zirm E: Eine erfolgreiche totale Keratoplastik *Graefes Arch Ophthalmol* 64:580, 1906.

Chapter 9

Preoperative Evaluation

Phakic eyes

S. LANCE FORSTOT

The most common diagnoses for which adult phakic penetrating keratoplasties are performed are:

1. Keratoconus
2. Corneal opacities secondary to infection or trauma
3. Fuchs' dystrophy
4. Hereditary stromal dystrophies (lattice, granular, and macular)

Aspects of the history and clinical examination that pertain to specific diagnoses are discussed.

HISTORY

The best previous visual acuity is important information worth obtaining. In most cases, there is a clear history of good vision before the development of the opacity or the progression of the corneal disease. However, the childhood onset of an opacity seen later in an adult may signify the presence of amblyopia. Previous macular or retinal problems, though less common in the phakic than the aphakic adult, may mean a less-than-optimal visual result despite a clear graft.

In Fuchs' dystrophy, a history of blurred vision may indicate corneal decompensation, particularly when signs of corneal edema are absent clinically. This is most likely the case when patients with early decompensation are examined in the late afternoon.

Patients with keratoconus may complain of distorted vision or multiple images despite their ability to read small letters on the Snellen chart. They may also have greatly diminished night vision and may have stopped driving at night.

History taking should document the use of topical medications, such as pressure-lowering agents for glaucoma. Poor control of intraocular pressure after keratoplasty may have a definite negative effect on graft survival. A history of allergy to topical medications should be noted. Allergy to an antiviral drug would preclude its use postoperatively if coverage or treatment of a recurrent herpetic infection was necessary. Similarly, an allergy to a preservative such as thimerosal (contained in Viroptic and Neosporin solutions) may also provoke unnecessary inflammation postoperatively.

A history of current and past medical disease and treatment is also vital. Cardiac or pulmonary disease may influence the decision to recommend surgery or the type of anesthesia (local versus general); cardiopulmonary disease may preclude the use of timolol or other nonselective topical beta-adrenergic receptor blockers for postoperative intraocular pressure control; a history of allergy to sulfonamides may preclude the use of carbonic anhydrase inhibitors; patients taking aspirin or blood-thinning medication may need a reduction in dosage or heparinization before surgery; and a patient receiving systemic corticosteroids may have wound healing significantly affected.

EXAMINATION

Visual Acuity. Assessment of visual acuity is paramount when trying to evaluate the risk-benefit ratio of surgery. Testing may be required in a lighted and a darkened room to evaluate a patient's symptoms. The availability of a glare-testing apparatus and contrast-sensitivity measurements may aid in the objective assessment of visual disability caused by keratoconus, corneal edema, scars, and stromal opacities.

In patients with dense corneal leukomas, ancillary testing of retinal and optic nerve function may be necessary. The pupils must be examined for an afferent defect. With a dense leukoma, the normal pupil may have to be observed for constriction using a swinging flashlight test. Color vision, Maddox-rod, and entopic phenomenon tests may be useful, indirect tests of retinal function. More sophisticated testing with potential acuity measurement machines and laser interferometers may be helpful in the evaluation of the prognosis of transplant surgery in patients with corneal edema and leukomas.

External Examination. Examination of the lids and skin may be important for graft prognosis. The face may provide a clue to the diagnosis of acne rosacea. Scarred lids from trauma, prior surgery, herpes zoster, or irradiation may influence the decision to perform surgery. Severe lid scarring may require lid surgery before grafting or a tarsorrhaphy at the time of the transplant to prevent exposure and graft melting.

Slitlamp Examination. The lids should be carefully examined for blepharitis and treated before surgery. The tear film should be observed for evidence of dry eye. Signs would include a decreased tear meniscus, floating debris, and a rapid tear breakup time. A Schirmer test and rose bengal staining may be performed to determine the severity of involvement.

The conjunctivae should be examined for scarring and symblepharon. The abnormal conjunctivae seen after chemical injuries and with ocular pemphigoid is an unhealthy setting for a corneal graft. Scarring of the conjunctivae may also be seen in those keratoconic patients with severe atopic keratoconjunctivitis.

The corneal examination is extremely important. The extent of the opacity may determine the graft size. Corneal vascularity will in part determine the prognosis and propensity for rejection. Superficial vessels are not as significant as their stromal counterparts.

The anterior chamber must be evaluated for evidence of inflammation. A transplant is best performed on a quiet, noninflamed eye. In those patients with scars from herpes simplex or herpes zoster, there should be no iritis present. Anterior synechiae are not usually a problem in the phakic patient. Exceptions may be leukomas from penetrating or chemical injuries or in patients with the iridocorneoendothelial syndrome. Preoperative planning for the intraoperative management of these synechiae often facilitates surgery.

Corneal Thickness. Corneal thickness is an important preoperative factor requiring careful study. Areas of corneal thinning may determine the size or placement of the graft. An eccentrically placed graft may be necessary. Severe, extensive thinning may indicate the need for a lamellar keratoplasty before a definitive penetrating graft. This may be the case in keratoglobus. Measurement of corneal thickness as

A

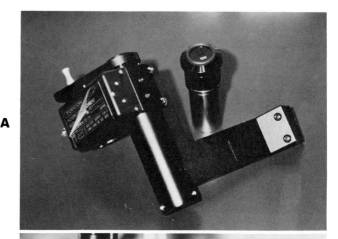

B

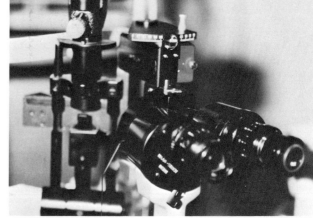

C

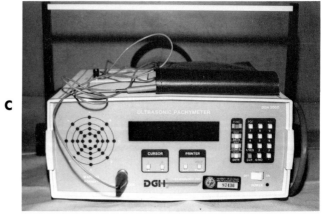

Fig. 9-1. A, Topcon optical pachymeter. **B,** Pachymeter mounted on slitlamp. **C,** Ultrasonic pachymeter.

opposed to a qualitative evaluation may be necessary. Pachymetry is useful in following eyes with Fuchs' dystrophy. This measurement of endothelial function is sometimes more useful than specular microscopy, especially when the guttate changes are severe or the edema precludes good endothelial visualization. Optical pachymeters (Fig. 9-1, *A*) as well as the newer ultrasonic pachymeters (Fig. 9-1, *C*) are useful.

Corneal Irregularity. There are several simple yet practical ways to assess corneal irregularity. A Placido disc or hand-held keratoscope (Fig. 9-2, *A*) will indicate irregular astigmatism. A hand-held van Loehnan keratoscope used at the slitlamp is also useful.[1] The corneoscope (Fig. 9-2, *B*) will photographically document irregularities (Fig 9-3). This instrument is useful in the assessment of scarring and the irregularity in keratoconus. Standard keratometry will also provide evidence of irregular astigmatism. If irregular astigmatism is present, a trial with a con-

tact lens may be necessary. A soft contact lens may mask small amounts of irregular astigmatism, but a rigid contact (gas permeable or hard) may be necessary for larger amounts of astigmatism.

Lens Status. If possible, one should determine the extent of lens opacity preoperatively, but occasionally this decision must be made during surgery after removal of the recipient corneal button. The type of extraction (intracapsular or extracapsular) should be determined. A dislocated lens may require an intracapsular procedure. Extracapsular extraction is routinely used in other situations. The decision for a lens implant is also better done before surgery. The decision for a "triple" (keratoplasty, lens extraction, and implant) will require an implant power calculation.

INTRAOCULAR PRESSURE AND RETINA

The intraocular pressure should be measured before surgery. Corneas with edema or severe scarring

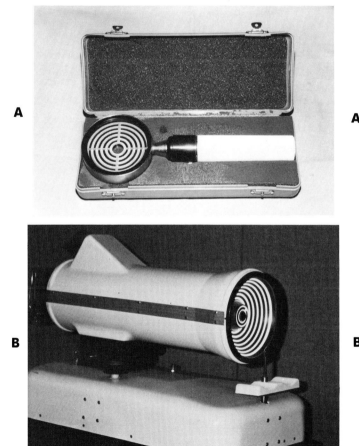

Fig. 9-2. A, Keeler keratoscope. **B,** Corneoscope.

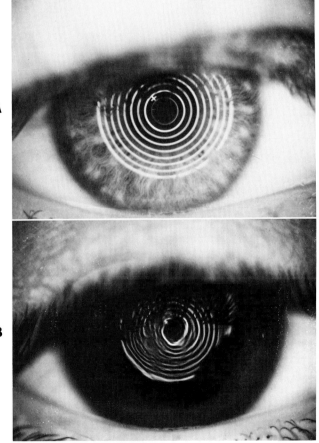

Fig. 9-3. A, Normal corneal topography. **B,** Advanced keratoconus.

may not be amenable to applanation tonometry. The MacKay-Marg, the pneumotonometer, and the Tono-Pen may be required for a more accurate pressure assessment in those instances.

If possible, the retina should be assessed with indirect ophthalmoscopy. The integrity of the retina and macula certainly are crucial for a good visual result after keratoplasty. Ultrasonography may be needed to rule out a retinal detachment. Electrophysiologic testing may be helpful. As previously mentioned, potential acuity meter testing or laser interferometry may be useful in the evaluation of retinal function.

PATIENT EVALUATION

Once all the pertinent information from the history and clinical examination has been obtained, an overall and individualized assessment of the patient must be made. Factors such as the age of the patient, the status of the other eye (cataractous, blind, good vision), need for binocularity, prognosis for the specific condition being operated, and the ability to comply with postoperative care and follow-up study, play a role in the decision to proceed with surgery. Ultimately, given as much information as possible, the patient and the family will need to make the final decision.

REFERENCES

1. Drews RC: The van Loehnan keratoscope at surgery. In Emery JM, Jacobson AC, editors: *Current concepts in cataract surgery,* St. Louis, 1980, Mosby–Year Book, pp 237-238.
2. Mannis MJ, Zadnik K, Johnson CA: The effect of penetrating keratoplasty on contrast sensitivity, *Arch Ophthalmol* 102:1513, 1984.
3. Paton D: *Penetrating keratoplasty: a symposium on medical and surgical diseases of the cornea,* Trans New Orleans Academy of Ophthalmology, St. Louis, 1980, Mosby–Year Book.
4. Rowsey JJ: Topographical analysis of the cornea: ten caveats in keratorefractive surgery. *Int Ophthalmol Clin* 23(4):1, 1983.
5. Steinert RF, Minkowski JS, Boruchoff SA: Pre-keratoplasty potential acuity evaluation: laser interferometer and potential acuity meter, *Ophthalmology* 91:1217, 1984.

Aphakic and pseudophakic eyes

ALAN SUGAR

Pseudophakic bullous keratopathy has become the leading indication for keratoplasty, accounting for more than 25% of grafts. When aphakic bullous keratopathy is added, more than one third of eyes are either aphakic or pseudophakic before keratoplasty.[23,24] The thorough preoperative evaluation of the aphakic or pseudophakic eye can help to prevent intraoperative and postoperative problems. Unlike the situation in the phakic eye, the surgeon must consider not only the corneal abnormality, but also the noncorneal complications of the previous cataract surgery. Such consideration can allow for appropriate planning of surgical technique and avoid disappointment for both patient and surgeon.

HISTORY

Taking a careful history is mandatory during the preoperative evaluation. Amblyopia, prior retinal disease, glaucoma, and optic neuropathy may be known to the patient but not be apparent on examination through an opaque cornea. Use of medications for control of inflammation or intraocular pressure must be known to avoid their exacerbation after keratoplasty. Often the history of the course of visual loss will be helpful in the determination of whether the decrease is solely related to the corneal problem. Knowledge of changes in vision throughout the day is often helpful in the evaluation of patients with corneal edema, especially when a patient examined late in the day has good vision despite poor vision much of the time. A history of the patient's past experience with and tolerance of contact lenses is helpful if future contact lens use is anticipated. A history of trauma and its sequelae should be sought. This historical evaluation should include an assessment of the patient's activities, employment, and avocations. Without this information, the relation of current visual function to visual needs cannot be evaluated.

A history of the best visual acuity obtained after the previous cataract surgery is critical. The corneal opacity may not be the only reason or even the major reason for poor vision. A history of visual loss from macular degeneration or cystoid macular edema may not contraindicate keratoplasty but will help in prognostication.

Perhaps the most critical historical information involves detailed information on the prior cataract surgery, including techniques of lens removal, status of the posterior capsule, and intraoperative and postoperative complications. The previous operative summaries should be read if possible. The type, power, and configuration of the intraocular lens used should be obtained from records or the patient registration card.

A history of general medical problems is helpful in planning anesthesia and preoperative and postoperative care. Management of medications is imperative in this generally elderly aphakic and pseudophakic population.

VISUAL FUNCTION

Assessment of best corrected visual acuity and best potential visual acuity are critical in decision making for keratoplasty. Keratometry will often make accurate refraction easier, especially if the corneal opacity limits retinoscopy. All corneal surgeons have had the experience of improving the vision of a patient referred for keratoplasty by careful refraction rather than surgery. In many cases, a hard contact lens will give unexpectedly good vision and, even if not practical for use in a given patient, may help in determining the potential postoperative acuity.[29] A pinhole may also help in determining visual potential.

When opacities of the cornea do not permit direct measurement of potential acuity, visual function must be inferred by indirect means. The relative afferent pupillary defect may be detected by the swinging-flashlight test if the pupil can be seen, or by the reverse test in the opposite eye.[19] A relative defect may indicate asymmetric glaucoma, optic nerve disease, or retinal disease and is a certain sign that the corneal problem does not account fully for the visual defect.

TESTS OF RETINAL FUNCTION

Various entoptic phenomena have been used to assess retinal function behind opacities in the ocular media.[9] Light perception and projection should be tested routinely in eyes with poor visual acuity. Occasionally, the bright light of the indirect ophthalmoscope must be used to obtain a response; in this case the prognosis is usually very poor and may preclude keratoplasty unless both eyes are similarly involved. Accurate light projection is not a guarantee of good retinal status, and poor projection may be present despite a normal retina and optic nerve when the corneal opacity is severe. Two-point light differentiation and color perception are also of only limited predictive value.

Entoptic images, visual images originating within the eye, may be of some value in the prediction of gross visual potential. A light moving over the closed lid will cast retinal vascular shadows detectable by most patients with normal retinas. When this pattern is detectable, there is likely to be at least perifoveal function. Detection of the normal avascular zone indicates that the fovea may be functioning.[12] The blue-field entoptic phenomenon allows assessment of the ability of the patient to detect white blood cells passing through the perifoveal capillaries when looking into bright blue light. This is a moderately good predictor of macular function in patients with anterior segment opacity.[28]

Laser interferometric visual acuity testing was introduced to assess potential visual acuity in patients with opacities of the media, particularly cataract. It has been shown to be of value in patients with corneal opacity, though less so than in cataract patients.[14,15]

This technique requires an adequate pathway for two laser beams to enter the pupil and is therefore of limited value in patients with severe opacities. Because the test is somewhat influenced by large refractive errors, the correction should be used during testing in aphakic patients.[6] Laser interferometry tends to overestimate acuity in eyes with amblyopia.[15] Unfortunately falsely optimistic readings are also obtained in eyes with cystoid macular edema, a frequent concern in eyes with pseudophakic bullous keratopathy.[7] They also tend to overread potential acuity in eyes with macular degeneration, another continual concern in this older population.[8] White-light interferometers, such as the Lotmar visometer (Haag-Streit, Waldwick, N.J.) and the IRAS interferometer, (Randwal, Southbridge, Mass.), use similar principles and are moderately accurate in postoperative vision prediction of patients with lens opacity.[13,17] These methods are limited by severe opacities. A good visual acuity response is more likely to be helpful than a poor response in clinical decision making.

The potential acuity meter (PAM) of Guyton and Minkowski projects a visual acuity chart through a tiny aerial aperture.[16] Like the interferometers, it requires at least a pinhole-sized clear pathway to allow the beam to reach the retina. Its predictive value before keratoplasty is less than in cataract patients.[34] This accuracy can be significantly increased by placement of a hard contact lens on the cornea during testing.[30] As with other methods the cystoid macular edema prevalent in eyes with pseudophakic bullous keratopathy may lead to false-positive results.[34]

The use of electrophysiologic methods to predict visual function is still not available or accurate enough for most routine uses. When, however, the psychophysiologic tests previously discussed are not helpful in making a decision and widespread retinal damage or degeneration must be ruled out, measurement of the electroretinogram may occasionally be of some value. Bright-flash electroretinogram (ERG) will give a response despite most medium opacities,[10] and transscleral ERG can be used to bypass the ocular media.[27] Both methods measure only gross retinal function. The visual evoked response (VER) is a better measure of central retinal function. Pattern stimuli can give a relatively precise measure of visual function when the media are clear, but flash stimuli or transscleral stimuli must be used when the cornea is opaque. The VER can be helpful in predicting the outcome in poor-prognosis cases.[3]

Visual field testing is important in the evaluation of visual function, especially when there is a history of glaucoma or optic nerve disease and the fundus cannot be well seen. Formal visual field testing is often not feasible. The use of a hand-held light can be very useful in gross evaluation of the field when vision is hand movements or light perception only. This penlight field usually will detect hemianopsia or the temporal island of advanced glaucoma. Generalized constriction, however, is not a reliable predictor of postoperative visual field limitation.

RETINAL STRUCTURE

The preoperative detection of retinal detachment is of particular concern in the aphakic eye with an opaque cornea because of the rate of detachment in such eyes, especially when they had complicated cataract extraction. The presence of detachment may contraindicate keratoplasty or may indicate the use of a temporary keratoprosthesis for combined keratoplasty and detachment surgery.[5,11] Knowledge of the presence of macular disease may not contraindicate surgery but may help in prognostication. The visual function tests discussed already are likely to indicate the presence of retinal detachment. Indirect ophthalmoscopy must be performed on all prekeratoplasty patients, but the view may be limited. Fortunately, contact B-scan ultrasonography can be performed easily and rapidly as a screening procedure for retinal detachments and intraocular tumors. Preoperative detection of a retinal detachment may save unnecessary grafting and postoperative disappointment and may also allow planning for a complex combined procedure. In the past, keratoplasty was performed first, and retinal detachment repair followed when the view was adequate. Landers and co-workers[21] and Eckardt[5] have developed temporary keratoprostheses for insertion after trephination of the recipient cornea. Vitrectomy and scleral buckling are then performed and followed by donor cornea placement at the same sitting. Experience with this method has been encouraging.[11] In our hands it has been especially useful in eyes after complex trauma.

SCREENING FOR CYSTOID MACULAR EDEMA

Cystoid macular edema (CME) is a major preoperative and postoperative problem in eyes with aphakic and pseudophakic bullous keratopathy.[1,4] CME occurs transiently in from none to 17% of eyes with intraocular lenses (IOLs) and appears to be more frequent in eyes with iris-supported IOLs and intracapsular cataract extraction than in eyes with posterior chamber IOLs after extracapsular cataract extraction.[31] It is more frequent when the cataract extraction was associated with vitreous loss or capsule rupture. Of critical importance is the association of late-developing CME with late pseudophakic corneal edema, possibly through the mediation of a common inflammatory process related to the IOL.

Although fluorescein angiography usually cannot be performed because of the corneal edema, fluorescein angioscopy with an indirect ophthalmoscope and blue filter will often allow a view of late macular fluorescein pooling.[4] The presence of CME does not preclude keratoplasty. It does, however, limit the visual prognosis. CME is the most frequent vision-threatening complication of pseudophakic keratoplasty, occurring in about one third of patients and almost two-thirds of those with less than 20/40 vision.[35] Many patients with CME after pseudophakic keratoplasty will have gradual improvement in vision and clearing of their CME over a period of 2 to 3 years.[25,32] Preoperative awareness of CME will avoid early disappointment and blame on the keratoplasty rather than on earlier procedures. Careful examination for vitreous in the anterior segment will help in the prediction of the need for vitrectomy, a risk factor for CME.[20]

CORNEAL EXAMINATION

Obviously the slitlamp examination is the essential feature of the diagnostic evaluation. Careful attention should be paid to the status of the lids, conjunctiva, and cornea. Good lid apposition is necessary because exposure or entropion can lead to epithelial defects, poor wound healing, and corneal graft melting. Infectious blepharitis should be treated preoperatively to prevent graft infection. Scarring of the conjunctiva increases the risk of graft surface problems, especially when it is a sign of ocular cicatricial pemphigoid.

Most aphakic and pseudophakic grafts are performed for bullous keratopathy. Because the extent of corneal edema may vary with humidity and time of day, the edema noted at examination late in the day may not appear adequate to warrant keratoplasty. Measurement of corneal thickness may document stromal edema when there is little epithelial edema or striate keratopathy, and a history of morning blurring or a repeat examination early in the day may be helpful. Serial pachymetry is often helpful in documenting progression. Specular microscopy of the corneal endothelium may be helpful in the evaluation of eyes with marginal vision and edema. Endothelial density below 500 to 600 cells/mm^2 indicates that the cornea, if beginning to decompensate, will likely become progressively more edematous over the next several months.[2] When the central cell count is 300 or less in a cornea with only peripheral edema, complete endothelial decompensation soon follows.

Documentation of the slitlamp examination should include variations in corneal thickness, degree and depth of vascularization, and location of opacities and edema. Waring and Laibson have described a helpful scheme for diagraming slitlamp findings with colored-pencil drawings.[36] The status of the anterior chamber, presence of peripheral synechiae, and position, type, and stability of the intraocular lens, vitreous, and capsule are important to observe preoperatively.

Routine considerations for all grafts should not be neglected in aphakic and pseudophakic eyes. One of the most important of these is intraocular pressure. There is a high prevalence of glaucoma in eyes with pseudophakic bullous keratopathy; about 35% of patients are using antiglaucoma therapy at the time of keratoplasty.[35] Measurement of intraocular pressure may not be accurate by applanation, and MacKay-Marg or pneumotonometry may be necessary. Intraocular pressure should be controlled before keratoplasty, if possible, though combining keratoplasty with trabeculectomy or Molteno valve filtering is increasingly done.

EVALUATION OF THE INTRAOCULAR LENS

In the pseudophakic patient about to have keratoplasty, usually for bullous keratopathy, special attention must be paid to the intraocular lens itself and to its relationships with surrounding structures. Several features must be observed. Was the cataract extraction intracapsular or extracapsular; is the capsule intact; is it clear? An intact capsule, even if not clear, is best preserved, and laser capsulotomy should be performed later. The iris must be examined for sutures to an intraocular lens, areas of erosion or dialysis, iridectomies, and peripheral anterior synechiae. Peripheral anterior synechiae are more likely to be present in complicated cases with anterior chamber lenses and should be inspected by gonioscopy if the view is adequate.[26] Their presence is of relevance to the prognosis for glaucoma, technical considerations for removal of anterior chamber lenses, and insertion of secondary lenses.

The type of IOL present is critically important. The evolving approach to the original IOL in eyes with pseudophakic bullous keratopathy has been influenced by the poor long-term results of keratoplasty in eyes with iris-supported and closed-loop anterior chamber IOLs. Despite rare dissent, clinical data support removal of all lenses other than posterior chamber lenses, except for stable, well-positioned semiflexible, one-piece anterior chamber lenses.[35] The closed-loop lenses, including the Azar 91Z, ORC Stableflex, Leiske Style 10, and the Hessburg lens, are particu-

larly likely to cause continued inflammation and endothelial cell loss. There is evidence, however, that the Kelman "Multiflex" type of lens may be safely retained, or used as a secondary lens.[22]

Although IOL removal, without replacement, was formerly considered a reasonable approach, it often led to a technically successful graft but an unused eye. Contact lens use is often unsatisfactory in the elderly aphakic population, though improved lenses are tolerated well by the grafted cornea. Usually, however, a replacement or secondary IOL is inserted at the time of grafting for pseudophakic or aphakic keratoplasty. There are several reports of large series of patients with clear grafts and good vision after exchange or secondary insertion of sutured posterior chamber IOLs or Multiflex-style anterior chamber IOLs.[37] Sutured lenses may be attached to the iris or the sclera.[32,33] There are currently no data available to convincingly show better results with any of these methods than with the others. When secondary or exchange lenses are used, the IOL power must be calculated based on axial length and an estimate of the postoperative corneal power and anterior chamber depth. The best approach to estimating keratometry is to use the average postoperative keratometry of previous cases. This value is influenced by graft size, donor-host disparity, suturing techniques, and surgeon; it is used in the standard theoretical or empirical formulas. Because the grafted cornea is often steeper than the original cornea, especially if an oversized donor is used, eyes with retained IOLs may end up more myopic than is desirable.[18]

CONCLUSIONS

The evaluation and preparation of the aphakic or pseudophakic patient for keratoplasty includes all the considerations given to phakic eyes and consideration of the effects of prior surgery. We are concerned about posterior-segment complications that affect prognosis and anterior-segment alterations that affect the surgical approach. Usually the most critical special consideration in these eyes is the plan for management of the original IOL and its retention or replacement. The patient must be involved in the planning process to allow an anatomic and functional outcome that best serves the patient's and surgeon's goals.

REFERENCES

1. Apple DJ, Mamalis N, Loftfield K, et al: Complications of intraocular lenses: a historical and histopathological review, *Surv Ophthalmol* 29:1-54, 1984.
2. Bates AK, Cheng H, Hiorns RW: Pseudophakic bullous keratopathy: relationship with endothelial cell density and use of a

predictive cell loss model, *Curr Eye Res* 5:363-366, 1986.

3. Binder PS, Ayazuddin M, Hintze R: Visual prognosis for corneal transplantation based on preoperative visual evoked potential and electroretinogram, *Ophthalmology* 89:661-666, 1982.

4. Brightbill FS, Dudley SS: Aphakic bullous keratopathy: preoperative fluorescein angiographic screening for macular edema, *Contact Intraocular Lens Med J* 7:144-149, 1981.

5. Eckardt C: A new temporary keratoprosthesis for pars plana vitrectomy, *Retina* 7:34-37, 1987.

6. Enoch JM, Bedell HE, Kaufman HE: Interferometric visual acuity testing in anterior segment disease, *Arch Ophthalmol* 97:1916-1919, 1979.

7. Faulkner W: Laser interferometric prediction of postoperative visual acuity in patients with cataracts, *Am J Ophthalmol* 95:626-636, 1983.

8. Fish GE, Birch DG, Fuller DG, et al: A comparison of visual function tests in eyes with maculopathy, *Ophthalmology* 93:1177-1182, 1986.

9. Fuller DG, Hutton WL: Presurgical evaluation of eyes with opaque media, New York, 1982, Grune & Stratton.

10. Fuller DG, Knighton RW, Machemer R: Bright-flash electroretinography for the evaluation of eyes with opaque vitreous, *Am J Ophthalmol* 80:214-223, 1975.

11. Gelender H, Vaiser A, Snyder WB, et al: Temporary keratoprosthesis for combined penetrating keratoplasty, pars plana vitrectomy, and repair of retinal detachment, *Ophthalmology* 95:897-901, 1988.

12. Goldmann H: Examination of the fundus of the cataractous eye, *Am J Ophthalmol* 73:309-320, 1972.

13. Goldstein J, Jamara RJ, Hecht SD, et al: Clinical comparison of the SITE IRAS hand-held interferometer and Haag-Streit Lotmar visometer, *J Cataract Refract Surg* 14:208-211, 1988.

14. Graney MJ, Applegate WM, Miller ST, et al: A clinical index for predicting visual acuity after cataract surgery, *Am J Ophthalmol* 105:460-465, 1988.

15. Gstalder RJ, Green DG: Laser interferometry in corneal opacifications, *Arch Ophthalmol* 87:269-274, 1972.

16. Guyton DL: Instruments for measuring retinal visual acuity behind cataract—1982, *Ophthalmology* 89(8S):34-39, 1982.

17. Hanna IT, Sigurdsson H, Baines PS, et al: The role of white light interferometry in predicting visual acuity following posterior capsulotomy, *Eye* 3:468-471, 1989.

18. Heidemann DG, Sugar A, Meyer RF, et al: Oversized donor grafts in penetrating keratoplasty, *Arch Ophthalmol* 103:1807-1811, 1985.

19. Kaback MB, Burde RM, Becker B: Relative afferent pupillary defect in glaucoma, *Am J Ophthalmol* 81:462-468, 1976.

20. Kramer SE: Cystoid macular edema after penetrating keratoplasty, *Ophthalmology* 88:782-787, 1981.

21. Landers MB, Foulks GN, Landers DM, et al: Temporary keratoprosthesis for use during pars plana vitrectomy, *Am J Ophthalmol* 91:615-619, 1981.

22. Lim ES, Apple DJ, Tsai JC, et al: An analysis of flexible anterior chamber lenses with special reference to the normalized rate of lens explanation, *Ophthalmology* 98:243-246, 1991.

23. Mamalis N, Craig MT, Coulter VL, et al: Penetrating keratoplasty 1981-1988: clinical indications and pathologic findings, *J Cataract Refract Surg* 17:163-167, 1991.

24. Mohamadi P, McDonnell JM, Irvine JA, et al: Changing indications for penetrating keratoplasty 1984-1988, *Am J Ophthalmol* 107:550-552, 1989.

25. Price FW, Whitson WE: Natural history of cystoid macular edema in pseudophakic bullous keratopathy, *J Cataract Refract Surg* 16:163-169, 1990.

26. Rowsey JJ, Gaylor JR: Intraocular lens disasters, peripheral anterior synechiae, *Ophthalmology* 87:646-663, 1980.

27. Schanzlin DJ, Pokorny J, Ernest JT, et al: Transscleral electroretinography, *Invest Ophthalmol Vis Sci* 17:58-60, 1978.

28. Sinclair SH, Loebl M, Riva CE: Blue field entoptic test in patients with ocular trauma, *Arch Ophthalmol* 99:464-467, 1981.

29. Smiddy WE, Hamburg TR, Kramer GP, et al: Contact lenses for visual rehabilitation after corneal laceration repair, *Ophthalmology* 96:293-298, 1989.

30. Smiddy WE, Horowitz TH, Stark WJ, et al: Potential acuity meter for predicting postoperative visual acuity in penetrating keratoplasty: a new method using a hard contact lens, *Ophthalmology* 94:12-16, 1987.

31. Smith SG, Lindstrom RL: *Intraocular lenses: complications and their management*, Thorofare, NJ, 1988, Slack Inc.

32. Soong HK, Musch DC, Kowal V, et al: Implantation of posterior chamber intraocular lenses in the absence of lens capsule during penetrating keratoplasty, *Arch Ophthalmol* 107:660-665, 1989.

33. Spigelman AV, Lindstrom RL, Nichols BD, et al: Implantation of a posterior chamber lens without capsular support during penetrating keratoplasty or as a secondary lens implant, *Ophthalmic Surg* 19:396-398, 1988.

34. Steinert RF, Minkowski JS, Boruchoff SA: Pre-keratoplasty potential acuity evaluation, *Ophthalmology* 91:1217-1220, 1984.

35. Sugar A: An analysis of corneal endothelial and graft survival in pseudophakic bullous keratopathy, *Trans Am Ophthalmol Soc* 87:762-801, 1989.

36. Waring GO, Laibson PR: A systematic method of drawing corneal pathologic conditions, *Arch Ophthalmol* 95:1540-1542, 1977.

37. Zaidman GW, Goldman S: A prospective study on the implantation of anterior chamber intraocular lenses during keratoplasty for pseudophakic and aphakic bullous keratopathy, *Ophthalmology* 97:757-762, 1990.

Chapter 10

Preoperative Measurements

Intraocular pressure

MARK J. WEINER

Glaucomatous damage to the optic nerve is one of the leading causes of poor visual results in patients with clear penetrating keratoplasties. The accurate measurement of intraocular pressure in the preoperative and postoperative periods is therefore essential for establishing prognosis and for the attainment of the best visual results. Indentation and applanation tonometers are the two general categories of instruments available for the assessment of intraocular pressure.

SCHIØTZ TONOMETER

The indentation device, which is classically represented by the Schiøtz tonometer, measures the depth of indentation of a plunger of given weight sliding through a curved footplate and correlates this with the pressure in the eye. Pressure readings are generally too low in eyes with high scleral rigidity and too high in those with low scleral rigidity. In addition, the calibration depends on a standard radius of corneal curvature, which may be altered in disease states. For patients with corneal disease, Schiøtz tonometry has proved grossly inaccurate, usually giving an underestimation of the intraocular pressure. Kaufman, Wind, and Waltman[4] compared Schiøtz results to anterior chamber cannulation studies in six patients with irregular, scarred, or edematous corneas and found both great variability and inaccuracy in the Schiøtz values. The inaccuracies were so great that not even a general indication of intraocular pressure could be obtained. Cannulation pressure as high as 50 mm Hg were recorded as normal or nearly normal with the Schiøtz. McMillan and Forster[7] confirmed these results in three cases.

APPLANATION TONOMETRY

In applanation tonometry the force required to flatten the segment of the sphere (in this case the cornea) is correlated to the pressure inside a sphere (the eye). According to the definition of pressure, pressure equals force divided by area:

$$P = \frac{F}{A}$$

Since the cornea has some structural resistance to deformation, a force, N, tends to push the applanating surface away from the eye. Counteracting that force are tears that tend to pull the applanator toward the eye by surface tension (force M). When these factors are taken into account:

$$P = \frac{F + M - N}{A}$$

At an applanating diameter between 3 and 4 mm, M and N are approximately equal.

GOLDMANN TONOMETER

In the Goldmann applanator, the most commonly clinically used device for the measurement of intraocular pressure, a diameter of 3.06 mm was chosen, since at that diameter the grams of force times 10 equal the pressure in millimeters of mercury.[9] Unfortunately, the Goldmann tonometer has also proved to be either unusable or inaccurate in scarred or edematous corneas. Kaufman, Wind, and Waltman[4] found Goldmann readings to be grossly inaccurate and not reproducible because the irregular corneal surface causes pooling of fluorescein dye and irregular optical images of the circles. McMillan and Forster[7] found that in owl monkey eyes the Goldmann tonometer tends to give a low reading in eyes with edematous corneas. Kaufman[3] suggests an easily flattened edematous epithelium as a mechanism for the artifactually low readings. The Perkins tonometer, a handheld device that operates in a fashion similar to the Goldmann, had readings lower than those manometrically determined in both normal and edematous corneas.[7]

MacKAY-MARG TONOMETER

The MacKay-Marg tonometer also measures intraocular pressure by applanation. A 1.5 mm flat plunger is mounted so that it protrudes 5 mm beyond the flat footplate. Movements of the plunger are sensed by a linear transducer and recorded electronically. As the cornea is flattened against the plunger, the plunger displacement rises to a crest, which represents intraocular pressure plus the bending forces of the cornea. As the cornea bends beyond the transducer area onto the surrounding footplate, the plunger is relieved from the corneal bending forces by the footplate, and its recoil produces a notch in the force record, which correlates with the intraocular pressure. Further pressure of this tonometer against the eye falsely elevates the intraocular pressure.[11] The back end of the slope of the reading is quite comparable to the front end in many readings (Fig. 8-1). Because of its smaller area of applanation and its reliance on electronic and not optical measurement techniques, one would theoretically expect the MacKay-Marg tonometer to prove more reliable than the Goldmann in scarred, edematous corneas. This has proved to be the case. Wind and Irvine[15] showed excellent correlation of MacKay-Marg tonometer results to anterior chamber cannulation manometry in rabbits with either severe corneal edema or a status of 24 hours after penetrating keratoplasty. Kaufman, Wind, and Waltman[4] compared MacKay-Marg tonometer results to cannulation studies in six patients with irregular, scarred, or edematous corneas and again found excellent correlation over a wide range of intraocular pressures. Wind and Kaufman[16] then compared MacKay-Marg tonometer results to anterior chamber manometry in two patients immediately after penetrating keratoplasty. They varied the intraocular pressure by injecting balanced saline solution into the graft wound and again found the MacKay-Marg readings to be accurate, reproducible, and comparable to cannulation studies over a wide range of intraocular pressures. McMillan and Forster[7] also found good correlation of MacKay-Marg tonometer values to cannulation in owl monkeys with normal edematous corneas and in four patients at the time of penetrating keratoplasty or trabeculotomy. The principal disadvantages of MacKay-Marg tonometry are that a good reproducible tracing must be obtained with the probe held perpendicular to the globe, and this must be correctly interpreted by an observer skilled in the use of the tonometer. Inaccurate placement of the tonometer and its use tend to

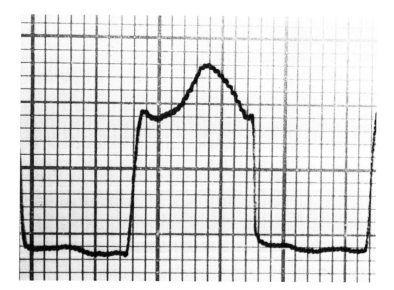

Fig. 10-1. MacKay-Marg tonometer tracing. Notch at front and back of recording indicates true intraocular pressure (IOP). To calculate IOP, count number of small spaces between upper notch and lower baseline, multiplied by 2. Spaces on left side of curve = $10.5 \times 2 = 21$ mm Hg. Spaces on right side of curve = $10 \times 2 = 20$ mm Hg.

result in falsely high readings because the bending force is not relieved from the cornea at the appropriate time.

The Tono-Pen. The Tono-Pen is a miniaturized digital electronic tonometer that operates on the same principle as the MacKay-Marg tonometer. A 1.02 mm diameter central plunger attached to the sensing element is surrounded by a nearly flush 3.22 mm diameter annulus. An onboard microprocessor analyses the wave form resulting from corneal applanation, determines its suitability, and then averages three to six samples. The mean pressure along with the range of the coefficient of variance are shown on a liquid crystal display.[8]

Several studies have compared the Tono-Pen to the Goldmann applanation tonometer in normal corneas.[1,5] In general, there was excellent correlation in the 11 to 20 mm Hg interval, with some degree of underestimation of the pressure in the 21 mm and higher range and overestimation of pressure in the 10 mm Hg and below range. An additional study[13] of 50 eyes that had recently undergone penetrating keratoplasty revealed excellent correlation between the Tono-Pen and the MacKay-Marg tonometer.

PNEUMOTONOMETER

The pneumotonometer was considered a form of applanation tonometry by its originators[6] though this has been disputed by others.[10] It utilizes a hollow plunger that rides in a porous sleeve (the handpiece). Gas flows both through the plunger to its tip and through the wall of the sleeve to form an air bearing, which propels the plunger outward. When the tip is applied to the cornea, escape of gas is impeded and the gas pressure within the handpiece rises. The pressure rise in turn propels the plunger toward the eye with greater force. The pressure in the gas flow system is recorded as proportional to the intraocular pressure.[10] In manometric studies of cadaver eyes, good correlation was found with pneumotonographic results.[6] Moses and Grodzki,[10] however, found the pneumotonograph scale to be compressed, giving an overestimation of intraocular pressure in a physiologic range. They also found further compression of the scale when the instrument was held vertically. Quigley and Langham[12] compared pneumotonographic and Goldmann tonometric results in eyes with normal corneas. They found good correlation with the two instruments, though the pneumotonograph gave slightly higher pressure results. West, Capella, and Kaufman[14] conducted the only large study up to now, utilizing the pneumotonogram in patients with normal and diseased corneas. In the normal group, readings correlated closely with Goldmann applanation values though the results were more variable. In the diseased or grafted corneas, there was good correlation with MacKay-Marg tonometer results but again with more variability. Additionally, although only a few patients with elevated intraocular pressures were recorded, the data showed that the readings could be falsely low with higher pressures.

The relative disadvantages of the pneumotonometer compared to the MacKay-Marg tonometer are its larger probe size, making it difficult to use in patients with smaller diameter grafts, the need to hold the probe in position for a longer period of time, and the maintenance required to replace the gas cylinders. Another device for determining intraocular pressure, the noncontact air puff tonometer, requires a large area of regular surface to obtain a reproducible result and is not believed to be accurate in irregular scarred corneas.

SUMMARY

It is important to measure the intraocular pressure before and after penetrating keratoplasty because of the high incidence of preoperative and postoperative glaucoma.[2] Schiøtz and Goldmann tonometry have proved to be either impossible or grossly inaccurate in the measurement of intraocular pressure, especially in the preoperative state. Particularly striking are the grossly low values obtained by these types of tonometry in eyes with epithelial edema. These techniques should be avoided in those cases despite the temptation to rely on them because of their general ease, availability, and reliability in normal corneas. MacKay-Marg tonometry, as proved by both experimental and human manometric studies, accurately represents the intraocular pressure measured by cannulation. Unfortunately these tonometers are no longer being manufactured, and repair is difficult. The Tono-Pen, an electronic miniaturized version of the MacKay-Marg tonometer, is an excellent substitute that is readily available. The pneumotonometer also seems to adequately reflect the intraocular pressure in eyes with diseased corneas, but its accuracy, especially at higher pressures, is not well documented.

ACKNOWLEDGMENT

I wish to thank Stephen R. Waltman, M.D., for his contributions as coauthor of the first edition of this chapter.

REFERENCES

1. Frankel REP, Hong YS, Shin DH: Comparison of the Tono-Pen to the Goldmann Applanation Tonometer, *Arch Ophthalmol* 106:750-753, 1988.

2. Irvine AR, Kaufman HE: Intraocular pressure following penetrating keratoplasty, *Am J Ophthalmol* 68:835-844, 1969.
3. Kaufman HE: Pressure measurement: Which tonometer? *Invest Ophthalmol* 11:80-85, 1972.
4. Kaufman HE, Wind CA, Waltman SR: Validity of MacKay-Marg electronic applanation tonometer in patients' scarred irregular corneas, *Am J Ophthalmol* 69:1003-1007, 1970.
5. Kao SF et al: Clinical comparison of the Oculab Tono-Pen to the Goldmann applanation tonometer, *Ophthalmology* 94:1541-1544, 1987.
6. Langham ME, McCarthy E: A rapid pneumatic applanation tonometer: comparative findings and evaluation, *Arch Ophthalmol* 79:389-399, 1968.
7. McMillan F, Forster RK: Comparison of MacKay-Marg, Goldmann, and Perkins tonometers in abnormal corneas, *Arch Ophthalmol* 93:420-425, 1975.
8. Minckler DS et al: Clinical evaluation of the Oculab Tono-Pen, *Am J Ophthalmol* 104:168-173, 1987.
9. Moses RA: *Adler's physiology of the eye: clinical application*, St. Louis, 1981, Mosby–Year Book, pp 242-248.
10. Moses RA, Grodzki WJ Jr: The pneumotonograph: a laboratory study, *Arch Ophthalmol* 97:547-552, 1979.
11. Moses RA, Marg E, Oechsli R: Evaluation of the basic validity and clinical usefulness of the MacKay-Marg tonometer, *Invest Ophthalmol* 1:78-85, 1962.
12. Quigley HA, Langham ME: Comparative intraocular pressure measurements with the pneumotonograph and Goldmann tonometer, *Am J Ophthalmol* 80:266-273, 1975.
13. Rootman DS et al: Accuracy and precision of the Tono-Pen in measuring intraocular pressure after keratoplasty and epikeratophakia and in scarred cornea, *Arch Ophthalmol* 106:1600-1700, 1988.
14. West CE, Capella JA, Kaufman HE: Measurement of intraocular pressure with pneumatic applanation tonometer, *Am J Ophthalmol* 74:505-509, 1972.
15. Wind CA, Irvine AR: Electronic applanation tonometry in corneal edema and keratoplasty, *Invest Ophthalmol* 8:620-624, 1969.
16. Wind CA, Kaufman HE: Validity of MacKay-Marg applanation tonometry following penetrating keratoplasty in man, *Am J Ophthalmol* 72:117-118, 1971.

Intraocular lens power

DAVID C. MUSCH
ROGER F. MEYER

The approach most commonly employed in treating patients who require corneal transplantation and cataract removal for visual rehabilitation involves a combined surgical procedure, termed the "triple procedure," in which penetrating keratoplasty (PK), extracapsular cataract extraction (ECCE), and intraocular lens (IOL) implantation are performed together. Although this procedure was initially viewed with caution, because of its complexity and unpredictability, and alternative approaches continue to be evaluated,[3,8,20] it is now accepted as a standard approach, with the support of multiple studies that have documented its success.* This success, however, has been tempered by the occurrence of refractive "surprises" (such as the "9-diopter surprise"[7]), which have resulted from problems with estimation of the appropriate IOL power for individual patients. The goal of this chapter is to describe the unique problems associated with IOL power estimation for the triple procedure, to review methods that are in use to estimate IOL power, and to provide guidance on practical approaches to this estimation for corneal surgeons.

THE PROBLEM

To determine the optimal IOL power for a particular patient, one must make some assumptions concerning the postoperative status of other important components of that patient's refractive system. For selection of an IOL power that optimizes the patient's postoperative refractive status, three factors are important to determine during the preoperative assessment—both axial length and corneal curvature of the eye to be operated upon and the refractive status of the fellow eye. Although the preoperative measurement of axial length provides a good approximation of the axial length after triple procedure surgery and the preoperative refractive state of the fellow eye is likely to remain stable, this is not the case for corneal curvature. The association between preoperative keratometry, when it can be measured, and postoperative keratometry values obtained after stabilization of curvature is at best weak.[17,26] Therefore the major problem with estimating IOL power for triple procedure surgery lies in the attempt to predict a specific patient's postoperative, stable, corneal curvature.

If the predicted corneal curvature is steeper than the actual postoperative result, the patient will require a plus spherical correction to account for the undercorrection of the IOL; conversely, if the prediction is flatter than the actual result, a minus lens will be required. In each case the resulting aniseikonia may be substantial and disruptive to the patient's visual function and life-style. To add to the prediction problem, it has been demonstrated that corneal curvature can change greatly and unpredictably upon suture removal,[14,34] and so knowledge of the expected curvature 1 year after surgery, when most patients have some sutures remaining, may be a poor approximation of sutures-out curvature.

SOME PROPOSED SOLUTIONS

Estimation methods for IOL power in triple procedure surgery can be placed within three general categories: clinical judgment, formulas from cataract/IOL surgery, and personalized regression approaches.

---

*References 2, 6, 13, 15-17, 22, 23, 28, 29, 32, 40-43.

Clinical Judgment. One of the first corneal surgeons to perform triple procedures utilized a standard 18.00 diopter (D) IOL for PK combined with intracapsular cataract extraction (ICCE) and an iris-fixated IOL because of the "unpredictability of the final refractive error."[40] This determination was likely based upon the fact that an 18.00 D iris-fixated IOL would produce about the same refractive power as the crystalline lens (which has an average power of 19.70 D[39]) because of the more forward position of the IOL.[25] In a subsequent report,[43] this surgeon varied the IOL power based upon "such factors as lens power prior to the onset of corneal disease whenever possible and refractive status of the fellow eye." It is evident from a review of this surgeon's results that his approach yielded refractive results that are within the range reported by others using different approaches.

Formulas from Cataract/IOL Surgery. Since the routine use of IOLs in cataract surgery preceded that in triple procedure surgery by many years, by the time that triple procedure surgery was introduced, several approaches to IOL power calculation in cataract surgery had been refined by the experience of thousands of cataract cases. Reports have provided results from use of two cataract/IOL formulas for triple procedure surgery, the Binkhorst[9,10] and Sanders-Retzlaff-Kraff (SRK)[36,38] formulas. Both formulas include the corneal curvature and axial length measurements; the Binkhorst equation requires the postoperative anterior chamber depth and the refractive index of the aqueous and vitreous, and the SRK formula requires knowledge of an "A" constant that is specific for the IOL style used. Since both are available on preprogramed or programable, hand-held calculators,[11,37] many corneal surgeons used one or both of these equations as guides to IOL power selection. The IOL power can be calculated for an emmetropic outcome or for matching the refractive status of the fellow eye.

Personalized Regression Approaches. The Binkhorst and SRK equations were developed by pooling of the results from large numbers of cataract surgeries and developing of a mathematical expression of the relationship between predictive preoperative factors and the refractive outcome. Such mathematical expressions take the form of a multiple regression equation, which can also be developed for IOL power prediction in the triple procedure. For example, after determining that axial length was the only preoperative factor that was significantly related to their patients' refractive outcome, Gabel and co-workers[19] prepared a linear regression equation that was then used to estimate the IOL power in subsequent patients. The necessary components for this approach are complete records of all patients' preoperative measurements, complete follow-up study to ascertain the refractive outcome, and access to statistical software or consultation to provide the regression equation that best characterizes the relationship between the preoperative factors and refractive outcome.

RESULTS OF REPORTED SERIES

Reports from series of triple procedures in which these approaches were used provide an indication of the average refractive outcome that can be anticipated. When we use as a criterion of success a spherical equivalent within 2 diopters of emmetropia, a successful refractive outcome has been reported in 26% to 67% of patient series of various sizes.* Using the clinical judgment approach, Taylor and co-workers[43] reported that 61% (25/41) of the eyes undergoing triple procedure (including 16 eyes undergoing PK/ICCE/IOL and 25 eyes undergoing PK/ECCE/IOL) with complete information and adequate follow-up study had a postoperative spherical equivalent within 2 diopters of emmetropia.

Katz and Forster,[26] using the SRK formula, reported that 26% of 53 consecutive triple procedures (51 PK/ECCE/IOL, 3 others) achieved a refractive outcome within 2 diopters of that predicted. Using a modified SRK formula in which the "A" constant was periodically adjusted to reflect outcomes from the author's growing series, Binder[7] most recently reported that 63% of eyes undergoing triple procedure with a posterior chamber IOL resulted in a refractive outcome within 2 diopters of emmetropia. This result was similar to the 57% refractive success reported by Gabel and co-workers,[19] using the Binkhorst formula in 94 consecutive eyes in which PK and ECCE were performed with insertion of either a posterior chamber ($n = 91$) or anterior chamber IOL ($n = 3$). Mattax and McCulley,[31] reporting on refractive results from 16 triple procedure patients who achieved 20/40 or better visual acuity, found that 62.5% were within 2 diopters of the desired refractive outcome. In the subset ($n = 11$) for whom the IOL power was calculated using the SRK formula and a standard postoperative keratometry value (43.00 D), 82% were within 2 diopters of the desired outcome.

Finally, in the two published reports of series in which a regression equation was developed and applied, the success rate was 62% (35/56) in Crawford and co-workers' series[17] and 67% (35/52) in Musch

---

*References 4, 6, 7, 15, 17, 19, 26, 32-33, 43.

and Meyer's report.[33] Although there have been no randomized studies of the different approaches to IOL power estimation, Musch and Meyer[33] evaluated the refractive outcome that would have resulted if the Binkhorst or SRK formulas were used and could not claim a significantly greater success rate produced by their regression approach.

FACTORS THAT CONTRIBUTE TO REFRACTIVE OUTCOME

The goal of triple procedure surgery is to restore effective visual function. Although multiple factors, such as macular degeneration and graft failure, can deny achievement of that goal, it is imperative that the optimal IOL power be selected for patients about to undergo the surgery. The first consideration is the refractive status of the fellow eye. If the fellow eye is visually functional, an attempt to match its refractive state is desirable; thereby, the evident aniseikonic problems created by differing image sizes are avoided. The desired endpoint of triple procedure surgery therefore is a refractive outcome that is similar enough to the functioning fellow eye that aniseikonia is avoided.

In order to achieve that outcome, the corneal surgeon must be aware of the influence that his or her surgical procedure has on the postoperative refractive status. Factors that must be considered are described below:

Axial Length. Axial length is an important refractive factor, and its preoperative measure is necessary for IOL power assessment. All the standard equations and regression approaches utilize this measure in IOL power calculation. Measurement of the fellow, unoperated eye's axial length is also advisable, since the close symmetry between eyes can serve as a reference for unusually long or short axial lengths that may result from an error in measurement.[24]

Postoperative Corneal Curvature. Multiple factors have an effect on post-PK corneal curvature. The amount of disparity between the diameter of the donor button and the tissue bed influences postoperative corneal curvature in a direct manner. If an oversized graft is used, steeper corneal curvature results than same-sized grafting has. In several studies that have addressed this effect,[12,18,21] 0.5 mm oversized grafts were on average three or more diopters steeper than same-sized grafts. As a general rule, Troutman[44] stated that for every 0.1 mm increase in donor button diameter over recipient bed diameter there will be a corresponding increase of 0.67 D in average keratometry. Use of an oversized graft therefore will reduce the IOL power necessary for triple procedure surgery.

Suture technique may have an important influence on post-PK astigmatism, and recent studies have explored the advantages of using combined running and interrupted sutures[5,35] or an adjustable, running suture[30] in reducing astigmatism after PK. Although these techniques may indeed be advantageous, until all sutures are removed, the post-PK corneal curvature cannot be assumed to be "final" or stabilized. Several studies have demonstrated that suture removal influences corneal curvature in an unpredictable manner, even when that removal occurs several years after surgery.[14,34] The ability to accurately predict sutures-out corneal curvature therefore is limited by both the unpredictable curvature change upon suture removal and the sparse information on sutures-out corneal curvature in large patient series.

Of course, knowledge of the "final" or stabilized post-PK corneal curvature would greatly benefit IOL power selection. Binder[7] has advocated use of the average postoperative keratometry value from a well-defined, recent series of surgeon-specific patients, for inclusion in the IOL power calculation. This practice has yielded relatively good reported overall refractive success.[7] The importance of using a standardized triple procedure technique along with an average postoperative keratometry value was stressed by Mattax and McCulley,[31] who found a high rate of refractive success (81.8%) within a small series of 11 patients. However, unexpected steepness, flatness, or astigmatic change has limited the ability to obtain a refractive endpoint within 2 diopters of that desired to a maximum of 60% to 70% in most series, which is far less than the 90% or better success rates reported for cataract surgery.

Other Factors. In some IOL power equations, it is necessary to enter the anterior chamber depth. Anterior chamber depth has been shown to increase when oversized grafts are used,[21] and the increase should relate closely to the amount of disparity between donor and host sizes. Since most surgeons do not vary graft-size disparity among triple procedure cases, this effect would be uniform within all patients of most surgeons. A recent report[1] has identified an association between donor corneal power and post-PK corneal power. Although the study was small and needs to be replicated, the association is intriguing. Several other factors, such as recipient diagnosis, preoperative keratometry in the operated eye, and fellow-eye keratometry, have been evaluated, but there is little to no relationship of these factors with post-PK corneal curvature.

CONCLUSIONS

One should select the optimal IOL power for a patient by considering the refractive status of the patient when his or her graft has healed and all sutures are out. If the fellow eye is not a consideration, for whatever reason, it would be desirable to provide a slightly minus spherical equivalent for the operated eye, so that the patient's near vision is suited to reading and other near-vision tasks. To this end, we routinely select a −1.5 diopter spherical equivalent as a refractive goal for such patients. Of course, if the fellow eye is a factor, its refractive state must be assessed, and the goal of IOL power selection is to match that refractive state as closely as possible.

Studies up to now have not provided evidence that allows us to advise use of one of the above-mentioned IOL power selection methods as superior to the others. What is evident, and advised by others as well,[7,27] is the need to have a good grasp of your specific surgical procedure and its effect on your patients' corneal curvature. In order to have this knowledge, consistent technique is important,[31] as well as complete records on the preoperative and postoperative refractive parameters outlined above. A new corneal surgeon who intends to perform triple procedure surgery may wish to initially use one of the cataract/IOL power formulas and then modify this based upon the results obtained. Although few surgeons in private practice have access to statistical consultation on personalized regression approaches, all have the ability to collect accurate measures of the effect of their surgical technique on their patients' refractive condition. The important step that then should be taken but often is neglected is to gain an overview of that information that will allow for a beneficial modification of the IOL power selection method and thereby decrease the refractive variability found in patients who have undergone triple procedure surgery.

REFERENCES

1. Abdel-Hakim ASE, Khalil A: Intraocular lens power calculations in the triple procedure, *Br J Ophthalmol* 73:709-713, 1989.
2. Aquavella JV, Shaw EL, Rao GN: Intraocular lens implantation combined with penetrating keratoplasty, *Ophthalmic Surg* 8:113-116, 1977.
3. Binder PS: Secondary intraocular lens implantation during or after corneal transplantation, *Am J Ophthalmol* 99:515-520, 1985.
4. Binder PS: Intraocular lens powers used in the triple procedure: effect on visual acuity and refractive error, *Ophthalmology* 92:1561-1566, 1985.
5. Binder PS: Selective suture removal can reduce postkeratoplasty astigmatism, *Ophthalmology* 92:1412-1416, 1985.
6. Binder PS: The triple procedure: refractive results, 1985 update, *Ophthalmology* 93:1482-1488, 1986.
7. Binder PS: Refractive errors encountered with the triple procedure. In *Cornea, Refractive Surgery and Contact Lens,* Transactions of the New Orleans Academy of Ophthalmology, New York, 1987, Raven Press, pp 111-120.
8. Binder PS: Intraocular lens implantation after penetrating keratoplasty, *Refract Corneal Surg* 5:224-230, 1989.
9. Binkhorst CD, Loones LH: Intraocular lens power, *Trans Am Acad Ophthalmol Otolaryngol* 81:70-74, 1976.
10. Binkhorst RD: The optical design of intraocular lens implants, *Ophthalmic Surg* 6:17-31, 1975.
11. Binkhorst RD: *Intraocular lens power calculation manual: a guide to the author's TI-8/51 IOL power module,* ed 2, New York, 1981, RD Binkhorst.
12. Bourne WM, Davison JA, O'Fallon WM: The effects of oversize donor buttons on postoperative intraocular pressure and corneal curvature in aphakic penetrating keratoplasty, *Ophthalmology* 89:242-246, 1982.
13. Bruner WE, Stark WJ, Maumenee AE: Combined keratoplasty, cataract extraction, and intraocular lens implantation: experience at the Wilmer Institute, *Ophthalmic Surg* 12:657-660, 1981.
14. Burk LL, Waring GO III, Radjee B, Stulting RD: The effect of selective suture removal on astigmatism following penetrating keratoplasty, *Ophthalmic Surg* 19:849-854, 1988.
15. Busin M, Arffa RC, McDonald MB, Kaufman HE: Combined penetrating keratoplasty, extracapsular cataract extraction, and posterior chamber intraocular lens implantation, *Ophthalmic Surg* 18:272-275, 1987.
16. Charlton KH, Binder PS, Perl T: Visual prognosis in pseudophakic corneal transplants, *Ophthalmic Surg* 12:411-419, 1981.
17. Crawford GJ, Stulting RD, Waring GO III, et al: The triple procedure: analysis of outcome, refraction, and intraocular lens calculation, *Ophthalmology* 93:817-824, 1986.
18. Duran JA, Malvar A, Diez E: Corneal dioptric power after penetrating keratoplasty, *Br J Ophthalmol* 73:657-660, 1989.
19. Gabel MG, Meyer RF, Musch DC: Intraocular lens power. In Brightbill FS, editor: *Corneal surgery. theory, technique, and tissue,* St. Louis, 1986, Mosby–Year Book.
20. Geggel HS: Intraocular lens implantation after penetrating keratoplasty: improved unaided visual acuity, astigmatism, and safety in patients with combined corneal disease and cataract, *Ophthalmology* 97:1460-1467, 1990.
21. Heidemann DG, Sugar A, Meyer RF, Musch DC: Oversized donor grafts in penetrating keratoplasty: a randomized trial, *Arch Ophthalmol* 103:1807-1811, 1985.
22. Hunkeler JD, Hyde LL: The triple procedure: combined penetrating keratoplasty, extracapsular cataract extraction and intraocular lens implantation: an expanded experience, *Am Intra-Ocular Implant Soc J* 9:20-24, 1983.
23. Hunkeler JD, Hyde LL: The triple procedure: combined penetrating keratoplasty, cataract extraction and lens implantation, *Am Intra-Ocular Implant Soc J* 5:222-224, 1979.
24. Insler MS: Liability for intraocular lens calculations, *Am J Ophthalmol* 110:578-579, 1990.
25. Jaffe NS, Jaffe MS, Jaffe GF: *Cataract surgery and its complications,* ed 5, St. Louis, 1990, Mosby–Year Book, p 146.
26. Katz HR, Forster RK: Intraocular lens calculation in combined penetrating keratoplasty, cataract extraction and intraocular lens implantation, *Ophthalmology* 92:1203-1207, 1985.
27. Kaufman HE: Corneal transplant optics, *Refract Corneal Surg* 5:213-215, 1989.
28. Lee JR, Dohlman CH: Intraocular lens implantation in combination with keratoplasty, *Ann Ophthalmol* 9:513-518, 1977.

29. Lindstrom RL, Harris WS, Doughman DJ: Combined penetrating keratoplasty, extracapsular cataract extraction, and posterior chamber lens implantation, *Am Intra-Ocular Implant Soc J* 7:130-132, 1981.

30. McNeill JI, Wessels IF: Adjustment of single continuous suture to control astigmatism after penetrating keratoplasty, *Refract Corneal Surg* 5:216-223, 1989.

31. Mattax JB, McCulley JP: The effect of standardized keratoplasty technique on IOL power calculation for the triple procedure, *Acta Ophthalmol* 67(suppl 192):24-29, 1989.

32. Meyer RF, Musch DC: Assessment of success and complications of triple procedure surgery, *Am J Ophthalmol* 104:233-240, 1987.

33. Musch DC, Meyer RF: Prospective evaluation of a regression-determined formula for use in triple procedure surgery, *Ophthalmology* 95:79-85, 1988.

34. Musch DC, Meyer RF, Sugar A: The effect of removing running sutures on astigmatism after penetrating keratoplasty, *Arch Ophthalmol* 106:488-492, 1988.

35. Musch DC, Meyer RF, Sugar A, Soong HK: Corneal astigmatism after penetrating keratoplasty: the role of suture technique, *Ophthalmology* 96:698-703, 1989.

36. Retzlaff J: Posterior chamber implant power calculation: regression formulas, *Am Intra-Ocular Implant Soc J* 6:268-270, 1980.

37. Retzlaff JA, Sanders DR, Kraff M: *Lens implant power calculation: a manual for ophthalmologists and biometrists*, ed 3, Thorofare, NJ, 1990, Slack, Inc.

38. Sanders DR, Kraff MC: Improvement of intraocular lens power calculation using empirical data, *Am Intra-Ocular Implant Soc J* 6:263-267, 1980.

39. Sorsby A, Leary GA, Richards MJ: Correlation ametropia and component ametropia, *Vision Res* 2:309-313, 1962.

40. Taylor DM: Keratoplasty and intraocular lenses, *Ophthalmic Surg* 7:31-42, 1976.

41. Taylor DM, Khaliq A: Keratoplasty and intraocular lenses: follow-up study, *Ophthalmic Surg* 8:49-57, 1977.

42. Taylor DM, Khaliq A, Maxwell R: Keratoplasty and intraocular lenses: current status, *Ophthalmology* 86:242-254, 1979.

43. Taylor DM, Stern AL, McDonald P: The triple procedure: 2 to 10 year follow-up, *Trans Am Ophthalmol Soc* 84:221-245, 1986.

44. Troutman RC: *Microsurgery of the anterior segment of the eye: the cornea, optics and surgery*, St. Louis, 1977, Mosby–Year Book, vol 2, p 107.

Chapter 11

Phakic Keratoplasty

Technique

JOEL SUGAR

The major difference between phakic keratoplasty and keratoplasty combined with lens removal or keratoplasty in the aphakic eye is the need for protection of the lens of the eye and, because of the shallower anterior chamber that is present, the need for protection of the graft endothelium from contact with intraocular structures.

ANESTHESIA WITH AKINESIA, AND HYPOTONY

In phakic patients where no lens procedure is intended it has been our standard approach to use miotics, usually 2% pilocarpine every 10 minutes for three doses starting 1 hour preoperatively. This dosage serves to sufficiently constrict the pupil so that the risk of injury to the anterior lens capsule is minimized. Once in the operating room, we prefer to use local anesthesia because of its greater convenience and because of the rapid postoperative patient mobilization that this allows. There is no evidence from a corneal standpoint that either approach, local or general anesthesia, is preferable. Adequate anesthesia and akinesia of both the eyelids and the globe are essential. An uncomfortable patient who is moving during the procedure or a patient whose eyelids squeeze or whose globe moves induces a greater risk of chamber shallowing and inexact suture placement. When local anesthetic is used, it is important to look for periocular hemorrhage. Retrobulbar hemorrhage or a pronounced preseptal hemorrhage causing increased pressure on the globe compromises the safety of the procedure. Preoperative hypotony can be obtained through digital massage or the use of a mechanical balloon pressure maintainer preoperatively. This lack of positive pressure appears to play a significant role in reducing endothelial and lens complications intraoperatively.[1]

FIELD PREPARATION AND DRAPING

The operative field should be prepared and draped appropriately with the goal of providing a sterile field that is protected from surrounding nonsterile areas. Draping should be carried out also to provide adequate access for monitoring of the patient and adequate ventilation for the patient. It is standard to have a cardiac monitor, a pulse oximeter, and an intravenous line in place to aid in this. The drape should be sufficiently loosely applied so that contact with the drapes by the surgeon and surgical assistants neither pulls on the eye nor transmits pressure to the orbit, increasing intraocular pressure.

EXPOSURE AND GLOBE FIXATION AND SUPPORT

Adequate exposure of the anterior segment of the eye and adequate fixation and support of the globe are exceedingly important and need to be established before one proceeds with keratoplasty. In unusual circumstances this may require lysis of symblepharons and excision of fibrotic scar to provide such exposure. Although a closed-bladed speculum and double adult or pediatric fixation ring (Fig. 11-1) may be used in phakic keratoplasty, I prefer to use a combined supporting ring and speculum, the McNeill-Goldman blepharostat,[10] to provide both globe support and exposure. This is fixated to the superficial sclera with four 5-0 Dacron sutures. Adequate studies have yet to be carried out to demonstrate the most appropriate suturing technique, many sur-

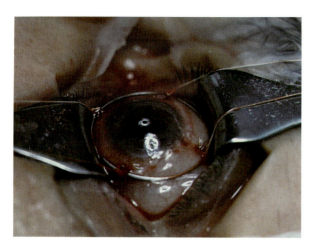

Fig. 11-1. Close-bladed lid speculum and double fixation ring held in place with four 5-0 Dacron sutures.

geons use more than four sutures, and many place sutures both on the anterior and posterior rings of the device. The effect of such sutures is uncertain, but sutures that are too long or too tight may certainly distort the globe, presumably leading to distortions in wound shape and ultimate postoperative astigmatism.[12] The presence of a supporting ring, however, appears to allow easier maintenance of the anterior chamber during both phakic and aphakic keratoplasties.

DONOR PREPARATION

A number of questions arise in choosing a technique of donor preparation. Brightbill and Polack[5] have demonstrated that punching the donor material from the endothelial side against a firm surface leads to less endothelial damage and cleaner cuts than corneal preparation from the epithelial surface. Various cutting blocks have been described[4,18] for this purpose, and they are discussed in Chapter 14. Various punches have been developed for holding the trephine blade, and a hand-held disposable trephine may also be used for cutting the donor (Fig. 11-2). Greater controversy has existed concerning the size of the donor material to be cut relative to the size of the recipient bed prepared. Troutman[20] and Olson[11] have demonstrated that a larger trephine is necessary to prepare tissue from the posterior surface than is needed to prepare the recipient bed. In aphakic eyes, a 0.5 mm larger donor led to less hyperopia in two out of three studies.[3,14,15] In a study comparing a relatively small number of phakic eyes, Perl, Charlton, and Binder[15] showed more myopia in eyes using oversized donor material than in same-sized donor material, but this difference was

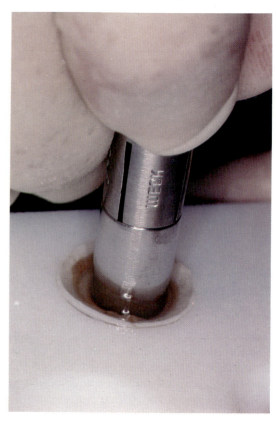

Fig. 11-2. Donor button is punched from endothelial side. Punch type of trephine holders appear to provide more reliably straight-edge cuts than hand-held trephine shown above.

not statistically significant. Based on this it has been our preference to use 0.25 mm larger trephines in preparing donor material in phakic eyes rather than 0.5 mm larger donor material in the hope of reducing myopia in these usually myopic persons. Others have used donor material of the same size as or even smaller than that of recipient material to reduce myopia in keratoconus patients.[8,23] The effect of varying donor size on glaucoma does not appear to be an important issue in phakic keratoplasty. An additional issue in preparing donor material for keratoplasty is the question of retaining epithelium on the donor tissue. Tuberville et al.[21] have suggested that removing donor epithelium reduces the frequency of immune graft reactions, but others have failed to confirm this.[17] I continue to maintain donor epithelium because of the greater ease of postoperative patient management.

PREPARATION OF RECIPIENT BED

The recipient bed is prepared with a trephine that is large enough to surround the diseased tissue and escape the pupillary axis while not being so large as to

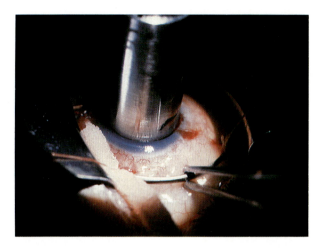

Fig. 11-3. Recipient bed is trephined using a new disposable trephine blade.

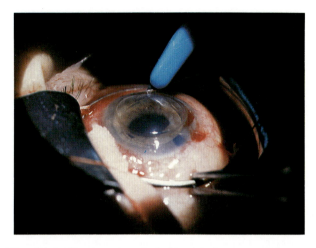

Fig. 11-4. Fixation ring is held with forceps while controlled anterior chamber entry is made with a sharp blade.

encroach upon the limbus. In eyes with keratoconus we attempt to surround the biomicroscopically abnormal cornea with the trephine. Numerous trephines have been developed—both manual and automated—that have varying degrees of complexity.[13] We prefer an open-bladed, disposable trephine for cutting the recipient bed. The advantages to this include the ability to directly sight down the barrel of the trephine to aid in accurate positioning and not having a central guard, which may distort tissue shape during trephination.[9] A forceps is used to grasp the fixation ring and the trephine blade is held in the opposite hand and first pressed onto the cornea and then gently rotated (Fig. 11-3). Experience allows one to reasonably estimate the depth of the cut being made. Automated trephines and suction trephines can be used as well. Interestingly, uniformity of cuts varies with the trephine type and the ideal trephine that provides straight cuts without tissue distortion has yet to be found though van Rij and Waring[22] found a nondisposable suction trephine and a free disposable blade the most uniform. Non-round cuts have been suggested in the past on astigmatic corneas,[20] but the ultimate utility of this remains to be determined.

CHAMBER ENTRY

One may enter the anterior chamber using the trephine while cutting the recipient bed. This is safe to do if the surgeon is aware of the need to immediately release pressure when the chamber is entered. This usually leads to a very perpendicular cut and allows easy removal of the host cornea. Many surgeons prefer the more controlled entry that is allowed when one trephines approximately three

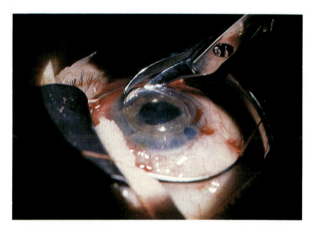

Fig. 11-5. Right-sided scissors cut through trephine groove avoiding iris touch.

fourths of the way into the recipient bed and then uses a sharp disposable blade to enter the anterior chamber (Fig. 11-4). This allows the surgeon to leave a posterior lip of Descemet's membrane if he so desires by sloping his scissors' cut.

HOST CUTTING AND REMOVAL

One then removes the host button by cutting with a curved, fine corneal scissors (Fig. 11-5). The recipient cornea is grasped with a fine forceps during this maneuver and the scissors are held perpendicularly or sloped to allow a posterior bevel of the tissue (Fig. 11-6). This creates a slightly smaller posterior than anterior opening in the recipient bed, which may allow for easier wound apposition. The disadvantage of this technique is that an uneven posterior lip may lead to tilting of the graft and resultant astigmatism.

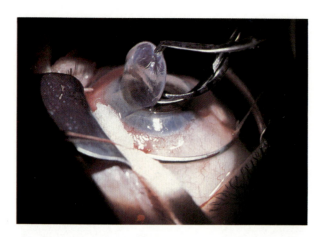

Fig. 11-6. Cornea is grasped with a forceps as it is being cut.

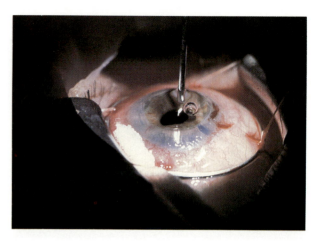

Fig. 11-7. Sodium hyaluronate is placed on lens capsule and iris.

When a posterior tag of stroma and Descemet's membrane is left in just one area, this area may be the site of graft displacement at the time of suture removal and subsequent induced astigmatism. For this reason I tend to remove tags perpendicularly when they are present. Pulling too strongly on a tag while cutting it out may lead to actual undercutting of the recipient bed, which may also lead to astigmatism.

IRIS MANAGEMENT

As mentioned earlier I prefer to constrict the pupil in phakic keratoplasty to protect the lens. During surgery our clinic does not routinely perform iridectomies because this has not appeared to be necessary. In patients who have a history of inflammation it may be necessary to lyse posterior synechiae by gentle sweeping with hyaluronate or a cyclodialysis spatula through the pupil. In such patients, as well as patients who are undergoing keratoplasty for herpes simplex keratitis or other disorders that may be associated with future anterior segment inflammation, I do perform a peripheral iridotomy. Extensive anterior synechiae may be lysed with a cyclodialysis spatula, but broadly adherent synechiae are often better managed when they are transected with a sharp scissors. Highly vascularized peripheral synechiae that do not extend to the region of the graft are often best left alone.

GRAFT PLACEMENT AND CHAMBER MAINTENANCE

The next step is to place the donor cornea onto the recipient bed for suturing in place. It has become my standard procedure to place a viscoelastic

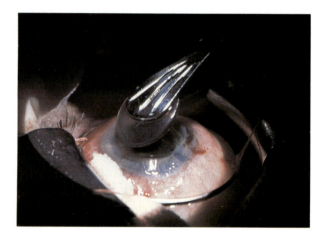

Fig. 11-8. Donor cornea is placed over recipient bed.

substance over the anterior lens capsule and the anterior iris surface first and then to place the donor cornea over this (Figs. 11-7 and 11-8). The combination of the preoperative massage, scleral fixation ring, and viscoelastic material appears to prevent forward movement of the iris-lens diaphragm and trauma to the donor corneal endothelium.[1] Saline solutions or air can be used for anterior chamber maintenance as well, but they are not so effective during the initial graft placement. Rotation of the graft for best alignment has been suggested in the past but has not been demonstrated to be effective (R.C. Troutman, personal communication, June 1985). During subsequent portions of the procedure much of the viscoelastic material may be lost from the chamber, but the chamber still is maintained. I remove this material after the first seven interrupted sutures have been placed because of pronounced

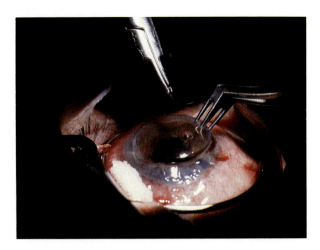

Fig. 11-9. Placement of initial interrupted fixation suture at 12 o'clock position using Polack double forceps.

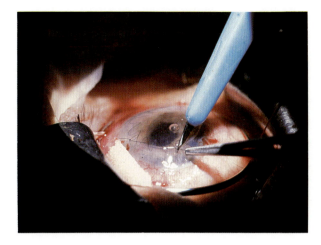

Fig. 11-10. Trimming suture with sharp blade and tying forceps.

pressure elevations, which we have demonstrated with retention of viscoelastic materials in keratoplasty.[6]

SUTURING

Suturing is an area of perhaps the greatest intersurgeon variation. Suturing techniques range from the use of multiple interrupted sutures to double running sutures and to combinations of running and interrupted sutures. With all techniques it is first necessary to place four initial interrupted sutures so as to achieve fixation. The first suture is placed at 12 o'clock (Fig. 11-9) followed by a suture at 6 o'clock. In placing the 6 o'clock suture it is important to attempt to align the donor tissue so that there is equal distribution to both sides of the suture. Additional sutures are then placed at 3 and 9 o'clock. Subsequent suturing may consist in the placement of 12 additional interrupted sutures, 4 or 8 additional interrupted sutures and a running suture, or a double running suture with removal of the initial interrupted sutures. It is my preference to use 10-0 nylon for all interrupted sutures and 11-0 nylon when interrupted sutures are followed by a continuous suture. When all the interrupted sutures are to be removed before the end of the procedure, the first continuous suture is of 10-0 nylon whereas the second is of 11-0 nylon. It is my intention to place the interrupted sutures as deep as possible without perforating Descemet's membrane. When a continuous suture is used in addition, this is placed more superficially. When a double continuous suture is placed, a 10-0 nylon suture is placed deep whereas the 11-0 is more superficial. We have tended to avoid through and through suturing, as described by

Troutman, because of the potential for endothelial damage.[19]

Suture tension also is an important issue. With interrupted sutures, tight suturing may provide a more secure wound but leads to more epithelial difficulties postoperatively and greater difficulty in achieving optical correction while the sutures are in. Sutures that are too loose may lead to wound displacement. Our tendency is to tighten interrupted sutures more than continuous sutures. I trim all sutures close to the knots and bury all the knots. The knots may be rotated into the host or the donor tissue. I prefer to leave the knots buried in host tissue so that vascularization, if it occurs to the knots, will be farther from the graft, though the opposite approach may make vascularization less likely. This area requires further study. For further discussion about suture materials, needles, and suturing techniques see Chapter 15.

FINAL CHECKS

Once suturing has been completed, the suture ends are trimmed short with a sharp blade (Fig. 11-10). The knot may be rotated into the stroma or left superficially where it is rapidly covered by epithelium. The more deeply placed knots are often difficult to remove postoperatively. One then checks the wound for its integrity by deepening the chamber with balanced salt solution (Fig. 11-11) and checking the wound margins for fluid leaks using sponges and gentle pressure on the globe (Fig. 11-12). When necessary, additional sutures are placed. If iris is adherent to the wound, it is either swept free with a cyclodialysis spatula placed through the wound 90 degrees from the adherent iris, or forced posteriorly by use of irrigation with sodium hyaluronate. At this

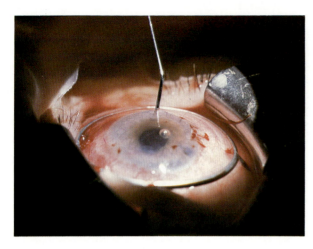

Fig. 11-11. Anterior chamber deepened using no. 27 gage irrigating tip and balanced salt solution.

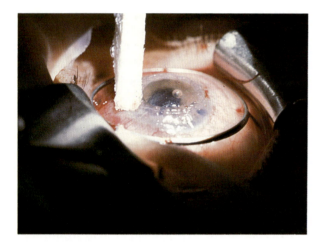

Fig. 11-12. Wound is checked for fluid leakage using gentle pressure with cellulose sponge.

point some surgeons recommend the use of intraoperative keratometry to ascertain anastigmatic positioning of the graft, but I am unaware of convincing evidence that this is of long-term benefit.

MEDICATIONS

At the end of the procedure it is our routine to inject subconjunctival antibiotics. Evidence for the benefits of this and for the optimal antibiotic to be used is as yet lacking.[16] Subconjunctival soluble corticosteroids may be injected as well, but the ultimate benefit of this is also undetermined.

REFERENCES

1. Bourne WM: Reduction of endothelial cell loss during phakic penetrating keratoplasty, *Am J Ophthalmol* 89:787-790, 1980.

2. Bourne WM: Current techniques for improved visual results after penetrating keratoplasty, *Ophthalmic Surg* 12:321-327, 1981.
3. Bourne WM, Davison JA, O'Fallon WM: The effects of oversize donor buttons in postoperative intraocular pressure and corneal curvature in aphakic penetrating keratoplasty, *Ophthalmology* 89:242-246, 1982.
4. Brightbill FS, Calkins B: New forceps and cutting block for donor corneas, *Am J Ophthalmol* 89:744-745, 1980.
5. Brightbill FS, Polack FM, Slappey T: A comparison of two methods for cutting donor corneal buttons, *Am J Ophthalmol* 75:500-505, 1973.
6. Burke S, Sugar J, Farber M: Comparison of the effects of two viscoelastic agents, Healon and Viscoat, on post-operative intraocular pressure after penetrating keratoplasty, *Ophthalmic Surg* 21:821-826, 1990.
7. Davison JA, Bourne WM: Results of penetrating keratoplasty using a double running suture technique *Arch Ophthalmol* 99:1591-1595, 1981.
8. Girard LJ, Egnez I, Esnaola N, et al: Effect of penetrating keratoplasty using grafts of various sizes on keratoconic myopia and astigmatism, *J Cataract Refract Surg* 14:541-547, 1988.
9. Kaufman HE: Astigmatism after keratoplasty—possible cause and prevention, *Am J Ophthalmol* 94:556-557, 1982.
10. McNeill JI, Goldman KN, Kaufman HE: Combined scleral ring and blepharostat, *Am J Ophthalmol* 83:592-593, 1977.
11. Olson RJ: Variation in corneal graft size related to trephine technique, *Arch Ophthalmol* 97:1323-1325, 1979.
12. Olson RJ: The effect of scleral fixation ring placement and trephine tilting on keratoplasty wound size and donor shape, *Ophthalmic Surg* 12:23-26, 1981.
13. Olson RJ: The contact lens corneal cutter: accuracy and reproducibility, *Ophthalmic Surg* 13:210-211, 1982.
14. Olson RJ, Mattingly TP, Waltman SR, Kaufman HE: Refractive variation and donor tissue size in aphakic keratoplasty, *Arch Ophthalmol* 97:1480-1481, 1979.
15. Perl T, Charlton KH, Binder PS: Disparate diameter grafting, astigmatism, intraocular pressure, and visual acuity, *Ophthalmology* 88:774-781, 1981.
16. Starr MB: Prophylactic antibiotics for ophthalmic surgery, *Surv Ophthalmol* 27:353-373, 1983.
17. Stulting RD, Waring GO III, Bridges WZ, Cavanagh HD: Effect of donor epithelium on corneal transplant survival, *Ophthalmology* 95:803-912, 1988.
18. Tanne E: A new donor cutting block for penetrating keratoplasty, *Ophthalmic Surg* 12:371-372, 1981.
19. Troutman RC: *Microsurgery of the anterior segment of the eye*, vol 1, St. Louis, 1974, Mosby–Year Book.
20. Troutman RC: Astigmatic consideration in corneal graft, *Ophthalmic Surg* 10:21-26, 1979.
21. Tuberville AW, Foster CV, Wood TO: The effect of donor cornea epithelium removal on the incidence of allograft rejection reactions, *Ophthalmology* 90:1351-1356, 1983.
22. van Rij G, Waring GO III: Configuration of corneal trephine opening using five different trephines in human donor eyes, *Arch Ophthalmol* 106:1228-1233, 1988.
23. Wilson SE, Bourne WM: Effect of recipient-donor trephine size disparity on refractive error in keratoconus, *Ophthalmology* 96:299-304, 1989.

Recipient diseases

KERATOCONUS

Clinical Manifestations

ROBERT S. FEDER

Definition. Keratoconus is a clinical term used to describe a condition in which the cornea assumes a conical shape because of thinning and protrusion. The process is noninflammatory. Cellular infiltration and vascularization do not occur. It is usually bilateral, and although it involves the central two thirds of the cornea, it is usually centered just below the visual axis. This disease process results in mild to pronounced impairment of the quality of vision.

Prevalence, Distribution, and Course. Reported estimates of the frequency of keratoconus vary widely. Commonly quoted figures range from 4[16] to 600[32] per 100,000. Most estimates fall between 50 and 230 per 100,000.[3,13,18,31] Keratoconus occurs in people of all races. A female preponderance has been observed in most studies; however, the ratio varies from 57% to 66.7%.[2,6,38,64]

Keratoconus usually occurs bilaterally. In a large series[2] only 14.3% had unilateral disease. Although unilateral cases do exist, the frequency might be even lower than reported if diagnostic criteria and examination techniques allowed the detection of very early keratoconus in the fellow eye. A diligent search for early signs, such as inferior corneal steepening or irregular astigmatism, might reveal the presence of very mild disease in the "normal" eye.

The onset of keratoconus occurs at about the age of puberty. The cornea begins to thin and protrude resulting in irregular astigmatism with what is usually a steep curvature. Usually, over a period of 10 to 20 years, the process continues until the progression gradually stops. If a faint broad iron ring was present, it becomes a thinner more discrete ring. The rate of progression is variable. The severity of the disorder at the time progression stops can range from very mild irregular astigmatism to severe thinning, protrusion, and scarring requiring keratoplasty.

Heredity. The etiologic role of heredity in the development of keratoconus has not been clearly established. The significance of heredity must be evaluated independently of other potential systemic or local risk factors for the disease. Studies in which relatives of keratoconus patients were examined are difficult to interpret if the proband was a long-term contact lens wearer or if the family member had a history of atopic disease.

Keratoconus certainly appears to be under genetic control in some instances. For example, a total of five sets of identical twins with conical cornea have been reported in the literature.[17,19,29,67] In a retrospective review Hallerman and Wilson[28] found that 22 of 304 patients had at least one blood relative with keratoconus. They concluded that the frequency of inheritance was at least 7% (22/304). The largest prospective study was performed by Hammerstein.[29] A total of 162 blood relatives of 52 keratoconus patients were examined, and 13 (8%) had the disease.

Rabinowitz and co-workers[51] have used computer-assisted corneal topography to examine family members of keratoconus patients. This sensitive technique uncovered abnormalities in clinically unaffected individuals. Whether these cases would progress to clinically significant disease is unknown.

Patients commonly ask if keratoconus is inherited and if their children will develop the disorder. Based on available information it seems reasonable to tell them the chances that a blood relative would have the disease is less than 1 in 10.

Associated Disease

SYSTEMIC DISEASE. Over the past half century much has been written linking keratoconus to atopic disease. Early papers described a limited number of patients with keratoconus who manifested atopic disease.[12,20,62] Ridley,[54] Gasset,[21] and Copeman[13] found atopic disease to be more common in a keratoconus population. The largest controlled study[15,53] found a positive history of atopic disease in 35% of 182 keratoconus patients as compared to 12% of 100 normal control patients.

The thorough evaluation of the keratoconus patient should include a complete history of atopic disease. Appropriate referrals can be made if significant atopic disease is newly revealed. Allergic lid and conjunctival disease can affect contact lens tolerance adversely. As a result, surgical intervention may be required earlier in the course of the disease to effect visual rehabilitation.

Rados[52] was the first to report an association between Down's syndrome and keratoconus. Most series report the incidence between 5.5% and 8%.[14,46,49] Corneal hydrops occurs with increased frequency in patients with Down's syndrome or other forms of mental deficiency. This may be attributable to habitual ocular massage.

Keratoconus is known to occur in noninflammatory connective tissue disorders.[1,65] Most notable among these are Ehlers-Danlos syndrome and osteogenesis imperfecta. Robertson found the prevalence of hypermobility of the joints to be 50% in 44 consecutive keratoconus patients.[56] Keratoconus has been associated with other disorders of connective tissue such as oculodentodigital syndrome, Rieger's syndrome,[27] anetoderma,[11] and focal dermal hypoplasia.[69] It has also been reported in nail-patella syndrome,[27] Apert's syndrome,[23] craniofacial dysostosis (Crouzon's syndrome),[68] and Marfan's syndrome.[4] Beardsley and Foulks have described an association of keratoconus with mitral valve prolapse.[7] Nucci and Brancato[48] recently reported two sisters with congenital hip dysplasia and keratoconus.

Isolated case reports appear in the literature associating keratoconus with other systemic diseases. These associations can be considered strong only after many confirmatory cases have been reported.

OCULAR DISEASE. Keratoconus can also appear in the presence of isolated ocular pathosis. A classic example is retinitis pigmentosa. Many authors, enumerated by Franceschetti[18] and Duke-Elder,[16] have reported this association.

Infantile tapetoretinal degeneration (Leber's congenital amaurosis) is frequently complicated by keratoconus and cataract. In a large study by Alstrom and Olson[1] more than one third of those patients over 45 years of age had keratoconus. Conical cornea has also been reported with retinopathy of prematurity[34,39] and aniridia.[16,18,37]

Finally, an association between vernal conjunctivitis and keratoconus is widely reported.[8,16,18,24,26] This relationship was statistically proved by Bietti and Ferraboschi.[8] Grayson[26] points out that keratoconus can also be seen in atopic keratoconjunctivitis.

Etiology. Over the years many theories have been postulated regarding the etiology of keratoconus. Nevertheless the cause of this corneal disorder remains an enigma. Results from both laboratory and clinical studies have provided useful clues as to the cause.

Based on histopathologic studies, Teng[63] concluded that keratoconus was primarily a disease of the ectodermal layer of the cornea and that the corneal stroma, of mesodermal origin, was affected secondarily. Sabiston[58] supported Teng's theory based on the histopathologic similarities between keratoconus and atopic disease, which is associated in some cases and also affects tissues of ectodermal origin. Mohan[47] suggested the possibility of an ectodermal syndrome to explain the coexistence of keratoconus with retinitis pigmentosa and macular coloboma (involving neuroectoderm).

At least in some instances keratoconus would appear to be caused by abnormalities of connective tissue.[45] These abnormalities would primarily affect tissues of mesodermal origin, such as the corneal stroma. This theory might explain the association of connective tissue diseases like osteogenesis imperfecta and Ehlers-Danlos syndrome with keratoconus.

Perhaps the structural changes that occur in the keratoconic cornea are under direct genetic control. The disease is certainly inherited in some families, and it is associated with some systemic diseases that are inherited, such as trisomy 21. The results of attempts to correlate certain HLA types with keratoconus[9,22,33,65] have been inconclusive. It is also possible that the genetic influence is more subtle, requiring the effects of environmental stimuli to produce the phenotypic characteristic of keratoconus.

Several reports have implicated eye rubbing as an important etiologic factor in the development of keratoconus.[13,21,35,53,55] The reported prevalence among keratoconus patients ranges from 66%[13] to 73%.[35] Eye rubbing may be the etiologic link between conical cornea and associated systemic and ocular diseases. Itching, ocular irritation, and eye rubbing are common features of vernal catarrh and atopic disease. Vigorous eye rubbing has frequently been observed in patients with Down's syndrome and may explain the high incidence of associated corneal hydrops. Finally, eye rubbing is said to be a habit commonly seen in poorly sighted patients with Leber's tapetoretinal degeneration[35] and retinopathy of prematurity, both of which are associated with keratoconus.

Contact lens wear is another form of corneal microtrauma that seems to be associated with keratoconus. Many authors have described isolated cases of conical cornea occurring unilaterally and bilaterally in the presence of hard contact lens wear.[5,10,30,31,44] Retrospective studies have found a history of contact lens wear before the diagnosis of keratoconus in 17.5%[33] and 26.5% of cases. These retrospective studies and anecdotal reports suggest a circumstantial association between contact lens wear and keratoconus, but they do not prove a cause-and-effect relationship.

Macsai and coauthors[40] in a retrospective review identified a subgroup of keratoconus patients that were not believed to have had the condition before the onset of contact lens wear. This group, when compared with keratoconus patients with no history of contact lens wear before the diagnosis, was older and tended to have central cones with a flatter corneal curvature. Although a cause-and-effect relationship may be impossible to prove, this is the most convincing evidence up to now of the strong association of keratoconus and long-term contact lens wear.

Diagnosis. Typically, an affected patient in the teens or twenties consults an ophthalmologist for symptoms of progressive visual blurring or distortion; however, reduction of visual function can be observed before visual acuity loss can be measured.[42] Photophobia, glare, and ocular irritation may also be

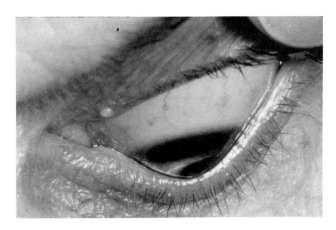

Fig. 11-13. Angulation of lower lid on downgaze caused by corneal protrusion in advanced keratoconus is referred to as Munson's sign.

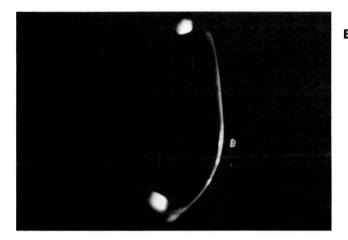

Fig. 11-14. An eccentric area of corneal protrusion and thinning is characteristic of keratoconus.

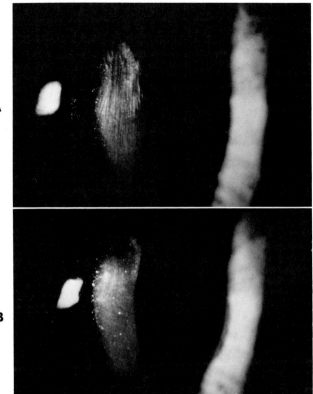

Fig. 11-15. Corneal striae in keratoconus. **A,** Striae occur in the posterior stroma and Descemet's membrane. **B,** Striae disappear when external pressure is applied to the globe.

noted. Examination reveals high, irregular myopic astigmatism. A scissoring reflex is commonly seen on retinoscopy. The irregular corneal astigmatism is confirmed when keratometry is performed and the central mires cannot be superimposed. In advanced keratoconus, the corneal protrusion may cause angulation of the lower lid on downgaze (Fig. 11-13). This has been referred to as "Munson's sign."[3] Usually the diagnosis of the disease is made long before Munson's sign is evident.

Slitlamp examination reveals characteristic findings. An eccentrically located ectatic protrusion of the cornea is noted (Fig. 11-14). The apex is usually inferior to a horizontal line through the pupillary axis. Corneal thinning from one half to one fifth of normal thickness is observed in the apex of the protrusion.[16] Corneal striae occur in the posterior stroma, just anterior to Descemet's membrane (Fig.

11-15, *A*).[3,16,25,59] When the intraocular pressure is transiently raised by application of external pressure to the globe, the folds disappear (Fig. 11-15, *B*).[36,57] The fine striae described are to be distinguished from the superficial linear scars seen at the corneal apex (Figs. 11-16 and 11-17). These are caused by ruptures in Bowman's layer.[3,16] Subtle anterior clear spaces (Fig. 11-17) were identified at the slitlamp in 38% of 69 consecutive keratoconus cases.[60] Light and electron microscopy revealed breaks in Bowman's layer in two corneal buttons of patients with this clinical finding.

In more advanced cases, deeper opacities can be seen at the apex of the cone resulting from ruptures in Descemet's membrane. Acute keratoconus or corneal hydrops results from stromal imbibition of aqueous through these defects (Figs. 11-18, *A* and *B*). The edema may persist for weeks or months, usually diminishing gradually. Eventually, it is replaced by scarring (Fig. 11-18, *C*), which in some cases may result in flattening of the conical contour.

Fleischer's ring is a partial or complete annular

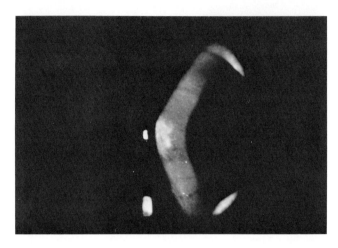

Fig. 11-16. Scars occurring in the corneal apex at Bowman's layer are characteristically seen.

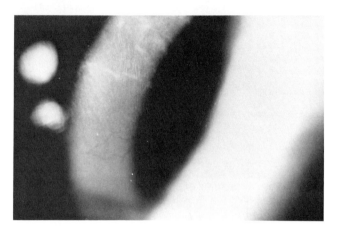

Fig. 11-17. An area of linear scars occurring at Bowman's layer is noted superiorly. Darker gray lines (inferior to scars) correspond to clear zones, which are ruptures in Bowman's layer.

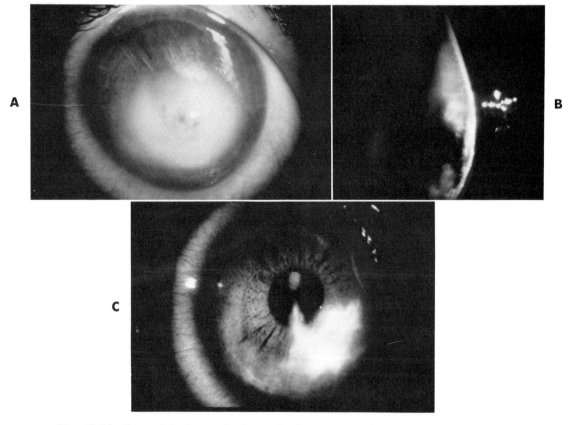

Fig. 11-18. Corneal hydrops. **A,** Corneal edema results from stromal imbibition of aqueous through ruptures in Descemet's membrane. **B,** Slit beam demonstrates the area of corneal thickening. **C,** In most cases the area is eventually replaced by scarring.

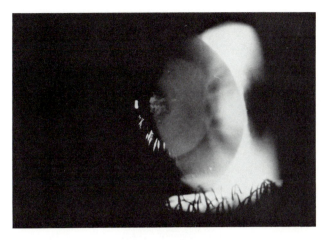

Fig. 11-19. Fleischer ring is a partial or complete, brown, annular, iron line found at base of cone.

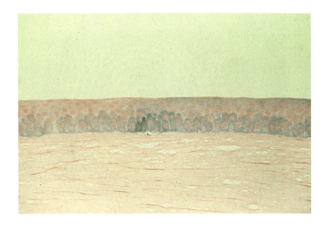

Fig. 11-20. Iron deposited in basal layer of epithelium is colored blue in this Prussian blue stain of a Fleischer ring. (Prussian blue, 288×.)

A

B

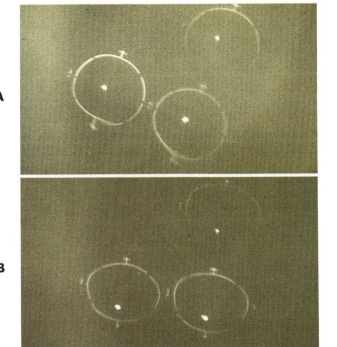

Fig. 11-21. Inferior steepening is characteristic finding in keratoconus. **A,** Central keratometry of a conical cornea. Notice central location of fixation light and mildly irregular mires. **B,** In this case on upgaze the curvature of inferior cornea steepened 8 diopters. Notice that fixation light is now reflected inferiorly. Superior mires splay apart, and mires become increasingly elliptical.

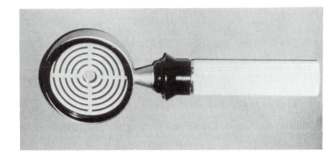

Fig. 11-22. Klein hand-held keratoscope.

ectasia progresses, the ring tends to become more densely pigmented, narrower, and may become complete. Cobalt blue illumination in the widest possible slit beam can be used in early cases to enhance the appearance of a subtle iron ring.

The diagnosis of early keratoconus depends on assessment of the topography of the central and paracentral cornea. The keratometer is an invaluable, readily available tool for measuring central corneal curvature. Inability to superimpose the central keratometric rings is suggestive of irregular corneal astigmatism, a hallmark of keratoconus.

Inferior corneal steepening, an early sign of keratoconus, can be detected earlier, and subtle progression is followed by use of topographic keratometry.[43] Special modifications to the keratometer have been described,[61] but inferior steepening can be detected without a topographic keratometer. By performing central keratometry followed by keratometry with the patient in upgaze (Fig. 11-21), one can identify contour abnormalities in the inferior area of the cornea.

line commonly seen at the base of the cone (Fig. 11-19). When identified it can aid the keratoplasty surgeon as a landmark for the peripheral edge of the cone. The ring is formed from hemosiderin pigment deposited in the basal epithelium (Fig. 11-20). As the

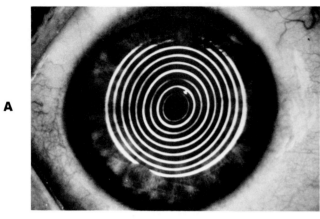

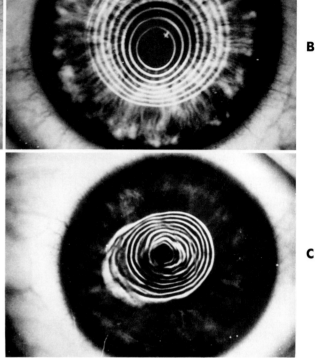

Fig. 11-23. Corneoscope aids in diagnosis of keratoconus. **A,** Steepening of inferior cornea, one of the earliest signs, is indicated by closer ring spacing inferiorly. **B,** With progression, steepening extends peripherally. **C,** With further progression, every quadrant may show involvement. (**A** to **C,** Courtesy J. James Rowsey, MD, Tampa.)

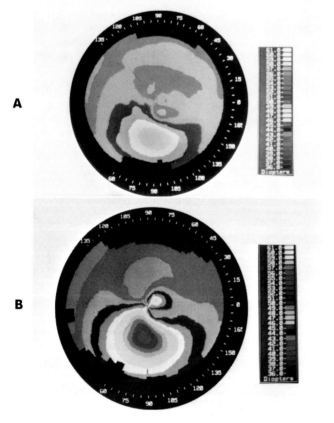

Fig. 11-24. Computer-generated color-contour maps. **A,** Inferior steepening of corneal contour is demonstrated. **B,** Serial topography of same eye revealed progressive steeping of inferior cornea. (From Maguire LJ, Lowry JC: *Am J Ophthalmol* 112:41-45, 1991.)

There is no keratometric value beyond which the diagnosis of keratoconus is definite. There are patients with steep corneas and high astigmatic errors who do not have keratoconus and, on the other hand, patients with keratoconus who have central corneas of normal steepness.

The hand-held keratoscope or Placido disc provides qualitative topographic information (Fig. 11-22). Closer ring spacing inferiorly indicates corneal steepening. Keratoscopes modified to fit in the slitlamp may eliminate error induced from poor alignment or tilt.

The photokeratoscope has undergone many modifications over the years.[50,57] Rowsey and co-workers[57] analyzed keratoconus and its progression in 827 patients using a topographic corneoscope. They concluded that with the corneoscope one could detect the earliest stages of the disease (Fig. 11-23).

The latest technological advance has been the development of computer-assisted corneal mapping systems that analyze data from a keratoscopic image to generate a color-coded contour map (Fig. 11-24). These systems have been used to detect and further characterize the topographic changes found in keratoconus,[41,42,66] particularly at the subclinical stage. The future role for these expensive systems in the early diagnosis and management of keratoconus is being evaluated.

The ophthalmologist should make use of all the available modalities to carefully evaluate the topography of the paracentral as well as the central cornea. A documented increase in corneal curvature over time remains a most sensitive indicator of keratoconus.

Treatment. Advances in contact lens technology, new surgical procedures, such as epikeratoplasty, and improvements in keratoplasty technique and tissue preservation have enhanced the ophthalmologist's ability to treat the patient with keratoconus.

The management of keratoconus must still be tailored to the individual patient. Patient vision needs and comfort tolerance may vary considerably. Good communication between the ophthalmologist and the patient is necessary to determine whether contact lens refit or surgical intervention is the best next step in managing a particular case of keratoconus.

REFERENCES

1. Alström CH, Olson O: Heredo-retinopathia congenitalis: monohybride recessiva autosomalis, *Hereditas Genetiskt Arkiv* 43:1-177, 1957.
2. Amsler M: Quelques données du problème, *Bull Soc Belge Ophtalmol* 129:331-354, 1961.
3. Appelbaum A: Keratoconus, *Arch Ophthalmol* 15:900-921, 1936.
4. Austin MG, Schaefer RF: Marfan's syndrome, with unusual blood vessel manifestations, *Arch Pathol* 64:205-209, 1957.
5. Barry WE, Tredici TJ: Keratoconus in USAF flying personnel, *Aerospace Med* 43:1027-1030, 1972.
6. Barth J: Statistisches über 300 Keratokonusfälle mit 557 befallenen Augen, Zürich, 1948, Druck von Gebrüder Josef und Karl Eberle Einsiedeln.
7. Beardsley TL, Foulks GN: An association of keratoconus and mitral valve prolapse, *Ophthalmology* 89:35-37, 1982.
8. Bietti GB, Ferrabosche C: Sur l'association du kératocone avec le catarrhe printanier et sur son évidence statistique, *Bull Mem Soc Fr Ophtalmol* 71:185-198, 1958.
9. Blagojević M, Szanojević-Paović A, Susaković N, et al: HLA antigens and keratoconus. In Trevor-Roper PD, editor: *VIth Congress of the European Society of Ophthalmology*, vol 40, London, 1981, The Royal Society of Medicine and Academic Press.
10. Brady HR: Keratoconus development in a contact lens wearer, *Contact Lens Med Bull* 5:23, 1972.
11. Brenner S, Nemet P, Legum C: Jadassohn-type anetoderma in association with keratoconus and cataract, *Ophthalmologica* 174:181-184, 1977.
12. Brunsting LA, Reed WB, Bair HL: Occurrence of cataracts and keratoconus with atopic dermatitis, *Arch Dermatol* 72:237-241, 1955.
13. Copeman PW: Eczema and keratoconus, *Br Med J* 2:977-979, 1965.
14. Cullen JF, Butler HG: Mongolism (Down's syndrome) and keratoconus, *Br J Ophthalmol* 47:321-330, 1963.
15. Davies PD, Lobascher D, Menon JA, et al: Immunological studies in keratoconus, *Trans Ophthalmol Soc UK* 96:173-178, 1976.
16. Duke-Elder S, Leigh AG: *System of ophthalmology. Diseases of the outer eye*, vol 8, London, 1965, Henry Kimpton (presently Mosby–Year Book).
17. Etzine S: Conical cornea in identical twins, *S Afr Med J* 28:154-155, 1954.
18. Franceschetti A: Keratoconus. In King JH, McTique JW, editors: *The Cornea World Congress*, Washington, DC, 1965, Butterworth.
19. Franceschetti A, Lisch K, Klein D: Zwei eineiige Zwillingspaare mit konkordantem keratokonus, *Klin Monatsbl Augenheilkd* 133:15-30, 1958.
20. Galin MA, Berger R: Atopy and keratoconus, *Am J Ophthalmol* 45:904-906, 1958.
21. Gasset AR, Hinson WA, Frias JL: Keratoconus and atopic diseases, *Ann Ophthalmol* 10:991-994, 1978.
22. Gasset AR, Richman AV, Frias JL: HLA antigens and keratoconus, *Ann Ophthalmol* 9:767-768, 1977.
23. Geerarts WJ: *Ocular syndromes*, ed 2, Philadelphia, 1969, Lea & Febiger.
24. Goldberg MF, Sugar J: Keratoconus. In Bergsma D, editor: *Birth defects compendium*, ed 2, New York, 1979, Alan R Liss Inc.
25. Grayson M, Keates RH: *Manual of diseases of the cornea*, Boston, 1969, Little, Brown, pp 87-93.
26. *Ibid*, pp 275-280.
27. Greenfield G, Romano A, Stein R, et al: Blue sclerae and keratoconus: key features of a distinct heritable disorder of connective tissue, *Clin Genet* 4:8-16, 1973.
28. Hallermann W, Wilson EJ: Genetische Betrachtungen über den Keratokonus, *Klin Monatsbl Augenheilkd* 170:906-908, 1977.
29. Hammerstein W: Zur Genetik des Keratoconus, *Albrecht von Graefes Arch Klin Exp Ophthalmol* 190:293-308, 1974.
30. Hartstein J: Corneal warping, *Am J Ophthalmol* 60:1103-1104, 1965.
31. Hartstein J: Keratoconus and contact lenses, *JAMA* 208:539, 1969.
32. Hofstetter H: A keratoscopic survey of 13,395 eyes, *Am J Optom Am Acad Optom* 36:3-11, 1959.
33. Karantinos D, Louletzoglou M, Stavropoulou K, et al: Histocompatibility antigens (HLA) in keratoconus. In Trevor-Roper P, editor: *VIth Congress of the European Society of Ophthalmology*, vol 40, London, 1981, The Royal Society of Medicine and Academic Press, pp 933-936.
34. Karel I: Akutní keratokonus jako komplikace retrolentární fibroplasie, *Česk Oftal* 25:347-351, 1969.
35. Karseras AG, Ruben M: Aetiology of keratoconus, *Br J Ophthalmol* 60:522-525, 1976.
36. Katz HH: A hypothesis for the formation of vertical cornmeal striae as observed in the wearing of soft contact lenses and in keratoconus, *Am J Optom Physiol Opt* 53:420-421, 1976.
37. Kenyon KA, Fogle JA, Grayson M: Dysgeneses, dystrophies, and degenerations of the cornea. In Duane TK, Yaeger EA, editors: *Clinical ophthalmology*, vol 4, ed 6, Philadelphia, 1982, Harper & Row, pp 1-55.
38. Laqua H: Hereditäre Erkrankungen beim Keratokonus, *Klin Monatsbl Augenheilkd* 159:609-618, 1971.
39. Lorfel RS, Sugar HS: Keratoconus associated with retrolental fibroplasia, *Ann Ophthalmol* 8:449-450, 1976.
40. Macsai MS, Varley GA, Krachmer JH: Development of keratoconus after contact lens wear: patient characteristics, *Arch Ophthalmol* 108:534-538, 1990.

41. Maguire LJ, Bourne WM: Corneal topography of early keratoconus, *Am J Ophthalmol* 108:107-112, 1989.

42. Maguire LJ, Lowry JC: Identifying progression of subclinical keratoconus by serial topography analysis, *Am J Ophthalmol* 112:41-45, 1991.

43. Maréchal-Courtois C: Topographic study of the corneal at different stages of development of keratoconus, *Bull Soc Belge Ophtalmol* 147:495-505, 1967.

44. Mark HH: Keratoconus appearing after contact lens wear, *Eye Ear Nose Throat Mon* 53:225-226, 1974.

45. Maumenee IH: Hereditary connective tissue diseases involving the eye, *Trans Ophthalmol Soc UK* 94:753-763, 1974.

46. Missiroli A, Vanni V: Sui segni oculari della sindrome di Down, *Boll Ocul* 49:123-139, 1970.

47. Mohan M: Ectodermal syndrome keratoconus and associated ocular abnormalities, *Orient Arch Ophthalmol* 4:229-237, 1966.

48. Nucci P, Brancato R: Keratoconus and congenital hip dysplasia, *Am J Ophthalmol* 111:775-776, 1991.

49. Pierse K, Eustace P: Acute keratoconus in mongols, *Br J Ophthalmol* 55:50-54, 1971.

50. Poster MG, Gelfer DM, Greenwald I, et al: An optical classification of keratoconus: a preliminary report, *Am J Optom Arch Am Acad Optom* 45:216-230, 1968.

51. Rabinowitz YS, Garbus J, McDonnell PJ: Computer-assisted corneal topography in family members of patients with keratoconus, *Arch Ophthalmol* 108:365-371, 1990.

52. Rados A: Conical cornea and mongolism, *Arch Ophthalmol* 40:454-478, 1948.

53. Rahi A, Davies P, Ruben M, et al: Keratoconus and coexisting atopic disease, *Br J Ophthalmol* 61:761-764, 1977.

54. Ridley F: Contact lenses in treatment of keratoconus, *Br J Ophthalmol* 40:295-304, 1956.

55. Ridley F: Eye-rubbing and contact lenses, *Br J Ophthalmol* 45:631, 1961.

56. Robertson I: Keratoconus and the Ehlers-Danlos syndrome: a new aspect of keratoconus, *Med J Aust* 1:571-573, 1975.

57. Rowsey JJ, Reynolds AE, Brown R: Corneal topography: corneascope, *Arch Ophthalmol* 99:1093-1100, 1981.

58. Sabiston DW: The association of keratoconus, dermatitis, and asthma, *Trans Ophthalmol Soc NZ* 18:66-72, 1966.

59. Schmidt M: Nature and genesis of the striae in keratoconus, *Klin Monatsbl Augenheilkd* 101:36-49, 1938.

60. Shapiro MB, Rodrigues MM, Mandel MR, et al: Anterior clear spaces in keratoconus, *Ophthalmology* 93:1310-1319, 1986.

61. Soper JW, Sampson WG, Girard LJ: Corneal topography, keratometry, and contact lenses, *Arch Ophthalmol* 67:91-98, 1962.

62. Spencer WH, Fisher JJ: The association of keratoconus with atopic dermatitis, *Am J Ophthalmol* 47:332-334, 1959.

63. Teng CC: Electron microscope study of the pathology of keratoconus: part I, *Am J Ophthalmol* 55:18-47, 1963.

64. Thomas CI: *The cornea*, Springfield, Ill, 1955, Charles C Thomas, Publisher, pp 233-248.

65. Wachtmeister L, Ingemansson SO, Möller E: Atopy and HLA antigens in patients with keratoconus, *Acta Ophthalmol (Copenh)* 60:113-122, 1982.

66. Wilson SE, Klyce SD: Advances in the analysis of corneal topography, *Surv Ophthalmol* 35:269-277, 1991.

67. Woillez M, Razemon PH, Constantinides G: A propos d'un nouveau cas de kératocone chez des jumeaux univitellins, *Bull Soc Ophtalmol Fr* 76:279-281, 1976.

68. Wolter FR: Bilateral keratoconus in Crouzon's syndrome with unilateral acute hydrops, *J Pediatr Ophthalmol* 14:141-143, 1977.

69. Zala L, Ettlin C, Krebs A: Fokale dermale Hypoplasie mit Keratokonus, Ösophaguspapillomen und Hidrokystomen, *Dermatologica* 150:176-185, 1975.

Results of Surgery

THOMAS O. WOOD

AUDREY W. TUBERVILLE

Corneal grafting for keratoconus has one of the highest success rates of any category of patients undergoing penetrating keratoplasty. Castroviejo reported successful grafting for keratoconus in 1937; since that time numerous reports have confirmed favorable long-term results.[2-4,8,13,20]

Although long-term graft clarity is achieved in 90% to 100% of eyes, postoperative myopia and astigmatism are still major problems.[2,8,13,20,25] Troutman recognized that grafts 7.5 mm or smaller were associated with a significant amount of myopia postoperatively. The myopia was reduced significantly when 8 mm or larger grafts were used. Astigmatism, however, was unaffected by graft size.[26]

Homograft rejection reactions vary in frequency in different series. In one long-term study of 326 grafts for keratoconus, the graft failure rate from endothelial rejection was 2.5%.[20] The incidence of grafts developing a rejection episode has been reported as high as 37.7%, with a graft loss rate of 25% in those eyes developing a rejection phenomenon.[5]

Although most surgeons prefer younger donor tissue for keratoconus patients, recent evidence indicates that donor age does not affect the long-term visual result or graft clarity.[16,20] The long-term endothelial cell count in patients with keratoconus seems to be related to the recipient's age not the donor cornea age.[16]

Surgical alternatives. Visual correction with spectacles or a contact lens is sufficient treatment for many patients with keratoconus. When a patient is unable to wear a contact lens, surgical intervention may be indicated. In addition to penetrating keratoplasty, other surgical procedures such as lamellar keratoplasty, thermokeratoplasty, and epikeratophakia have been advocated for visual rehabilitation.[6,9,10,22,29]

Thermokeratoplasty has been abandoned for the most part in this country because of alternative treatments that appear more satisfactory.[1,12] In Japan thermokeratoplasty results are more acceptable. In a series of 1700 Japanese patients with keratoconus, 800 eyes underwent thermokeratoplasty, averaging a final contact lens visual acuity of 20/30. The goal of this study was to convert patients intolerant to contact lenses to satisfactory contact lens wearers. Only

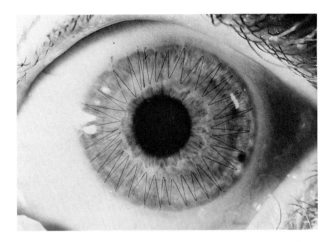

Fig. 11-25. One year after 8 mm penetrating keratoplasty, vision 20/50 with sutures. Final vision 7 years after operation 20/25 − 3.

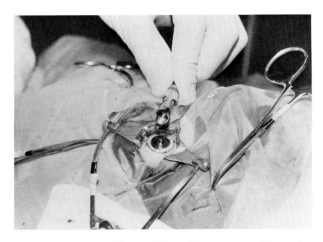

Fig. 11-26. Disposable trephine without a guard is used to prevent flattening of the cone during trephination. This photo shows a reusable trephine with obturator retracted in blade. This prevents flattening of cone during trephination, thereby avoiding a distorted or smaller recipient cut. Notice single Flieringa ring attached to drape with four fixation sutures. Adjustable bladed lid speculum prevents direct pressure on globe.

7% of the eyes undergoing thermokeratoplasty eventually required penetrating keratoplasty. The high success rate in this series was attributed to the spatial location of the cone, which appears to be lower in the Japanese population, and to the use of a cool temperature probe resulting in less tissue destruction at the time of thermokeratoplasty.[11]

Study group and methods. We reviewed 204 corneal transplants (penetrating and lamellar) that we performed in eyes with keratoconus with regard to the effect of graft size on the final refractive error; the incidence of rejection relative to (1) graft size and (2) removal of the donor button epithelium; type of optical correction required after keratoplasty; and the effect of suture removal on visual acuity and final refraction.

SURGICAL TECHNIQUE. All grafts in this series had a single running 10-0 nylon closure (Fig. 11-25). Initially some patients were operated on under general anesthesia, but most were done with local anesthesia. Most of the grafts had a small posterior bevel cut on the recipient cornea to ensure a tight wound closure with superficial suture bites.

Pilocarpine is instilled topically approximately 30 minutes before the local anesthesia. A peribulbar block is given using 2 ml of lidocaine (Xylocaine) 2%, 5 minutes before the bupivacaine injection. The Honan balloon is then placed on the eye for a minimum of 30 minutes, preferably 45 to 60 minutes, before the surgery is begun. This assures a soft eye, in most cases, with the iris well away from the cornea. The small pupil protects the lens. A single Flieringa ring is sutured to the episclera. The ring is usually 16 to 17 mm in diameter. An evenly distributed upward and outward pull is exerted by four sutures at-

tached to the Flieringa ring and clipped to the drape. A lid speculum is used to hold the eyelids away from the eye. The combination of the upward pull of the ring and the retraction of the lids from the globe assures, in most cases, negative pressure when the eye is opened.

The trephine of choice is selected, usually 8.0 mm. A disposable trephine without a guard is used to avoid flattening of the cone during trephination. If the cone is inadvertently flattened during trephination, a smaller cut will be made in the recipient corneal bed (Fig. 11-26). The trephine is centered over the pupil. A trephine cut is made to approximately nine tenths of the depth of the cornea. A round Beaver knife blade (no. 64) is used to make a lamellar dissection in the depth of the trephine mark approximately 1 mm toward the center of the cornea. The donor button is then cut the same size as the recipient. When the recipient button is removed, care is taken to offset the scissors centrally approximately 0.25 mm so that a small posterior lip is made on the recipient cornea. A peripheral iridotomy is cut. The donor button is placed into the recipient bed. A small air bubble is placed in the anterior chamber to protect the macula from the direct light of the microscope. The four cardinal interrupted sutures are placed, with care being taken to center the graft, and then an additional eight interrupted sutures are placed. When the graft is seated and a watertight wound is formed, the anterior segment is irrigated until the eye has a normal tactile tension. A running

10-0 nylon suture with 24 to 30 bites is placed. After proper tension on the running suture has been achieved, all the interrupted sutures are removed. The knot on the running suture is then buried in the corneal stroma. The ring is removed, and a final suture adjustment is made to make certain there is equal distribution of pressure on the sutures for 360 degrees. At the conclusion of surgery the air bubble is aspirated and the anterior segment is again irrigated to ensure that there are no iris adhesions to the wound and that the pressure is normal. Dexamethasone, 2 mg, gentamicin, 10 mg, and vancomycin hydrochloride, 10 mg, are injected subconjunctivally.

Postoperatively the patient receives topical steroids six times daily and antibiotic drops twice daily. The steroid is tapered one drop per week until a dosage of one drop every 2 or 3 days is reached. This regimen is continued for about 1 year postoperatively. The running sutures are left in place unless they become exposed.

Results. Two hundred and four corneal transplants for keratoconus have been examined retrospectively. Twelve eyes received 7.5 mm grafts, 116 eyes had 8.0 mm grafts, 48 eyes had 8.5 mm grafts,

and 18 eyes had lamellar keratoplasty 8.0 mm or larger in size. One eye received a 7.0 mm graft, and nine eyes had disparate-sized donor material (five with a 7.5 mm bed size/8.0 mm donor size and four with 8.0/8.5).

Three transplants have lost clarity, two from endothelial rejection (Fig. 11-27), one of which was associated with an episode of pupillary block glaucoma and iris adherence to the cornea. The third graft that lost transparency was associated with a pupillary supported intraocular lens after a triple procedure. Five of the transplants were combined with a cataract extraction (Table 11-1).

GRAFT SIZE AND REFRACTIVE ERROR. The effect of graft size on final refractive error after suture removal was determined in 108 corneal transplants (Table 11-2). The follow-up time ranged from 0.7 to 10 years. Graft size had no effect on the best corrected visual acuity. Most of the patients with 7.5 mm grafts have high myopic refractive errors.

Progressing from 7.5 to 8.0 mm, we found that 8 mm penetrating corneal transplantation provided significant improvement in the myopic refractive error but did not reduce the astigmatic error significantly. When comparing 8.0 with 8.5 mm transplants, we noted no significant difference in the refraction or visual acuity. Lamellar corneal transplants resulted in the lowest mean refractive error, but this was not significantly different from 8.0 or 8.5 mm penetrating grafts (Fig. 11-28[29] and Table 11-2).[25,29]

SUTURES AND REFRACTIVE ERROR. To determine the effect of sutures on the final refractive error and vision, we compared 83 8.0 mm and 35 8.5 mm grafts with either retained or removed sutures (Table 11-3). There was no significant difference in the final refractive errors in either group of transplants with or without sutures. Recently we have begun reducing astigmatism 4 to 8 weeks postoperatively by adjusting the single

Table 11-1. Graft Sizes

Size (mm)	Number
7.0	1
7.5	12
8.0	116
8.5	48
7.5/8.0	5 with cataract
8.0/8.5	4
Lamellar keratoplasty	18
TOTAL	204

Table 11-2. Effect of Size on Refraction

Size (mm)	Number	Time (years)	Refraction (Average Sphere; Average Minus Cylinder)		Visual Acuity
7.5	11	7	−5.38	−4.61	20/30+
8.0	67	3.8	+0.43*	−3.66	20/25−
8.5	12	2.9	−0.02	−3.17	20/25−
L 8>	18	4.5	−0.50	−2.75	20/40
TOTAL	108 grafts				

*sph p = 0.000009 (8.0)
sph p = 0.004 (8.5)
sph p = 0.002 (L 8>)
The p value allows comparison of sphere (sph) of 8.0 and 8.5 mm and lamellar grafts with that of 7.5 mm grafts.
The cylinder difference in each category was not significant.
L8>, Lamellar grafts 8.0 mm or larger.

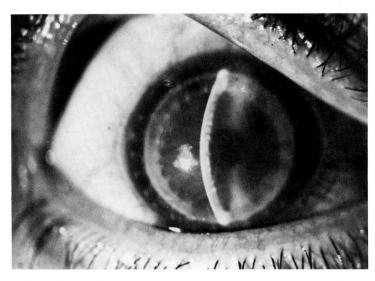

Fig. 11-27. Endothelial rejection 7 months after surgery with generalized stromal thickening treated with topical steroids. Vision 3 years after operation 20/20−2.

Table 11-3. Final Refractive Error in 8.0 and 8.5 mm Grafts With Sutures Retained or Removed

Sutures	Number	Time (years)	Refraction (Average Sphere; Average Minus Cylinder)		Visual Acuity
8.0 mm grafts Sutures in (SEM, 0.58 0.34)	16	1.1	+1.38	−2.83	20/30−
Sutures out (SEM, 0.47 0.33)	67	3.8	+0.43	−3.66	20/25−
8.5 mm grafts Sutures in (SEM, 0.39 0.39)	23	0.98	−0.36	−2.77	20/30−
Sutures out (SEM, 0.88 0.78)	12	2.92	−0.02	−3.17	20/25−

SEM, Standard error of the mean, in diopters (first number, sphere; second number, cylinder).

Table 11-4. Rejection Incidence in 7.5 and 8.0 mm Grafts

Size (mm)	Rejection (%)	Donor epithelium (off-on)	Mean Time to Rejection
7.5	8.3% (1 of 12)	Off	
8.0	23% (25 of 108)	Off	1.7 years
8.0	26% (11 of 42)	Off	
8.0	21% (14 of 66)	On	

running 10-0 nylon suture to flatten the steep axis of the cornea.[15,19,23]

BILATERAL GRAFTS. Nine eyes that underwent bilateral 8.0 mm transplants had final refractions available. We found no significant ($p = 0.36$) anisometropia in these cases.

GRAFT REJECTION AND DONOR SIZE. We examined the incidence of graft rejection in 7.5, 8.0, and 8.5 mm transplants (Table 11-4). Removal of the epithelium had no beneficial effect in preventing graft rejection in these patients. In 8 mm grafts 25 rejections occurred, 23 were endothelial and 2 were superficial stromal. Factors associated with the rejection episodes included loose sutures in 7 eyes, pregnancy in

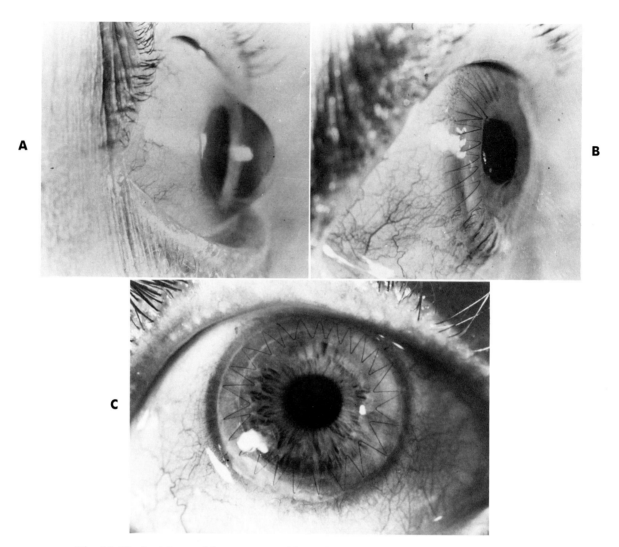

Fig. 11-28. A, Advanced keratoconus with total corneal thinning. **B,** Same eye postoperatively with 10 mm lamellar tectonic graft. **C,** A penetrating graft was eventually required to achieve useful vision.

3, and 1 associated with pupillary block glaucoma and iris adherence to the cornea.

Data were available on 20 of the 8 mm grafts that underwent rejection episodes for determination of postoperative time to rejection. The mean time to rejection episode was 1.7 years with a range of 0.2 to 8.0 years. The rejection episode occurred at a mean of 2.3 years postoperatively in 6 eyes with donor epithelium removed and 1.47 years postoperatively in 11 eyes with the donor epithelium transplanted.

In patients undergoing 8.5 mm grafts, the overall rejection rate was 29% (12 of 41 eyes) (Table 11-5). Endothelial rejection occurred in 11 eyes and stromal rejection in one eye, but none of the grafts lost transparency. Factors associated with rejection occurred in 25% of eyes with 8.5 mm transplants. One had a rejection in association with a loose suture, 2 with pregnancy, and 1 after an influenza shot. Graft size and the presence of donor epithelium had no significant effect on the rejection rate.

VISUAL CORRECTION AFTER KERATOPLASTY. In the 8.0 and 8.5 mm transplants, there were large enough numbers to compare the type of correction required in each size of graft. One hundred three 8.0 mm grafts and 42 8.5 mm grafts were included in this analysis. In the 8.0 mm transplants, 81.5% (84 eyes) accepted spectacle correction, 14.5% (15 eyes) required contact lenses, and 3.9% (4) wore no correc-

Table 11-5. Rejection Incidence in 8.5 mm Grafts

	Rejection (%)	Donor Epithelium (off-on)	Mean Time to Rejection
	30% (10 of 23)	Off	9 months
	25% (2 of 8)	On	1.5 years
TOTAL	29% (12 of 41)	Off and on	0.87 years

tion. In 42 8.5 mm grafts, the type of correction is as follows: 76% (32) accepted a spectacle correction, 9.5% (4) wear contact lenses, and 14.3% (6) require no correction. In the 10 uncorrected eyes the median vision was 20/40 and the range was 20/30 to 20/60 with only 3 eyes seeing 20/50 or less. The difference in patients requiring no correction with 8.5 mm versus 8.0 mm transplants was statistically significant ($p = 0.05$, χ^2).

Discussion. For many years it has been recognized that corneal transplantation for keratoconus has a high success rate. Penetrating keratoplasty improves the measurable visual acuity as well as the quality of vision.[17] Troutman[25,26] pointed out that obtaining a clear graft must be accompanied by a satisfactory refractive error for the patient to obtain useful vision.

The advent of the running 10-0 nylon suture closure has improved the visual prognosis as well as the postoperative spherical refractive error in penetrating keratoplasty for keratoconus.[26] A persistent problem with running 10-0 nylon closure occurs in the occasional patient who has satisfactory visual acuity with the running suture in place but develops a high astigmatic correction when the suture is removed. However, the reverse may also occur with patients having high astigmatic erors with the suture in place but improved refraction when the suture is removed. Suture removal in the 8.0 and 8.5 mm grafts in this series had no significant effect on the mean cylindrical correction.[25]

Most patients who have been grafted for keratoconus can wear a spectacle correction. In many cases the refractive astigmatic correction is much lower than the astigmatic error measured on the keratometer.[25]

Most of the graft recipients received the same-sized donor button. Nine of the eyes had disparate-sized grafts, five associated with cataract extraction. This series was not large enough to determine the effect of disparate-sized donor tissue on the refractive error. Troutman and Gaster found that with 8 mm recipients using same-sized, 0.1 mm and 0.2

mm larger donors for keratoconus had no significant effect on the postoperative refractive error.[25] A significant increase in myopia occurs using 7.5 mm recipients with 7.5 and 8.0 mm donors.[21,26]

In 8.5 mm grafts, using the same-sized donor button as recipient cut, we found that the refractive error stabilized by the sixth postoperative week giving useful vision. The mean refractive error did not significantly change 1.5 years postoperatively with the sutures still in place or by the third postoperative year with the sutures removed. Although graft size in the penetrating keratoplasty group did not significantly affect final visual acuity, there was a significant decrease in the myopic refractive error going from 7.5 to 8.0 mm and larger penetrating keratoplasties.[26] Grafts larger than 8.5 mm (8.7 to 10 mm) seem to reduce astigmatism but increase the possibility of rejection.[24,25] An alternative to large penetrating keratoplasties in eyes with peripheral thinning is to first perform a tectonic lamellar graft then a smaller penetrating graft[24] (Fig. 11-28).

The overall rejection rate in penetrating keratoplasties in this series was approximately 25%; however, only 1.2% of the eyes lost graft clarity as a result of endothelial rejection. The association of exposed sutures, pregnancy, and flu shots as precipitating factors in graft rejection is important to recognize.[28]

Removal of the donor epithelium did not have a significant effect on the graft rejection rate in the 7.5, 8.0, and 8.5 mm grafts. The rejection phenomenon usually resolved with therapy and may be more related to graft size (that is, larger than 8.5 mm) than transplantation of the donor epithelium.[24,25,27] The low incidence of graft loss and the improved spherical refraction warrants the use of the grafts larger than 7.5 mm in obtaining a more functional eye postoperatively.

Two of the patients in this series developed cataracts postoperatively—one in an elderly patient with bilateral cataracts and the other in a young man on prolonged high-dose topical steroids. Cataracts have been reported in almost one third of cases in one series after keratoconus keratoplasty.[7] Although cataracts are recognized as occurring after penetrating keratoplasty for keratoconus, they rarely require removal or interfere with visual acuity.[20] They have a direct relationship with the amount of steroids used after keratoplasty.[7]

Hydrops was seen in several patients in this series (Fig. 11-29), but none required acute surgical intervention.[14] Medical management with cycloplegics and hypertonic saline ointment was usually sufficient to allow healing. Stromal neovascularization was

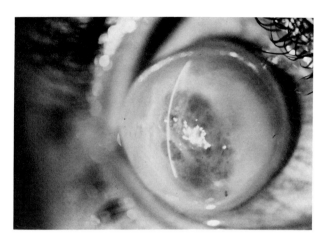

Fig. 11-29. Severe hydrops that resolved over several months. Topical steroids were eventually used to reduce stromal neovascularization. A penetrating keratoplasty was done after complete resolution of the hydrops.

treated with topical steroids to try to minimize vascular ingrowth. Penetrating keratoplasty was necessary in most cases of resolved hydrops because of corneal scarring and decreased vision.

Visual acuity in lamellar transplants is not as predictable as in penetrating grafts. Therefore we reserve lamellar transplants for patients who are not good candidates for penetrating transplants.

Summary. Eight millimeter or larger penetrating keratoplasties for keratoconus have a significantly better postoperative spherical correction than 7.5 mm grafts. Most patients with 8.0 and 8.5 mm grafts were able to wear spectacle correction postoperatively. Rejection episodes occurred in the 8.0 and 8.5 mm group at a rate of 25% and in the 7.5 mm group, 8.3%, yet only 1.2% of the grafts were lost as a consequence of endothelial rejection.

REFERENCES

1. Arentsen JJ, Laibson PR: Thermokeratoplasty for keratoconus, *Am J Ophthalmol* 82:447-449, 1976.
2. Buxton JN, Schuman M, Pecego J: Graft reactions after unilateral and bilateral keratoplasty for keratoconus, *Ophthalmology* 88:771-773, 1981.
3. Castroviejo R: Surgery of the cornea, *Int Abstr Surg* 65:489-505, 1937.
4. Castroviejo, R.: Keratoplasty in treatment of keratoconus, *Arch Ophthalmol* 42:776-800, 1949.
5. Chandler JW, Kaufman HE: Graft reactions after keratoplasty for keratoconus, *Am J Ophthalmol* 77:543-547, 1974.
6. Dietz TR, Durrie DS: Indications and treatment of keratoconus using epikeratophakia, *Ophthalmology* 95(2):236-246, 1988.

7. Donshik PC, Cavanaugh HD, Boruchoff SA, et al: Posterior subcapsular cataracts induced by topical corticosteroids following keratoplasty for keratoconus, *Ann Ophthalmol* 13:29-32, 1981.
8. Ehlers N, Olsen T: Long term results of corneal grafting in keratoconus, *Acta Ophthalmol* 61:918-926, 1983.
9. Frantz JM, McDonald MB, and Kaufman HE: Results of penetrating keratoplasty after epikeratophakia for keratoconus in the nationwide study, *Ophthalmology* 96(8):1151-1159, 1989.
10. Gasset AR, Kaufman HE: Thermokeratoplasty in the treatment of keratoconus, *Am J Ophthalmol* 79:226-232, 1975.
11. Itoi M, Nakaji Y, Nakae T: Keratoconus: the Japanese experience, *CLAO J* 9:254-256, 1983.
12. Keates RH, Dingle J: Thermokeratoplasty for keratoconus, *Ophthalmic Surg* 6:89-92, 1975.
13. Keates RH, Falkenstein S: Keratoplasty in keratoconus, *Am J Ophthalmol* 74:442-444, 1972.
14. Krachmer JH, Feder RD, Belin NW: Keratoconus and related noninflammatory corneal thinning disorders, *Surv Ophthalmol* 28:293-322, 1984.
15. Lin DTC, Wilson SE, Reidy JJ, et al: An adjustable single running suture technique to reduce postkeratoplasty astigmatism: a preliminary report, *Ophthalmology* 97(7):934-938, 1990.
16. Linn JG, Stuart JC, Warnicki JW, et al: Endothelial morphology in long-term keratoconus corneal transplants, *Ophthalmology* 88:761-770, 1981.
17. Mannis MJ, Zadnik K, Johnson CA: The effect of penetrating keratoplasty on contrast sensitivity in keratoconus, *Arch Ophthalmol* 102:1513-1516, 1984.
18. McDonald MB, Kaufman HE, Durrie DS, et al: Epikeratophakia for keratoconus: the nationwide study, *Arch Ophthalmol* 104:1294-1300, 1986.
19. McNeill JI, Wessels IF: Adjustment of single continuous suture to control astigmatism after penetrating keratoplasty, *Refract Corneal Surg* 5:216-223, 1989.
20. Paglen PG, Fine M, Abbott RL, et al: The prognosis for keratoplasty in keratoconus, *Ophthalmology* 89:651-654, 1982.
21. Perry HD, Foulks GN: Oversize donor buttons in corneal transplantation surgery for keratoconus, *Ophthalmic Surg* 18(10):751-752, 1987.
22. Richard JM, Paton D, Gasset AR: A comparison of penetrating keratoplasty and lamellar keratoplasty in the surgical management of keratoconus, *Am J Ophthalmol* 86:807-811, 1978.
23. Roper-Hall MJ: Control of astigmatism after surgery and trauma, *Br J Ophthalmol* 66:556-559, 1982.
24. Speaker MG, Arentsen JJ, Laibson PR: Long-term survival of large diameter penetrating keratoplasties for keratoconus and pellucid marginal degeneration, *Acta Ophthalmol* 67(suppl 192):17-19, 1989.
25. Troutman RC, Gaster RN: Surgical advances and results of keratoconus, *Am J Ophthalmol* 90:131-136, 1980.
26. Troutman RC, Meltzer M: Astigmatism and myopia in keratoconus, *Trans Am Ophthalmol Soc* 70:265-277, 1972.
27. Tuberville AW, Foster CS, Wood TO: The effect of donor cornea epithelium removal on the incidence of allograft rejection reactions, *Ophthalmology* 90:1351-1356, 1983.
28. Tuberville AW, Wood TO: Corneal ulcers in corneal transplants, *Curr Eye Res* 1(8):479-485, 1981.
29. Wood TO: Lamellar transplants in keratoconus, *Am J Ophthalmol* 83:543-545, 1977.

FUCHS' DYSTROPHY

S. ARTHUR BORUCHOFF
ANTHONY P. ADAMIS

Corneal edema in association with corneal guttae characterizes Fuchs' dystrophy. First reported in 1910 by the Viennese ophthalmologist Ernst Fuchs,[9] the condition was described as a bilateral corneal clouding in elderly patients, primarily affecting the central cornea. Six years later, having studied the condition with a slitlamp, Koeppe described focal endothelial changes in patients with Fuchs' dystrophy.[5] Vogt noted these changes and called them "guttae" (Latin: n. droplets; *guttatum*, adj. droplike).[9] Ultrastructural studies performed years later confirmed that the disease was the result of a primary dysfunction of the corneal endothelium.[4]

Corneal guttae are focal excrescences of Descemet's membrane deposited by morphologically and physiologically altered endothelial cells. The significance of the abnormal excrescences is not known; however they are the precursors of full blown Fuchs' dystrophy.

Although guttae are common, only a small percentage of corneas with corneal guttae progress to corneal edema. The incidence of corneal guttae without edema has been studied in several large series. Lorenzetti and co-workers studied 2002 patients and found central corneal guttae in 31% of eyes between 20 and 39 years of age and in 70% of eyes older than 40.[6] The inheritance pattern is autosomal dominant with 100% penetrance. There is a variable expressivity that is more pronounced in females.[8] The association of Fuchs' dystrophy and open-angle glaucoma remains a matter of debate.[2,7]

The clinician must address the clinical relevance of guttae in the individual patient. The presence of corneal guttae does not necessarily imply that a specific cornea will become edematous. An analysis of a series of patients followed by one of us for over 10 years has determined that only 10% of patients with readibly observed confluent guttae on initial examination developed corneal edema within 10 years.[3] Furthermore, only 10% of patients with corneal guttae who underwent cataract extraction developed corneal edema within 10 years.

The surgeon's dilemma lies in trying to predict which corneas with guttae will decompensate. In our experience, the *clinical symptoms* of early dysfunction are the best predictors of postoperative corneal decompensation. The early symptoms associated with endothelial dysfunction and corneal edema are (1) halos around lights and (2) decreased vision upon awakening that improves during the waking state. These symptoms are attributable to epithelial edema that develops during the night when the lids are closed. Upon awakening, the epithelium loses some of its excess fluid through evaporation of the tear film. Halos occur when the fine epithelial microcysts on the surface of the cornea refract light as if passing through multiple small convex lenses.

Clinical examination of a patient with symptoms of corneal edema may not at a given time reveal corneal edema. The time of day of the examination is important, since examinations late in the day may miss the epithelial edema that occurs in the morning. The biomicroscopic *signs* of corneal edema include an increased thickness of the corneal stroma, Descemet's folds, and epithelial edema.

Clear, compact, nonedematous corneas with confluent guttae can also diminish visual acuity. Although there are no studies documenting exactly how much vision is lost from endothelial guttae alone, the impression of many experienced corneal surgeons is that the loss of a line or two on the Snellen chart may be attributable to corneal guttae *per se*.

Specialized instrumentation can be used to characterize objectively the status of the cornea. The corneal thickness can be accurately measured by a variety of pachymeters (pachometers). Measurements of 0.70 mm or greater are often associated with clinically evident edema.

It is known that during a person's lifetime there is a natural attrition of endothelial cells. The cell density, which may be as high as 4000 cells/mm^2 in youth, diminishes with time so that the adult may have a cell density in the range of 2000 cells/mm^2. The aged may have a cell count that is significantly less.

Specular microscopy permits the clinician to analyze the endothelial mosaic. The size and uniformity of the cellular components along with the endothelial cell density can be determined and documented. Specular microscopy also permits documentation of progressive cell loss in an individual patient; however it must be emphasized that the cell density does not necessarily correlate with the functioning of the endothelium. It is our experience that some patients with cell densities in the range of 400 to 500 cells/mm^2 have undergone cataract surgery with retention of a clear compact cornea and no evidence of endothelial dysfunction postoperatively. On the other hand, some corneas with much higher cell counts have decompensated with time or after surgery.

Specular microscopy alone does not allow one to be able to predict which patients with corneal guttae will develop corneal edema. Furthermore, specular microscopy has limited application in advanced Fuchs' dystrophy because by the time the dystrophy is clinically evident (that is, corneal edema is present), the ability to visualize the endothelium becomes diminished. One particularly important use of specular microscopy is the documentation of cell loss after various intraocular procedures, giving some index as to the amount of trauma involved in the surgery itself.

In summary, the majority of corneas with guttae will remain clear over time. Furthermore, intraocular surgery in eyes with clear corneas and confluent guttae is successful 90% of the time if there are no symptoms of corneal edema and care is taken intraoperatively to protect the cornea (such as endocapsular phacoemulsification and use of viscoelastic substances). The decision whether to do a cataract operation together with a corneal transplant or a cataract operation alone should be determined by the presence or absence of the *symptoms* of corneal edema. This necessarily requires careful history taking with attention directed to the symptoms of decreased vision upon awakening or halos around lights. Biomicroscopic examination should confirm the presence of corneal guttae to account for the corneal edema. Pachymetry and specular microscopy are not absolutely necessary but do provide useful objective evidence of the presence and progression of Fuchs' dystrophy.

REFERENCES

See also Chapter 6, pp. 55-56, for additional discussion and figures on Fuchs' dystrophy.
1. Boruchoff SA: Unpublished data.
2. Buxton JN, Preston RW, Reichers R, et al: Tonography in cornea guttata: a preliminary report, *Arch Ophthalmol* 77:602-603, 1967.
3. Fuchs E: Dystrophia epithelialis corneae, *Albrecht von Graefes Arch Klin Ophthalmol* 76:478-508, 1910.
4. Hogan MJ, Wood I, Fine M: Fuchs' endothelial dystrophy of the cornea: 29th Sanford Gifford Memorial Lecture, *Am J Ophthalmol* 78:363-383, 1974.
5. Koeppe L: Klinische Beobachtungen mit der Nernstspaltlampe und dem Hornhautmikroskop, *Albrecht von Graefes Arch Klin Ophthalmol* 91:363-379, 1916.
6. Lorenzetti DWC, Votila MH, Parikh N, Kaufman HE: Central cornea guttata, *Am J Ophthalmol* 64:1155-1158, 1967.
7. Roberts CW, Steinert RF, Thomas JV, Boruchoff SA: Endothelial guttata and the facility of aqueous outflow, *Cornea* 3:5-9, 1984.
8. Rosenblum P, Stark WJ, Maumenee IH, et al: Hereditary Fuchs' dystrophy, *Am J Ophthalmol* 90:455-462, 1980.
9. Vogt A: Weitere Ergebnisse der Spaltlampenmikroskopie des vordern Bulbusabschnitts, *Albrecht von Graefes Arch Klin Ophthalmol* 106:63-103, 1921.

INTERSTITIAL KERATITIS
MARK R. SAWUSCH
RONALD E. SMITH

Interstitial keratitis (IK) is a term that denotes any nonsuppurative inflammatory process of the corneal stroma that does not primarily involve the epithelium or endothelium. Although IK was formerly a common cause of corneal blindness, the number of patients requiring keratoplasty for this condition fell at least 60% with the introduction of antibiotics to treat the most common etiologic agents.[5] In recent studies from the United States, only 2% to 4% of patients undergoing penetrating keratoplasty had a diagnosis of interstitial keratitis.[6,8]

Etiology. Interstitial keratitis may be caused by numerous pathologic conditions (Table 11-6), but the majority of cases are secondary to congenital syphilis. Other common causes include bacterial in-

Table 11-6. Conditions Associated with Interstitial Keratitis

Bacterial infections
Syphilis—congenital or acquired
Tuberculosis
Relapsing fever
Leprosy
Lymphogranuloma venereum
Lyme disease
Viral infections
Herpes simplex—types I and II
Herpes zoster
Mumps
Vaccinia
Rubeola
Infectious mononucleosis
Influenza
Rubella
Epstein-Barr
Protozoan and helminthic infections
Onchocerciasis
Cysticercosis
Leishmaniasis
Trypanosomiasis
Schistosomiasis
Malaria
Systemic disease
Cogan's syndrome
Sarcoidosis
Mycosis fungoides
Hidradenitis suppurativa
Incontinentia pigmenti
Kaposi's sarcoma
Psoriasis
Systemic lupus erythematosus
Polyarteritis nodosa
Chemical poisons
Arsenic
Gold

fections such as tuberculosis and acquired syphilis, viral infections such as herpes, and parasitic infections.

Interstitial keratitis usually represents an allergic response to systemic infection, resulting in an antigen-antibody-complement or delayed-hypersensitivity reaction. Occasionally, direct invasion of organisms into the corneal stroma may produce IK.

IK may also be seen in association with systemic inflammatory diseases of unknown cause, such as sarcoidosis, polyarteritis nodosa, and systemic lupus erythematosus. Cogan[2] described a rare syndrome of interstitial keratitis associated with vestibuloauditory symptoms, including vertigo, hearing loss, and tinnitus.[4] This condition is idiopathic but probably represents a form of hypersensitivity reaction.

In some cases, the cause of IK is difficult to determine and can be assumed only by an association with systemic disease. When the cause is not apparent, useful studies include the VDRL (Venereal Disease Research Laboratories), FTA-ABS (fluorescent titer antibody absorption), PPD (purified protein derivative) skin test, chest x-ray, and serology for connective tissue disease.

Although interstitial keratitis may be caused by a wide variety of agents, the corneal responses are nonetheless similar and best illustrated by a description of the response to syphilis.

Bacterial Interstitial Keratitis. Congenital syphilis is much more commonly associated with IK than acquired syphilis is, and it accounts for approximately 90% of all cases of IK.[9] The condition represents an antigen-antibody-complement reaction to *Treponema pallidum*. The onset of findings may be delayed several years and typically occurs between 5 and 25 years of age. Hutchinson's triad for congenital syphilis consists in interstitial keratitis, deafness, and malformed incisor teeth. IK is typically bilateral in congenital cases and unilateral in cases of acquired syphilis.

It is unusual to see cases of acute interstitial keratitis today because the incidence of congenital syphilis has greatly decreased since the introduction of penicillin. The acute stage presents with intense photophobia, severe pain, tearing, conjunctival injection, and decreased vision. The stroma is variably cloudy and edematous with a ground-glass appearance and single or multiple dense white infiltrates, particularly in the deep layers. Stromal opacification is often in a feathery or patchy distribution but may become diffuse and reduce vision to light perception. Miosis, keratitic precipitates, and uveitis may be associated or masked by corneal inflammation. After several weeks, deep or superficial neovascularization

proceeds radially from the limbus to the central cornea; in advanced cases this produces a pink, "salmon-patch" appearance. If untreated, this acute inflammatory stage may persist for 2 to 4 months and then spontaneously resolve over 1 to 2 years. Treatment with corticosteroids and appropriate antibiotic agents usually results in earlier resolution of the acute inflammatory phase and improved visual prognosis.

IK more commonly presents as the late, inactive stage in adults, when the residual effects of previously active inflammation are first seen. The corneal infiltrates and edema of the acute phase resolve, leaving behind diffuse or patchy, deep stromal scarring and opacification and nonperfused "ghost" vessels (Figs. 11-30 and 11-31). The cornea clears over

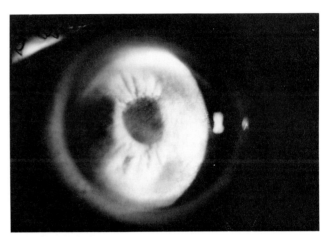

Fig. 11-30. Corneal scarring and mild lipid keratopathy with vertical ghost vessels in 68-year-old male. Diagnosis: mild luetic, inactive interstitial keratitis.

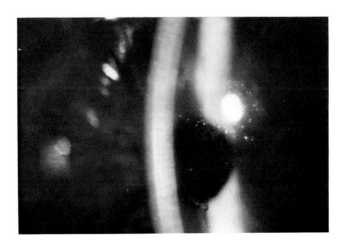

Fig. 11-31. Deep stromal horizontal ghost vessels seen in slitlamp beam of patient with diffuse corneal leukoma in both eyes secondary to inactive interstitial keratitis.

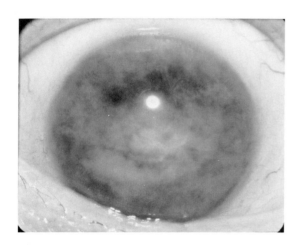

Fig. 11-32. Visual acuity 20/200 in eye with dense leukoma from luetic interstitial keratitis.

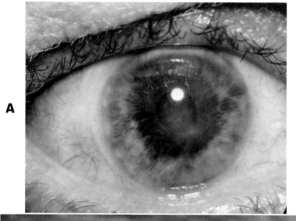

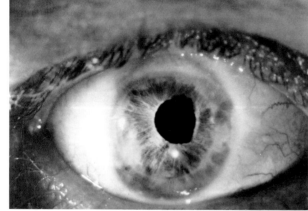

Fig. 11-33. Preoperative and postoperative views of eye having combined procedure for leukoma and cataract for inactive interstitial keratitis. Patients with mild corneal scarring and visual acuity of 20/40 to 20/60 may not present for surgery until late-onset senile cataract further diminishes ability to function.

several weeks to months from the periphery to the center, which may long remain for an extended period. The scarring is usually more noticeable in patients who did not receive early treatment with corticosteroids (Fig. 11-32). Scarring and thinning can also produce clinically significant irregular astigmatism.

The uveitis resolves but may result in posterior synechiae, areas of iris atrophy (Fig. 11-33, *A*), and secondary glaucoma.[3] Descemet's membrane may become folded or split and the endothelium destroyed, producing bullous keratopathy.[10] Other less common late sequelae include corneal thinning and ectasia, band keratopathy, lipid keratopathy (Fig. 11-30), Salzman's nodular degeneration, and cataract. A history of severe childhood ocular inflammation that persisted for several months or prior treatment for syphilis are helpful in making the diagnosis. The presence of prior syphilitic infection can be confirmed by a positive FTA-ABS test.

IK secondary to tuberculosis presents with symptoms and signs similar to those of syphilitic IK but is more commonly sectorial, peripheral, unilateral, and more superficial. It is believed to represent an immunologic reaction to tuberculoprotein in patients with systemic tuberculosis. A positive tuberculin skin test and negative FTA-ABS test are helpful in establishing the diagnosis.

Treatment. Antibiotic therapy should be initiated if there is active underlying systemic disease. However, since interstitial keratitis usually represents a hypersensitivity reaction, antibiotic therapy has proved to be of little value in treatment of the ocular disease. In fact, it is possible to exacerbate the ocular inflammation by antibiotic therapy because of an increase in the available antigen (Jarisch-Herxheimer reaction).

Topical steroids and cycloplegics are the mainstays of therapy and are used to prevent anterior and posterior synechiae, provide comfort, and improve the visual outcome by lessening scarring from inflammation. Maintenance steroid therapy (such as one or two drops of prednisolone daily) must be continued for at least 1 to 2 years, since steroids may prolong the clinical course. Corneal transplantation should generally not be considered during the acute stages of IK, since vision usually improves and there is a higher risk of graft failure.

After resolution of the acute inflammation, the corneal scarring of the late stage is variable and may or may not be visually significant. When keratitis has been quiescent on little or no steroid therapy for several months, penetrating keratoplasty may be indicated for visually significant corneal scarring.

The results of penetrating keratoplasty for interstitial keratitis have been relatively good (Fig. 11-33). Significant improvement in vision and clear grafts were reported by Rabb and Fine[5] in 49 (80%) of 61 keratoplasties for IK. Graft rejection episodes have been reported to occur in 9% to 18% of patients with IK, particularly in those having patent stromal neovascularization.[1,5] A major complication of keratoplasty is poor union between donor and recipient in areas of thinning of the recipient bed.[5] This can result in wound dehiscence after suture removal or in graft override. The graft size or centering may have to be adjusted so that the line of union is within the thickest stroma available. However, grafts larger than 8.0 mm are rarely advisable because of the risk of rejection and of angle compromise from synechiae. Postoperative uveitis may also be more common in patients with interstitial keratitis who undergo keratoplasty.[5] Postoperative glaucoma develops in about 12% of cases but can usually be controlled medically.[5] Interstitial keratitis may recur in a corneal graft, particularly in patients with herpetic IK.[7]

When interstitial keratitis is associated with cataract, simple cataract surgery may suffice if the patient had relatively good visual acuity before the development of cataract. However, excellent results from the triple procedure have been reported for patients with IK and cataract.[4]

REFERENCES

1. Boisjoly HM, Bernard PM, Dube I, et al: Effect of factors unrelated to tissue matching on corneal transplant endothelial rejection, *Am J Ophthalmol* 107:647, 1989.
2. Cogan DG, Dickerson GR: Nonsyphilitic interstitial keratitis with vestibuloauditory symptoms, *Arch Ophthalmol* 71:172, 1964.
3. Lichter PR, Shaffer RN: Interstitial keratitis and glaucoma, *Am J Ophthalmol* 68:241, 1969.
4. Pedersen OO: Combined corneal transplantation, extracapsular cataract extraction, and artificial lens implantation (triple procedure), *Acta Ophthalmol* 182(suppl):83, 1987.
5. Rabb MF, Fine M: Penetrating keratoplasty in interstitial keratitis, *Am J Ophthalmol* 67:907, 1969.
6. Rapuano CJ, Cohen EJ, Brady SE, et al: Indications for and outcomes of repeat penetrating keratoplasty, *Am J Ophthalmol* 109:689, 1990.
7. Rice NSC, Jones BR: Problems of corneal grafting in herpetic keratitis, *Ciba Found Symp* 15:221, 1973.
8. Robin JB, Gindi JJ, Koh K, et al: An update of the indications for penetrating keratoplasty: 1979 through 1983, *Arch Ophthalmol* 104:87, 1986.
9. Smith JL: Testing for congenital syphilis in interstitial keratitis, *Am J Ophthalmol* 72:816, 1971.
10. Waring GO, Font RL, Rodrigues MM, Mulberger RD: Alterations of Descemet's membrane in interstitial keratitis, *Am J Ophthalmol* 81:773, 1976.

NONHERPETIC CORNEAL LEUKOMA
MICHAEL W. BELIN

The major causes of nonherpetic corneal leukomas are shown in Table 11-7. This chapter is a discussion of some of the unique properties when one is treating vascularized corneas, classic corneal dystrophies, and traumatic scars.

Prognosis. The goal in treating any patient is visual improvement and rehabilitation. The prognosis in patients with nonvascularized, central, corneal scars is very good. Graft clarity should be obtained in more than 95% of patients.[12] Vascularized scars, scars crossing the limbus, and corneal trauma associated with other major ocular disturbances are indicators of a poorer outcome. Long-standing childhood trauma should raise the suspicion of irreversible amblyopia.

Most patients with corneal dystrophies do not require transplantation. Both mild-to-moderate granular, lattice, and posterior polymorphous dystrophies (PPMD) are compatible with good visual functioning.[9] Many of these dystrophies including Reis-Bücklers' will have a significant improvement in vi-

Table 11-7. Major Causes of Nonherpetic Corneal Leukoma

Congenital
Peters' anomaly
Congenital hereditary corneal dystrophy (CHED)
Posterior circumscribed keratoconus
Classic dystrophies (rarely present at birth)
    Macular
    Lattice
    Granular
    Reis-Bücklers'
    Central crystalline
    Posterior polymorphous (PPMD)
Traumatic
Stromal scarring secondary to corneal laceration
Breaks in Descemet's (birth trauma)
Metabolic
Mucopolysaccharidoses
Band keratopathy
Fabry's keratopathy
Lipid keratopathy
Environmental
Band keratopathy secondary to exposure
Spheroidal degeneration
Pterygium
Inflammatory/infectious
Corneal ulcer
Band keratopathy
Keratic precipitates
Interstitial keratitis
Rosacea keratitis
Neoplastic
Carcinoma (in situ)

sion with the use of a contact lens.[10] Because these corneas are typically nonvascularized, when patients do require keratoplasty, the prognosis for immunologic acceptance is good. However, all cases of corneal dystrophies may recur in the graft. The incidence is probably highest in Reis-Bücklers' where recurrences can occur after penetrating or lamellar keratoplasty and keratectomy and lowest in macular dystrophy.[1,5-8]

In the majority of corneal transplants, the host's lack of previous sensitization and vascularization allow for an unusually high success rate.[11] In high-risk vascularized corneas, surgery may be complicated by excessive bleeding and early suture erosion, and long-term graft survival may be threatened by immunologic graft rejection. The use of topical 2% cyclosporin A ointment in initial studies[3,4] appears to have a favorable effect on allograft rejection and is currently the subject of a national collaborative study in the United States.

Preoperative Evaluation. The initial evaluation of any patient begins with a history and thorough eye examination. Key points in the history to elucidate are the age at which the opacity was noted (to rule out amblyopia), previous surgeries, and the most recent level of acceptable visual functioning. A past history of useful vision is one of the best preoperative prognostic indicators.

The eye exam should always include a spectacle refraction to determine best corrected vision. We often utilize the keratometer to determine our initial cylinder and axis. In addition the keratometer relates whether the astigmatism is regular or irregular, and by quantifying the clarity of the mires, it indicates the degree of surface irregularity. If any degree of surface irregularity is noted, the spectacle refraction is followed by a diagnostic rigid lens fitting. The lens is fit to minimize any central air bubbles or lens flexure. I find that a large-diameter (9.3 to 9.7 mm) lens fits approximately 1 to 1.5 diopters flatter than flattest K with a central thickness of at least 0.15 mm being acceptable. An overrefraction is then performed, with any residual astigmatism being noted. Contact lens–corrected best visual acuities are often dramatically better than the spectacle-corrected best visions. This is particularly true after trauma where irregular astigmatism may be the major impediment to vision and with some of the classic dystrophies where surface distortion contributes heavily to the visual loss. In those patients, alternatives to full-thickness penetrating keratoplasty should be entertained. These include both soft and rigid lens wear, frequent use of ocular lubrication, superficial keratectomy, and lamellar keratoplasty.

One also needs to rule out medical conditions such as rosacea, blepharitis, and chronic exposure, which may be contributing to the corneal surface abnormality.

Central pachymetry is measured to rule out increased corneal thickness indicative of endothelial dysfunction. It is not uncommon to see diffuse stromal haze with surface irregularity misdiagnosed as corneal edema. Although significant stromal haze makes specular examination of the endothelium difficult, a normal corneal thickness would imply normal functioning endothelium. This distinction is important because anterior stromal scarring may be amenable to lamellar keratectomy or keratoplasty, which would be contraindicated in endothelial dysfunction. Currently newer devices are available (Steinway/Barraquer microkeratome, Steinway Instrument Co, San Diego, Calif., and Draeger rotokeratome, Storz Ophthalmics, Inc., St. Louis, Mo.), which allow for precise lamellar sections. These devices are capable of preparing both the donor lamellar transplant and the recipient bed. Lamellar dissections that leave less than 0.25 to 0.3 mm residual recipient corneal thickness are hazardous and not recommended. Although I routinely utilize ultrasonic pachymetry to determine corneal thickness, optical pachymetry must be utilized to determine the level of stromal opacification and whether a lamellar dissection can safely remove all the overlying stromal opacification.

The cornea is examined for evidence of vascularization. Deep stromal vascularization is one of the major poor prognostic indicators. Patients who are candidates for corneal transplantation and exhibit significant stromal vascularization may be treated with typed corneal tissue or with systemic or topical immunomodulators. It is my practice to treat these patients with topical cyclosporin 2% in addition to our normal preoperative and postoperative regimen. Occasionally patients are seen with a few isolated large vessels (Fig. 11-34). These patients are occasionally pretreated with argon-laser corneal photocoagulation. Typical settings are 0.1 msec, 100 to 200 μm spot size, and approximately 500 mW power. A contact lens is usually not utilized. For maximum heat absorption blue-green light is employed (with dye lasers yellow may be used). It is impossible to close off all the vessels and often the collateral vessels subsequently enlarge requiring multiple treatments. Better results are found with localized vascularization and lipid keratopathy, where I have had dramatic results with absorption of the lipid and considerable improvement in visual acuities.

Operative Considerations. In corneas with nor-

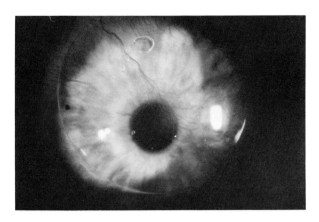

Fig. 11-34. Area of deep stromal vascularization encroaching on visual axis. This clinical presentation of a localized feeder system is amenable to laser corneal photocoagulation.

mal functioning endothelium or in those with significant vascularization, my selected trephines are typically 0.25 mm smaller than those used in endothelial dysfunction. A slightly smaller graft is technically easier and further removes the graft-host junction from the vascular limbus. With endothelial dysfunction one of the goals is to transplant as much viable endothelium as possible and my typical graft is 7.75/8.0 mm or 8.0/8.25 mm (recipient/donor). With traumatic scars, vascularized corneas and (nonendothelial) corneal dystrophies, I typically utilize 7.5/7.75 mm or 7.75/8.0 mm.

In vascularized corneas, bleeding can be controlled by partial-thickness trephinization and allowance for the vessels to coagulate. Alternatively, phenylephrine (Neo-Synephrine) soaked cellulose sponges can be directly applied to the cut vascular bed. In cases (such as phakic keratoplasty) where pupillary constriction is desired, phenylephrine (Neo-Synephrine) should be used judiciously and never dropped directly onto the cornea. Extensive vascularization can be treated with wet-field cautery applied to the scleral bed after a peritomy is performed. This is more successful for conjunctival and episcleral vessels than deep stromal vessels. Cautery should never be applied directly to the transplant wound because it can cause collagen shrinkage, wound distortion, and persistent wound leaks.

Wound closure in nonvascularized corneas is typically with 12 interrupted 10-0 nylon sutures followed by either a running 10-0 or 11-0 nylon. Vascularized corneas have a high incidence of early suture erosion and vascular ingrowth. Here, an all-interrupted closure allows for the necessary selective removal.

Lamellar Keratoplasty. Lamellar corneal grafting may be indicated in patients who present with opacities not involving the full thickness of the cornea. Subepithelial scars and anterior stromal dystrophies may be amenable to lamellar keratoplasty. The advantages of lamellar grafting over penetrating keratoplasty are the avoidance of entering the anterior chamber, the shorter wound healing and convalescence, and the reduced incidence of allograft reactions. In addition, donor tissue not suitable for penetrating keratoplasty may successfully be used in lamellar surgery because preservation of viable endothelium is not necessary. The major disadvantages include the greater technical difficulty and potential opacification and vascularization of the stromal interface limiting visual function. The microkeratome is capable of making the lamellar dissection for both the recipient and the donor material. The precision of these instruments and meticulous irrigation and cleaning of the lamellar bed has greatly reduced opacification at the host-donor interface.

Superficial Keratectomy. This procedure consists in excision of the superficial layers of the cornea (epithelium, Bowman's layer, and superficial stroma) without tissue replacement. The primary indications are the removal of hyperplastic or necrotic tissue (such as corneal dermoid, pterygium); obtaining tissue for diagnosis (histopathology, microbiology); and excision of a tumor, scarring, or portions of the cornea affected by Reis-Bücklers' dystrophy. The area of dissection can be marked freehand with an adjustable depth blade, or a trephine can be used to superficially mark the area. A lamellar dissection can be carried out with either a sharp or dull blade. Although a sharp blade is quicker, care must be taken to maintain the surgical plane to avoid inadvertent perforation. A lamellar keratectomy can also be performed using a microkeratome or a diamond burr on a surgical drill (such as the Hall drill, Zimmer Inc., Warsaw, Indiana).

Postoperative Management. The postoperative management of the nonvascularized recipients does not differ significantly from other keratoplasty patients. One needs to observe any trauma patient for glaucoma and retinal complications. Patients grafted for corneal dystrophies need to be examined for recurrences.

Vascularized recipients, however, need more frequent monitoring. Suture erosion is very common. If left untreated, an eroded suture is a stimulus for vascularization and a potential nidus for infection. Once vessels cross the graft-host junction, the wound can be assumed secure in that region and the corresponding sutures can be removed. Because of the increased incidence of graft reactions, the postoperative visits are more frequent. Minor indicators of early immunologic reaction such as background cell and flare or subepithelial infiltrates[2] should be treated aggressively, whereas major indicators such as keratitic precipitates, stromal thickening, or an endothelial rejection line almost always require systemic or periocular steroids.

REFERENCES

1. Akova YA et al: Recurrent macular corneal dystrophy following penetrating keratoplasty, *Eye* 4:698, 1990.
2. Aldredge OC, Krachmer JH: Clinical types of corneal transplant rejection: their manifestations, frequency, preoperative correlates and treatment, *Arch Ophthalmol* 99:599, 1981.
3. Belin MW, Bouchard CS, Frantz S, Chmielinska J: Topical cyclosporine in high risk corneal transplants, *Ophthalmology* 96(8):1144, 1989.
4. Belin MW, Bouchard CS, Phillips TM: Update on topical cyclosporin A: background, immunology, pharmacology, *Cornea* 9(3):184, 1990.
5. Boruchoff SA, Weiner MJ, Albert DA: Recurrence of posterior polymorphous corneal dystrophy after penetrating keratoplasty, *Am J Ophthalmol* 109:323, 1990.
6. Caldwell DR: Postoperative recurrence of Reis-Bücklers' corneal dystrophy, *Am J Ophthalmol* 85:577, 1978.
7. de Felice GP, Carta S: Lattice dystrophy of the cornea: a clinical and histopathologic study, *Ophthalmologica* (Basel) 192:135, 1986.
8. Klintworth GK et al: Recurrence of macular corneal dystrophy within grafts, *Am J Ophthalmol* 95:60, 1983.
9. Möller HU: Granular corneal dystrophy Groenouw type I: clinical aspects and treatment, *Acta Ophthalmolog* 68:384, 1990.
10. Musco PS, Aquavella JV: Therapeutic contact lenses. In Dabezies OH, editor: *Contact lenses—the CLAO guide to basic science and clinical practice,* Boston, 1984, Little, Brown.
11. Smolin G, O'Connor GR: Corneal graft reaction. In *Ocular immunology,* Boston, 1986, Little, Brown, pp 282-283.
12. Zauberman H: Corneal graft transparency: Is 100% an achievable goal? *Isr J Med Sci* 2:101, 1984.

HERPES SIMPLEX LEUKOMA
Surgical Considerations
JEFFREY DAY LANIER

Herpes simplex keratitis may be the most common cause of infectious blindness in the United States[4,15,19] and in other developed countries. The clinical classification of ocular herpes infections can be confusing because of the great variety of clinical presentations and terms used to describe these variations.

Primary herpes simplex is designated as the first infection with *Herpesvirus hominis.* Primary infections are usually mild and seen in children, with ocular involvement being a relatively uncommon presenting sign. When ocular involvement does occur, a follicular conjunctivitis may be observed and at times with a membranous formation. The keratitis is usually minimal, with transitory dendrites lasting 1 or 2 days occurring 7 to 10 days after the onset of symptoms. Residual corneal scarring is unusual.

CLASSIFICATION OF RECURRENT HERPETIC KERATITIS. Recurrent herpes simplex infections develop after the patient has had previous exposure and has developed some immunity to the virus. Recurrent herpes simplex keratitis can be classified simply as:
1. Active epithelial keratitis
2. Disciform stromal keratitis
3. Infiltrative stromal keratitis

Active epithelial keratitis most commonly presents as a dendrite, but many other forms may be seen. Most active herpetic epithelial keratitis heals spontaneously without sequelae in a natural course from a few days to 28 days. Topical antiviral agents may or may not alter this natural course of healing.

Disciform stromal keratitis is a disc-shaped stromal edema with minimal or no infiltration of white cells. It is considered an immunologic response to antigens of live virus, viral particles, or both. The term "disciform" was originally described before the advent of the slitlamp (biomicroscope) and may have several causes, one of which is herpes simplex keratitis. The natural course of a disciform stromal keratitis caused by herpes simplex is 2 to 6 months' duration. Topical corticosteroids decrease the stromal edema in the majority of disciform stromal keratitis, but the true ultimate benefit of topical steroids is still unknown.

Infiltrative (white blood cells) stromal keratitis (Fig. 11-35) is the sight-threatening form of herpes simplex keratitis. The natural course of healing is 2 to 12 months' duration with possible significant residual scarring. No therapeutic approach up to now has eliminated this major cause of infectious blindness; therefore penetrating keratoplasty has become a surgical approach to attempt visual rehabilitation.

Preoperative considerations. The reported success rate of penetrating keratoplasty in herpes simplex keratitis has been somewhat variable, but all reports concur that it is not in the most favorable category.[2,3,5,7,11,16,18] The optimal preoperative condition required in an eye with herpetic keratitis before penetrating keratoplasty remains speculative. There are, however, some guidelines that seem to have merit both clinically and theoretically.

SUPPRESSING INFLAMMATION. A common denominator prevailing in the reported cases of penetrating keratoplasty for herpetic disease is that of increased success rate when the eye is free of inflammation for an extended period of time. This may be the single most important variable in determining success or failure. Several questions remain unanswered from a scientific standpoint in relation to the treatment

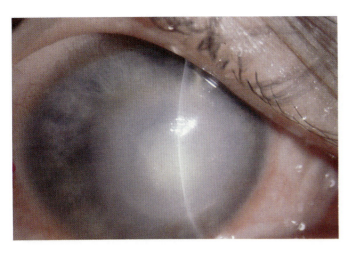

Fig. 11-35. Herpes simplex stromal keratitis with chronic inflammation, pain, photophobia, and increased intraocular pressure. Patient had been treated with topical corticosteroids.

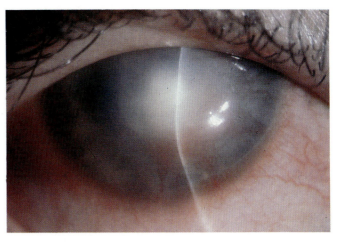

Fig. 11-36. Same patient 1 month after discontinuation of corticosteroids. Ocular inflammation has increased.

needed to quiet these eyes: (1) Should the inflammation simply be controlled with topical corticosteroids and for how long? (2) Should topical corticosteroids be discontinued completely and for how long? (3) How long should antiviral therapy, if used, be continued with corticosteroid treatment? (4) Should systemic antiviral therapy be used preoperatively or postoperatively in penetrating keratoplasty for herpes simplex keratitis?

It is generally considered advantageous if the eye is free of inflammation without corticosteroid therapy for a period of 6 to 24 months, but this is also speculative.

A common regimen used when treating infiltrative stromal herpetic keratitis is to slowly taper corticosteroid usage (and antiviral therapy if used) by a decrease in the frequency of application and eventually complete discontinuance of the corticosteroids. At times the concentration of the corticosteroid must be reduced by less than is commercially available. This can be accomplished by dilution of the commercial 1/8% corticosteroid to 1/16% and 1/32%, with the addition of artificial tears or other similar ophthalmic solutions.

It may take months or years to totally discontinue use of corticosteroids. As the frequency and concentration are decreased, the ocular inflammation usually increases. Seldom does an eye remain noninflamed as corticosteroids are reduced. It is important that patients understand this when tapering dosage. Allowing the eye to have some inflammation may be necessary to obtain an eventual noninflamed state.

ANTIVIRAL MEDICATION. The concomitant use of antiviral medications along with topical corticosteroids

has been advocated[15] and used by some, but not by all. Antiviral medications are toxic to the corneal epithelium, especially when used frequently or for longer than 10 to 20 days. A common regimen is to follow the corticosteroid drop with an antiviral medication, drop for drop, until the frequency of corticosteroid drops is reduced to less than four times a day, and then the antiviral is discontinued. The potential toxicity of antiviral medications must always be kept in mind.

Acyclovir orally has shown beneficial effect as adjunct therapy in recalcitrant cases of herpes simplex viral keratouveitis and stromal keratitis, but chronic acyclovir therapy appears to be necessary to reduce the recurrence rate in this group.[20] Of most concern is the possible severe rebound recurrence that may occur with cessation of oral acyclovir as reported by Schwab[20] in 3 of 27 patients. The National Eye Institute is presently sponsoring the Herpetic Eye Disease Study involving eight clinical centers to evaluate the efficacy of oral acyclovir in the treatment of herpetic stromal keratitis and iridocyclitis.

CESSATION OF STEROID TREATMENT. Corticosteroids can be discontinued abruptly (Figs. 11-35 to 11-38), but this approach is not routinely advocated. The abrupt cessation of corticosteroids may lead to an acute inflammatory rebound response that is characterized by increased vascularity and infiltration of the corneal stroma, uveitis, and secondary glaucoma lasting 1 to 3 months but rarely longer. During this inflammatory period intraocular pressure must be monitored and controlled if necessary and the pupil moved to prevent anterior and posterior synechiae.

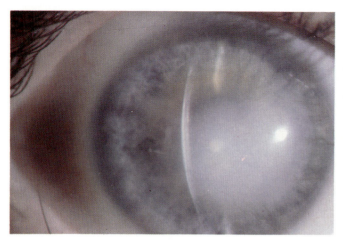

Fig. 11-37. Same eye 6 months after discontinuation of corticosteroids. Symptoms have subsided, eye quieted, and intraocular pressure was controlled.

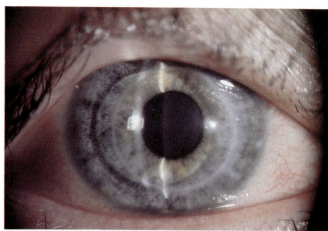

Fig. 11-38. Same eye 2 years after discontinuation of corticosteroids and 16 months after penetrating keratoplasty.

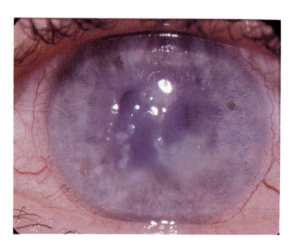

Fig. 11-39. Twenty-eight-year-old farmer with 5-year history of recurrent herpes simplex epithelial and stromal keratitis unresponsive to medical treatment. Preconjunctival flap OS. Visual acuity OD was 20/15.

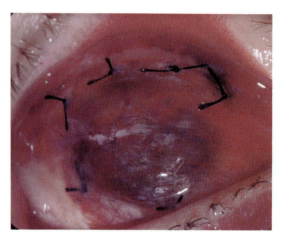

Fig. 11-40. Same eye 2 weeks after Gunderson conjunctival flap in 1972. 8-0 silk sutures used to anchor flap were supplemented with 10-0 nylon to close a small rent centrally.

The acute inflammation will begin receding in 1 to 3 months; intraocular pressure becomes controlled without medication, vascularization is reduced, active stromal infiltration diminishes, and the patient becomes comfortable. Once this stage is reached, the remaining months of rehabilitation are usually well tolerated by the patient. The advantage of this approach to treatment is in reducing the time necessary to achieve a noninflamed eye, usually less than 12 months. The disadvantages, however, are the initial 1 to 3 months of acute inflammation.

The decision to initiate the tapering versus the abrupt method of eliminating corticosteroids is very complex and involves the philosophy of the physi-

cian, the specific clinical situation, and the informed consent of the patient.

CONJUNCTIVAL FLAP. Along with the above therapeutic approaches, a total or partial thin conjunctival flap[9] is an effective means of managing advanced cases of herpetic keratitis. The conjunctival flap can be used as a temporary measure (usually 8 to 10 months) or can remain permanently in place for treatment of herpetic corneal ulcers resistant to therapy.

The surgical technique for conjunctival flap formation[9,14] is reviewed in Chapter 30. There are three vital features of the procedure: (1) thinness of the flap exclusive of Tenon's tissue, (2) absence of

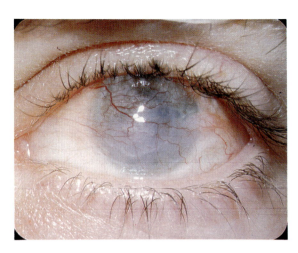

Fig. 11-41. Same eye 6 months later. Patient off all medication and symptom free. Twelve-year follow-up check: patient asymptomatic with visual acuity of 20/200 and refused corneal transplant.

buttonholes to avoid tissue separation, and (3) absence of traction from the base of the flap. The dramatic beneficial effects of decreased pain, photophobia, and epiphora, characteristic of chronic inflammatory disease, usually decrease or exclude the need for continued use of topical medications to control inflammation (Figs. 11-39 to 11-41).

CORNEAL SENSATION. Corneal sensation is commonly diminished by chronic herpes simplex keratitis. This decreased sensation can be minimal to totally absent, and the duration can be short to permanent. If the sensation is diminished, neurotrophic keratitis may occur, resulting in poor healing of the overlying corneal epithelium.[5,7] A return of corneal sensation preoperatively may be of benefit in promoting epithelial healing in the postoperative period, but it is not necessary to have a return of normal corneal sensation before proceeding with keratoplasty. Unfortunately a return of corneal sensation may take years to occur if it returns at all.

VASCULARIZATION. Attempting to control corneal vascularization before penetrating keratoplasty by various means has been advocated over the years, though the ultimate benefit of this has never been elucidated. Most corneal surgeons will simply control bleeding at the time of surgery with light cautery or irrigation.

An increased survival rate of clear grafts in severely vascularized corneas has recently been reported by the use of HLA-DR (class II) antigen matching.[12]

Surgical considerations. Most corneal surgeons do not alter their surgical technique specifically for herpetic keratitis. An exception is the use of interrupted sutures in vascularized corneas[8] where more rapid healing and loosening permits selective suture removal.

A basic principle in corneal transplant surgery is to place stitches into the healthiest recipient tissue possible. This principle is important when one is determining graft size and centration. When extremely thin or necrotic recipient tissue is present or areas of stromal scarring extend to the paracentral cornea, large-diameter or eccentric grafts may be necessary.

Stromal necrosis and perforation are rare complications and can usually be treated with tissue adhesive and a therapeutic soft contact lens when the perforation is 2 mm or less. One should avoid doing a penetrating keratoplasty in a severely inflamed eye. This may be necessary, however, in acute perforations of 3 mm or greater. One must be aware that this condition results in a much more difficult surgical procedure. The orbit cannot be adequately decompressed, resulting in possible orbital pressure pushing the lens and iris forward. Bleeding from the wound and the iris surface may be more extensive. Fibrin formation during and after surgery may be excessive, resulting in synechia and pupillary block. Wound closure may be more difficult. All these adversities must be considered before one attempts the surgical skills in a potentially very difficult procedure.

Postoperative considerations. The postoperative course of keratoplasties for herpetic keratitis can be extremely variable. Healing is more rapid where significant vascularization is present, but at times healing may be delayed by the frequent use of corticosteroids. Healing of the epithelium may be very poor because of a neurotrophic cornea, dryness, or recurrent herpetic keratitis in the graft. If the epithelial defect persists, rebound inflammation with surface fibrosis or loss of the normal Bowman's surface may occur.

MEDICATIONS. Most surgeons advocate titrating topical corticosteroids as necessary to control postoperative inflammation. The inflammation may be minimal or extensive. Some have reported an increase in the incidence of recurrent herpes simplex keratitis with the use of high-dosage corticosteroids,[2] whereas others have not.[3]

The concomitant use of antiviral medications along with topical corticosteroids are used by some surgeons postoperatively[3,11] but not routinely by others.[5] Most corneal surgeons will use antiviral medications only when topical corticosteroids are used frequently (such as every 1 to 2 hours) and use the antiviral medications only for a 10- to 20-day period. The literature neither supports the theoretical postulation that the use of antiviral medications reduces the incidence of recurrent herpes simplex in postoperative keratoplasties[3,5,11] nor supports the theory that the use of high doses of topical corticosteroids increases the incidence of recurrent herpes simplex in postoperative keratoplasties.[2,3] Since there is no definitive therapeutic regimen for the use of antiviral and corticosteroid medications in postoperative keratoplasties, the corneal surgeon must use his clinical judgment in the use of these drugs, keeping in mind the potential toxic and detrimental effects of each.

Beyer and co-workers[21] reported that systemic acyclovir administered prophylactically immediately before and after keratoplasty reduced herpes simplex virus shedding, epithelial geographic ulcers, and stromal keratitis in rabbits latently infected with HSV-I. The results of the National Eye Institute Herpetic Eye Disease Study and other well-controlled clinical trials are needed to determine the efficacy of oral acyclovir for both herpetic infections and prophylactic use in penetrating keratoplasty for herpes simplex. The concern of severe rebound recurrence after cessation of acyclovir must also be elucidated.

COMPLICATIONS. The major complications of grafting eyes with herpes are (1) recurrent herpes simplex keratitis and (2) homograft reaction. Differentiating the two problems can be a diagnostic dilemma, but observation of clinical signs may be helpful (Table 11-8). The most specific clinical sign is a classical herpetic dendrite of the epithelium, best appreciated by staining with fluorescein or rose bengal. The first recurrence within a graft has been reported to be epithelial in 74.7%.[5] Positive cultures are most likely to be obtained during the active herpetic dendritic stage. Any epithelial defect can heal in a dendritic shape and mimic a herpetic dendrite. Geographic epithelial defects are not a specific clinical sign for herpes simplex keratitis. If a geographic epithelial defect is associated with recurrent herpes, there are usually superficial focal granular stromal infiltrates present.

The homograft reaction is usually associated with a more evenly distributed stromal edema even though only a sector of the cornea may be involved. The inferior portion of the cornea is the most common site of initial involvement in graft reactions, whereas recurrent herpetic keratitis occurs at the line of union between the graft and the recipient in 61.5% of cases.[5] A Khodadoust keratic precipitate line would signify that a graft reaction was occurring.

Decreased corneal sensation is an unreliable dif-

Table 11-8. Clinical Signs Helpful in Differentiating Recurrent Herpes Simplex Keratitis from Allograft Reaction

Recurrent Herpes Simplex Keratitis	Allograft Reaction
Epithelial dendrite	Nonspecific
Geographic defect	Nonspecific
Stromal focal, granular infiltrates	Evenly distributed stromal edema
Most common in graft-wound junction	Most common in inferior graft
No Khodadoust line	Khodadoust line
Sensation is an unreliable sign	Sensation is an unreliable sign

ferentiating clinical sign because corneal sensation within a corneal graft is normally diminished. Decreased or absent corneal sensation would not help differentiate a homograft reaction from recurrent herpes simplex keratitis.

The recurrence rate of herpes simplex keratitis postoperatively depends on the duration of follow-up time and criteria of diagnosis. The range of reported recurrence is from 6% to 47% and can occur immediately postoperatively or years later.[2,5,7,11] A recurrence of herpes simplex keratitis within a graft does not necessarily result in an opaque graft. Central scars or completely opaque grafts have been reported to occur in only 23.8% of herpetic recurrences.[5]

Corneal homograft reaction has been reported as high as 79%[2] and 71%,[7] whereas others have reported a much lower incidence of 20.6%.[3] Preoperative vascularization has commonly been related to increased homograft reaction in herpes keratitis[2,7,11] as well as in corneal transplantation in general.[1,10,13] Others did not find vascularization statistically significant for increase homograft reaction in herpes keratitis[3] or in corneal transplantation in general.[6]

Even though herpes keratitis is not in the most favorable category for successful keratoplasty, clear grafts with good visual rehabilitation can be obtained if surgery is performed in quiet eyes and postoperative complications are anticipated and treated appropriately.

REFERENCES

1. Cherry PMH, Pashby RC, Tradros ML, et al: An analysis of corneal transplantation. I. Graft clarity, *Ann Ophthalmol* 11:461, 1979.
2. Cobo LM, Coster DJ, Rice MSC, Jones BR: Prognosis and management of corneal transplantation for herpes keratitis, *Arch Ophthalmol* 98:1755, 1980.

3. Cohen EJ, Laibson PR, Arentsen JJ: Corneal transplantation of herpes simplex keratitis, *Am J Ophthalmol* 95:645-650, 1983.
4. Dawson CR, Togni B: Herpes simplex eye infections: clinical manifestations, pathogenesis and management, *Surv Ophthalmol* 21:121, 1976.
5. Fine M, Cignetti FE: Penetrating keratoplasty in herpes simplex keratitis, *Arch Ophthalmol* 95:613, 1977.
6. Fine M, Stein M: The role of corneal vascularization in human corneal graft reaction. In Porter R, Knight J, editors: Corneal graft failure, *Ciba Found Symp* 15:193, Amsterdam/New York, 1973, Elsevier Publishing Co./Associated Scientific Publications.
7. Foster CS, Duncan J: Penetrating keratoplasty for herpes simplex keratitis, *Am J Ophthalmol* 92:336, 1981.
8. Friedlaender M: *Contemporary profiles in corneal transplant surgery,* San Francisco, 1985, Alcon Laboratories.
9. Gundersen T: Conjunctival flaps in the treatment of corneal disease with reference to a new technique of application, *AMA Arch Ophthalmol* 60:880, 1958.
10. Hogan MJ, Kimura SJ, Thygeson P: Pathology of herpes simplex kerato-iritis, *Am J Ophthalmol* 57:551-564, 1964.
11. Khodadoust AA: The allograft rejection reaction: the leading cause of late graft failure of clinical corneal grafts. In Porter R, Knight J, editors: Corneal graft failure, *Ciba Found Symp* 15:151-168, Amsterdam/New York, 1973, Elsevier Publishing Co./Associated Scientific Publications.
12. Mayer DJ, Martin GK, Casey TA: *The value of HLA-DR (class II) antigen matching in corneal transplantation,* Presented at the American Academy of Ophthalmology, San Francisco, Oct 1985.
13. Moore TE Jr, Arundson SB: The corneal graft: a multiple variable analysis of the penetrating keratoplasty, *Am J Ophthalmol* 72(suppl):205, 1971.
14. Paton D, Milauskas AT: Indications, surgical technique, and results of thin conjunctival flaps on the cornea, *Int Ophthalmol Clin* 10:329-345, 1970.
15. Patterson A, Jones B: The management of ocular herpes, *Trans Ophthalmol Soc UK* 87:537, 1967.
16. Polak FM, Kaufman HE: Penetrating keratoplasty in herpes keratitis, *Am J Ophthalmol* 73:908, 1972.
17. Valenton MJ, Tau R, Abendanio R, Nievera L: Causes of corneal ulceration, *Philippine J Ophthalmol* 10:64, 1978.
18. Völker-Dieben HJ, Kok-van Alphen CC, D'Amaro J, de Lange P: The effect of prospective HLA-A and B matching in 288 penetrating keratoplasties for herpes simplex keratitis, *Acta Ophthalmol* 62:513-523, 1984.
19. Workshop on the treatment and prevention of herpes simplex virus infection: News from the National Institute of Health, *J Infect Dis* 127:117, 1973.
20. Schwab I: Oral acyclovir in the management of herpes ocular infections, *Ophthalmology* vol 95, April 1988.
21. Beyer CF, Arens MQ, Hill GA, et al: Oral acyclovir reduces the incidence of recurrent herpes simplex keratitis in rabbits after penetrating keratoplasty, *Arch Ophthalmol* 107:1200-1205, 1989.

Results of Surgery
JOHN W. CHANDLER

The corneal sequelae of herpes simplex and herpes zoster keratitis are a major infectious cause for corneal transplantation in the United States. Many centers have reported their results after penetrating keratoplasty for scars caused by herpes sim-

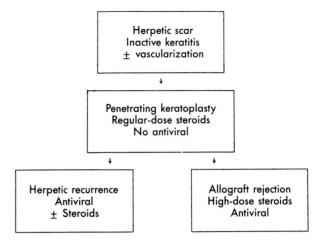

Fig. 11-42. Schema of management of patients with inactive herpetic scars.

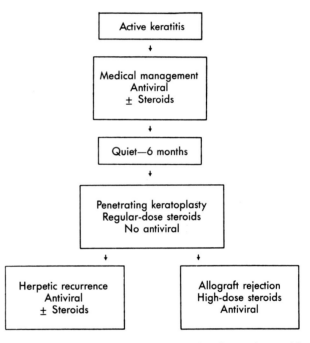

Fig. 11-43. Schema of management plan for patients with active herpetic keratitis who need a corneal transplant.

plex keratitis.[1-7,9,11,12] Although less frequently reported, some series now report reasonably good results after penetrating keratoplasty for the scarring caused by herpes zoster viral keratitis.[10,13,14]

Penetrating keratoplasty after herpes simplex keratitis. In the reviews of penetrating keratoplasty for herpetic keratitis, the following three groups seem to include virtually all patients: (1) inactive scarring with or without vascularization, (2) active herpetic keratitis, and (3) stromal keratitis with or without perforation. These groups present different intraoperative and postoperative problems, but the group with inactive herpetic disease is the most likely to have successful results. Improved management of cataracts, recurrent herpetic attacks, and graft rejection have improved the long-term results. As a basic tenet, it is best to get the process to an inactive state for at least 6 months before performing penetrating keratoplasty (Figs. 11-42 and 11-43).

INACTIVE SCARRING (GROUP I). Patients with histories or findings consistent with herpetic keratitis and scars that decrease vision are good candidates if there has been an absence of active disease for 6 months or longer. The presence of varying degrees of vascularization do not preclude success but may predispose to allograft rejection. Foster and Duncan[7] report clear grafts in 90% of patients with scars without active inflammation, ulceration, or vascularization, and 80% clear grafts in eyes with disciform edema. Cobo and co-workers[1] used life tables to demonstrate that 69% of grafts remained clear at 2 years when surgery was performed when inflammation was inactive. In contrast, the 2-year survival of clear grafts performed while the recipient eye was actively inflamed was reduced to 44%.

In this same report, at 5 years the rejection rates were 16% in avascular recipient corneas but rose to 30% in those with partially vascularized host beds. Cohen and co-workers[2] were unable to find significant differences in rejection rates between patient groups with varying degrees of vascularization. The trends were similar to those reported by Cobo and co-workers.[1] In all these series[1,2,6,7,9,11] clear grafts were obtained in 69% to 86% of recipients with inactive inflammation at the time of surgery. Although the visual acuities in these patients were generally good, other ocular abnormalities precluded excellent vision in the entire group. These results indicate that patients with inactive herpetic keratitis and corneal opacities are good candidates for corneal transplantation (Fig. 11-42). Recurrent herpetic keratitis and allograft rejection can occur concomitantly or separately. Ficker and associates[4,5] recently demonstrated that survival of grafts during rejection episodes was significantly improved by concomitant antiviral and corticosteroid therapy (even in the absence of conclusive clinical evidence of recurrent herpetic disease). Likewise, immediate removal of any loose sutures improved results. It appears as though the frequency of allograft rejection is approximately the same for herpetic keratitis and keratoconus recipients. However, herpetic keratitis recipients are about three times as likely to go on to develop irreversible rejection.[3]

The medical management after surgery should in-

clude the usual corticosteroid therapy, such as topical prednisolone acetate, dexamethasone, or an equivalent steroid four times daily. The routine use of topical antivirals is controversial but may be contraindicated, since 44% will develop epithelial toxicity and persistent epithelial defects.[7] Antiviral use also appears to delay wound healing,[8] especially when used with corticosteroids.[12] The rate of recurrence of active herpes simplex keratitis in this group is in the range of 5% to 8%.[1,2] The appearance of active herpetic disease mandates a full course of therapy with topical antiviral medication. The potential role of oral acyclovir in this situation has yet to be established. If corticosteroids are in use at the time of recurrence, they should be continued. If not, the antiviral should be instituted alone and the subsequent clinical course monitored in case corticosteroids are needed. Allograft rejection is the largest cause of graft failure in this group. When a rejection episode is detected on clinical grounds, aggressive corticosteroid therapy is required, including frequent topical drops and possibly an intravenous single bolus of 125 mg of methylprednisolone or its equivalent with or without a short, intensive course of prednisone given orally. The aggressive use of corticosteroids may predispose to recurrent epithelial herpetic keratitis, necessitating concomitant topical antiviral therapy.

ACTIVE HERPETIC KERATITIS (GROUP II). The second group of patients facing penetrating keratoplasty are those with active herpetic keratitis, but results of surgery in these eyes are less impressive, having only a 44% success[1] contrasted with a 69% to 86% rate in grafts for inactive disease.[1,2,6,7,9,11] The report of Polack and Kaufman suggests that penetrating keratoplasty is far more successful in patients who have had inactive disease for at least 6 months. Therefore medical management may be required to achieve a 6-month period of inactive disease before corneal transplantation (Fig. 11-43). Both antiviral drugs to stop active viral replication and topical corticosteroids to suppress secondary inflammation may be needed. The management of eyes in the postoperative period including allograft rejections is similar to that in group I cases.

STROMAL HERPES SIMPLEX KERATITIS (GROUP III). The final category includes patients with herpetic keratitis with stromal ulceration with or without perforation. Although most of these patients give a definite history of antecedent herpetic keratitis, one should keep this diagnosis in mind when the corneal surgeon is faced with a corneal perforation of unknown cause. Although a penetrating keratoplasty can be performed in this situation, the results are very poor

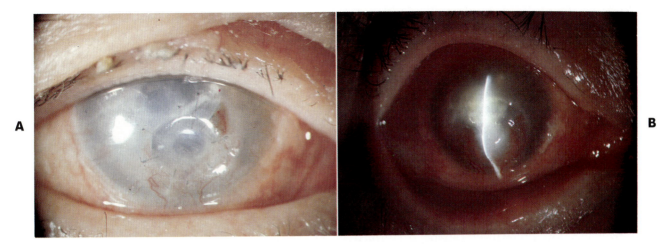

Fig. 11-44. A, Sixty-year-old man with chronic stromal herpes simplex after penetrating patch graft anchored by interrupted 10-0 nylon sutures. Linear stromal infiltration seen superior to graft along with prominent deep vascularization inferiorly. **B,** Same eye 6 months later with diffuse stromal infiltration of entire cornea. Keratitis could not be controlled, and enucleation was performed.

(Fig. 11-44). The preferred treatment is to restore corneal integrity, allow the inflammation to become quiescent, and thus convert the eye to a more favorable prognosis group (Fig. 11-45).

When the area of ulceration or perforation is small, it is often possible to stabilize the situation with tissue adhesive and a therapeutic bandage soft contact lens (see Chapter 30). If the ulceration does not appear to be in danger of perforation, a conjunctival flap may be used. Once the eye has been repaired, medical management can commence with antiviral drugs using corticosteroids as dictated by the clinical course. Larger stromal ulcerations and perforations must be approached in a slightly different way. If there is no threat of perforation, a conjunctival flap may be adequate. However, if perforation is present or impending, the stroma must be reinforced. Although some people argue for immediate penetrating keratoplasty,[11] others advocate a lamellar keratoplasty.[7] Neither approach is likely to lead to a good visual outcome, and both may risk spreading infection beyond control (Fig. 11-44). These measures must be considered as temporizing and the first step in achievement of inactive inflammation before definitive grafting later.

There are other factors that may lead to the failure of penetrating keratoplasty in patients with herpetic keratitis. Cataracts and glaucoma, as well as primary donor failure, are occasionally observed. Microbial keratitis from bacteria and fungi may occur. Technical problems associated with surgery are not infrequent. For example, segmental peripheral corneal thinning is sometimes present in eyes with

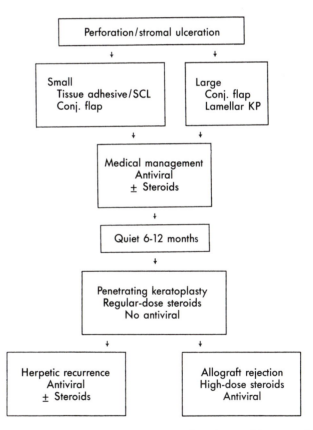

Fig. 11-45. Schema of treatment of patients with stromal ulceration or perforation caused by herpes simplex keratitis. *Conj.,* Conjunctival; *KP,* keratoplasty; *SCL,* soft contact lens.

previous herpetic stromal keratitis. Failure to recognize and plan surgery around these problems can lead to poor wound apposition and subsequent graft failure.

Penetrating keratoplasty after herpes zoster keratitis. The group of patients having penetrating keratoplasty after herpes zoster keratitis presents unique challenges to the corneal transplant surgeon. Approximately 40% of patients with herpes zoster ophthalmicus develop keratitis. Many of them develop corneal scarring and reduced visual acuity. Several concomitant sequelae can predispose penetrating grafts to failure. Chief among these are trichiasis, neuroparalytic keratitis, glaucoma, and anterior segment ischemia. Lid procedures can be performed once the active disease is quiescent. If everything else is optimal, neuroparalytic keratitis is a surmountable problem. However, anterior segment ischemia is a poor prognostic sign.

Soong and co-workers,[14] have achieved clear grafts in nine patients with scarred corneas caused by herpes zoster infections by selecting them on the basis of no active disease of the eyelids, cornea and conjunctiva, well-controlled intraocular pressures, and no active keratouveitis. In another series, 10 of 12 patients had clear grafts an average of 36 months after surgery.[13] In this series[13] and another,[10] tarsorrhaphies proved beneficial in the management of epithelial defects related to the neuroparalytic keratitis after penetrating keratoplasty.

These patients are very difficult to manage, and careful selection of surgical patients along with monitoring of the other sequelae of the infection must continue in the postoperative period. Successful management begins with early recognition of problems and immediate aggressive therapy. Allograft rejection is quite common and is managed as outlined above. The recurrence of active herpes zoster infection after grafting is uncommon.

REFERENCES

1. Cobo LM et al: Prognosis and management of corneal transplantation for herpetic keratitis, *Arch Ophthalmol* 98:1755, 1980.
2. Cohen EJ, Laibson PR, Arentsen JJ: Corneal transplantation for herpes simplex keratitis, *Am J Ophthalmol* 95:645, 1983.
3. Epstein RJ, Seedor JA, Driezen NG, et al: Penetrating keratoplasty for herpes simplex keratitis and keratoconus, *Ophthalmology* 94:935, 1987.
4. Ficker LA, Kirkness CA, Rice NS, Steele AD: Longterm prognosis for corneal grafting in herpes simplex keratitis, *Eye* 2:400, 1988.
5. Ficker LA, Kirkness CM, Rice NS, Steele AD: The changing management and improved prognosis for the corneal grafting in herpes simplex keratitis, *Ophthalmology* 16:1587, 1989.
6. Fine F, Cignetti FE: Penetrating keratoplasty in herpes simplex keratitis: recurrence in grafts, *Arch Ophthalmol* 95:613, 1977.
7. Foster CS, Duncan J: Penetrating keratoplasty for herpes simplex keratitis, *Am J Ophthalmol* 92:336, 1981.
8. Langston RHS, Pavan-Langston D, Dohlman CH: Antiviral medication and corneal wound healing, *Arch Ophthalmol* 92:509, 1974.
9. Langston RHS, Pavan-Langston D, Dohlman CH: Penetrating keratoplasty for herpetic keratitis: prognostic and therapeutic determinants, *Trans Am Acad Ophthalmol Otolaryngol* 79:577, 1975.
10. Marsh RJ, Cooper M: Ocular surgery in ophthalmic zoster, *Eye* 3:313, 1989.
11. Polack FM, Kaufman HE: Penetrating keratoplasty in herpetic keratitis, *Am J Ophthalmol* 73:908, 1972.
12. Puelhorn G, Sosath G, Thiel HJ: The effects of 5-iodo-2-deoxyuridine (IDU) and dexamethasone on corneal wound healing in the rabbit, *Acta Ophthalmol* 56:40, 1978.
13. Reed JW, Joyner SJ, Knauer WJ III: Penetrating keratoplasty for herpes zoster keratopathy, *Am J Ophthalmol* 107:257, 1989.
14. Soong HK, Schwartz AE, Meyer RF, Sugar A: Penetrating keratoplasty for corneal scarring due to herpes zoster ophthalmicus, *Br J Ophthalmol* 73:19, 1989.

Chapter 12

Aphakic and Pseudophakic Keratoplasty

Technique

RICHARD L. ABBOTT

Corneal edema in aphakic and pseudophakic eyes has become the leading indication for penetrating keratoplasty during the past decade.[1,13,17,18] The reasons for this are several: (1) There is an overall increase in cataract surgery and the ages of the patients.[2,12,20] (2) The combination of new cataract surgical techniques and intraocular lens implantation may cause increased intraocular trauma to the corneal endothelium. (3) There may be an accelerated rate of corneal endothelial cell loss after surgery, related to the lens implant style.[6,8,11,12,14] (4) There is more donor tissue available and surgeons trained to perform keratoplasty surgery. (5) The techniques and instrumentation for aphakic and pseudophakic keratoplasty have significantly improved resulting in a more favorable prognosis for a clear graft and possibly improved vision.[3,16]

This chapter is a review of the current surgical techniques and instruments used for aphakic and pseudophakic keratoplasty.

SURGICAL CONSIDERATIONS FOR APHAKIC KERATOPLASTY

Before one performs keratoplasty on a patient with aphakic or pseudophakic corneal edema, careful preoperative planning and attention must be given to the following potential problems:

1. Presence of irregular thinning or thickening and neovascularization of the host cornea
2. Presence of loose vitreous in the anterior chamber
3. Presence of anterior and posterior synechiae
4. Status of pupil and size and location of peripheral iridectomy

5. Increased incidence of elevated intraocular pressure
6. Increased incidence of cystoid macular edema
7. Status of opposite eye (phakic, aphakic, or pseudophakic)

The surgical technique of aphakic keratoplasty may vary depending on many of these findings. It is the obligation of the corneal surgeon to recognize these potential problems preoperatively so that the surgical approach can be appropriately tailored for best results. In addition, thorough familiarization with anterior vitrectomy techniques and instrumentation should be accomplished before this type of surgery is performed.

TECHNIQUE IN APHAKIC KERATOPLASTY

Surgery may be done under general endotracheal anesthesia or with retrobulbar and seventh-nerve regional anesthesia combined with intravenous analgesic and hypnotic medication administered by a standby anesthesiologist. If general anesthesia is employed, a nonpolarizing muscle relaxant (such as pancuronium bromide) may be used to prevent any "bucking" or possible movement of the patient during surgery. Before draping, attention should be given to the positioning of the patient on the operating table. Tilting the table in a slight reverse Trendelenburg position and avoiding significant hyperextension of the neck help to decrease positive vitreous pressure in the aphakic eye. Turning the patient's head slightly to the side opposite the eye to be operated on increases exposure and helps decrease any interference from the patient's nose during surgery (Fig. 12-1). Applying compression to the globe be-

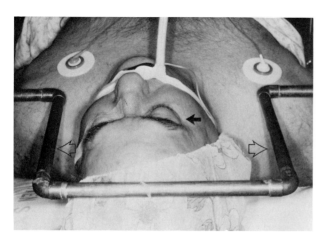

Fig. 12-1. Slight rotation of patient's head to side opposite the eye to be operated *(dark arrow)* improves exposure. *Light arrows,* Surgeon's wrist rest.

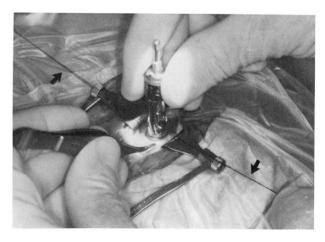

Fig. 12-2. Bridle sutures *(arrows)* placed beneath superior and inferior rectus muscles help provide stabilization during trephination.

fore surgery either with a mechanical device or digital massage lowers the intraocular pressure. In some cases, intravenous mannitol may be started 1 hour before surgery to minimize vitreous bulging once the cornea has been trephined. The operating microscope is then positioned over the patient and adjusted to the surgeon's need for height and surgical field. A microsurgical vitrectomy instrument is brought into the operating room and prepared for possible use during the surgery. After a routine sterile washing and draping of the patient are performed, the operation is ready to be begun.

A wire or solid blade lid speculum is inserted between the lids and carefully checked to ensure that there is no pressure on the globe. Either a single or double Flieringa ring may be fixed to the globe with sutures of 6-0 vicryl on a spatula type of needle. The 12 and 6 o'clock sutures are left long for stabilization of the globe by the assistant during the trephination. Extreme care must be taken in the placement of the scleral support ring, since unequal placement of the fixation sutures can cause irregularity in the graft recipient bed and considerable graft astigmatism. Because of this problem, many corneal surgeons have discontinued using the Flieringa ring and simply place a bridle suture beneath the superior and inferior rectus muscles using 5-0 silk suture. These two sutures provide a means for stabilization of the globe during trephination (Fig. 12-2). If proper care has been taken in the preoperative positioning of the patient and placement of the lid speculum, there seems to be less need for the scleral support ring.

At this time the eye is carefully inspected through the operating microscope. Attention is specifically directed to the status of the cornea and presence of

neovascularization or anterior synechiae. The anterior chamber and iris are examined to confirm preoperative findings of vitreous involvement, secondary membranes, posterior synechiae, and the status of the pupil. Using a handheld trephine of suitable diameter (either disposable or reusable), one makes a mark on the surface of the cornea that will serve as a guide to help choose the appropriate graft size. This mark is best seen if the cornea is blotted dry. If the epithelium is edematous and loose, it may be removed with a cellulose sponge at this time. The graft size should be large enough to replace a significant portion of the edematous cornea, but not so large that peripheral anterior synechiae and secondary glaucoma become an increased postoperative risk. In addition, attention must be paid to other important findings (position of the pupil, presence of peripheral iridectomy, location of deep corneal neovascularization) in the determination of the final size and position of the new corneal graft. Almost all trephine incisions in aphakic cases have been 7.5 to 8.5 mm in diameter.

At this point attention is directed away from the recipient eye to a separate table where the donor cornea is prepared (Fig. 12-3). A corneal protector is placed over the patient's eye and the microscope light is turned off. The donor cornea with scleral rim is transferred from a small vial containing either Dexsol or Optisol (both from Chiron Intraoptics, Irvine, Calif.) (Fig. 12-4) and placed on a Teflon cutting block with the epithelial surface facing down. Extreme care is taken to minimize trauma to the endothelial cells. The donor cornea is carefully centered on the Teflon block beneath the punch trephine to avoid cutting an oval button or creating a shelved edge (Fig. 12-5). A disposable trephine blade

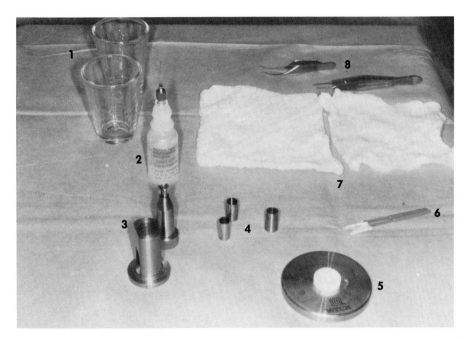

Fig. 12-3. Donor preparation table includes the following: *1*, two medicine glasses; *2*, balanced salt solution; *3*, corneal punch; *4*, disposable trephine blades (different sizes); *5*, Teflon block and punch base; *6*, cellulose sponges; *7*, moistened gauze pads; *8*, 0.12 and 0.3 mm forceps.

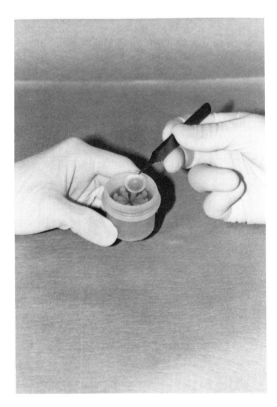

Fig. 12-4. Donor corneal tissue is removed from its storage vial for transfer to cutting block.

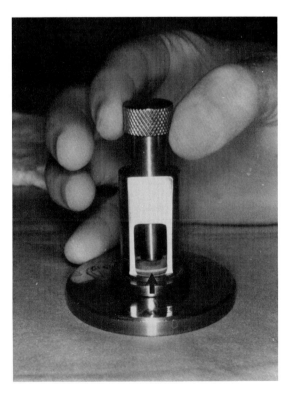

Fig. 12-5. Donor corneal tissue *(arrow)* is centered on the Teflon block before button is cut.

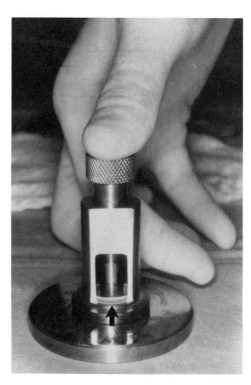

Fig. 12-6. Firm pressure is applied downward on punch trephine to allow it to pass through corneal tissue *(arrow)* and engage the Teflon block.

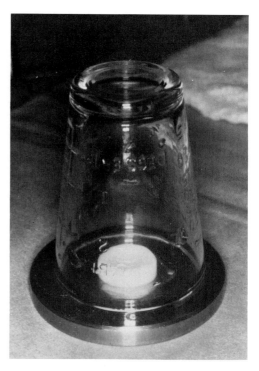

Fig. 12-8. Medicine glass is moistened with balanced salt solution and placed over corneal button and Teflon block for temporary storage of donor tissue.

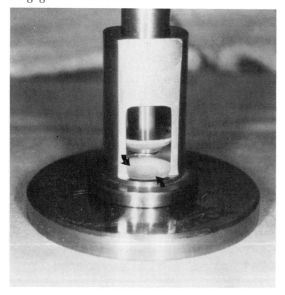

Fig. 12-7. If a clean cut has been made, donor button should remain on Teflon block *(arrows)* when punch trephine is withdrawn.

is used usually 0.2 to 0.5 mm larger than the recipient graft bed. A slightly larger donor button is punched to avoid the disparity that is created by trephination of the recipient from the epithelial surface and donor from the endothelial surface with

the same size blade.[5,10] Firm, steady pressure is applied to the punch trephine to allow it to pass through the donor tissue into the Teflon block (Fig. 12-6). When the trephine has passed through the donor corneal tissue and engages the cutting block, there is a sudden change in resistance and a distinct "crunching" sound is heard. If a clean through-and-through cut has been made, the donor button should remain on the Teflon block when the punch trephine is removed (Fig. 12-7). A drop of balanced salt solution, donor storage medium, or viscoelastic material is carefully placed on the endothelial surface to prevent drying. One then puts the donor button into a moist chamber for temporary storage by covering the Teflon block with a moistened medicine glass or transferring the donor tissue into a moistened petri dish (Fig. 12-8). The tissue is then brought back to the recipient table for later use.

Attention is now directed back to the patient where the corneal protector is removed from over the eye and the recipient cornea is once again carefully inspected. If a guarded trephine is used, it should be set for cutting at 80% depth. The assistant holds the superior and inferior rectus sutures and the surgeon grasps the horizontal limbal tissue at the 9 or 3 o'clock position with 0.12 or 0.13 mm tooth

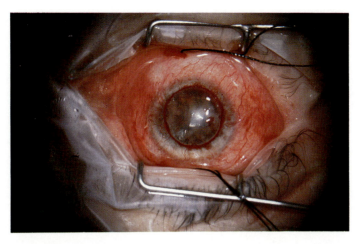

Fig. 12-9. Initial partial-thickness trephination in vascularized corneas avoids hemorrhage into anterior chamber. Bleeding stops spontaneously within a few minutes.

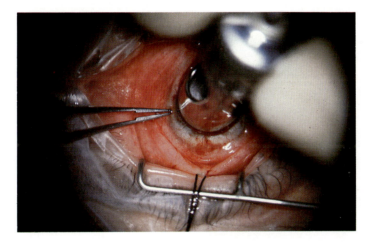

Fig. 12-10. Hand-held trephine may be placed within previous cut to deepen incision. Three-point fixation is used to stabilize globe.

forceps to stabilize the globe (Fig. 12-2). The trephine blade is then set within the previous mark on the corneal surface. After ensuring that there is not any undue pressure on the globe and the trephine is perpendicular to the corneal surface, the cutting of the corneal tissue is carefully begun. The surgeon gently rotates the trephine in a circular motion attempting to apply equal pressure on all edges of the cutting surface so that uniform depth is obtained. Care should be taken to avoid uncontrolled entry into the anterior chamber at this time.

The trephine is removed, and the depth of the incision checked with the microcyclodialysis spatula. In vascularized corneas, partial-thickness trephination allows bleeding and rapid spasm of the superficial and midstromal blood vessels, avoiding hemorrhage into the anterior chamber (Fig. 12-9). If the incision

depth is found to be unequal one may place the trephine within the previous cut by "skating" the trephine on the corneal surface and feeling the blade enter into the deeper portions of the incision (Fig. 12-10). Extreme care must be taken to avoid creating a "double cut" in the corneal tissue. This step can be repeated as often as necessary until a deep cut is obtained in all areas. Beveling of the incision through the stroma should be avoided to allow precise fitting of the donor button within the recipient bed.

The anterior chamber is slowly entered with a microsharp blade within the incision close to the point of fixation. A 3 to 4 mm incision is made to allow easy entrance of the angulated curved microcorneal scissors. The blades of the scissors are kept perpendicular to the plane of the iris, leaving a narrow rim of endothelium and Descemet's membrane on the

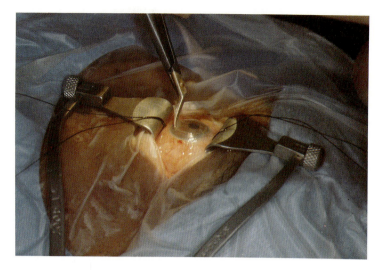

Fig. 12-11. Blades of angulated curved microcorneal scissors are kept perpendicular to plane of iris to avoid creating a large posterior bevel in wound.

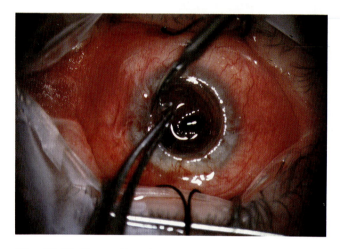

Fig. 12-12. Excess lip of Descemet's membrane may be trimmed from wound with curved Vannas scissors.

posterior margin of the recipient bed (Fig. 12-11). As the cutting of the cornea is completed, attention should be directed to its endothelial surface where vitreous attachments or iris adhesions may have to be cut before removal of the corneal tissue. In addition, any adventitious tissue should be removed from the wound with the Vannas scissors (Fig. 12-12). If the hyaloid face is intact and away from the cornea, the pupil may be constricted with acetylcholine to help maintain this state. Once the recipient cornea has been removed from the eye, several different approaches may be taken depending on the preoperative and intraoperative findings. These may be divided into four separate groups and are discussed separately:

1. Aphakia with hyaloid face intact
2. Aphakia with loose vitreous in the anterior chamber
3. Pseudophakia with hyaloid face intact
4. Pseudophakia with loose vitreous in the anterior chamber

APHAKIA WITH HYALOID FACE INTACT

If the hyaloid face is intact and away from the cornea, the pupil may be constricted with acetylcholine to help maintain this state. A decision must be made whether to insert an intraocular lens into this eye and is based on the following factors:

1. Phakic or intraocular lens in other eye
2. Aphakic and contact lens in other eye
3. Physical needs and activities of patient
4. Inability to wear a contact lens
5. Overall health of involved eye to tolerate a secondary implant
6. Relative risk of insertion and possible vitreous involvement

If an intraocular lens is to be inserted into the eye, a small amount of viscoelastic material is first placed over the pupil and on the surface of the iris to help act as a "cushion" for the underlying vitreous. Using a flexible anterior-chamber style of lens with 3-point fixation, one can perform the insertion through a 7.5 mm or larger recipient bed opening without difficulty. Once the lens is in an adequate position, additional viscoelastic material as well as balanced salt solution are used to fill the remainder of the anterior chamber. The donor button is then transferred to the recipient bed and sutured in place.

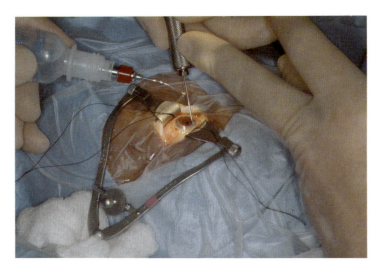

Fig. 12-13. "Open-sky" vitrectomy is performed with a mechanical vitreous cutting and aspirating instrument held within pupil or in peripheral iridectomy. Balanced salt solution may be dripped into anterior chamber during vitrectomy.

APHAKIA WITH LOOSE VITREOUS IN ANTERIOR CHAMBER

During the preoperative evaluation of the patient, attempts should be made to determine the presence of loose vitreous in the anterior chamber. If this is present or highly suspected, plans should be made before one begins the surgical procedure to prepare and have ready the use of a guillotine type of vitreous cutting and aspirating instrument. The employment of a mechanical vitreous cutting instrument in these cases reduces vitreous traction and iris inflammation associated with the technique of removal by cellulose sponge absorption.[4] Some surgeons have also advocated the evacuation of fluid vitreous through the pars plana before entry into the anterior chamber.[7]

If formed vitreous is encountered in the anterior chamber at the time of removal of the corneal button, care must be taken to cut any adhesions from the posterior surface of the cornea. Once the cornea has been removed, an "open-sky" vitrectomy is performed with the mechanical vitreous instrument held within the center of the pupil or in the peripheral iridectomy using low suction (4 to 6 mm Hg) and a rapid cutting rate (300 to 400 cuts per minute) (Fig. 12-13). Balanced salt solution may be gently dripped into the anterior chamber as needed during vitrectomy. The vitrectomy is considered adequate when the iris has dropped posteriorly well back from the recipient bed and there is no formed vitreous left in the anterior chamber. One can check this with a cellulose sponge, carefully touching the surface of the iris. Attempts should be made to free the pupil from vitreous adhesions and secondary membranes and to remove as well any strands of vitreous to the peripheral cornea. After this has been completed, the anterior chamber is filled with balanced salt solution before placement of the donor tissue within the recipient bed. If indicated, consideration for a secondary lens implant may be given before placement of the donor graft tissue.

A vitrectomy should not be performed if the vitreous face is unbroken and does not protrude anteriorly, since there is a definite increased risk of cystoid macular edema and retinal detachment occurring after this procedure.[9]

PSEUDOPHAKIA WITH HYALOID FACE INTACT

The presence of an intraocular lens in a patient with corneal edema requires careful clinical examination and planning of the surgery before one goes to the operating room. There are several important factors that must be considered when one performs surgery on these patients. If the hyaloid is unbroken or the posterior capsule is intact, the style of the implant and its effect on the eye primarily determine the surgical approach. Following are the indications for removing the intraocular lens at the time of keratoplasty:

1. Patient history of pain and signs of recurrent hyphema, uncontrolled glaucoma, or persistent uveitis.
2. Endothelial touch
3. Dislocated loops and unstable lens
4. Metal haptic materials

5. Presence of chronic cystoid macular edema

6. Iris sphincter erosion

If the pseudophakos must be removed, plans for an anterior vitrectomy must be made even if the hyaloid face is undisturbed.

Depending on the lens style and length of time that it has been in place, frequently there are strong adhesions to the angle, iris, vitreous, capsular bag, or ciliary sulcus. Removal of these lenses can be extremely difficult and traumatic to the eye and requires familiarity with the many styles of lenses that have been available for insertion over the years.[19] Various forms of iris clips and loops must be opened or cut before lysis of iris and vitreous adhesions that surround the implant. The use of blunt and sharp dissection in the removal of these lenses is required, and care must be taken to preserve as much iris tissue as possible. In some cases, supporting haptics must be cut from the lens optic and then carefully rotated free from dense fibrous tissue in the angle or ciliary sulcus. After removal of the implant, the anterior vitrectomy is performed in a similar fashion as described in the previous section. Consideration for implantation of a different style of pseudophakos can be given.

If the pseudophakos can be retained, the operation in some regards may actually be less complicated than the usual aphakic keratoplasty. The miotic pupil and intraocular lens help provide a barrier to the prolapse of vitreous through the pupil when the posterior capsule is not intact. The more recent use of posterior chamber lenses has decreased the incidence of uveitis, secondary glaucoma, and cornea-related problems and frequently allows the implant to remain in place at the time of keratoplasty.[21] Considerations for leaving the intraocular lens in place are summarized as follows:

1. Lens is in excellent position and appears stable.
2. Eye is quiet.
3. There is no low-grade inflammation.
4. Pupil is mobile.

PSEUDOPHAKIA WITH LOOSE VITREOUS IN ANTERIOR CHAMBER

In patients with pseudophakic corneal edema and loose vitreous involving the anterior segment, the course of action is mainly determined by the type of implant present. In most cases, plans should be made for removal of the pseudophakos combined with a partial anterior vitrectomy at the time of keratoplasty. The style of the implant and its position in the eye will help determine the surgical approach.

In general, iris plane lenses should be removed; however anterior chamber lenses that appear stable

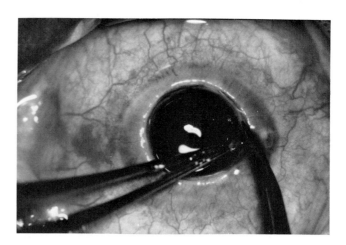

Fig. 12-14. "Open-sky" vitrectomy may be performed beneath a pseudophakos that will be left within eye.

frequently can be left in place, with the vitrectomy being performed beneath the lens (Fig. 12-14). Similar problems are encountered in the removal of these lenses as discussed in the previous section; however vitreous involvement may be more extensive and may require a partial vitrectomy before lens removal. Placement of a different style of lens implant in these eyes should be considered.

SUTURING OF DONOR BUTTON

The donor graft, which has been temporarily stored in a moist chamber on the Mayo stand, is now transferred by the surgeon to the recipient bed. [Editor's note: Many surgeons prefer cutting the donor button *immediately* before suturing rather than storing it during the preparatory surgical phases outlined.] This transferral is accomplished either by grasping of the anterior edge of the button with a fine 0.12 mm forceps (Fig. 12-15) or by use of a corneal spatula to invert the graft onto the recipient bed. Depending on the condition of the anterior chamber, either a large air bubble, balanced salt solution, or a viscoelastic substance will be present beneath the graft. If a pseudophakos is present, it is imperative that the endothelium not come into contact with it during the suturing of the graft. Care must be taken in the placement of the first corneal suture at the 12 o'clock position, since the graft is freely mobile and can easily be displaced so that possible damage to the endothelium is caused. It is recommended therefore that this first suture be placed primarily to anchor the graft in position and can easily be removed and replaced with a deeper suture if necessary. All sutures should be placed deeply

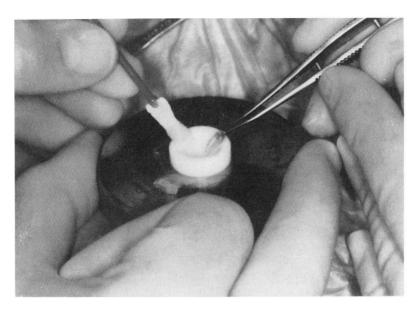

Fig. 12-15. Donor button is transferred from moist chamber to recipient bed using a 0.12 mm forceps.

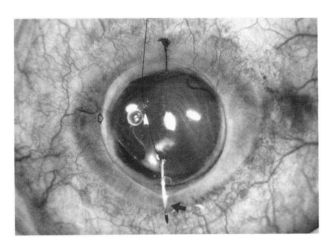

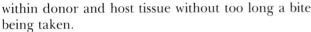

Fig. 12-16. After 6 o'clock suture, *dark arrow*, is placed, graft edges are checked at 3 and 9 o'clock for override or gaping of wound. In this case there is overriding of graft at 9 o'clock, *white arrow.*

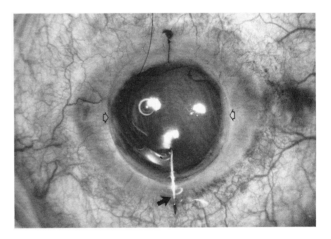

Fig. 12-17. The 6 o'clock suture is removed and placed slightly to the right, *dark arrow*. New position of graft at 3 and 9 o'clock, *white arrow*, is now better aligned.

within donor and host tissue without too long a bite being taken.

The most important suture to be placed by the surgeon is the second cardinal suture at 6 o'clock. It is this suture that most affects the final position of the donor graft within the recipient bed, and careful attention should be paid to the alignment of this suture. It is recommended that the surgeon leave the needle in place after it has been passed through both the donor and host tissue to check the graft edges at 3 and 9 o'clock positions for override or gaping of the wound (Fig. 12-16). If this is detected, the needle

can easily be backed out of the wound and repositioned; thus one can correct the possible wound disparity (Fig. 12-17). The 3 and 9 o'clock sutures are then placed equidistant between the 12 and 6 o'clock sutures. The graft surface is dried to better observe the diamond crease that forms between the four cardinal sutures. If the sutures have been placed equidistant from each other, each side of the diamond will be equal and additional sutures may now be placed. Cardinal sutures may have to be repositioned, however, if the sides of the "diamond" are not aligned, causing malposition of the donor graft

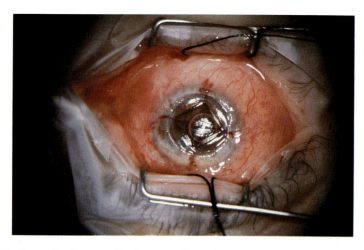

Fig. 12-18. Once the four cardinal sutures have been placed, a diamond crease will be apparent on graft surface. Wound alignment should be checked at this point before additional placement of sutures.

(Fig. 12-18). Once satisfactory placement of the initial four cardinal sutures has been completed, the anterior chamber should be redeepened with either balanced salt solution or viscoelastic material using a 2 ml syringe attached to a 30-gage angulated cannula. Closure of the wound is now complete with either additional interrupted sutures of 10-0 nylon or with a continuous suture of the same or finer nylon suture.

On completion of suturing, the anterior chamber is carefully examined to make sure that there are no synechiae present, the pseudophakos is in good position (if present), and large amounts of air or visoelastic substance have been removed. The integrity of the wound is checked by application of gentle pressure with a dry cellulose sponge between each suture on the host cornea. If any fluid escapes, either a suture is added or replaced to achieve satisfactory wound closure. They eye is left normotensive at the completion of the case. The bridle sutures are removed, and the subconjunctival injections of antibiotic (tobramycin and cefazolin) are given inferiorly. Subconjunctival injection of a corticosteroid is given when there has been a vitrectomy or significant manipulation of the iris at the time of surgery. If interrupted sutures have been used, a bandage therapeutic soft contact lens may be placed over the cornea to help promote epithelialization of the graft and provide additional patient comfort. Several drops of a combined antibiotic-corticosteroid medication are given, the lids are closed, and a monocular bandage is applied.

REFERENCES

1. Arentsen JJ, Morgan B, Green WR: Changing indications for keratoplasty, *Am J Ophthalmol* 81:313-318, 1976.
2. Bernth-Petersen, P.: A change in indictions for cataract surgery? A 10 year comparative epidemiologic study, *Acta Ophthalmol* 59:206-210, 1981.
3. Binder PS: Secondary intraocular lens implantation during or after corneal transplantation, *Am J Ophthalmol* 99:515-520, 1985.
4. Boruchoff SA: Therapeutic keratoplasty. In Smolin G, Thoft RA, editors: *The cornea*, Boston, 1983, Little, Brown.
5. Casey TA, Mayer DJ: *Corneal grafting: principles and practice*, Philadelphia, 1984, Saunders.
6. Fenzel RF, Hab SG: Evaluation of semiflexible and flexible anterior chamber intraocular lenses, *Am Intraocular Implant Soc J* 9:42, 1983.
7. Fine M: Keratoplasty in aphakia. In King JM, McTigue JW, editors, *The Cornea World Congress*, Washington, DC, 1965, Butterworth, pp 538-552.
8. Kraff MC, Sanders DR, and Lieberman HL: Monitoring for continuing endothelial cell loss with cataract extraction and intraocular lens implantation, *Ophthalmology* 89:30-34, 1982.
9. Kramer SG: Cystoid macular edema after aphakic penetrating keratoplasty, *Ophthalmology* 88:782-787, 1981.
10. Kramer SG: Keratoplasty techniques, *Trans Pacific Coast Oto-Ophthalmol Soc* 64:39-43, 1983.
11. Liesegang TJ, Bourne WM, and Ilstrup, DM: Short- and long-term endothelial cell loss associated with cataract extraction and intraocular lens implantation, *Am J Ophthalmol* 97:32-39, 1984.
12. Liesegang, TJ, Bourne, WM, Ilstrup, DM: Prospective 5-year postoperative study of cataract extraction and lens implantation, *Trans Am Ophthalmol Soc* 87:57-75; discussion 76-78, 1990.
13. Mamalis N, Craig MT, Coulter VL, et al: Penetrating keratoplasty 1981-1988: clinical indications and pathologic findings, *J Cataract Refract Surg* 17:163-167, 1991.
14. Matsuda M, Miyake K, Inaba M: Long-term corneal endothelial changes after intraocular lens implantation, *Am J Ophthalmol* 105:248-252, 1988.
15. Nadler DJ, Schwartz B: Cataract surgery in the United States 1968-1976: a descriptive epidemiologic study, *Ophthalmology* 87:10-18, 1980.

16. Olson RJ et al: Visual results after penetrating keratoplasty for aphakic bullous keratopathy and Fuchs' dystrophy, *Am J Ophthalmol* 88:1000-1004, 1979.
17. Robin JB, Gindi JJ, Koh K, et al: An update of the indications for penetrating keratoplasty, *Arch Ophthalmol* 104:87-89, 1986.
18. Smith RE et al: Penetrating keratoplasty: changing indications, 1947-1978, *Arch Ophthalmol* 98:1226-1229, 1980.
19. Stamper RL, Sugar A: *The intraocular lens,* San Francisco, 1982, American Academy of Ophthalmology.
20. Stark WJ et al: Update of intraocular lenses implanted in the United States, *Am J Ophthalmol* 98:238-239, 1984.
21. Taylor DM et al: Pseudophakic bullous keratopathy, *Ophthalmology* 90:19-24, 1983.

Penetrating Keratoplasty for Pseudophakic Bullous Keratopathy

MARK G. SPEAKER
PETER R. LAIBSON
ELISABETH J. COHEN

Pseudophakic bullous keratopathy (PBK) represents one of the most challenging as well as the most frequent[4,24] indications for penetrating keratoplasty in the United States. The challenges in many of these patients are often not limited to performing a keratoplasty with minimal postoperative astigmatism but include atraumatic removal of an intraocular lens from fibrous encasement in delicate uveal tissue, restoration of normal anterior segment anatomy, and implantation of an intraocular lens that will remain stable and not engender further inflammation. Numerous advances in tissue preservation, instrumentation, and surgical technique over the past decade have produced improved results in the treatment of intraocular lens–related corneal edema. Despite all these advances, pseudophakic bullous keratopathy is responsible for irreversible visual loss in some eyes because of persistent macular dysfunction,[5] glaucoma, or other complications such as retinal detachment.

Pseudophakic bullous keratopathy is an important chapter in the history of the development of intraocular lenses. It has been treated at great cost to patients and society[37] but has also motivated in part the advances in lens design that we enjoy today. Familiarity with the design flaws and complications of each type of intraocular lens is important in managing patients with PBK. This subject has previously been extensively reviewed by David Apple[1] and will not be reviewed here.

Medical management of pseudophakic bullous keratopathy is usually limited to controlling intraocular pressure, inflammation, and vascularization before definitive surgery. If corneal endothelial damage related to an intraocular lens can be identified before the onset of clinically significant corneal edema, surgery directed at correcting the intraocular lens problem without keratoplasty may be appropriate but is not within the scope of this chapter. If the intraocular pressure cannot be satisfactorily controlled with medications, filtration or seton surgery should be performed and stabilization of intraocular pressure achieved before keratoplasty.

The definitive therapy for pseudophakic bullous keratopathy is penetrating keratoplasty, and the principal long-term goals in penetrating keratoplasty for PBK are to achieve a clear graft with minimal astigmatism, uncomplicated pseudophakia, controlled intraocular pressure and to restore or preserve macular function. In the past, failure of grafts for PBK occurred principally in the absence of rejection, implicating intraocular lens–mediated inflammation or endothelial trauma as the cause of endothelial failure. Along with endothelial failure, glaucoma, macular edema, and macular degeneration are the principal factors responsible for poor vision after surgery for pseudophakic bullous keratopathy. The relationship between intraocular lens–mediated inflammation and the development of synechiae and glaucoma has been well established. A direct relationship between inflammation, vitreous traction from adhesion to anterior segment structures, and macular edema is strongly suspected.[19] Evidence has accumulated over the last few years that successful long-term restoration of vision is dependent in large part on successful management of the intraocular lens at the time of surgery.[5,30] Successful surgery for pseudophakic bullous keratopathy requires careful preoperative planning.

The three intraocular lens (IOL) management options that are available at the time of keratoplasty are to retain, remove without replacement, or exchange the lens. Removal of the IOL is generally not a satisfactory option in these patients because most are elderly and are not able to handle a contact lens successfully. Contact lens wear after keratoplasty also carries some risks such as infectious ulceration and, in the case of poly(methyl methacrylate), or PMMA, and probably soft contact lenses as well, hypoxic damage to the graft endothelium.[18] Gas-permeable contact lenses are relatively well tolerated by the graft endothelium[31] but are still difficult for most elderly patients to wear.

The major disadvantage of retaining the existing IOL at the time of keratoplasty is the risk of propagating the same problems to the transplanted cornea in the postoperative period. In the early 1980s the options for replacement of the lens were limited, and there was no compelling evidence that removal

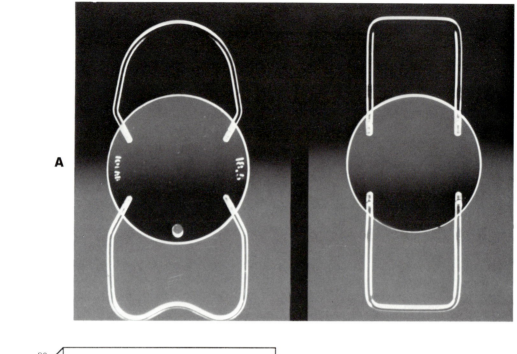

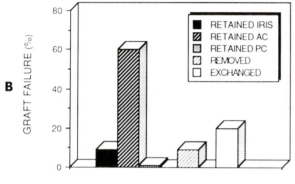

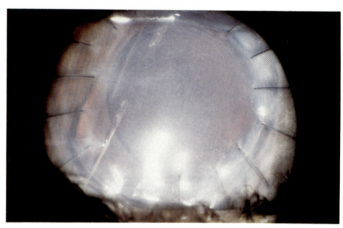

Fig. 12-19. A, Azar 91Z, *left,* and Leiske, *right,* were most popular of closed-loop semi-flexible anterior chamber lenses. **B,** Retention of these lenses at time of penetrating keratoplasty was associated with early graft failure (see reference 7), as demonstrated in **C,** clinical photograph of failed graft with retained Leiske lens.

or retention of the IOL affected the outcome.[29] In 1987, we reported that 60% of the grafts had failed at 1 year postoperatively in eyes in which a closed-loop anterior chamber IOL had been retained at surgery, prompting the recommendation that all closed-loop anterior chamber IOLs be removed at the time of penetrating keratoplasty[30] (Fig. 12-19). The indications for removal of an IOL at the time of penetrating keratoplasty for pseudophakic bullous keratopathy can be summarized as follows:

1. Any unstable IOL

2. Presence of significant uveitis, poorly controlled glaucoma, or recurrent hyphema (the UGH syndrome)
3. Metal clips or loops on the IOL
4. Any closed-loop anterior chamber IOL, such as Leiske, Azar 91Z, Stableflex, Americal 100-AC, Optiflex, Hessburg, CooperVision 600, Dannheim
5. A rigid Choyce style of anterior chamber IOL
6. Most iris-supported IOLs with the optic in front of the iris

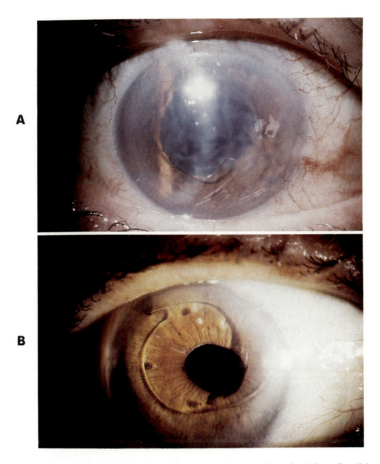

Fig. 12-20. A, Pseudophakic bullous keratopathy associated with a flexible open-loop anterior chamber lens. **B,** Haptic of undersized multiflex lens has dislocated through iridectomy, causing chronic iritis.

There are no clear indications in the literature concerning the management of PBK associated with a modern open-loop flexible anterior chamber lens. If the lens is loose or dislocated because of improper sizing or excessively large iridectomies (Fig. 12-20), the lens should be exchanged for an anterior chamber lens of the proper size, or the iris repaired. If an open-loop anterior chamber lens appears to be stably fixated but the anterior chamber is shallow, or if the eye is inflamed or tender, it should be exchanged for a suture-fixated posterior chamber lens.

Keratoplasty for pseudophakic bullous keratopathy associated with a posterior chamber lens has an excellent prognosis, and the intraocular lens should be retained unless it is unstable.[3] When pseudophakic bullous keratopathy occurs after extracapsular cataract extraction with posterior chamber lens implantation, the onset of corneal edema is quite rapid, often immediately after surgery and on average within 4 months.[3] The onset of corneal decompensation after posterior chamber lens implantation can be considered relatively rapid in contrast to anterior chamber and older iris-supported lenses. The average postoperative interval between lens implantation and the onset of corneal edema was 24 months with anterior chamber lenses and 47 months with iris-supported lenses. Preoperative endothelial dystrophy has been documented by histology in the affected eyes[16] and clinically in the fellow eyes[3] of patients with bullous keratopathy after posterior chamber lens implantation. The presence of endothelial dystrophy preoperatively implies a limited endothelial functional reserve and predisposes these patients to rapid endothelial failure after surgical trauma. These observations indicate that a careful preoperative slitlamp examination looking for guttate changes and especially signs of early corneal edema such as loss of the normal bow-shaped corneal contour in the slit beam and striae would help to identify patients at risk. Patients who report poor vision upon awakening that improves with time during the day should be examined carefully and patched overnight so that they can be examined upon eye opening when corneal edema is most apparent. Great care should be taken with these patients to perform cataract extraction as atraumatically as possible.

When an intraocular lens is removed, vitrectomy is usually necessary. The notion that vitrectomy promotes cystoid macular edema has not been supported by the series reported up to now.[12,30,39] In fact, the importance to a successful outcome of re-

storing normal anatomic relationships in the anterior segment through meticulous removal of vitreous, synechiolysis, and restoration of a central pupil with adequate iris tension, so-called anterior segment reconstruction, has been generally acknowledged.[36] Additional support for this concept was provided by the study of Price and Whitson,[21] who reported resolution after keratoplasty, vitrectomy, and IOL exchange of clinical and angiographic cystoid macular edema related to an anterior chamber lens in 75% of patients with cystoid macular edema and PBK.

The technique employed for explanation of an intraocular lens is important in order to prevent dam-

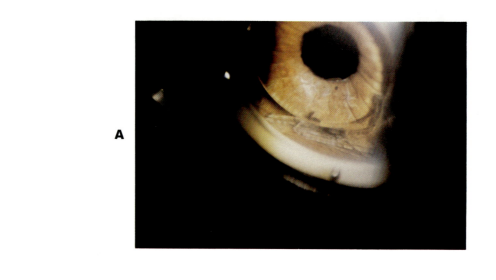

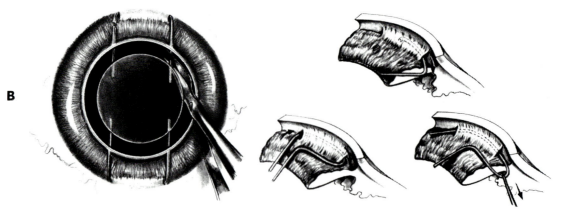

Fig. 12-21. A, Gonioscopic photo showing cocoons around haptic of closed-loop anterior lens. **B,** Removal of closed-loop lens involves amputating the haptics from the optic. One arm is left longer to facilitate manipulation, and the other is cut close to angle to facilitate rotation out of cocoon. **C,** Long arm is grasped and rotated out of cocoon. **D,** In the case of a Stableflex lens, peripheral arm of haptic is pushed into cocoon, exposing "toe" of haptic, which would otherwise be hidden from view in angle. **E,** Toe of Stableflex haptic can then be grasped with a lens hook and extracted from the cocoon. (Adapted from Epstein RJ et al: *Ophthalmic Surg* 20:599, 1989.)

age to the iris and ciliary body. The technique for removal of closed-loop anterior chamber lenses depends on the lens design and whether the haptics are embedded in fibrous tissue in the angle, so-called cocoons, or have eroded through the iris or into the wound. Therefore it is important to identify the type of lens and inspect the haptics with gonioscopy preoperatively when visibility permits (Fig. 12-21, *A*). A distinction should be made between anterior chamber lenses of a single closed-loop (Leiske, Azar 91Z), versus double closed-loop (Stableflex), and open-loop design, since the proper techniques for removal of these lenses are different and are not interchangeable without risk of significant trauma and bleeding. The appropriate technique for removal of anterior chamber lens styles involves testing the haptics for incarceration in the angle. Frequently, the superior haptic of a vertically oriented lens is not fixed in the angle and can be removed without special maneuvers. Haptics embedded in a cataract wound can be amputated and left in the eye if necessary. Those haptics that are fixed in the angle must be amputated from the optic and rotated out of the fibrous cocoons in which they are encased, as illustrated in Fig. 12-21, *C* to *E*. If bleeding occurs, it can usually be controlled by the application of viscoelastic material or cautery to the area.

Restoration of the pupil to a central, round configuration by gonioplasty and iridoplasty serves several important functions. These include prevention of glaucoma and allograft rejection related to synechia formation through restoration of symmetric centripetal tension on the iris, improvement of the support for an anterior chamber lens if it is to be used, and improvement of the optical performance of the eye. A typically employed technique is illustrated in Fig. 12-22; however, familiarity with variations of this technique as described by Waring[36] is useful.

Improved longevity of grafts, with reports of greater than 90% graft clarity after 1 year, and improved visual outcome with greater than 50% achieving a vision of 20/40 or better[11,12] can likely be attributed to the use of these techniques as well as oversized donor buttons, the availability of viscoelastic materials, improved vitrectomy instruments, and modern anterior chamber IOLs for lens exchange. These developments have provided a compelling rationale for IOL exchange combined with penetrating keratoplasty for pseudophakic bullous keratopathy.

The options for intraocular lens replacement have expanded in recent years with the development of suture fixation techniques for implantation of posterior chamber lenses in the absence of capsular support. Fig. 12-23 summarizes our approach to this problem. Before surgery, the pupil should be dilated as widely as possible, and after the application of glycerin to improve visibility, the space behind the iris should be inspected with the slitlamp for the presence of an intact posterior capsule or remnants of one. Gonioscopy may be helpful in identifying these remnants. If an adequate examination cannot be performed preoperatively, the iris should be retracted at the time of surgery to determine whether suffient capsular remnants exist. It is often necessary to dissect the iris free from the remaining capsule, and this is best accomplished with a combination of

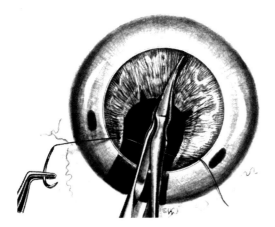 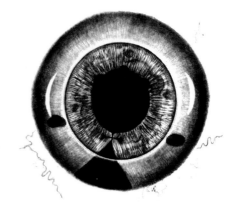

Fig. 12-22. Reconstruction of updrawn pupil after removal of corneal button. Multiple sphincterotomies, iridotomies, and a 10-0 polypropylene (Prolene) suture are used to restore a central round pupil.

MANAGEMENT OPTIONS: IOL EXCHANGE

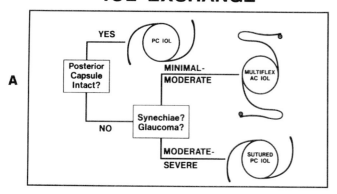

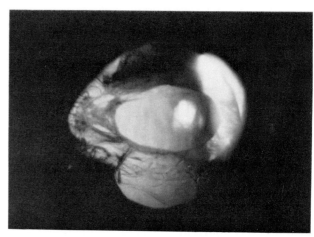

Fig. 12-23. A, Algorithm used in evaluating patients for intraocular lens exchange. When sufficient posterior capsule is present, as in **B** shown in retroillumination, access to ciliary sulcus is created by a combination of viscodissection and sharp dissection. If sufficient posterior capsular support is not available and anterior segment abnormalities such as synechiae (≤90 degrees) and glaucoma are minimal to moderate, we recommend the use of a Multiflex anterior chamber lens. When there are moderate to severe anterior segment abnormalities or glaucoma, we recommend use of a suture-fixated posterior chamber lens.

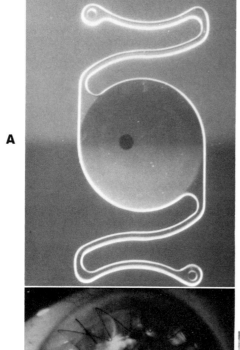

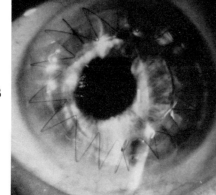

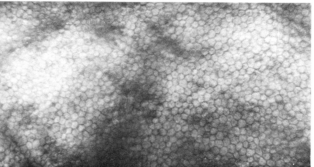

Fig. 12-24. A, Multiflex open-loop flexible anterior chamber lens. **B,** Clinical photograph and, **C,** specular microscopic view 20 months after penetrating keratoplasty and intraocular lens exchange with a Multiflex anterior chamber lens demonstrating a stable endothelial morphology (pachymetry 0.497 mm; cell density 1531/mm²; coefficient of variation 0.225; 61% hexagonal cells; figure coefficient 0.872).

viscodissection and sharp dissection. If the posterior capsule is intact or if remnants remain as is increasingly the case after complicated extracapsular surgery, a posterior chamber IOL can be implanted in the ciliary sulcus[25] (Fig. 12-23). Small remnants of posterior capsule are often sufficient for stable secondary implantation of a posterior chamber IOL, because the capsule becomes quite rigid from fibrosis within several weeks after cataract extraction. One can test the stability of lens fixation in the standard fashion by watching for immediate recentration of the optic after displacing the optic toward each haptic with a hook.

If there isn't adequate capsular support for a posterior chamber IOL, one must decide between an anterior chamber lens and suture fixation of a posterior chamber lens. The Kelman Omnifit (3-point fixation) or Multiflex (4-point fixation) style of lenses are modern open-loop, flexible anterior chamber IOLs with excellent records in primary implantation and lens exchange,[11,12,14,30,36,39] as discussed above. The advantages of these lenses compared to previous anterior chamber lenses are an excellent finish making them extremely biocompatible, an oval haptic cross section that prevents anterior vaulting, and discrete point fixation making fibrosis in the angle unlikely and facilitating explanation should it be necessary, in addition to flexible haptics, which eliminate most sizing problems.

Specular microscopy is of great value in evaluating the effects of intraocular lenses on the corneal endothelium. The development of quantitative techniques for assessing endothelial morphology has led to the observation that the phakic graft endothelium achieves a stable morphology after the first postoperative year, despite a continued decline in density through the third year.[17] Therefore the compatibility of a particular style of intraocular lens with long-term endothelial survival and graft clarity can be assessed. Specular microscopic evaluation of corneal

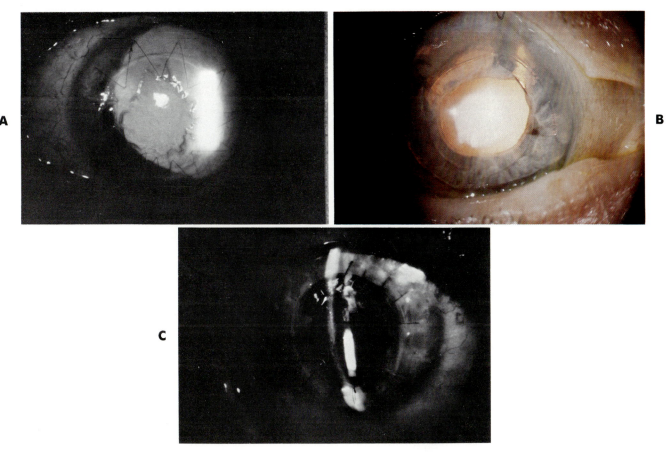

Fig. 12-25. A, Multiflex anterior chamber lens has dislocated into vitreous because of inadequate iris support. **B,** Multiflex lens has been implanted backwards so that it vaults posteriorly against iris, causing chafing and iritis. **C,** Multiflex lens is seen in proximity to graft endothelium in an eye with extensive synechiae. Graft failed 3 months after photograph was taken.

donor endothelium in eyes with a Multiflex lens found no evidence of significant intraocular lens–mediated trauma,[13,32,34] indicating a good long-range prognosis for graft clarity with these lenses in the anterior chamber (Fig. 12-24).

There are several situations in which premature graft failure or a problematic postoperative course can be anticipated after implantation of a modern anterior chamber lens. If insufficient iris tissue is available for support of the lens, the lens may be dislocated into the vitreous, or if it is too small, it may rotate through large iridectomies (Fig. 12-25). The intermediate-size Multiflex style of lens is suitable for most eyes, and the footplates should be implanted in portions of the angle that are not already compromised by synechiae. Care must be taken to avoid placing the footplates over iridectomies and to repair them if they are too large. Once implanted, the haptics should be drawn toward the optic and elevated with a lens hook to ensure that the footplates are not snagged in the peripheral iris and are properly seated in the angle. In addition, attention must be paid to implanting the lens so that it vaults in the proper direction (Fig. 12-25); otherwise the optic abrades the iris and causes significant inflammation. Patients with glaucoma contolled on more than one medication may require additional medication or glaucoma surgery after implantation of an anterior chamber lens into an already damaged angle. When anterior chamber lenses are implanted into eyes whose anterior chamber depth could not be adequately restored, the grafts develop early endothelial failure from being placed in close apposition to the lens (Fig. 12-25). Therefore, if one implants the flexible anterior chamber lens properly and avoids these problematic situations either through anterior segment reconstruction when possible or the use of a suture-fixated posterior chamber lens, the results obtained with Multiflex anterior chamber lenses for lens exchange should be quite satisfactory.

Suture fixation of posterior chamber intraocular lenses is an option for lens exchange that we prefer in patients who are not good candidates for an anterior chamber lens as described above. In the absence of adequate capsular support for a posterior chamber lens, suture fixation can be accomplished in two different ways. The optic or the haptics of the lens can be secured to the posterior surface of the iris, or the haptics can be sutured transsclerally through the ciliary sulcus.[26] Both techniques have advantages and disadvantages that have been described. It is somewhat ironic that after abandoning iris-supported lenses in the early 1980s we have come back to iris-supported posterior chamber lenses in the early 1990s.

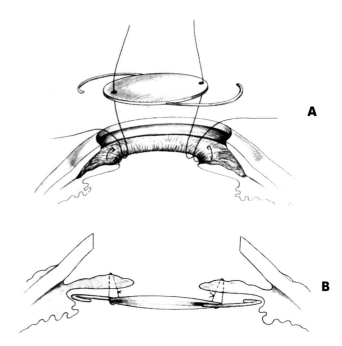

Fig. 12-26. A, Fixation of posterior chamber lens to iris using two polypropylene (Prolene) sutures passed through two positioning holes. **B,** Suture knots are tied under surface of iris. (Adapted from Price FW, Whitson WE: *Ophthalmology* 96:1234-1240, 1989.)

The iris-fixation technique is technically the most straightforward and least time consuming. Fixation of the lens haptics to the iris is not favored because of difficulties in assuring adequate fixation. Fixation of the optic to the iris is preferred, and in this technique (Fig. 12-26) 10-0 polypropylene (Prolene) sutures are passed through the positioning holes in a 4-hole[7] or 2-hole lens.[20] This technique does not require haptic fixation in the sulcus and postmortem studies have shown that the haptics do not remain there.[2] Chafing of the iris is not clinically apparent, and inflammatory complications similar to those seen with older pupil-supported lenses have not been reported up to now. One of the disadvantages of this technique is that a sufficient amount of iris tissue to support the lens is sometimes not available. In addition, use of this technique for secondary intraocular lens implantation through a limbal incision is limited by the technical difficulty of suturing within the anterior chamber.

The technique of transscleral fixation of a posterior chamber lens requires longer surgical time and more intraoperative manipulation than iris fixation or placement of an anterior chamber lens. Many surgeons believe, however, that the advantages of

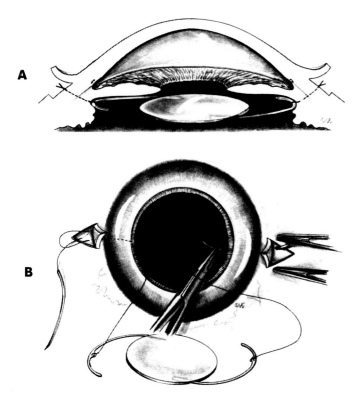

Fig. 12-27. A, Preferred position of posterior chamber lens after transscleral fixation with both haptics in ciliary sulcus. **B,** Preferred posterior chamber lens for transscleral fixation is a smaller diameter (≤12.5 mm), 7 mm optic all-PMMA lens with manufactured holes in the midpoint of the haptics. Single-armed 10-0 polypropylene (Prolene) sutures are attached through holes to haptics, and the needles are passed through keratoplasty opening, under iris, and through ciliary sulcus, *right.* Polypropylene suture exits in bed of partial-thickness scleral flap. One secures it under flap by making a superficial pass through bed of flap and tying loop that is created to tail of suture, *left.*

transscleral fixation of a posterior chamber lens outweigh these disadvantages. Favorable clinical results have been reported,[10,33] yet intraoperative and postoperative complications such as hemorrhage and lens decentration and tilt can occur.[9,10,22] Long-term stability of the lens is enhanced, and complications are minimized when fixation of both haptics in the ciliary sulcus is achieved (Fig. 12-27). With current surgical techniques, transscleral suture fixation necessitates blind passage of needles with the objective of traversing the ciliary sulcus (Fig. 12-27). We have demonstrated that the difficulty inherent in verifying intraoperatively the placement of the needles and lens haptics in the ciliary sulcus explains many of the observed complications of the procedure.[28]

Transscleral suture placement based solely on external measurements from the limbus[8] frequently misses the sulcus and leads to haptic fixation outside the sulcus.[28] It is likely that in cases performed without the benefit of direct visualization of the sulcus, neither the haptics nor the sutures are located in the ciliary sulcus, as observed in autopsy eyes.[15] Anterior placement of a suture needle through the iris root may cause intraoperative hemorrhage and postoperative synechial angle closure (Fig. 12-28, *A*). Our in vitro studies and clinical observations indicate that posterior placement of a needle can lead to asymmetric haptic fixation and subsequent decentration of the optic of the lens (Fig. 12-28, *B* and *C*). This phenomenon is analogous to the decentration reported after implantation of a posterior chamber lens in the presence of capsular support, with one haptic in the capsular bag and one in the ciliary sulcus. Clearly these complications would negate the advantages of suture fixation of a posterior chamber lens but can be avoided in part by use of techniques for direct visualization of the sulcus. Dental mirrors have been used intraoperatively with some success; however we have found that the use of an intraoperative endoscope to guide suture and haptic placement provides the best visibility and flexibility (Fig. 12-28, *D*).

We have found that in order for the surgeon to insert a haptic in the sulcus any vitreous blocking the entrance to the sulcus must be removed (Fig. 12-28, *E*). We sweep the sulcus with a cyclodialysis spatula after a thorough vitrectomy that includes the area of the sulcus before attempting placement of the needles through the sulcus and implantation of the lens. The haptics of the lens must be guided into the sulcus with lens hooks because simply pulling the sutures taut does not guarantee that the haptics will be guided into the sulcus. A smaller overall diameter posterior chamber lens (12.0 or 12.5 mm) with a 7.0 mm optic and manufactured holes in the midpoint of the haptics for attachment of sutures is preferred for transscleral fixation. The advantages of a smaller lens compared to a 13.5 mm lens is their greater stability when implanted in the sulcus because of a closer approximation of the actual sulcus dimensions and less potential for damage to ciliary processes, optic decentration and tilt, and erosion of haptics into uveal tissues.

One must fix the polypropylene (Prolene) sutures on the external surface of the sclera by tying the suture to itself (Fig. 12-28, *A* and *B*). The Prolene suture knot can erode through conjunctiva (Fig. 12-28, *F*) and cause a localized episcleritis and foreign-body sensation and pose a risk of endophthalmitis. There-

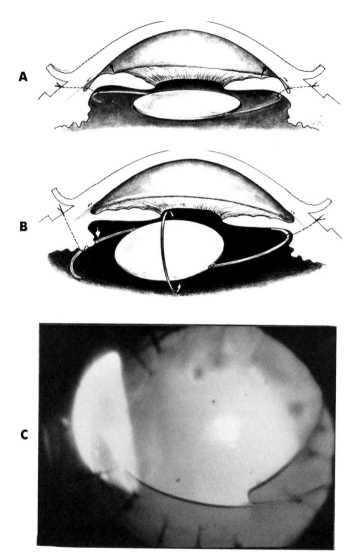

Fig. 12-28. A, Placement of transscleral sutures anterior to ciliary sulcus creates peripheral anterior synechiae and chronic angle closure glaucoma. **B,** Asymmetric transscleral fixation of haptics of a posterior chamber lens with one haptic in ciliary sulcus and one fixated posterior to sulcus causes tilting and decentration of lens. Sliding of haptic through suture loop causes progressive decentration, as demonstrated in **C,** clinical photograph showing decentered transsclerally fixated posterior chamber lens in retroillumination. **D,** Photograph taken from video monitor of intraocular endoscope showing a suture needle passing through ciliary processes during transscleral fixation. **E,** Implantation of haptics in sulcus requires removal of vitreous adherent to posterior surface of iris that is blocking the entrance to sulcus. Failure to perform adequate peripheral vitrectomy results in fixation of haptic posterior to ciliary sulcus on pars plicata. **F,** Three months after keratoplasty with transscleral fixation of posterior chamber lens. Graft is clear, visual acuity is 20/30, and posterior chamber lens and intraocular pressure are stable; however, knot of one of the polypropylene sutures has eroded through the conjunctiva and is causing a localized episcleritis. (**E** from Speaker MG et al: Complications of transscleral fixation of posterior chamber intraocular lenses outside the ciliary sulcus, *Am J Ophthalmol* [in press].)

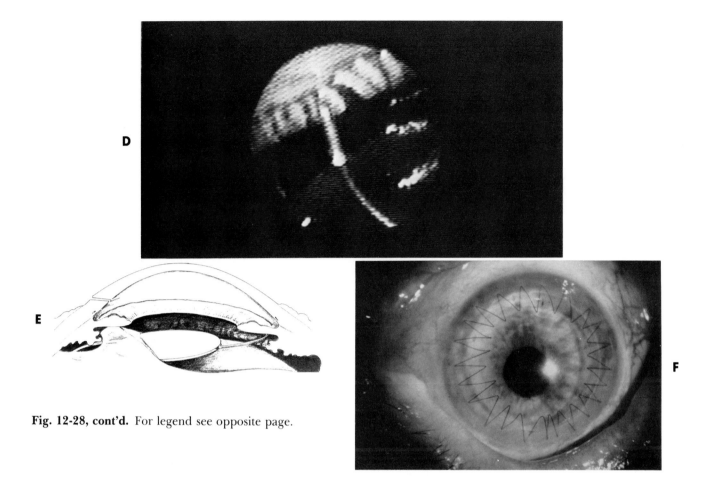

Fig. 12-28, cont'd. For legend see opposite page.

fore partial-thickness scleral flaps should be prepared before the eye is opened, under which the Prolene knots are buried. The scleral flaps and the sutures must be placed exactly 180 degrees apart; otherwise the optic of the lens will be fixed in a decentered position. Tension on the sutures should be avoided when the transscleral sutures are being tied externally because necrosis of ciliary processes with resulting intraocular inflammation, increased intraocular pressure, and cystoid macular edema may result from overtightening. Exposure of the suture knot may occur from erosion through the conjunctiva or scleral flap, in which case it may be covered with tissue such as sclera or cornea. Cutting the Prolene sutures externally should probably be avoided because our experience with two cases in

which sutured lenses were removed showed that the lenses were not fibrosed into position.

The visual results obtained with suture-fixated posterior chamber lenses have been encouraging.[20,26,35] Cohen and associates[5] pointed out that recovery of vision after penetrating keratoplasty for pseudophakic bullous keratopathy may take 1 or more years, possibly because of resolution of cystoid macular edema. Delayed resolution of cystoid macular edema would explain the observation in one series that the percentage of patients achieving 20/40 vision or better increases from 30% at 6 months to 63% at 2 years postoperatively[27] (Fig. 12-29). The early results of suture fixation of posterior chamber lenses and implantation of Kelman open-loop anterior chamber lenses combined with keratoplasty ap-

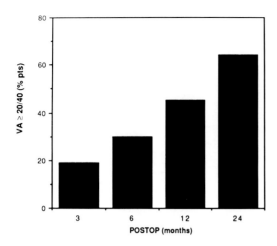

Fig. 12-29. Progressive increase with time in percentage of patients achieving a visual acuity of 20/40 or better is seen after penetrating keratoplasty and suture fixation of a posterior chamber lens. (Adapted from Soong HK et al: *Arch Ophthalmol* 107:660-665, 1989.)

pear to be similar with respect to graft survival and endothelial stability, intraocular pressure, and visual acuity.[6,13,34] Long-term results of iris versus transscleral fixation of posterior chamber lenses will be required to decide which technique is preferred and whether the results are better than those obtained with modern anterior chamber lenses. We prefer to use iris fixation over transscleral fixation of a posterior chamber lens in patients who have an existing trabeculectomy in order to avoid conjunctival manipulation that might compromise filtration postoperatively. Until more information is available, careful preoperative evaluation and choice of intraocular lens management options using the guidelines presented in this chapter should be helpful in obtaining optimal results.

A successful keratoplasty for pseudophakic bullous keratopathy should have a good long-term prognosis. Long-term follow-up studies on keratoplasties have demonstrated that once the initial endothelial remodeling and cell loss of 30% to 50% has been completed over the first 3 to 5 years after surgery, the rate of endothelial cell loss stabilizes at 2% to 3% per year.[38] This rate of cell loss is compatible with several decades of graft clarity if the initial cell density is over 2000 cells/mm², since graft clarity is compatible with cell densities under 500/mm². However, repeat keratoplasty is sometimes necessary after rejection or endothelial failure. The same principles apply to repeat surgery as to the original procedure, and the prognosis appears to be good.[23]

REFERENCES

1. Apple DJ, Mamalis N, Olson RJ, Kincaid MC: *Intraocular lenses: evolution, design, complications, and pathology,* Baltimore, 1989, Williams & Wilkins.
2. Apple DJ, Price FW, Gwin T, et al: Sutured retropupillary posterior chamber intraocular lenses for exchange or secondary implantation, *Ophthalmology* 96:1241-1247, 1989.
3. Arentsen JJ, Donoso R, Laibson PR, Cohen EJ: Penetrating keratoplasty for the treatment of pseudophakic corneal edema associated with posterior chamber lens implantation, *Ophthalmic Surg* 18:514-517, 1987.
4. Brady SE, Rapuano CJ, Arentsen JJ, et al: Clinical indications for and procedures associated with penetrating keratoplasty, 1983-88, *Am J Ophthalmol* 108:118-22, 1989.
5. Cohen EJ, Brady SE, Leavitt K, et al: Pseudophakic bullous keratopathy, *Am J Ophthalmol* 106:264-269, 1988.
6. Davis RM, Best D, Gilbert GE: Comparison of intraocular lens fixation techniques performed during penetrating keratoplasty, *Am J Ophthalmol* 111:743-749, 1991.
7. Drews RC: Posterior chamber lens implantation during keratoplasty without posterior capsule support, *Cornea* 6:30-40, 1987.
8. Duffey RJ, Holland EJ, Agapitos PJ, Lindstrom RL: Anatomic study of transsclerally sutured intraocular lens implantation, *Am J Ophthalmol* 108:300, 1989.
9. Heidemann DG, Dunn SP: Visual results and complications of transsclerally sutured intraocular lenses in penetrating keratoplasty, *Ophthalmic Surg* 21:609, 1990.
10. Johnson SM: Results of exchanging anterior chamber lenses with sulcus-fixated posterior chamber IOLs without capsular support in penetrating keratoplasty, *Ophthalmic Surg* 20:465, 1989.
11. Koenig SB, McDermott ML, Hyndiuk RA: Penetrating keratoplasty and intraocular lens exchange for pseudophakic bullous keratopathy associated with a closed-loop anterior chamber intraocular lens, *Am J Ophthalmol* 108:43-48, 1989.
12. Kornmehl EW, Steinert RF, Odrich MG, Stevens JB: Penetrating keratoplasty for pseudophakic bullous keratopathy associated with closed-loop anterior chamber lenses, *Ophthalmology* 97:407-412, discussion 413-414, 1990.
13. Lass JH, DeSantis DM, Reinhart WJ, Hossain TS, Hom DL: Clinical and morphometric results of penetrating keratoplasty with one piece anterior chamber or suture-fixated posterior chamber lenses in the absence of lens capsule, *Arch Ophthalmol* 108:1427-1431, 1990.
14. Lim ES, Apple DJ, Tsai JC, et al: An analysis of flexible anterior chamber lenses with special reference to the normalized rate of lens explantation, *Ophthalmology* 98:243-246, 1991.
15. Lubniewski AJ, Holland EJ, Van Meter WS, et al: Histologic study of eyes with transsclerally sutured posterior chamber intraocular lenses, *Am J Ophthalmol* 110:237, 1990.
16. Lugo M, Cohen EJ, Eagle RC Jr, et al: The incidence of preoperative endothelial dystrophy in pseudophakic bullous keratopathy, *Ophthalmic Surg* 19:16-19, 1988.
17. Matsuda M, Bourne WM: Long-term morphologic changes in the endothelium of transplanted corneas, *Arch Ophthalmol* 103:1343-1346, 1985.
18. Matsuda M, MacRae SM, Inaba M, Manabe R: The effect of contact lens wear on the keratoconic corneal endothelium after penetrating keratoplasty, *Am J Ophthalmol* 107:246-251, 1989.
19. Milch FA, Yannuzzi LA: Medical and surgical treatment of aphakic cystoid macular edema, *Int Ophthalmol Clin* 27:205-217, 1987.

20. Price FW, Whitson WE: Visual results of suture-fixated posterior chamber lenses during penetrating keratoplasty, *Ophthalmology* 96:1234-1240, 1989.

21. Price FW Jr, Whitson WE: Natural history of cystoid macular edema in pseudophakic bullous keratopathy, *J Cataract Refract Surg* 16:163-169, 1990.

22. Price FW, Whitson EW: Suprachoroidal hemorrhage after placement of a sclera-fixated lens, *J Cataract Refract Surg* 16:514, 1990.

23. Rapuano CJ, Cohen EJ, Brady SE, et al: Indications for and outcomes of repeat penetrating keratoplasty, *Am J Ophthalmol* 109:689-695, 1990.

24. Robin JB, Gindi JJ, Koh K, Schanzlin DJ, et al: An update of the indications for penetrating keratoplasty, 1979 through 1983, *Arch Ophthalmol* 104:87-89, 1986.

25. Smith RE, Beatty RF, Clifford WS: Pseudophakic keratoplasty: posterior chamber lens implantation in the presence of ruptured posterior capsule, *Ophthalmic Surg* 18:344-348, 1987.

26. Soong HK, Meyer RF, Sugar A: Techniques of posterior chamber lens implantation without capsular support during penetrating keratoplasty: a review, *Refract Corneal Surg* 5:249-255, 1989.

27. Soong HK, Musch DC, Kowal V, et al: Implantation of posterior chamber intraocular lenses in the absence of lens capsule during penetrating keratoplasty, *Arch Ophthalmol* 107:660-665, 1989.

28. Speaker MG, Raskin EM, Menikoff JA: Complications of transscleral fixation of posterior chamber intraocular lenses outside the ciliary sulcus, *Am J Ophthalmol.* (In press.)

29. Speaker MG, Laibson PR, Cohen EJ, Arentsen JJ: Pseudophakic bullous keratopathy. In Cavanaugh HD, editor: *The cornea*, New York, 1988, Raven Press.

30. Speaker MG, Lugo M, Laibson PR, et al: Pseudophakic bullous keratopathy: management of the intraocular lens, *Ophthalmology* 95:1260-1268, 1988.

31. Speaker MG, Cohen EJ, Edelhauser HF, et al: Effect of gas permeable contact lenses on the endothelium of corneal transplants, *Arch Ophthalmol* 109:1703, 1991.

32. Speaker MG, Cohen EJ, Edelhauser HF, et al: Effect of intraocular lens management on the endothelium of corneal transplants, *Arch Ophthalmol.* (In press.)

33. Spigelman AV, Lindstrom RL, Nichols BD: Implantation of posterior chamber lens without capsular support during penetrating keratoplasty or as a secondary lens implant, *Ophthalmic Surg* 19:396, 1988.

34. Sugar A: An analysis of corneal endothelial and graft survival in pseudophakic bullous keratopathy, *Trans Am Ophthalmol Soc* 87:762-801, 1989.

35. van der Schaft TL, van Rij G, Renardel de Lavalette JGC, Beekhuis WH: Results of penetrating keratoplasty for pseudophakic bullous keratopathy with the exchange of an intraocular lens, *Br J Ophthalmol* 73:704-708, 1989.

36. Waring GO III: Management of pseudophakic corneal edema with reconstruction of the anterior ocular segment, *Arch Ophthalmol* 105:709-715, 1987.

37. Waring GO III: The 50-year epidemic of pseudophakic corneal edema, *Arch Ophthalmol* 107:657-659, 1989.

38. Zacks CM, Abbott RL, Fine M: Long-term changes in corneal endothelium after keratoplasty: a follow-up study, *Cornea* 9:92-97, 1990.

39. Zaidman GW, Goldman S: A prospective study on the implantation of anterior chamber intraocular lenses during keratoplasty for pseudophakic and aphakic bullous keratopathy, *Ophthalmology* 97:757-762, 1990.

Lens replacement in pseudophakic bullous keratopathy

ANTERIOR CHAMBER INTRAOCULAR LENSES

JONATHAN H. LASS

The choice of an intraocular lens (IOL) for IOL exchange in pseudophakic penetrating keratoplasty or secondary IOL implantation in aphakic penetrating keratoplasty remains controversial. The poor graft and endothelial survival observed with closed-loop anterior chamber IOLs[17,19] has led to a strong interest in the use of sutured posterior chamber IOLs, either iris or scleral fixated, in these settings.[2-5,7,8,12,14-16,18,20,24] This interest has been based on the assumed advantages of an IOL situated posterior to the pupil: improved visual results because of less cystoid macular edema from a possible barrier effect on the vitreous, less secondary glaucoma because of less trabecular meshwork damage, and, most importantly, reduced endothelial cell loss because of posterior pupillary IOL location. There are disadvantages, however: the operating time is longer, vitrectomy is needed in all cases, iris or ciliary body suturing is required, and there is increased potential for endophthalmitis, retinal detachment, and vitreous hemorrhage.

Experimental[1] and clinical evidence* indicates that the Kelman-style, one-piece, open-loop poly(methyl methacrylate) (PMMA) IOL performs more favorably than the closed-loop IOL for anterior chamber insertion and is associated with long-term graft survival. The major advantages over the sutured posterior chamber IOL technique are ease and speed of IOL insertion and fixation, lack of suturing for IOL fixation, and avoidance of vitrectomy in many cases. In patients with extensive peripheral anterior synechiae, however, there is potential for greater development of the synechiae, as well as secondary glaucoma and endothelial cell loss. These potential greater risks for the anterior chamber technique, however, have not been borne out in two comparative studies of these two IOL techniques.[6,12,16] Therefore, based on retrospective experience and appealing advantages, the anterior chamber IOL technique in pseudophakic keratoplasty remains a feasible alternative in eyes with 90 degrees or less of peripheral anterior synechiae and controlled intraocular pressure.

Technique—Pseudophakic. The technique for pseudophakic keratoplasty with IOL exchange for a

---

*References 6, 7, 9, 11-13, 17, 19, 22, 23, 25.

Kelman-style, one-piece, open-loop PMMA anterior chamber lens has been well described.* Preoperatively, a Honan pressure balloon is applied. The pupil is constricted with 1% pilocarpine hydrochloride applied three times, 5 minutes apart, 1 hour before surgery. Surgery is performed under local anesthesia. A single Flieringa ring is sutured to the episclera with six interrupted 6-0 black silk sutures. The lid speculum is subsequently removed, and the silk sutures are anchored to the drape. Before trephination of the recipient bed, the size of the new anterior chamber IOL is determined by measurement of the horizontal limbal diameter and the addition of 1 mm. My method for determining power of the new anterior chamber IOL is to take the original anterior chamber IOL power and subtract 1.5 diopters, based on the assumption of an average of 1 to 2 diopters of corneal steepening postoperatively. If the original IOL is an iris-plane style, 2.5 diopters are subtracted. The graft is cut from the endothelial side, 0.25 mm larger than the recipient bed, most commonly an 8.25 mm donor in an 8.0 mm recipient bed. After partial trephination to two-thirds depth with a Hessburg-Barron trephine, the anterior chamber is entered with a no. 67 Beaver blade, and the host corneal button is excised with Castroviejo scissors, with a small shelf of Descemet's membrane being left. Lysis of any anterior or goniosynechiae is then performed in areas apart from the old anterior chamber IOL with a Barraquer cyclodialysis spatula.

Multiple techniques have been described for removal of closed-loop anterior chamber IOLs, most commonly the Stableflex lens.[9,10,17,23] Briefly, one first removes the optic by cutting each double closed-loop haptic two thirds of the distance from the optic to the angle with Vannas scissors. The haptics are then gently removed with McPherson forceps without the fibrous tissue surrounding the haptics being disturbed. Any bleeding is controlled by use of sodium hyaluronate (Healon) in the angle or compression with a Weck-Cel sponge soaked with epinephrine 1:1000. If excessive bleeding is encountered, one leaves any residual haptic material within the angle, severing any exposed material at the iris root. Once the original anterior chamber IOL is removed, if the vitreous presents in the anterior chamber, an anterior vitrectomy is performed with a disposable vitrector. Rigid, PMMA anterior chamber IOLs (such as that of Choyce) are either left in place, if there is no history of cystoid macular edema, or re-

*References 6, 7, 9-13, 17, 19, 22, 23, 25.

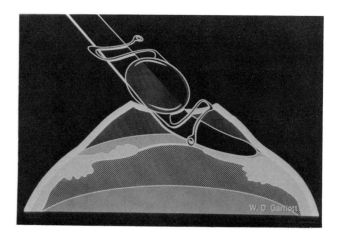

Fig. 12-30. Insertion of Kelman-style, one-piece, open-loop PMMA anterior chamber intraocular lens with lens guide during pseudophakic penetrating keratoplasty.

moved through a scleral incision before corneal trephination. All iris plane IOLs are removed. Iridoplasty is performed to repair pupillary deformities, if necessary, with a 10-0 polypropylene (Prolene) suture on a tapered needle. The pupil is then further constricted with intraocular acetylcholine, and the angle is deepened with Healon.

Positioning of the new anterior chamber IOL is determined by the presence of residual peripheral anterior synechiae and peripheral or sector iridectomies. Most commonly the new anterior chamber IOL is positioned horizontally usually from 3 to 9 o'clock within the angle with or without a disposable lens guide (Figs. 12-30 and 12-31). Either an all-PMMA, tripod-fixation anterior chamber IOL (such as the American Medical Optics Model AC 21) or an all-PMMA, open-loop, four-point-fixation anterior chamber IOL (such as the Cilco Kelman Multiflex II) is suitable for implantation. With proper placement, the pupil should remain round, with no tenting of the iris. If residual peripheral anterior synechiae are believed to be greater than 90 degrees, sutured, sclera-fixated, posterior chamber IOL implantation is performed, or the eye is left aphakic. After implantation, the anterior chamber is filled with Healon, and the donor button is sewn in place.

Technique—Aphakic. The technique for aphakic keratoplasty with secondary anterior chamber IOL implantation is essentially the same as that described above, except that anterior vitrectomy is required in all cases and IOL power calculation and positioning differ. Power calculation can be determined based on the keratometry and axial-length measurement of the fellow eye along with comparison of the previous spectacle correction of both eyes, or it may be based on the axial length measurement of the operative eye and an average keratometry reading (such as 43 D) determined from one's own previous keratoplasty experience. If, as often, a sector iridectomy is present, the anterior chamber IOL will have to be positioned horizontally.

Anterior Chamber IOL versus Sutured Posterior Chamber IOL in Pseudophakic Keratoplasty. Reports concerning these two procedures in pseudophakic keratoplasty have described the clinical results of a retrospective, nonrandomized series of cases for either procedure at a given center. Table 12-1 shows graft survival ranging from 88% to 100% for the published anterior chamber IOL series and from 76% to 98% for the published sutured posterior chamber IOL series, with follow-up observation as long as 5 years for either IOL technique. Eyes with a postoperative best-corrected visual acuity of 20/40 have ranged from 18% to 58% for the anterior chamber IOL series and from 7% to 60% for the sutured posterior chamber IOL series.

There have been, however, few studies performed at the same center comparing graft clarity, visual results, control of intraocular pressure, and endothelial survival with these two IOL types after penetrating keratoplasty. Our center has reported such data on 25 patients with an open-loop anterior chamber IOL and 24 patients with a posterior chamber IOL sutured to the iris 1 year after penetrating keratoplasty.[12] At this endpoint, we found that average best-corrected visual acuity was comparable between the two groups. Similarly, 29% of the eyes were 20/40 or better best corrected in the anterior chamber IOL group and 25% in the sutured posterior chamber IOL group. The Michigan center similarly found no difference in the percentage of patients with 20/40 or better best-corrected visual acuity at 1 year: 39% in their anterior chamber IOL group and 45% in their sutured posterior

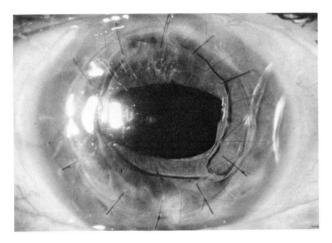

Fig. 12-31. Horizontally placed Cilco Multiflex II anterior chamber intraocular lens 6 months after pseudophakic penetrating keratoplasty.

Table 12-1. Results of Penetrating Keratoplasty in Pseudophakic Bullous Keratopathy with Intraocular Lens (IOL) Exchange

Study	Number of Eyes	Follow-up (months)	Clear Grafts (%)	Visual acuity* (≥20/40)	New Cases of Glaucoma (%)	Average Endothelial Cell Loss at 1 Year (%)
Sutured posterior chamber IOL						
Busin et al.[3]	14	3-18	93	7	29	NR
Cowden and Hu[4]	14	2-14	93	7	NR	NR
Hall and Muenzler[5]	53	6-63	88	37	6	NR
Johnson[8]	47	5-30	98	27	NR	NR
Lass et al.[12]	24	12	96	29	4	27
Price and Whitson[14]	233	12-68	96	60	2	NR
van der Schaft et al.[20]	215	12-56	76	45	24	NR
Soong et al.[15]	53	3-13	96	43	NR	NR
Soong et al.[16]	133	3-24	97	45	16	19
Sugar[19]	701	NR	92	NR	NR	19
Open-loop anterior chamber IOL						
Hassan et al.[6]	40	4-51	95	39	23	11
Koenig et al.[9]	20	4-45	100	35	25	NR
Kornmehl et al.[11]	40	7-59	95	58	10	NR
Lass et al.[12]	25	12	88	25	0	32
Polack[13]	99	12-60	94	18	NR	NR
Sugar[19]	19	NR	95	NR	NR	17
Zaidman and Goldman[25]	36	3-32	89	31	14	NR

NR, Not reported or not specified.
*Last examination.

chamber IOL group.[6,16] Differences in visual results between these two centers may be attributable to patient differences in preexisting cystoid macular edema and macular degeneration.

Both centers have provided detailed intraocular pressure data, demonstrating comparable control for the two IOL types, contrary to previous postulation. In our study, average intraocular pressure did not differ for the two groups at 1 year.[12] In addition, no new cases of glaucoma occurred in our anterior chamber IOL group and only one new case (4%) in the sutured posterior chamber IOL group. Compared with our results, those of the Michigan center showed a higher percentage of new glaucoma cases in both their anterior chamber IOL group (23%)[6] and their sutured posterior chamber IOL group (16%)[18]; however, the two IOL groups at the Michigan center were comparable to ours.

Most importantly, both centers found that the two IOL groups experienced the same average endothelial cell loss at 1 year (Table 12-1), disputing the assumed advantage of the posterior pupillary location of the IOL in protecting the endothelium, at least when the posterior capsule is absent. In fact, the Michigan center has extended their observations to 2 years on 35% of their initial patient population and, surprisingly, found 38% cell loss in their sutured posterior chamber IOL,[18] compared with 21% in their anterior chamber IOL group.[6] Whether a similar difference in cell loss between the two IOL groups beyond 1 year will be found with a greater number of patients in each group remains to be determined.

Conclusions. Based on the simplicity of performance and comparable long-term clinical success and endothelial survival, the open-loop anterior chamber IOL technique is a feasible alternative to the sutured posterior chamber IOL technique in pseudophakic penetrating keratoplasty. However, deficiencies in study design (that is, retrospective, nonrandomized) of the published reports (Table 12-1) on the clinical performance and endothelial survival for either IOL type preclude a definitive determination of which IOL technique is favorable when there is sufficient angle to accommodate an anterior chamber IOL. The conclusions of these reports may have been influenced by case-selection bias, varying follow-up observation, and incomplete data retrieval. A prospective, randomized trial clearly addresses these deficiencies and would provide a definitive conclusion on the advantages of one IOL type over the other in regard to graft clarity, best-corrected acuity, development of new glaucoma, and other complications (such as hemorrhage,

endophthalmitis), and endothelial cell survival.

A prospective study of this question should control for differing donor characteristics by the use of paired donors. The exclusion of those eyes in which an anterior chamber IOL could not be positioned (peripheral anterior synechiae greater than 90 degrees) should allow for proper randomization of eyes with equal risk for cystoid macular edema and new glaucoma development. An anterior vitrectomy should also be performed on all eyes, since this procedure may affect development of cystoid macular edema. Finally, the study should be of sufficient duration (3 to 5 years) to allow detection of any long-term differences between the two IOL types in terms of (1) best-corrected visual acuity, including any improvement attributable to resolution of chronic cystoid macular edema, (2) development of new glaucoma attributable to progressive secondary angle closure glaucoma, and (3) any progression in endothelial cell loss beyond 1 year. Only such a trial, suggested by numerous authors,[2,6,11-12,16,21,25] will resolve the management of pseudophakic bullous keratopathy, the most common indication for penetrating keratoplasty today.

REFERENCES

1. Apple DJ et al: Anterior chamber lenses. Part II: A laboratory study, *J Cataract Refract Surg* 13:175, 1987.
2. Apple DJ et al: Sutured retropupillary posterior chamber intraocular lenses for exchange or secondary implantation, *Ophthalmology* 96:1241, 1989.
3. Busin M et al: Complications of sulcus-supported intraocular lenses with iris sutures, implanted during penetrating keratoplasty after intracapsular cataract extraction, *Ophthalmology* 97:401, 1990.
4. Cowden JW, Hu BV: A new surgical technique for posterior chamber lens fixation during penetrating keratoplasty in the absence of capsule or zonular support, *Cornea* 7:231, 1988.
5. Hall JR, Muenzler WS: Intraocular lens replacement in pseudophakic bullous keratopathy, *Trans Ophthalmol Soc UK* 104:541, 1985.
6. Hassan TS et al: Implantation of Kelman-style, open-loop anterior chamber lenses during keratoplasty for aphakic and pseudophakic bullous keratopathy: a comparison with iris-sutured posterior chamber lenses, *Ophthalmology* 98:875, 1991.
7. Insler MS, Kook MS, Kaufman HE: Penetrating keratoplasty for pseudophakic bullous keratopathy associated with semi-flexible, closed-loop anterior chamber intraocular lenses, *Am J Ophthalmol* 107:252, 1989.
8. Johnson SM: Results of exchanging anterior chamber lenses with sulcus-fixated posterior chamber IOLs without capsular support in penetrating keratoplasty, *Ophthalmic Surg* 20:465, 1989.
9. Koenig SB, McDermott ML, Hyndiuk RA: Penetrating keratoplasty and intraocular lens exchange for pseudophakic bullous keratopathy associated with a closed-loop anterior chamber intraocular lens, *Am J Ophthalmol* 108:43, 1989.
10. Koenig SB, Solomon JM: Removal of closed-loop anterior

chamber intraocular lenses during penetrating keratoplasty, *Cornea* 6:207, 1987.

11. Kornmehl EW et al: Penetrating keratoplasty for pseudophakic bullous keratopathy associated with closed-loop anterior chamber intraocular lenses, *Ophthalmology* 97:407, 1990.

12. Lass JH et al: Clinical and morphometric results of penetrating keratoplasty with one-piece anterior chamber or suture-fixated posterior chamber lenses in the absence of lens capsule, *Arch Ophthalmol* 108:1427, 1990.

13. Polack FM: Results of keratoplasty for aphakic or pseudophakic corneal edema with intraocular lens implantation or exchange, *Cornea* 7:239, 1988.

14. Price FW Jr, Whitson WE: Visual results of suture-fixated posterior chamber lenses during penetrating keratoplasty, *Ophthalmology* 96:1234, 1989.

15. Soong HK, Meyer RF, Sugar A: Posterior chamber IOL implantation during keratoplasty for aphakic or pseudophakic corneal edema, *Cornea* 6:306, 1987.

16. Soong HK et al: Implantation of posterior chamber intraocular lenses in the absence of lens capsule during penetrating keratoplasty, *Arch Ophthalmol* 107:660, 1989.

17. Speaker MG et al: Penetrating keratoplasty for pseudophakic bullous keratopathy: management of the intraocular lens, *Ophthalmology* 95:1260, 1988.

18. Spiegelman AV et al: Implantation of a posterior chamber lens without capsular support during penetrating keratoplasty or as a secondary lens implant, *Ophthalmic Surg* 19:396, 1988.

19. Sugar A: An analysis of corneal endothelial and graft survival in pseudophakic bullous keratopathy, *Trans Am Ophthalmol Soc* 87:762, 1989.

20. van der Schaft TL et al: Results of penetrating keratoplasty for pseudophakic bullous keratopathy with the exchange of an intraocular lens, *Br J Ophthalmol* 73:704, 1989.

21. Waring GO III: The 50-year epidemic of pseudophakic corneal edema, *Arch Ophthalmol* 107:657, 1989.

22. Waring GO III, Kenyon KR, Gemmill MC: Results of anterior segment reconstruction for aphakic and pseudophakic corneal edema, *Ophthalmology* 95:836, 1988.

23. Waring GO III, Stulting RD, Street D: Penetrating keratoplasty for pseudophakic corneal edema with exchange of intraocular lenses, *Arch Ophthalmol* 105:58, 1987.

24. Wong SK et al: Use of posterior chamber lenses in pseudophakic bullous keratopathy, *Arch Ophthalmol* 105:856, 1987.

25. Zaidman GW, Goldman S: A prospective study on the implantation of anterior chamber intraocular lenses during keratoplasty for pseudophakic and aphakic bullous keratopathy, *Ophthalmology* 97:757, 1990.

POSTERIOR CHAMBER INTRAOCULAR LENSES—IRIS FIXATED

W. STANLEY MUENZLER
J. ROGER HALL

Pseudophakic bullous keratopathy (PBK) continues to be one of the leading indications for penetrating keratoplasty.[2] Because of the large numbers of closed-looped anterior chamber lenses previously implanted, along with other styles now discontinued, PBK will likely remain one of the major reasons for penetrating keratoplasty for some time.[21] Whenever

possible, PBK should be treated with exchange of the lens implant. Exceptions to this would be well-positioned posterior chamber lenses and, rarely, a well-positioned anterior chamber lens. In the unusual cases of recurrent hemorrhage or uncontrolled uveitis, the lens should be removed and not exchanged. Glaucoma must be controlled before keratoplasty though some advocate the addition of trabeculectomy at the time of penetrating keratoplasty.[8]

This section deals with lens replacement in PBK utilizing sutured posterior chamber lenses, suturing through four positioning holes. Other authors have described suturing the lens in the retrocorneal space using two positioning holes,[15] suturing the haptic to the iris,[5] and sulcus-to-sclera suture fixation.[4,9,18]

Technique. Most cases are performed under local anesthesia, though general anesthesia may be indicated in some situations or at the surgeon's preference. A soft globe is mandatory, at times requiring intravenous agents.

Lid and scleral support are provided by the McNeill-Goldman ring. The outer ring is sutured loosely to the sclera so that there is minimal distortion of the globe and minimal pressure from the lids. This ring also provides excellent stabilization of the eye for trephination. One of us (J.R.H.) does not use a ring.

The donor cornea is then transferred to the Brightbill block where it is punched from the endothelial surface with a disposable trephine blade. In cases with normal anterior chamber depth, the donor is trephined with a blade 0.25 mm larger than the recipient. In cases with a shallow anterior chamber or with glaucoma, a donor 0.5 mm larger is used. The corneal button is then transferred to a Fine corneal storage box and covered with media from the donor cornea.

Before the recipient eye is entered, the posterior chamber lens is prepared. The lens generally used is a nonangulated J- or C-loop lens with four positioning holes. The lens is placed on a tissue wipe under the operating microscope. Two 10-0 polypropylene sutures with tapered needles are used (BV100-4, Ethicon). One suture is placed up through the positioning holes on each side (Fig. 12-32). The suture is stretched slightly and covered with viscoelastic material to make it more manageable. The tissue wipe is folded over the implant with its preplaced sutures and placed aside.

The recipient cornea is trephined to a depth of about 80% with a disposable blade. The anterior chamber is then entered and the globe slowly decompressed. The implant is removed after inspection of the angle with a dental mirror according to

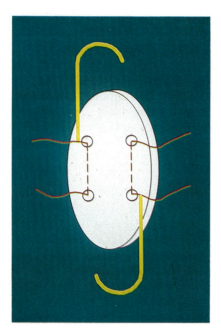

Fig. 12-32. Before entering recipient eye, 4-hole posterior chamber lens is prepared on a tissue wipe with use of two 10-0 polypropylene sutures double armed with tapered needles. Two needle ends of the first suture passed upwards through positioning holes on one side, and then second suture is similarly placed through the opposite side holes. Later, lens with needles and sutures transferred to the eye and viewed against iris for best positioning.

the method described by Waring.[20] Some rigid anterior chamber lenses and Copeland style of lenses may be removed without disturbance to the vitreous, but most other lenses will require vitrectomy after removal from their entrapment in the angle. Gonioplasty and iridoplasty may be needed and can be performed at this time. Bleeding from the angle is controlled with cellulose sponges soaked in 1:1000 epinephrine. Viscoelastic materials are also beneficial to control bleeding. In rare cases, a bipolar cautery is used. Vitrectomy is then accomplished with a mechanical vitrectomy instrument until the iris falls posterior to its normal plane and no further strands are found with dry cellulose sponges. The pupil is contracted with acetylcholine, and the posterior segment is refilled with normal saline.

The lens implant is then held over the iris to determine the best position for its placement, with avoidance of any atrophic areas. Two small tying forceps are used to handle the lens and suture. The first suture is placed up through the iris in the lower quadrant, emerging at approximately the midperipheral iris (Fig. 12-33). The second suture is then placed in the upper quadrant. The sutures are then

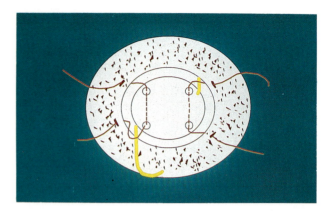

Fig. 12-33. First needle is placed up through the midperipheral iris in lower quadrant and other end through midperipheral upper iris. Similar maneuvers are then carried out on opposite side. Inferior loop is then placed behind iris, and superior loop is last to be positioned behind iris. Two ends of right suture and two ends of left suture are tied together with knots in front of iris.

inserted on the opposite side. The inferior haptic and then the entire optic is placed behind the iris. The two ends of the right suture and then the two ends of the left suture are tied with knots, which are placed in front of the iris. A double-throw square knot with one separate throw is tied on each side of the anterior surface of the iris so that any pinching of the tissue is avoided. The suture ends are cut flush to the knot. Saline is once again used to fill the globe, and dry cellulose sponges are utilized to detect any vitreous that might present around the implant or through the iridectomies. A small amount of viscoelastic material is used to coat the implant and the iris. The donor cornea is then sutured in place with 12 interrupted 10-0 nylon sutures. The edges are aligned with a 25-gage bent needle, and the knots are buried in the stroma. A running 10-0 nylon suture is then placed between each of the single sutures. The edges are realigned once again, the anterior chamber is filled with saline, and after the wound is found to be watertight, subconjunctival injections of antibiotic and steroid are given. Physostigmine sulfate 0.25% ointment is instilled in the cul-de-sac, and a patch and shield are applied.

Postoperative Care. Postoperative care must be tailored to each individual case, and no case can be considered as routine. Special attention to the epithelium and intraocular pressure are important. Patching, frequent lubrication, tarsorrhaphy, and punctal occlusion may all be necessary in cases of delayed epithelialization. The intraocular pressure must be monitored closely, especially during the first few weeks, and any changes are treated appropriately.

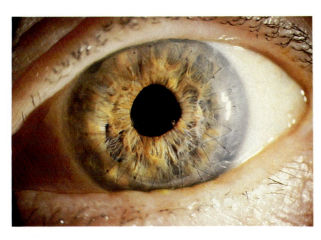

Fig. 12-34. Recent postoperative. Sutures at 2 and 8 o'clock positions. Some gathering of iris at 8 o'clock. Small iris tag at 4 o'clock.

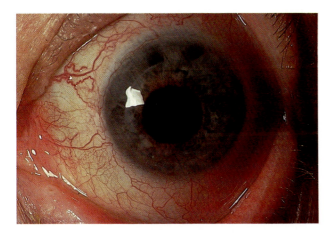

Fig. 12-35. Four years' postoperative view. Sutures at 12 and 6 o'clock positions. Pupil round and regular.

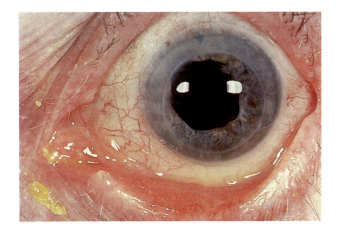

Fig. 12-36. Nine years' postoperative view. Sutures at 4 and 10 o'clock positions. Pupil dilates well.

Table 12-2. Types of Preoperative Visual Acuity

Preoperative Visual Acuity	Number of Eyes
Light perception and projection	1
Hand movements	4
Finger counting	24
20/400	27
20/200	8
20/60-100	3
	67

Table 12-3. Types of Postoperative Visual Acuity

Postoperative Visual Acuity	Number of Eyes	Percent of Total
No light perception	1	
Hand movement	2	
Finger counting	6	28%
20/400	4	
20/200	6	
20/50-100	20	30%
20/20-40	28	42%
	67	

Results. We have presented the initial[7,13,22] and long-term[14] results of this procedure (Figs. 12-34 to 12-36). Others have reported similar findings.[12,17,19] Long-term results in 42 cases showed all eyes with clear thin grafts at 2 years. Three cases developed typical homograft rejections. The visual acuity was stable in 34 of the 42, had improved in 4 cases because of clearing of cystoid macular edema, and had decreased in 4 cases. One of the cases that lost vision was from an irreversible graft rejection, and 3 cases were worse from age-related macular degeneration. There were no new cases of glaucoma. Pachymetric readings were stable, and gonioscopy revealed no changes in the angle. Pseudophakodonesis was minimal.

An additional unreported 67 cases have been followed for a minimum of 2 years. The range of follow-up observation was 32 months to 5 years. Preoperative acuity was less than 20/200 in all but 3 cases (Table 12-2). Postoperatively, acuity improved in 80% at the 2-year level with only 3 cases being worse than the preoperative level (Table 12-3). Cystoid macular edema improved clinically in eight cases. Grafts were clear in 88%. In the 8 cases with edematous grafts, 5 of these were from homograft rejections and 3 were from ocular surface failures. Ninety-five percent of the cases showed visual acuity of 20/200 or worse preoperatively. Postoperatively,

80% were better than 20/200, with 42% between 20/20 and 20/40, 30% between 20/50 and 20/100, and 28% at 20/200 or worse. Additional glaucoma medications were required in 5 cases, with one patient requiring trabeculectomy and one eye being lost from uncontrollable glaucoma and requiring a retrobulbar alcohol injection.

Discussion. The major theoretical advantage of this technique is in the avoidance of the anterior chamber structure such as the trabecular meshwork, the angle recess, and the endothelium of the cornea. Of course, the lens is closer to the nodal point of the eye. The use of posterior chamber lenses sutured to the sclera have shown nearly equal short-term results[4,9,18] and have the theoretical advantage of less contact with the iris. Also, they may be inserted in cases where there is complete absence or severe loss of iris tissue. They have the potential disadvantage of infection hemorrhage, and erosion into the uveal tissue.[3,10] Open-loop anterior chamber lenses have been recently utilized with long-term follow-up study[11] with comparable results. It would appear that the only real advantage of the flexible tripod anterior chamber lens is its ease of insertion. With the method described here, it is believed that insertion of a sutured posterior chamber intraocular lens may be accomplished with no greater difficulty than one in the anterior chamber and with no increased operating time. Results have generally been predictable, and one is able to tell the patient that (1) the pain or irritation that many have will almost always be relieved, (2) the vision will almost always be improved, and (3) in many instances the vision will gradually improve.[16]

Are these lenses more than iris supported? One cannot be certain of that except in pathologic specimens, where they do not appear to be.[1] However, they appear to be stable with little movement, which makes one believe that there may be some fixation beyond that provided by the sutures. Which of these approaches is the preferred one? Perhaps only multicenter prospective studies will answer this question.[21] In the meantime, each method has its merits, and one should be prepared to utilize or modify these procedures at the time of surgery. Results have been similar but varied, perhaps because of the art so succinctly stated in Eisner:[6] "The underlying cause of success or failure remain obscure. This may be why the operative methods described by one author are often less successful in other hands: although the method has been learned, the craftsmanship has not. The experience, dexterity, and intuition are not conscious processes and are thus difficult to transfer to others."

In summary, a method of suturing posterior chamber lenses at the time of penetrating keratoplasty with lens exchange is presented. Long-term results of this procedure have been reasonably predictable and generally improve the overall status of the eye.

REFERENCES

1. Apple DJ, Price FW, Gwin T, et al: Sutured retropupillary posterior chamber intraocular lenses for exchange or secondary implantation, *Ophthalmology* 96:1241-1247, 1989.
2. Brady SE, Rapuano CJ, Arentsen JJ, et al: Clinical indications for and procedures associated with penetrating keratoplasty, *Am J Ophthalmol* 108:118-122, 1989.
3. Busin M, Brauweiler P, Böker T, Spitznas M: Complications of sulcus-supported intraocular lenses with iris sutures, implanted during penetrating keratoplasty after intracapsular cataract extraction, *Ophthalmology* 97:401-406, 1990.
4. Cowden JW, Hu BV: A new surgical technique for posterior chamber lens fixation during penetrating keratoplasty in the absence of capsular or zonular support, *Cornea* 7(3):231-235, 1988.
5. Drews RC: Posterior chamber lens implantation during keratoplasty without posterior chamber lens capsule support, *Cornea* 6:38-40, 1987.
6. Eisner G: *Eye surgery*, ed 2, Berlin, 1990, Springer-Verlag; see its introduction.
7. Hall JR, Muenzler WS: Intraocular lens replacement in pseudophakic bullous keratopathy, *Trans Ophthalmol Soc UK* 104:541-545, 1985.
8. Insler MS, Cooper HD, Kastl PR, Caldwell DR: Penetrating keratoplasty with trabeculectomy, *Am J Ophthalmol* 100:593-595, 1985.
9. Johnson SM: Results of exchanging anterior chamber lenses with sulcus-fixated posterior chamber IOLs without capsular support in penetrating keratoplasty, *Ophthalmic Surg* 20(7):465-468, 1989.
10. Koch DD: The dilemma of pseudophakic bullous keratopathy, *Ophthalmol Surg* 20(7):463-464, 1989.
11. Kornmehl EW, Steinert RF, Odrich MG, et al: Penetrating keratoplasty for pseudophakic bullous keratopathy associated with closed-loop anterior chamber intraocular lenses, *Ophthalmology* 97:407-414, 1990.
12. Lass JH, DeSantis DM, Reinhart WJ, et al: Clinical and morphometric results of penetrating keratoplasty with one-piece anterior chamber or suture-fixated posterior chamber lenses in the absence of lens capsule, *Arch Ophthalmol* 108:1427-1431, 1990.
13. Muenzler WS, Hall JR: Lens replacement in pseudophakic bullous keratopathy. In Brightbill FS editor: *Corneal surgery*, St. Louis, 1986, Mosby–Year Book.
14. Muenzler WS, Hall JR: Long-term evaluation of sutured-in posterior chamber lenses. In Cavanaugh HD, editor: *The cornea: Trans World Congress on the Cornea III*, New York, Raven Press, pp 365-366.
15. Price FW Jr, Whitson WE: Visual results of suture-fixated posterior chamber lenses during penetrating keratoplasty, *Ophthalmology* 96:1234-1240, 1989.
16. Price FW Jr, Whitson WE: Natural history of cystoid macular edema in pseudophakic bullous keratopathy, *J Cataract Refract Surg* 16:163-169, 1990.
17. Soong HK, Musch DC, Kowal V, et al: Implantation of posterior chamber intraocular lenses in the absence of lens capsule

during penetrating keratoplasty, *Arch Ophthalmol* 107:660-665, 1989.

18. Stark WJ, Gottsch JD, Goodman DF, et al: Posterior chamber intraocular lens implantation in the absence of capsular support, *Arch Ophthalmol* 107:1078-1083, 1989.
19. Sugar A: An analysis of corneal endothelial and graft survival in pseudophakic bullous keratopathy, *Trans Am Ophthalmol Soc* 87:762, 1989.
20. Waring GO III: Management of pseudophakic corneal edema with reconstruction of the anterior ocular segment, *Arch Ophthalmol* 105:709-715, 1987.
21. Waring GO III: The 50-year epidemic of pseudophakic corneal edema, *Arch Ophthalmol* 107:657-659, 1989.
22. Wong SK, Stark WJ, Gottsch JD, et al: Use of posterior chamber lenses in pseudophakic bullous keratopathy, *Arch Ophthalmol* 105:856-857, 1987.

POSTERIOR CHAMBER INTRAOCULAR LENSES—SCLERA FIXATED
PETER A. RAPOZA

The number of penetrating keratoplasties performed yearly continues to increase in frequency. In a review of 2299 penetrating keratoplasties performed between 1983 and 1988, 526 cases (22.9%) were performed for the indication of pseudophakic bullous keratopathy (PBK).[3] Over this 5-year period the percentage of cases of PBK grew from 43 (12.1%) to 108 (27.4%), becoming the most common indication for corneal transplantation. The majority of the intraocular lenses (IOLs) present within eyes requiring penetrating keratoplasty were anterior chamber lenses (AC IOL) 62.9%, followed by posterior chamber (PC IOL) 12.0%, iris fixated (IF IOL) 9.3%, and unknown 2.6%. By 1988, penetrating keratoplasty was performed in association with IOL removal and IOL exchange in 10% and 58% of cases respectively.

At the time of penetrating keratoplasty for PBK, a decision must be made regarding the management of the previously implanted lens. IOLs may be left in place, removed, or exchanged. Clinical strategies involving the extraction or exchange of IOLs are derived from reports citing a high rate of complications with closed-loop AC IOLs and IF IOLs.[1,32] Graft-failure rates 2 years after penetrating keratoplasty are 60% in eyes with retained AC IOLs (primarily closed-loop or rigid AC IOLs), 20% for exchanged IOLs, 9% for removed IOLs and retained IF IOLs, and 0 for retained PC IOLs.[36] The current choice of replacement IOLs include open-loop AC IOLs or PC IOLs placed in the ciliary sulcus with support from the zonular-capsular diaphragm or fixated by sutures passing through the iris or sclera and ciliary body.

Intraocular Implantation in Pseudophakic Bullous Keratopathy

Anterior Chamber Intraocular Lenses (AC IOL). A variety of theoretical and practical considerations guide the ophthalmic surgeon in selecting a technique of IOL replacement in the individual patient.[33,42] The exchange of a closed-loop AC IOL or IF IOL for an open-loop AC IOL is the most rapidly accomplished procedure requiring minimal manipulation of the eye. Only vitreous anterior to the pupil need be excised. The technique requires adequate support in the anterior chamber angle for the IOL haptics. No sutures are necessary to fixate the implant, and so the potential for intraoperative hemorrhage or postoperative endophthalmitis along a suture track is small. The positioning of the haptics on the trabecular meshwork, however, increases the risk of developing peripheral anterior synechiae, which could compromise aqueous outflow.[19] The proximity of the AC IOL to the corneal endothelium may result in greater endothelial cell loss than with PC IOL implantation if the situation is analogous to that found in cataract extraction.[26]

Retrospective reviews of patients undergoing penetrating keratoplasty with implantation of an open-

Table 12-4. Results of Penetrating Keratoplasty with Anterior Chamber Intraocular Lens Implantation for Pseudophakic Bullous Keratopathy

Authors	Number of Eyes	Visual Acuity (20/40)	Clear Grafts	Cystoid Macular Edema	Glau-coma	Retinal Detachment	Endoph-thalmitis	Graft Rejection	Intraoperative Hemorrhage	Follow-up Study (months)
Insler et al.[16]	32	41%	84%	25%	16%	3%	3%	22%	16%	13
Koenig et al.[18]	20	75%	100%	25%	25%	0	5%	NA	15%	15
Kornmehl et al.[20]	40	58%	95%	10%	13%	3%	0	5%	5%	24
Lass et al.[21]	25	24%	88%	NA	NA	NA	NA	NA	NA	12
Hassan et al.[11]	40	63%	95%	33%	23%	3%	NA	13%	NA	25
Waring et al.[40]	25	32%	88%	36%	28%	0	4%	NA	28%	19
Zaidman et al.[42]	46	31%	89%	20%	11%	2%	0	7%	≤7%	15

NA, Not answered or not addressed in article.

loop AC IOL either as a correction for aphakia or in exchange for a closed-loop AC IOL report visual acuities of 20/40 or better in 24% to 75% of eyes and clear grafts in 84% to 100% of cases during average follow-up periods ranging from 12 to 25 months (Table 12-4).[16,18,20,21,40] Adverse outcomes included cystoid macular edema (10% to 36%), new onset of glaucoma or a "significant" rise in intraocular pressure (11% to 28%), endophthalmitis (0 to 4%), and retinal detachment (0 to 3%). In a prospective series, 11 patients with aphakic bullous keratopathy (ABK) and 35 patients with PBK underwent penetrating keratoplasty with exchange of closed-loop AC IOLs for open-loop AC IOLs. The results were similar with a visual acuity of 20/40 or better in 31% and clear grafts in 89% of cases with an average follow-up observation of 15 months. Cystoid macular edema was found in 20% and glaucoma developed postoperatively in 11% of patients.[42]

Iris-Fixated Posterior Chamber Intraocular Lenses (IF-PC IOL). PC IOLs implanted at the time of cataract extraction have been associated with less cystoid macular edema, pupillary block glaucoma, uveitis-glaucoma-hyphema syndrome, and PBK than other implant styles.[1] In the context of penetrating keratoplasty, PC IOLs may be implanted at the time of cataract extraction as part of a "triple procedure" with haptics in the capsular bag or anterior to the lens zonules at the ciliary sulcus. If the zonular-capsular diaphragm is deficient, partial or complete fixation of the IOL may be accomplished by suture fixation of the optic or haptics to the iris or to the ciliary sulcus and sclera.

Potential advantages of IF-PC IOLs include their greater distance from the corneal endothelium, less potential for inducing peripheral anterior synechiae, and their location at the nodal point of the eye.[33,42] Potential disadvantages involve the need for a vitrectomy and intraoperative suture placement increasing the duration of the surgical procedure. The technique also demands the development of additional surgical skills, which requires more manipulation of the eye than in the implantation of an AC IOL. The technique may not be appropriate in eyes with large iris colobomas not allowing adequate iris support for the IOL, in eyes with extensive peripheral anterior synechiae, or in eyes with prior significant iridocorneal adhesions because the IOL may reside anteriorly to its optimal position. Postoperatively, dilatation of the pupil may be limited, the contact of the IOL with the iris may cause uveitis or pupillary block glaucoma, and fixation sutures could degrade or untie resulting in damage to the corneal endothelium or dislocation of the IOL.

The technique of implantation of IF-PC IOLs was first described utilizing polypropylene (Prolene) sutures passed through the four positioning holes of an IOL optic and then tied over the iris overlying the positioning holes.[11] Passing sutures through only two positioning holes or around the haptics allowed the fixation sutures to be tied in the peripheral iris, permitting greater pupil dilatation after surgery and a lessened zone of compression of iris between sutures and the IOL, reducing uveal inflammation and iritis.[7,41]

The placement of IF-PC IOLs during penetrating keratoplasty for PBK has been retrospectively studied with resultant best-corrected visual acuities of 20/40 or better in 7% to 60% of eyes and with clear grafts in 88% to 97% of cases with an average follow-up observation between 8 and 37 months (Table 12-5).[4,12,21,27,32] Adverse outcomes included cystoid macular edema (3% to 36%), new onset of glaucoma (4% to 29%), endophthalmitis (0% to 5%), and retinal detachment (0 to 2%).

Endothelial cell loss at 1 year after penetrating keratoplasty with implantation of AC IOLs or IF-PC IOLs was found to be 32% and 27% respectively.[20] A larger case series, however, reported endothelial cell loss of 12% versus 19% at 1 year and 21% versus

Table 12-5. Results of Penetrating Keratoplasty with Anterior Chamber Intraocular Lens Implantation for Pseudophakic Bullous Keratopathy

Authors	Number of Eyes	Visual Acuity (20/40)	Clear Grafts	Cystoid Macular Edema	Glaucoma	Retinal Detachment	Endophthalmitis	Graft Rejection	Intraoperative Hemorrhage	Follow-up Study (months)
Busin et al.[4]	14	7%	93%	29%	29%	0	0	7%	NA	8
Lass et al.[21]	25	29%	96%	NA	NA	NA	NA	NA	NA	12
Hall et al.[12]	53	38%	88%	23%	4%	2%	0	12%	NA	37
Price et al.[28]	233	60%	96%	3%	12%	1%	5%	1%	1%	26
Soong et al.[34]	133	45%	97%	36%	16%	2%	2%	4%	NA	12

NA, Not answered or not addressed in article.

38% at 2 years for AC IOLs and PC IOLs respectively.[11,34,39] Visual acuity of ≥20/40 was attained in over 63% of the patients in both groups.[11]

A report of four eyes obtained post mortem with IF-PC IOLs found that seven of the eight haptics were not located in the ciliary sulcus but rather suspended behind the iris and ciliary body, an implication that the iris sutures were instrumental in keeping the IOLs in stable positions.[2]

Transsclerally Sutured Posterior Chamber Intraocular Lenses (TS-PC IOL). The implantation of a transsclerally sutured PC IOL provides the advantages already discussed as well as greater surgical flexibility. The technique may be utilized in conjunction with either penetrating keratoplasty or through a limbal wound regardless of the preoperative anatomy of the iris and anterior chamber angle.[22,33,38] Lack of iris-fixation sutures permits maximal pupillary dilatation and minimizes contact between the IOL and the iris. As in IF-PC IOLs, the haptics are ideally located in the ciliary sulcus, and so contact with the ciliary body is no greater than with IF-PC IOL implantation. Passing needles through the ciliary body and sclera, however, may increase the risks of intraoperative hemorrhage from the ciliary body into the vitreous or within the suprachoroidal space.[29] In addition, a route for microbial invasion of the eye may be created.[14] The technique is slightly more difficult to perform than IF-PC IOL implantation and often requires a longer intraoperative period than the alternative techniques, but the actual time the globe is "open" is similar in both PC IOL procedures.

The surgical approach was first described as a technique for implanting a specially designed closed-loop PC IOL through pars plana with anchoring sutures at the sclera after pars plana cataract extractions.[9] The use of a hypodermic needle suture guide with a transport guide suture was described as a means to use a TS-PC IOL during penetrating keratoplasty for PBK.[24] Results of its utilization were not provided. In another series, 14 patients underwent penetrating keratoplasty for PBK with TS-PC IOL implantation utilizing one double-armed suture for each haptic with needles passed 1 mm posterior to the limbus through full-thickness sclera.[5] Although 93% of grafts were clear at 6 months, visual acuity was ≥20/40 in only a single eye. In a separate series, 15 patients underwent similar surgery with average visual acuity of 20/76 at ≥3 months of follow-up observation.[37] The only complication noted was exposed polypropylene fixation-suture ends. The addition of partial-thickness scleral flaps to cover the polypropylene suture knots was reported for limbal implantation of TS-PC IOLs but not applied to keratoplasty.[15] Utilization of a specially designed needle,

similar to that used by cobblers, in conjunction with an IOL with control tips on the haptics was suggested, but no results were presented.[27]

IOL tilt was estimated to be the most common postoperative complication of TS-PC IOL implantation in a mail survey of corneal surgeons in the United States.[31] Three-point fixation of the TS-PC IOL was introduced as a means to prevent rotation of the IOL around the potential axis of rotation created by the two-point fixation procedure.[17] A cadaver eye model demonstrated that three-point fixation produced less IOL tilt and decentration than two-point fixation.[35] An alternative means to prevent intraocular lens tilt was four-point fixation with the two sutures from each haptic tied together and buried in a partial-thickness scleral groove.[25]

A persistent concern with implantation of TS-PC IOLs is accurate localization of haptics and suture exit sites through the ciliary sulcus. A cadaver model demonstrated that transscleral sutures should exit the sclera less than 1 mm posterior to the corneoscleral limbus for true ciliary sulcus fixation.[5] With use of a cadaver eye model and attempts to pass sutures less than 1 mm posterior to the surgical limbus, only 25% of haptics were ciliary sulcus fixated, whereas the remainder were fixated to pars plicata.[30]

Variable reports exist concerning the propensity of TS-PC IOLs to remain in position or dislocate after removal or cutting of fixation sutures.[14,17] In two eyes studied histologically after penetrating keratoplasty with TS-PC IOL implantation, only 1 of 4 haptics were located in the ciliary sulcus. IOL stability was studied up to 6 months postoperatively and found to be primarily a result of continued integrity of the fixation sutures rather than such integrity by development of scarring encapsulating the haptics.[23] In addition, if polypropylene fixation suture ends remain exposed, they can be lightly cauterized to shrink the polypropylene into a smooth mass along the sclera or covered by a scleral patch graft.[33]

Accurate localization of the ciliary sulcus is potentially more difficult in eyes where limbal landmarks are obscured by scarring. Miniature dental mirrors have been introduced to allow direct inspection, but they are difficult to use and require additional manipulation of the iris.[17,40] Using transillumination to determine the location of the ciliary sulcus in cadaver eyes has proved successful. Needles that were passed "open sky" through the eye wall came out at the marked site. All sutures traversed the ciliary sulcus even in eyes with obscuration of limbal landmarks.[10] The technique has been successfully employed with three-point fixation of TS-PC IOLs with no decentration of IOLs and no induced IOL tilt (Fig. 12-37).

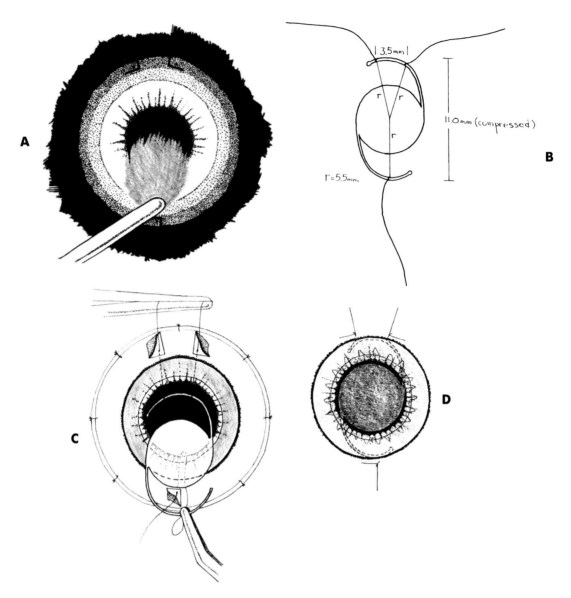

Fig. 12-37. A, Prepare radial partial-thickness sclerotomies. Inferior sclerotomies are centered 4.0 mm apart. Transilluminate the ciliary sulcus with a posterior segment or Finhoff transilluminator (with microscope light off) straddling the limbus 180 degrees from the area of interest. Mark desired exit sites within sclerotomies at junction of anterior and middle thirds of (yellow-brown) band just anterior to dark ciliary body shadow and just posterior to sclerotic scatter-induced bright illumination band at surgical limbus. **B,** Fixate 10-0 polypropylene (Prolene) suture swaged to a curved spatula needle to the haptics of an all-PMMA posterior chamber IOL preferably with an optic of ≥6.0 mm diameter and an overall length of ≤13.0 mm. Tie 3-1-1-1 knots in all locations with knots of two-point fixated haptic being 3.5 mm apart. **C,** Suture Flieringa ring to eye. Perform trephination of recipient bed. Pass each needle from internally through ciliary body and sclera to exiting at marks within sclerotomies. Introduce haptics while applying gentle traction on their attached sutures. **D,** Anchor the polypropylene suture to sclerostomy bed by taking an additional scleral bite adjacent to exit site and tie suture to itself with a 3-1-1-1 knot. Suture ends can be cut, or needle can be passed posteriorly in sclera with suture cut flush at scleral exit site. Donor button is sutured into recipient bed. Partial-thickness sclerostomies are sutured closed with 8.0 polyglactin 910 (Vicryl) suture. Conjunctiva is closed by cauterization or suture.

Table 12-6. Results of Penetrating Keratoplasty with Transscleral Posterior Chamber Intraocular Lens Implantation for Pseudophakic Bullous Keratopathy

Authors	Number of Eyes	Visual Acuity (20/40)	Clear Grafts	Cystoid Macular Edema	Glaucoma	Retinal Detachment	Endoph-thalmitis	Graft Rejection	Intraoperative Hemorrhage	Intraoperative Choroidal Detachments	Follow-up Study (months)
Cowden et al.[5]	14	7%	93%	NA	8%	0	0	NA	NA	NA	6
Heidemann et al.[13]	56	31%	89%	36%	29%	5%	0	7%	14%	5%	11
Johnson[17]	47	27%	98%	31%	NA	0	0	NA	10%	2%	13

NA, Not answered or addressed in article.

The two largest series of patients undergoing implantation of a TS-PC IOL in conjunction with penetrating keratoplasty for PBK report visual acuities of ≥20/40 in 27% to 31% of eyes with clear grafts in 89% to 98% of cases with an 11- to 13-month range in follow-up observation (Table 12-6).[13,17] Adverse outcomes included cystoid macular edema (31% to 36%), glaucoma (0 to 29%), retinal detachment (0 to 5%), intraoperative hemorrhage (10% to 14%), and intraoperative choroidal detachment (2% to 5%). No cases of endophthalmitis were reported. A single retrospective study compared AC IOL, IF-PC IOL, and TS-PC IOL in a total of 41 eyes and found no significant difference in postoperative visual acuity, central corneal thickness, or intraocular pressure among the groups.[6]

Summary. Intraocular lens implantation during penetrating keratoplasty for pseudophakic bullous keratopathy continues to increase in frequency. Advances made in surgical techniques and design modifications in IOLs and suture materials allow the surgeon to perform efficiently while reducing the operative risks to the eye. Because the reported surgical series are primarily retrospective with the inherent biases of retrospective trials, an objective comparison of AC IOL, IF-PC IOL, and TS-PC IOL implantation cannot be generated. An informal comparison of each surgical technique reporting similar average periods of follow-up observation reveals no clinically significant differences in outcome or any adverse effects.[13,16,17,21,34] Randomized clinical trials are necessary to provide appropriate guidance for assessment of currently available surgical modalities.

REFERENCES

1. Apple DJ, Mamalis N, Loftfield K, et al: Complications of intraocular lenses: a historical and histopathological review, *Surv Ophthalmol* 29:1, 1984.
2. Apple DJ, Price FW, Gwin T, et al: Sutured retropupillary posterior chamber intraocular lenses for exchange or secondary implantation, *Ophthalmology* 96:1241, 1989.
3. Brady SE, Rapuano CJ, Arentsen JJ, et al: Clinical indications for and procedures associated with penetrating keratoplasty, 1983-1988, *Am J Ophthalmol* 108:118, 1989.
4. Busin M, Brauweiler P, Boeker T, et al: Complications of sulcus-supported intraocular lenses with iris sutures, implanted during penetrating keratoplasty after intracapsular cataract extraction, *Ophthalmology* 97:401, 1990.
5. Cowden JW, Hu BV: A new surgical technique for posterior chamber lens fixation during penetrating keratoplasty in the absence of capsular or zonular support, *Cornea* 7:231, 1988.
6. Davis RM, Best D, Gilbert GE: Comparison of intraocular lens fixation techniques performed during penetrating keratoplasty, *Am J Ophthalmol* 111:743, 1991.
7. Drews RC: Posterior chamber lens implantation during keratoplasty without posterior lens capsule support, *Cornea* 6:38, 1987.

8. Duffey RJ, Holland EJ, Agapitos PJ, et al: Anatomic study of transsclerally sutured intraocular lens implantation, *Am J Ophthalmol* 108:300, 1989.

9. Girard LJ: Pars plana phacoprosthesis (aphakic intraocular implant), a preliminary report, *Ophthalmic Surg* 12:19, 1981.

10. Groos EB, Rapoza PA: Transillumination for accurate transscleral suture placement through the ciliary sulcus, *Invest Ophthalmol Vis Sci* 32(suppl):796, 1991 (ARVO Abstracts).

11. Hassan TS, Soong HK, Sugar A, et al: Implantation of Kelman-style open-loop anterior chamber lenses during keratoplasty for aphakic and pseudophakic bullous keratopathy: a comparison with iris-sutured posterior chamber lenses, *Ophthalmology* 98:875, 1991.

12. Hall JR, Muenzler WS: Lens replacement in pseudophakic bullous keratopathy, *Trans Ophthalmol Soc UK* 4:541, 1985.

13. Heidemann DG, Dunn SP: Visual results and complications of transsclerally sutured intraocular lenses in penetrating keratoplasty, *Ophthalmic Surg* 21:609, 1990.

14. Heilskov T, Joondeph BC, Olsen KR, et al: Late endophthalmitis after transscleral fixation of a posterior chamber intraocular lens, *Arch Ophthalmol* 107:1427, 1989.

15. Hu BV, Shin DH, Gibbs KA, et al: Implantation of posterior chamber lens in the absence of capsular and zonular support, *Arch Ophthalmol* 106:416, 1988.

16. Insler MS, Kook MS, Kaufman HE: Penetrating keratoplasty for pseudophakic bullous keratopathy associated with semiflexible, closed-loop anterior chamber intraocular lenses, *Am J Ophthalmol* 107:252, 1989.

17. Johnson SM: Results of exchanging anterior chamber lenses with sulcus-fixated posterior chamber IOLs without capsular support in penetrating keratoplasty, *Ophthalmic Surg* 20:465, 1989.

18. Koenig SB, McDermott ML, Hyndiuk RA: Penetrating keratoplasty and intraocular lens exchange for pseudophakic bullous keratopathy associated with a closed-loop anterior chamber intraocular lens, *Am J Ophthalmol* 108:43, 1989.

19. Kooner KS, Dulaney DD, Zimmerman TJ: Intraocular pressure following secondary anterior chamber lens implantation, *Ophthalmic Surg* 19:274, 1988.

20. Kornmehl EW, Steinert RF, Odrich MG, et al: Penetrating keratoplasty for pseudophakic bullous keratopathy associated with closed-loop anterior chamber intraocular lenses, *Ophthalmology* 97:407, 1990.

21. Lass JH, DeSantis DM, Reinhart WJ, et al: Clinical and morphometric results of penetrating keratoplasty with one-piece anterior-chamber or suture-fixated posterior-chamber lenses in the absence of lens capsule, *Arch Ophthalmol* 108:1427, 1990.

22. Lindquist TD, Agapitos PJ, Lindstrom RL, et al: Transscleral fixation of posterior chamber intraocular lenses in the absence of capsule support, *Ophthalmic Surg* 20:769, 1989.

23. Lubniewski AJ, Holland EJ, Van Meter WS, et al: Histologic study of eyes with transsclerally sutured posterior chamber intraocular lenses, *Am J Ophthalmol* 110:237, 1990.

24. Malbran ES, Malbran E Jr, Negri I: Lens guide suture for transport and fixation in secondary IOL implantation after intracapsular extraction, *Int Ophthalmol* 9:151, 1986.

25. Mannarino AP, Hannush SB: A new technique for transscleral fixation of a posterior chamber intraocular lens in the absence of capsular support during penetrating keratoplasty, *Refract Corneal Surg* 6:353, 1990.

26. Matsuda M, Miyake K, Inaba M: Long-term corneal endothelial changes after intraocular lens implantation, *Am J Ophthalmol* 105:248, 1988.

27. Pannu JS: A new suturing technique for ciliary sulcus fixation in the absence of posterior capsule, *Ophthalmic Surg* 19:751, 1988.

28. Price FW, Whitson WE: Visual results of suture-fixated posterior chamber lenses during penetrating keratoplasty, *Ophthalmology* 96:1234, 1989.

29. Price FW, Whitson WE: Suprachoroidal hemorrhage after placement of a scleral-fixated lens, *J Cataract Refract Surg* 16:514, 1990.

30. Robin SB, Rubenstein JB, Kay MD, et al: Haptic location of transsclerally sutured posterior chamber intraocular lenses in the cadaver eye, *Invest Ophthalmol Vis Sci* 32(suppl):796, 1991 (ARVO Abstracts).

31. Sen HA, Smith PW: Current trends in suture fixation of posterior chamber intraocular lenses, *Ophthalmic Surg* 21:689, 1990.

32. Smith PW, Wong SK, Stark WJ, et al.: Complications of closed-loop anterior chamber intraocular lenses, *Arch Ophthalmol* 105:52, 1987.

33. Soong HK, Meyer RF, Sugar A: Techniques for posterior chamber lens implantation without capsular support during penetrating keratoplasty: a review, *Refract Corneal Surg* 5:249, 1989.

34. Soong HK, Musch DC, Kowal V, et al: Implantation of posterior chamber intraocular lenses in the absence of lens capsule during penetrating keratoplasty, *Arch Ophthalmol* 107:660, 1989.

35. Sossi NP, Frueh BE, Feldman ST: Reducing tilt and decentration of sutured intraocular lens implants, *Invest Ophthalmol Vis Sci* 32(suppl):796, 1991 (ARVO Abstracts).

36. Speaker MG, Lugo M, Laibson PR, et al: Penetrating keratoplasty for pseudophakic bullous keratopathy: management of the intraocular lens, *Ophthalmology* 95:1260, 1988.

37. Spigelman AV, Lindstrom RL, Nichols BD, et al: Implantation of a posterior chamber lens without capsular support during penetrating keratoplasty or as a secondary lens implant, *Ophthalmic Surg* 19:396, 1988.

38. Stark WJ, Gottsch JD, Goodman DF, et al: Posterior chamber intraocular lens implantation in the absence of capsular support, *Arch Ophthalmol* 107:1078, 1989.

39. Sugar A: An analysis of corneal endothelial and graft survival in pseudophakic bullous keratopathy, *Trans Am Ophthalmol Soc* 87:762, 1989.

40. Waring GO, Stulting RD, Street D: Penetrating keratoplasty for pseudophakic corneal edema with exchange of intraocular lenses, *Arch Ophthalmol* 105:58, 1987.

41. Wong SK, Stark WJ, Gottsch JD, et al: Use of posterior chamber lenses in pseudophakic bullous keratopathy, *Arch Ophthalmol* 105:856, 1987.

42. Zaidman GW, Goldman S: A prospective study on the implantation of anterior chamber intraocular lenses during keratoplasty for pseudophakic and aphakic bullous keratopathy, *Ophthalmology* 97:757, 1990.

Chapter 13

Combined Procedures

Long-term observations

GREGORY J. PAMEL
DANIEL M. TAYLOR

HISTORICAL BACKGROUND AND REVIEW OF THE LITERATURE

Corneal disease and opacification combined with cataract formation have presented a therapeutic challenge to corneal surgeons since the advent of penetrating keratoplasty. From 1906, when the first successful penetrating keratoplasty was performed by Zirm,[60] to the early 1960s, the prevailing opinion was that keratoplasty had to be performed separately from cataract extraction. If the keratoplasty was performed first, subsequent cataract extraction led to a high incidence of graft decompensation, ranging from 10% to 61%.[14,28,39,47,54] If the cataract was performed before keratoplasty or corneal disease developed subsequently (such as aphakic bullous keratopathy, keratitis, or traumatic scarring), the graft-failure rate was high, ranging from 57% to 100%.[23,31,59] This was largely attributable to vitreous contact with donor endothelium. This problem was eventually solved by aspiration of liquid pockets of vitreous through the pars plana as advocated by Fine[20-22] and Barraquer[5] and subsequently by either cellular sponge removal of formed vitreous from the anterior chamber or through the use of vitreous suction cutter devices. The overall success rate with multiple procedures was thus greatly improved, but convalescence remained prolonged, requiring a year or more before useful vision could be restored.

In 1960, Hughes[28] reported a 31% success rate in 13 cases of combined penetrating keratoplasty with intracapsular cataract extraction. In 1966 Katzin and Meltzer[34] reported on 10 combined procedures with seven grafts remaining clear. Casey,[17] Kaufman,[35] Arentsen and Laibson,[4] Olson and Waltman,[46] Brightbill[11] and others also reported successful results with combined procedures. Not only was the possibility of maintaining a clear graft enhanced, but also the time required for rehabilitation was greatly reduced.

From 1966 through the early 1970s the combined procedure of penetrating keratoplasty and intracapsular cataract extraction remained the method of choice for a majority of corneal surgeons to treat combined corneal opacification and cataract formation. However, a major problem remained, that is, aphakic visual rehabilitation using contact lenses often on highly astigmatic graft surfaces when the fellow eye was relatively normal. With the reintroduction and gradual acceptance of intraocular lens (IOL) implants for cataract surgery, it was only a matter of time before this sight-restoring procedure would be embraced by pioneering corneal surgeons. In 1967 Byron and Reshmi performed a penetrating keratoplasty, cataract extraction, and IOL insertion but failed to document their accomplishments in the literature. Hunkeler and Hyde[29] began performing the procedure in 1973 and have used it with considerable success. Lee and Dohlman[38] began their series in 1974. I (D.M.T.)[56-58] began my series in 1975 and in 1976 first called attention to the utility of the triple procedure in a report of 6 cases. Critics held that the surgery was much too radical and unpredictable to be given serious consideration.[36] However, by the late 1970s, several reports confirming

Table 13-1. Published Results of Triple Procedures from 1976 to 1991

Study	Number of Eyes	Mean Follow-up Time (months)	Clear Grafts (%)	Visual Acuity 20/20 to 20/40 (%)
Taylor[55]	6	7.7	100	33.3
Aquavella et al.[3]	5	15.0	80.0	Not reported
Lee and Dohlman[38]	10	15.9	60.0	50.0
Alpar[2]	18	21.0	94.0	77.7
Taylor et al.[57]	22	Unknown	77.0	36.3
Gould[25]	11	Not reported	72.0	54.5
Lindstrom et al.[40]	18	21.0	89.0	55.5
Hunkeler and Hyde[30]	177	>6.0	89.0	88.7
Crawford et al.[18]	56	15.8	90.0	65.2
Binder[6]	60	24.5	91.6	61.6
Bruner[12]	12	27.3	90	80
Polack[44]	60	6-48	98.3	35
Taylor[58]	66	24-120	95.4	54
Katz and Forster[33]	53	8.9	96	64
Gabel et al.[24]	94	Not reported	Not reported	82
Binder[9]	78	24.5	97	71.8
Meyer et al.[43]	166	17	98	83
Busin et al.[13]	22	4	95	64
Skorpik et al.[51]	21	22	100	71
Mattax et al.[42]	21	11.8	95.2	76

Table 13-2. Published Indications for Triple Procedures, 1976 to 1991[9,12,14,18,33,38,40,43,58]

Corneal Disease	Range of Incidence (%)
Fuchs' endothelial dystrophy	31-80
Leukoma	19-35
Keratoconus	5-21
Herpes simplex keratitis	4.5-14
Interstitial keratitis	4-14

benefits of the combined technique were published[29,30,38,57,58] (Table 13-1). In the 1980s, reports on the triple procedure addressed the issues of visual and refractive results, graft clarity, IOL calculations, and intraoperative and postoperative complications further supporting the effectiveness of this procedure.[6,9,12,13,17,18,24,25,30,33,40,42,43,51,58]

INDICATIONS

By far the leading indication for the triple procedure is Fuchs' endothelial dystrophy. A review of the literature shows that this condition has been present in 31.3% to 77% of the eyes undergoing the triple procedure from 1976 to 1991 (Table 13-2). Since Fuchs' dystrophy is more common among females, there is a larger percentage of females reported who have undergone the triple procedure. The second most common cause reported has been corneal leukoma (18% to 33.3%) and interstitial keratitis (8.3% to 18.7%). Herpes simplex is the third most common condition cited (7.2% to 13%).[9,12,14,18,33,38,40,43,58]

GRAFT CLARITY

Early reported series of triple procedures between 1976[55] and 1980[15] showed a range of clear grafts from 60% to 94%. However, the range of clear grafts increased in the series reported by Lindstrom and co-workers[40] (1981) through most recently the series reported by Skorpik and co-workers[50] (1988) from 89% to 100%. Taylor's series[58] published in 1986 has the longest follow-up observation of any published series and showed a graft-clarity rate of 95.8%. The initial reported series either combined results of both intracapsular and extracapsular technique or were strictly results of intracapsular cataract extraction with keratoplasty. The inferior results of the intracapsular technique versus the extracapsular technique on graft clarity are well known. Furthermore, these earlier series included implantation of iris-plane and iris-fixated lenses, which can adversely affect graft clarity and ultimately cause graft failure. The later series involved primarily the extracapsular technique with posterior chamber lens implantation and showed graft clarity results of 95% to 100% similar to results seen in penetrating keratoplasty in phakic eyes[9,13,17,42,43,51] (Table 13-3).

Table 13-3. Reported Series on Triple Procedures Involving Posterior Chamber Lenses

Study	Posterior Chamber Intraocular Lenses (%)	Mean Follow-up (months)	Clear Grafts (%)	Visual Acuity 20/20 to 20/40 (%)
Lindstrom et al.[40]	100	21	89	55.5
Crawford et al.[18]	91	15.8	>90	>77
Katz and Forster[33]	96	8.9	96	64
Binder[9]	100	6-72	97	75
Gabel et al.[24]	100	Not known	100	82
Meyer et al.[43]	100	17	98	83
Busin et al.[13]	100	4	95	64
Skorpik et al.[51]	100	22	100	71

VISUAL AND REFRACTIVE RESULTS

The percentage of eyes achieving 20/40 vision or better with the triple procedure has increased from the initial reported series by Taylor of 33%[55] to 88.7%[30] reported in the largest series by Hunkeler and Hyde (see Table 13-1). The improvement in results has been attributable in part to better surgical technique, improved donor-storage media, and the evolution from anterior chamber and iris clip lenses to posterior chamber lenses.

In Taylor's series[58] with the longest follow-up observation, 54% of eyes had 20/40 vision or better though in the subset of eyes with posterior chamber IOLs this increased to 64%. When eyes with posterior segment disorder were eliminated in this subset, 92% of eyes saw 20/40 or better. This compares favorably with Crawford's results[18] who reported that 76.8% of eyes saw 20/40 or better, and Skorpik's results,[51] who reported 84% of eyes without posterior segment disorder saw 20/40 or better. Meyer,[43] in the largest series of triple procedures with posterior chamber lenses, reported 83% of eyes achieving 20/40 vision or better after an average of 17 months of follow-up observation (see Table 13-3).

The potential for early visual rehabilitation in eyes undergoing the triple procedure has been one of the main reasons behind its near universal acceptance by corneal surgeons. Binder[9] reported the average time to a stable refraction in his series to be 6.2 months, whereas Crawford and co-workers[18] reported this average time to be 7 months. In Meyer's series[43] of 166 consecutive eyes, the average time to providing a stable refraction was 4 months even though the average time at which a subset of eyes (*n* = 52) achieved 20/40 visual acuity was 2 months. Mattax and co-workers[42] reported that 81.3% of their patients without posterior segment disorder saw 20/40 or better 6 months after surgery. The most frequent posterior segment conditions that have been found to limit visual outcome in the triple procedure are

---

FACTORS ASSOCIATED WITH POSTKERATOPLASTY ASTIGMATISM[8]

Presurgical factors

Donor astigmatism, scars
Recipient corneal condition (thickness, edema, vascularization)
Previous keratoplasty
Recipient astigmatism
Donor age (pediatric cornea)

Surgical factors

Trephination error
Suture technique
Donor/recipient disparity

Postsurgical factors

Focal wound vascularization
Donor/recipient melting
Suture erosion, compression, torque
Timing of suture removal and technique
Wound dehiscence, override
Wound healing

---

age-related macular degeneration and glaucomatous optic atrophy.

Postoperative corneal astigmatism can limit visual outcome significantly after penetrating keratoplasty. The numerous factors influencing postkeratoplasty astigmatism have been discussed in detail elsewhere[8] (see Box). Mean astigmatism has ranged from 2.66 to 5.4 diopters in reported triple procedure series[6,9,18,24,32,42,43,58] (see Table 13-3) and does not differ significantly from astigmatism after keratoplasty performed for other indications.

CALCULATION OF LENS POWER

Preoperative prediction of intraocular implant power needed to achieve the desired postoperative refractive error in eyes undergoing the triple proce-

Table 13-4.   Refractive Results from the Triple Procedure

Study	Intraocular Lens Type	Intraocular Lens Formula	Mean Postoperative Spherical Equivalent (Range)	Astigmatism: Diopters (Range)	±2.00 Emmetropia or Desired Power (%)
Taylor et al.[58]	I,P	None used	−1.31 (−8.00/6.25)	3.6 (plano to 7.5)	60.9
Katz and Forster[33]	A,P	SRK	−0.61 (−6.88/7.89)	5.4	26
Gabel et al.[24]	A,P	Binkhorst	−0.77 (−14/4.5)	NR	57
Crawford et al.[18]	A,I,P	NR	−0.33 (−5.5/6.62)	3.23 (plano to 8.0)	62
Binder[6]	A,I,P	Binkhorst-SRK	−1.78 (−14.7/5.25)	3.1 (plano to 10.0)	58
Binder[9]	A,I,P	Binkhorst-SRK	−1.57 (−14.7/5.25)	2.98 (plano to 11.4)	57.9
Meyer et al.[43]	P	Binkhorst-SRK	NR	4.39 (0.25 to 11.5)	57 B 67 SRK
Mattax et al.[42]	A,P	Binkhorst	NR	2.66 (0.78 to 4.54)	62.5

A, Anterior chamber; I, iris-fixated; P, posterior chamber.
B, Binkhorst; NR, not reported; SRK, Sanders, Retzlaff, Kraff.

dure has met with limited success. A review of the literature shows that 26% to 67% of eyes have obtained postoperative refractive errors within ±2 diopters of emmetropia[6,9,18,24,33,42,43,58] (Table 13-4). In contrast, 90% or more of postoperative refractions fall within ±2 diopters of emmetropia in eyes that have undergone cataract extraction and intraocular lens implantation alone.[26,27]

In order for IOL power prediction to be accurate, the determinants of IOL power, which include keratometry, anterior chamber depth, and axial length must remain fairly constant after surgery. Or, if they do change, they must do so in a predictable manner. Since penetrating keratoplasty alters the preoperative keratometry readings and even the axial length and anterior chamber depth, the accuracy of IOL power calculations diminishes with this procedure. The corneal surgeon is faced with the difficulty of attempting to predict postoperative keratometry when calculating the implant power. Furthermore, postoperative keratometry may be influenced by many preoperative, surgical, and postoperative factors[8] (see Box, p. 179). Using multiple regression analysis, Crawford and co-workers[18] demonstrated that there is a poor correlation between preoperative and postoperative keratometry readings. Axial length was found to be the single most important factor contributing to the prediction of the IOL power. They were unable to develop a single formula to accurately predict lens power for every surgeon in their series because of the variability of postoperative keratometry readings from surgeon to surgeon.

Corneal surgeons have used several approaches to determining IOL power with keratoplasty. Taylor[57] attempts to acquire the refractive information of each eye before the onset of corneal disease. If this is unavailable, he estimates IOL power by determining the refractive status, keratometry reading, and axial length of the fellow eye bearing in mind that A-scan measurements of eyes with diseased corneas can be unreliable. If the preoperative data are not obtainable, he then uses a standard biconvex implant averaging 19.5 diopters. With this method, he has been able to obtain desired IOL power similar to other methods.[58]

Katz and co-workers[33] using the (Sanders, Retzlaff, Kraff) formula have used keratometry readings from the fellow eye or the recipient eye or used average keratometry readings from a recent, concurrent series of penetrating keratoplasties. Gabel and colleagues[24] calculated implant power in a similar manner using the Binkhorst formula. Binder[6,9] estimated lens implant power in his triple procedure cases based on estimated postkeratoplasty keratometry readings from a consecutive series of patients in whom the same donor/recipient diameter combination as well as the same suturing technique were used.

In the Mattax and McCulley series,[42] a standarized *k* value was used to calculate IOL power based on one surgeon's average postkeratoplasty keratometry values after recent transplants. They showed that if one surgeon controlled for suturing technique, donor size, and donor/recipient size disparity the predictive value of IOL calculations with use of the SRK formula was over 80% in those eyes that achieved 20/40 vision or better.

There is still no universal way corneal surgeons can achieve accurate IOL calculations in the triple procedure. Refractive surprises will always be a potential problem so long as the preoperative keratometry of the donor cornea remains unknown. Placing the implant within the capsular bag versus within the sulcus can decrease or increase the effective power of the lens from 0.5 to 1 diopter.[9] By using the same donor/recipient combination, lens implant style, and suturing technique as well as continually updating his series of transplants to determine an estimated postoperative keratometry reading, the corneal surgeon will be able to maximize his chances of achieving IOL accuracy. Alternatively, if refractive information of the eye before the onset of corneal disease is available, I (D.M.T.) have shown that IOL accuracy can be as effective as other methods.

INTRAOPERATIVE COMPLICATIONS

Intraoperative complications that occur with the triple procedure include capsule rupture with vitreous loss as well as suprachoroidal hemorrhage. Capsule rupture with vitreous loss has been found to be very low in reported triple procedure series. Hunkeler and Hyde[30] reported an incidence of 1.1%. In my (D.M.T.) series, no cases of capsular rupture occurred. Crawford and co-workers[18] reported an incidence of 16% though most of these capsular ruptures occurred in the early cases of the series presumably when the technical learning curve was still rising. In Meyer's series,[43] 4% of the cases had had capsular rupture with vitreous loss. This complication does not appear to be more prevalent than routine extracapsular cataract surgery.[32]

Expulsive hemorrhage was found in two cases (3.3%) in Taylor's series.[58] Other series did not report this complication. Speaker and colleagues[53] found a higher incidence of suprachoroidal hemorrhage in patients undergoing penetrating keratoplasty compared to other procedures and attributed this to the open-sky technique. Presumably, since keratoplasty with cataract extraction traditionally involves a more prolonged open-sky procedure, the risk should be higher. However, the reported series on triple procedures clearly indicates that this complication is as infrequent as in penetrating keratoplasty alone.

POSTOPERATIVE COMPLICATIONS

In addition to corneal astigmatism, other postoperative complications include graft rejection and failure, postoperative glaucoma, posterior capsule opacification, cystoid macular edema, and retinal detachment (Table 13-5). *Graft rejection* and failure are important complications when one is evaluating the triple procedure. The reported incidence of rejection ranges from 0 to 11% during the first-year follow-up observation. It is difficult to interpret graft rejection or failure rates from different reported series, since the earlier reports included a larger proportion of anterior chamber and iris clip lenses not found in later series. Furthermore, follow-up periods varied considerably. Meyer[43] reported an incidence of graft rejection of 16.2% at a 2-year fol-

Table 13-5. Incidence of Postoperative Complications in Reported Series of Triple Procedures, 1976 to 1988[2,3,13,18,33,38,40,42,44,51,58]

Complication	Range of Incidence (%)
Graft rejection	0-11
Graft failure	6-20
Postoperative glaucoma	1.5-19
Posterior capsule opacification	7-10
Cystoid macula edema	0-6
Retinal detachment	0-2
Endophthalmitis	<1

low-up period in his series of posterior chamber implants but no graft failures. In a subset of Taylor's series[58] of eyes that had undergone triple procedures with a 5- to 10-year follow-up study, only one eye out of 20 (5%) developed graft failure. This occurred in a patient with an iris-supported lens. There were no failed grafts in patients who underwent a triple procedure with a posterior chamber lens. The presence of a posterior chamber lens has not been shown to increase the incidence or severity of rejection.[9,13,17,33,42,43,51]

Endothelial cell loss after penetrating keratoplasty alone as well as cataract extraction with posterior chamber lens implantation alone have been shown to occur over time.[1,19,45,50] Meyer and co-workers[43] have documented endothelial cell loss over time after the triple procedure: 14% after 1 year, 20% after 2 years, and 23% after 3 years. Although the amount does appear to be greater than cataract extraction with posterior chamber lens implantation alone, it does not appear to be greater than penetrating keratoplasty alone.[1,41,49] In Taylor's series[58] involving extracapsular–posterior chamber triple procedures with a 2- to 5-year follow-up study specular microscopy showed a remarkably high average cell count of 2278 cells/mm^2, with a range of 700 to 3300 cells/mm^2. Sixty-eight percent had 2000 cells or more per square millimeter. These high counts are in part attributable to the age of the donors, which averaged 28. Secure (in-the-bag) fixation with minimal uveal contact may greatly reduce the incidence of chronic low-grade inflammation and secondary endothelial cell loss.

Postoperative glaucoma defined as elevated intraocular pressure developing in eyes with normal preoperative intraocular pressures and requiring long-term medical and surgical therapy has been reported in 1.5% to 19% of eyes undergoing triple procedures.[18,29,30,33,40,43,58] Some authors do not mention what level of intraocular pressure they decided to treat, or, if in fact glaucomatous optic nerve damage occurred. Lee and Dohlman[38] reported that 60% of their patients had elevated intraocular pressure at some time postoperatively though most pressure increases were temporary and secondary to steroid treatment. Meyer[43] used strict criteria of treating elevated intraocular pressure greater than 21 on two consecutive visits and attributes this to his higher incidence of postoperative glaucoma compared to other series. Peripheral anterior synechiae developed in 5% of eyes in his series, and three eyes required laser peripheral iridectomy for pseudophakic pupillary block glaucoma. This latter complication was first reported by Taylor[56] in 1977 but has been reported only three other times since then. Meyer[43] believed it occurred often enough after his third case that he subsequently began performing peripheral iridotomies in the remaining eyes in his series.

Posterior capsule opacification has been found in 7% to 10% of eyes in reported series of triple procedures.[9,12,14,18,33,38,40,43,58] This complication should increase in frequency as the follow-up period increases. There does not appear to be a higher incidence of posterior capsule opacification in the triple procedure compared to routine extracapsular cataract surgery alone.[32]

Cystoid macular edema (CME) has been reported to occur from 0 to 6% in eyes undergoing the triple procedure.[16,18,33,37,38,40,43] Some studies defined clinically significant CME as that causing vision loss to 20/40 or worse.[43] Other reports do not clearly define the criteria used to diagnose CME.[37,38] Nonetheless, the incidence does not appear to be any higher than that reported with routine extracapsular cataract surgery.[32] Kramer[37] reported no cases of CME in his series of combined keratoplasty and extracapsular cataract extraction compared to an incidence of 35% and 27% in his aphakic and pseudophakic keratoplasties respectively.

Retinal detachment has been reported to occur between 0 and 2% of eyes undergoing the triple procedure.[30,58] The frequency of this complication is similar to that reported in phakic keratoplasty eyes as well as eyes that have undergone extracapsular cataract extraction with posterior chamber lens implantation with intact posterior capsules.[52] There appears to be no additive risk for retinal detachment when one is performing these procedures simultaneously.

Endophthalmitis is a rare complication of the triple procedure that has been reported only in Meyer's series[43] of eyes undergoing this procedure.

CONCLUSION

Penetrating keratoplasy combined with extracapsular cataract extraction and intraocular lens implantation is an effective procedure for dealing with combined corneal disease and cataract. There is a faster visual rehabilitation with this procedure compared with a staged approach without an increase in the complication rate or added risk to graft survival. Patients who require corneal transplant who have early cataracts should be considered candidates for the triple procedure, since the postoperative course of a corneal graft alone will worsen the cataract. This will ultimately delay visual rehabilitation until the cataract is removed leading to patient dissatisfaction. A second procedure will lead to additional endothelial cell loss, placing the graft at risk for failure.

Although there is no universal formula to provide complete accuracy of intraocular lens power, several methods exist to provide consistently predictable results. Several patients in Taylor's series[58] who received a triple procedure 15 years ago continue to have clear grafts and useful vision testifying to the long-term stability of the procedure.

REFERENCES

1. Abbott RL, Fine M, Guillet E: Long term changes in corneal endothelium following penetrating keratoplasty, *Ophthalmology* 90:676-685, 1983.
2. Alpar JJ: Keratoplasty with primary and secondary lens implantation, *Ophthalmic Surg* 9(4):58-66, 1978.
3. Aquavella JV, Shaw EL, Gullapalli RN: Intraocular lens implantation combined with penetrating keratoplasty, *Ophthalmic Surg* 8(3):113-116, 1977.
4. Arentsen JJ, Laibson PR: Penetrating keratoplasty and cataract extraction, *Arch Ophthalmol* 96:75-76, 1978.
5. Barraquer J: Present status of corneal transplant surgery, *Highlights of Ophthalmology* 5:320, 1962.
6. Binder PS: Intraocular lens power used in the triple procedure, *Ophthalmology* 92:1561-1566, 1985.
7. Binder PS: Secondary intraocular lens implantation during or after corneal transplantation, *Am J Ophthalmol* 99:515-520, 1985.
8. Binder PS: Surgical correction of astigmatism. In *Cornea, refractive surgery, and contact lens*, Transactions of the New Orleans Academy of Ophthalmology, New York, 1987, Raven Press, p 7.
9. Binder PS: Refractive errors encountered with the triple procedure. In *Cornea, refractive surgery, and contact lens*, Transactions of the New Orleans Academy of Ophthalmology, New York, 1987, Raven Press, pp 111-120.
10. Bourne WM: One year observation of transplanted human corneal endothelium, *Ophthalmology* 87:673-679, 1980.
11. Brightbill FS, Stainer GA, Hunkeler JD: A comparison of intracapsular and extracapsular lens extraction combined with keratoplasty, *Ophthalmology* 90:34-37, 1983.
12. Bruner WE, Stark WJ, Maumenee AE: Combined keratoplasty, cataract extraction, and intraocular lens implantation: experience at the Wilmer Institute, *Ophthalmic Surg* 12(9):657-660, 1981.
13. Busin M, Arffa RC, McDonald MB, Kaufman HE: Combined

penetrating keratoplasty, extracapsular cataract extraction, and posterior chamber lens implantation, *Ophthalmic Surg* 18(4):272-275, 1987.

14. Buxton J: Non simultaneous and simultaneous corneal graft and cataract extraction. In Welsh RC, Welsh J, editors: *The new report on cataract surgery*, Miami, 1969, Miami Educational Press, p 196.

15. Buxton J: The triple procedure (corneal graft, intracapsular cataract extraction and intraocular lens), *Contact and IOL Med J* 6:409-412, 1980.

16. Buxton JN, Jaffe NS: Combined keratoplasty, cataract extraction and intraocular lens implantation, *Am Intra-Ocular Implant Soc J* 4:110, 1978.

17. Casey TA: The combined operation of cataract and corneal graft, *Trans Ophthalmol Soc UK* 89:659-668, 1969.

18. Crawford GJ, Stulting RD, Waring GO, et al: The triple procedure, *Ophthalmology* 93:817-824, 1986.

19. Culbertson WW, Abbott RL, Forster RK: Endothelial cell loss in penetrating keratoplasty, *Ophthalmology* 89:600-604, 1982.

20. Fine M: Therapeutic keratoplasty, Symposium: Corneal Surgery, *Trans Am Acad Ophthalmol Otolaryngol* 64:786-806, 1960.

21. Fine M: Keratoplasty in aphakia. In King JM, McTigue JW, editors: *The Cornea World Congress*, Washington, DC, 1965, Butterworth, pp 538-552.

22. Fine M: Penetrating keratoplasty in aphakia, *Arch Ophthalmol* 72:50-56, 1964.

23. Franceschetti A: Corneal grafting, *Trans Ophthalmol Soc UK* 69:17, 1949.

24. Gabel MG, Meyer RF, Musch DC: Calculation of intraocular lens implant power for the triple procedure surgery. In Brightbill FS, editor: *Corneal surgery: theory, technique, and tissue*, St. Louis, 1986, Mosby–Year Book.

25. Gould HL: Keratoplasty and intraocular lenses, *Am Intra-ocular Implant Soc J* 6:42-44, 1980.

26. Holliday JT, Prager TC, Ruiz RS, et al: Improving the predictability of intraocular lens power calculations, *Arch Ophthalmol* 104:539-541, 1986.

27. Holliday JT, Musgrove KH, Prager TC, et al: A three-part system for refining intraocular lens power calculations, *J Cataract Refract Surg* 14:17-24, 1988.

28. Hughes WF: Keratoplasty for corneal dystrophies, *Am J Ophthalmol* 50:1100-1114, 1960.

29. Hunkeler JD, Hyde LL: The triple procedure: combined penetrating keratoplasty, cataract extraction and lens implantation, *Am Intra-Ocular Implant Soc J* 5(3):222-224, 1979.

30. Hunkeler JD, Hyde LL: The triple procedure: combined penetrating keratoplasty, extracapsular cataract extraction and lens implantation: an expanded experience, *Am Intra-Ocular Implant Soc J* 9:20-24, 1983.

31. Iliff CE, Castroviejo R, Hughes WF, et al: Present status of corneal transplant surgery, *Trans Am Acad Ophthalmol Otolaryngol* 67:308-309, 1963.

32. Jaffe NS, Jaffe MS, Jaffe GF, editors: *Cataract surgery and its complications*, Philadelphia, 1990, Lippincott.

33. Katz HR, Forster RK: Intraocular lens calculation in combined penetrating keratoplasty, cataract extraction and intraocular lens implantation, *Ophthalmology* 92:1203-1207, 1985.

34. Katzin HM, Meltzer JF: Combined surgery for corneal transplantation and cataract extraction, *Am J Ophthalmol* 62:556-560, 1960.

35. Kaufman HE: Combined keratoplasty and cataract extraction, *Am J Ophthalmol* 77:824-829, 1974.

36. Kaufman HE: Intraocular lenses combined with keratoplasty

and cataract extraction, *Highlights of Ophthalmology* 5:4-5, 1977.

37. Kramer SG: Penetrating keratoplasty combined with extracapsular cataract extraction, *Am J Ophthalmol* 100:129-133, 1985.

38. Lee JR, Dohlman CH: Intraocular lens implantation in combination with keratoplasty, *Ann Ophthalmol* 9:513-518, 1977.

39. Lemp MA, Pfister RR, Dohlman CH: The effects of intraocular surgery on clear corneal grafts, *Am J Ophthalmol* 70:719, 1970.

40. Lindstrom RL, Harris WS, Doughman DJ: Combined penetrating keratoplasty, extracapsular cataract extraction, and posterior chamber lens implantation, *Am Intra-Ocular Implant Soc J* 7:130-132, 1981.

41. Linn JG Jr, Stuart JC, Warnicki JW: Endothelial morphology in long term keratoconus corneal transplants, *Ophthalmology* 88:761-769, 1981.

42. Mattax JB, McCulley JP: The effect of standarized keratoplasty technique on IOL power calculation for the triple procedure, *Acta Ophthalmol* 67(suppl 192):24-29, 1989.

43. Meyer RF, Musch DC: Assessment of success and complications of triple procedure surgery, *Trans Am Acad Ophthal Soc* 85:350-367, 1987.

44. Polack FM: The triple procedure—use of Healon in preserved donor tissue, *Cataract* 2(5):15-22, 1985.

45. Olsen T: Postoperative changes in the endothelial cell density of corneal grafts, *Acta Ophthalmol* 59:863-870, 1981.

46. Olsen RJ, Waltman SR, Mattingly TP, Kaufman HE: Visual results after penetrating keratoplasty for aphakic bullous keratopathy and Fuchs' dystrophy, *Am J Ophthalmol* 88:1000-1004, 1979.

47. Paton RT, Swartz G: Keratoplasty for Fuchs' dystrophy, *Arch Ophthalmol* 61:366, 1969.

48. Polack FM: The triple procedure—use of Healon in preserved donor tissue, *Cataract* 2(5):15-22, 1985.

49. Rao GN, Stevens RE, Harris JK, Aquavella JV: Long term changes in corneal endothelium following intraocular lens implantation, *Ophthalmology* 88:386-397, 1981.

50. Ruusuvaara P, Setala K: The triple procedure penetrating keratoplasty, extracapsular cataract extraction and posterior chamber lens implantation, *Acta Ophthalmol* 65:433-443, 1987.

51. Skorpik C, Menapace R, Gnad HD, Grasl M: The triple procedure—results in cataract patients with corneal opacity, *Ophthalmologica* 196(1):1-6, 1988.

52. Smith PW, Stark WJ, Maumenee AE, et al: Retinal detachment after extracapsular cataract extraction with posterior chamber lens implantation, *Ophthalmology* 94:495-504, 1987.

53. Speaker MG, Guerriero PN, Met JA, et al: A case-controlled study of risk factors for intraoperative suprachoroidal expulsive hemorrhage, *Ophthalmology* 98:202-210, 1991.

54. Stark WJ, Maumenee AE: Cataract extraction after successful penetrating keratoplasty, *Am J Ophthalmol* 75:751-754, 1973.

55. Taylor DM: Keratoplasty and intraocular lenses, *Ophthalmic Surg* 7(1):31-42, 1976.

56. Taylor DM, Khaliq A: Keratoplasty and intraocular lenses: follow-up study, *Ophthalmic Surg* 8:49-57, 1977.

57. Taylor DM, Khalig R, Maxwell R: Keratoplasty and intraocular lenses: current status, *Ophthalmology* 86:242-254, 1979.

58. Taylor DM, Stern AL, McDonald P: The triple procedure: 2-10 year follow-up, *Trans Am Acad Ophthalmol Soc* 84:221-249, 1986.

59. Thomas JWT: Technique and results in keratoplasty, *Trans Ophthalmol Soc UK* 75:473, 1955.

60. Zirm E: Eine erfolgreiche totale Keratoplastik, *Arch Ophthalmol* 64:580-593, 1906.

Surgical Technique: the Triple Procedure

JOHN D. HUNKELER
DANIEL S. DURRIE
TIMOTHY B. CAVANAUGH

Combined penetrating keratoplasty, cataract extraction, and lens implantation is the currently accepted treatment of choice for older patients with combined corneal and cataract disease. As with lens implantation alone, the lower age limits for this procedure are steadily being lowered. Logic dictates the efficacy of the procedure with the reduction of surgical and visual morbidity versus performing surgery two or more times. Clinical results have been extremely encouraging, as reported by Lee and Dohlman,[11] Alpar,[1] Buxton and Jaffe,[5] Hunkeler and Hyde,[8] Buxton,[4] and Lindstrom, Harris and Doughman.[12] The long-term results continue to be encouraging, as reported by Hunkeler and Hyde[9] in 1983. Casey reports the surgical technique in the triple procedure, describing the implantation of the anterior chamber lens, the iris-supported lens, or the posterior chamber lens.[6]

ADVANTAGES OF EXTRACAPSULAR TECHNIQUE AND POSTERIOR CHAMBER INTRAOCULAR LENSES

Acceptance of the triple procedure as the treatment of choice for patients with combined corneal and cataract disease has been gradual in coming. Certainly the success of penetrating keratoplasty and long-term graft survival have improved dramatically as has our understanding of the corneal function as it relates to graft survival. Furthermore, the refinement of extracapsular surgical techniques combined with posterior chamber lens implantation has served as a breakthrough to allow more surgeons to consider performing the triple procedure. With the extracapsular technique, the posterior capsule functions not only as a protective barrier between the anterior and posterior compartments of the eye, but also as a platform of support for a posterior chamber lens.[16] With the optic of the posterior chamber lens behind a small pupil of a constricted iris, the endothelium is naturally protected during corneal suturing, an advantage that makes the operation much simpler. With both anterior chamber and iris-supported lens implants, more intraocular lens material is exposed to the endothelial surface with the attendant risk of endothelial damage. With the flexible anterior chamber lenses, there is a greater risk of forward vaulting than with the less flexible, solid, polymethylmethacrylate lenses.

VISCOELASTIC SUBSTANCES

In discussing the evolution and advancement of the techniques in the triple procedure, it is also extremely important to recognize the role of viscosurgery. Before the advent of viscoelastic substances like sodium hyaluronate, the triple procedure was much more difficult to perform from a technical standpoint. We have learned to use viscoelastic substances to coat the endothelium and the implant, allowing us to maintain tissue-plane separation throughout the surgical procedure. This is critical in the prevention of endothelial cell trauma during graft suturing. It is difficult to recall the days when we performed surgery without viscoelastic substances, utilizing a two-plane intraocular lens with mild-to-moderate pressure on the posterior lens capsule threatening to force the implant forward against the endothelium of the donor cornea. When this happened, the lens implant portion of the operation was abandoned, necessitating either spectacle or contact lens fitting postoperatively, or secondary intraocular lens implantation later.

COMBINED VERSUS SINGLE PROCEDURES

The indications for the triple procedure are relatively straightforward. Those patients with combined corneal and cataract disease who require improvement in vision within their own reasonable life-style are excellent candidates for the procedure. If the improvement in visual function can be achieved by either cataract and lens implant surgery or corneal surgery separately, the simpler procedure should be the procedure of choice. The assessment of the extent of corneal disease and lens opacity is based upon the surgeon's preoperative evaluation. Occasionally, however, the surgeon may have to delay the final decision about the severity of the cataract until the time of surgery when the cloudy cornea has been removed and the lens can be inspected directly. If the cataract appears to be dense enough to decrease the vision to 20/50 or worse postoperatively and a clear cornea is in place, the lens should be removed at the time of keratoplasty. When the patient with a cataract disease is being assessed, if the surgeon believes the vision will be 20/50 or worse because of corneal opacification postoperatively, a triple procedure should be performed. On the other hand, some patients with mild nonprogressive regular corneal scarring, as in eyes with inactive interstitial keratitis of luetic origin, may regain excellent visual activity after cataract surgery alone. The opinion of a corneal specialist regarding single versus combined procedures in such cases is invaluable.

Be cautioned, however, that the prolonged operating time associated with the combined procedure is potentially associated with the devastating complication of expulsive choroidal hemorrhage. Although the complication can occur with either corneal transplant or cataract surgery alone, it is more likely to occur in triple procedures. Most cases seem to occur in patients that move, cough, or squeeze the eyelids during the "open-sky" portion of the operation. The importance of an adequate lid block cannot be overemphasized. In patients that have risk factors for expulsive choroidal hemorrhage (advanced age, glaucoma) or are likely to be restless during surgery, the surgeon may be wise to stage the procedures. Good results have been obtained with an initial penetrating keratoplasty followed later by phacoemulsification and posterior chamber lens implantation. Another advantage to the staged method is the improved accuracy in lens-implant power calculations using stable postkeratoplasty keratometry readings.

INDICATIONS FOR SURGERY—FUCHS' DYSTROPHY

The majority of patients who undergo the triple procedure have Fuchs' corneal endothelial dystrophy combined with cataract. Evaluation of the patient with Fuchs' dystrophy is a little more complex. In the patient with severe cornea guttata and cataract formation, a critical evaluation is necessary to assess the need for combined corneal and cataract surgery. When the cataract is severe enough to warrant extraction and possible lens implantation, a critical evaluation of the endothelial function is necessary. Symptoms and manifestations of early morning corneal edema certainly indicate endothelial decompensation, and epithelial edema in the contralateral eye should arouse suspicion of impending corneal decompensation in the eye under scrutiny. An increase in the corneal thickness beyond 0.62 mm indicates possible impending corneal decompensation, as does the presence of Descemet's folds and central epithelial edema. Certainly, when there is generalized epithelial edema, gross thickening of the cornea, extensive formation of bullae, and peripheral corneal vascularization, the diagnosis and suggested management are straightforward. It is the subtle case that requires good clinical judgment to avoid corneal decompensation after cataract extraction with or without lens implantation and without corneal transplantation. The presence of cornea guttata alone is not an indication for the triple procedure. However, with corneal thicknesses over 0.62 mm, evidence of prior corneal decompensation and the presence of obvious corneal changes on slitlamp examination are indications to proceed with keratoplasty. Corneal scarring caused by prior injury or infection, keratoconus, and hereditary corneal dystrophy make up the bulk of the remaining indications.

CONTRAINDICATIONS

If a simple corneal transplant is contraindicated, for example, in an eye with ocular pemphigoid or infiltrative keratitis with corneal melting, then a triple procedure also should not be performed. Patients with proliferative diabetic retinopathy, uncontrolled glaucoma, and recurrent episodes of moderately severe or severe uveitis and patients with abnormal anterior segment anatomy that is not supportive of a lens implant are poor candidates for the triple procedure. Furthermore, patients with a history of severe herpetic stromal keratitis or prior active keratouveitis may have complicated postoperative courses afterward. Based on clinical experience, these patients may do better with separate procedures.

INTRAOCULAR-LENS POWER CALCULATIONS

After the decision has been made to proceed with the triple procedure, the lens-implant power calculation should be performed. Binder[2] and Crawford and co-workers[7] have attempted to evaluate the parameters that assist in proper lens-implant power selection. They have developed linear-regression formulas based on their clinical experience. Retzlaff reported a linear-regression formula that has been used for cataract extraction with lens implantation.[13] It has been our experience to use this published regression formula utilizing the standard *A* constant for the particular intraocular lens to be used in inserting a prospective, postoperative keratometric value into the formula. After reviewing a series of 100 patients, the mean keratometric value was 44.0 diopters in patients at least 1 year after operation and sutures out. The measurements were taken at least 1 month after suture removal. The formula is as follows:

$$\text{Intraocular lens power} = A \text{ constant (usually 116 diopters)}$$

$$-2.5 \times \text{Axial length} -0.9 \times 43.5 \text{ diopters}$$

Each corneal surgeon should individualize his or her own IOL power calculations by noting the average keratometry readings for a series of patients after keratoplasty.

SURGICAL TECHNIQUE

Softening the Globe. Once suitable corneal donor tissue has been obtained, the intraocular lens power has been calculated and the correct lens has been ordered, the surgeon is ready to proceed. On the day of surgery, either a local or general anesthetic may be used. In our practice, the majority of cases are done under local anesthesia. If general anesthesia is selected, endotracheal anesthesia is preferred. For local anesthesia, minimal preoperative sedation is necessary. We first achieve ocular and orbital compression using the Honan pressure cuff to soften the eye for 20 to 30 minutes preoperatively at the pressure level of 20 to 25 mm Hg. Routinely a soft eye is obtained with minimal orbital pressure. We typically use peribulbar anesthesia along with a facial nerve block followed by placement of the Honan balloon for 10 minutes at 30 mm Hg. The anesthetic is usually given during the latter stages of ocular compression to lengthen the duration of the anesthetic for the entire procedure. Giving the anesthetic before ocular compression takes effect allows much of it to wear off before the end of the surgical procedure. We prefer a combination of Marcaine (bupivacaine) and Xylocaine (lidocaine) anesthetics. Equal parts of 4% lidocaine and 0.75% bupivacaine are mixed to give a solution that is 0.375% bupivacaine and 2% lidocaine. Wydase (hyaluronidase) is also incorporated with the anesthetic to aid in tissue spread. This local anesthesia gives a rapid onset with the lidocaine, long staying power with the bupivacaine, and few adverse reactions. The eye is anesthetized topically using tetracaine 0.5% on admission. Topical polymyxin B sulfate, neomycin, gramicidin is instilled onto the surface of the cornea 30, 45, and 60 minutes before surgery. Pupillary dilatation is achieved with 1% cyclopentolate, and 2.5% phenylephrine is given in the same time interval preoperatively (30, 45, and 60 minutes).

Preparation. The patient is brought to the operating room and placed on the operating table in a supine position with the head and drapes supported by the Chan wrist rest system. In the space between the patient's head and the wrist, excess irrigating fluids from the operation can be pooled so that the foot controls of the microscope will be protected. The operating microscope should have excellent coaxial illumination, preferably with a motorized focus and zoom lens and an *x-y* translation system, which allows optimal utilization of the microscope throughout the operation. Final positioning of the patient is important, and it is our preference to have the facial features in a flat plane and the head in an apparently comfortable position. We also prefer to have the body relatively flat with some break at the knees for patient comfort.

We prefer to prepare the donor tissue before prepping and draping the patient and to cut the donor tissue endothelial side up with an Iowa or Troutman corneal trephine punch. The disposable trephine selected is 0.25 mm greater than the opening to be made in the recipient cornea. The donor button is placed in a sterile petri dish in balanced saline solution and covered before transplantation. The eye is prepared with povidone-iodine (Betadine) solution and saline irrigation. A paper drape is used to cover the body, and a separate paper drape is further utilized to cover the head with a solid patch of adhesive plastic in the center. The facial drape is prepared by removal of the adhesive protecting patch, and the lids are retracted by the scrubnurse assistant. The adhesive surface is applied directly to the retracted lids and exposed host cornea. The sticky adhesive will not adhere to the cornea but adheres nicely to the lids and lashes. A central cut is made in the drape adhesive plastic to allow the insertion of a wire lid speculum. The lashes remain everted and out of the surgical field. A single Flieringa ring is then secured into place with four interrupted 6-0 silk sutures placed at 1:30, 4:30, 7:30, and 10:30 o'clock positions. The rest of the suture can be passed under the ring at 6 and 12 o'clock in order to maneuver the Flieringa ring and globe during the operation, as needed. The speculum and Flieringa ring are inspected to ensure minimal pressure effects upon the globe throughout the operation.

Before actually starting the operation, one would be wise to have vitrectomy instrumentation available. Certainly the equipment does not need to be set up but should be available if a vitrectomy becomes necessary.

Removal of Epithelium. By the time of surgery, several pathologic changes may have occurred in eyes with Fuchs' corneal dystrophy (Fig. 13-1). Epithelial edema, bullae, and striate keratopathy may result in significant corneal thickening. Frank corneal decompensation may have occurred in addition to dense, nuclear cataract formation. It is our preference to remove edematous corneal epithelium with or without micropannus with a No. 15 Bard-Parker blade. This decreases the chance for slippage of the trephine and irregular cutting of Bowman's membrane and the anterior lamellae of the cornea. Occasionally, some cautery is required for prolific vessels, but this is unusual because the bleeding normally ceases on its own. Where no minimal peripheral epithelial edema exists, removal of healthy pe-

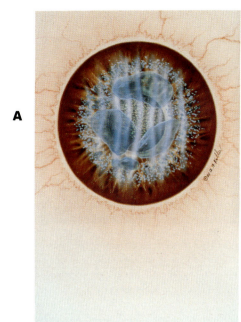

A

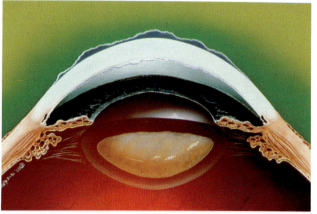

B

Fig. 13-1. A, Cornea with advanced Fuchs' dystrophy showing microcystoid and bullous epithelial edema, striate keratopathy, and circumciliary flush. **B,** Dense nuclear cataract in eye with advanced Fuchs' corneal dystrophy. Slit-lamp evaluation of lens changes may be difficult when significant corneal edema is present.

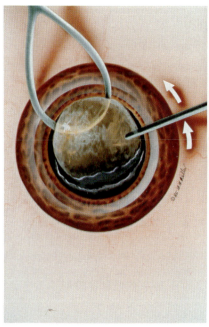

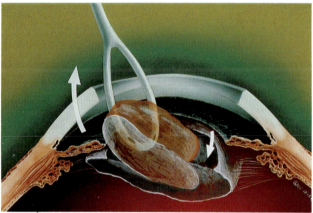

Fig. 13-2. Lens loop and irrigating cannula used to deliver nucleus after anterior capsulotomy.

ripheral recipient epithelium is unnecessary.

Cutting the Recipient Wound. A Barron-Hessburg vacuum trephine is used to incise the recipient cornea. The blade is aligned with the edge of the trephine housing under operating microscope guidance, and the blade is then retracted 3 quarter turns. The cross hairs in the trephine are centered on the cornea with the syringe plunger held in. When we are certain that the trephine is in the proper posi-

tion, the plunger is released and the resultant vacuum suctions the trephine mechanism in place. The blade is then advanced 6½ quarter turns, which corresponds to a corneal incision of approximately 300 μm. The incision depth is checked with 0.12 mm tooth forceps. The dissection is carried deeper with a slight inward beveling by use of either a diamond knife or a disposable 22-degree blade. The anterior chamber is then entered, and the incision is ex-

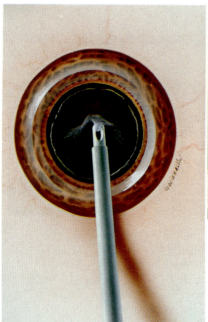

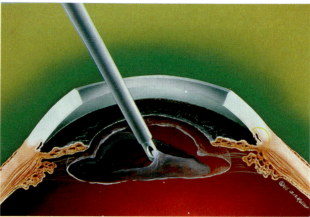

Fig. 13-3. Aspiration of residual lens cortex after removal of nucleus. Stripping is best accomplished when peripheral anterior cortex is engaged and gently pulled toward center with improved red reflex being noted.

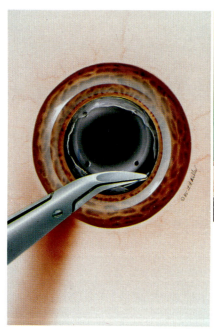

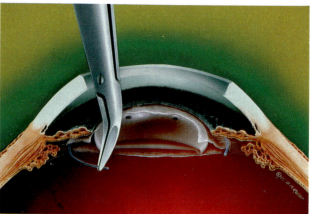

Fig. 13-4. In-the-bag placement of posterior-chamber intraocular lens using needle-holder guidance of superior loop.

tended 360 degrees with corneal transplant microscissors. There is a slight obvious inner bevel to the incision.

Capsulotomy and Lens Removal. A round capsulotomy is performed with scissors or capsulorrhexis. It is wise to avoid contact with the iris to prevent premature myosis before removal of the nucleus. The central piece of anterior capsule is removed, and any excess tags of peripheral anterior capsule can also be removed at this point. A nice, round

opening is preferred. The lens nucleus is removed by placement of a lens loop under the inferior pole of the elevated nucleus (Fig. 13-2). The nucleus is raised superiorly and anteriorly with a 25-gage irrigating cannula placed just above the inferior pole, which is then forced superiorly and anteriorly. The cleavage plane develops, allowing insertion of the lens loop with or without an irrigating component. Once this cleavage plane has been established, a counterclockwise rotary movement is used with a 25-

gage irrigating cannula to spin the nucleus out of the capsule bag. If this fails, for whatever reason, the nucleus can be brought forward with posterior pressure on the peripheral cornea in the 5 o'clock meridian, which raises the intraocular pressure, bringing the nucleus forward. At this point, the 25-gage irrigating cannula can fix the nucleus, and the lens loop can be slipped underneath the nucleus before its removal. It is also possible to remove the nucleus by application of a cryoprobe to the dried central nucleus and to gently pull it up.

Irrigation and Aspiration. The remainder of the lens cortex can be removed with conventional cortical cleanup, irrigation, and aspiration systems (Fig. 13-3). Our preference is the use of mechanical irrigation and aspiration; however, manual technique can be equally effective. It is important to use relatively little fluid irrigation because excess fluid obscures the surgeon's view of the red reflex and creates multiple-mirrored images from the fluid surface, obscuring a good view of the cortex and posterior lens capsule. The anterior cortical tissue is engaged with the aspirator and stripped toward the center. There is no special technique required for cortical stripping in the soft eye. Occasionally, with positive posterior pressure and a convex posterior lens capsule, aspiration in the fornix of the capsule bag is difficult, but this can be facilitated by gentle posterior pressure on the peripheral posterior lens capsule while one strips away the cortical material. The gentle posterior pressure develops the cleavage plane, allowing engagement of the anterior cortex peripherally. Once the majority of cortex has been removed, a Kratz sandblasted capsule polisher is used to clean off the central posterior capsule.

Intraocular Lens Insertion. Ultraviolet-absorbing posterior chamber IOLs are our choice for placement within the capsular bag (Fig. 13-4). Sodium hyaluronate may be used to separate the anterior and posterior lens capsules to facilitate "in-the-bag" loop placement. If necessary, the lens position can be inspected with a hook, and the lens implant rotated to achieve centration. A small peripheral iridotomy is optional. After the IOL is positioned, acetylcholine chloride (Miochol) is used for miosis and to ensure final placement of the lens behind the iris. Viscoelastic material is then placed into the anterior chamber and along the corneal incision.

Suturing the Graft. The donor cornea is removed from the petri dish containing the balanced saline solution and placed over the recipient hole where it is secured with four cardinal 10-0 monofilament nylon sutures, placed sequentially at 12, 6, 3, and 9 o'clock positions. The chamber can be deepened with balanced saline solution at this point and supplemented with air or viscoelastic material. With a nice coat of viscoelastic material, it is possible to use air, which minimizes the amount of viscoelastic material and gives a firmer eye for excellent suture placement. Recently, we have changed to Viscoat and have not experienced significant postoperative intraocular pressure rises despite often leaving much of the material in the anterior chamber at the close of surgery.

Eight additional interrupted sutures (Fig. 13-5, *A*) are placed equally spaced between the four cardinal sutures, and all the knots are buried in the peripheral host cornea. Suture depth placement is at the 50% or greater level. Short bites are preferred to minimize tissue compression centrally, with a larger central optical zone being left. Between each of the 12 bites of permanent interrupted suture, one places continuous sutures, also utilizing 10-0 monofilament nylon (Fig. 13-5, *B*) with the knot buried on the host side. Tying the continuous suture more gently than the interrupted sutures allows for effective reduction of graft astigmatism by selective removal of the interrupted sutures.

Adjustment of Sutures. The anterior chamber air and excess viscoelastic substance are removed from the anterior chamber, and the wound tightness is inspected. With a tight wound at this point, the Flieringa ring is removed. Attention is now paid to adjustment of the suture tension to minimize postkeratoplasty astigmatism.

In lieu of sophisticated instrumentation, a simple instrument such as the Hyde astigmatic ruler can be used to project a circular keratoscopic image onto the cornea.[10] The coaxial light of the operating microscope is directed toward the vertically aligned eye. A circular image is created as the coaxial light reflects off the inner circular ring of the astigmatic ruler, projecting such a ring onto the corneal surface, which can be monitored by the surgeon viewing through the oculars of the microscope system. The continuous suture can be relaxed in the steep meridian and tightened in the flat meridian. The oval mire can be converted to a circular configuration, which is the desired end point. Although this doesn't solve the long-term problems, it helps to minimize postkeratoplasty astigmatism until selective suture removal can be performed[14] and may obviate the need for such suture removal. This allows earlier visual rehabilitation for the patient with much less cylindric correction in the short term, the intermediate term, and, one would hope, in the long term.

Recently, we have been conducting a study using 24 interrupted 11-0 Mersilene sutures for closure.

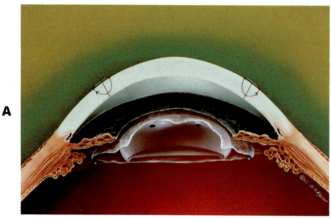

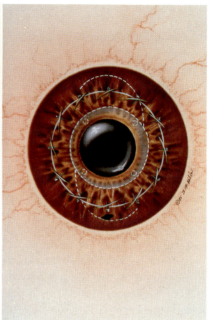

Fig. 13-5. A, Corneal button held in place with interrupted nylon suture placed at three-fourths depth and knots buried on recipient side. **B,** Closure with 12 interrupted nylon sutures with each continuous suture bite between each clock hour.

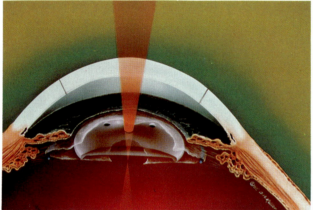

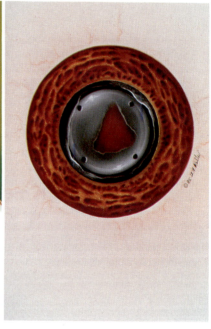

Fig. 13-6. YAG laser capsulectomy through graft. Any secondary iritis or glaucoma must be controlled to avoid graft failure and rejection.

We have been pleased with the control we have over postkeratoplasty astigmatism with early selective suture removal and like the added insurance for long-term wound integrity that permanent sutures provide. We have been impressed how little graft incisions heal even over the period of years. Wound dehiscence after suture removal or trauma is not an uncommon occurrence even years postoperatively. In addition, at the time of regraft, most wounds can easily be separated using minimal blunt dissection with jewelers' forceps. Our hope is that the 11-0 Mersilene sutures will be well tolerated on a perma-

nent basis and thereby provide a lifetime of wound security for transplant patients.

Inadvertent Capsular Rupture. If the posterior lens capsule is inadvertently broken during the procedure either with a small tear centrally or peripherally in a small sector, a posterior chamber lens may still be inserted. Provided that there is a stable capsular platform, the lens can be gently inserted within the capsular bag or in the ciliary sulcus. If, however, extensive vitreous surgery is required, it is advisable to insert a flexible anterior chamber lens. One can accomplish this through the keratoplasty opening,

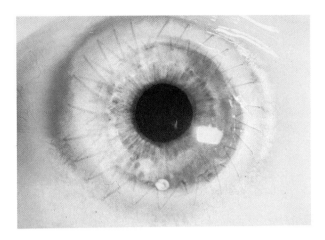

Fig. 13-7. Eye 8 months after operation by triple procedure with continuous suture alone.

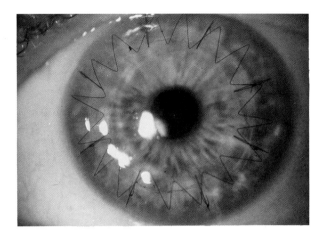

Fig. 13-8. Eye 7 months after operation by triple procedure with interrupted 10-0 and continuous 11-0 nylon suture.

avoiding a second incision at the limbus. It is rarely necessary to do this, but a backup lens and the appropriate power should be available. Sizing can present a problem, and so flexibility is important.

Once the suture has been adjusted to minimize astigmatism, the procedure is essentially complete. The Flieringa ring is removed, and subconjunctival injections of 0.5 ml of betamethasone (Celestone) and 0.5 ml of gentamicin are then give in the inferior temporal quadrant. A patch and Fox shield is applied to the eye after instillation of an antibiotic steroid ointment. The procedure can be performed on an outpatient basis, and the patient is then prepared for discharge. Otherwise, a 2-day hospital stay is usually all that is necessary.

POSTOPERATIVE CARE

The patient is examined on the first postoperative day for wound integrity, anterior chamber inflammation, and measurement of the intraocular pressure. With current suturing techniques, a pronounced elevation of the intraocular pressure may occur, especially if excess viscoelastic material is left inside the eye. This is best controlled with oral carbonic anhydrase inhibitors such as acetazolamide (Diamox) or methazolamide (Neptazane). The remainder of the postoperative care and treatment is similar to that outlined in Chapter 18.

Following the aforementioned protocol, excellent clinical results can be obtained. Rapid visual rehabilitation with minimal postkeratoplasty astigmatism gives the patient a good functional result. Posterior capsular opacification occurs with about the same frequency as in simple extracapsular cataract extraction and is treated by YAG-laser capsulectomy (Fig. 13-6) without threat to the graft.

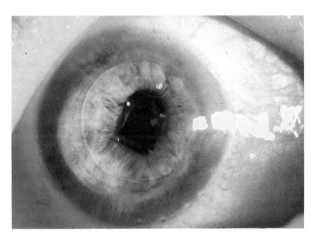

Fig. 13-9. Eye 4 years after operation by triple procedure with medallion style of intraocular lens inserted into capsular bag for fixation.

Certainly, variations on this technique can give equally good results. Different suturing techniques with continuous or interrupted sutures alone (Fig. 13-7) or in combination with 11-0 nylon (Fig. 13-8) work very nicely. However, in our hands, the 12 interrupted 10-0 nylon sutures with a continuous suture of 10-0 nylon has been most effective up to now. As reported previously, the long-term results in our expanded series of triple procedures report 80% 20/40 or better. The graft survival rate is comparable to the results with keratoplasty in the absence of a lens implant (Fig. 13-9). The triple procedure continues to be the treatment of choice for the majority of patients with combined corneal and cataract disease requiring surgery to restore functional vision.

REFERENCES

1. Alpar JJ: Keratoplasty with primary and secondary lens implantation, *Ophthalmic Surg* 9:58-66, 1978.
2. Binder PS: Intraocular lens powers used in the triple procedure: effect on visual acuity and refractive error, *Ophthalmology* 92:1561-1566, 1985.
3. Bourne WM: Morphologic and functional evaluation of the endothelium of transplanted human corneas, Trans *Am Ophthalmol Soc* 81:403-450, 1983.
4. Buxton JN: The triple procedure: corneal graft, intracapsular cataract extraction and intraocular lens, *Contact Intra-Ocular Lens Med J* 6:409-412, 1980.
5. Buxton JN, Jaffe MS: Combined keratoplasty, cataract extraction with intraocular lens implantation, *Am Intra-Ocular Implant Soc J* 4(3):110, 1978.
6. Casey TA: *Corneal grafting*, Philadelphia, 1984, Saunders, pp 208-217.
7. Crawford GJ, Stulting RD, Waring GO III, et al: The triple procedure: analysis of the outcome, refraction and intraocular lens power calculation, *Ophthalmology* 91:88, 1984. (Abstract.)
8. Hunkeler JD, Hyde LL: The triple procedure: combined penetrating keratoplasty, cataract extraction and lens implantation, *Am Intra-Ocular Implant Soc J* 5(3):222-224, 1979.

9. Hunkeler JD, Hyde LL: The triple procedure: combined penetrating keratoplasty, extracapsular cataract extraction and lens implantation: an expanded experience, *Am Intra-Ocular Implant Soc J* 9:20-24, 1983.
10. Hyde LL: The surgical astigmatic ruler, *Am Intra-Ocular Implant Soc J* 10:84-86, 1984.
11. Lee JR, Dohlman CH: Intraocular lens implantation in combination with keratoplasty, *Ann Ophthalmol* 9:58-66, 1978.
12. Lindstrom RL, Harris WS, Doughman DJ: Combined penetrating keratoplasty, extracapsular cataract extraction and posterior chamber lens implantation, *Am Intra-Ocular Implant Soc J* 7:130-132, 1981.
13. Retzlaff J: Posterior chamber implant power calculation: regressive formula, *Am Intra-Ocular Implant Soc J* 6:268-273, 1980.
14. Stainer GA, Perl T, Binder PS: Controlled reduction of postkeratoplasty astigmatism, *Ophthalmology* 89:668-676, 1982.
15. Sugar A, Meyer R, Heidemann D, et al: Specular microscopic followup of corneal grafts for pseudophakic bullous keratopathy, *Ophthalmology* 92:325-330, 1985.
16. Worst J: Extracapsular surgery in lens implantation (Binkhorst Lecture). Part IV. Some anatomical and pathophysiological implications, *Am Intra-Ocular Implant Soc J* 4(1):7-14, 1978.

Chapter 14

Corneal Trephines and Cutting Blocks

EMANUEL TANNE

The most common complication of corneal transplantation remains excessive postoperative astigmatism. Its creation intraoperatively is related to several events but primarily to host-graft disparity.[5,33] Troutman estimates from clinical measurements that a 0.1 mm disparity in host-graft size results in approximately 1 diopter of astigmatism,[34] and Olson's mathematical model predicted significant meridional astigmatism in the presence of relatively small host-graft differences.[22] Since the perfect fit of a donor button in its recipient bed is dependent on equality of size and similarity of shape, it behooves the corneal surgeon to seek out those trephines and cutting blocks that achieve the most accurate and reproducible cuts.

HISTORY

The concept of a circular cutting trephine was conceived by Erasmus Darwin in 1796, but the first trephine was actually constructed by Arthur von Hipple in 1886.[37] The von Hipple trephine consisted of a circular cutting edge on a long shaft and an obturator and depth guide. The shaft was rotated mechanically by a wind-up clocklike mechanism at the opposite end. In 1906 Eduard Konrad Zirm performed the first successful human corneal transplant with the von Hipple trephine. For many years to come the circular trephine would remain the basic instrument for trephination, and its development ushered in the era of present-day keratoplasty.

CLASSIFICATION OF TREPHINES

1. Traditional circular cutting trephines
2. Single-point cutting trephines
3. Combination trephines
4. Noncontact trephines (lasers)

Traditional Circular Cutting Trephines. There are three types of circular cutting trephines:
Motorized
Suction-fixation type
Special-purpose type
Initially circular cutting trephines with solid handles, such as the early Castroviejo models, did not have disposable cutting edges and therefore required continual resharpening, which in turn often led to alterations of the original circular dimensions. Improvements came in the form of disposable blades thus eliminating dullness and distortion. The solid-handled device with an adjustable inner core obturator permitted the surgeon to select the depth of corneal cut and afforded a limited opportunity for controlled entry into the anterior chamber. Nevertheless, actual entry is a surgically learned experience that has a potential for nightmarish results. With the advent of the surgical microscope and its restricted field, the once advantageous obturator became a liability, for it obstructed visualization of the central cornea beneath the trephine and made centration difficult. As microsurgical keratoplasty procedures became the order of the day, see-through trephines gained popularity and ingenious models appeared. Drews,[10] Donaldson,[8] Miller,[20] Doughman,[9] and many other names are associated with their introduction (Fig. 14-1). Drews created a cone type of trephine, Donaldson added a handle for stability, Miller an open "branding-iron" configuration, and Doughman a hollow tube holder accepting varying size blades. Now for the first time the microsurgeon

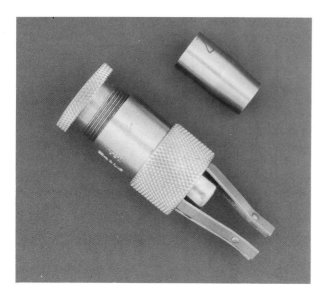

Fig. 14-1. See-through handle and disposable trephine blade.

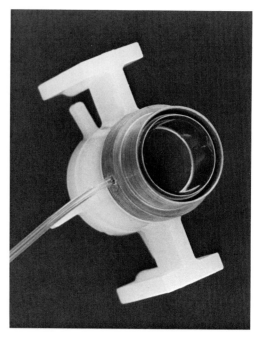

Fig. 14-2. Hessburg-Barron disposable trephine with outer corneal suction ring and inner circular cutting blade.

not only was able to view his direct entry into the anterior chamber, but also he did so assuredly without changing the angle of his vision.

The see-through instruments provide a microscope view of the central cornea through the hollow circular blade, but since they require the surgeon's hand to rotate the trephine, some obstruction of the microscope field is inevitable. Smirmaul and Casey[30] addressed this problem. The large main body of their trephine is fixated by one hand outside the microscopic field. The nonfixating hand, also remote from the field, turns a flexible shaft connected at right angles to the circular cutter by a bevel gear. A clear view of the entire cornea and the corneoscleral limbus is possible with this instrument.

Motorized. Motorized trephines, though especially popular in Germany and Switzerland, have not received wide acceptance in America. Early models by Rizzuti,[27] Arato,[2] and Kadesky[16] and a later model by Barraquer and Mateus had in common an electric motor in the main body and a circular trephine at the motor shaft end. The Rizzuti and Arato model had, in addition, a wire ring extension around the blade to serve as a stable centering device and to permit anterior chamber entry without jeopardizing anterior chamber structures. Cohen's and Benko's[6] concern about anterior chamber injury led them to develop a protective corneal clamp over which motorized trephining took place. However, a T-shape penetrating corneal incision was required for clamp placement. The Hoffmann[15] motorized trephine

makes use of a limbal suction ring to assist in anterior chamber maintenance and protection during trephination.

Besides potential anterior chamber damage, some surgeons have complained about the corkscrew type of edge created by some motorized trephines. However, Schanzlin, Robin, and Spence[28] reported less stromal lamellar disruption and a smoother interface using a variable-speed trephine (Micro-Keratron, Hans Geuder, Heidelberg) at 800 rpm than with manual trephinations. This finding of better stromal preservation led those authors to speculate that a better opportunity for wound healing may occur. The Micro-Keratron unit not only allows for variation of rotation velocity, but also has rapid braking within a tenth of a second.

Suction Fixation. Despite the improvement in sharpness and see-through viewing, the elusive goal of a truly perpendicular cut has not been completely attainable. Trephine tilting results in ovaling of the recipient bed as well as undercutting and posterior lip formation of the wound.[23] Hessburg and Barron,[14] utilizing the suction-fixation principle of the Guyton-Bahan motorized corneal trephine, developed a simplified disposable trephine. The trephine consists of an outer corneal suction ring for fixation and an inner circular cutting blade (Fig. 14-2). A spring-loaded disposable syringe (Fig. 14-3) creates the required negative pressure, and the suction fixa-

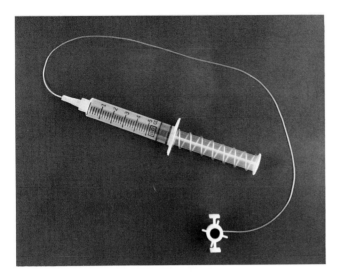

Fig. 14-3. Hessburg-Barron disposable trephine with spring-loaded syringe for creating suction.

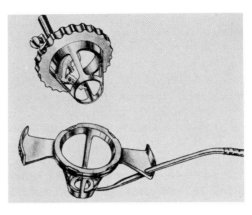

Fig. 14-4. Lieberman single-point, cam-guided corneal cutter. (From Troutman RC: *Microsurgery of the anterior segment of the eye.* Vol. 2, *The cornea: optics and surgery*, St. Louis, 1977, Mosby–Year Book.)

tion provides stability and an opportunity to cut perpendicularly to the limbal plane regardless of the angle or tilt of the trephine. Phillips[26] has reported the instrument useful for extremely soft or perforated eyes. Duffin and co-workers[12] reported accurate, spherical cuts in the anterior stroma but with a tendency toward outward beveling in the posterior layers. Although the Hessburg-Barron trephine appears to be a vast improvement over the other circular cutting trephines, corneal distortion still remains a problem.

Special-Use Trephines. The conventional corneal "cookie-cutter" trephine was modified by Moses and Holm[21] to perform a definitive transplant in cases of optical zone lacerations. This instrument would consolidate two separate surgical procedures, that of initial repair and later transplantation, into one. To avoid lens and iris damage during trephining, they supported the lacerated cornea from behind by a protective plate placed in the anterior chamber, a principle originally reported by Wiener and Alvis[38] in 1940. The Moses unit incorporates a buttonlike footplate on a vertical shaft. After footplate introduction into the anterior chamber an upper plate is brought down toward the buttonlike footplate until the cornea is securely clamped between the two plates. The trephine descends along the vertical shaft completing the cut without damage to the iris or lens.

Single-Point Cutting Trephines. In the quest for reduced corneal distortion, the single point cutter evolved. Since fixation takes place at the limbus or on the sclera, the problem of corneal distortion is

greatly reduced. The Lieberman[18] single-point cutter uses limbal suction fixation and is composed of two cones, one revolving within the other (Fig. 14-4). The outer cone is held by the fixating hand and contains the suction ring (10 to 15 mm Hg). The inner cone revolves and carries a disposable razor blade knife and is capable of making both circular and oval perpendicular cuts if desired with diameters from 2.0 to 8.5 mm. For 20-degree-angle cuts the surgeon may use an interchangeable cutter for lamellar transplants. After each rotation of the blade an adjusting screw is turned to lower the blade a few thousandths of an inch. The trephine cuts 360 degrees, and after cutting approximately 60 degrees of Descemet's membrane and endothelium Lieberman discontinues trephine rotation and completes the wound with corneal scissors. This instrument is for whole-eye trephination only and cannot be used in the popular endothelial punch technique on preserved corneas.

Crock and co-workers[7] have produced a similar single-point cutter that uses serrated edges for friction fixation at the limbus, an angle-cutting blade, and a quartz contact lens at the base of the inner cone. The serrated edge footplate on the outer cone is reversible for purposes of adjusting the contact lens to steeper conical corneas. A retractable control rod projects upwards from the body and is coupled with a micrometer screw to set the depth of the cutting blade. Each complete rotation of the rod produces a 0.3 mm change in blade depth. A second control rod is used to rotate the cutting blade. The instrument is not adjustable for different diameters, and therefore additional cutters must be used. The cutters are available in 1 mm variations ranging from 7 to 10 mm. Since the blade is angled, the instrument must be used on both the donor and the recipient to have similar edge configuration. Olson[24] experimentally found considerable variability in corneal opening size, which he attributed to cases in which uniform corneal contact with the contact lens was not achieved. However, the single-point corneal cutters do provide superior visibility under the microscope, the least corneal distortion, and a potential for reproducible controlled cutting.

Combination Trephines. As would be expected with the passage of time, new trephine systems that combine the best features of previous trephines have emerged. For example, the Hanna trephine system,[39] though using a circular razor cutting blade, incorporates many of the advantageous features characteristic of earlier single-point cutters (Lieberman and Crock). The instrument consists of two separate parts: a limbal suction ring system and a mechanical trephine fitted within the suction ring. The limbal suction fixates the trephine perpendicular to the cornea regardless of eye position. Cutting with the trephine is achieved by rotation of an external curled knob that is ultimately connected to the blade through a series of gears. A preset depth of cut is selected, and by rotation of the gear system the cut is obtained at the desired depth. Once the depth is reached there is no further descent of the blade despite continued knob rotation. An additional feature is the use of corneal support surfaces on either side of the trephine blade to enhance verticality of the cut. To aid in centration there is a gunsight alignment hole in the center of the trephine obturator.

In 1988 Krumeich and co-workers[17] described a trephine that also employs a circular cutting blade and a limbal suction fixation. The device, known as the Guided Trephine System (GTS), does not distort corneal curvature or raise intraocular tension with its unique suction-ring design. Centration is obtained by use of a cross-hair device placed initially within the suction-ring opening before positioning of the trephine. Unlike the Hanna trephine, the GTS uses a fixed-glass obturator for corneal support and thus trephines the cornea in an applanated state. The authors believe this enhances perpendicularity of the corneal cuts.

Noncontact Trephines (Lasers). In search for the ideal cutting device, the potential use of lasers for noncontact trephination must be considered. Laser noncontact trephination eliminates corneal topography distortion, provides complete corneal visualization, and improves centration. Comparative corneal edge studies have shown excimer laser (193 nm) noncontact trephination to be superior to mechanical trephination.[29] However, significant problems re-

main in equipment design, safety, corneal wound size,[32] potential for endothelial injury,[19] and mutagenicity, as well as cost.

In summary, the theoretical ideal trephine should have several features. Accurate and reproducible centration is a requirement.[35] Visualization of the circumference of the cutting edge, limbal area, and the central pupillary zone under the operating microscope is mandatory, and the instrument must be sharp, cut perpendicularly, and avoid corneal topography distortion and damage to anterior chamber structures. In addition, it must have stable fixation to avoid slipping and false cuts.

CUTTING BLOCKS AND CORNEAL PUNCHES

Before the present decade preparation of the donor graft was accomplished by the same technique applied to the recipient. The same inherent difficulties encountered in cutting the recipient were duplicated in cutting donor tissue. The anterior approach consisted in either trephination only or anterior chamber entry by trephine and wound completion by scissors. With the introduction of McCarey-Kaufman medium and the verification of better endothelial edge survival,[4] the posterior punch technique came into vogue. Cutting the donor tissue from the posterior surface has eliminated many of the aforementioned difficulties encountered in cutting the recipient from the anterior surface. Producing a circular button with an even edge profile is achievable with presently available instruments. Early descriptions of punch cutting of the graft from the endothelial side, usually over a paraffin block, exist in the ophthalmic literature.[1,36] The present-day cutting blocks attempt to approximate the corneal shape and reduce tissue distortion. More recently Teflon was used for cutting blocks, and early models consisted of several concavities of a single radius of curvature usually around 7.5 mm. The Brightbill[3] Teflon cutting block utilizes three wells, each with a different radius of curvature and diameter along with an 8 mm red centering dot. The Tanne[31] cutting block has a single well with multiple radii of curvature and a central air-escape hole (Fig. 14-5). This polycarbonate disposable block has a central 8 mm zone with a 7.85 mm (43.00-diopter) radius of curvature, a peripheral 2 mm wide zone of 8.23 mm, and a 3 mm wide parascleral zone of 12.25 mm radius (Fig. 14-6). A new version of this cutting block includes two concentric inlays of colored Teflon (polytef). The outer black Teflon zone has a 12.5 mm chord length and corresponds to the limbus, whereas a second white Teflon inlay with an 8

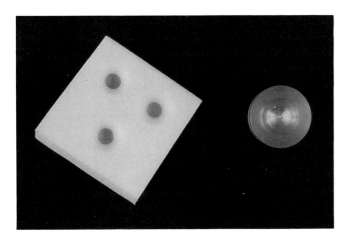

Fig. 14-5. *Left,* Brightbill Teflon cutting block containing three wells of varying diameter and base curve. *Right,* Tanne polycarbonate block with single multiple-curved well.

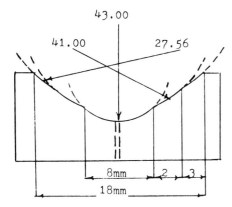

Fig. 14-6. Polycarbonate cutting block with three radii of curvatures. Design resembles posterior concave surface of a hard contact lens.

mm chord length identifies the central zone of the donor cornea.

Several cutting blocks make use of suction to both hold in place and mark the epithelial surface of the donor. Marking of the donor and the host improves alignment of host-donor circumference and facilitates suture placement according to the designers.[13,25]

Despite the development of improved cutting blocks freehand punching is an obstacle to accurate cutting and being off center will produce incomplete cuts, as well as eccentric cuts with an elliptical configuration. A preferred method is to combine a disposable multiple-radius cutting block with a vertical piston assembly containing the cutting edge. Troutman, Polack, Steele, Van Rij, Casey (East Grinstead), Cardona-Roskothen, Tanne, Hanna, Allarakhia

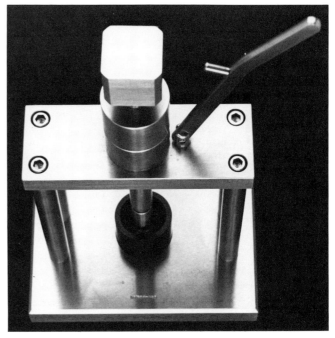

Fig. 14-7. Lieberman corneal punch.

(3M), and Lieberman among others have designed this type of cutting instrument. The Lieberman corneal punch illustrates the common features of these devices (Fig. 14-7). Accurate cutting is possible with the Lieberman punch, particularly in the 7.5 and 8 mm sizes.[11] As is the case with all punches, the punch itself, the tissue, and the block must be in perfect alignment.

With continual technical improvement in cutting methods the reduction and eventual elimination of excessive postkeratoplasty astigmatism can be anticipated in the not-too-distant future.

REFERENCES

1. Amsler M, Verry F: The removal of the graft for keratoplasty, *Arch Ophthalmol* (Paris) 8:150, 1948.
2. Arato S: A new electro-motor cornea trephine for keratoplasty, *Ophthalmologica* 121:38, 1951.
3. Brightbill FS: New forceps and cutting block for donor corneas, *Am J Ophthalmol* 89:744, 1980.
4. Brightbill FS, Polack FM, Slappey T: A comparison of two methods for cutting donor corneal buttons, *Am J Ophthalmol* 75(3):500, 1973.
5. Cohen LK, Tripoli NK, Pelton AC, et al: Effect of tissue fit on corneal shape after transplantation, *Invest Ophthalmol* 25:1226, 1984.
6. Cohen SW, Benko W: Automated motorized penetrating keratoplasty, *Ann Ophthalmol* 14:1461-1466, 1977.
7. Crock GW, Pericic L, Chapman-Smith JS, et al: A new system of microsurgery for human and experimental corneal grafting. I. The contact lens corneal cutter, stereotaxic eye holder, donor disc chuck, and frame, *Br J Ophthalmol* 62:74-80, 1978.

8. Donaldson WBM, Haining WM: A new corneal trephine, *Trans Ophthalmol Soc UK* 98:14-15, 1978.

9. Doughmann DJ: Corneal trephine holder, *Ophthalmology* 85(8):875-876, 1978.

10. Drews RC: Corneal trephine, *Trans Am Acad Ophthalmol Otolaryngol* 78:op223-224, 1974.

11. Duffin MR, Olson RJ: Laboratory analysis of the Lieberman corneal punch, *Ophthalmic Surg* 14:153, 1983.

12. Duffin MR, Olson RJ, Ohrloff C: Analysis of the Hessburg-Barron vacuum trephine, *Ophthalmic Surg* 15:51-54, 1984.

13. Gilbard JP, Rothman RC, Kenyon KR: A new donor cornea marker and punch for penetrating keratoplasty, *Ophthalmic Surg* 18:908-911, 1987.

14. Hessburg PC, Barron M: A disposable corneal trephine, *Ophthalmic Surg* 11:730, 1980.

15. Hoffmann F: Keratoplastik mit neuem Rotor-trepan, *Fortschr Ophthalmol* 79:552-554, 1983.

16. Kadesky D: An electric automatic trephine, *Am J Ophthalmol* 49:1038, 1960.

17. Krumeich J, Binder PS, Knuelle A: The theoretical effect of trephine tilt on post keratoplasty astigmatism, *CLAO J* 14(4):213-219, 1988.

18. Lieberman DM: A new corneal trephine, *Am J Ophthalmol* 81:684, 1976.

19. Marshal J, Trakel S, Rothery S, Schubert H: An ultrastructural study of corneal incisions induced by an excimer laser at 193nm, *Ophthalmology* 92:749-758, 1985.

20. Miller D: A new microsurgical corneal trephine, *Ophthalmic Surg* 10(7):55-58, 1979.

21. Moses RA, Holm O: A trephine for primary corneal transplant in repair of corneal laceration, *Am J Ophthalmol* 72(6):1147, 1971.

22. Olson RJ: Corneal curvature changes associated with penetrating keratoplasty: a mathematical model, *Ophthalmic Surg* 11:838, 1980.

23. Olson RJ: The effect of scleral fixation ring placement and trephine tilting on keratoplasty wound size and donor shape, *Ophthalmic Surg* 12(1):23-26, 1981.

24. Olson RJ: The contact lens cutter: accuracy and reproducibility, *Ophthalmic Surg* 13(3):210, 1982.

25. Pflugfelder S, Parel JM: A suction trephine block for marking donor corneal buttons, *Arch Ophthalmol* 106(2):276-281, 1988.

26. Phillips RL: Vacuum trephination of the hypotonus eye, *Ophthalmic Surg* 14:513-514, 1983.

27. Rizzuti BA: Automatic corneal trephine with special centering device, *Trans Am Acad Ophthalmol Otolaryngol* 68:894-898, 1964.

28. Schanzlin DJ, Robin JB, Spence DJ: Clinical and ultrasture analysis of variable speed corneal trephination, *Ophthalmic Surg* 14:755, 1983.

29. Serdarevic ON, Hanna K, Gribomont AC, et al: Excimer laser trephination in penetrating keratoplasty, *Ophthalmology* 95(4):493-505, 1988.

30. Smirmaul H, Casey TA: A clear view trephine and lamellar dissector for corneal grafting, *Am J Ophthalmol* 90:92-94, 1980.

31. Tanne E: A new donor cutting block for penetrating keratoplasty, *Ophthalmic Surg* 12:371, 1981.

32. Thompson K, Barraquer E, Parel JM, et al: Potential use of lasers for penetrating keratoplasty, *J Cataract Refract Surg* 15:397-403, 1989.

33. Troutman RC: *Microsurgery of the anterior segment of the eye. II. The cornea: optics and surgery,* St. Louis, 1977, Mosby–Year Book.

34. Troutman RC: Astigmatic considerations in corneal graft, *Ophthalmic Surg* 10(5):21-26, 1979.

35. Uozato H, Guyton DL: Centering corneal surgical procedures, *Am J Ophthalmol* 103:264-275, 1987.

36. Vannas M: A study of corneal transplantation and operative technique, *Albrecht von Graefes Arch Klin Exp Ophthalmol* 140:709, 1939.

37. von Hipple, A: Eine neue Methode der Hornhauttransplantation, *Arch Ophthalmol* 34(I):108, 1888.

38. Wiener M, Alvis BY: Transplantation of cornea by means of a mechanically obtained bevelled edge segment, *Am J Ophthalmol* 23:877, 1940.

39. Waring GO, Hanna KD: The Hanna suction punch block and trephine system for penetrating keratoplasty, *Arch Ophthalmol* 107(10):1536-1539, 1989.

Chapter 15

Suture Materials and Techniques

RICHARD C. TROUTMAN

DAVID H. HAIGHT

SANDRA BELMONT

The success of modern penetrating keratoplasty must be judged both on graft clarity and postoperative refractive error. The advent of topical steroids and nonabsorbable monofilament suture material has greatly improved the ability to obtain clear grafts, but minimizing refractive error has been a more vexing problem. Despite exacting microsurgical techniques, a high degree of post–penetrating keratoplasty astigmatism exists in as many as 10% to 20% of patients.[18,23,26,27,32,33] Some contributing factors for this irreducible astigmatism include poorly fitting fixation rings, mismatch between donor and recipient configuration because of poor trephination techniques, recipient pathosis, undetected donor astigmatism, the prolonged use of steroids, and the variation in suture material, pattern, and removal.[2,3,10,24,25,31,34] Most of these issues are addressed elsewhere in the book. Here we discuss the role of suture material and techniques as it relates to successful wound closure with minimal astigmatism.

SUTURE MATERIALS

Before the 1970s, absorbable suture materials or braided silk sutures were commonly employed for keratoplasty closures. Since that time, they have been almost completely abandoned in favor of nonabsorbable monofilament materials. At the present time, the only role for absorbables and silk are ancillary ones involving conjunctival closure or traction and scleral ring fixation, respectively.

Nylon. In the past two decades, 10-0 nylon has become the most popular suture material for keratoplasty closure. The monofilament construction permits smooth passage through corneal tissue, and the level of tissue reaction is greatly reduced. Over the years, improvements in manufacturing techniques have produced stronger and more consistent threads, thus reducing inadvertent breakage during surgery. One characteristic of nylon is its elasticity, which must be considered when one is tensioning and tying the suture. Sutures that may appear tight by visual inspection may actually be too loose and lead to wound leaks, whereas excessive tensioning can lead to cheese-wiring of the suture through corneal tissue or to an excessively flattened wound with a drumhead configuration. The elastic properties of the nylon also contribute to shifts in corneal curvature that take place postoperatively. Additionally, nylon undergoes a gradual process of hydrolysis resulting in late relaxation of wound tension and suture fragmentation that can lead to irritation, vascular ingrowth, infection, or graft reaction. For these reasons, it is most desirable to remove nylon sutures at an appropriate postoperative interval.

Despite these inherent difficulties, nylon remains the standard for keratoplasty closure because of its low tissue reactivity and relative ease of handling. 10-0 is the most frequently used size, though 9-0 and 11-0 are sometimes employed, with the latter most often used in combination with a mixed running-interrupted pattern or in combination with other suture materials.

Polypropylene. Polypropylene (Prolene) suture is a truly nonabsorbable material, not subject to the hydrolysis of nylon, and possessing high tensile strength. In theory, it could offer permanent wound support in keratoplasty; in practice it is a stiff material suffering from the elasticity of nylon but lacking its ease in handling. It is rarely used as a single suture in keratoplasty but is used by some surgeons when combining a running and interrupted pattern. In this scenario the interrupted ones are usually 10-0 nylon and the running ones are polypropylene; the intent is to selectively remove the interrupted ones to modify postoperative astigmatism while leaving the polypropylene in place to provide long-term or permanent wound support. In addition to this application, polypropylene is often the suture of choice for ancillary procedures including iris repair or the sclera or iris fixation of a posterior chamber lens in the absence of capsular support.[30]

Polyester (Mersilene). 10-0 and 11-0 polyester (Mersilene) suture was developed as another alternative material that would not be biodegraded and thus allow for permanent tension to be maintained in a keratoplasty incision. Mersilene is stronger than nylon and also is much less elastic. These properties should enable the surgeon to control wound tension more precisely intraoperatively. Once the tension is set and reaches an equilibrium in the tissue, it should not change, thereby resulting in stable corneal curvature and refraction. This suture would seem to permit astigmatism control by intraoperative or immediate postoperative suture adjustment leading to a permanent result and obviating the need for suture removal or secondary astigmatism surgery.

Early experience with this material has not realized these ideals. The suture is stiff, and in its present form has a pale green color not easily seen. Thus its handling is not as easy as that of nylon. In addition, its tissue reactivity seems somewhat greater. One of us (S.B.) has performed about 20 keratoplasties with 11-0 Mersilene, and, of these, 6 developed sterile suture infiltrates. In a much larger study, Waring and co-workers compared Mersilene to nylon in two techniques.[5] In the first a combined running and interrupted pattern with selective removal of the interrupteds postoperatively was employed (*n* = 45). In the second a single running Mersilene with postoperative adjustment was employed (*n* = 23). Tissue complications such as infiltration, infection, and neovascularization and handling complications such as exposed knots, loose and tight sutures, and wound leaks were compared. They found

a fivefold increase in handling-related complications and a threefold increase in tissue-related complications when comparing Mersilene to nylon. Thus, although the properties of Mersilene are promising, early experience has shown it to be problematic. Perhaps modification of the material will improve its usefulness, but at the present time nylon remains the suture of choice in keratoplasty.

NEEDLES

To begin a discussion of needles in keratoplasty, it may be useful to review briefly some basic nomenclature:

Length. Total distance of the needle from point to swage before bending.

Cord Length. Straight-line distance from point to swage after bending.

Curvature. That portion of a circle to which the needle is bent (that is, ½ circle = 180 degrees).

Diameter. Diameter of the original wire from which the needle is made measured in thousandths of an inch or mils (1 mil = 0.001 inches).

Regular cutting. Cross section of a triangle with the base down.

Reverse cutting. Cross section of a triangle with the apex down.

Spatulated. A flattened reverse cutting point with the third cutting edge on the bottom removed (also known as *side cutting*).

Tapered. Circular cross section.

Needle and point configurations are outlined in Figs. 15-1 and 15-2.

Most needles supplied with the aforementioned

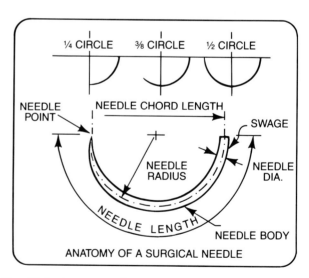

Fig. 15-1. Anatomy of a surgical needle. (Courtesy Ethicon, Inc, 1992, Somerville, NJ.)

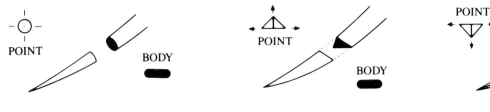

TAPER POINT
For soft, easily penetrated tissues.

CONVENTIONAL CUTTING
Two opposing cutting edges, with a third on inside curve. Change in cross-section from a triangular cutting tip to a flattened body.

REVERSE CUTTING
Cutting edge on outer curve. For tough, difficult-to-penetrate tissues.

Fig. 15-2. Geometry of stainless steel surgical needles. (Courtesy Ethicon, Inc, Somerville, NJ, 1992.)

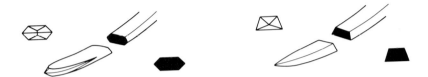

Fig. 15-3. CS (concave spatula) design of Ethicon surgical needle. (Courtesy Ethicon, Inc, Somerville, NJ, 1992.)

suture materials are either 6-mil or 4-mil size, with the latter usually appearing with 11-0 materials. These relatively small-diameter needles allow for easier tissue penetration and produce small needle tracts, which are less prone to leakage. In recent years, the major ophthalmic suture companies (Alcon and Ethicon) have developed needle configurations to maintain rigidity despite small wire sizes as well as to facilitate knot burial in the presence of small needle tracts. All keratoplasty needles are of the spatulated reverse-cutting type. This design permits the needle to split lamellae, rather than cutting through them, and offers a smaller less traumatic point. Ethicon has recently introduced its CS design, which features a concave-spatula configuration (Fig. 15-3). This needle displaces more mass in a horizontal direction and in effect slices a wider, thinner tissue opening. Alcon's Excalibur S series needles are also spatulated but feature a deeper triangular cross section creating a more even, overall cross section to the tract. Our preliminary experience with both of these designs show improvement in penetration and ease of knot burial compared with earlier designs. The ultimate choice of point design will probably remain a matter of individual preference for each surgeon.

Full-Curve Needles. Full-curve needles are the most frequently used in keratoplasty as well as in most other anterior segment surgeries. The bend of the needle is circular and the curvature typically ranges from 140 degrees to 180 degrees. These needles achieve long and somewhat shallow bites and afford the same handling characteristics as found in cataract wound closures. This familiarity has kept this needle design popular among graft surgeons, and it may be the best choice for those who use a no-torque suture pattern in which the bites are intentionally nonradial. Care must be taken, however, to achieve a deep enough bite, especially in the presence of edematous tissue. With this configuration, in order to achieve deeper bites, the bites must be made longer, and this can lead to a reduced optical zone for the graft as well as an enhancement of the effect on tissue compression and resultant corneal distortion when the suture is tensioned. The exact length and depth of the bite achieved with these needles will depend on their curvature and length; in general, short cord lengths and large curvatures result in short and deep bites.

Examples of full-curve needles include Ethicon's CS-160-6 and Alcon's CU-5 and SU-5 (Fig. 15-4, *A*).

Minicurve. In an attempt to facilitate shorter and deeper bites, the minicurve needles were developed. They share with the full-curve needles a continuous nonchanging radius, and their curvature may be specified in degrees (such as 160 degrees). However,

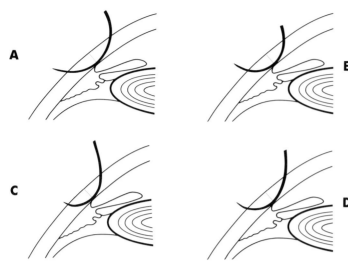

Fig. 15-4. Examples of curvature of surgical needles. **A,** Full-curve needle. **B,** Minicurve needle. **C,** Bicurve needle. **D,** Compound-curve needle. (Courtesy Ethicon, Inc, Somerville, NJ, 1992.)

the cord length and radius of curvature is significantly smaller than that of their full-curve counterparts. This allows for a deeper bite while it traverses less distance across the wound. In practice, these needles are difficult to handle because of their small size and tight radii and are not commonly employed. They may. however, be useful when suture placement must take place in a very confined space such as repair of corneal lacerations or suturing of keratotomy incisions. Examples of these needles include Ethicon's CS-M-6 and Alcon's SUM-5 (Fig. 15-4, *B*).

Bicurve. A further development to achieve short, deep bites while improving handling is the bicurve needle. This design features an average to flat radius of curvature from the swage to the midportion and a much steeper or tighter radius from midportion to point.

The initial flat portion toward the swage facilitates handling, and the tighter radius toward the tip permits rapid turnout after a deep bite is achieved. In practice, these needles allow for more efficient placement of deep or penetrating bites equidistant from both sides of the wound without requiring excessively long bites. The short bite avoids compromise of the optical zone, and the depth provides more secure closure. These needles are best driven with a short, straight-jawed needle holder. The technique involves grasping the flatter portion of the needle, placing the point perpendicular to the corneal surface, driving the needle down to the desired depth, and then rotating the point out by rolling the needle holder in the fingertips. This manipulation is sub-

stantially different from that employed for full-curve needles but is easily learned and affords efficient, reproducible closures. Examples of these needles include Ethicon's CS-B-6 and Alcon's SU-6 and SU-8 (Fig. 15-4, *C*).

Compound Curve. The compound curve needle available from Ethicon is a further modification of a bicurve design. The needle has an initial flat curve changing to a steeper curve, and this is terminated by a sharp, straight point. The straight portion further facilitates initial entrance and penetration to depth, and rapid turnout is assured by the steep curve immediately behind the point. This needle is available as the TGW-6-C plus and the CS-C-6 (Fig. 15-4, *D*).

Ultimately the choice of needle is a matter of individual preference, but certain principles must be observed. Suture bites must be of sufficient depth to afford secure closure without posterior wound gape. This is especially important if secondary astigmatism surgery such as wedge resection or relaxing incisions are required. Suture bites should not be excessively long so as to avoid reduction in effective optical zone size and excessive and perhaps unequal tension across the wound. We prefer full-thickness suturing and routinely employ bicurve or compound curve needles.

Selected needles and sutures for keratoplasty from Alcon and Ethicon are listed in Tables 15-1 and 15-2.

SUTURE TECHNIQUES

There is a variety of suture techniques employed at this time in the field of corneal transplantation. These include single continuous (radial placement versus no-torque), double continuous (same direction versus opposing pattern), interrupted, and a combination of interrupted and continuous.[6-8,14,16,20-22,29,38] The advantages of a continuous suture include ease of placement and removal, fewer knots to stimulate vascularization, and the ability to adjust loop tension under intraoperative keratometric control and postoperatively at the slitlamp. The disadvantage of the continuous technique includes the potential for loss of wound integrity if the suture should break (that is, inadvertently or during suture adjustment postoperatively). This is especially hazardous with a single continuous. In addition, there is the inability to modulate the post–penetrating keratoplasty astigmatism by a selective suture-removal technique.

The advantage of the interrupted technique is sequential suture removal in cases of highly vascularized corneas and in manipulation of post–penetrat-

Table 15-1.   Selected Sutures for Keratoplasty: Ethicon

Needle	Curvature	Cord Length (mm)	Radius (mm)	Wire (mils)	Length (mm)	Suture
CS-160-4*	160°	4.00	2.00	4	5.50	10-0 nylon
CS-M-4	160°	3.00	1.50	4	4.27	10-0 nylon
CS-160-6*	160°	4.00	2.00	6	5.50	10-0 nylon
						9-0 nylon
CS-160-6	160°	4.00	2.00	6	5.50	10-0 nylon
						10-0 Mersilene
						10-0 Prolene
CS-175-6*	175°	4.57	2.28	6	6.98	10-0 nylon
CS-140-6*	140°	4.75	2.54	6	6.19	10-0 nylon
						9-0 nylon
CS-140-6	140°	4.75	2.54	6	6.19	10-0 nylon
						10-0 Mersilene
						11-0 Mersilene
CS-M-6*	160°	3.00	1.52	6	4.27	10-0 nylon
CS-B-6*	Bicurve	NA	1.39/2.54	6	4.82	10-0 nylon
						9-0 nylon
CS-C-6*	Compound curve	NA	1.39/2.54	6	4.82	10-0 nylon
						9-0 nylon
TG160-4-3M*	160°	3.00	1.52	4	4.27	10-0 Mersilene
						11-0 Mersilene
TG160-4*	160°	4.00	2.00	4	5.50	10-0 nylon
						11-0 nylon
						10-0 Mersilene
						11-0 Mersilene
						10-0 Prolene
TG140-4*	140°	4.75	2.54	4	6.19	11-0 Mersilene
TG4-S*	Bicurve	NA	1.39/2.54	4	4.82	10-0 nylon
						11-0 Mersilene
TG4-C*	Compound curve	NA	1.39/2.54	4	4.82	10-0 nylon
TG160-6-3M*	160°	3.00	1.52	6	4.27	11-0 Mersilene
TG160-6*	160°	4.00	2.00	6	5.50	10-0 Mersilene
						11-0 Mersilene
						10-0 Prolene
TG140-6*	140°	4.75	2.54	6	6.19	10-0 Mersilene
						11-0 Mersilene
						10-0 Prolene
TG6-S*	Bicurve	NA	1.39/2.54	6	4.82	10-0 Mersilene
						11-0 Mersilene
						10-0 Prolene
TG6-C*	Compound curve	NA	1.39/2.54	6	4.82	10-0 Mersilene
						11-0 Mersilene
						10-0 Prolene

NA, Not applicable; polypropylene (Prolene); polyester (Mersilene).
*Double-armed suture.

ing keratoplasty astigmatism. They also seem to promote more rapid wound healing. However, the disadvantages include a tendency toward greater reaction at each suture site, especially if the knots become exposed, more tedious placement and removal, and inability to adjust, intraoperatively utilizing the surgical keratometer. The following is a description of the most commonly used suture patterns in penetrating keratoplasty today. Each surgeon must have a rationale for choosing the suture pattern that he or she believes works best for obtaining secure anatomic closure, minimal final sutures-out astigmatism, and average corneal curvature.

Initial Graft Placement and Suturing. We have shown a statistically significant decrease in postoperative all-sutures-out astigmatism using a technique of rotation of the donor cornea within the recipient bed before suturing.[2] Therefore we advocate that after placement of the donor button into the recipient bed it should be rotated into a position of best fit using a surgical keratometer as a guide. When a spherical reflex is obtained with the keratometer, the first

Table 15-2. Selected Sutures for Keratoplasty: Alcon

Needle	Curvature	Cord Length (mm)	Radius (mm)	Wire (mils)	Length (mm)	Suture
CU-1	140°	4.75	2.54	6	6.19	9-0 nylon 10-0 nylon
CU-2	175°	4.57	2.28	6	6.98	9-0 nylon 10-0 nylon
CU-5	160°	4.01	1.98	6	5.51	9-0 nylon 10-0 nylon 11-0 nylon
Cu-6	105°-85°	NA	0.86/ 3.10	6	6.17	9-0 nylon 10-0 nylon
CU-8	90°-50°	3.71	1.52/ 2.79	6	4.83	9-0 nylon 10-0 nylon
CUM-5	160°	3.00	1.52	6	4.22	10-0 nylon 11-0 nylon
CU-11	140°	4.75	2.54	4	6.19	10-0 nylon 11-0 nylon
CU-15	160°	4.01	1.98	4	5.51	9-0 nylon 10-0 nylon 11-0 nylon
CUM-15	160°	3.00	1.52	4	4.22	9-0 nylon 10-0 nylon
AU-1	140°	4.75	2.54	6	6.19	10-0 nylon 10-0 polypropylene
AU-2	175°	4.57	2.28	6	6.98	10-0 nylon
AU-5	160°	4.01	1.98	6	5.51	9-0 nylon 10-0 polypropylene
AU-6	105°-85°	NA	0.86/ 3.10	6	6.17	10-0 nylon
AU-8	90°-50°	3.71	1.52/ 2.79	6	4.83	9-0 nylon 10-0 nylon 10-0 polypropylene
AUM-5	160°	3.00	1.52	6	4.22	10-0 nylon
AU-15	160°	4.01	1.98	4	5.51	10-0 nylon
AUM-15	160°	3.00	1.52	4	4.22	9-0 nylon 10-0 nylon
AU-18	90°-50°	3.71	1.52/ 2.79	4	4.83	9-0 nylon 10-0 polypropylene
SU-5	160°	4.01	NA	6	NA	9-0 nylon 10-0 nylon 10-0 polypropylene
SU-2	175°	4.57	NA	6	NA	10-0 nylon
SU-6	105°-85°	NA	NA	6	NA	10-0 nylon
SU-8	90°-50°	3.71	NA	6	NA	10-0 nylon
SUM-5	160°	3.00	NA	6	NA	10-0 nylon
SU-18	90°-50°	3.71	NA	4	NA	10-0 nylon

NA, Not applicable.
*All the above sutures are double armed.

fixation suture is placed. A cupped forceps is used to grasp the donor approximately 1 mm from the wound edge at the 6 o'clock position. A 10-0 nylon suture on a compound-curve needle is used for all fixation sutures. This configuration assures short deep bites. We are proponents of a through-and-through suture technique. It has been shown that sutures placed at the level of Descemet's membrane migrate anteriorly within a few days and may result in a posterior wound gape or lambda effect[36] (Fig. 15-5). The net effect is poor healing of the posterior aspect of the wound leading to instability and possible increased astigmatism when all sutures are removed. We utilize the slip-knot technique for all suturing in keratoplasty for optimum titration of tension across the wound.[28] The second suture is the most critical. Care must be taken to place the suture 180 degrees from the first suture with constant attention to the keratometry to assure maintenance of a spherical reflex. We believe that the use of six in-

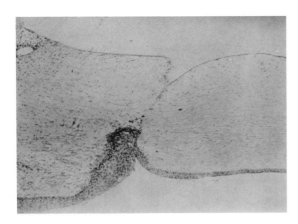

Fig. 15-5. Posterior wound gape, or lambda effect. Sutures placed at level of Descemet's membrane migrate anteriorly within a few days and therefore result in a posterior wound gape.

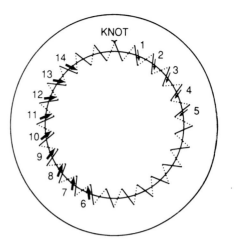

Fig. 15-6. Exposed part of suture is gently but firmly grasped with Tennant tying forceps at its crossing of donor interface. With a careful tug a small amount of slack is moved toward tight semimeridian. Adjoining suture, which received the slack, is then grasped, and slack is moved toward tight semimeridian.

terrupted sutures provides optimum wound apposition and fixation of the donor, which facilitates the subsequent placement of additional interrupted or continuous sutures. Regardless of which suture technique is employed, we advocate burying all knots on the donor side. Burying the knot in the recipient increases the rate of vascularization at that site with the inherent complications of graft rejection and can lead to difficulties in suture removal. After placement of the six fixation sutures the surgeon must choose from one of the following closure techniques.

Continuous (Single-Radial Placement) Technique. Many surgeons use a single continuous technique (see Fig. 15-11, *A*), which is done by placement of 17 to 26 equally spaced bites. Theoretically a radially placed single continuous suture will torque the wound in the direction of the suture. This may contribute to a higher degree of sutures-in astigmatism necessitating adjustment as compared to an antitorque technique, though this has not been documented. The timing of suture adjustment is optimized in the early postoperative period (1 to 6 weeks) before the suture starts to degrade and the possibility of breakage increases. In a recently reported series by McNeil and Wessels[21] of 330 eyes there was a 2.4% breakage rate. When breakage occurs, the suture has to be spliced together with the additional knots, potentially complicating further suture adjustment. The technique consists in the use of either a keratometer or, if available, a corneal topographic analysis unit[15] to guide suture adjustment evaluation. The suture is adjusted at the slitlamp using a Tennant tying forceps and topical anesthesia. Alternatively the adjustment may be made using a

surgical microscope and keratometer with the patient in a supine position. This affords better access to the cornea and a greater degree of control. Generally suture adjustment can begin as early as the first postoperative visit in patients with 3.00 D or greater of regular astigmatism. Starting at the flattest meridian (Fig. 15-6) one grasps the suture with gentle traction and progressively pulls up on a loop-by-loop basis toward the steep meridian. If epithelialization has already occurred, it is necessary to free all loops before adjustment. We have found a thin spatula (such as the Johnson) to be useful in sliding under each loop to break the epithelium. Prophylactic antibiotics are recommended to decrease the risk of infection, since suture adjustment does result in epithelial defects. Current proponents of the single continuous suture adjustment technique espouse the theory of early visual rehabilitation while sutures are in after suture modulation. Recently reported sutures-in data (Lin and co-workers[20]; Figs. 15-7 to 15-10) found a 1.7 ± 0.7 D postadjustment astigmatism in the study group versus a 5.4 ± 2.4 D astigmatism in a double running control group. Some published reports do state that a sutures-out astigmatism of approximately 3.5 D occurred in the adjusted group.[21] This range is similar to a variety of techniques when all sutures are removed.[3,7,17,27] It is our belief that for evaluation of any suturing technique in terms of affecting postoperative astigmatism, all sutures must be out. Our current suture materials must eventually be removed

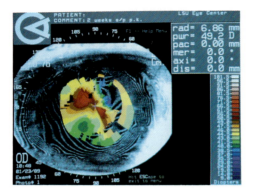

A

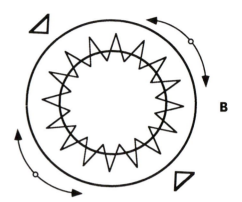

B

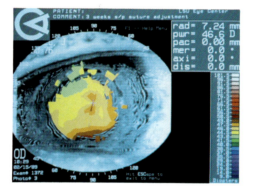

C

Fig. 15-7. A, Absolute-scale color-coded topographic map of a cornea in test group 2 weeks after penetrating keratoplasty. Map shows 8.5 D of astigmatism and paracentral surface irregularity superotemporal to visual axis. Color-coded dioptric scale is on right. **B,** Schema demonstrates method of suture adjustment used to reduce astigmatism shown in above map. *Open arrows* point to steepest meridian *(warm colors* in Fig. 15-7, *A).* Suture is grasped with Tennant tying forceps at flatter meridian approximately represented by midpoints of *curved double-headed arrows* on both sides of cornea *(cool figures* in Fig. 15-7, *A).* On opposite sides of flattest meridian, suture is gently pulled up perpendicular to corneal surface to tighten and create slack in suture. Slack is moved toward steeper meridian by redistributing it in direction of *small arrows* along suture bites in both directions. **C,** Absolute-scale color-coded topographic map of same cornea 1 month after suture adjustment. Residual astigmatism is 1.8 D. Axis has shifted approximately 60 degrees from location of axis before suture adjustment. (From Lin DT et al: *Ophthalmology* 97:934-938, 1990.)

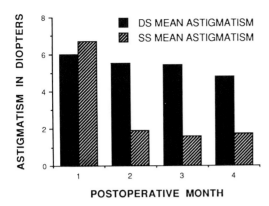

Fig. 15-8. Mean astigmatism of test group with single-running suture *(SS; striped bar)* compared to that of control group with double-running suture *(DS; solid bar)* at 1, 2, 3, and 4 months after penetrating keratoplasty. (From Lin DT et al: *Ophthalmology* 97:934-938, 1990.)

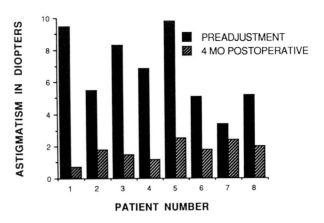

Fig. 15-9. Corneal astigmatism for each patient in test group before suture adjustment *(solid bar)* and 4 months after keratoplasty *(striped bar)*. (From Lin DT et al: *Ophthalmology* 97:934-938, 1990.)

because of biodegradation. Polyester sutures, as previously pointed out, are not suitable because of difficulty in handling, a greater tissue reactivity, and a tendency to "cheese-wire." We look forward to the future when techniques of suture adjustment are used with a material that is nonreactive, easily manipulated, and resistant to biodegradation.

Continuous (Single, No-Torque) Technique. To circumvent torsion of the wound when using a single continuous pattern (Fig. 15-11, *A*) some surgeons are attempting to place a single continuous no-torque suture. The classic no-torque suture involves eight bites placed at 45 degrees from the radial plane angled in the direction of suture advancement. This pattern creates a series of isosceles triangles, which negates wound torsion. This technique was originally developed for use in lamellar refractive keratoplasty procedures. It has been modified by some surgeons to be used in a single continuous pattern with an increased number of bites. Each bite is again directed at 45 degrees from the radial plane. Advocates of this technique believe that it is also effective in reducing wound torsion.[13]

Double Continuous (Torque-Antitorque). To have the advantage of an antitorque technique and the benefit of a double suture, the double continuous torque-antitorque suture technique was developed (Fig. 15-11, *B*). This is our current preference. The first continuous 10-0 nylon is placed clockwise in a radial pattern. The second 10-0 nylon is run counterclockwise paralleling the torqued bites of the tightened and tied-clockwise suture. The second suture is given tension to compensate for the torque, and the suture loops are adjusted by use of the surgical keratometer to approximate corneal sphericity.

Using this technique with a full-thickness closure allows all sutures to be removed at 6 months in keratoconus and 12 months in disorders such as Fuchs' dystrophy and pseudophakic bullous keratopathy. We strongly believe that all sutures should be removed as expeditiously as possible and any significant astigmatism dealt with secondarily with either relaxing incisions, wedge resection, or combinations thereof.[1,12,19,35] The possibility of the excimer laser as a treatment modality for secondary postkeratoplasty astigmatism awaits future investigation.

A new technique to correct postkeratoplasty astigmatism using the double continuous torque-antitorque suture pattern has recently been described.[9] This involves placement of additional sutures based on photokeratoscopic identification of peripheral abnormalities or "microdehiscences." The theory behind the technique is that placement of additional sutures will stabilize areas of "microdehiscence" and stimulate the normal progression of corneal wound healing. Again sutures-out data in this study group were reported in the 3-diopter range.

Double Continuous (Same Direction) Technique. Some surgeons favor a double continuous pattern (Fig. 15-11, *C*) using a 10-0 nylon and 11-0 nylon run in the same direction.[38] The 10-0 nylon is placed at the level of Descemet's, and the 11-0 nylon is one half to two thirds the depth of the cornea. The 10-0 nylon is removed as early as 2 months, whereas the 11-0 nylon is left in for up to 15 to 20 months. The advocates believe that this technique permits early visual rehabilitation, though recent reports in the literature have shown unpredictable changes in astigmatism after removal of the 11-0 nylon.[11,22,38]

A

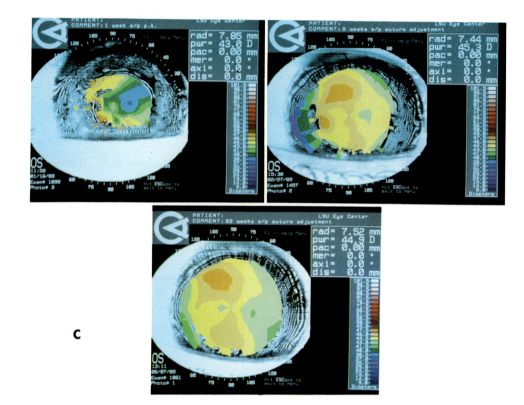

B

C

Fig. 15-10. A, Absolute-scale color-coded topography map of a cornea in test group before suture adjustment shows 6.8 D of astigmatism with steep meridian at approximately 125 degrees (simulated keratometry [that is, Sim K] = [46.3 × 125°]/[39.5 × 35°]). There also is central irregular astigmatism. **B,** Topographic map of same cornea 1 month after suture adjustment shows 1.4 D of astigmatism (Sim K = [46.1 × 97°]/[44.7 × 7°]). **C,** Topographic map of same cornea approximately 3 months after suture adjustment shows 1.8 D of astigmatism (Sim K = [45.7 × 93°]/[43.9 × 3°]). These three figures demonstrate that there was little change in the topographic pattern over the 3-month observation period after suture adjustment. (From Lin DT et al: *Ophthalmology* 97:934-938, 1990.)

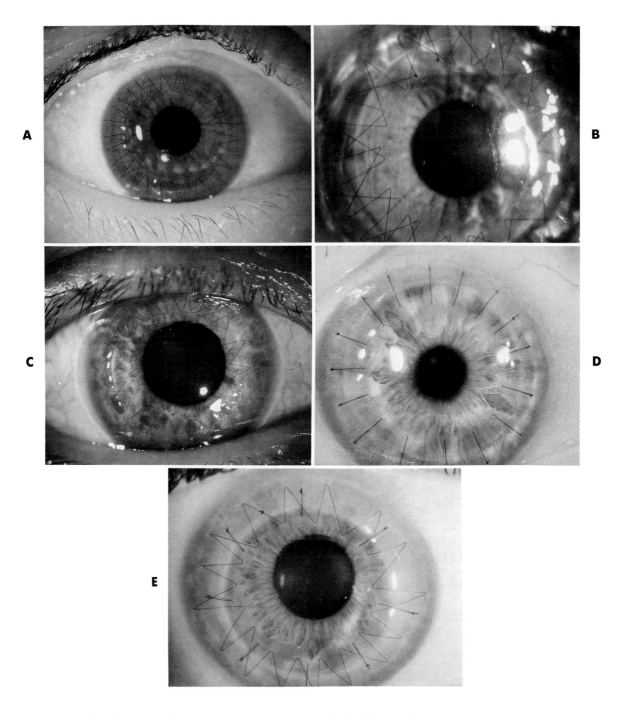

Fig. 15-11. A, Single continuous, no torque. **B,** Double continuous torque, antitorque pattern. **C,** Double continuous, 10-0 and 11-0 nylon placed in same clockwise direction. **D,** All interrupted pattern. **E,** Combination interrupted and single continuous sutures.

Interrupted Technique. Some surgeons prefer to close their corneal transplants totally with interrupted sutures (Fig. 15-11, *D*). This technique is advisable in children whose wound healing rate is rapid. It is also the technique of choice in heavily vascularized corneas and in corneas with segmental vascularization because of variability in wound heal-

ing. This method has the potential to afford greater wound security because of the multiplicity of sutures. It is difficult to modulate the astigmatism intraoperatively with this technique though it does have the advantage of modification of postoperative astigmatism by selective suture removal.

Interrupted Combination Technique. Currently

many corneal surgeons are using a combination of interrupted and a single continuous suture (Fig. 15-11, *E*) to selectively remove the interrupted sutures in an attempt to control postoperative astigmatism.[6-8,23,29] There are published reports that demonstrate that selective suture removal can reduce astigmatism after corneal transplantation while sutures are in place. The theory behind the technique is to selectively remove sutures early in the postoperative period to allow the cornea to heal in a given configuration of least sutures-in astigmatism. The proponents believe that additional suture removal will not affect final corneal curvature if the cornea is "fixed" in one position for 1 year or more. One series in the literature evaluating this technique does give sutures-out data on 188 eyes.[7] The mean astigmatism before suture removal was 3.7 D, and the mean astigmatism after suture removal was 3.5 D.

The technique consists in placing eight interrupted 10-0 nylon sutures in the cardinal positions combined with a continuous 11-0, 16-bite nylon suture. Based on either central keratometry readings or corneal topographic analysis the interrupted sutures in the steep meridian are selectively removed at the slitlamp beginning at 6 weeks postoperatively. The main disadvantage is the time-consuming number of postoperative visits to remove sutures that remain in place for up to 18 months. In addition, other complications include wound dehiscence, suture-induced irritation, vascularization, and the potential for suture-associated bacterial corneal infection.

CONCLUSION

There is currently a variety of needles, sutures, and suture patterns available as previously described. We are proponents of a full-thickness closure using 10-0 nylon on a compound-curve needle in a double continuous antitorquing pattern. Using this pattern of suture placement and removal, one subjects the patient to only two changes in postkeratoplasty refraction, the first with sutures in and the second with sutures out unless corrective surgery for high astigmatism is required. We believe this is less time consuming and more beneficial to the patient than the numerous changes in refraction occasioned by selective removal of interrupted sutures in an attempt to reduce or eliminate postoperative astigmatism. As previously discussed the double continuous torque-antitorque suture patterns as well as postoperative selective suture modulation by adjustment, removal, or addition are obtaining a final suture-out astigmatism of approximately 3 diopters. This represents significant progress toward moving kerato-

plasty wound closure from a purely anatomic act to one that deliberately attempts modification of the important refractive errors of ametropias and astigmatism in corneal transplantation.

REFERENCES

1. Belmont SC, Troutman RC: Compensating compression sutures in wedge resection, *J Refract Surg* 1(3):104-107, 1985.
2. Belmont SC, Zimm JL, Troutman RC, Gilwit PH: The triple procedure: reliability of keratometry readings in predicting final refractive error, *Cornea*. (Submitted.)
3. Belmont SC, Troutman RC, Buzard KA: Control of astigmatism aided by intraoperative keratometry, *Cornea*. (Submitted.)
4. Belmont SC, Zimm JL, Storch RL, et al: *Postpenetrating keratoplasty astigmatism using the Krumeich guided trephine system*, Bethesda, Md, 1990, Association for Research in Vision and Ophthalmology.
5. Bertram B, Waring G, et al: Complications of Mersilene sutures in penetrating keratoplasty. (In press.)
6. Binder PS: Selective suture removal can reduce post-keratoplasty astigmatism, *Ophthalmology* 92(10):L1412-1416, 1985.
7. Binder PS: The effect of suture removal on postkeratoplasty astigmatism, *Am J Ophthalmol* 105:637-645, 1988.
8. Burk LL, Waring GO, Radjee B, Stulting RD: The effect of selective suture removal on astigmatism following penetrating keratoplasty, *Ophthalmic Surg* 19:849-854, 1988.
9. Buzard KA: Repair of the "microdehiscence" to correct postkeratoplasty astigmatism, *Ophthalmic Surg* 20:876-882, 1989.
10. Cohen KL, Holman RE, Tripoli MK, et al: Effect of trephine tilt on corneal button dimensions, *Am J Ophthalmol* 101:722-725, 1986.
11. Davison JA, Bourne WM: Results of penetrating keratoplasty using double running suture technique, *Arch Ophthalmol* 99:1591-1595, 1981.
12. Draga A, Belmont SC, Troutman RC: *Combination relaxing incisions and corneal wedge resection for postkeratoplasty astigmatism*, poster exhibit, Sarasota, Fla, 1990, Association for Research in Vision and Ophthalmology.
13. Eisner G: Compression sutures. In *Eye surgery*, Berlin, 1980, Springer-Verlag.
14. Eliason JA, McCulley JP: A comparison between interrupted and continuous suturing techniques in keratoplasty, *Cornea* 9(1):10-16, 1990.
15. Gormley DJ, Gersten M, Koplin RD, Lubkin V: Corneal modeling, *Cornea* 7:30-35, 1988.
16. Haight DH, Troutman RC: The use of disparate diameter corneal grafts to obtain average postoperative keratometry readings, *J Refract Surg* 1:161, 1985.
17. Insler MS, Cooper DH, Caldwell DR: Final surgical results with a suction trephine, *Ophthalmic Surg* 18:23, 1987.
18. Jensen AD, Maumanee AE: Refractive errors following keratoplasty, *Trans Am Ophthalmol Soc* 72:123-131, 1974.
19. Krachmer JH, Fenzl RE: Surgical corection of high postkeratoplasty astigmatism, *Arch Ophthalmol* 98:1400-1402, 1980.
20. Lin DT, Wilson SE, Reidy J, et al: An adjustable single running suture technique to reduce post-keratoplasty astigmatism, *Ophthalmology* 97:934-938, 1990.
21. McNeill JI, Wessels IF: Adjustment of single continuous suture to control astigmatism after penetrating keratoplasty, *Refract Corneal Surg* 5:216-223, 1989.
22. Musch DC, Meyer RF, Sugar A, Soong HK: Corneal astigmatism after penetrating keratoplasty, *Ophthalmology* 96:698-703, 1988.

23. Musch DC, Meyer RF, Sugar A: The effect of removing running sutures on astigmatism after penetrating keratoplasty, *Arch Ophthalmol* 106:488-492, 1988.
24. Olson RJ: Variation in corneal graft size related to trephine technique, *Arch Ophthalmol* 97:1323-1325, 1979.
25. Olson RJ: The effect of scleral fixation ring placement and trephine tilting on keratoplasty wound size and donor shape, *Ophthalmic Surg* 12:23-26, 1981.
26. Perl T, Charlton KH, Binder PS: Disparate diameter grafting: astigmatism, intraocular pressure and visual acuity, *Ophthalmology* 88:774-781, 1981.
27. Perlman EM: An analysis and interpretation of refractive errors after penetrating keratoplasty, *Ophthalmology* 88:39-45, 1981.
28. Rabkin SS, Troutman RC: A clinical application of the slip-knot tie in corneal surgery, *Ophthalmic Surg* 12:571-573, 1981.
29. Stainer GA, Perl T, Binder PS: Controlled reduction of post-keratoplasty astigmatism, *Ophthalmology* 89:668-676, 1982.
30. Stark WJ, Goodman G, Goodman D, Gottsch J: Posterior chamber intraocular lens implantation in the absence of posterior capsular support: *Ophthalmic Surg* 19(4):240-243, April 1988.
31. Troutman RC, Gaster RM: Surgical advances and results in keratoconus, *Am J Ophthalmol* 90:131-136, 1980.
32. Troutman RC: Astigmatic considerations in corneal graft, *Ophthalmic Surg* 10(5):21-26, 1979.
33. Troutman RC, Meltzer M: Astigmatism and myopia in keratoconus, *Trans Am Ophthalmol Soc* 70:265-277, 1972.
34. Troutman RC, Swinger CA, Belmont SC: Selective positioning of the donor cornea in penetrating keratoplasty for keratoconus: postoperative astigmatism, *Cornea* 3:135-139, 1984.
35. Troutman RC, Swinger CA: Relaxing incision for control of post-operative astigmatism following keratoplasty, *Ophthalmic Surg* 11:117-120, 1980.
36. Troutman RC: *Microsurgery of the anterior segment of the eye.* II. *The cornea,* St. Louis, 1977, Mosby–Year Book.
37. Van Rij G, Cornell FM, Waring GO III, et al: Postoperative astigmatism after central vs. eccentric penetrating keratoplasties, *Am J Ophthalmol* 99:317-320, 1985.
38. Young SR, Olson RJ: Results of a double running suture in penetrating keratoplasty performed on keratoconus patients, *Ophthalmic Surg* 16(12):779-786, 1985.

Chapter 16

Viscoelastic Materials

JEREMY E. LEVENSON

PAUL S. IMPERIA

Viscoelastic materials have added a new dimension to corneal surgery. Although originally introduced into anterior segment surgery as a means of protecting the corneal endothelium during intraocular lens implantation,[33] these materials have now found an ever-expanding role in corneal transplantation. They offer an exquisite tool for both coating and protecting surfaces, for separating tissue spaces and avoiding adhesions postoperatively. These features make viscoelastics an ideal addition to the modern corneal surgeon's armamentarium, for they assist in the surgeon's overall goal of maximizing the survival of donor graft endothelium.

Fechner[17] has listed the following features for suitable viscoelastic materials:

1. They must be inert and isosmotic, sterile, nonpyrogenic, and nonantigenic.
2. They must be free of corpuscular elements (clumps) and be optically clear.
3. They must be viscous enough to satisfy clinical needs.
4. They must be hydrophilic and be able to be diluted so that:
   a. It is possible to irrigate most of the material out of the eye at the end of the operation.
   b. The remains can leave the anterior chamber through the natural outflow channels.

The first commercially available viscoelastic material was sodium hyaluronate (Healon, Pharmacia, Piscataway, N.J.), introduced in 1980; it remains the standard by which newer materials are judged. Currently there are several formulations of sodium hy-

Table 16-1. Viscoelastic materials

Generic name	Trade name
Sodium hyaluronate	Healon, Healon Yellow (Pharmacia) Ial (Fidia), Vitrax (Edward Weck)
Hydroxypropyl meth-ylcellulose	Occucoat (Storz)
Sodium hyaluronate/ chondroitin sulfate:	Viscoat (Alcon)
Hydroxypropyl methylcellulose/ chondroitin sulfate	Ocugel (Surgidev)
Polyacrilamide	Orcolon (ORC)
Proprietary	Cellugel (Vision Biology)

aluronate and several other types of viscoelastic substances and combinations available (Table 16-1).

Each commercial preparation varies in (1) the chemical properties of molecular structure, molecular weight, concentration, pH, buffering agent, and osmolality and (2) the rheologic properties of viscosity, pseudoplasticity, viscoelasticity, and surface tension.[7,27,30] Viscosity is a solution's resistance to flow. Viscoelasticity is the ability of a solution, when deformed, to return to its original shape. Pseudoplasticity is the ability to transform, when under pressure, from a semisolid to a liquid state. Surface tension relates to molecular cohesiveness and retards a solution from coating solid objects. These properties affect the clinical behavior of a material in terms of endothelial protection, tendency to increase intraoc-

Table 16-2. Clinical properties of some viscoelastics (best to worst: *5* to *1*)

Property	Healon	Viscoat	Occucoat	Orcolon	Ocugel
Chamber maintenance	5	5	2	4	3
Intraocular lens/tissue coating	2	5	5	3	5
Ease of removal	5	2	2	4	2
Intraocular pressure rise	3	4	4	4	4
Endothelial protection	4	5	4	4	5
Optical clarity	5	4	5	5	5

Modified from Lane SS, Lindstrom RL: Viscoelastic agents: formulation, clinical applications, and complications. (Course handout.)

Table 16-3. Properties of some viscoelastic materials

Trade name	Manufacturer	Components	Molecular weight	Viscosity (centipoises)	Source	Osmolality (mOsm/kg water)
Healon	Pharmacia	NaHA	$2.5\text{-}3.8 \times 10^6$	26-50,000	Rooster combs	309
Viscoat	Alcon	NaHA/CDS	6.0×10^5	30-50,000	Bacterial fermentation; shark-fin cartilage	360
Occucoat	Storz	HPMC	0.9×10^5	4000	Wood pulp	319
Orcolon*	ORC	Polyacrilamide	1×10^6	40,000	Synthetic	340
Ocugel*	Surgidev	HPMC/CDS	1.4×10^5	125,000	Wood pulp; shark-fin cartilage	310
						310

Modified from Lane SS, Lindstrom RL: Viscoelastic agents: formation, clinical applications, and complications. (Course handout.)
CDS, chondroitin sulfate; *HPMC*, Hydroxypropyl methylcellulose; *NaHA*, sodium hyaluronate.
*Not yet commercially available.

ular pressure, ease of removal, space maintenance, coating ability, and flow characteristics[27,30] (Tables 16-2 and 16-3).

An ideal viscoelastic would have a viscosity inversely proportional to the rate it was being deformed. This would allow good space maintenance at rest and easy flow when put in motion. No one material is universally ideal. The unique properties of each material make it more or less suitable for a particular surgical application. In addition, air has some of the features described above and has been used during corneal transplantation.

SODIUM HYALURONATE

Sodium hyaluronate was introduced into ophthalmic surgery as a vitreous substitute.[4] It is a high-molecular-weight polysaccharide composed of sodium glucuronate and *N*-acetylglucosamine. Sodium hyaluronate is found ubiquitously throughout the body and is present in high concentrations in the vitreous humor. It is obtained from several sources including the dermis of rooster combs, umbilical cords, and cultures of streptococci. Each commercial preparation has the same structure but may vary in molecular weight and osmolality.

It has the highest molecular weight, in excess of 1 million, of the available viscoelastic molecules. It is relatively viscous and pseudoplastic, allowing for good space maintenance, ease of removal, and endothelial protection. It is nonantigenic, nontoxic, and relatively noninflammatory and does not interfere with wound healing. Some studies indicate that it may actually facilitate wound healing through the modulation of various inflammatory cells.[3]

The disadvantages are its low coating ability, tendency to elevate intraocular pressure, need for refrigeration, and high drag force on removal, which can damage endothelium.[12,21] All the viscoelastic materials tend to elevate intraocular pressure. Sodium hyaluronate elevates intraocular pressure as much as other viscoelastic materials and by some accounts more so.[5,15]

Healon Yellow, consisting of sodium hyaluronate and 0.005 mg/ml sodium fluorescein, has been formulated to enhance the visibility of the material in the eye. Ial (Fidia Research Laboratories, Padua, Italy) is a low-molecular-weight sodium hyaluronate preparation undergoing clinical trials in the United States. Vitrax (Edward Weck, Research Triangle Park, N.C.) is a hyaluronic acid extract dissolved in balanced salt solution with a low molecular weight and high concentration. It is the only sodium hyaluronate preparation not requiring refrigeration. Sodium hyaluronate has gained widespread acceptance by corneal surgeons as attested by the many published reports of its use in corneal transplantation.[1,34,37,38,40,45]

CHONDROITIN SULFATE

Chondroitin sulfate is a mucopolysaccharide found naturally in human tissues and is a normal constituent of the cornea. Unlike sodium hyaluronate, it is sulfated, resulting in an extra negative charge. This negative charge allows chondroitin sulfate to better coat the positively charged tissue, intraocular lenses, and surgical instruments and thus decrease the electrostatic interaction between the implant and endothelium.[22,44] Safety and efficacy have been documented for the human eye.[10]

Chondroitin sulfate 20% was initially used successfully in coating intraocular lenses but because of low viscosity was poor in space maintenance.[44] Increasing the concentration to 50% resulted in a hyperosmotic solution that caused endothelial dehydration and damage.[31,44] A 1:3 mixture of 4% chondroitin sulfate derived from shark-fin cartilage and 3% sodium hyaluronate (Viscoat, CooperVision-Cilco, Huntington, W.Va.) seeks to combine the advantageous properties of each individual material. Clinically, ease of removal remains a problem. A combination of chondroitin sulfate and hydroxypropyl methylcellulose called Ocugel (Surgidev, Goleta, Calif.) is being developed to offer better coating ability and space maintenance than Viscoat does. However, it is less pseudoplastic requiring a large-bore cannula and is more difficult to remove.[30]

METHYLCELLULOSE

Methylcellulose 1% was introduced into anterior segment surgery by Fechner[16] as a coating for intraocular lenses. A 2% solution was found more effective in space maintenance[17] and is available as Occucoat (Storz, St. Louis, Mo.). The main ingredient is a highly purified brand of hydroxypropyl methylcellulose derived from wood pulp. Although the human enzyme systems supposedly cannot metabolize methylcellulose, this does not appear to be of any clinical significance when used in small quantities in the eye. It has been used in many cataract extraction–lens implantation operations without deleterious results.[17,19] The use of methylcellulose in keratoplasty with equally satisfactory results also has been reported.[45]

Methylcellulose has a low surface tension, which increases coating ability, but a lack of elasticity, which makes it more of a "viscoadherent" than viscoelastic. It has been shown not to damage the endothelium.[31] Other advantages are its ready avail-

ability, ability to be autoclaved, low cost, and ability to be stored and shipped at room temperature. Disadvantages include poor pseudoplasticity requiring a large cannula, difficulty in removal, and poorer space maintenance. Other concerns at present include the lack of extensive research and clinical experience, the nonuniformity of source material, and impurities.

POLYACRYLAMIDE

Orcolon (Optical Radiation Corporation, Azusa, Calif.) is a viscoelastic material having synthetic polyacrylamide as its active ingredient. Viscosity and coating ability are both comparable to 1% sodium hyaluronate. No refrigeration is required, and it is cleared rapidly with a half-life of less than 2 hours in the anterior chamber. There is some question of inflammatory potential, but in animal studies it compared favorably with 1% sodium hyaluronate in terms of safety and efficacy.[41] It is currently being evaluated in clinical trials.

OTHER VISCOELASTIC MATERIALS

Human placental collagen, type IV, may have promise as a viscoelastic material in ocular surgery.[41] It differs from other viscoelastics in being a protein rather than a polysaccharide. Clinical trials outside the United States are underway. Complications asso-

---

APPLICATIONS OF VISCOELASTIC MATERIAL IN CORNEAL SURGERY

Fill anterior chamber of whole donor globe to facilitate trephination.
Fill anterior chamber of recipient globe to prevent tissue damage and loss of aqueous.
Firm whole eye before lamellar dissection.
Coat donor button to retard swelling.
Synechiolysis.
Tampon hemorrhage.
Fill anterior chamber before placing donor cornea to protect endothelium, prevent donor from falling into vitreous, and aid in suture placement.
Leave in eye postoperatively to help avoid synechiae and prevent keratolenticular touch.
Aid in placement of posterior or anterior chamber intraocular lens.
Tampon vitreous.
Assist in sealing corneal perforations by reforming anterior chamber before tissue adhesive is applied.
Protect epithelium while suturing.

ciated with an intraocular protein preparation are a concern.

Cellugel (Vision Biology, Santa Barbara, Calif.) is a proprietary synthetic carbohydrate polymer similar to polyacrylamide. Advantages include no need for refrigeration and ability to be autoclaved. Clinical trials outside the United States are in progress.

AIR

Intraocular air has some of the features of a viscoelastic material, and before the introduction of sodium hyaluronate, air was used to move tissues and separate spaces within the anterior chamber. It can be sterilized when it is passed through a Millipore filter. However, air passes much more readily through a partially sutured wound and cannot maintain the anterior chamber against even moderate posterior pressure. It has been shown to have at least a slightly detrimental effect on the endothelium.[28,35,36] Although potential uses for air during corneal transplantation will be pointed out, its use has been largely superseded by other viscoelastic materials.

SURGICAL APPLICATIONS OF VISCOELASTIC MATERIALS

An ideal viscoelastic for penetrating keratoplasty would chiefly protect the new donor endothelium, maintain the space between the donor tissue and the rest of the anterior segment, and be able to be left in at the end of surgery without producing a rise in intraocular pressure.

Although the use of the above viscoelastics in corneal transplant surgery has been reported in the literature, most of the experience in this country has been with sodium hyaluronate. The following potential application for these materials during surgery are based on published reports and our experience and are summarized in the Box.

Trephination and Preparation of Donor Corneal Button. Although it is much less common to trephine the donor button from a fresh, whole eye since the widespread use of preservation media, a viscoelastic material can assist in the maneuver. Filling the anterior chamber with a viscoelastic (less ideally air) through a paracentesis opening will allow more complete trephination without involving the underlying intraocular tissues. Alternatively, placing a viscoelastic material in the anterior chamber through the wound after initial trephination will assist in the final cutting of the donor button with corneal scissors or a diamond knife.[45] In like manner, a viscoelastic material can be used to firm up a whole eye before one dissects a lamellar corneal button.

Before one punches out the donor button from

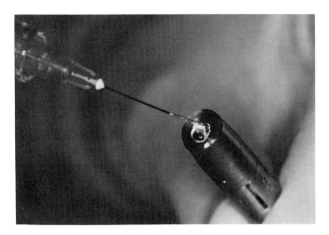

Fig. 16-1. Placing viscoelastic material in barrel of trephine.

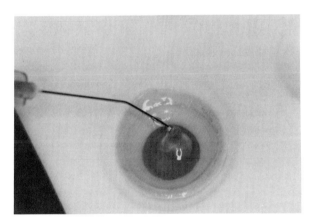

Fig. 16-2. Protecting donor button in cutting block with layer of viscoelastic.

the endothelial surface of an excised cornea, a viscoelastic material used to coat the barrel of the trephine after the obturator has been retracted 4 to 5 mm from the cutting edge of the blade will provide a protective cushion as well as a coating for the endothelium[24] (Fig. 16-1). If a viscoelastic material has not been used on the trephine, one may place it directly on the donor button after punching and before placing the balanced saline solution (Fig. 16-2). The viscoelastic material will retard swelling of the button and will thus assist in approximating tissues accurately during the suturing procedure, particularly if there has been a significant delay while the recipient eye is prepared.

Trephination of Recipient Eye. After the initial trephination and just after the anterior chamber is entered, a viscoelastic material can be placed through the wound (Fig. 16-3). By helping to main-

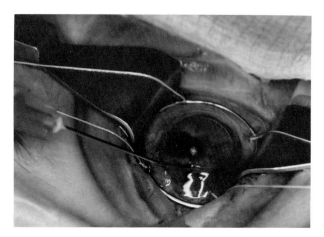

Fig. 16-3. Injecting viscoelastic through small anterior chamber entry point after initial trephination.

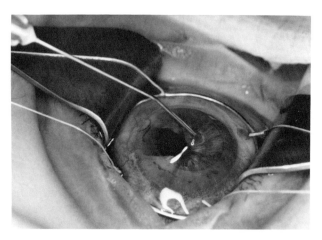

Fig. 16-4. Filling anterior chamber with viscoelastic before placement of donor button in recipient bed.

tain the anterior chamber, the material also helps in making completion of the excision of the recipient button with scissors or a diamond blade easier as well as safer by offering some protection to the underlying iris and lens. Such a technique is particularly helpful in cases such as keratoconus where the floppy cornea tends to collapse posteriorly, distorting the wound.

Gruber and co-workers[20] have recommended filling the entire anterior chamber through a paracentesis opening before trephination. They suggest that initially an air bubble be placed in the anterior chamber to force all the aqueous out the paracentesis opening. The air can then be replaced with a viscoelastic material. It is important to remember to place the cannula of the syringe containing the material across the anterior chamber so that the filling process can be begun from the opposite side. Otherwise, the material will trap the air bubble in the anterior chamber and not replace it. With the chamber filled with a viscoelastic material it is now much safer to do a through-and-through 360-degree trephination with less risk of damaging the underlying tissues.

A relative disadvantage in placing a viscoelastic in the anterior chamber at this stage of the procedure arises in an aphakic eye where one is not certain beforehand that vitrectomy will be necessary. Although, in general, formed vitreous can be distinguished from a viscoelastic by the tendency of the former to adhere to a cellulose sponge producing signs of traction whereas the latter drops away, a small prolapsing vitreal strand in the anterior chamber might be hidden, giving a false impression that a partial vitrectomy is not needed.

Phakic Grafts. Studies have shown that the manip-

ulation of the donor button during suturing and the rubbing of the button against the iris diaphragm cause endothelial cell loss, especially in phakic grafts.[8,9] Filling the anterior chamber with a viscoelastic material before placement of the donor button in the recipient bed (Fig. 16-4) has a beneficial effect on postsurgical graft edema and therefore presumably on endothelial survival.[1,34,37,38,40,45] A viscoelastic material tends to stabilize the donor button, making suturing easier and preventing contact with the iris.

Pseudophakic Grafts. Corneal transplantation over a previously implanted intraocular lens, particularly of the anterior chamber variety, requires special precautions, since even transient contact between a polymethylmethacrylate lens and the posterior surface of the graft will produce immediate damage to the endothelium because of the adherence of the cell membranes to the plastic.[25,26] The use of various trans–anterior chamber struts and stay sutures to hold the intraocular lens posteriorly and allow an air bubble to be maintained between the lens and the endothelium of the graft have proved helpful in these cases.[43] A much simpler and more effective method involves coating the lens with a layer of a viscoelastic material before placement of the donor button in the recipient bed[38,40,45] (Fig. 16-5). Alpar[1] has shown that the use of sodium hyaluronate in pseudophakic corneal transplants produced thinner grafts with less cell loss when compared to a control group in which air and balanced saline solution were used. In our experience, a viscoelastic material placed over an intraocular lens has allowed successful corneal transplantation even when the anterior chamber has collapsed because of posterior pressure, a situation that might otherwise

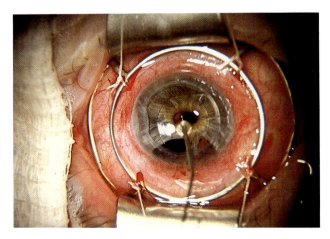

Fig. 16-5. Coating anterior chamber IOL with viscoelastic before suturing in donor button.

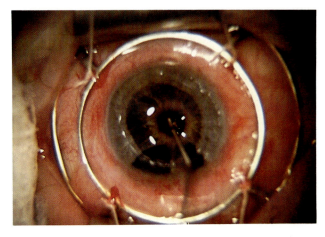

Fig. 16-6. Viscoelastic placed over pupil and iridectomy sites.

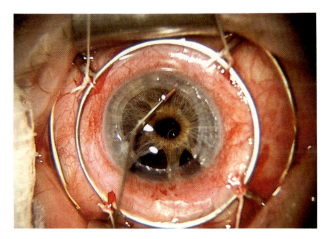

Fig. 16-7. Viscoelastic placed into chamber angle.

require removal of the implant if a viscoelastic material had not been used.

Triple Procedures. Cataract extraction with intraocular lens implantation at the time of corneal transplantation can be facilitated by a viscoelastic material, both to protect the graft from the lens once it is in place and to assist with the lens implantation itself. As in a standard cataract operation, in-the-bag placement of an intraocular lens at the time of keratoplasty is greatly facilitated by use of a capsulorrhexis procedure to make the anterior capsulotomy. If the opening cannot be made large enough to safely allow expression of the nucleus, an open-sky emulsification can be done. A viscoelastic material can be helpful in assisting in removal of the nuclear fragments once the nucleus has been fractured into smaller pieces. After removal of the nucleus and cortical cleanup, a viscoelastic material can be used to elevate the anterior capsular flaps, facilitating in-the-bag insertion of the posterior chamber lens. If sulcus fixation is considered desirable or if too much posterior pressure causing anterior displacement of the posterior capsule makes sulcus fixation the safest alternative, a viscoelastic material can be used as a tool to separate the iris from the posterior capsule. This will make lens insertion easier and safer. Other uses in cataract extraction are reviewed elsewhere and include tamponing breaks in the posterior capsule to place an intraocular lens, removal of intraocular lenses, preventing and repositioning iris prolapse, hydrodelineation of nucleus and cortex, keeping the pupil dilated, and repositioning or repairing a detachment of Descemet's membrane.[4,39]

Aphakic Keratoplasty With and Without Secondary Lens Implantation. In aphakic keratoplasty with an intact, posteriorly positioned vitreous face, place-

ment of a viscoelastic material in the anterior chamber either before trephination, through a paracentesis opening, or just after trephination, will help to reduce the chances of vitreous prolapse and the need for an anterior vitrectomy. When an anterior vitrectomy has been performed, a viscoelastic material can be placed over the pupil and iridectomy sites (Fig. 16-6). The weight and viscosity of the material acts like a cork in a bottle, pushing back and keeping the vitreous posterior to the iris, thus preventing a stray strand of vitreous from prolapsing into the anterior chamber and possibly adhering to the wound during suturing of the graft. An air bubble in the anterior chamber can be used for the same purpose. However, care must be taken, since accidentally trapping a large air bubble in the posterior chamber behind a constricted pupil can make adequate reformation of the anterior chamber impossible.

If secondary lens implantation is performed, a viscoelastic material in the posterior chamber will help prevent vitreous prolapse and traction during the maneuvers necessary in the placement of an anterior chamber lens through the central trephine opening. This maneuver is also helpful before one sutures a posterior chamber lens to avoid vitreous traction and prolapse. A small amount of a viscoelastic material placed in the chamber angle will assist in the proper placement of the "feet" of the anterior chamber lens and in prevention of entrapment of the iris with consequent pupillary distortion (Fig. 16-7). A layer of the material should also be placed over the implant before placement and suturing of the donor button.

SPECIAL SITUATIONS

A viscoelastic material can be helpful in several special situations that may arise during the operative procedure. Bleeding may occur in such situations as lysing synechiae or removing an intraocular lens, particularly a flexible anterior chamber lens whose haptics have become enmeshed in fibrous adhesions. Viscoelastic substances will tend to localize blood in the angle and keep it from passing through the pupil into the vitreous in aphakic eyes. They also appear to tampon oozing from capillaries though it is not effective against more pronounced bleeding.[42] Such bleeding should be controlled before one introduces a viscoelastic material, since blood mixed with sodium hyaluronate has its presence in the anterior chamber prolonged.

When anterior synechiae to the wound are noted after suturing of the graft and filling of the anterior chamber with balanced saline solution, it is important to release these adhesions before surgery is finished because they may be progressive and lead to compromise of the angle. A fine cyclodialysis spatula or a cannula attached to a syringe filled with balanced saline solution or air can be used to sweep away the synechiae, but this is not without some risk to the endothelium of the graft as well as to the lens. A much more elegant method is to use a viscoelastic material introduced through the wound or through a paracentesis opening as a tool to push the iris away from the back of the cornea.

A situation that involves elements of both the aforementioned problems and where a viscoelastic material may make the difference between successful surgery and a disaster arises when a graft is done on an inflamed eye. The irides of such eyes tend to ooze blood and more significantly fibrin, which causes the iris to adhere to the peripheral area of the cornea. If not released, these adhesions will lead to difficulty in controlling glaucoma. A viscoelastic material can be used to separate the "sticky" iris from the corneal rim and reform the angle before placement of the donor button in the recipient bed. Although not completely effective, a layer of such a material between the iris and the cornea in the immediate postoperative period may decrease the incidence of late-forming anterior synechiae. Usually, it is best to leave the material in the eye at the end of surgery and deal with any secondary glaucoma medically.

A viscoelastic material combined with a cyanoacrylate tissue adhesive can be used to restore the anterior chamber after a corneal perforation.[23] Introducing the material through a paracentesis tract, if possible, or directly through the wound allows repositioning of the iris, releasing of anterior synechiae, and the reformation of the anterior chamber. After removal of any excess material appearing about the surface of the cornea, which would interfere with adherence, the opening is sealed with a tissue adhesive. Maguen and co-workers[19] have used this technique to obtain normotensive eyes after perforation. A primary corneal transplant can then be safely performed, giving a better tectonic result and shorter visual rehabilitation. Other uses of viscoelastic materials in anterior segment trauma have been reviewed[13] and include restoring the pressure and shape of the globe, evacuating hyphemas, foreign-body removal, controlling bleeding, and manipulation of tissues to restore anatomy.

PROTECTION OF EPITHELIUM

Placement of a viscoelastic material on the donor button during suturing is very effective in protecting

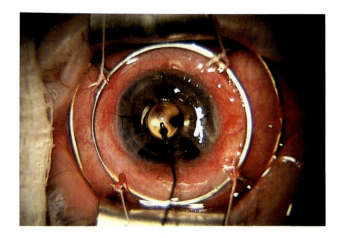

Fig. 16-8. Coating donor epithelium for protection during suturing.

the epithelium (Fig. 16-8). Although it may make suture material more difficult to manipulate and decrease visualization, it relieves the need for constant irrigation of the donor button with balanced saline solution, which can be traumatic to the epithelium.

GENERAL PRINCIPLES AND TECHNIQUES

Materials with poorer elasticity, such as Viscoat, will require a larger cannula (such as $\geq$ 25 gage) for injection. These are generally supplied commercially with the material. Only syringes with a Luer-Lok system should be used to avoid the cannula being inadvertently propelled into the eye. The material should be flowing and all air bubbles expressed from the syringe before entry into the eye. A slow injection will tend to avoid trapping air, fluid, or debris. If an air bubble is desired, it should be placed anterior to the material. Intraocular medications should be instilled posterior to the viscoelastic material to minimize endothelial toxicity. Avoid overfilling the eye and placing the viscoelastic where it cannot be removed easily.

POSTOPERATIVE COMPLICATIONS AND REMOVAL OF VISCOELASTIC MATERIALS

The major complication from the use of viscoelastic materials is the development of postoperative glaucoma.[38,40] The mechanism is complex and related to decreased outflow facility.[3] It may be modulated by individual variations in trabecular pore size and charge, by the amount of fibrin and inflammatory debris present that are pushed into the trabecular meshwork, or by simple mechanical blockage.[30] An overload of glycosaminoglycans in the trabecular meshwork similar to the situation believed to contribute to primary open-angle glaucoma may also be a factor.[30]

Clinically, intraocular pressure peaks at 4 to 7 hours and generally returns to preoperative levels by 24 hours.[3,31] Alpar[1] reported an average pressure rise of 10 mm Hg in a group of cases in which sodium hyaluronate had been used when compared to a control group. This amount of intraocular pressure elevation is fairly typical of most viscoelastics. The manufacturers of Viscoat claim a minimal elevation of intraocular pressure and no need for removal at the end of surgery. Numerous studies support this claim but are either anecdotal reports or lack frequent enough pressure monitoring to evaluate the early and common 4- to 7-hour elevation. In two studies using frequent pressure monitoring and directly comparing Healon with Viscoat results showed both to elevate intraocular pressure—equally in one study[5] and greater with Healon in the other.[15]

The volume of a viscoelastic material left in the eye appears to be one of the factors influencing the postoperative pressure response. If 0.3 ml of sodium hyaluronate or less are used in the anterior chamber, the occurrence of postoperative pressure elevation is rare.[38,40] As a general rule, the smallest amount of a viscoelastic material as possible, consistent with clinical objectives, should be used. In a phakic patient where coating of the iris is the only objective, as little as 0.1 ml of viscoelastic may be all that is needed. In addition, excessive sodium hyaluronate in the anterior chamber can give the false impression of a watertight wound closure, resulting in a postoperative wound leak.[6]

Another factor influencing the postoperative response of an eye to a viscoelastic material is the preoperative status of its outflow capacity. An eye with diminished outflow and pressure problems preoperatively is very likely to have postoperative glaucoma problems even without the use of such a material. Such patients and all in whom a viscoelastic is not removed, unless medically contraindicated, should be given a carbonic anhydrase inhibitor prophylactically in the immediate postoperative period and have their intraocular pressures closely monitored. This can blunt but may not eliminate the increased intraocular pressure.[29] Using topical hypotensives alone or in addition to a carbonic anhydrase inhibitor may provide equal or superior blunting of intraocular pressure elevation but has not been studied extensively.

Removal of a viscoelastic material at the end of surgery is technically more difficult after keratoplasty than after cataract surgery. However, in cases where relatively large amounts have been used, it is advisable to remove at least some of the material. Removing a viscoelastic material may only reduce or shorten the rise in intraocular pressure and not eliminate it.[19] The earlier in the suturing process that this can be done, the easier it is to remove the material. In cases where there is relatively little posterior pressure, after the anterior chamber is stabilized with four to six cardinal sutures, a cannula with balanced saline solution placed deep into the chamber in each of the quadrants while the wound is slightly separated will allow a good proportion of the material to be irrigated from the eye. Healon is more easily removed than other less cohesive materials such as Viscoat, which require direct aspiration at the site of the viscoelastic.[18] Placement of an air bubble in the anterior chamber before tying a running suture has been suggested as a way of pushing a viscoelastic material into the chamber angle from where it can be directly aspirated.[20] The air bubble can then be replaced with balanced saline solution. Maneuvers to remove a viscoelastic material should not be too vigorous, especially with the more viscous materials such as sodium hyaluronate, so as to avoid shear stress on the endothelium.[21]

REFERENCES

1. Alpar JJ: The use of Healon in corneal transplant surgery with and without intraocular lenses, *Ophthalmic Surg* 15:757, 1984.
2. Alpar JJ: Viscoelastic surgery, *Ann Ophthalmol* 19:350, 1987.
3. Balazs EA: Viscosurgery, features of a true viscosurgical tool and its role in ophthalmic surgery. In Miller D, Stegmann R, editors: *Treatment of anterior segment ocular trauma*, Montreal, 1986, Medicopea, pp 121-128.
4. Balazs EA, Gibbs DA: *The rheological properties and biologic function of the intercellular matrix*, London, 1970, Academic Press, pp 1241-1254.
5. Barron BA, Busin M, Page C, et al: Comparison of the effects of Viscoat and Healon on postoperative intraocular pressure, *Am J Ophthalmol* 100:377, 1985.
6. Berkowitz PJ: Surgical wound leaks associated with sodium hyaluronate (Healon), *Am J Ophthalmol* 95:714, 1983.
7. Bothner H, Wik O: Rheology of intraocular solutions. In Rosen ES, editor: *Viscoelastic material: basic science and clinical applications*, New York, 1989, Pergamon Press, pp 3-22.
8. Bourne WM, Kaufman HE: The endothelium of clear corneal transplants, *Arch Ophthalmol* 94:1730, 1976.
9. Bourne WM, O'Fallon WM: Endothelial cell loss during penetrating keratoplasty, *Am J Ophthalmol* 85:760, 1978.
10. Carty JB: Chondroitin sulfate in anterior segment surgery, *Trans Ophthalmol Soc UK* 103:263, 1983.
11. Charleux J, Dupont D, Charleux M, et al: *Human placental collagen type IV: an alternative as viscoplastic solution in ocular microsurgery*, Proc XXV International Congress of Ophthalmology, Rome, 1986, Amsterdam, 1987, Kugler & Ghedini, pp 1066-1067.
12. Cherfan GM, Rich WJ, Wright G: Raised intraocular pressure and other problems with sodium hyaluronate and cataract surgery, *Trans Ophthalmol Soc UK* 103:277, 1983.
13. Drews RC: Sodium hyaluronate (Healon®) in the repair of perforating injuries of the eye, *Ophthalmic Surg* 17:23, 1986.
14. Eisner G: General consideration concerning viscous material in ophthalmic surgery, *Trans Ophthalmol Soc UK* 103:247, 1983.
15. Embriano PJ: Postoperative pressure after phacoemulsification: sodium hyaluronate vs. sodium chondroitin sulfate–sodium hyaluronate, *Ann Ophthalmol* 21:85, 1989.
16. Fechner PU: Methylcellulose in lens implantation, *Am Intra-Ocular Implant Soc J* 3:180, 1977.
17. Fechner PU: Methylcellulose, a viscous cushioning material in ophthalmic surgery, *Trans Ophthalmol Soc UK* 103:259, 1983.
18. Glaser DB, Katz HR, Boyd JE, et al: Protective effects of viscous solutions in phacoemulsification and traumatic lens implantation, *Arch Ophthalmol* 107:1047, 1989.
19. Glaser DB, Matsuda M, Edelhauser HF: A comparison of the efficacy and toxicity of and intraocular pressure response to viscous solutions in the anterior chamber, *Arch Ophthalmol* 104:1819, 1986.
20. Gruber PF, Schipper I, Kern R: Use of Healon for corneal trephination in penetrating keratoplasty, *Ophthalmic Surg* 15:773, 1984.
21. Hammer ME, Burch TG: Viscous corneal protection by sodium hyaluronate, chondroitin sulfate, and methylcellulose, *Invest Ophthalmol Vis Sci* 25:1329, 1984.
22. Harrison SE, Soll DB, Shayegan M, Clinch T: Chondroitin sulfate: a new and effective protective agent for intraocular lens insertion, *Ophthalmology* 89:1254, 1982.
23. Hirst LW, De Juan E Jr: Sodium hyaluronate and tissue adhesives in treating corneal perforations, *Ophthalmology* 89:1250, 1982.
24. Insler MD: A new use for sodium hyaluronate (Healon®) in penetrating keratoplasty, *Ann Opthalmol* 17:106, 1985.
25. Kaufman H, Katz J: Endothelial damage from intraocular lens insertion, *Invest Ophthalmol* 15:996, 1976.
26. Kaufman H, Katz J: Endothelial damage from intraocular lens insertion, *Invest Ophthalmol* 16:265, 1977.
27. Lane SS et al: Prospective comparison of the effects of Occucoat, Viscoat and Healon on intraocular pressure and endothelial cell loss, *J Cataract Refract Surg* 17(1):21-26, 1991.
28. Leibowitz HM, Loring RA: Corneal endothelium, the effect of air in the anterior chamber, *Arch Ophthalmol* 92:227, 1974.
29. Lewen R, Insler MS: The effect of prophylactic acetazolamide on the intraocular pressure rise associated with Healon-aided intraocular lens surgery, *Ann Ophthalmol* 17:315, 1985.
30. Liesegang TJ: Viscoelastic substances in ophthalmology, *Surv Ophthalmol* 34:268, 1990.
31. MacRae SM, et al: The effects of sodium hyaluronate, chondroitin sulfate, and methylcellulose on the corneal endothelium and intraocular pressure, *Am J Ophthalmol* 95:332, 1983.
32. Maguen E, Nesburn AB, Macy JI: Combined use of sodium hyaluronate and tissue adhesive in penetrating keratoplasty of corneal perforations, *Ophthalmic Surg* 15:55, 1984.
33. Miller D, O'Connor P, Williams J: Use of Na-hyaluronate during intraocular lens implantation in rabbits, *Ophthalmic Surg* 8:58, 1977.
34. Miller D, Stegmann R: Use of Na-hyaluronate in auto-corneal transplantation in rabbits, *Ophthalmic Surg* 11:19, 1980.
35. Muir MGK, Sherrard ES, Andrews V, et al: Air, methylcellulose, sodium hyaluronate and the corneal endothelium—endothelial protective agents, *Eye* 1:480, 1987.
36. Olson RJ: Air and the corneal endothelium, *Arch Ophthalmol* 98:1283, 1980.
37. Pape LG, Balazs EA: The use of sodium hyaluronate (Healon®) in anterior segment surgery, *Ophthalmology* 87:699, 1980.
38. Polack FM: Penetrating keratoplasty using MK stored corneas and Na hyaluronate (Healon), *Trans Am Ophthalmol Soc* 80:248, 1982.
39. Polack FM: Healon® (Na hyaluronate): a review of the literature, *Cornea* 5:81, 1986.
40. Polack FM, Demong T, Santaella H: Sodium hyaluronate (Healon) in keratoplasty and IOL implantation, *Ophthalmology* 88:425, 1981.
41. Roberts B, Peiffer RL Jr: Experimental evaluation of a synthetic viscoelastic material on intraocular pressure and corneal endothelium, *J Cataract Refract Surg* 15:321, 1989.
42. Roper-Hall MJ: Visco-elastic material in the surgery of ocular trauma, *Trans Ophthalmol Soc UK* 103:274, 1983.
43. Simcoe CW: Retaining devices for protection of corneal endothelium, *Am Intra-Ocular Implant Soc J* 5:234, 1979.
44. Soll DB, et al: Evaluation and protection of corneal endothelium, *Am Intra-Ocular Implant Soc J* 6:239, 1980.
45. Steele AD: Visco-elastic material in keratoplasty, *Trans Ophthalmol Soc UK* 103:208, 1983.

Chapter 17

Expulsive Hemorrhage

JOHN J. PURCELL, JR.

The most devastating complication that can occur during penetrating keratoplasty is an expulsive choroidal hemorrhage. Since the eye is in an open-sky position during penetrating keratoplasty, an expulsive hemorrhage is more difficult to control and is managed differently from those occurring in other forms of intraocular surgery.

BACKGROUND

Expulsive hemorrhage has been reported in cataract surgery,[7] glaucoma surgery,[13] retinal detachment surgery,[15] and spontaneously.[14] Expulsive choroidal effusion[10] may cause vitreous loss and mimic an early expulsive choroidal hemorrhage. In a prospective study, limited choroidal hemorrhage associated with intracapsular cataract extraction was found in 3.07% of 521 eyes.[6] Delayed nonexpulsive suprachoroidal hemorrhage can occur after filtering surgery.[5]

Early reports of expulsive hemorrhage with penetrating keratoplasty were of isolated cases,[4,12] until a collaborative review of 14 cases[9] indicated the complexity of the problem. Most corneal surgeons who perform a large number of penetrating keratoplasties have had to deal with expulsive hemorrhages.

PREDISPOSING CONDITIONS

The incidence of expulsive hemorrhage may be increasing as newer and more sophisticated surgical techniques have developed. Eyes that would have been considered lost in the past are now operable (Fig. 17-1). In our review of 14 cases of expulsive hemorrhage[10] 10 were eyes that had sustained injury, were infected or inflamed, or had previous in-

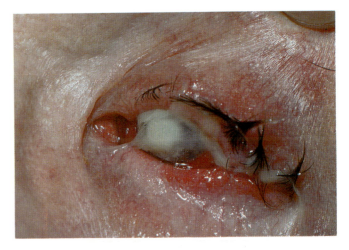

Fig. 17-1. Preoperative photograph of a *Proteus* corneal abscess with perforation.

traocular surgery. Inflammation, hypotonia, or previous trauma predisposes eyes to expulsive hemorrhages.

The incidence during intracapsular cataract extraction is estimated at 0.21%.[7] In 852 consecutive penetrating keratoplasties, I have had 4 expulsive hemorrhages, which is an incidence of 0.47%. This is higher than in cataract extraction. The cornea surgeon must be prepared for an expulsive hemorrhage, especially when operating on an inflamed eye. Hypotonia alone cannot produce experimental choroidal detachment,[2,3] but venous congestion or inflammation with hypotonia can produce an effusion into the ciliochoroidal space. Other predisposing factors include vascular fragility associated with age,[11] glaucoma,[8] and myopia.[6]

221

INTRAOPERATIVE DEVELOPMENT

Preoperatively, the reduction of intraocular pressure, shrinkage of aqueous and vitreous volume, and presumably a decrease in choroidal blood flow may be beneficial in preventing expulsive choroidal hemorrhage. This can be achieved with a Honan balloon or other similar apparatus.

The trephination should be performed so that there is no increase in the intraocular pressure by excessive pressure with the trephine. Gentle pressure with the trephine blade and then a gradual scratch-down incision to gradually decompress the globe should prevent rapid changes in intraocular pressure.

Intraoperatively, the use of viscoelastic materials may by their weight and volume increase the resistance to the progression of choroidal detachment and possible expulsive hemorrhage.

Through the microscope the corneal surgeon is in a unique position to observe choroidal detachments developing during intraocular surgery (Fig. 17-2). This is especially true during anterior vitrectomy. These are usually small and self-limited and resolve after surgery. They can be seen (especially with a dilated pupil) as brownish masses or ridges and folds that develop during the open-sky technique. Large choroidal detachments often are present in perfo-

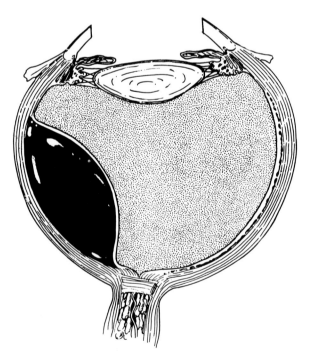

Fig. 17-2. Choroidal detachments developing during keratoplasty often are seen through operating microscope.

rated eyes before surgery and may progress during the procedure. Rapidly developing choroidal detachments can occur at any time during the procedure and may be a forerunner of expulsive choroidal hemorrhage. In our series, Valsalva maneuvers by patients during general anesthesia led to the occurrence of an expulsive hemorrhage in two patients.[9] The rate of blood flow in the choroid is the highest per unit volume of any tissue, and the capillaries of the choroid are four times the diameter of the other capillaries.[1] Valsalva maneuvers rapidly raise the pressure in these vessels; with anesthesia, no forced lid closure is present to protect the eye from transiently elevated venous pressure and an expulsive hemorrhage can ensue.

A choroidal hemorrhage may start gradually, with vitreous bulge, and then expulse with massive hemorrhage and loss of the intraocular contents. The corneal surgeon must be prepared to redirect the hemorrhage posteriorly, attempt to restore normal ocular architecture, and close the wound. During a penetrating keratoplasty the eye is in an open-sky position, a unique and very difficult situation for managing the hemorrhage.

Preoperatively, those eyes with inflammation, previous surgery, glaucoma, or myopia should be suspected as potential cases of expulsive hemorrhage.

MANAGEMENT

Intraoperatively the management of an expulsive hemorrhage depends on when it occurs. After a lamellar trephination, most surgeons enter the anterior chamber with a scratch-down incision. An expulsive hemorrhage that occurs immediately when the globe is entered is usually easier to manage because an open-sky situation is not present. Once the expulsive hemorrhage is recognized, an immediate stab incision should be made into the choroidal space. A knife blade capable of making such an opening should be available on the instrument trays. Most fine diamond knives are not suitable, and a larger blade should be available. This is a direct stab (not a dissection) through conjunctiva and sclera. Usually the most accessible area for the sclerotomy is the inferotemporal quadrant. The opening should be large enough to allow blood and clots to be redirected posteriorly. It is often necessary, while the corneal wound is being closed, to reopen this area and expel clots. If the initial stab is not productive, other quadrants should be opened. Once the posterior sclerotomy has been performed, the corneal opening should be closed. Prolapsed iris, lens, vitreous, or retina may by appropriately handled in a slow bleed or after a posterior sclerotomy, but in an

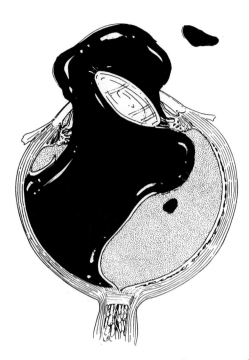

Fig. 17-3. Expulsive choroidal hemorrhage occurring after removal of diseased cornea.

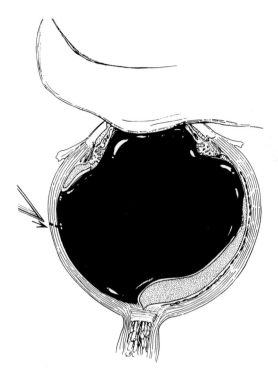

Fig. 17-4. Closure of wound with fingertip and posterior sclerotomy for expulsive choroidal hemorrhage.

expulsive situation these should be ignored and the wound closed. Fine 10-0 nylon sutures will not hold the wound if a serious hemorrhage has occurred, and 6-0 or 7-0 silk sutures should be available. After wound closure, clots and prolapsed material can be managed if the posterior sclerotomy is functioning and the hemorrhage is redirected posteriorly.

The most difficult expulsive hemorrhage to manage is the one that occurs when an open-sky situation exists (Figs. 17-3 to 17-6). This can occur at any time after the cornea has been removed, including during lens extraction or anterior vitrectomy. In this situation, the tip of the thumb or a finger is placed into the opening and a posterior sclerotomy performed. A cornea must be available to be sutured in place immediately; therefore the donor tissue should be prepared and ready to be used before removal of the host cornea. In addition, the host cornea should be placed in saline solution or the storage medium, rather than formalin, and should be available for immediate use. Silk sutures are used to close the wound.

Even after a severe expulsive hemorrhage, the visual outcome can be surprisingly good,[9] and it is probably best not to eviscerate these eyes primarily but to secure the wound and evaluate them postoperatively.

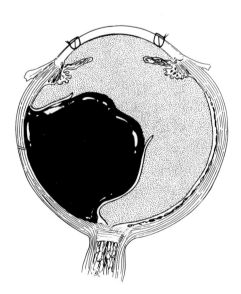

Fig. 17-5. Cornea sutured in place, normal anterior segment architecture restored, and posterior sclerotomy left open.

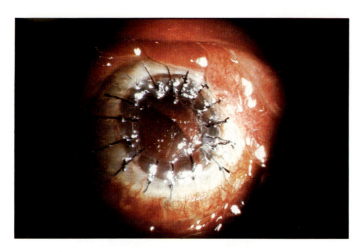

Fig. 17-6. Donor cornea secured in place with silk sutures after posterior sclerotomy for an expulsive choroidal hemorrhage.

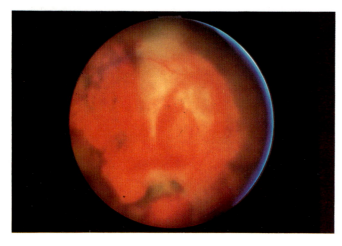

Fig. 17-7. View of resolving expulsive hemorrhage after repeat keratoplasty.

The postoperative management includes systemic antibiotic coverage, assessment of vision, and management of intraocular pressure and inflammation. Evacuation of the hyphema, vitrectomy, repair of a retinal detachment, and a regraft may yield good vision in a few cases (Fig. 17-7). Other eyes require evisceration or enucleation.

The corneal surgeon should be aware of the increased risk of expulsive hemorrhage during kerato-plasty in certain eyes and be prepared to manage this immediately when it occurs. Proper knives and suture material should be available on the instrument tray preoperatively for immediate use.

Because of newer techniques and more aggressive attempts to save extremely sick eyes, today's corneal surgeon is bound to experience expulsive hemorrhage and must be prepared to manage this dreaded experience.

REFERENCES

1. Alm A, Bill A: Ocular and optic nerve blood flow at normal and increased intraocular pressures in monkeys *(Macaca irus):* a study with radioactively labelled microspheres including flow determinations in brain and some other tissues, *Exp Eye Res* 15:15-29, 1973.
2. Capper SA, Leopold IH: Mechanisms of serious choroidal detachment, *Arch Ophthalmol* 55:101-113, 1956.
3. Collins ET: Intraocular tension: I. An experimental investigation as to some of the effects of hypotony in rabbits' eyes, *Trans Ophthalmol Soc UK* 38:217-227, 1918.
4. Girard LJ, Spak KE, Hawkins RS, Caldwell D: Expulsive hemorrhage during intraocular surgery, *Trans Am Acad Ophthalmol Otolaryngol* 77:119-125, 1973.
5. Gressel MG, Parrish RK, Heuer DK: Delayed nonexpulsive suprachoroidal hemorrhage, *Arch Ophthalmol* 102:1757-1760, 1984.
6. Hoffman P, Pollack A, Oliver M: Limited choroidal hemorrhage associated with the intracapsular cataract extraction, *Arch Ophthalmol* 102:1761-1765, 1984.
7. Jaffe NS: *Cataract surgery and its complications,* St. Louis, 1972, Mosby–Year Book.
8. Manschot WA: Glaucoma—vascular necrosis—expulsive hemorrhage, *Acta Ophthalmol* 23:309-342, 1945.
9. Purcell JJ, Krachmer JH, Doughman DJ, Bourne WA: Expulsive hemorrhage in penetrating keratoplasty, *Ophthalmology* 89:41-43, 1982.
10. Ruiz RS, Salmonsen PC: Expulsive choroidal effusion: a complication of intraocular hemorrhage, *Arch Ophthalmol* 94:69-70, 1976.
11. Samuels B: Postoperative nonexpulsive subchoroidal hemorrhage, *Arch Ophthalmol* 8:840-851, 1931.
12. Taylor DM: Expulsive hemorrhage: some observations and comments, *Trans Am Ophthalmol Soc* 92:33-35, 1974.
13. Verhoeff FH: Scleral puncture for expulsive subchoroidal hemorrhage following sclerostomy—scleral puncture for postoperative separation of the choroid, *Ophthalmic Rec* 24:55-59, 1915.
14. Winslow RL, Stevenson W III, Yanoff M: Spontaneous expulsive choroidal hemorrhage, *Arch Ophthalmol* 92:33-35, 1974.
15. Wolter JR: Expulsive hemorrhage during retinal detachment surgery, *Am J Ophthalmol* 51:264-266, 1961.

Chapter 18

Routine Postoperative Management

WILLIAM R. SULLIVAN

Modern suturing techniques have greatly simplified the postoperative care of the keratoplasty patient. A watertight wound secured with a suture that will be rapidly covered with epithelium usually ensures a smooth postoperative course and permits the patient to resume normal daily activities very quickly.

Each corneal surgeon has his own guidelines for managing the routine keratoplasty patient, and there are few studies to demonstrate the superiority of one approach over another. Rather than attempt to catalog all the variations in successful management techniques, this section presents the current approach of one surgeon, the author.

IMMEDIATE POSTOPERATIVE CARE

After the final knot has been tied and buried and the wound checked for leakage by depression of the scleral edge with a cellulose sponge, an antibiotic and steroid combination is given, either as a topical ointment or as a subconjunctival injection. If the surgery was performed under general anesthesia, a 4 ml retrobulbar injection of one of the long-acting local anesthetics, such as 0.75% Marcaine (bupivacaine hydrochloride), is given to prevent postoperative pain. Two gauze pads are used to patch the eye, and a metal shield is applied.

Whether the surgery was done on an inpatient or outpatient basis, the patient is encouraged to resume normal diet and activity patterns immediately, with the only warning being that he should avoid direct trauma to the eye. The traditional warnings about bending, stooping, sleeping position, and so on are probably outmoded with modern wound closure and only tend to make the patient unnecessarily anxious. The trend toward outpatient surgery has considerable merit, in that patients are less likely to injure themselves in the familiar surroundings of their own home than they are in the hospital.

With the use of a long-acting retrobulbar anesthetic, pain during the first night is greatly reduced, and patients seldom require anything stronger than acetaminophen for analgesia. For the occasional patient with more severe pain, a prescription for one of the oral narcotic medications, such as Percocet (an oxycodone and acetaminophen preparation), is given. Stronger medications are almost never needed after the first 24 hours, and the need for them should alert the surgeon to the presence of possible complications.

FOLLOW-UP CARE

Frequency of Examination. Even in the uncomplicated keratoplasty, patients should be seen daily for the first 2 or 3 days after surgery. Careful attention is given to the integrity of the wound, epithelial defects, the intraocular pressure, the amount of iritis, and the possibility of infection. Visits should continue two or three times weekly until the epithelium is healed and the sutures are covered, or as long as there is any uncertainty about control of the other factors mentioned above.

After this initial period, patients should be followed every week or two for the first 6 to 8 weeks and then every month to 6 weeks for the first year. In the absence of complications, visits are then scheduled at increasing intervals, ultimately once or twice a year. Since most complications can be successfully treated with early intervention, patients should be repeatedly warned to be seen within a day or two with any unusual symptoms, no matter how long it has been since the surgery.

Early Wound Problems. The patch is removed on the first postoperative day, and the patient is advised to wear glasses during daytime and the metal shield at night for the first 8 weeks. If an epithelial defect is persistent, patching may be resumed, though this situation is more often managed with direct taping of the eyelids or a bandage soft contact lens.

Wound leaks are rare with current suturing techniques but should be looked for carefully. Unusual stromal swelling, a shallow anterior chamber, or low intraocular pressure should make the surgeon especially alert. Patching and a soft contact lens may be sufficient treatment for minor leaks. A leak that persists for more than 4 or 5 days or results in a constantly flat chamber for 2 days should be repaired with additional interrupted sutures. Iris or vitreous prolapse through the wound should be repaired promptly.

Medications. Topical steroid drops, such as prednisolone acetate 1%, are prescribed four times a day. The frequency is decreased as inflammatory signs subside, usually to a level of two or three drops a day by the end of the first month. They are usually continued once or twice a day through the first 3 months. The risk-to-benefit ratio after this is not clear, but an argument can be made for continuing the drops once or twice a day as a hedge against late graft failure in the aphakic patient with normal intraocular pressure. If the patient is phakic or there is any elevation of the pressure, the risks of steroid-induced cataract or glaucoma probably preclude continuing topical steroid once 3 months have passed and inflammatory signs have disappeared.

Topical antibiotics, usually in the form of an antibiotic-steroid combination ointment, are started twice a day on the first postoperative day and continued once or twice a day for about 3 weeks. This is discontinued once the epithelium is intact and there is no suspicion of infection.

After topical antibiotics and steroids have been tapered or stopped, patients who live or travel in areas where they cannot reach ophthalmic care within a day or two should keep on hand one of the antibiotic-steroid combination agents. They should start using this hourly until they can reach an ophthalmologist if they develop significant pain, photophobia, blurring, or discharge in the operated eye. The risk of this is small compared with the importance of prompt treatment for corneal rejection or infection problems.

Many surgeons routinely use cycloplegics in the early postoperative period. This is probably unnecessary except with extraordinary iritis and can result in the loss of a small pupil if the iris becomes stuck in a dilated position. If the surgeon believes that use of a cycloplegic is essential, a short-acting drug, such as cyclopentolate 1%, is preferred. The goal is to keep the pupil moving so that posterior synechiae won't have time to form. One should be especially cautious about dilating the pupil in patients with keratoconus, where there may be an increased risk of persistent pupillary dilatation.

The intraocular pressure should be monitored closely throughout the entire postoperative period and treated aggressively if it becomes elevated. The routine use of timolol for the first postoperative week should be considered if there is any uncertainty about the pressure, especially if one of the viscoelastic materials was used at surgery or there is blood in the anterior chamber.

When timolol alone is not adequate to control the pressure, carbonic anhydrase inhibitors, such as acetazolamide, are preferable to the miotics because the miotics may aggravate iritis in the early postoperative period. Pressure elevations after the first week arouse suspicion of a steroid effect, and switching to fluoromethalone may be helpful in controlling the pressure. When the pressure continues to be a problem despite the aforementioned measures, miotics should be tried before one resorts to surgical intervention.

Visual Rehabilitation. Efforts at refraction before 6 to 8 weeks are seldom productive but should begin about 2 months after surgery. Selective removal of interrupted sutures to alter astigmatism can begin at this time and is continued at each visit until the astigmatism is reduced below about 2.5 diopters or until there are no more appropriate sutures to remove. If excessive astigmatism is still present at 8 to 9 months, removal of the running suture is sometimes helpful, though the running suture is ordinarily left in place until it spontaneously breaks and has to be removed.

A prescription for appropriate glasses or contact lenses is given as soon as the refraction seems to be stabilizing. This occurs occasionally as early as 2 to 3 months after surgery, but patient discouragement can be minimized if one warns the patient that it may take 6 or more months before a useful prescription can be given.

Resumption of Activities. Patients are usually quite concerned about resumption of their ordinary activities. It can be helpful to discuss with them the two major considerations involved—infection and trauma. The risk of introducing an infectious agent is present until the epithelium is firmly healed, and so it is wise to avoid contaminating situations such as dusty environments and swimming until this has occurred.

Patients with keratoplasty should be aware that the surgical incision will always be the weakest part of the eye and could be ruptured by direct trauma months or years later. Situations with a high risk of blunt injury to the eye, such as contact sports, diving, racket sports, and skiing, should be avoided completely for 6 to 12 months after surgery. After that time, caution and protective eye wear are essential for the person who badly wants to resume such activities.

The most common questions confronted by the surgeon relate to such activities as reading, hair washing, driving, and returning to work. These ac-

tivities may be safely resumed as soon as the patient's comfort and the vision in the unoperated eye permit. Guidelines in these matters must be tailored to the individual patient, based on his occupation and the status of the other eye.

CONCLUSION

The success of keratoplasty, more than any other ophthalmic surgery, depends on careful and diligent postoperative care. Both the patient and the surgeon must be constantly alert to changes in the eye so that problems can be promptly treated. Most complications can be reversed if therapy is started within a few days but may be irreversible if several weeks are allowed to elapse. Educating the patient and the referring physician to contact the surgeon immediately about any change in the condition of the eye may be the most important factor in the success or failure of the corneal transplant.

Chapter 19

Suture Removal

EDWARD L. SHAW

FREDERICK S. BRIGHTBILL

The decision to remove a corneal transplant suture is complex yet critical to final visual outcome and is based primarily on sound clinical judgment.

CRITERIA FOR SUTURE REMOVAL

A crystal-clear corneal transplant with high astigmatism and poor vision does not constitute a successful case. Almost any well-prepared ophthalmologist can tie a nylon suture and close a wound, but the expertise comes in knowing when to remove the suture.

Several criteria for considering suture removal are as follows:

1. A loose suture
2. A tight suture
3. Vascularization of the suture tract
4. Vascularization of the recipient stroma
5. Pronounced inflammation or infiltration around a suture
6. Contraction of the wound
7. A thin fibrous wound scar

When the graft-host interface shows a visible, fine wound scar or there is obvious vascularization around a suture, removal is necessary. A loose suture that was not seen previously usually reflects scar formation with wound contracture and should be taken out. Otherwise, mucus and debris may become trapped around the suture and provoke a foreign-body reaction or act as a nidus of infection. This can also act as an immunologic stimulus leading to graft rejection.[2,19]

Numerous problems may be caused by loose sutures or exposed knots:

1. Foreign-body sensation and pain
2. Epithelial erosions and ulcers
3. Corneal vascularization
4. Dellen
5. Conjunctival injection
6. Tarsal ulcers
7. Giant papillary hypertrophy or conjunctivitis, or both
8. Blepharospasm or blepharoptosis, or both
9. Photophobia
10. Iritis
11. Infection
12. Graft failure

A loose suture may cause severe pain, photophobia, blepharospasm, and even blepharoptosis.[29,31] Upper tarsal conjunctival ulcers and giant papillary hypertrophy[32] may occur from loose or irritating sutures, and if conjunctival injection and corneal epithelial trauma continue, iritis may follow, leading to graft rejection and possible failure.

If a suture is too tight, severe corneal flattening occurs in the same meridian as the interrupted suture. Extreme flattening of the center of the cornea in a plateau configuration can be seen with a tight running suture. The impression of a tight suture may be easily confirmed by slitlamp examination. One may see "stress" lines in the deep stroma and Descemet's membrane as well as a "cheese-wiring" effect as the suture cuts through the corneal tissue. The keratometer and corneometer further confirm the astigmatic effect and irregular corneal surface.

If the knot of an interrupted suture has a long end causing significant foreign-body symptoms but the suture cannot be removed because of inadequate wound healing, either cutting or cauterization of the suture end using a low-temperature disposable cautery is warranted. With slitlamp observation, the tip of the cautery is brought to the immediate vicinity of the suture end and activated momentarily. After release of the on button, the tip is touched to the suture end, melting it into a small, smooth ball. Care must be taken not to burn too close to the epithelium because ulceration can occur.

Cutting the exposed suture end is also possible by use of one hand to grasp the suture with a jewelers' forceps and the other hand to cut it, utilizing a razor knife. This can be accomplished under slitlamp control with an assistant holding the eyelids open.

WOUND HEALING

The majority of modern-day grafted corneas heal without obvious vascularization of the graft-host interface. The practice of burying suture knots either on the donor or recipient sides of the wound has limited the growth of limbal vessels into the donor and resulted in white, quiet eyes with minimal irritation. These transplants with buried sutures require less corticosteroid than in earlier times when surface knots stimulated vascular ingrowth to the graft-host interface and threatened rejection. The object of corticosteroid treatment should probably be to use as low a dose as possible to limit iritis and vascularization but not interfere with wound healing. After the first few weeks of treatment, that may be as little as one or two drops daily of 1% prednisolone acetate.

Although corneal vascularization is usually a definitive sign of wound healing and an indication for suture removal, it may not be a foolproof sign. In fact, one may often be misled if vascularization alone is used as the sole measure of healing. One must be sure that in cases of corneal scarring and edema, keratoconus with wound-thickness disparity, and chemical burns, that adequate time has elapsed for full wound healing and maximal wound tensile strength.[6,22] This is especially true when one is administering antibiotics, topical and systemic steroids, antivirals, and bandage contact lenses, all of which may significantly alter wound healing while modifying the vascular response. It is well documented that some antibiotics prolong epithelial repair, which is known to be essential for proper wound healing. Idoxuridine, trifluorothymidine, and arabinoside monophosphate (the monophosphate ester of vidarabine) cause toxic changes in regenerating epithelium. Interestingly, only the last actually retards closure of corneal wounds while increasing stromal wound strength.[10,14,24] The first two antivirals reduce tensile wound strength by 50%.[20,24]

Corticosteroids have been implicated both clinically and experimentally in delayed corneal wound healing and in decreased tensile strength.[1,16,27] This effect is believed to be attributable to the direct reduction in fibroblastic activity at the wound edge. These fibroblasts are derived from the stromal keratocytes, which migrate from the limbal area.[15] The steroid effect, studied with DNA-synthesis inhibition techniques, showed 73% to 82% reduction of cells incorporating isotope and a 50% reduction in the area of healing.[21,25]

The use of a bandage soft contact lens after keratoplasty to treat an epithelial defect, ameliorate poor surface wetting, or alleviate suture irritation may lead to superficial vascularization, which may give the impression of deep wound edge vascularization. This effect would be very much like that seen when conjunctiva covers a poorly apposed cataract wound. If sutures are removed too soon, wound dehiscence may occur. On the other hand, a thick bandage lens or a lens fitting too tightly can cause deep vascularization and provoke graft rejection.[19]

The ultimate dilemma therefore occurs in the treatment of flagrant vascularization of the suture tract (Fig. 19-1). Graft rejection is of great concern requiring increased dosage of corticosteroid. With more steroid use, wound healing is slowed. If the sutures seem to be provoking vascularization, one may

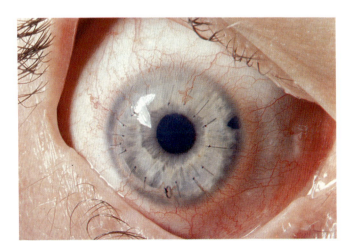

Fig. 19-1. Forty-year-old white woman with long history of herpes simplex keratitis with pronounced vascularization. Three months postoperatively there is exuberant vessel growth over and through suture tracts. Notice single 9-0 silk suture needed at time of surgery because of persistant leaking through needle tracts. Six sutures have already been removed.

need to remove them, keeping in mind the possibility for wound separation. If maintenance of the vascularized suture is imperative, injection of depot corticosteroid (such as triamcinolone, 20 mg) subconjunctivally around the area of donor-recipient vascularization may solve both problems by causing regression of vessels and allowing suture retention.

The use of argon laser to specifically close a particularly large vessel leading to an obvious area of the graft or to a suture has been advocated and may be helpful in preventing secondary lipid keratopathy or potential rejection. One of us (E.L.S.) has had better success with conjunctival recession and cautery than with the laser. Using either method, the offending vessels have either remained inactive or have slowly returned but with far less aggressiveness.

NYLON SUTURES

Since its introduction in 1968, the 10-0 monofilament nylon (22 μm) suture has become the overwhelming choice of transplant surgeons. Some authorities advocate the use of 11-0 monofilament nylon (16 to 18 μm) suture combined with the 10-0 nylon,[7,15,27] and 8-0 white silk anchoring sutures are used still but by only a few surgeons.

The development of this extremely fine, consistent, elastic, and minimally tissue-reactive suture has revolutionized corneal transplantation. The rate of corneal rejection has dropped because of diminished inflammation and vascularization of the wound. The negative side effect of controlled healing is that significantly more time is now needed to achieve complete wound healing. Whereas silk sutures require only a few weeks to a few months for wound healing, nylon sutures take months and often a year to achieve the same effect. Wound override and late wound dehiscence may still occur[11,26] but with diminished frequency because most transplant surgeons now wait 7 to 12 months to remove the final nylon sutures. This contrasts with studies of wound dehiscence reported in the early and middle seventies when experience was first being gained in their use.[3,4,7,9,11,31]

Other complications related to suture removal[9,12,23] may include:

1. Wound gape
2. Wound override
3. High astigmatism
4. Rapid graft edema
5. Graft failure
6. Endophthalmitis
7. Glaucoma
8. Hyphema with vitreous hemorrhage
9. Retinal detachment
10. Epithelial downgrowth

WHEN TO REMOVE SUTURES

Given the effect of factors such as recipient age, method of suturing, and medication on graft wound healing, an exact timetable for suture removal is of limited value and only general guidelines follow:

1. In grafts sutured with both interrupted and running sutures, the usual sequence for removal of the cardinal (anchoring) 9-0 or 10-0 nylon sutures (if not removed at the end of surgery) begins around the fourth to sixth postoperative week.

2. When 10-0 nylon suture in interrupted fashion alone (usually 16) is used, suture removal is initiated at about 3 months and completed between 6 and 12 months.

3. For 10-0 nylon running suture alone, in the majority of cases it is left in place for 7 to 12 months.

4. When used with 11-0 nylon suture (double running technique), the ophthalmologist has several choices: (1) the 10-0 running nylon suture may be removed between 2 and 4 months and the 11-0 left in place indefinitely,[8,16,30] (2) both sutures may be left in place indefinitely if spectacle refraction provides good vision, or (3) when scar formation is noted (6 to 12 months), either the 10-0 or 11-0 suture is removed while retaining the other and refraction done 4 to 6 weeks later.

5. Remove all broken or loose sutures protruding through or above the epithelium (except when no healing has occurred) to prevent induced infection, chronic irritation (which may lead to rejection), and frequent return visits for removal of suture remnants.

In infants and children, where wound healing may occur rapidly (weeks to just a few months), the timing of suture removal becomes extremely critical. Rapid new vessel formation, wound contraction, and loosening of sutures[28] may lead to rejection at a much earlier time than in the adult eye. Parents should be encouraged to inspect the eye frequently for increased injection, discharge, or accumulation of mucus around loosened sutures. Often, weekly visits are needed so that suture removal can be carried out and inflammation leading to rejection avoided.

TECHNIQUE

Many instruments and techniques can be used to remove sutures. They are as follows:

1. Vannas scissors
2. Westcott scissors (sharp points)
3. Razor blade knife (blade breaker)
4. Beaver blade no. 75
5. 20-gage needle
6. Argon or YAG (yttrium-aluminum-garnet) laser

7. Jewelers' forceps
8. Tying forceps

Topical anesthesia is used with either proparacaine hydrochloride or tetracaine hydrochloride. Suture removal may be carried out with the patient seated at the slitlamp, or a microscope may be used with the patient reclined in the office chair. In the former method, an assistant holds the upper eyelid against the supraorbital rim with a sterile Q-Tip applicator so that no pressure is exerted against the eye. A razor blade knife is used to cut the sutures in host tissue (when knots are buried in the donor cornea) and a jewelers' forceps remove the sutures by grasping the knot. The suture is rotated so that the force is directed toward the periphery. This protects against the graft being pulled away from the host. For recipient buried suture knots, the opposite technique is performed.

Our preferred technique is to cut sutures at the curve of the suture and then use the blade of the knife to tease the suture free of epithelium so that there is a long piece of suture to grasp with a jewelers' forceps. A 45-degree Alcon I-Knife or a 75 Beaver Microsharp blade, originally used at surgery and then resterilized for one or two more uses, usually suffices.

With running 10-0 nylon sutures, every other loop in the host cornea is first cut, leaving an intact loop that is also grasped in the host tissue and pulled peripherally. E.L.S. routinely uses no antibiotic prophylaxis, but F.S.B. uses Polysporin ointment, b.i.d., for 3 days. Patients are instructed to contact the office if there is pain, excessive redness, decreased visual acuity, or photophobia. Significant change in vision is very common after suture removal, and patients need to be forewarned of this. Most patients are then examined 24 to 48 hours after suture removal for epithelial defects, wound override, or dehiscence.

Children or patients with severe photophobia or blepharospasm may need general anesthesia, mask-assisted oxygen with deep intravenous sedation, or peribulbar blocks to facilitate wound inspection and suture removal.

COMPLICATIONS OF SUTURE REMOVAL

The four most commonly encountered problems after suture removal are (1) retained suture material, (2) infection, (3) wound dehiscence, and (4) induced astigmatism.

Retained Suture Material. Chronic low-grade inflammation (Fig. 19-2), visual fluctuation caused by changes in astigmatism, and late suture erosion through the graft surface may occur with retained

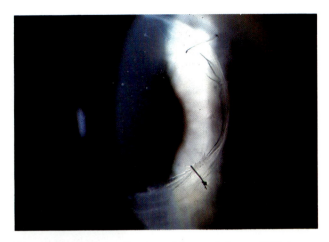

Fig. 19-2. White, active keratitic precipitates (KP) in eye with retained, broken, buried 10-0 nylon sutures 8 months after penetrating keratoplasty for keratoconus.

nylon sutures. With running suture wound closure, this is usually not a problem except at the position of the buried knot (usually 12 o'clock). With multiple interrupted buried suture knots, however, suture breakage in attempted knot removal may occur, especially if the knot has not been placed close to the graft surface or if a significant amount of stromal fibrosis has occurred around the knot.

Bourne and Maguire[5] have suggested using the argon laser to cut the knot free of the suture in the cases where the bulky knot and trailing suture cannot be removed with the usual technique. They use a laser setting of 300 to 500 mW, 50 μm spot size and a 0.2-second duration pulse. Although this technique seems like overkill, it may serve unique situations and should be considered.

Infection. Harris and associates[13] reported a large series of 108 bacterial and fungal ulcers in patients having penetrating keratoplasties 1 to 72 months before "an exposed suture having been noted and/or removed." Thirty-three eyes (31% of total number of infections) occurred within 10 days of suture removal. The majority of infections (89%) occurred in eyes receiving corticosteroids and maintenance antibiotics.

It is apparent clinically that the act of suture removal is a potentially dangerous time. This occurs presumably because the epithelial surface is broken and mucoid debris and bacterial organisms are introduced into the graft as the nylon suture is rotated out of the stroma. The surgeon needs to show particular care when cutting and removing loose sutures so as to avoid introducing debris into the graft. After suture removal, the topical instillation of antibiotics for several days would seem justified and is advised.

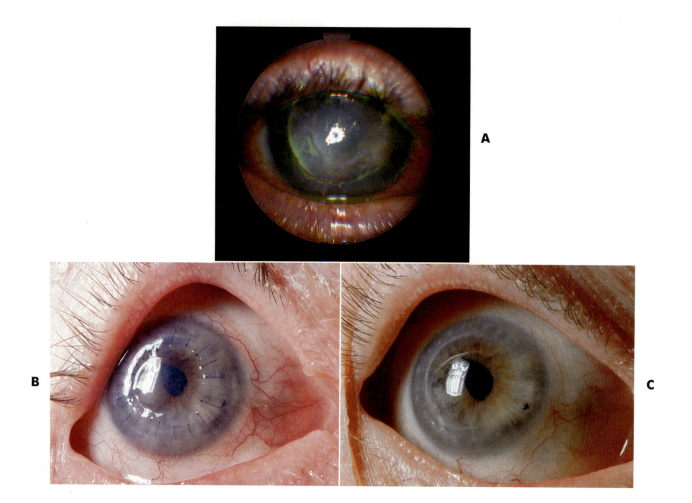

Fig. 19-3. A, Temporal-half wound dehiscence 4 days after running 10-0 nylon suture removal; 9½ months postoperatively in a 72-year-old white man. **B,** Appearance of same patient 4 months after wound revision and placement of interrupted sutures. Notice that nasal sutures are placed in apparently healed wound as a precaution to further wound separation. **C,** Same patient 13 months after wound revision with vision corrected to 20/40 with a +8.50 +2.00 × 120 aphakic spectacle.

Wound Dehiscence. In the event of wound dehiscence, wound override, or wound rupture (Figs. 19-3, *A,* and 19-4, *A*) the patient is scheduled for immediate surgical repair. Most of E.L.S.'s adult patients are repaired under topical anesthesia only. F.S.B. prefers peribulbar injection before repair. A small percentage of patients (usually children) have intravenous sedation or anesthesia standby, or both. If there is only anterior wound dehiscence, interrupted 10-0 nylon sutures are placed in the center of the wound and past the obvious limits of poor wound healing to prevent further wound separation (Fig. 19-3, *B* and *C*). One should take care to pass the needle through the apparently intact wound without touching the wound edges, thereby lessening chances of further dehiscence. As many sutures as needed are used. If there has been inordinate amounts of wound edema, instead of 10-0 nylon E.L.S. uses 9-0 polypropylene (Prolene) or rarely 8-0 silk for wound approximation. If there is a broken running suture, it is spliced to a new 10-0 nylon after the graft is aligned with interrupted 10-0 nylon sutures (Fig. 19-4). In those cases of complete wound dehiscence or rupture when there is a flat chamber, the anterior chamber is redeepened with air or sodium hyaluronate to separate the iris from the wound during suturing. Subconjunctival gentamicin sulfate and Celestone are used. The new sutures are considered as if they were initially placed, and wound healing is judged as previously described.

The overall incidence of wound dehiscence has

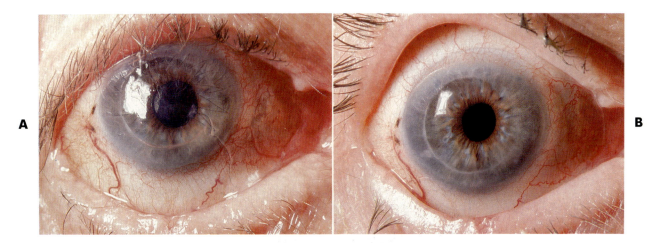

Fig. 19-4. A, Traumatic dehiscence between 5 and 7 o'clock 3 months postoperatively in 79-year-old white woman. Running suture was spliced onto new running 10-0 nylon for wound repair. **B,** Same case 8½ months with all sutures removed. Vision was 20/25 with a soft contact lens.

been estimated at 2% to 9%.[3,8,21,26] Some cases in earlier reports occurred in the first months after surgery and were attributable to poor healing or necrotic recipient tissue and were not directly related to suture removal.[3,7] Graft failure rates of 50% after wound dehiscence were reported in the older literature[3] but have declined significantly in our experience in recent years.

Induced Astigmatism. Nylon sutures may induce wound compression when tightened because of their inherent elasticity and the need to achieve watertight wound closure at surgery. Many grafted eyes before suture removal have flatter K readings and become steeper (that is, more myopic) after suture removal. Significant changes in astigmatism (either greater or less) may also accompany suture removal.

■   ■   ■

A word of caution is advisable. Some corneal surgeons advocate observation rather than suture removal in quiet grafted eyes that are without progressive vascularization and have minimal postoperative astigmatism (less than 3.5 diopters). Many grafted eyes, particularly when the knots are buried, individual sutures are selectively removed, or the double running technique is utilized, have regular mires on keratometry and very acceptable distance and near visual acuity at the 20/30 level. Too many corneal surgeons have shared the unnerving experience of inducing large amounts of astigmatism and patient annoyance by removing compressive sutures in low astigmatic grafts. An evolving concept regarding suture removal in an otherwise quiet eye that is re-

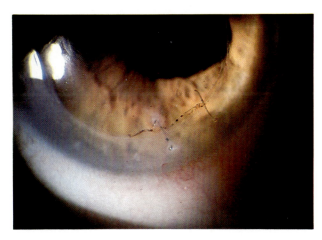

Fig. 19-5. Late breakage of interrupted 10-0 nylon suture 3 years after penetrating keratoplasty for Fuchs' dystrophy in 80-year-old man. Notice whitish subepithelial reaction surrounding both protruding ends of 5:30 o'clock suture and secondary perilimbal inflammation.

fractable using a spectacle or a contact lens to an acceptable level of vision is to "allow the wound to heal as it is with the suture in place."

The trade-off in some eyes where suture retention is the decided course of action seems to be chronic changes in refractive error (that is, a mildly unstable wound) and very subtle inflammation, particularly surrounding the retained suture with subepithelial fibrosis, and ultimately in many eyes late suture breakage with accompanying inflammation (Fig. 19-5).

REFERENCES

1. Aquavella JV, Gasset A, Dohlman CH: Corticosteroids in corneal wound healing, *Am J Ophthalmol* 58:621, 1964.
2. Aronson SG et al: The pathogenesis of suture toxicity, *Arch Ophthalmol* 84:641, 1970.
3. Binder PS et al: Keratoplasty wound separations, *Am J Ophthalmol* 80:109, 1975.
4. Boruchoff SA, Jensen AD, Dohlman CH: Comparison of suture techniques in keratoplasty, *Ann Ophthalmol* 7:433, 1975.
5. Bourne WM, Maguire LJ: Use of the argon laser to avoid complications from incomplete removal of corneal sutures with deeply buried knots, *Am J Ophthalmol* 110:310-311, 1990.
6. Brown SI: Results of corneal transplantation in diffuse corneal edema, *Am J Ophthalmol* 70:20, 1970.
7. Brown SI, Tragakis MP: Wound dehiscence with keratoplasty, *Am J Ophthalmol* 72:115, 1971.
8. Davison JA, Bourne WM: Results of penetrating keratoplasty using a double running suture technique, *Arch Ophthalmol* 99:1591, 1981.
9. Forstot SL, Abel R Jr, Binder PS: Bacterial endophthalmitis following suture removal after penetrating keratoplasty, *Am J Ophthalmol* 80:509, 1975.
10. Foster CS, Pavan-Langston D: Corneal wound healing and antiviral medication, *Arch Ophthalmol* 95:2062, 1977.
11. Friedman AH: Late traumatic wound rupture following successful partial penetrating keratoplasty, *Am J Ophthalmol* 75:117, 1973.
12. Goldberg DB et al: Graft edema after suture removal, *Am J Ophthalmol* 88:165, 1979.
13. Harris DJ, Stulting RD, Waring GO III, Wilson LA: Late bacterial and fungal keratitis after corneal transplantation, *Ophthalmology* 95:1450-1457, 1988.
14. Langston RH, Pavan-Langston D, Dohlman CH: Antiviral medication and corneal wound healing, *Arch Ophthalmol* 92:509, 1974.
15. Matsuda H, Smelser GK: Electron microscopy of corneal wound healing, *Exp Eye Res* 16:427, 1973.
16. McDonald TO et al: Corneal wound healing. 1. Inhibition of stromal healing by three dexamethasone derivatives, *Invest Ophthalmol* 9:730, 1970.
17. McNeill JI, Kaufman HE: A double running suture technique for keratoplasty: earlier visual rehabilitation, *Ophthalmic Surg* 8:58, 1977.
18. Nirankari VS, Karesh JW, Richards RD: Complications of exposed monofilament sutures, *Am J Ophthalmol* 95:515-519, 1983.
19. Paque J, Poirier RH: Corneal allograft reaction and its relationship to suture site neovascularization, *Ophthalmic Surg* 8:71, 1977.
20. Payrau P, Dohlman CH: IDU in corneal wound healing, *Am J Ophthalmol* 57:999, 1964.
21. Polack FM: *Corneal transplantation,* New York, 1977, Grune & Stratton, p 45.
22. Polack FM: Keratoplasty in aphakic eyes with corneal edema: results in 100 cases with 10-year followup, *Ophthalmic Surg* 11:701, 1980.
23. Polack FM, Binder PS: Detachment of Descemet's membrane from grafts following wound separation: light and scanning electron microscope study, *Ann Ophthalmol* 7:47, 1975.
24. Polack FM, Rose J: The effect of 5-iododeoxyuridine (IDU) in corneal wound healing, *Arch Ophthalmol* 71:520, 1964.
25. Polack FM, Rosen P: Topical steroids and tritiated thymidine uptake, *Arch Ophthalmol* 77:400, 1967.
26. Raber IM, Arentsen JJ, Laibson PR: Traumatic wound dehiscence after penetrating keratoplasty, *Arch Ophthalmol* 98:1407, 1980.
27. Sanchez J, Polack FM: Effect of topical steroids on the healing of corneal endothelium, *Invest Ophthalmol* 13:17, 1974.
28. Schanzlin DJ, Goldberg DB, Brown SI: Transplantation of congenitally opaque corneas, *Ophthalmology* 87:1253, 1980.
29. Shahinian L Jr, Brown SI: Postoperative complications with protruding monofilament nylon sutures, *Am J Ophthalmol* 83:546, 1977.
30. Stainer GA, Perl T, Binder PS: Controlled reduction of post keratoplasty astigmatism, *Ophthalmology* 89:668, 1982.
31. Stark WJ et al: The results of 102 penetrating keratoplasties using 10-0 monofilament and nylon suture, *Ophthalmic Surg* 3:11, 1972.
32. Sugar A, and Meyer RF: Giant papillary conjunctivitis after keratoplasty, *Am J Ophthalmol* 91:239, 1981.

Chapter 20

Epithelial Problems

J. DANIEL NELSON

The integrity of the corneal epithelium after keratoplasty is vital for graft survival. The normal intact corneal epithelium provides an optical interface with the tear film as well as a barrier to the external environment, noxious substances, and microorganisms. The presence of an epithelial defect (Fig. 20-1) not only interferes with vision, but may also increase the risk of rejection, infection, thinning, and perforation.[6] Epithelial defects have been shown to occur on the first postoperative day in approximately 70% of donor corneas stored in McCarey-Kaufman (MK) medium[18] and in approximately 80% of corneas stored in organ culture medium.[19] This chapter examines the problem of epithelial defects after keratoplasty and their etiology, prevention, and treatment.

ETIOLOGY

The causes of epithelial defects can be divided into (1) those occurring during storage of the donor cornea before keratoplasty, (2) those occurring intraoperatively, and (3) those occurring postoperatively.

Epithelial Cell Loss During Donor Cornea Storage. The energy source for corneal epithelial cell maintenance and wound healing is provided mainly from glycogen stores within the corneal epithelial cells. Survival of donor epithelium before and during storage is dependent on the maintenance of the metabolic requirements of the epithelium. Therefore epithelial cell survival is directly related to and dependent on the method of donor storage (Table 20-1). Epithelial glycogen stores decrease rapidly after 1 hour in situ. Cooling the ocular surface with ice packs after death reduces the epithelial metabolic requirements and preserves glycogen stores.[39] Storage in a moist chamber at 4° C stabilizes cellular glycogen levels for 49 hours.[37] Intact epithelium can be maintained for as long as 79 hours with storage in MK medium at 4° C.[18] However, viability of the epithelium may be less than optimal because approximately 35% of corneas stored in this manner will have 5% to 100% of the epithelium missing after storage before keratoplasty.[18]

The epithelia of corneas stored under organ culture conditions maintain a normal ultrastructural appearance for at least 35 days and, after 11 days in culture, actually show an increase in glycogen stores within the epithelial cells.[6] Although corneas stored in organ culture reveal sloughing of the more superficial epithelium after about 14 days, electron microscopy studies document that three or four layers of epithelial cells still persist.[44] Newer media such as K-Sol, CSM, Dexsol, and Optisol (Chiron Intraoptics, Irvine, California) are now available. In general, these media, though adequate for corneal endothelial preservation, are inadequate for prolonged cor-

Table 20-1. Length of Time Corneal Epithelial Glycogen Stores Are Maintained Under Various Types of Storage Conditions and Temperatures

Storage Method	Length of Time
Room temperature	1 hour
4° C	48 hours
McCarey-Kaufman medium (4° C)	79 hours
Organ culture medium (34° C)	35 days

235

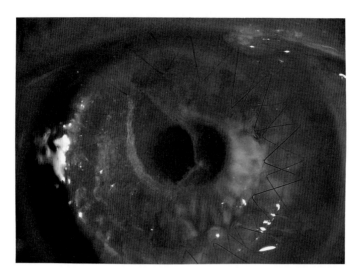

Fig. 20-1. Central corneal epithelial defect after penetrating keratoplasty.

neal epithelial preservation. A recent study evaluating corneal storage over 20 days in K-Sol and MK media found that the integrity of the epithelium was erratic with respect to media and time.[7] In a study of epithelial defects after penetrating keratoplasty, 6 of 21 (29%) Optisol-stored and 7 of 23 (30%) Dexsol-stored corneas (1 to 6 days of storage time) had epithelial defects more than 75% on the first postoperative day after penetrating keratoplasty (unpublished data). The addition of dextran to the media may prolong epithelial survival.[15]

To preserve donor corneal epithelium, one should tape donor eyes shut to prevent desiccation and should apply ice packs to the closed lids immediately after death to decrease the metabolic activity of the corneal epithelium. Postmortem and postenucleation times should be as short as possible to prevent epithelial stress and preserve glycogen stores. Storage in MK medium may prevent loss of glycogen stores for at least 3 days. This is probably true for newer types of storage media also. Storage in organ culture medium on a long-term basis may allow the epithelium to build up depleted glycogen stores and aid in preserving epithelial integrity. The stress of prolonged donor corneal storage in presently available media can lead to depletion of glycogen stores, epithelial cell loss, epithelial defects, and deficient epithelial wound healing postoperatively. Storage in organ culture medium for less than 14 days may not allow the epithelium time to replenish glycogen stores lost during the stress of early storage.

Intraoperative Epithelial Cell Loss. The most obvious reason for loss of the corneal epithelium during surgery is purposeful removal by the surgeon. It

has been shown that removal of corneal epithelium from donor corneas taken from fresh whole globes or from donor eyes stored in MK medium reduced the incidence of corneal rejection from 26.0% to 7.5%.[41] A more recent study in 228 corneal transplants compared the rate of corneal transplant rejection in corneas that had the epithelium removed after suture placement against corneas where the epithelium was left intact.[35] Corneas were stored in modified MK media at 4° C and transplanted within 4 days. No statistical difference was found in the rejection rates between the two groups. Removal of the donor epithelium must be balanced against a higher rate of postoperative epithelial defects.[42] The probability of long-term graft survival is probably greatest when the epithelium is left intact. It is interesting to note that the rate of donor corneal rejection of tissue stored in organ culture medium before keratoplasty is 28.9%[6] even though there are no Langerhans' cells present in the epithelium of organ-cultured corneas after 7 to 14 days.[10]

Cutting of the donor corneal button can also lead to loss of the epithelium, especially if the button is cut with the epithelial side down against the cutting block.

Intraoperative trauma from manipulation of the donor corneal button during suturing can lead to peripheral epithelial defects along the donor-host interface (Fig. 20-2). The drying effect of the operation microscope light as well as environmental dryness can lead to desiccation of the epithelium and sloughing.

Postoperative Epithelial Cell Loss. The usual causes of immediate postoperative cell loss are re-

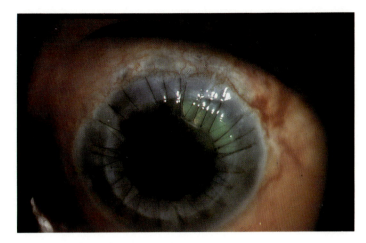

Fig. 20-2. Corneal epithelial defect along donor-host interface caused by surface trauma during suturing.

lated to trauma. An open eye beneath the eye dressing, lashes pressed onto or rubbing on the donor corneal surface, and traumatic removal of the epithelium by the lids when the eye is first opened can all lead to epithelial cell loss.

Local environmental abnormalities, such as entropion, trichiasis, lid scarring, and blepharitis can lead to epithelial irregularities and defects. Loose or exposed sutures or knots will result in epithelial defects caused by mechanical abrasion.

Topical medications and preservatives may have an adverse effect on epithelial wound healing (Fig. 20-3) because of inhibition of epithelial migration, epithelial mitosis, or epithelial attachment to the underlying basement membrane.[8,13,26,29,37,38,45]

Abnormalities of the tear film from decreased aqueous secretion, rapid evaporation, mucin deficiency, blepharitis, poor lid position or movement, and lagophthalmos (Fig. 20-4) can influence epithelial health[20,21] and wound healing. Some systemic medication may exert an indirect effect on the corneal epithelium through their effects on tear secretion and epithelial cell wound healing.[3]

Local primary ocular surface disease caused by ocular pemphigoid (Fig. 20-5), Stevens-Johnson syndrome, or chemical burns may prevent normal epithelial wound healing because of lid scarring and symblepharon, entropion, trichiasis, goblet cell deficiencies,[20,21] or intrinsic epithelial abnormalities.[40]

Morphology changes of the epithelium have been noted after denervation of the cornea. Cornea nerves are probably required for corneal mitotic ac-

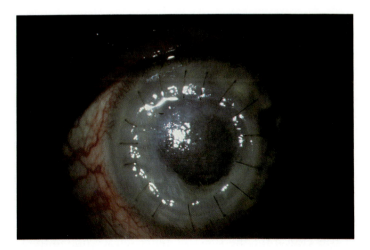

Fig. 20-3. Epithelial irregularity after penetrating keratoplasty attributable to medication toxicity (keratitis medicamentosa).

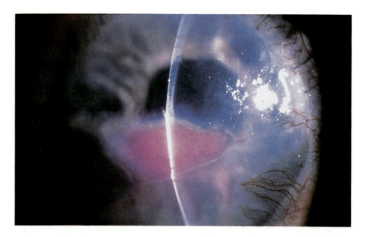

Fig. 20-4. Corneal epithelial defect caused by incomplete blinking and lagophthalmos.

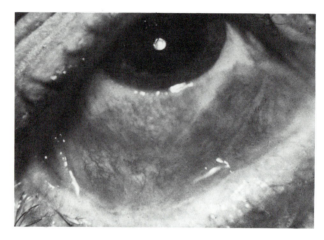

Fig. 20-5. Chronic keratoconjunctivitis with symblepharon formation caused by active cicatricial ocular pemphigoid.

tivity and wound healing.[4,32] It may be, at least in the early postoperative period, that denervation of the donor corneal epithelium may retard epithelial wound healing (Figs. 20-6 and 20-7).

Finally, patients may induce self-inflicted epithelial damage through mechanical trauma with fingernails, mascara brushes, or curling irons as well as through the abuse of topical medications.

PREVENTION OF EPITHELIAL DEFECTS

Preoperative Prevention. It is critical for the survival of the donor corneal epithelium that preexistent dry-eye conditions and local ocular surface dis-

ease, such as ocular pemphigoid, be recognized and treated or, at the very least, controlled before surgery. Aberrant lashes (trichiasis) should be eliminated either by electrolysis or cryotherapy. Ectropion, entropion, lagophthalmos, and lid scarring may require prior surgical repair (Figs. 20-4 and 20-8). Blepharitis, whether from local or systemic disease, such as rosacea (Fig. 20-9), must be controlled through the use of lid hygiene, topical lubrication, antibiotics, and steroids if needed. The value of systemic tetracycline in the treatment of rosacea should not be forgotten.[17]

Intraoperative Prevention. To prevent postopera-

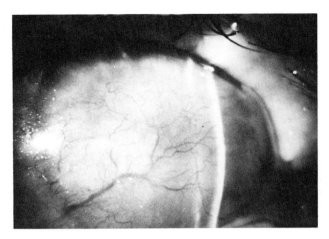

Fig. 20-6. Scarred and vascularized cornea caused by a chronic neurotrophic keratitis before keratoplasty.

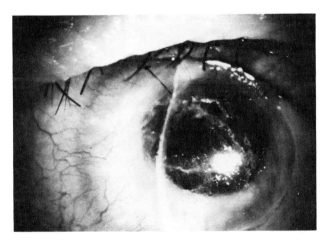

Fig. 20-7. Same eye as in Fig. 20-6 after penetrating keratoplasty. Corneal epithelium is irregular with several small epithelial defects.

tive epithelial defects the epithelium should not be removed at the time of surgery. Although some studies[12,41] document its value in decreasing rejection, others do not.[1] The epithelium must be protected from the external environment at the time of surgery. Manipulation of the epithelium during the cutting of the donor button and suturing should be minimized. Viscoelastic substances are very useful in protecting the epithelium from the external environment.

Experimental studies in chick embryo corneas have shown that sodium hyaluronate (0.1%) better protected the epithelium against dryness than either hydroxymethyl cellulose (1%) or physiologic balanced saline solution (PBS).[46] In addition, sodium hyaluronate (0.1%) was not toxic to the corneal epithelium

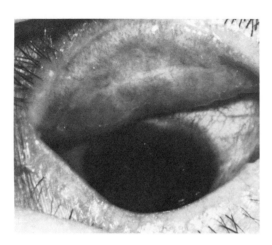

Fig. 20-8. Upper lid scarring caused by a chronic atopic keratoconjunctivitis.

and reduced the toxic effects of benzalkonium chloride on the epithelium. It has been shown that the rate of epithelial defects after keratoplasty using tissue stored under organ-culture conditions decreased from 82% to 36% when sodium hyaluronate was used to protect the epithelium during suturing.[19] Another study showed that corneal epithelium healed faster after keratoplasty when sodium hyaluronate (0.1%) was used intraoperatively.[30] Sodium

hyaluronate should be placed on the cutting block to protect the epithelium during the cutting of the donor button as well as on the ocular surface of the host eye to protect host corneal and conjunctival epithelium during suturing. Although the suturing technique is at times tedious with sodium hyaluronate coating the ocular surface, its benefits to the epithelium far outweigh its disadvantages. When the surgical procedure is finished, the ocular surface including host and donor tissue, should be coated with sodium hyaluronate before the lids are closed and the dressing is applied. Taping the lids closed will prevent exposure of the eye beneath the dressing.

Collagen shields have been placed on the cornea at the conclusion of keratoplasty to protect the donor epithelium. The use of a 24-hour shield (Bausch and Lomb) significantly reduced the rate of epithelial staining and epithelial defects on the first postoperative day compared to those eyes that did not have a collagen shield placed.[31] However, by postoperative day 8, there was no difference between the two groups. The authors commented that if longer acting shields are used they must be well hydrated.

Postoperative Prevention. All loose sutures should be removed and replaced if necessary. Loose sutures may lead to epithelial defects through their mechanical abrading effect (Fig. 20-10). The surface should be kept well lubricated with artificial tears and ointments. If artificial tears are required more than 4 to 6 times daily, it is generally best to use one of the commercially available unpreserved solutions. Ointments may also be used but should be unpre-

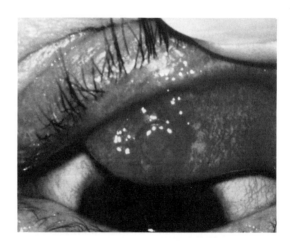

Fig. 20-9. Chronic rosacea blepharitis with resultant chalazion and granulation tissue formation.

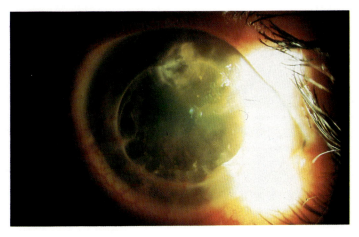

Fig. 20-10. Corneal ulcer initiated by a loose suture at 12 o'clock position on donor cornea.

served. Patients with sensitivity to lanolin or wool should avoid the lanolin-containing ointments. Topical antibiotics,[28,34] antivirals,[11] timolol,[26] and steroids may exert a toxic effect on the epithelium and should not be used indiscriminately. Experimental studies, using tissue culture models, indicate that tobramycin may have less effect on corneal epithelial wound healing than gentamicin.[14,22]

Patients must be instructed in the correct and careful placement of topical medications to avoid trauma to the epithelium. Finally, any epithelial defects that do occur must be treated rapidly to prevent further complications of corneal ulceration, thinning, and perforation.

THERAPY OF EPITHELIAL DEFECTS

If an epithelial defect does occur after keratoplasty, it must be treated promptly and vigorously to preserve the donor cornea. Without an intact corneal epithelium the risks of infection, thinning, and perforation increase.[6] The main objectives in treating an epithelial defect are as follows:

1. Prevention of further loss of epithelial cells
2. Promotion of epithelial cell wound healing
3. Protection of the epithelium once it has healed to allow it to attach to the underlying basement membrane.

Prevention of Further Epithelial Cell Loss. To prevent further loss of the epithelium, one must give careful attention to the cause of the defect. Careful clinical examination for lash and lid abnormalities and abnormalities of the ocular surface is mandatory. Aberrant lashes and loose sutures should be removed, poor lid movement and position corrected, lubrication instituted, and epithelial toxic medications eliminated in favor of less toxic medications.

Aberrant lashes may be removed by epilation, electrolysis, or cryotherapy. Epilation is temporary because the lashes will normally regrow within 2 to 3 weeks. Electrolysis works well only for removing a few lashes. Cryotherapy is probably the treatment of choice. A double freeze-thaw-freeze technique at −80° C for 40 to 60 seconds is required (Fig. 20-11).

Promotion of Epithelial Wound Healing. To promote epithelial wound healing, topical preparations that promote wound healing may be of use. Fibronectin has been believed to promote epithelial wound healing.[24,25] A more recent study indicates that, in a rabbit epithelial defect model, topical fibronectin might not promote wound healing.[23] There is evidence that topical vitamin A may promote epithelial wound healing.[43] Topical preparations of epidermal growth factor have not proved helpful.[11] Promotion of epithelial wound healing requires an environment that will provide the epithelium with nutrients and oxygen. An important concept in relation to this is the tear volume–to–surface area (TVSA) ratio. The goal of any therapy as it relates to the tear film is to increase the TVSA ratio. For example, in the case of keratoconjunctivitis sicca (KCS) there is a decrease in the TVSA ratio because of a decrease in aqueous tears. Topical lubrication increases the TVSA ratio by increasing the tear volume. Other treatment modalities will also increase the TVSA ratio.

Punctal occlusion may be of benefit in patients with KCS both before and after keratoplasty to prevent and treat epithelial defects. The therapeutic affect is attributable to an increased tear retention and resultant increase in the TVSA ratio. Punctal occlusion may be accomplished on a temporary basis through the use of punctal plugs, collagen plugs, or

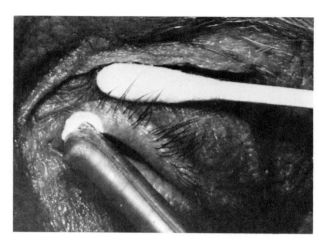

Fig. 20-11. Cryotherapy for trichiasis. A regular retinal probe is used. The aberrant lashes are frozen to $-80°$ C for 40 to 60 seconds and allowed to thaw for 2 minutes. The area is then refrozen at $-80°$ C for an additional 40 seconds.

punctal sutures (Fig. 20-12). Permanent punctal closure can be achieved using laser, cautery, or diathermy (Fig. 20-13).

Collagen shields may also be used to promote postkeratoplasty epithelial wound healing. A recent study compared the use of a 24-hour collagen shield (Bausch and Lomb) to the use of a bandage contact lens (Bausch and Lomb, Plano O_4) in patients with epithelial defects after keratoplasty and found collagen shields not to be useful.[9] In the bandage lens–treated group, 16 of 22 (73%) corneal epithelial defects healed, whereas none of 7 in the collagen shield–treated group healed. In these 7 patients, 5 epithelial defects healed when a bandage contact lens was placed. No adverse effects were noted in either group.

Protection of the Healing Epithelium. Several treatment modalities are available to protect the ocular surface and aid wound healing of the epithelium. These include pressure patching, bandage soft contact lenses, and lateral tarsorrhaphy. Pressure patching has not been shown to promote epithelial wound healing and may actually retard it.[36] The adage should be, "Patch for comfort, not for epithelial healing."

Bandage soft contact lenses. The use of bandage soft contact lenses for the treatment of epithelial defects after keratoplasty is a "two-edged sword." Bandage soft contact lenses function to protect the epithelial surface from the mechanical trauma of the

lashes and lids. They allow for nutrient and oxygen transfer as well as provide an optically clear interface for vision. However any changes in hydration state of the lens will change the fit of the lens, which may result in decreased oxygen diffusion across the lens to the corneal epithelium and lead to a tight lens syndrome. Keep in mind that epithelial wound healing requires oxygen from the tear film and any compromise in oxygen diffusion will inhibit wound healing. A lens fit that is too tight (steep) as well as too loose (flat) can result in further trauma to the epithelium. The former is caused by anoxia, the later by mechanical trauma.

The complication rate, especially with secondary bacterial corneal ulcers can be high (Fig. 20-14). In a recent study[33] 9 of 39 eyes that required a bandage soft contact lens for epithelial defects after keratoplasty developed corneal ulcer infiltrates (23% incidence). *Staphylococcus epidermidis* was the most frequently isolated organism. Previously authors have described the occurrence of corneal ulcers after penetrating keratoplasty: Lemp, 11% incidence in 9 cases of bandage contact lens use;[16] Purcell, 16% incidence in six cases;[29] and Cowden, 11.5% incidence in 26 cases.[5] Other authors have reported no episodes of infectious complications in relation to bandage lenses after keratoplasty.[2,27] However most of the lenses in those studies were placed for reasons other than persistent epithelial defects.

Lateral tarsorrhaphy. Another therapeutic modal-

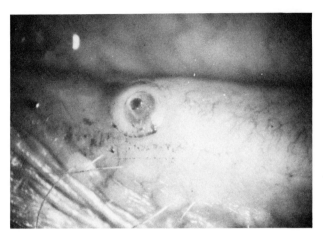

Fig. 20-12. Punctal plug occlusion of inferior canaliculus. Punctal occlusion functions to increase the tear volume relative to exposed ocular surface area.

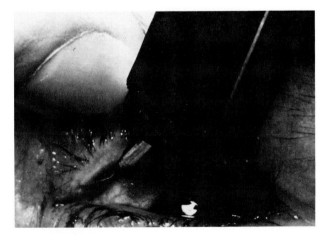

Fig. 20-13. Permanent punctal occlusion using diathermy. Epithelium lining canaliculus is first removed by a dental burr. Diathermy needle is then passed 4 to 6 mm into canaliculus. While needle is slowly withdrawn, canaliculus is cauterized.

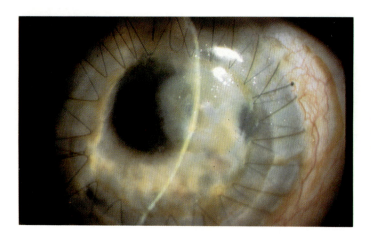

Fig. 20-14. *Staphylococcus epidermidis* corneal ulcer occurring in early postoperative period after placement of a soft-bandage contact lens for a nonhealing epithelial defect.

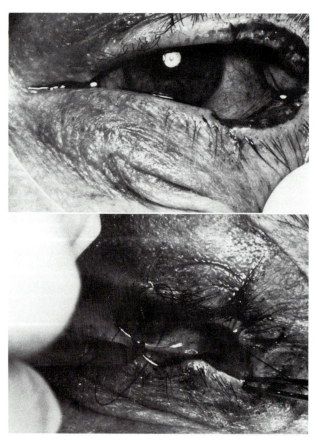

A

B

Fig. 20-15. Lateral tarsorrhaphy. **A,** Posterior margins of lateral portions of upper and lower lids are carefully removed. **B,** Single 6-0 nylon suture is passed through debrided margin and tarsus of both lids.

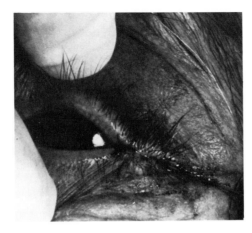

Fig. 20-15, cont'd. C, Suture is tied with knot laterally to avoid trauma to cornea.

ity that is very helpful in the treatment of epithelial defects is lateral tarsorrhaphy. Its therapeutic effect is attributable to the decrease in exposed ocular surface area, which increases the TVSA ratio. It also functions to protect the epithelial surface as well as promote the spreading of the tear film. At the preset time a lateral tarsorrhaphy is preferable to a bandage contact lens in instances of nonhealing epithelial defects. Our rule is, "If an epithelial defect does not heal with a tarsorrhaphy, it probably will not heal with any other treatment modality." A single-suture technique is preferable. A 6-0 nylon suture passed through the abraded posterior margins of the lateral upper and lower lids works quite well (Fig. 20-15).

SUMMARY

The maintenance of an intact epithelium after keratoplasty is of utmost importance for the survival of the donor cornea. Great care must be taken to eliminate any host problems that may prevent the maintenance of a normal epithelial surface. Storage of the donor cornea must take into consideration the maintenance of an intact epithelium on the donor cornea. Intraoperatively the corneal epithelium of both the donor and the host must be protected from trauma and desiccation. Finally, careful management of the ocular surface is required to maintain an intact epithelium postoperatively, and when epithe-

lial defects do occur, they must be treated appropriately to minimize risk to the donor cornea.

REFERENCES

1. Alldredge OC, Krachmer JH: Clinical types of corneal transplant rejection: their manifestations, frequency, preoperative correlates, and treatment, *Arch Ophthalmol* 99:599, 1981.
2. Aquavella JV, Shaw FL: Hydrophilic bandages in penetrating keratoplasty, *Ann Ophthalmol* 8:1207, 1976.
3. Bergmann MT, Newman BC, Johnson NC: The effect of a diuretic (hydrochlorothiazide) on tear production in humans *Am J Ophthalmol* 99:173, 1985.
4. Beuerman RW et al: Modulation of latency and velocity in corneal epithelial wound healing, *Invest Ophthalmol Vis Sci* 26(suppl):91, 1985, ARVO abstracts.
5. Cowden JW: Continuous wear aphakic soft contact lenses following keratoplasty, *Ann Ophthalmol* 12:579, 1980.
6. Doughman DJ: Prolonged donor corneal preservation in organ culture: long-term clinical evaluation, *Trans Am Ophthalmol Soc* 78:567, 1980.
7. Farge EJ, Font RA, Wilhelmus KR, et al: Morphological changes of K-Sol preserved human corneas, *Cornea* 8:159, 1989.
8. Friedenwald JS, Buschke W: Mitotic and wound healing activities of the corneal epithelium, *Arch Ophthalmol* 32:410, 1944.
9. Groden LR, White W: Porcine collagen corneal shield treatment of persistent epithelial defects following penetrating keratoplasty, *Cornea* 16:95, 1990.
10. Holland EJ et al: The effect of organ culture corneal preservation on Langerhans cells, *Invest Ophthalmol Vis Sci* 26(suppl):236, 1985, ARVO abstracts.
11. Kandarakis AS, Page C, Kaufman HE: The effect of epidermal growth factor on epithelial healing after penetrating keratoplasty in human eyes, *Am J Ophthalmol* 98:411, 1984.

12. Khodadoust AA, Silverstein AM: The survival and rejection of epithelium in experimental corneal transplants, *Invest Ophthalmol Vis Sci* 8:169, 1969.
13. Lass JH et al: Antiviral medications and corneal wound healing, *Antiviral Res* 4:143, 1984.
14. Lass JH, Mack RJ, Imperia PS et al: An *in vitro* analysis of aminoglycoside corneal epithelial toxicity, *Curr Eye Res* 8:299, 1989.
15. Lass JH, Reinhart WJ, Skelnik DL: An *in vitro* and clinical comparision of corneal storage with chondrotin sulfate corneal storage media with and without dextran, *Ophthalmology* 971:96, 1990.
16. Lemp MA: The effect of extended-wear aphakic hydrophilic contact lenses after penetrating keratoplasty, *Am J Ophthalmol* 90:331, 1980.
17. Marmion UJ: Tetracyclines in the treatment of ocular rosacea, *Proc R Soc Med* 62:11, 1969.
18. Meyer RF, Bobb KC: Corneal epithelium in penetrating keratoplasty, *Am J Ophthalmol* 90:142, 1982.
19. Miller RA et al: Healon use for the prevention of donor epithelial cell loss during keratoplasty, *Invest Ophthalmol Vis Sci* 25(suppl):171, 1984, ARVO abstracts.
20. Nelson JD, Havener VR, Cameron JD: Cellulose acetate impressions of the ocular surface: dry eye states, *Arch Ophthalmol* 101:1869, 1983.
21. Nelson JD, Wright JC: Conjunctival goblet cell densities in ocular surface disease, *Arch Ophthalmol* 102:1049, 1984.
22. Nelson JD, Silverman V, Lima PH, Beckman G: Corneal epithelial wound healing: a tissue culture assay on the effect of antibiotics, *Curr Eye Res* 9:277, 1990.
23. Newton C, Hatchell DL, Klintworth GK, Brown CF: Topical fibronectin and corneal epithelial wound healing in the rabbit, *Arch Ophthalmol* 106:1277, 1988.
24. Nishida T et al: Fibronectin: a new therapy for cornea trophic ulcer, *Arch Ophthalmol* 101:1046, 1983.
25. Nishida T et al: Fibronectin enhancement of corneal epithelial wound healing of rabbits *in vivo*, *Arch Ophthalmol* 102:455, 1984.
26. Nork TM et al: Timolol inhibits corneal epithelial wound healing in monkeys and rabbits, *Arch Ophthalmol* 102:1224, 1984.
27. Paglan PG, Webster RG, Abbott RL: The advantages of interrupted sutures and therapeutic lens in keratoplasty, *Ophthalmic Surg* 12:95, 1981.
28. Petroutsos G et al: Antibiotics and corneal epithelial wound healing, *Arch Ophthalmol* 101:1335, 1983.
29. Purcell JJ Jr: Extended-wear contact lenses after corneal grafts, *Am J Ophthalmol* 91:119, 1981.
30. Reed DB, Mannis MJ, Hills JF, Johnson CA: Corneal epithelial healing after penetrating keratoplasty using topical Healon versus balanced salt solution, *Ophthalmic Surg* 18:525, 1987.
31. Ruffini JJ, Aquavella JV, LoCascio JA: Effect of collagen shields on corneal epithelialization following penetrating keratoplasty, *Ophthalmic Surg* 20:21, 1989.
32. Schimmelpfennig B, Beuerman R: Sensory deprivation of the rabbit cornea affects epithelial properties, *Exp Neurol* 69:196, 1980.
33. Smith SG et al: Corneal ulcer-infiltrate associated with soft contact lens use following penetrating keratoplasty, *Cornea* 3:131, 1984.
34. Stern GA, Schemmer GB, Farber RD, Gorovoy MS: Effects of topical antibiotic solutions on corneal epithelial wound healing, *Arch Ophthalmol* 101:644, 1983.
35. Stulting RD, Waring GO, Bridges W, Cavanaugh HD: Effects of donor epithelium on corneal transplant survival, *Ophthalmology* 95:803, 1988.
36. Sugar AA, Meyer RF, Bahn CF: A randomized trial of pressure patching for epithelial defects after keratoplasty, *Am J Ophthalmol* 95:637, 1983.
37. Thoft RA, Friend J: Corneal epithelial changes during midterm storage, *Invest Ophthalmol Vis Sci* 15:82, 1976.
38. Thoft RA, Friend J: The XYZ hypothesis of corneal epithelial maintenance, *Invest Ophthalmol Vis Sci* 24:1442, 1983.
39. Thoft RA, Friend J, Dohlman CH: Corneal epithelial preservation, *Arch Ophthalmol* 93:357, 1975.
40. Thoft RA et al: Cicatricial pemphigoid associated with hyperproliferation of the conjunctival epithelium, *Am J Ophthalmol* 98:37, 1984.
41. Tuberville AW, Foster CS, Wood TO: The effect of donor corneal epithelium removal on the incidence of allograft rejection reactions, *Ophthalmology* 90:1351, 1983.
42. Tuberville AW, Wood TO: Corneal ulcers in corneal transplants, *Curr Eye Res* 1:479, 1981.
43. Ubels JL, Edelhauser HF, Austin KH: Healing of experimental corneal wounds treated with topically applied retinoids, *Am J Ophthalmol* 95:353, 1983.
44. Van Horn DL et al: The ultrastructure of human organ cultured cornea. II. Stroma and epithelium, *Arch Ophthalmol* 94:1791, 1976.
45. Wilson FM: Adverse external ocular effects of topical ophthalmic medications, *Surv Ophthalmol* 24:57, 1979.
46. Wysenbeek YS, Loya N, Sira IB, et al: The effect of sodium hyaluronate on corneal epithelium, *Invest Ophthalmol Vis Sci* 29:194, 1988.

Chapter 21

Glaucoma

CATHERINE NEWTON

LINDA L. BURK

One of the major causes of graft failure is inadequate control of elevated intraocular pressure. Although the endothelium may tolerate modest elevations of intraocular pressure, as seen in chronic open-angle glaucoma,[36] Bigar and Witmer[8] have shown significant endothelial cell loss as result of acute and greatly elevated intraocular pressure. It is imperative to recognize and treat glaucoma after keratoplasty so that graft clarity is preserved.

DIAGNOSIS

Glaucoma is defined as elevated intraocular pressure sufficient to cause injury to the optic nerve as evidenced by characteristic loss of the visual field or glaucomatous cupping of the optic nerve disc. Often it is not possible to assess adequately the optic nerve and visual field preoperatively or in the immediate postoperative period because of preoperative media opacification and postoperative corneal distortion. The intraocular pressure, however, can and must be determined.

In a landmark article by Irvine and Kaufman,[31] attention was called to the association of elevated intraocular pressures with penetrating keratoplasty and the need for the accurate assessment of the postkeratoplasty intraocular pressure. It has been shown that the intraocular pressure in the early postoperative period can be measured most precisely with either the Mackay-Marg electronic applanation tonometer[31], the pneumatic applanation tonometer,[62] or the Tono-Pen.[49]

INCIDENCE

The incidence of moderately to greatly elevated intraocular pressure after penetrating keratoplasty is yet unknown. There are reports ranging from 13%[33] and 38%[31] in phakic eyes to 42%[33] and 89%[21] in aphakic eyes, with an overall incidence of 33.6%.[54]

PATHOGENESIS

In addition to preexisting glaucoma, new onset of postoperative glaucoma may develop as a result of any number of mechanical problems, including sequelae of inflammatory conditions, wound closure technique, and paraoperative pharmacologic agents.

The causes of elevated intraocular pressure after penetrating keratoplasty are listed below:

Inflammatory sequelae
  Fibrinous iritis
  Peripheral anterior synechiae
  Posterior synechiae
Suturing technique
  Compression of angle
  Trabecular meshwork collapse
  Wound leak with loss of anterior chamber volume
  Posterior wound gape with iridocorneal adhesions
Drug-induced elevation
  Alpha-chymotrypsin
  Corticosteroid
  Viscoelastic substances

Other

   Ghost-cell glaucoma
   Misdirected aqueous or ciliary block (malignant) glaucoma
   Preoperative angle recession
   Preoperative glaucoma

Many investigators consistently noted an increased incidence of postoperative glaucoma in aphakic patients. Zimmerman and co-workers[65] postulated the mechanism to be that of loss of trabecular meshwork support, that is, the lens and zonules. In a study by Brightbill and co-workers[13] patients undergoing combined procedures involving intracapsular cataract extractions had a 74% incidence of postoperative elevated intraocular pressure compared with a 43% incidence in patients undergoing combined procedures with extracapsular cataract extraction. This result may lend further credibility to Zimmerman's theory of glaucoma arising from loss of trabecular meshwork support.

Bourne and co-workers[10] corroborated the findings of Zimmerman and co-workers[65] showing that using a 0.5 mm. larger donor (punched from the endothelial side) resulted in significant decrease in the incidence of postoperative glaucoma in aphakic patients. The need for disparate-sized grafting is predicated on the use of tight wound closure with resultant tissue compresion. Some authors have noted no elevation of intraocular pressure by utilizing more shallow suturing techniques in same-sized grafts.[44] Still others[47] were unable to appreciate any significant elevation of intraocular pressure between same-sized and disparate-sized grafting. Troutman[58] and Olson[45] have demonstrated that donor corneas fashioned by trephination from the epithelial side have larger diameters than those that are cut with the same-sized trephine but from the endothelial side.

Extracapsular cataract extraction has eliminated the need for alpha-chymotrypsin, which was implicated in the early postoperative intraocular pressure rise after intracapsular cataract extraction. The use of viscoelastic substances to protect the corneal endothelium in extracapsular cataract extraction has resulted in new problems with early, yet often quite elevated, postoperative intraocular pressures. In a primate study, MacRae and co-workers[41] documented the intraocular pressure peak of 67 mm Hg, 90 minutes after intracameral injection of 1% sodium hyaluronate. Many surgeons advocate replacement of the viscoelastic substance with balanced saline solution at the conclusion of the operation to avoid the high elevations in postoperative intraocular pressures. In a clinical study comparing the effects of Viscoat (3.8% sodium chondroitin sulfate and 3% sodium hyaluronate), and Healon (1% sodium hyaluronate), 4 eyes of 24 had pressures greater than or equal to 50 mm Hg despite the surgeon's attempted removal of the viscoelastic substance at the conclusion of the operation.[2] These pressures occurred at 24 hours or less postoperatively. Unacceptably high pressures may be sustained for several hours if no treatment is given.

MANAGEMENT

Preventive Measures. Thoft and colleagues,[56] as well as most corneal surgeons, advocate the liberal use of topical corticosteroids in the early postoperative period to prevent the sequelae of severe ocular inflammation.[56] François[25] and Goldmann[27] have demonstrated that long-term use of corticosteroids can cause glaucoma in susceptible patients. Therefore consideration should be given to using fluorometholone in patients at risk for steroid-responsive glaucoma.

As previously mentioned, for the surgeon who tends to use tight suturing techniques resulting in tissue compression, the use of 0.5 mm larger donor grafts for the recipient beds is advised.[10,65] Cohen and co-workers advocate iridoplasty to create a mechanically rigid iris diaphragm in patients at risk for progressive peripheral anterior synechiae.[19]

Preexisting peripheral anterior synechiae may progress to 360-degree involvement of the anterior chamber angle.[56] For this reason, some surgeons advise using a dental mirror to inspect the anterior chamber angle at operation and also as an aid for goniosynechiolysis.[16,60,61]

Medical Treatment. Depending on the cause of the elevated intraocular pressure after keratoplasty, medical management in the form of beta-adrenergic blocking agents, epinephrine and dipivefrin (a prodrug of epinephrine), miotics, and topical and systemic carbonic anhydrase inhibitors may be useful. Dailey and co-workers[21] demonstrated the additive effect of topical timolol maleate and systemic acetazolamide on decreasing the rate of aqueous formation in normal humans. Barron and co-workers[2] found viscoelastic substance–induced postoperative elevated intraocular pressure responded to systemic acetazolamide and topical timolol maleate. Even in secondarily closed angles after penetrating keratoplasty, Lass and Pavan-Langston were able to control intraocular pressures in many patients by adding timolol maleate to the regimen of carbonic anhydrase inhibitors and miotics.[37] Shrader and colleagues[53] found that 45% of the patients over 65 years of age treated with systemic acetazolamide developed a malaise symptom complex consisting in fatigue, depression, anorexia, and weight loss. Therefore systemic carbonic anhydrase inhibitors must be used with great caution in the elderly keratoplasty patient population.

Recent promising clinical results have been obtained with topical carbonic anhydrase inhibitors. Most notably MK-507 appears to be very well tolerated and to precipitate a significant decrease in intraocular pressures. Soon these drugs should be available for clinical use.[39]

Because postoperative elevated intraocular pressure appears to be a greater problem in the aphakic and pseudophakic eyes, the use of epinephrine and dipivefrin must be used with great caution because they are known to produce transient though often reversible cystoid macular edema.

Miotics are known to dilate the ocular blood vessels and break down the blood aqueous barrier, and they may induce chronic iridocyclitis. Therefore they are used with caution in eyes that are already inflamed. Additionally, consideration must be given to use of miotics in aphakic patients because there is an associated increased risk of retinal tear and subsequent retinal detachment with use of miotics in aphakic eyes. When there are significant synechiae, miotics may be of little benefit.

Apraclonidine hydrochloride (Iopidine) is a relatively selective alpha$_2$-adrenergic agonist. Because apraclonidine is a potent anterior segment vasoconstrictor, it is useful in cases such as hemolytic glaucoma and where pressure is secondarily elevated after an intraoperative anterior segment bleed. It is most useful in the paraoperative period, since it is a relatively short-term intraocular pressure–lowering drug. Suggested dosing would be one hour preoperatively and 12 hours postoperatively.[48]

Argon-Laser Trabeculoplasty. Van Meter and co-workers[59] have reported on control of intraocular pressure in 10 of 14 eyes treated with adjuvant argon-laser trabeculoplasty (ALT) after penetrating keratoplasty. Six of the 10 required only 180 degrees of treatment. Two additional patients were controlled with a combination of 180 degrees of ALT and argon-laser cyclophotocoagulation of up to six ciliary processes. ALT was performed with a blue-green argon laser unit with a 50 μm spot size, a 0.1-second duration, and 300 to 1350 milliwatts (mW) of power. It was the impression of Van Meter and co-workers[59] that postkeratoplasty eyes required slightly more energy to produce blanching of the trabecular meshwork than nonpostkeratoplasty eyes.

In addition, they noted that because of the optics in treating postkeratoplasty patients the resultant laser burn appeared larger than what they routinely observed in nonpostkeratoplasty patients.

Argon-laser trabeculoplasty should be considered when a dramatic decrease in intraocular pressure is not required. Postoperative intraocular pressure rises have greatly decreased in number with the introduction of Apraclonidine (Iopidine).[45] However, the amount of trabecular meshwork available for treatment may be limited by peripheral anterior synchiae and anterior chamber intraocular lens haptics.

Holmium-laser trabeculectomy has received FDA approval. This is an *ab externo* approach and has been described by Hoskins and colleagues.[29] *Ab interno* laser sclerostomies have also been advocated and have had limited success.[7,42,64] All these filtration procedures have similar problems with postoperative scarring though the less invasive procedures seem to have fewer intraoperative complications with concomitantly fewer risks.

Misdirected Aqueous, Ciliovitreal Block, or Malignant Glaucoma. In cases of misdirected aqueous resulting in ciliovitreal block, so-called malignant glaucoma, Epstein and co-workers[23] have advocated neodymium:YAG laser therapy to the intact hyloid face. The theory is that the pathogenesis of ciliovitreal block is total obliteration of the posterior chamber by the vitreous body, which comes forward into apposition with the posterior surface of the iris and ciliary body because aqueous humor filters behind the vitreous body. In this situation a peripheral iridectomy is of no help. They have reported successful therapy with rupture of the hyaloid face using the YAG laser. Indeed misdirected aqueous may occur even in the presence of a posterior chamber lens and intact posterior capsule. Tomey and co-workers[57] describe the use of the Nd:YAG with 3 to 10 mW energy for a total of as much as 375 mJ. Others have reported similar success with argon laser to the intact hyaloid face.[55]

Cyclodestructive Procedures. Today there are multiple new alternatives to ciliary body ablation. In addition to cyclocryotherapy, transpupillary argon cyclophotocoagulation, argon endolaser cyclophotocoagulation (transpupillary or endoscopic), and therapeutic ultrasound, both contact and noncontact transscleral Nd:YAG cyclophotocoagulation are available. Because cyclodialysis for postkeratoplasty glaucoma was rarely successful (22%), the procedure virtually has been abandoned.[18] Therapeutic ultrasound[15] has been reported as effective in refractory glaucomas but not without significant complications including scleral thinning, iritis, hypotony, corneal decompensation, and vitreous hemorrhage. It is limited to only a few investigators and is not widely available.

The mainstay of surgical intervention for intractable glaucoma after penetrating keratoplasty has been that of cyclocryotherapy. West, Wood, and Kaufman[63] found that control of intraocular pressure could be obtained in 15 of 23 eyes sustaining intractable glaucoma after keratoplasty. They recommended that the safest effective method was a one-time freeze. A cryoprobe was applied for 60 seconds, three spots per quadrant, at a temperature of −50° C. It was their experience that the freeze-thaw-refreeze technique represented too vigorous a therapy and resulted in significantly more complications.[63] Binder and colleagues[9] found that 82% of transplants remain clear after cyclocryotherapy for intractable postkeratoplasty glaucoma, despite a complication rate of 14%. Bellows and Grant[6] found that freezing the inferior 180 degrees of the globe at six equidistant points for 1 minute each to a temperature of −60° to −80° C resulted in a 92% success rate in patients with chronic open-angle glaucoma and surgical aphakia. In addition to the cryotherapy, patients were often continued on their pretreatment topical medications. Caprioli and co-workers[17] reported pressure control in 76% of eyes with aphakic open-angle glaucoma and 68% of eyes with aphakic angle-closure glaucoma after treatment with 180 degrees of cyclocryotherapy. Some required additional treatment totaling 360 degrees. In addition to loss of vision and considerable discomfort, complications of cyclocryotherapy include phthisis bulbi, persistent inflammation, corneal decompensation, cystoid macular edema, and hemorrhage.

Lee[38] found that transpupillary argon-laser photocoagulation of the ciliary processes could reduce intraocular pressure in direct proportion to the number of ciliary processes that were ablated. The technique requires a Goldmann three-mirror lens or a facsimile. The laser was set with a 50 to 100 μm spot size for a duration of 0.1 to 0.2 second and with a power of 1000 mW. Care was taken to avoid large ciliary process capillaries. Hemostasis was obtained with repeated application of the laser with larger (200 μm) spot size, 0.2-second duration, and lower power (250 mW). Ciliary processes were ablated one at a time. Since preliminary data indicated that, if possible, at least one fourth of the total ciliary processes should be coagulated, Lee treated an average of 16 ciliary processes (range, 8 to 27) in the first treatment. Half of the 14 patients required additional treatment, four required one additional treatment, and two required two additional treatments. The largest number of ciliary processes treated was 43. A limiting factor of transpupillary argon-laser cyclophotocoagulation is visualization of the processes. Therefore a widely dilated pupil or a specialized contact lens with scleral indentor are helpful. When visualization of the ciliary processes is limited, argon-laser endophotocoagulation of the ciliary processes using either transpupillary or endoscopic visualization has been described.[46,52] However, both are invasive procedures requiring a pars plana incision, aphakia, or lensectomy at the time of the procedure and anterior vitrectomy.

In the early 1970s Beckman[3,4] used high-energy pulses emitted from ruby and Nd:YAG lasers to successfully lower intraocular pressure. The commercial availability of the Lasag Microruptor 2 in 1984 made this procedure more widely available. In this non-contact mode, the laser energy is delivered by a slit-lamp. The helium-neon (HeNe) aiming beam is focused on the conjunctiva, and the Nd:YAG laser beam is maximally defocused to reach the ciliary body. Although treatment parameters varied among the early investigators, the overall success rate ranged from 56% in neovascular glaucoma to 86% in aphakia. In a cadaver study, Hampton and Shields[28] concluded that a tangential beam 1 to 1.5 mm posterior to the limbus and an energy level of 8 joules were optimal parameters for ciliary body destruction. Using these parameters and 30 laser spots, they obtained successful lowering of intraocular pressure in 69% after one treatment and 83% after a second treatment. Although iritis and hyphema were not uncommon, subjectively the patients had less pain and inflammation. The rate of phthisis appears to be lower than with cyclocryotherapy. Sympathetic ophthalmia was seen 5 months after Nd:YAG laser therapy in a congenital glaucoma patient who had multiple surgeries and the complication of uveal tissue to the wound.[22]

Cohen[20] reported intraocular pressure control in 67% at 1 year after Nd:YAG laser photocoagulation for postkeratoplasty glaucoma. Multiple treatments were required in 13 eyes (46%). Of the 14 eyes with clear pretreatment grafts, six (43%) became edematous during follow-up observation. All the failed grafts had multiple treatments. It was difficult to ascertain whether these grafts failed as a result of endothelial damage secondary to previously elevated intraocular pressure, inflammation caused by the cyclophotocoagulation, or endothelial rejection. No graft demonstrated classic signs of endothelial rejection. Shields'[52] preliminary experience has been encouraging in postkeratoplasty glaucoma, especially in aphakic cases. In my (L.L.B., unpublished) series of 10 patients treated with transscleral Nd:YAG laser photocoagulation for glaucoma after penetrating keratoplasty, 9 eyes were controlled. Of 8 eyes with clear grafts before treatment, 6 remain clear at mean follow-up study of 19 months.

Nd:YAG energy may also be delivered to the ciliary body by a fiberoptic sapphire-tipped probe (SLT CLMD [Surgical Laser Technologies, Malvern, PA 19355]). In this contact mode, 70% to 80% of eyes were lower than 25 mm Hg.[1,11,12,51] Complications were fewer, an indication that the method may have more precise localization and less adjacent tissue injury than without that probe.

Continuous-wave Nd:YAG lasers used in general surgical, urologic and gynecologic procedures are often available at full-service hospitals. These can be modified with the fiberoptic sapphire-tipped probe (Medical Energy, Pensacola, FL 32504). It is important to remember that some of the "general surgical" lasers do not have stable delivery at the very low power settings needed for cyclodestructive procedures.

Both delivery systems of transscleral Nd:YAG cyclophotocoagulation are effective methods of lowering intraocular pressure in the refractory glaucomas and may offer the advantage of less inflammation and visual loss over conventional cyclocryotherapy.

Seton Surgery. Modern seton devices have shown promise in the treatment of refractory glaucoma. The Molteno implant is the most commonly used seton. It is a one-piece drainage system that employs a nonvalved silicone tube that is placed into the anterior chamber and is connected to a rimmed polypropylene episcleral plate (single or double). The plate or plates stimulate a fibrous reaction that encapsulates the entire system. Aqueous flow creates a filtering bleb by separation of the capsule off the surface of the plate or plates.

Molteno[43] reported control of intraocular pressure in 26 of 27 aphakic eyes. Subsequent reports by other authors reported a 63% to 65% success rate in pseudophakia with refractory glaucoma. The main complication of these shunt devices is overfiltration in the early postoperative period, leading to prolonged hypotony, suprachoroidal hemorrhage, and choroidal effusion. Other complications include obstruction of the tube by vitreous or uveal tissue and implant exposure. Temporary tube ligation, anterior vitrectomy, and scleral patch graft have decreased the incidence of these complications.

In postkeratoplasty glaucoma, the intraocular pressure has responded well to the use of a silicone drainage tube, though the rate of complications was high.[26] McDonnell[40] reported 71% of eyes controlled after insertion of single-plate Molteno implant for medically uncontrolled glaucoma after keratoplasty. Unfortunately, corneal allograft rejections occurred in 7 of 17 eyes. In Beebe's[5] study of 35 eyes with seton surgery 86% were judged successful from a glaucoma standpoint. However, graft rejection occurred in 34% and nonimmunologic failure was seen in 26%. Increased inflammation may result from the presence of the implanted foreign body. Kirkness[34] suggested that inflammatory cells may transverse the altered blood-ocular barrier into the anterior chamber from the area surrounding the subconjunctival seton, causing increased rate of graft rejection and failure. Meticulous attention must be made to the level of anterior segment inflammation in the postoperative period. Low-grade inflammation may improve intraocular pressure control but may also herald an early graft rejection.

Conventional Surgical Intervention. Reports on trabeculectomy for medically unresponsive glaucoma after penetrating keratoplasty are extremely rare. Scarring of the conjunctiva from previous surgery may limit the successful formation of an avascular filtering bleb. In a retrospective study of 502 penetrating keratoplasty cases, Foulks[24] reported that surgical therapy of glaucoma was required in 22 eyes. Trabeculectomy was performed in five eyes. Four patients had intraocular pressure controlled, whereas three had complications of clouding of the graft, choroidal detachment, vitreous hemorrhage and phthisis bulbi. In a study of 35 eyes undergoing trabeculectomy for postkeratoplasty glaucoma, Gilvarry[26] had 70% of eyes controlled at 9 months and only 50% at 2 years. Eighty-three percent of the successful eyes required glaucoma medication to achieve intraocular pressure control. This success rate in comparable to results of trabeculectomy in aphakia. Grafts remained clear in 89% of successful trabeculectomies compared to only 41% in the trabeculectomy failures. Adverse prognostic factors include multiple grafts and synechial closure of the angle.

In addition to standard filtering procedures, ab interno procedures, which eliminate the usual conjunctival dissection, have been advocated. These involve mechanical trephines as well as the previously mentioned laser modalities.[14]

Gilvarry considers trabeculectomy in eyes with little conjunctival scarring because there is a relatively low rate of complications. The use of adjunctive 5-fluorouracil (5-FU) with trabeculectomy has been widely investigated. It is known to produce large and persistent epithelial defects, which predispose to microbial keratitis and stromal scarring and thinning.[35] It should be used with caution in the recently grafted eye. The occurrence of postoperative flat chamber has been decreased with the use of delayed argon-laser suture lysis of the scleral flap.[50]

Insler[30] described combining trabeculectomy with penetrating keratoplasty. Five of seven eyes had an intraocular pressure less than or equal to 22 mm Hg at mean follow-up examination of 16 months. Although a combined procedure is technically possible, it is generally believed that glaucoma should be controlled before penetrating keratoplasty.

SUMMARY

Inadequate control of intraocular pressure after penetrating keratoplasty is one of the leading causes of graft failure. For avoidance of this complication it is mandatory that intraocular pressure be assessed accurately, early, and often. Careful paraoperative evaluation of the keratoplasty patient, if one keeps in mind risk factors such as inflammation, mechanical problems, and drug-induced side effects, will lead to better management. Glaucoma is a final outcome, but its pathogenesis is multifactorial. It is incumbent upon the keratoplasty surgeon to attempt to elucidate the pathogenesis of the postoperative glaucoma so that one or more appropriate therapies can be instituted to remedy the problem.

Surgical intervention is often necessary although significant risks to the graft exist with any proposed intraocular procedure. The surgeon must decide which procedure is appropriate on an individual basis. Argon-laser trabeculoplasty may be considered in eyes where a dramatic improvement in intraocular pressure is not necessary. Trabeculectomy with or without 5-FU when the conjunctiva is mobile and not heavily scarred may be indicated. Seton devices are successful, but the rate of graft failure and complications are significant. With fewer complications and ease of initial and repeat treatment, transscleral Nd:YAG laser cyclophotocoagulation is preferred over conventional cyclocryotherapy and may be preferred over the more invasive seton surgery. Further study is needed to determine which of the recently available treatments will be the surgical procedure of choice in postkeratoplasty glaucoma. No matter what treatment is chosen, the glaucoma subspecialist, in addition to the cornea subspecialist, must always be alert for graft reactions. Graft reactions are often reversible if diagnosed and treated promptly and appropriately.

REFERENCES

1. Allingham RR, deKater AW, Bellows AR, Hsu J: Probe placement and power levels in contact transscleral neodymi-um:YAG cyclophotocoagulation, *Arch Ophthalmol* 108:738, 1990.
2. Barron BA, Busin M, Page C, et al: Comparison of the effects of Viscoat and Healon on postoperative intraocular pressure, *Am J Ophthalmol* 100:377, 1985.
3. Beckman H, Sugar HS: Neodymium laser cyclocoagulation, *Arch Ophthalmol* 90:27, 1973.
4. Beckman H, Waterman J: Transscleral ruby laser cyclocoagulation, *Am J Ophthalmol* 98:788, 1984.
5. Beebe WE, Starita RJ, Fellman RL, et al: The use of Molteno implant and anterior chamber tube shunt to encircling band for the treatment of glaucoma in keratoplasty patients, *Ophthalmology* 97:1414, 1990.
6. Bellows AR, Grant WM: Cyclocryotherapy of chronic open-angle glaucoma in aphakic eyes, *Am J Ophthalmol* 85:615, 1978.
7. Berlin, MS: Excimer laser applications in glaucoma surgery, *Ophthalmol Clin North Am* 1:255, 1988.
8. Bigar F, Witmer R: Corneal endothelial changes in primary acute angle closure glaucoma, *Ophthalmology* 89:596, 1982.
9. Binder PS, Abel R Jr, Kaufman HE: Cyclocryotherapy for glaucoma after penetrating keratoplasty, *Am J Ophthalmol* 79:489, 1975.
10. Bourne WM, Davison MA, O'Fallon WM: The effects of oversize donor buttons on postoperative intraocular pressure and corneal curvature in aphakic penetrating keratoplasty, *Ophthalmology* 89:242, 1982.
11. Brancato R, Giovanni L, Trabucchi G, Pietroni C: Contact transscleral cyclophotocoagulation with Nd:YAG laser in uncontrolled glaucoma, *Ophthalmic Surg* 20(8):547, 1989.
12. Brancato R, Leoni G, Trabucchi G, Cappellini A: Probe placement and energy levels in continuous wave neodymium-YAG contact transscleral cyclophotocoagulation, *Arch Ophthalmol* 108:679, 1990.
13. Brightbill FS, Stainer GA, Hunkeler JD: A comparison of intracapsular and extracapsular lens extraction combined with keratoplasty, *Ophthalmology* 90:34, 1983.
14. Brown RH, Lynch MG: Ab interno filtering surgery, *Ophthalmol Clin North Am* 1:199, 1988.
15. Burgess SE, Silverman RH, Coleman DJ, et al: Treatment of glaucoma with high-intensity focused ultrasound, *Ophthalmology* 93:831, 1986.
16. Campbell DG, Vela A: Modern goniosynechiolysis for the treatment of synechial angle-closure glaucoma, *Ophthalmology* 91:1052, 1984.
17. Caprioli J, Stang SL, Spaeth GL, Poryzees EH: Cyclocryotherapy in the treatment of advanced glaucoma, *Ophthalmology* 92:947, 1985.
18. Casey TA, Gibbs D: Complications in corneal grafting, *Trans Ophthalmol Soc UK* 92:517, 1972.
19. Cohen EJ, Kenyon KR, Dohlman CH: Iridoplasty for prevention of post-keratoplasty angle closure and glaucoma, *Ophthalmic Surg* 13:994, 1982.
20. Cohen EJ, Schwartz LW, Luskind RD, et al: Neodymium:YAG laser transscleral cyclophotocoagulation for glaucoma after penetrating keratoplasty, *Ophthalmic Surg* 20:713, 1989.
21. Dailey RA, Brubaker RF, Bourne WM: The effects of timolol maleate and acetazolamide on the rate of aqueous formation in normal human subjects, *Am J Ophthalmol* 93:232, 1982.
22. Edward DP, Brown SV, Higginbotham E, et al: Sympathetic ophthalmia following neodymium:YAG cyclotherapy, *Ophthalmic Surg* 20(8):544, 1989.
23. Epstein DL, Steinert RF, Puliafito CA: Neodymium:YAG laser therapy to the anterior hyaloid in aphakic malignant (ciliovitreal block) glaucoma, *Am J Ophthalmol* 98:137, 1984.

24. Foulks GN: Glaucoma associated with penetrating keratoplasty, *Ophthalmology* 94:871, 1987.

25. François, J.: Cortisone et tension oculaire, *Ann Ocul* 187:805, 1954.

26. Gilvarry AME, Kirkness CM, Steele AD, et al: Management of post-keratoplasty glaucoma by trabeculectomy, *Eye* 3:713, 1989.

27. Goldmann H: Cortisone glaucoma, *Arch Ophthalmol* 68:621, 1962.

28. Hampton C, Shields MB: Transscleral neodymium-YAG cyclophotocoagulation, *Arch Ophthalmol* 106:1121, 1988.

29. Hoskins HD Jr, Iwach AG, Drake MV, et al: Subconjunctival THC:YAG laser limbal sclerostomy *ab externo* in the rabbit, *Ophthalmic Surg* 21:589, 1990.

30. Insler MS, Cooper HD, Kastl PR, Caldwell DR: Penetrating keratoplasty with trabeculectomy, *Am J Ophthalmol* 100:593, 1985.

31. Irvine AR, Kaufman HE: Intraocular pressure following penetrating keratoplasty, *Am J Ophthalmol* 68:835, 1969.

32. Jampel H: Questions and answers: Failed filtering operations, *Arch Ophthalmol* 108:495, 1990.

33. Karesh JW, Nirankari MS: Factors associated with glaucoma after penetrating keratoplasty, *Am J Ophthalmol* 96:160, 1983.

34. Kirkness CM, Ling Y, Rice NSC: The use of silicone drainage tubing to control post-keratoplasty glaucoma, *Eye* 2:583, 1988.

35. Knapp A, Heuer DK, Stern GA, et al: Serious corneal complications of glaucoma filtering surgery with postoperative 5-fluorouracil, *Am J Ophthalmol* 103:183, 1987.

36. Korey M, Gieser D, Kass MA, et al: Central corneal endothelial cell density and central corneal thickness in ocular hypertension and primary open angle glaucoma, *Am J Ophthalmol* 94:610, 1982.

37. Lass JH, Pavan-Langston D: Timolol therapy in secondary angle-closure glaucoma post penetrating keratoplasty, *Ophthalmology* 86:51, 1979.

38. Lee PF: Argon laser photocoagulation of the ciliary processes in cases of aphakic glaucoma, *Arch Ophthalmol* 97:2135, 1979.

39. Lippa EA, Schuman JS, Higginbotham EJ, et al: MK-507 versus Sezolamide, *Ophthalmology* 98:308, 1991.

40. McDonnell PJ, Robin JB, Schanzlin DJ, et al: Molteno implant for control of glaucoma in eyes after penetrating keratoplasty, *Ophthalmology* 95:364, 1988.

41. MacRae SM, Edelhauser HF, Hyndiuk RA, et al: The effects of sodium hyaluronate, chondroitin sulfate, and methylcellulose on the corneal endothelium and intraocular pressure, *Am J Ophthalmol* 95:332, 1983.

42. March WF: The principles of laser sclerostomy, *Ophthalmol Clin North Am* 1:239, 1988.

43. Molteno ACB, Bon Biljon G, Ancker E: Two stage insertion of glaucoma drainage implants, *Trans Ophthalmol Soc NZ* 31:17, 1979.

44. Nissenkorn I, Wood TO: Intraocular pressure following aphakic transplants, *Ann Ophthalmol* 15:1168, 1983.

45. Olson RJ: Variation in corneal graft size related to trephine technique, *Arch Ophthalmol* 97:1323, 1979.

46. Patel AC, Thompson JT, Michels RG, Quigley HA: Endophotocoagulation of ciliary body for refractory glaucoma in aphakes, *Ophthalmology* 92(suppl 2):65, 1985.

47. Perl T, Charlton KH, Binder PS: Disparate diameter grafting: astigmatism, intraocular pressure, and visual acuity, *Ophthalmology* 88:774, 1981.

48. Robin AL: Questions and answers: apraclonidine uses, *Arch Ophthalmol* 108:337, 1990.

49. Rootman DS, Insler MS, Thompson HW, et al: Accuracy and precision of the Tono-Pen® in measuring intraocular pressure after keratoplasty and epikeratophakia and on scarred corneas, *Arch Ophthalmol* 106:1697, 1988.

50. Savage JA, Condon GP, Lytle RA, et al: Laser suture lysis after trabeculectomy, *Ophthalmology* 95:1631, 1988.

51. Schubert HD: Noncontact and contact pars plana transscleral neodymium:YAG laser cyclophotocoagulation in postmortem eyes, *Ophthalmology* 96:1471, 1989.

52. Shields MB, Chandler DB, Hickingbotham DW, Klintworth GK: Histopathology of endoscopic cyclophotocoagulation in primates, *Invest Ophthalmol Vis Sci* 26(suppl):158, 1985, ARVO abstracts.

53. Shrader CE, Thomas JV, Simmons RJ: Relationship of patient age and tolerance to carbonic anhydrase inhibitors, *Am J Ophthalmol* 96:730, 1983.

54. Simmons RB, Stern RA, Teekhasaenee C, Kenyon KR: Elevated intraocular pressure following penetrating keratoplasty, *Tr Am Ophthalmol Soc* 87:79, 1989.

55. Strasser G: Neodymium YAG laser therapy to the anterior hyaloid in aphakic malignant (ciliovitreal block) glaucoma, *Am J Ophthalmol* 99:368, 1985 (Letter to editor).

56. Thoft RA, Gordon JM, Dohlman CH: Glaucoma following keratoplasty, *Trans Am Acad Ophthalmol Otolaryngol* 78:op352, 1974.

57. Tomey KF, Senft SH, Antonios SR, et al: Aqueous misdirection and flat chamber after posterior chamber implants with and without trabeculectomy, *Arch Ophthalmol* 105:770, 1987.

58. Troutman RC: *Microsurgery of the anterior segment of the eye: the cornea: optics and surgery*, vol 2, St. Louis, 1977, Mosby—Year Book.

59. Van Meter WS, Allen RC, Waring GO III, Stulting RD: Laser trabeculoplasty for glaucoma in aphakic and pseudophakic eyes after penetrating keratoplasty, *Arch Ophthalmol* 106:185, 1985.

60. Vela A: Personal communication, Emory University, Atlanta, Georgia, 1985.

61. Weiss JS, Waring GO III: Dental mirror for goniosynechiolysis during penetrating keratoplasty, *Am J Ophthalmol* 100:331, 1985.

62. West CE, Capella JA, Kaufman HE: Measurement of intraocular pressure with a pneumatic applanation tonometer, *Am J Ophthalmol* 74:505, 1972.

63. West CE, Wood TO, Kaufman HE: Cyclocryotherapy for glaucoma pre- or postpenetrating keratoplasty, *Am J Ophthalmol* 76:485, 1973.

64. Wilson RP, Javitt JC: *Ab interno* laser sclerostomy in aphakic patients with glaucoma and chronic inflammation, *Am J Ophthalmol* 110:178, 1990.

65. Zimmerman T, Olson R, Waltman S, Kaufman H: Transplant size and elevated intraocular pressure, *Arch Ophthalmol* 96:2231, 1978.

Chapter 22

Rejection

Clinical forms, diagnosis, and treatment

MICHAEL B. SHAPIRO
MARK R. MANDEL
JAY H. KRACHMER

Since the advent of more rigid eyebanking procedures and greatly improved microsurgical techniques, the most frequent cause of corneal graft failure after an initial period of clarity is the allograft-rejection reaction. Episodes of corneal allograft rejection complicate from 2.3%[9] to 68%[12] of cases of penetrating keratoplasty. Approximately 12% of these reactions in good prognosis cases, and up to 40% in complicated cases eventually lead to corneal transplant failure.[16]

The corneal graft rejection was first described by Paufique, Sourdille, and Offret[15] in 1948. These authors used the term *maladie du greffon* (graft sickness) to characterize a clouding of the graft from no apparent clinical reason after an initial period of a clear graft. An allergic reaction by the recipient to foreign protein in the transplanted tissue was the proposed pathogenesis. Maumenee[12] in 1951 provided experimental evidence that a graft reaction in rabbits was caused by sensitization of the host to donor tissue. In 1969 Khodadoust and Silverstein[10] demonstrated that the corneal epithelium, stroma, and endothelium may be rejected separately or together. Maumenee[13] described the clinical aspects of the corneal homograft reaction in 1962. Polack and Kanai[18] subsequently showed morphologically that sensitized lymphatic tissue is responsible for the rejection reaction with subsequent destruction of the donor endothelium resulting in edema of the graft.

The corneal allograft rejection is a complex immune response composed of a sequence of events. Initiation of this cascade is with the recognition of foreign histocompatibility antigens on cells of corneal allografts by the host immune system. This is known as host sensitization. It is followed by the generation of a specific efferent immune response to these antigens, the localization of these foreign cells, and the subsequent destruction of the corneal allograft.

The diagnosis of corneal allograft rejection can be made only if the corneal graft remains clear for at least 10 days after penetrating keratoplasty. Graft rejections can be classified into three types—epithelial, subepithelial infiltrates, and endothelial.

EPITHELIAL REJECTION

An epithelial rejection is characterized by the presence of an epithelial rejection line. This is a well-demarcated elevated line in the epithelium that stains with either fluorescein or rose bengal (Fig. 22-1). It often begins in the periphery and progresses to the center of the graft during the course of several days to a few weeks. The epithelium behind the rejection line may appear hazy and irregular.

Examination of the rejected area under high-power magnification shows destroyed epithelial cells on the graft side of the rejection line and large cells with prominent microvilli on the host side of the rejection line. These cells are believed to correspond to host cells migrating across the transplant behind the rejection line and replacing destroyed donor epithelial cells. Transmission electron microscopy shows lymphocytes present within the rejected epithelial cell layer.[17] Epithelial rejection usually takes place in a quiet or mildly inflamed eye. The true frequency of epithelial rejection is hard to determine because it

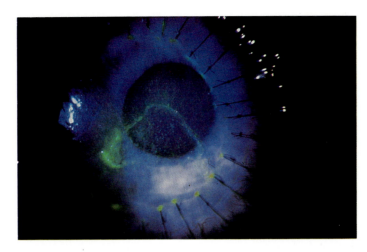

Fig. 22-1. Epithelial rejection line 9 weeks after penetrating keratoplasty for alkali burn.

can easily take place without symptoms between examinations. Alldredge and Krachmer[1] reported epithelial rejection in 15 of 156 grafts (10%). In their study the average onset of an epithelial line was 3 months, with a range of 1 to 13 months. They found epithelial rejection to be more common in patients younger than 50 years. Arentsen[2] found epithelial rejection lines in only 12 of 869 grafts (14%).

Of the total 27 epithelial rejection episodes reported in the above two studies, 20 (74%) presented before or with other forms of rejection (subepithelial infiltrates with or without endothelial rejection). This has lead to the vigorous treatment of epithelial rejections because, even though in themselves they do not result in loss of vision or destruction to the cornea, they may represent a smoldering graft rejection process with possible endothelial rejection to follow.

SUBEPITHELIAL INFILTRATES

Subepithelial infiltrates as a sign of corneal transplant rejection were first described by Krachmer and Alldredge[11] in 1978. These infiltrates appear as whitish deposits immediately beneath Bowman's layer and are from 0.2 to 0.5 mm in diameter (Fig. 22-2). The lesions are not unlike those seen in epidemic keratoconjunctivitis; however they are seen in the absence of conjunctivitis. They are found only in the donor cornea and are randomly positioned on the graft rather than being confined to the periphery or to a segment of the graft. Subepithelial infiltrates are best observed with the broad oblique beam of the slitlamp. They disappear promptly with topical corticosteroid treatment and sometimes leave faint subepithelial scars.

The exact frequency of subepithelial infiltrates is hard to ascertain because the lesions can be very subtle and easily be missed. Alldredge and Krachmer[1] reported the occurrence of subepithelial infiltrates in 23 of 156 grafts (15%). The average onset of these subepithelial infiltrates was 10 months after the transplant, with a range of 6 weeks to 21 months. They were more often observed in patients younger than 50 years. Arentsen[2] found subepithelial infiltrates in 21 of 869 grafts (2.4%).

Subepithelial infiltrates can be seen concurrently with endothelial or epithelial rejection lines, but they may also occur with only a few keratic precipitates, with a slight anterior chamber reaction, or with no other inflammatory changes. The importance of finding subepithelial infiltrates in a corneal transplant is similar to that of finding epithelial rejection. The subepithelial infiltrates themselves do not cause decreased vision or graft failure but rather may signal a smoldering reaction in the host. Aggressive treatment of these lesions with topical corticosteroids is indicated, since they may be a harbinger of a more severe rejection reaction.

Immunopathologic and histopathologic correlates of subepithelial infiltrates have not been reported.

ENDOTHELIAL REJECTION

Endothelial rejection is characterized by conjunctival hyperemia, an anterior chamber reaction, keratic precipitates on the donor tissue, and graft edema occurring after at least a 2-week period of graft clarity. Patients undergoing an endothelial rejection usually present with any combination of the following symptoms—pain, redness, and decreased vision. The anterior chamber reaction is usually mild but may be-

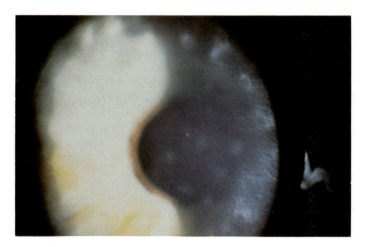

Fig. 22-2. Subepithelial infiltrates 4 months after penetrating keratoplasty for herpes simplex keratitis.

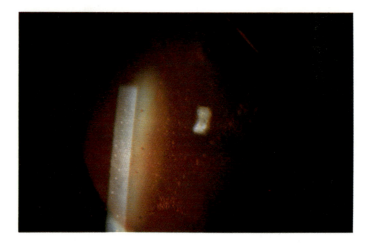

Fig. 22-3. Endothelial graft rejection 6 months after penetrating keratoplasty for keratoconus. Diffuse keratic precipitates can be seen in retroillumination.

come moderate. The keratic precipitates can be diffusely scattered (Fig. 22-3) or lined up in a chainlike configuration on the endothelial surface of the graft, forming the pathognomonic endothelial rejection line (Khodadoust line). This line starts in the periphery of the graft, often near a focus of corneal vascularization, and moves toward the center of the graft (Figs. 22-4 and 22-5). In 77 cases of endothelial rejection seen by Arentsen,[2] 35 (45%) were observed to have typical endothelial rejection lines. The stromal edema and folds in Descemet's membrane that form in the graft can be diffuse or segmental, as between the edge of the graft and an endothelial rejection line (Figs. 22-6 and 22-7). Histopathologic studies of endothelial rejection reveal lymphocytes of various shapes found free or between endothelial

cells, often forming a line between the rejected and normal area. Rejected endothelial cells appear elongated or rounded with loss of their cell junctions and destruction of many of their cytoplasmic processes.[17]

Reports in the literature vary widely on the incidence of endothelial rejection. The discrepancies can in part be accounted for in these retrospective studies by such uncontrolled factors as the use of corticosteroids after keratoplasty. In a series of 600 transplants, Gibbs and co-workers[7] reported a rejection rate of 44%. Offret and co-workers[14] found the frequency of rejection to be 30% and Polack reported 12%. Alldredge and Krachmer[1] reported a frequency of endothelial graft rejection to be 21%. In their series, the average onset after the transplant was 8 months, with a range of 2 weeks to 29 months.

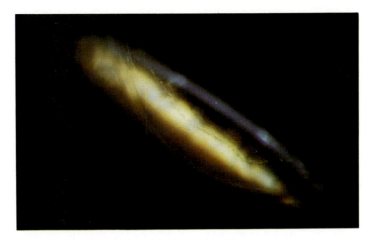

Fig. 22-4. Endothelial rejection line seen in periphery of keratoplasty performed 17 months previously for keratoconus.

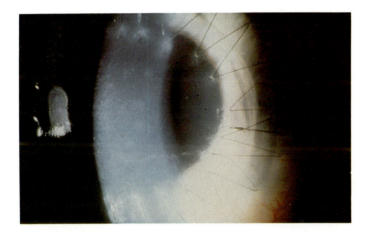

Fig. 22-5. Endothelial rejection 10 months after penetrating keratoplasty for keratoconus. Notice concomitant subepithelial infiltrates.

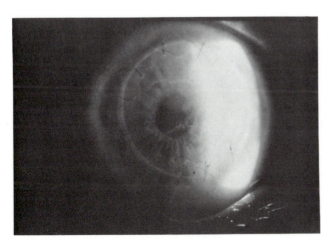

Fig. 22-6. Endothelial rejection 3 months after penetrating keratoplasty for keratoconus. Notice concomitant rejection lines.

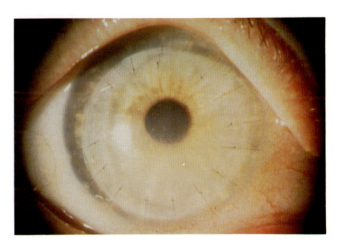

Fig. 22-7. Endothelial graft rejection 8 months after penetrating keratoplasty for Fuchs' dystrophy. Inferior half of cornea is edematous.

As with epithelial rejection and subepithelial infiltrates, endothelial rejection episodes were found to be more common in patients under 50 years compared to those who were 50 years of age and older. Perhaps this can be attributed to the more active immune system in younger patients.

Many reports divide their cases of penetrating keratoplasty into avascular and vascular categories with an almost uniform finding of an increase in endothelial rejections when a donor cornea is placed into a vascularized bed. Khodadoust[9] reported a series of 400 transplants and classified the frequency according to the degree of vascularity. He found rejection reactions in 3.5% of avascular cases, 13.3% of mildly vascular cases, 28% of moderately vascular cases, and 65% of heavily vascular cases, with the frequency for all cases being 23%. Gibbs and co-workers[7] found an increased rate of rejection in more vascularized corneas and also found that the reversibility of rejection was affected by the vascularization. The studies of Alldredge and Krachmer,[1] Cherry and co-workers[4] and Arentsen[2] all confirm the finding that the more there are of preoperative corneal vessels, the higher the frequency of graft rejection.

It is the clinical impression of many transplant surgeons that peripherally placed corneal grafts and larger corneal grafts have an increased incidence of rejection; however there are no data to confirm this. A possible explanation for this finding is the closeness of these grafts to limbal blood vessels.

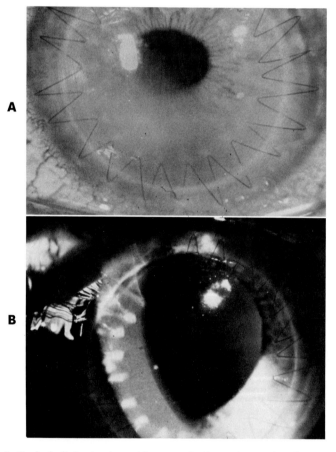

Fig. 22-8. A, Endothelial rejection with corneal edema 6 months after penetrating keratoplasty for keratoconus. **B,** Greatly improved 4 days after use of intensive corticosteroid therapy and cycloplegia.

To our knowledge, the longest period of time between a cornea transplant and the first episode of graft rejection is 35 years.[3] The incidence of patients experiencing recurrent episodes of endothelial rejection has been reported to be 20%.[2]

Donshik and co-workers[5] found a statistically significant increase in endothelial rejection episodes in bilateral grafts versus unilateral grafts for keratoconus (27% and 13% respectively). However the reports by Arentsen[2] and Alldredge and Krachmer[1] do not support this finding.

Arentsen[2] reported a statistically significant increase of endothelial rejections in cases that had postoperative synechiae. He recommends that every attempt should be made to prevent the formation of synechiae at the time of surgery.

DIFFERENTIAL DIAGNOSIS

Several other postkeratoplasty complications can be confused with graft rejection. Late graft failure caused by chronic progressive nonspecific endothelial decompensation is characterized by the gradual onset of graft edema. This entity, however, is not accompanied by inflammation or keratic precipitates.

The inflammation seen with a sterile or infectious endophthalmitis is usually more severe. Often there is an hypopyon and infiltrate in the vitreous, both of which are not seen in graft rejections.

Epithelial downgrowth can present with a posterior corneal line that mimics the classic endothelial rejection line. This entity can usually be differentiated from graft rejection by (1) clumps of cell-like material in the anterior chamber that are larger than the typical white blood cells seen in iritis and do not diminish with steroid use, (2) a faint white membrane seen on the surface of the iris that whitens upon argon-laser applications, and (3) glaucoma that can be abrupt in onset and rapidly becomes unresponsive to medical therapy. The prognosis in epithelial downgrowth is much poorer than that in graft rejection.

A confusing clinical picture is that of the appearance of inflammation and keratic precipitates in an eye that has had a transplant for herpes simplex. The differentiation between a rejection and recurrent herpetic uveitis is further confused when the corneal graft becomes edematous because of endothelial dysfunction secondary to inflammation. A careful search is made for an endothelial rejection line to help make the diagnosis. Often it is virtually impossible to differentiate these two entities. Intensive topical steroids, but no subconjunctival steroids, are used along with antiviral medications such as Viroptic (trifluorothymidine).

TREATMENT AND PROGNOSIS

The cornerstone of treatment for corneal allograft rejection is corticosteroids. The route of administration and dosage of corticosteroids is dependent on the type of rejection and its severity.

Epithelial rejections and subepithelial infiltrates do not result in decreased vision or graft damage but rather indicate that an immunologic reaction is occurring and endothelial rejection may soon follow. Treatment with topical prednisolone acetate 1% every 3 hours while the patient is awake is instituted. The patient is reexamined in 5 to 7 days. If the signs of rejection have regressed, the prednisolone is tapered to one half the previous dose every 3 days.

Endothelial rejection, if not treated early and vigorously, can often lead to rapid irreversible graft failure. If a patient has endothelial rejection without evidence of graft edema occurring 6 months or longer after surgery, topical prednisolone 1% drops are prescribed every hour while the patient is awake. Dexamethasone ointment is applied at night, and scopolamine 0.25% is used twice a day. The patient is examined in 3 days, and medications are tailored according to clinical findings at that time. If the patient has endothelial rejection accompanied by corneal edema or if the endothelial rejection occurs within 6 months after transplantation, then, in addition to hourly topical prednisolone 1% drops, scopolamine 0.25% twice a day, and dexamethasone ointment at night, a subconjunctival injection of 12 to 24 mg of dexamethasone sodium phosphate and orally administered prednisone 80 mg daily for an average adult are given (Fig. 22-8). The necessary precautions are taken with diabetics and patients with gastrointestinal ulcer disease. The use of a single pulsed intravenous injection of methylprednisolone, 125 to 500 mg, instead of prolonged oral administration of steroids has been advocated. This treatment regimen has the potential of improvement in graft survival, simplicity of administration, and decreased systemic side effects.[8]

Within 1 week to 10 days patients with severe rejection can be categorized into one of three groups. If the reaction has substantially improved as evidenced by less anterior chamber reaction, fewer keratic precipitates, and less edema, oral steroids can be abruptly stopped and intense topical medications continued. Alternatively, if the corneal edema and the anterior chamber inflammatory status are not significantly changed since the initial visit, it is unlikely that continued oral steroid use will be effective in abating the reaction. In this situation oral steroids should also be abruptly discontinued. However, if the inflammatory reaction and edema have partially subsided, systemic steroids should be tapered off over the ensuing weeks as intense topical medications are continued.

Patient education and open communication between patient and physician are just as important in preventing and treating corneal allograft rejection as medication is. The symptoms of corneal graft rejection include redness, decreased vision, and pain. In communicating with the patient, one refers to these symptoms as the three "danger signals" of rejection. Throughout the postoperative period the three major symptoms of rejection are continually reviewed with the patient. Because decreased vision is the most sensitive indicator, patients are instructed to test their vision daily by examining a familiar household object from the same distance. If the patient experiences any decrease in vision or increased redness or pain for more than 24 hours, he or she is instructed to contact a physician immediately. Strong impressions are that this form of patient education decreases the proportion of rejection reactions that would otherwise result in graft failures.

When a graft fails because of rejection, it is invariably caused by the endothelial type of reaction. Alldredge and Krachmer[1] found that 76% of grafts with endothelial rejection were successfully treated. The percentage probably would have been even higher if the series did not include a small number of patients who presented with rejections a week or longer in duration. Khodadoust[9] reported that half of the rejections in his series could be reversed with corticosteroids. Fine and Stein[6] found that 50% of vascular cases with rejection and 66% of avascular cases cleared with medical treatment. The prognosis for a repeat penetrating keratoplasty after a graft failure caused by rejection reaction probably relates more to factors such as corneal vascularization than the fact that a previous immune reaction has taken place.

Even though the treatment of corneal allograft rejection is often successful with corticosteroids, the ultimate goal is prevention of rejection. Further investigation into modifications of the complex immune mechanisms involved such as HLA matching and immunosuppressive drugs (such as cyclosporin A) is strongly indicated.

REFERENCES

1. Alldredge OC, Krachmer JH: Clinical types of corneal rejection: their manifestations, frequency, preoperative correlates, and treatment, *Arch Ophthalmol* 99:599, 1981.
2. Arentsen JJ: Corneal transplant allograft reaction: possible predisposing factors, *Trans Am Ophthalmol Soc* 81:361, 1983.
3. Arentsen JJ: Personal communication, Philadelphia, 1985.
4. Cherry PMH et al: An analysis of corneal transplantation: I. Graft clarity, *Ann Ophthalmol* 11:461, 1979.
5. Donshik PC et al: Effect of bilateral and unilateral grafts on the incidence of rejections in keratoconus, *Am J Ophthalmol* 87:823, 1979.
6. Fine M, Stein M: The role of corneal vascularization in human corneal graft reactions. In Porter R, Knight J, editors: Corneal graft failure, *Ciba Found Symp* 15:193, Amsterdam/New York, 1973, Elsevier Publishing Co./Associated Scientific Publishers.
7. Gibbs DC et al: The influence of tissue-type compatibility on the fate of full-thickness corneal grafts, *Trans Ophthalmol Soc UK* 94:101, 1974.
8. Hill JD, Maske R, Watson P: Corticosteroids in corneal graft rejection, *Ophthalmology* 98:329, 1991.
9. Khodadoust AA: The allograft rejection reaction: the leading cause of late failure of clinical corneal grafts. In Porter R, Knight J, editors: Corneal graft failure, *Ciba Found Symp* 15:151, Amsterdam/New York 1973, Elsevier Publishing Co./Associated Scientific Publishers.
10. Khodadoust AA, Silverstein AM: Transplantation and rejection of individual cell layers of the cornea, *Invest Ophthalmol Vis Sci* 8:180, 1969.
11. Krachmer JH, Alldredge OC: Subepithelial infiltrates: a probable sign of corneal transplant rejection, *Arch Ophthalmol* 96:2234, 1978.
12. Maumenee AE: The influence of donor-recipient sensitization on corneal grafts, *Am J Ophthalmol* 34:142, 1951.
13. Maumenee AE: Clinical aspects of the corneal homograft reaction, *Invest Ophthalmol Vis Sci* 1:244, 1962.
14. Offret G, Pouliquen Y, Guyot D: Aspects cliniques des réactions immunitaires après kératoplasties transfixiantes chez l'homme, *Arch Ophthalmol* 30:209, 1970.
15. Paufique L, Sourdille GP, and Offret G: *The grafts of the cornea (keratoplasties)*, Paris, 1948, Masson et Cie.
16. Polack FM: Editorial on recent advances: Corneal transplantation, *Invest Ophthalmol Vis Sci* 12:85, 1973.
17. Polack FM: *Corneal transplantation*, New York, 1977, Grune & Stratton, pp 201.
18. Polack FM, Kanai A: Electron microscopic studies of graft endothelium in corneal graft rejection, *Am J Ophthalmol* 73:711, 1972.

Immunosuppression in high-risk corneal transplantation

EDWARD J. HOLLAND
TIMOTHY W. OLSEN

Although corneal allografts are the most frequently performed and the most successful tissue allograft, immune-mediated rejection remains the leading cause of graft failure. The incidence of graft failure in routine penetrating keratoplasty is approximately 10%. Up to 30% of penetrating keratoplasty patients will have at least one episode of rejection.[1] These usually occur between 4 and 18 months postoperatively but may occur many years after successful transplantation and has been reported as late as 20 years postoperatively.[64] Approximately 50% to 70% of the rejection episodes can be reversed with topical steroids though some require the use of systemic steroids.

Several host factors have been shown to increase the risk of immune-mediated graft rejection. The most important factor seems to involve the degree of corneal vascularization. Repeat grafts, bilateral grafts, the presence of synechiae or inflammation, and younger recipients[1,2] are also factors that increase the risk of graft rejection. "High-risk" grafts are those grafts that have two or more quadrants of neovascularization or are failed because of rejection. The incidence of graft failure from allograft rejection in high-risk keratoplasty is 25% to 50%[2,24,27,41] and therefore the management of these patients is a significant challenge.

MECHANISM OF REJECTION

Immune-mediated rejection of an allogeneic cornea should be thought of as a complex cascade of cellular events that must be controlled early and aggressively in order to preserve graft function. Because new agents that show promise in controlling various components of the immunologic cascade are currently being investigated, a basic understanding of the rejection process is essential in treating corneal graft rejection.

Tissue allograft rejection can be divided into the afferent and efferent arms of the immune response. The afferent arm involves the sensitization of the host to foreign-tissue antigens. Human leukocyte antigens (HLA) are cell-surface glycoproteins whose structure is determined by four genes located on chromosome 6 (HLA-A, B, C, and D). Class I (HLA-A, B, and C) antigens are expressed on almost every nucleated cell in the body including corneal epithelium, stromal keratocytes, and endothelial cells, whereas class II (HLA-DR, DQ, DP) antigens are found selectively on B-lymphocytes, macrophages,[55] and other cells such as Langerhans' cells and interstitial dendritic cells. Under the influence of interferon-gamma (IFN-gamma), epithelial and endothelial cells have also been shown to express class II antigen.[79] These donor tissue antigens are processed by antigen-presenting cells (APCs) of either the host or more likely the donor cornea at or near the donor-host interface.[28,78] The modified foreign antigens are then externalized on the APC and presented to the host immune system in conjunction with HLA class II and interleukin-1 (IL-1).[7] Donor class I cell surface antigens are recognized by host cytotoxic T cells (CD8+), whereas donor class II antigens are recognized by helper T (T-helper, Th) cells (CD4+).[46]

The efferent arm of the immune response involves the host's response to foreign antigen. The activated Th cells release interleukin-2 (IL-2), inter-feron-gamma (IFN-gamma), macrophage activation factor (MAF), migration inhibiting factor (MIF), and many other lymphokines and cytokines. IL-2 stimulates the activation and proliferation of other T- and B-lymphocytes, whereas IFN-gamma induces class II antigen expression on donor tissue. Class II antigen expression is a potent stimulator of the cell-mediated allograft response. Cytotoxic T-lymphocytes (Tc) are the primary allograft effector cells and they attack corneal cells expressing class I antigen. Tc cells are activated by and proliferate in response to IL-2, which is produced by activated Th cells. B-cells produce antibody against the foreign antigen, which in turn attracts nonspecific inflammatory cells (macrophages), compliment, and natural killer cells or antibody-dependent cell-mediated cytotoxic cells (ADCC). T-suppressor cells (Ts) provide an immunoregulatory mechanism over Th cells, and the interaction and ratio of these two cell types is important in balancing the magnitude of the cell-mediated immune response.[47]

PREVENTING IMMUNE-MEDIATED GRAFT REJECTION

Three approaches in preventing immune-mediated allograft rejection are possible: (1) reduce the antigenicity of donor tissue, (2) minimize antigenic differences between host and donor, and (3) control of host immune response to foreign tissue.

REDUCE THE ANTIGENICITY OF THE DONOR TISSUE

Immunomodulation of corneal grafts during eye bank processing or through various tissue preservation techniques may be a methodology to reduce rejection in the future. For example, removal of the corneal epithelium was believed to decrease the risk of rejection because the epithelium was a source of class I antigen and class II antigen (Langerhans' cells); however, a recent study did not show a clinical benefit from this procedure.[69] Pretreatment of corneal grafts with ultraviolet light has been demonstrated to reduce the rejection rate in animal studies presumably by altering the immunogenicity of the graft.[50,56,80] Endothelial cell transplantation is also being evaluated in an attempt to decrease the antigenicity of the donor graft.[5,49,59] Although these techniques show promise for the future, at the present time they are not useful clinically.

MINIMIZE ANTIGENIC DIFFERENCES BETWEEN HOST AND DONOR

The value of tissue typing in corneal transplantation is an unresolved issue. It has been demonstrated in some studies that HLA typing is beneficial in high-risk vascularized corneal allografts, whereas it has shown little benefit in low-risk groups.[4,13,60,75] However, a more recent study has shown a strong association of endothelial allograft reactions and HLA-A or HLA-B incompatibility in low-risk recipients.[10] Although several studies have been conducted, a decision regarding the benefits of HLA tissue typing has not been clearly made. The HLA matching process does delay surgery and increases the expense of corneal transplantation, which may detract from its potential benefits. The Collaborative Corneal Transplant Study (CCTS) is an ongoing randomized multicenter trial that one would hope will resolve this issue.

CONTROL OF THE HOST IMMUNE RESPONSE

Currently, control of the host immune response through the use of pharmacologic agents remains the mainstay of preventing corneal allograft rejection.

Glucocorticosteroids. Glucocorticosteroids are the drugs of choice for treating acute graft rejection because no other agent has as great an effect on the acute-phase reactants of graft rejection as they do; therefore glucocorticosteroids represent a very important and useful though nonspecific immunomodulator.

Corticosteroids provide a variety of pharmacotherapeutic effects in treating eye disease. They have been shown to inhibit phospholipase-A2, responsible for initiating the prostaglandin cascade, decrease cellular and fibrinous exudation and tissue infiltration, inhibit fibroblastic and collagen-forming activity, retard epithelial regeneration, diminish postoperative neovascularization, restore the excessive permeability of inflamed capillaries,[18] and stabilize polymorphonuclear leukocyte lysosomal membranes, which have dramatic effects on diminishing acute inflammation.

Corticosteroids may also have an effect on T-cells involved with allograft rejection based on their ability to diminish the quantity of circulating T-lymphocytes, which then accumulate in the bone marrow.[14,22] Corticosteroids decrease the ratio of Th/Ts cells, inhibit T-cell replication in response to antigenic stimuli, and inhibit T-cell growth factor produced by macrophages and other T-cells.[29]

Drug delivery. In high-risk keratoplasty patients, frequent topical steroid use is extremely helpful in the perioperative period followed by continuous, long-term indefinite use when no contraindications exist. Corticosteroids can be administered topically,

subconjunctivally, and systemically. Topical application provides good corneal drug penetration and is relatively well tolerated by the graft while it avoids the complications of systemic therapy. Topical application has obvious side effects such as cataracts, glaucoma, and surface immunosuppression, which predisposes to infections or recrudescence of herpes simplex virus.

In high-risk recipients, relatively large doses of systemic corticosteroids, oral or intravenous, may be used in the immediate perioperative period followed by chronic low-dose oral steroids when no contraindications exist. The use of long-term, low-dose systemic corticosteroid (7.5 to 10 mg of prednisone per day), similar to the treatment protocol for solid-tissue grafts, may be beneficial in preventing graft rejection in this population of patients. Brief periods of systemic corticosteroid use have minimal side effects, whereas longer term therapy has been associated with a long list of adverse effects including (1) exacerbation of peptic ulcer disease, (2) mental changes and psychosis, (3) increasing severity of diabetes and hypertension, (4) osteoporotic changes, (5) delayed wound healing, (6) reactivation of latent infection such as tuberculosis, (7) electrolyte imbalance and edema, and (8) cushingoid changes.[16] High-risk recipients who require chronic systemic corticosteroids may benefit from alternate-day therapy, which seems to substantially reduce undesirable side effects. Double the daily dosage is administered on an alternate-day basis, which seems to offer equivalent immunosuppression against graft rejection while causing less adrenal suppression.[16]

Although corticosteroids may be efficacious when used alone in preventing rejection of high-risk grafts, rejection may still occur. In addition, optimal dosages of steroid may not be possible in many patients because of the adverse effects listed above. Therefore, more specific and less toxic agents are needed in the management of corneal transplant rejection in high-risk keratoplasty.

Azathioprine (Imuran). Azathioprine is a phase-specific cytotoxic agent that is rapidly converted after ingestion to mercaptopurine, which competitively inhibits purine synthesis. The mechanism of phase-specific cytotoxic agents is inhibition of cell replication during a specific phase of the cell cycle and is active only when cells are replicating. Clinically, this means that azathioprine exerts its effect on lymphocytes when given immediately after antigenic challenge or very early in the rejection process and will have little effect on established graft rejection or secondary responses.[26,35,63]

Azathioprine is currently used in most renal transplantation antirejection protocols in combination with corticosteroids and cyclosporin A. Three to 5 mg/kg/day are used to prevent rejection in solid-tissue allografts with a maintenance dosage of from 1 to 2 mg/kg/day. One to 2 mg/kg/day of oral azathioprine in combination with topical dexamethasone and oral prednisone has been reported to successfully treat rejection in high-risk corneal grafts and when used early in recurring rejection episodes.[3,45] Attempts should be made to slowly taper and eventually discontinue azathioprine. As seen with other tissue grafts, the simultaneous use of steroids and azathioprine may help to prevent rejection of high-risk corneal grafts and also allows for a lower dosage of systemic steroid to be used, thus allowing one to avoid the complications of excessively high dosages.

Continuation of azathioprine at a lower maintenance dosage should be accompanied by cautious monitoring of complete blood counts and liver function tests because significant side effects may occur with this agent including bone marrow suppression, anemia, thrombocytopenia, leukopenia, gastrointestinal tract toxicity, hepatocellular necrosis, an increased risk of neoplasia, and alopecia. These systemic effects restrict the use of azathioprine for prevention of corneal graft rejection and should only be considered in high-risk patients with one eye who are dependent on graft survival for functional vision. Each individual patient deserves a thorough explanation of all possible adverse effects and alternatives available.

Cyclosporin A. As the complexities of the immune system become better understood, newer agents are being developed to target specific actors in the immune system and allow for a more specific modulation of events involved with allograft rejection. Cyclosporin A (CsA) represents a new generation of immunosuppressive agent that has had a major impact on solid organ transplantation and has been shown to prolong hepatic,[68] renal,[38,67] and cardiac allografts[54] in addition to corneal allografts.

CsA is a hydrophobic, cyclic, undecapeptide metabolite from the fungus *Tolypocladium inflatum gans* isolated from a soil sample in southern Norway[15] that was later found by Borel and co-workers in 1977 to have inhibitory effects on lymphocyte function and antibody production.[11] CsA's unique property lies in its ability to selectively and reversibly interfere with certain populations of immunocompetent cells with no generalized cytotoxic effects, thus making it the first drug of a new generation of specific immunosuppressive agents.[25]

Mechanism of action. The mechanism of action of CsA has been studied intensively. It seems to act at a subcellular level by binding an intracellular peptide known as "cyclophilin,"[32] which has "PPIase" (peptidyl-prolyl isomerase) activity, which in turn regulates the rate-limiting step of intracellular protein synthesis. Cyclophilin and other cytoplasmic proteins with PPIase activity are believed to be a novel class of cytoplasmic regulatory proteins involved with activation of T-cells[33,62] and are now known as "immunophilins." The result of the subcellular activity of CsA is an inhibition of transcriptional activation of lymphokine genes[25] thereby inhibiting the proliferation and function of T-cytotoxic cells (Tc) by inhibiting the production of interleukin-2 (IL-2) and interferon-gamma (IFN-gamma) produced by T-helper cells (Th).[12,30,57,62] It has been suggested that T-suppressor cell (Ts) function, which is important for graft survival, is not inhibited by CsA and may actually be enhanced.[34] CsA also has an effect on humoral immunity based on both indirect (by its T-cell inhibition) and direct inhibition of B-cells responding to T-cell–independent antigens.[43] Finally, early reports in the literature indicate that CsA may have an inhibition on the expression of the high-affinity IL-2 receptor;[73] therefore, if present early in the sensitization stage of the immune response, CsA has the ability to minimize initiating events that lead to graft failure.

Systemic CsA. Even though CsA acts as a relatively specific immunomodulator directed at T-lymphocytes, the systemic administration of CsA has a significant list of adverse effects. The potential toxicity therefore restricts the use of systemic CsA to high-risk allografts in patients dependent on graft survival for functional vision. CsA has been shown in solid tissue allografts to be most beneficial when used in combination with azathioprine and corticosteroids, which minimizes renal dysfunction and allows for graft survival even in high-risk patients.[73]

CsA is available as an intravenous (50 mg/ml) or oral solution (100 mg/ml). The systemic dosage to prevent rejection of high-risk corneal allografts is not known; however, in solid-tissue allografts initial dosing begins preoperatively at from 12 to 15 mg/kg/day, which is then tapered to a maintenance dosage of 5 mg/kg/day[31] while the dosage for various autoimmune diseases ranges from 2 to 5 mg/kg/day.[17,40] When CsA is used with corticosteroids and azathioprine, the initial dose of CsA is 8 to 10 mg/kg/day and is then tapered to 2 to 4 mg/kg/day.[73]

Because of variable absorption, monitoring blood levels of CsA is recommended to minimize the systemic side effects, which include nephrotoxicity, hepatotoxicity, hypertension, neurotoxicity, thromboembolism, hirsutism, and gingival hyperplasia.[17] Ideal trough blood levels in renal transplantation are from 80 to 250 ng/ml as measured by high-performance liquid chromatography (HPLC).[53] Monitoring serum creatinine, blood urea nitrogen, and liver enzymes, complete blood counts, and blood pressure should be considered in patients on systemic CsA.

Although initiating systemic immunosuppression with CsA is difficult to justify in corneal transplantation, it has the following advantages: (1) CsA has a proved efficacy in solid-tissue allografts as compared to corticosteroids alone, (2) it acts as a specific immunomodulator, and (3) systemic therapy avoids ocular surface complications. We believe that systemic CsA, like azathioprine, should be reserved for high-risk corneal allografts in monocular patients who have no contraindications to the drug, are dependent on graft survival for functional vision, and are well informed as to the risks involved.

Topical CsA. Theoretically, to prevent allograft rejection, the lymphoid tissue and infiltrating lymphocytes capable of recognizing foreign antigen should be the "target" of immunosuppressive agents. With local immunosuppression, the regional lymphoid tissue corresponding to the allograft is targeted while other uninvolved sites are not affected by therapy. With regard to a vascularized corneal bed, it is conceivable that early rejection could be arrested by continuous, relatively low doses of immunosuppressive agents, which prevent T-cell activation and the rejection cascade. A vascularized graft always has access to the systemic circulation and the possibility of splenic or thymic T-cell activation. The efferent arm of the immune response would then become the target of therapy. CsA is presumed to initiate local immunosuppression by the same mechanism as it does for systemic immunosuppression, that is, inhibition of IL-2, IFN-gamma, IL-2 receptor (IL-2R) expression, and downregulation of class II antigen expression.

Several investigators have demonstrated successful topical immunosuppression with CsA. Foets and co-workers[23] evaluated the use of topical CsA on eccentric corneal allografts in the rabbit model and found that all treated grafts remained clear whereas nontreated grafts were rejected. Interestingly, when topical CsA was administered only in the unoperated eye (allograft eye untreated), the grafts were rejected even though systemic levels, determined by radioimmunoassay, were similar between each group. Significant serum levels of systemic CsA might have accounted for the immunosuppression

in this study; however, it indicates that local immunosuppression may be responsible for graft survival.

CsA is a neutral hydrophobic peptide that easily penetrates the intact hydrophobic corneal epithelium; however, the stroma is hydrophilic and is not easily penetrated by lipophilic substances. Various lipophilic carrier solutions have been used with CsA. A standard topical solution that has shown efficacy is 2% CsA in a lyophilic carrier (that is, sterile olive oil).

Patients generally tolerate topical CsA without difficulty. In a recent report of 11 high-risk keratoplasty subjects treated with 2% CsA in sterile olive oil, 10 corneas remained clear at a 16-month follow-up examination.[6] All patients were reported to have transient epithelial keratitis, which was self-limiting. In a review of 27 patients treated at the University of Minnesota with topical CsA for a variety of anterior-segment inflammatory conditions, we found two patients who experienced severe ocular discomfort because of the topical CsA. The remaining 25 patients tolerated the medication well including several patients receiving hourly application (unpublished data).

An unresolved issue in the use of topical CsA is the potential risk of systemic absorption and toxicity. One study reported a significant systemic absorption of topical CsA because whole blood levels were detectable by HPLC measurements.[6] Currently, most investigators have not been able to detect measurable whole blood levels from topical CsA in human trials despite frequent topical administration. The 27 patients treated at the University of Minnesota with topical CsA were monitored for renal function and serial whole blood levels for CsA. None of the patients had a significant elevation of serum creatinine, and whole blood CsA levels were nondetectable as determined by HPLC.

To support the argument that low-dose CsA therapy does not result in significant systemic toxicity, a recent study of psoriatic patients receiving low-dose oral CsA (2.5 mg/kg/day) concluded that CsA monitoring is not needed.[44] The total amount of drug in drops administered from the use of topical CsA would be less than that of the psoriatic patients treated with 2.5 mg/kg/day. However, because future studies are necessary to address the possible long-term effects of topical CsA administration, clinicians using CsA should consider monitoring whole blood levels of CsA, serum creatinine, liver function tests, and blood pressure.

Based on current animal studies and early clinical results, it is possible that topical CsA will be a valuable drug in preventing corneal allograft rejection and may be extremely beneficial in high-risk patients. Hopefully, the question of topical CsA's safety and efficacy will be answered from a prospective, randomized, multicenter trial of topical CsA in high-risk penetrating keratoplasty patients.

EXPERIMENTAL AGENTS

A variety of new immunoregulatory agents that have impressive effects in solid-tissue allografts are currently being studied. The obvious goal in preventing corneal allograft rejection is to utilize these agents to specifically target immune-mediated rejection without causing systemic toxicity. Although the cornea has been described as having an immunologically "privileged" site, which allows for such successful results in uncomplicated allografts, the cornea also has an anatomically "privileged" site by residing on the surface, which allows for direct and closely monitored management of the rejection process. We will briefly describe the agents that show promise in the future of penetrating keratoplasty.

FK-506. FK-506 is a macrolide first described in 1987 and isolated from the fungus *Streptomycetes tsukubaensis*.[42] It was later shown to prevent allograft rejection in various animal models.[36,51] FK-506 has been reported to be approximately 10 to 100 times more potent than CsA,[71] whereas its mechanism of action seems to be very similar to that of CsA. As mentioned earlier, immunophilins are intracytoplasmic receptors that regulate gene expression. CsA binds to one immunophilin known as cyclophilin (CyP), whereas FK-506 binds to a separate immunophilin known as FK-506-binding protein (FKBP).[9] The result is an inhibition of transcriptional activation of lymphokine genes; therefore T-cells lack the stimulus to replicate. FK-506 has been shown to be effective in preventing allograft rejection in dosages as low as 0.16 mg/kg/day in animal models.[52] Although toxicity of this new agent has not been clearly defined, it has been suggested to have diabetogenic and neurotoxicity similar to CsA but does not seem to display nephrotoxicity, hypertensive effects, or the many other side effects associated with CsA.[66]

Because CsA and FK-506 act at different receptor sites yet by a similar mechanism, one would expect a synergism when these two agents are used together. Indeed, FK-506 and CsA have been shown to act synergistically in preventing allograft rejection in animal models.[72,81] Since CsA has been clearly shown in experimental animal models to minimize corneal allograft rejection, the next logical step is to study combinations of FK-506 and CsA in animal models of corneal transplantation. FK-506 is highly lipophilic in nature, a characteristic that may allow for a corneal penetration similar to that of CsA.

Rapamycin. Rapamycin is also a macrolide that is structurally very similar to FK-506 and was first described in 1975 by Sehgal and colleagues and found to have antifungal activity.[61] Rapamycin has also been shown to prolong allografts in animal models, seems to be far more potent than CsA, and may be more potent than FK-506.[48] As one might assume, one site of action may be very similar to that of FK-506. It has been shown that rapamycin binds to FKBP and inhibits the immunophilin activity; however, although FK-506 appears to inhibit the antigen receptor–induced signals, rapamycin interferes with the IL-2–induced signal.[8] CsA and FK-506 have been shown to suppress T-cell activation at the level of lymphokine production, whereas rapamycin seems to act to prevent the T-cell response to lymphokines.[19] Because rapamycin and FK-506 bind at a common immunophilin, they inhibit each other's action, and it is therefore unlikely that these two agents will be useful together clinically. However, synergy between rapamycin and CsA has been demonstrated in the rat heart allograft model.[66] Rapamycin is also lipophilic in nature, a characteristic that may allow for a corneal penetration similar to that of CsA.

15-Deoxyspergualin. 15-Deoxyspergualin (DSG) is a new immunosuppressive agent, synthesized by Iwasawa[37] in 1982 from the antitumor antibiotic spergualin, derived from *Bacillus laterosporus*.[70] Umezawa[74] demonstrated that spergualin was found to reduce delayed hypersensitivity in mice and prolong skin allografts in rats. DSG has recently been shown to prolong other animal-model solid-organ allografts and has also been shown to prolong xenograft survival in renal and cardiac animal models.[21,58,76] Far less is known about the mechanism of action of DSG; however, it appears to act much differently from CsA, FK-506, or rapamycin and involves both lymphocyte and monocyte/macrophage inhibition. DSG has been shown to inhibit lysosomal enzyme release and superoxide production by monocytes, inhibit class II induction on monocytes in response to immunologic stimuli,[82,83] and inhibit human lymphocyte proliferation in response to mitogens or allogeneic stimulation. DSG may specifically attack lymphocyte clonal expansion during the acute phase of graft rejection while sparing T-suppressor cells.[84] We have shown that DSG successfully prevents corneal allograft rejection in the rat penetrating keratoplasty model and have also shown a synergistic effect between DSG and CsA in this same animal model.[85]

Toxicity is a limiting factor with the use of systemic DSG. The gastrointestinal tract and bone marrow seem to be the primary sites of toxicity. Ideally, the topical application of DSG would alleviate many of the systemic side effects as well as minimize systemic immunosuppression. Several biochemical constraints exist to limit topical application, and if future studies solve these constraints to topical delivery, DSG may prove to be another valuable tool in the growing list of more specific immunomodulating drugs used to prevent corneal allograft rejection.

The future management of corneal transplant patients will utilize more specific and less toxic immunosuppressive agents. In addition, new techniques for the immunomodulation of donor tissue to reduce corneal antigenicity may be possible. These methodologies will lead to improved success of high-risk penetrating keratoplasty.

REFERENCES

1. Aldredge OC, Krachmer JH: Clinical types of corneal transplant rejection, *Arch Ophthalmol* 99:599-604, 1981.
2. Arentsen JJ: Corneal transplant allograft reaction: possible predisposing factors, *Trans Am Ophthalmol Soc* 81:361-402, 1983.
3. Barraquer C, Zeman A: Imuran in penetrating keratoplasties, *Arch Soc Am Ophthalmol Optom* 17:97, 1983.
4. Batchelor JR, Casey TA, West A, et al: HLA matching and corneal grafting, *Lancet* 1:551, 1976.
5. Baum, JL, Neidra R, Davis D, Yue B: Mass culture of human corneal endothelial cells, *Arch Ophthalmol* 97:1136-1140, 1979.
6. Belin MW, Bouchard CS, Frantz BS, Chmielinska MS: Topical cylcosporine in high risk corneal transplants, *Ophthalmology* 96:1144-1150, 1989.
7. Belin MW, Bouchard CS, Phillips TM: Update on topical cyclosporin A: background, immunology, and pharmacology, *Cornea* 9(3):184-195, 1990.
8. Bierer BE, Mattila PS, Standaert RF, et al: Two distinct signal transmission pathways in T lymphocytes are inhibited by complexes formed between an immunophilin and either FK506 or rapamycin, *Proc Natl Acad Sci USA* 87:9231-9235, 1990.
9. Bierer BE, Schreiber SL, Burakoff SJ: The effect of the immunosuppressant FK-506 on alternate pathways of T cell activation, *Eur J Immunol* 21:439-445, 1991.
10. Boisjoly HM, Roy R, Bernard PM, et al: Association between corneal allograft reactions and HLA compatibility, *Ophthalmology* 97:1689-1698, 1990.
11. Borel JF, Feurer C, Magnée C, Stähelin H: Effects of the new anti-lymphocytic peptide cyclosporin A in animals, *Immunology* 32:1017, 1977.
12. Britton S, Palacios R: Cyclosporin A—usefulness, risks and mechanism of action, *Immunol Rev* 65:5, 1982.
13. Casey TA, Mayer DJ: *Corneal grafting*, San Francisco, 1984, Saunders.
14. Cohen JJ: Thymus-derived lymphocytes sequestered in bone marrow of hydrocortisone-treated mice, *J Immunol* 108:841-844, 1972.
15. Dreyfuss M, Harri E, Hoffmann H, et al: *Eur J Appl Microbiol* 3:125, 1976.
16. *Drug Evaluations*, ed 6, Adrenal corticosteroids in nonendocrine diseases, pp 1093-1104, Chicago, 1986, American Medical Association.
17. *Drug Evaluations*, ed 6, Immunomodulators: cytotoxic drugs, pp 1151-1152, Chicago, 1986, American Medical Association.
18. Duke-Elder S, Ashton N: Action of cortisone on tissue reactions of inflammation and repair with special reference to the eye, *Br J Ophthalmol* 35:695, 1951.
19. Dumont FJ, Staruch SL, Koprak MM, Sigal NH: Distinct mechanisms of suppression of murine T cell activation by the related macrolides FK506 and rapamycin, *J Immunol* 144:251, 1990.
20. Emmel EA, Verweij CL, Durand DB, et al: Cyclosporin A specifically inhibits function of nuclear proteins involved in T cell activation, *Science* 246:1617-1620, 1989.
21. Engemann R, Gassel HJ, Lafrenz E, et al: Transplantation tolerance after short-term administration of 15-deoxyspergualin in orthotopic rat liver transplantation, *Transplant Proc* 19:4241-4243, 1987.
22. Fauci AS: Mechanism of corticosteroid action on lymphocyte subpopulations: I. Redistribution of circulating T and B lymphocytes to the bone marrow, *Immunology* 38:669-680, 1975.
23. Foets B, Missotten L, Vanderveeren, Goossens W: Prolonged survival of allogeneic corneal grafts in rabbits treated with topically applied cyclosporine A systemic absorption and local immunosuppressive effect, *Br J Ophthalmol* 69:600-603, 1985.
24. Foulks GN, Sanfilippo F: Beneficial effects of histocompatibility in high risk corneal transplantation, *Am J Ophthalmol* 94:622-629, 1982.
25. Foxwell BMJ, Ruffel B: The mechanisms of action of cyclosporine, *Cardiol Clin* 8(1):107-117, 1990.
26. Fries D et al: Prospective study of triple association: cyclosporine, corticosteroids, and azathioprine in immunologically high-risk renal transplant, *Transplant Proc* 27:1231-1234, 1985.
27. Gibbs DC, Batchelor JR, Werb A, et al: The influence of tissue-type compatibility on the fate of full-thickness corneal grafts, *Trans Ophthalmol Soc UK* 94:101-126, 1974.
28. Gillette TE, Chandler JW, Greiner JV: Langerhans cells of the ocular surface, *Ophthalmology* 89:700, 1982.
29. Gillis S, Crabtree GR, Smith KA: Glucocorticoid-induced inhibition of T-cell growth factor production; I. The effect on mitogen-induced lymphocyte proliferation, *J Immunol* 123:1624-1631, 1979.
30. Granelli-Piperno A, Andrus L, Steinman RM: Lymphokine and nonlymphokine mRNA levels in stimulated human T cells: kinetics, mitogen requirements, and effects of cyclosporin A, *J Exp Med* 163:922, 1986.
31. Griffin PJA, Da Costa G, Salaman JR: A controlled trial of steroids in cyclosporine-treated renal transplant patients, *Transplantation* 43:505, 1987.
32. Harding MW, Handschumacher RE: Cyclophilin, a primary target molecule for cyclosporine: structural and functional implications, *Transplantation* 46:29S, 1988.
33. Harding MW, Galat A, Uehling DE, et al: A receptor for the immunosuppressant FK506 is a *cis-trans* peptidyl-prolyl isomerase, *Nature* 341:758-760, 1989.
34. Hess AD, Colombani PM: Mechanism of action: in vitro studies, *Prog Allergy* 38:198-221, 1986.
35. Illner W-D et al: Cyclosporine in combination with azathioprine and steroids in cadaveric renal transplant, *Transplant Proc* 27:1181-1184, 1985.
36. Inamura N, Nakahara K, Kino T, et al: Prolongation of skin allograft survival in rats by a novel immunosuppressive agent, FK 506, *Transplantation* 45:206-209, 1988.

37. Iwasawa H, Shinichi K, Daishiro, et al: Synthesis of (−)-15-deoxyspergualin and (−)-spergualin-15-phosphate, *J Antibiot* 12:1665, 1982.

38. Kahan BD et al: Cyclosporine immunosuppression mitigates immunologic risk factors in renal allotransplantation, *Transplant Proc XV*, 4:2469-2478, 1983.

39. Kaufman HE: Practical considerations in the selection of anti-inflammatory agents, *Trans Am Acad Ophthalmol Otolaryngol* 79:89, 1975.

40. Keown PA: Optimizing cyclosporine therapy: dose, levels and monitering, *Transplant Proc* 20(suppl 2):382-389, 1988.

41. Khodadoust AA: The allograft rejection reaction: the leading cause of late failure of clinical corneal grafts. In Porter R, Knight J, editors: *Corneal graft failure,* Amsterdam, 1973, Elsevier, pp 151-167.

42. Kino TH, Hatanaka M, Hashimoto M, et al: FK-506, a novel immunosuppressant isolated from a *Streptomyces.* I. Fermentation, isolation, and physico-chemical and biological characteristics, *J Antibiot* 40(9):1249, 1987.

43. Klaus GGB, Hawrylowicz CM: Activation and proliferation signals in mouse B cells II. Evidence for activation (G0 to G1) signals differing in sensitivity to cyclosporine, *Eur J Immunol* 14:250, 1984.

44. Lindholm A, Zachariae H, Reitamo HH, et al: Is cyclosporine blood concentration monitoring necessary in patients treated for severe chronic plaque form psoriasis? *Transplant Proc* 22:1293-1295, 1990.

45. MacKay IR, Bignel JL, Smith PH, et al: Prevention of corneal-graft failure with the immunosuppressive drug azathioprine, *Lancet* 7514:479, 1967.

46. Male D, Champion B, Cooke A: *Advanced immunology:* antigen processing and presentation; and cytotoxic lymphocytes, Philadelphia, 1987, Lippincott, pp 6.1-7.9.

47. Male D, Champion B, Cooke A: *Advanced immunology:* immunoregulation, Philadelphia, 1987, Lippincott, pp 10.1-10.17.

48. Morris RE, Wu J, Shorthouse R: A study of the contrasting effects of cyclosporine, FK 506, and rapamycin on the suppression of allograft rejection, *Transplant Proc* 22(4):1638-1641, 1990.

49. Nayak SK, Binder P: The growth of endothelium from human corneal rims in tissue culture, *Invest Ophthalmol Vis Sci* 25:1213-1216, 1984.

50. Niederkorn JY, Callanan D, Ross JR: Prevention of the induction of allospecific cytotoxic T lymphocyte and delayed-type hypersensitivity responses by ultraviolet irradiation of corneal allografts, *Transplantation* 50:281-286, 1990.

51. Ochiai T, Nagata M, Nakajima K, et al: Studies of the effects of FK506 on renal allografting in the beagle dog, *Transplantation* 44:729, 1987.

52. Ochiai T, Sakamoto K, Nagata M, et al: Studies on FK506 in experimental organ transplantation, *Transplant Proc* 20(suppl 1):209-214, 1988.

53. Uchida D, Yamada N, Orihara A, et al: Minimal low dosage of cyclosporine therapy in renal transplantation by careful monitoring of high-performance liquid chromatography whole blood trough levels, *Transplant Proc* 20(suppl 2):394-401, 1988.

54. Oyer PE et al: Cyclosporin in cardiac transplantations: a 2.5 year follow-up, *Trans Proc XV* 4:2552-2564, 1983.

55. Ray-Keil L, Gillette TE, Chandler JW: Murine heterotopic corneal transplantation: reduction in rejection rates by pretreatment of donor corneas with ultraviolet light, *Invest Ophthalmol Vis Sci* 26(3 suppl):78, 1985.

56. Ray-Keil L, Chandler JW: Reduction in the incidence of rejection of heterotopic murine corneal transplants by pretreatment with ultraviolet radiation, *Transplantation* 42:403-406, 1986.

57. Reem GH, Cook LA, Vilček JV: Gamma interferon synthesis by human thymocytes and T lymphocytes inhibited by cyclosporin A, *Science* 221:63-65, 1983.

58. Reichenspurner H, Hildebrandt A, Human PA, et al: 15-Deoxyspergualin for induction of graft nonreactivity after cardiac and renal allotransplantation in primates, *Transplantation* 50:181, 1990.

59. Samples JR, Binder PS, Nayak SK: Propagation of human corneal endothelium in vitro effect of growth factors, *Exp Eye Res* 52:121-128, 1991.

60. Sanfilippo F, MacQueen JM, Vaughn WK, Foulks GN: Reduced graft rejection with good HLA-A matching in high-risk corneal transplantation, *N Engl J Med* 315:29-35, 1986.

61. Sehgal SN, Baker H, Vezina C: Rapamycin (AY-22, 989), a new antifungal antibiotic II: fermentation, isolation, and characterization, *J Antibiot* 28:727-732, 1975.

62. Siekierka JJ, Hung SHY, Poe M, et al: A cytosolic binding protein for the immunosuppressant FK506 has peptidyl-prolyl isomerase activity but is distinct from cyclophilin, *Nature* 341:755-757, 1989.

63. Slapak M, Geoghegan T, Digard N, et al: The use of low-dose cyclosporine A in combination with azathioprine and steroids in renal transplantation, *Transplant Proc* 19(2 suppl 2):41-45, 1987.

64. Smith RS: Corneal transplantation. In Cerilli GJ, editor: *Organ transplantation and replacement*, Philadelphia, 1988, Lippincott, pp 625-628.

65. Sommer BG, Henry M, Ferguson RM: *Transplantation* 43:85, 1987.

66. Starzl TE, Fung JJ: Transplantation, *JAMA* 263:2686-2687, 1990.

67. Starzl TE et al: The Colorado-Pittsburgh cadaveric renal transplantation study with cyclosporine, *Trans Proc XV* 4:2459-2462, 1983.

68. Starzl TE et al: Report of Colorado-Pittsburgh liver transplantation studies, *Trans Proc XV* 4:2582-2585, 1983.

69. Stulting, RD, Waring, GO, Bridges, WZ Cavanagh, HD: Effect of donor epithelium on corneal transplant survival, *Ophthalmology* 95:803, 1988.

70. Takeuchi T, Iinuma H, Kunimoto S, et al: A new antitumor antibiotic, spergualin: isolation and antitumor activity, *J Antibiot* 34:1619, 1981.

71. Thomson AW: Interspecies comparison of the immunosuppressive efficacy and safety of FK 506, *Transplant Proc* 22(suppl 1):100-105, 1990.

72. Todo S, Ueda Y, Demetris JA, et al: Immunosuppression of canine, monkey and baboon allografts by FK-506, with special reference to synergism with other drugs and to tolerance induction, *Surgery* 104:239, 1988.
Uchida D et al, see reference 53.

73. Ueda H, Wayne HW, Yuk-Chun C, et al: The mechanism of synergistic interaction between anti-interleukin 2 receptor monoclonal antibody and cyclosporine therapy in rat recipients of organ allografts, *Transplantation* 50:545-550, 1990.

74. Umezawa H, Hayashi M, Abe F, et al: Immunosuppressive activities of 15-deoxyspergualin in animals, *J Antibiot* 38:283, 1985.

75. Völker-Dieben, HJ, Kok-van Alphen CC, Krut PJ: Advances and disappointments, indications and restrictions regarding HLA matched corneal grafts in high risk cases, *Doc Ophthalmol* 46:219, 1979.

76. Walter P, Thies J, Harbauer G, et al: Allogeneic heart transplantation in the rat with a new antitumoral drug—15-deoxyspergualin, *Transplant Proc* 21:530, 1986.

77. Walter P, Bernhard U, Seitz G, et al: Xenogeneic heart transplantation with 15-deoxyspergualin: prolongation of graft survival, *Transplant Proc* 19:3993, 1987.

78. Williams KA, Coster KJ: The role of the limbus in corneal allograft rejection, *Eye* 3:158, 1989.

79. Winman K, Cunman B, Forsum V, et al: Occurance of Ia (II) antigen on tissue of non-lymphoid origin, *Nature* 276:711, 1978.

80. Young E, Olkowski ST, Dana M, et al: Pretreatment of donor corneal endothelium with ultraviolet-B irradiation, *Transplant Proc* 21:3145-3146, 1989.

81. Zeevi A, Duquesnoy R, Eiras G, et al: Immunosuppressive effect of FK-506 on in vitro lymphocyte alloactivation: synergism with cyclosporine A, *Transplant Proc* 19(supp 6):40, 1987.

82. Dickneite G, Schorlemmer HU, Sedlacek HH: Decrease of mononuclear phagocyte cell functions and prolongation of graft survival in experimental transplantation by (±)-15-deoxyspergualin, *Int J Immunopharmacol* 9:559-565, 1987.

83. Dickneite G, Schorlemmer HU, Sedlacek HH, et al: Suppression of macrophage function and prolongation of graft survival by the new guanidinic-like structure, 15-deoxyspergualin, *Transplant Proc* 19:1301-1304, 1987.

84. Suzuki S, Kanashiro M, Watanabe H, Amemiya H: Therapeutic effect of 15-deoxyspergualin on acute graft rejection detected by ^{31}P nuclear magnetic resonance spectrography, and its effect on rat heart transplantation, *Transplantation* 46:669, 1988.

85. Olsen TW, Holland EJ, et al: Suppression of graft rejection using deoxyspergualine in the allogeneic rat penetrating keratoplasty model, *ARVO Abstracts*, pp 780, 1991.

Chapter 23

Postkeratoplasty Infections

JEFFREY D. ROBINSON

ROBERT A. HYNDIUK

The major objectives of this chapter are (1) to review the incidence and microbiologic spectrum of infectious keratitis and endophthalmitis among patients after penetrating keratoplasty, (2) to discuss the risk factors in the development of these infections, and (3) to emphasize techniques for prevention of these serious complications.

INFECTIOUS KERATITIS

Multiple retrospective studies and case reports regarding infectious keratitis after penetrating keratoplasty have been published.* The reported incidence rates range from 1.8% to 4.9% in the United States[41,73] to 11.9%[2] in Saudi Arabia. Approximately 40% of infections occurred within the first 6 months after transplantation, with the majority occurring within the first year.[18,27] The median interval between penetrating keratoplasty and infection varied from 5.5 to 10 months.[5,73]

The studies we reviewed showed a predominance of gram-positive bacterial infections, especially *Staphylococcus* species, despite a wide distribution of geographic locations. The most common organism isolated from several of the larger, more recent series are summarized in Table 23-1. In the majority of studies we reviewed, the incidence of fungal keratitis was uncommon (0 to 14%), with *Candida albicans* being the most frequent organism isolated.[5,18,73] The high incidence (34 cases) of fungal keratitis in the series reported by Harris and colleagues was attrib-

uted to possible geographic variation and higher risk patients with significant ocular surface disease or altered immune function.[27] Several cases of infectious crystalline keratopathy and *Acanthamoeba* keratitis have also been reported.[24,36,40,51,58,71]

Penetrating keratoplasties are often performed on eyes with compromised ocular defense mechanisms, rendering them more susceptible to infection. The preoperative indications for penetrating keratoplasty before infection in the series of studies we reviewed was highly variable. No increased risk was associated with any preoperative diagnosis except possibly herpes simplex keratitis[73] and grafts performed for complications of previous infectious keratitis.[5] As a rule, healthier eyes, such as those with keratoconus, were more resistant to infection than debilitated eyes with ongoing inflammatory or infectious processes.

Infectious keratitis that occurs in the early postoperative period may arise from intraoperative contamination, recurrent host disease, or infected donor material. Multiple possible risk factors were identified for developing late postoperative infection[2,5,18,27,73] (see Box, p. 270). Harris and co-workers reported 108 ulcers and 92 (85%) were associated with three factors: exposed sutures, contact lens wear, and epithelial defects.[27] Al-Hazzaa and co-workers found evidence of trachoma in 85% of cases of keratoplasty-related infections.[2]

Suture-related problems were a common predisposing factor. All studies we reviewed used standard interrupted or continuous 10-0 nylon sutures. A higher incidence of infection with interrupted su-

---

*References 2, 5, 14, 18, 25, 27, 31, 41, 45, 73, 77, 78.

Table 23-1. Organisms Isolated (number of cases)

	Fong et al.[18] Massachusetts, 1988	Harris et al.[27] Georgia, 1988	Hyndiuk et al.[31] Wisconsin, 1991	Al-Hazzaa,[2] Saudi Arabia, 1988
Gram positive				
Staphylococcus aureus	14	12	2	5
Coagulase-negative staphylococci	12	20	20	24
Corynebacterium diphtheriae	—	1	5	—
Streptococcus pneumoniae	5	6	1	29
β-Hemolytic streptococci	4	—	2	—
α-Hemolytic streptococci	3	2	4	5
Gram negative				
Serratia marcescens	8	9	2	—
Pseudomonas aeruginosa	7	7	5	13
Klebsiella species	3	3	1	—
Proteus mirabilis	1	6	1	—
Haemophilus species	1	1	1	5
Moraxella species	—	5	—	5
Fungi				
Candida species	3	33	3	—
Penicillium species	1	1	1	—

PREDISPOSING FACTORS

GRAFT PROBLEMS

Epithelial defects
Exposed sutures
Contact lens wear
Graft failure
Recent rejection episode
Wound dehiscence

OOCULAR SURFACE DISEASE

Dry eye syndrome
Mucosal scarring diseases (cicatricial pemphigoid, Stevens-Johnson syndrome, alkali burns)
Trichiasis/trachoma

TOPICAL MEDICATION

Corticosteroids

SYSTEMIC DISEASES

Diabetes mellitus
Systemic immunosuppression
Atopic disease

---

tures has been reported.[56] Fong and colleagues reported suture abscesses in 50% of their cases the first year after keratoplasty.[18]

It is important in reducing the risk of infection to ensure that all sutures are secure, the knots are buried, and the suture is covered by epithelium postoperatively. Exposed sutures breach the epithelial surface and normal barrier function, thus providing for initiation of the infection cascade with adhesion of the organism, penetration, and invasion into the corneal stroma.[30,70] Lint, suture fragments, and foreign debris may also be trapped by sutures and act as an "infectious wick." To this end, we avoid the use of cotton patches after the first postoperative day. We routinely check all patients with fluorescein to document an intact wound surface in the first week postoperatively before extending the length between follow-up visits. All loose sutures should be replaced and any foreign material (lint, debris, and so forth) removed from the suture tract. Unfortunately, wound remodeling, scar contracture, and cheese-wiring of inflamed stroma may loosen and expose previously secure sutures. Nylon suture biodegradation and rupture can also occur, frequently within 2 to 5 years postoperatively. Patients should be warned of the risks of suture abscess with loose or ruptured sutures and instructed to report any foreign-body sensation or irritation within 24 to 48 hours.

We manage loose or ruptured sutures aggres-

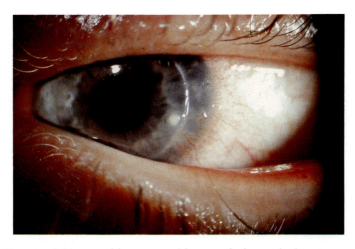

Fig. 23-1. Twenty-eight-year-old woman with wound abscess in keratoconus graft observed 1 day after suture removal. Heavy coagulase-positive *Staphylococcus aureus* was isolated and prompt treatment with gentamicin, 8 mg/ml, topically resulted in rapid resolution.

sively, as if the exposed suture represented a microabscess. After suture removal, we recommend a short aggressive course of prophylactic topical antibiotic for 2 days with initial and morning loading doses to maximize peak antibiotic concentrations, that is, tobramycin 0.3% or ciprofloxacin 0.3%—one drop every 5 minutes 5 times for a loading dose and then every 2 hours while awake for approximately 2 days or until the barrier function is normalized and no evidence of infection is noted. If a suture abscess is present (Fig. 23-1), we remove the offending suture and initiate early aggressive topical antibiotic treatment following standard protocols for infectious keratitis.[32,33] The choice of initial antibacterial or antifungal therapy should be based on gram stain if definitive, but usually broad-spectrum therapy is the most appropriate. Frequent fortified topical antibiotics that cover a broad spectrum of bacterial pathogens or frequent ciprofloxacin 0.3% solution should be used. Hospitalization may be required depending on the frequency of drops needed, severity of infection, and patient compliance.

Contact lens–associated microbial keratitis is another common risk factor for postkeratoplasty infection.[18,27,57,69] Fong and co-workers[18] reported 18 cases; 6 of 10 (60%) bandage contact lens infections were associated with gram-positive bacterial infection *(Staphylococcus epidermidis, S. aureus)*. In contrast, 6 of 8 (75%) aphakic hydrophilic extended-wear contact lens infections had gram-negative isolates *(S. marcescens, Pseudomonas aeruginosa)*. This was similar to results obtained in other extended-wear contact lens–associated microbial keratitis studies.[1,9] In contrast, Harris and co-workers reported 33 cases with

no increased incidence of gram-negative infections.[27] To prevent infection, patients should be educated on contact lens care and instructed to report early warning signs of infection immediately. Fortunately the use of aphakic contact lenses has diminished because of the use of intraocular lenses. Therapeutic bandage contact lenses are used by many surgeons for surface problems, and caution in their use is necessary because of the known risk factors in contact lens–related infectious keratitis.[57]

Punctate epithelial erosions or *epithelial defects* are another important predisposing factor. Harris and colleagues reported that these factors predated the ulcer in 55% of their cases.[27] Prophylactic preoperative treatment of preexisting factors such as exposure, dry eyes, and trichiasis is important. Every attempt should be made to improve the ocular environment with tear substitutes, punctal occlusion (plugs or permanent), lid margin hygiene, and lid surgery such as partial tarsorrhaphy and repair of spastic entropion. We routinely document preoperative Schirmer's testing on all keratoplasty and cataract patients and implant punctal plugs at the time of surgery if significant dryness exists. We also warn patients of the possibility of occlusion therapy being necessary postoperatively. We manage epithelial defects with aggressive lubrication or conservative occlusive therapy with antibiotic ointment. If this fails, Frost sutures or temporary suture lid closure may be necessary for 2 to 8 weeks. We do not routinely use or recommend bandage contact lenses or collagen shields in postgraft surface problems. Again, regular close follow-up examinations and patient education are important for detection of early infection.

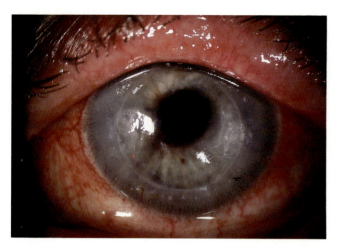

Fig. 23-2. Seventy-year-old woman with double wound abscess at 3 and 9 o'clock positions 10 months after penetrating keratoplasty in Fuchs' dystrophy. Smears showed gram-positive cocci and yeastlike organisms with *Candida* grown on culture. Treatment with natamycin (Pimaracin), neosporin, and erythromycin resulted in slow but complete healing and maintenance of graft clarity.

Topical corticosteroids are necessary in most keratoplasty patients but are a two-edged sword. They may impair host defense mechanisms allowing microbial superinfection. A high incidence of *Staphylococcus epidermidis* and *Candida* infections (Fig. 23-2) were reported in many series.[18,27,31] In a study of corneal ulcers in nonoperated eyes in South Florida by Liesegang and colleagues, they reported *S. epidermidis* as the etiologic agent in only 8% and *Candida albicans* in 7% of fungal cases.[46] These organisms are opportunistic in compromised tissues such as corneal grafts undergoing chronic immunosuppressive therapy. Corticosteroids sometimes mask the early signs of infection and enhance tissue invasion making early detection and treatment of infection an initial challenge. Corticosteroid usage has improved the overall prognosis of patients undergoing corneal transplants, and their risk in usage is known by all. Caution in their use should be practiced by all physicians, especially in long-term moderate or high-dose need situations.

The visual sequelae of graft infections may be devastating. Driebe and co-workers reported that only 14% of their patients achieved a final visual acuity greater than 6/60.[14] In Saudi Arabia, of 113 cases reported, only 27 (24%) had a final visual acuity of 20/400 or better.[2] In the studies we reviewed, corneal perforation or wound dehiscence occurred in approximately 10% to 20%.[5,18,27] Infection progressed to endophthalmitis in 4% to 13%, with many of

these eyes losing light perception.[5,18,27] The ocular morbidity was also serious, with a large proportion of affected patients losing graft clarity and requiring emergency or elective regrafting (30% to 60%).[18,27]

In summary, the overall prognosis for postoperative infectious keratitis may be poor. Infections are frequently far advanced because of early signs of infection being masked by poor graft innervation and of topical corticosteroid usage. This complication, though not common, carries high ocular morbidity and therefore demands early recognition and aggressive treatment. Careful attention to high-risk factors such as loose, broken, or debris-catching sutures, epithelial defects, and contact lens wearers will aid in prevention. All patients should be advised to seek treatment immediately if they feel a persistent foreign-body sensation or see a "white spot" on their eye, or if any abnormality persists for more than 24 hours. The incidence of postoperative bacterial keratitis can be minimized by appropriate patient education as well as good postoperative management of associated ocular conditions.

ENDOPHTHALMITIS

Endophthalmitis after penetrating keratoplasty may occur early or late postoperatively often with disastrous consequences. Fortunately, there is a relatively low incidence reported ranging from 0.1%[59] to 2%.[26] It has been estimated that the incidence of postkeratoplasty endophthalmitis from all causes is about the same as that after cataract extraction.[44] Despite the low incidence, however, study of postkeratoplasty endophthalmitis is important because this complication both is potentially preventable and has devastating visual consequences.

Endophthalmitis in the immediate postoperative period can usually be attributed to contamination of donor material or breaks in surgical technique. Reported incidences of bacterial contamination in donor eyes range from 12.4% to 100%.[59,62] Although the most common organism cultured from donor corneas is *Staphylococcus epidermidis*, no one organism is responsible for most infections.[59,62] Multiple gram-positive and gram-negative bacteria and fungi have been reported.[6,17,23,26,35,42-44,54,65,66,75]

Endophthalmitis has been documented from the use of tissue from donors with previous bacterial sepsis. Keates and colleagues found 7 of 20 corneas obtained from donors with systemic infections at the time of death to be culture positive, whereas none of the 25 eyes obtained from the nonseptic donors was positive.[38] Likewise, Khodadoust and colleagues reported 2 cases of *Escherichia coli* endophthalmitis after the use of tissue from a septic patient dying from peritonitis.[39] We have also experienced two cases of *P. aeruginosa* endophthalmitis after the use of tissue from an automobile accident ICU patient and two cases of pneumococcal endophthalmitis after the use of tissue from a patient dying from unexplained septicemia. To reduce the risk of transmission, potential donors are routinely screened by eye bank personnel and rejected if recent infection was a possibility.

Contaminated donor tissue is a commonly reported cause for postkeratoplasty infection. Multiple gentamicin-resistant organisms and streptococcal species have been reported to cause donor-to-host transmission of infection.* Currently gentamicin sulfate is still the most common antibiotic added to most storage media. However, it has poor activity against most streptococci and anaerobic organisms. In fact, gentamicin-based media has been used to isolate many types of streptococci, including β-hemolytic streptococci and pneumococci.[7,13] Fortunately, despite a relatively high incidence of culture-positive donor rims, the incidence of infection is still very low. Leveille and colleagues reviewed 1876 penetrating keratoplasties; 230 had positive donor rim cultures, and this resulted in only three cases of endophthalmitis.[44] In most cases, organisms transmitted by donor corneas are probably destroyed by host defenses or postoperative antibiotics.

To minimize this serious complication, we routinely screen all donor tissue preoperatively to evaluate for microbial infiltrates and prophylactically treat patients with broad-spectrum intraoperative subconjunctival and topical antibiotics, along with postoperative topical antibiotics. Postoperatively we routinely use topical ciprofloxacin 0.3% q.i.d. for 1 to 2 weeks, because of its broad spectrum and good tolerance by the stressed epithelium, and antibiotic ointment at bedtime (erythromycin or bacitracin-polymyxin) until significant ocular surface disease has resolved. Overall, infection occurring early after penetrating keratoplasty should raise the suspicion of a possible aminoglycoside-resistant organism playing a role. Current research is being done to identify alternative antibiotics to add to storage media to further reduce the risk of donor-transmitted infection. Vancomycin has recently been reported to be a promising addition to corneal storage media because of its efficacy and safety.[37,47,50]

Despite treatment, the prognosis for postkeratoplasty endophthalmitis is extremely poor. Guss and co-workers[26] reported 11 cases with the following posttreatment visual acuities: 20/200 (1), 20/400 (1), light perception (3), and no light perception (6). Gi-

rard and co-workers[23] reported five cases: 20/40 (1), 20/200 (1), light perception (1), and no light perception (2). Similar poor results were reported in multiple other case reports.

In conclusion, multiple causes for postoperative endophthalmitis after penetrating keratoplasty have been reported. Early cases within the first 72 hours usually result from donor-to-media contamination, or poor aseptic technique. Preoperatively, patients should be screened for significant ocular surface disease, and factors such as lid margin disease and dacryocystitis should be treated appropriately. At the time of surgery all donor rims should be cultured and broad-spectrum antibiotics administered. If a donor rim culture is positive, the patient may need to be observed more closely in follow-up examination (even though positive rim cultures are rarely a problem in our experience). Endophthalmitis in the late postoperative period is usually secondary to infectious keratitis but may complicate suture removal or relaxing incisions.[4,10,19,76] Again, the short-term aggressive use of prophylactic antibiotics and close follow-up observation is warranted after these procedures. Despite the low incidence, it is imperative to minimize the risk for infection by maintaining stringent screening and decontamination procedures in the eye bank, monitoring corneoscleral rim cultures, and developing new antimicrobials to supplement or replace gentamicin.

OTHER INFECTIONS

Sporadic transmission of viral infections including rabies[29,72] and Creutzfeldt-Jakob virus[15] has been reported. Transmission of these organisms can be avoided by rejection of tissue from patients dying of unknown neurologic or central nervous system diseases. Two systemic viral illnesses with a greater potential for contagion are hepatitis B and acquired immunodeficiency syndrome. Recovery of both viruses from ocular tissue has been reported.[8,11,12,20,21,60,64] There are no documented cases of donor-to-host transmission of either infection despite actual transplantation of corneas from seropositive donors.[61] Again to reduce the possibility of transmission, all potential donors with known high-risk behaviors should be rejected, and donor serum should be screened for antibodies against the hepatitis B and human immunodeficiency virus antigens.

SUMMARY

The overall prognosis for serious postkeratoplasty infectious keratitis and endophthalmitis may be poor. Fortunately the incidence of both infections is relatively uncommon. Early recognition of infection

---

*References 3, 16, 23, 28, 34, 44, 49, 52, 63, 67, 68.

and prompt treatment is of crucial importance. Careful attention to preoperative, operative, and postoperative factors will potentially reduce the risk of these devastating complications.

REFERENCES

1. Alfonso E, Mandelbaum S, Fox MJ, Forster RK: Ulcerative keratitis associated with contact lens wear, *Am J Ophthalmol* 101:429-433, 1986.
2. Al-Hazzaa SAF, Tabbara KF: Bacterial keratitis after penetrating keratoplasty, *Ophthalmology* 95:1504-1508, 1988.
3. Baer JC, Nirankari VS, Glaros DS: Streptococcal endophthalmitis from contaminated donor corneas after keratoplasty: clinical and laboratory investigations, *Arch Ophthalmol* 106:517-520, 1988.
4. Barak MH, Shapiro MB: Bacterial endophthalmitis following postkeratoplasty relaxing incisions, *Refract Corneal Surg* 6:271-272, 1990.
5. Bates AK, Kirkness CM, Ficker LA, et al: Microbial keratitis after penetrating keratoplasty, *Eye* 4:74-78, 1990.
6. Beyt BE, Waltman SR: Cryptococcal endophthalmitis after corneal transplantation, *N Engl J Med* 298:825, 1978.
7. Black WA, Van Buskirk F: Gentamicin as a selective agent for the isolation of beta haemolytic streptococci, *J Clin Pathol* 26:154-156, 1973.
8. Cantrill HL, Henry K, Jackson B, et al: Recovery of human immunodeficiency virus from ocular tissues in patients with acquired immune deficiency syndrome, *Ophthalmology* 95:1458-1462, 1988.
9. Cohen EJ, Laibson PR, Arentsen JJ, Clemons CS: Corneal ulcers associated with cosmetic extended wear soft contact lenses, *Ophthalmology* 94:109-114, 1987.
10. Confino J, Brown SI: Bacterial endophthalmitis associated with exposed monofilament sutures following corneal transplantation, *Am J Ophthalmol* 99:111-113, 1985.
11. Conway MD, Insler MS: The identification and incidence of human immunodeficiency virus antibodies and hepatitis B virus antigens in corneal donors, *Ophthalmology* 95:1463-1467, 1988.
12. Doro S, Navia BA, Kahn A, et al: Confirmation of HTLV-III virus in cornea, *Am J Ophthalmol* 102:390, 1986.
13. Dilworth JA, Stewart P, Gwaltney JM Jr, et al: Methods to improve detection of pneumococci in respiratory secretions, *J Clin Microbiol* 2:453-455, 1975.
14. Driebe WT, Stern GA: Microbial keratitis following corneal transplantation, *Cornea* 2:41-45, 1983.
15. Duffy P et al: Possible person-to-person transmission of Creutzfeldt-Jakob disease, *N Engl J Med* 290:692-693, 1974.
16. Escapini H Jr, Olson RJ, Kaufman HE: Donor cornea contamination with McCarey-Kaufman medium preservation, *Am J Ophthalmol* 88:59, 1979.
17. Fong LP, Gladstone D, Casey TA: Corneo-scleral rim cultures: donor contamination a case of fungal endophthalmitis transmitted by K-Sol stored cornea, *Eye* 2:670-676, 1988.
18. Fong LP, Ormerod LD, Kenyon KR, Foster CS: Microbial keratitis complicating penetrating keratoplasty, *Ophthalmology* 95:1269-1275, 1988.
19. Forstot SL, Abel R, Binder PS: Bacterial endophthalmitis following suture removal after penetrating keratoplasty, *Am J Ophthalmol* 80:509-512, 1975.
20. Fujikawa LS, Salahuddin SZ, Ablashi D, et al: HTLV-III in the tears of AIDS patients, *Ophthalmology* 93:1479-1481, 1986.
21. Fujikawa LS, Salahuddin SZ, Palestine AG, et al: Isolation of human T-lymphotropic virus type III from the tears of a patient with the acquired immunodeficiency syndrome, *Lancet* 2:529-530, 1985.
22. Gandhi SS, Lambert DW, Perry HD: Donor to host transmission of disease via corneal transplantation, *Surv Ophthalmol* 25:306-311, 1981.
23. Girard LJ: Bacterial endophthalmitis following the use of contaminated preserved corneal tissue, *Cornea* 1:255-257, 1982.
24. Gorovoy MS, Stern GA, Hood I, Allen MS: Intrastromal non-inflammatory bacterial colonization of a corneal graft, *Arch Ophthalmol* 101:1749, 1983.
25. Gross ND, Meyer RF: *Enterobacter cloacae* ulceration in a failed corneal graft: a case report, *Br J Ophthalmol* 69:542-544, 1985.
26. Guss RB, Koenig S, De La Pena W, et al: Endophthalmitis after penetrating keratoplasty, *Am J Ophthalmol* 95:651-658, 1983.
27. Harris DJ, Stulting RD, Waring GO, Wilson LA: Late bacterial and fungal keratitis after corneal transplantation, *Ophthalmology* 95:1450-1457, 1988.
28. Heidemann DG, Dunn SP, Haimann M: *Streptococcus salivarius* endophthalmitis from contaminated donor cornea after keratoplasty, *Am J Ophthalmol* 107:429-430, 1989.
29. Houff SA, Burton RC, Wilson RW, et al: Human-to-human transmission of rabies virus by corneal transplantation, *N Engl J Med* 300:603-604, 1979.
30. Hyndiuk RA: Experimental *Pseudomonas* keratitis. I. Sequential electron microscopy. II. Comparative therapy trials, *Trans Am Ophthalmol Soc* 79:540-624, 1981.
31. Hyndiuk RA, Kummerfeld KR, Wilmer Z: *Etiologic agents causing keratitis in Wisconsin.* Residents' Day Meeting, Medical College of Wisconsin, Milwaukee, Wisc, May 17, 1991.
32. Hyndiuk RA, Skorich D, Burd E: Bacterial keratitis. In Tabbara K, Hyndiuk R, editors: *Infections of the eye: diagnosis and management,* Boston, 1986, Little, Brown.
33. Hyndiuk RA, Snyder RW: Infectious diseases: bacterial keratitis. In Thoft R, Smolin G, editors: *The cornea,* ed 2, Boston, 1987, Little, Brown.
34. Insler MS, Cavanagh HD, Wilson LA: Gentamicin resistant *Pseudomonas* endophthalmitis after penetrating keratoplasty, *Br J Ophthalmol* 69:189-191, 1985.
35. Insler MS, Kook MS, Mani H, Peyman GA: *Citrobacter diversus* endophthalmitis following penetrating keratoplasty, *Am J Ophthalmol* 106:632-633, 1988.
36. James CB, McDonnell PJ, Falcon MG: Infectious crystalline keratopathy, *Br J Ophthalmol* 72:628-630, 1988.
37. Kattan HM, Pflugfelder SC: Corneal endothelial toxicity of vancomycin in corneal preservation media, *Invest Ophthalmol Vis Sci* 32(suppl):1063, 1991.
38. Keates RH, Misher KE, Rudinger D: Bacterial contamination of donor eyes, *Am J Ophthalmol* 84:617, 1977.
39. Khodadoust AA, Franklin RM: Transfer of bacterial infection by donor cornea in penetrating keratoplasty, *Am J Ophthalmol* 87:130-132, 1979.
40. Kincaid MC, Snip RC: Antibiotic resistance of crystalline bacterial ingrowth in a corneal graft, *Ophthalmic Surg* 18:268, 1987.
41. Lamensdorf M, Wilson LA, Waring GO, Cavanagh HD: Microbial keratitis after penetrating keratoplasty, *Ophthalmology* 89(suppl):124, 1982.
42. Larson PA, Lindstrom RL, Doughman DJ: *Torulopsis glabrata* endophthalmitis after keratoplasty with an organ cultured cornea, *Arch Ophthalmol* 96:1019, 1978.
43. LeFrancois M, Baum JL: *Flavobacterium* endophthalmitis following keratoplasty: use of a tissue culture medium—stored cornea, *Arch Ophthalmol* 94:1907-1909, 1976.

44. Leveille AS, McMullan FD, Cavanagh HD: Endophthalmitis following penetrating keratoplasty, *Ophthalmology* 90:38-39, 1983.

45. Levenson JE, Duffin RM, Gardner SK, Pettit TH: Dematiaceous fungal keratitis following penetrating keratoplasty, *Ophthalmic Surg* 15:578-582, 1984.

46. Liesegang TJ, Forster RK: Spectrum of microbial keratitis in South Florida, *Am J Ophthalmol* 90:38-47, 1980.

47. Lindquist TD, Roth BP, Fritsche TR: Safety and efficacy of vancomycin in corneal storage media, *Invest Ophthalmol Vis Sci* 32(suppl):1063, 1991.

48. Manuelidis EE, Angelo JN, Goygacz EJ, et al: Experimental Creutzfeldt-Jakob disease transmitted via the eye with infected cornea, *N Engl J Med* 296:1334-1336, 1977.

49. Matoba A, Moore MB, Merten JL, et al: Donor-to-host transmission of streptococcal infection by corneas stored in McCarey-Kaufman medium, *Cornea* 3:105-108, 1984.

50. Mavle M, Granus V, Snyder I, Macsai M: The effect of gentamicin, ciprofloxacin and vancomycin on gentamicin-resistant organisms in Optisol corneal storage medium, *Invest Ophthalmol Vis Sci* 32(suppl):1063, 1991.

51. Meisler DM, Langston RHS, Naab TJ, et al: Infectious crystalline keratopathy, *Am J Ophthalmol* 97:337-343, 1984.

52. Moore PJ, Linnemann CC Jr, Sanitato JJ, Binnion B: Pneumococcal endophthalmitis after corneal transplantation: control by modification of harvesting techniques, *Infect Control Hosp Epidemiol* 10:102-105, 1989.

53. Musch DC, Sugar A, Meyer RF: Demographic and predisposing factors in corneal ulceration, *Arch Ophthalmol* 101:1545-1548, 1983.

54. Nelson JD, Mindrup EA, Chung CK, et al: Fungal contamination in organ culture, *Arch Ophthalmol* 101:280-283, 1983.

55. Ormerod LD, Smith RE: Contact lens-associated microbial keratitis, *Arch Ophthalmol* 104:79-83, 1986.

56. Paglen PG, Webster RG Jr, Abbott RL: The advantages of interrupted sutures and a therapeutic lens in keratoplasty, *Ophthalmic Surg* 12:95-97, 1981.

57. Palmer ML, Hyndiuk RA: Contact lens–related infectious keratitis, *Curr Opin Infect Dis* 3:542-548, 1990.

58. Palmer ML, Lewis MT, Hyndiuk RA: Infectious crystalline keratopathy successfully treated with ciprofloxacin: a case report. (Publication pending.)

59. Pardos GJ, Gallagher MA: Microbial contamination of donor eyes, *Arch Ophthalmol* 100:1611-1613, 1982.

60. Pepose JS, Pardo F, Kessler JA, Kline R, et al: Screening cornea donors for antibodies against human immunodeficiency virus: efficacy of ELISA testing of cadaveric sera and aqueous humor, *Ophthalmology* 94:95-100, 1987.

61. Pepose JS, MacRae S, Quinn TC, Ward JW: Serologic markers after the transplantation of corneas from donors infected with human immunodeficiency virus, *Am J Ophthalmol* 103:798-801, 1987.

62. Polack FM, Locatcher-Khorazo D, Gutierrez E: Bacteriologic study of "donor" eyes, *Arch Ophthalmol* 78:219-225, 1987.

63. Poole T, Insler M: Contamination of donor cornea by gentamicin-resistant organisms, *Am J Ophthalmol* 97:560-564, 1984.

64. Raber IM, Freedman HM: Hepatitis B surface antigens in corneal donors, *Am J Ophthalmol* 104:255-258, 1987.

65. Rao GN, Aquavella JV: *Cephalosporium* endophthalmitis following penetrating keratoplasty, *Ophthalmic Surg* 10:34-37, 1979.

66. Saggau DD, Bourne WM, Sinkeldam IR, Roberts GD: Replication of fungi in K-Sol corneal preservation medium at 4° C, *Arch Ophthalmol* 104:1362-1363, 1986.

67. Schein OD, Miller JW, Wagoner MD: Panophthalmitis after penetrating keratoplasty, *Arch Ophthalmol* 107:21, 1989.

68. Shaw EL, Aquavella JU: Pneumococcal endophthalmitis following grafting of corneal tissue from a (cadaver) kidney donor, *Ann Ophthalmol* 9:435-440, 1977.

69. Smith SG, Lindstrom RL, Nelson JD, et al: Corneal ulcer infiltrate associated with soft contact lens use following penetrating keratoplasty, *Cornea* 3:131-134, 1984.

70. Snyder RW, Hyndiuk RA: Mechanisms of bacterial invasion of the cornea. In Duane TD, Jaeger EA, editors: *Biomedical foundations of ophthalmology*, Philadelphia, 1988, Lippincott.

71. Solomon JM, Hyndiuk RA, Koenig SB, Gradus MS: *Acanthamoeba* keratitis masquerading as corneal homograft rejection: a case report, *Arch Ophthalmol* 105:1326-1327, 1987.

72. Thongcharoen P et al: Human-to-human transmission of rabies via corneal transplant—Thailand, *MMWR* 30(37):473-474, 1981.

73. Tuberville AW, Wood TO: Corneal ulcers in corneal transplants, *Curr Eye Res* 1:479-485, 1981.

74. Viti A, Seetharama S, Snyder I, Schwab IR: Bacterial growth and the use of ciprofloxacin in MK media, *Invest Ophthalmol Vis Sci* 29(suppl):444, 1988.

75. Waltman SR, Beyt BE Jr: Cryptococcal endophthalmitis after corneal transplantation, *N Engl J Med* 298:825, 1978.

76. Weiss JL, Nelson JD, Lindstrom RL, Doughman DJ: Bacterial endophthalmitis following penetrating keratoplasty suture removal, *Cornea* 3:278-280, 1984-1985.

77. Wunsh SE, Boyle GL, Leopold IH, Littman ML: *Mycobacterium fortuitum* infection of the corneal graft, *Arch Ophthalmol* 82:602-607, 1969.

78. Zabel RW, Winegarden T, Holland EJ, Doughman DJ: *Acinetobacter* corneal ulcer after penetrating keratoplasty, *Am J Ophthalmol* 107:677-678, 1989.

Chapter 24

Astigmatism

Preoperative and operative factors

THOMAS A. CASEY

If rejection is the limiting factor in corneal transplantation, postoperative astigmatism causes the greatest disappointment to the patient, particularly in "simple" cases such as keratoconus where the patient expects more than a clear graft. The patient expects to be emmetropic and is surprised if spectacles with a large astigmatic error are prescribed, or if he has to resort to contact lenses. He or she may be disillusioned if refractive surgery has to be performed.

There are approximately 10 factors to be considered in reducing the risk of astigmatism. The *donor cornea* is usually ignored because this is outside our control. However, we know that statistically we occasionally graft an astigmatic cornea, just as we assume that we occasionally graft a cornea that has been infected with the herpes virus—possibly sometime in the distant past—otherwise how can we explain the rare instances of a central dendritic ulcer in a patient who has a graft for keratoconus. We have two sources of information about the donor cornea: the eye bank technician could check the spectacles worn by the deceased or inquire from the family, or corneoscopy or computerized corneoscopy could be performed (Fig. 24-1).

The second factor to be considered is perhaps a utopian ideal, but it is possible. This is the *method of cutting the graft*. Few surgeons nowadays cut from the whole eye, but when this method is used, varying edge shapes are formed. They are never vertical. They usually slope outwards; that is, the "endothelial" diameter is greater than the "epithelial," and this is considered to be attributable to the greater re-

sistance from Descemet's membrane. The graft edge also has a characteristic corkscrew edge. This method of cutting the graft is no longer advised.

Which of the many punches on the market are recommended, and do they all give a circular graft with a regular edge?

Apart from the ideal shape and edge, not all punches perform perfectly all the time. Some with fancy names, such as the guillotine, have a 50% failure rate, and the gymnastics of releasing a cut disc from the barrel of the trephine or trying to cut an incompletely severed corneal button are bound to lead to an irregular edge and astigmatism. I recommend three systems: the Hanna-Moria (Fig. 24-2), a French system that is expensive but very well engineered, my own simple punch (of no proprietary interest), which has been in use for 18 years, and the Krumeich system. It is somewhat disappointing that Pouliquen, in whose department the Hanna-Moria trephine was designed, has not produced a significant decrease in astigmatism. Is a punch necessary? Yes. It is difficult to match the centration and regular edge using the conventional trephine.

It is important to remember that the punched corneal disc is smaller than one cut from the whole eye. An 8 mm punched cornea emerges as 7.8 mm in diameter. *The size of the corneoscleral disc that is placed in the trephine* is important: the width of the scleral rim must be regular, and so it is probably preferable for the technician to use, say, a 15 mm trephine rather than cutting a freehand scleral rim. One of the many problems in using infant donor corneas is that of obtaining centration because the infant cornea may be less than 10 mm in diameter. In the special case of the infant donor, the keratometry reading may be 55 K, whereas the "well" of the punching system may be designed for a cornea of 42 K.

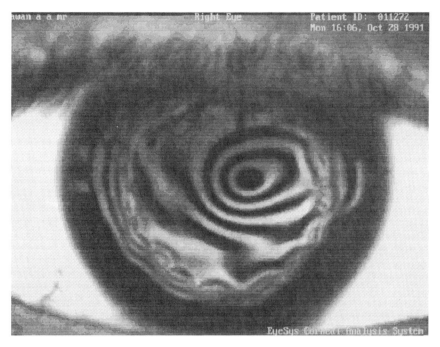

Fig. 24-1. Attempted corneal analysis on donor cornea.

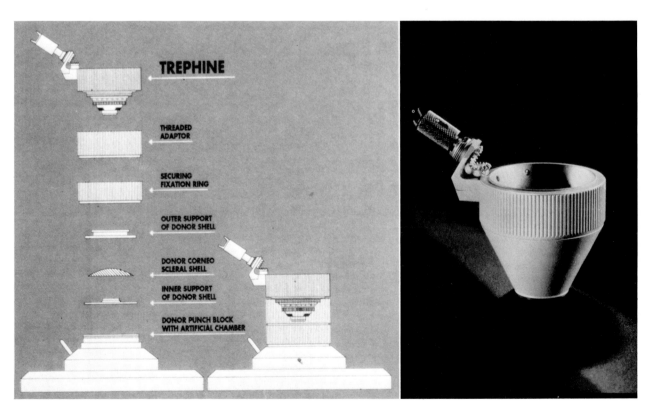

Fig. 24-2. Hanna-Moria trephine system.

The *recipient corneal disease* is an important factor. In herpetic keratitis, with vascularization and possibly thinning in the periphery, there will be a differential healing rate, and so a case may be made for interrupted sutures. However, it is in keratoconus, where these factors are absent, that there may be pronounced astigmatism, which leads to so much patient dissatisfaction.

The *intraocular pressure* is important: if it is too low, the corneal shape will mirror that found in trephining hypotonous donor eyes. In such cases of very low intraocular pressure, the trephine is used as a marker and the remainder of the dissection is with a blade or diamond knife. On the other hand, if the pressure is too high, trephination will result in early opening of the anterior chamber but in a small area only.

External compression factors. An elliptical opening is the most common error in grafting (Fig. 24-3). Why does this occur? One factor is the speculum, no matter how delicate. Another factor is the use of superior and inferior recti sutures, which may cause distortion of the globe. But exposure is essential; therefore lid sutures are possibly best. A further factor is the fixation forceps: this undoubtedly causes distortion. The circular fixation used by radial keratotomy surgeons is probably an advantage. The Flieringa type of scleral support ring can cause distortion and resultant astigmatism unless it is evenly fixated and ring sutures are cut before final tying of the transplant sutures.

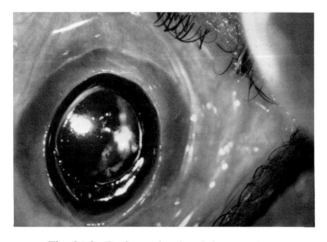

Fig. 24-3. Oval opening in triple procedure.

Eccentric trephination can cause astigmatism. It may be possible to judge the optic axis, and so one must reach a compromise by identifying the center of the cornea and marking it with a cautery. However, with the conventional trephine eccentration may still occur. The new Hessberg trephine overcomes some of these problems, and the Hanna trephining system is even better.

Most surgeons now use *disparate-sized donor and recipient* trephine systems to reduce the risk of glaucoma, with 0.25 to 0.3 mm being probably the maximum if astigmatism is to be avoided. Even this may cause an increase in the already existing myopia of keratoconus patients.

Tissue malapposition is a major factor. Malapposition of donor and host may occur in several ways. There may be a disparity in thickness, either because the host is excessively thin in conditions such as pellucid marginal degeneration, or in pseudophakic bullous keratopathy, where there is often an increase in thickness of 50% (in which case preoperative glycerol drops may help). Eye bank corneas (as compared with those taken from the whole eye) are usually of a standard thickness, and so the only exception is that of corneas stored in a tissue culture medium (widely used in Europe).

Suturing is without doubt the major cause of astigmatism, and there is no agreement on any particular type of suturing. Good results can be achieved by several techniques. Beginners are usually taught to take a 1.5 mm "bite" on the donor and a 2.5 mm "bite" on the recipient. They are told that the depth should be to the level of Descemet's membrane and that sutures that pass through the endothelium are bad. Nevertheless many surgeons make a "through-and-through" suture without any untoward effects. The placement of the four cardinal sutures is important, and placement of the second at 6 o'clock is vital. If this suture is not exactly in line with the first, there will be a torsion and astigmatism in the graft.

The sutures must be equidistant, and various methods of assisting the surgeon's eye have been devised. Charleux of Lyon had "prongs" attached to his trephine, but the fluorescein marks are difficult to see. The various radial keratotomy (RK) marks are simple and helpful. In the Storz system there are holes in the "nest" of the punch, making 16 punctate marks on the disc (with methylene blue). I have found this method very disappointing. The point marks on the donor are virtually invisible. I insert the four cardinal sutures and then mark the donor and recipient with the RK marker. I have found it less messy to use the marking pen of the plastic surgeons rather than dipping the marker in methylene blue. Of course, if the cardinal sutures are not in good position, there is an inbuilt error, but these four sutures can be removed once the donor and recipient have been marked.

Interrupted sutures are the most rational sutures to insert, since removal of the odd suture can be done later to help reduce the astigmatism in the postoperative period. But why do most corneal surgeons use a continuous suture? Speed is an important factor if the surgeon has to perform three or four transplants in a session. Surgeons also know that knots—no matter how well buried—may attract vessels. A combination of the two is a reasonable compromise.

The double continuous antitorque suture of Troutman is elegant and rational but probably makes little difference to astigmatism.

Operative keratometry is a significant advance. Which keratometer is best? I and others believe that the Smirmaul (Fig. 24-4) has certain advantages, though its mires may be difficult to see. Surgeons have raised the objection that a regular cornea at the end of the operation is no guarantee that it will remain

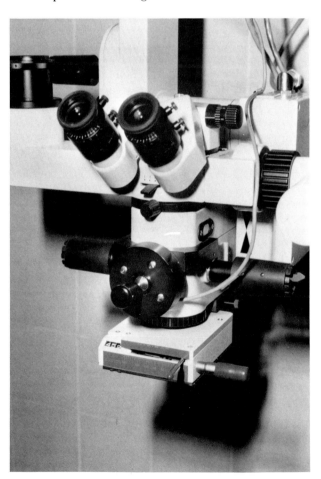

Fig. 24-4. Smirmaul intraoperative keratometer.

like this in the postoperative period. It is important that the running suture is tied (with a running knot) and that the chamber is reformed with balanced saline solution before an attempt is made to tighten parts of the cirumference where sutures are lax and to relax areas that are too tight.

The Krumeich trephine, an automated trephination system, is the newest and most exciting concept in reducing astigmatism. The donor button and the recipient opening are cut in exactly the same way and so are a perfect match. The corneoscleral disc is converted into a replica of the anterior chamber and is cut *externally*. The recipient eye is fixated with a suction system, and so there is no deformation of the globe.

Alas, the system costs 24,000 American dollars.

SUMMARY

Many factors are responsible for the development of astigmatism, and attention must be given in particular to the following aspects:

1. The intraocular pressure.
2. Avoiding distortion of the globe with the speculum, rectus sutures, and fixation forceps.
3. A suction trephine system is best, but if a conventional Franceschetti trephine is used, it should be perpendicular to the cornea, the minimum of pressure should be used, and the penetration depth should be controlled. The trephine should be sharp! Controlling perpendicularity is difficult. If any excess tissue occurs, it must be removed with scissors perpendicular to the wound.
4. Suturing must be meticulous, and some system of operative keratometry must be used to ensure that at the end of the operation, at least, there is minimal astigmatism. Other factors outside the operator's control may arise in the postoperative period.

REFERENCE
1. Casey TA, Mayer DJ: *Corneal grafting: principles and practice,* Philadelphia, 1984, Saunders.

Postkeratoplasty correction

SELECTIVE SUTURE REMOVAL
LINDA L. BURK

Astigmatism remains a significant obstacle in visual rehabilitation after penetrating keratoplasty. Important intraoperative factors related to postkeratoplasty astigmatism include trephination, wound configuration, wound healing, and suturing technique. New trephines, such as the suction trephine, have been advocated to obtain a round host bed and donor button with vertical edges. Wound healing is the most difficult to control because it depends on the individual patient. Modulation of wound healing with growth factors appears promising.

The surgeon may choose from a variety of suturing patterns[11] including single or double continuous running sutures, multiple interrupted sutures, or a combination of interrupted sutures and a running suture. Multiple interrupted sutures and a single interrupted suture require complete wound healing before suture removal. McNeill[12] described the adjustment of a single running 10-0 nylon with resultant significant decrease in postoperative astigmatism. Removal of either suture in the double running pattern can result in wide fluctuations in astigmatism.[4,13] The combination of multiple interrupted sutures and a continuous running suture allows for subsequent selective removal of interrupted sutures.[1-8,14] This technique permits early removal with minimal risk of wound dehiscence because the wound is supported by the continuous suture.

History. Selective suture removal to reduce postoperative astigmatism was first proposed by Cottingham[6,7] at the American Academy of Ophthalmology meeting in 1980. He used a combination of 12 interrupted 10-0 nylon sutures combined with a single continuous 12-bite nylon suture. With early selective removal of the interrupted suture he obtained a very low value of 1.5 diopters (D) of astigmatism. This method was attractive because of the quick rehabilitation time. It was believed that this was setting the cornea in a more spherical shape for long-term wound healing, thus reducing the final astigmatism when all sutures were removed. Subsequently, Stainer and co-workers[14] described a reduction in astigmatism using only 8 interrupted sutures and a 16-bite running suture. Binder[1] demonstrated that this technique could modify corneal curvature to reduce astigmatism. The majority of patients were stable in 7 months with about 3 D of residual astigmatism.

In 1986 Burk and colleagues[3,4] presented results on a retrospective study of 154 eyes that had selective suture removal. Seventy-five percent of patients required 5 of the 12 sutures removed to achieve less than or equal to 3 D of astigmatism. This occurred at about 5 months after penetrating keratoplasty. This led to a subsequent study[5] involving the timing of suture removal. The goal was to identify the offending tight sutures in the early postoperative period and remove them as early as possible. Two separate groups of consecutive patients with different timing of suture removal were studied. One group had multiple interrupted sutures removed during a single clinic visit; the other had only one suture removed on each successive clinical visit. The two series of patients reported indicate that removal of one interrupted suture on a series of sequential visits probably gives better control over the final amount of astigmatism than attempting to remove all the tight sutures required to achieve 3 D or less of astigmatism at a single visit. Patients in the sequential group achieved 1.9 D of astigmatism at 1 year compared to 3.1 D in the group in which sutures were removed in a single visit. The major drawback in attempting to remove all the tight sutures at a single visit was the large change in astigmatism that occurred between the end of the first visit and the next clinical visit; this was particularly true when four or more sutures were removed. Burk and co-workers[5] concluded that only one or two sutures at a single visit should be removed to allow the cornea time to reshape itself between visits, setting the stage for the next, more controlled suture removal.

The theory of the selective suture removal technique is based on the assumption that the corneal curvature can be modified in the early postoperative period and then allowed to remain in a given configuration for 2 to 3 years. It is unknown whether the early reduction of astigmatism by suture manipulation can set the cornea in a more spherical configuration during wound healing. Although Binder[2] has demonstrated a greater reduction in astigmatism when sutures are selectively removed less than 1 year after surgery as compared to more than 1 year after surgery, there is no statistical proof that holding the cornea in an ideal configuration will ultimately lower astigmatism. Late removal of a single running nylon suture can result in a 6 diopter change in astigmatism.[4,13] However, selective suture removal for postkeratoplasty astigmatism has been shown to hasten visual rehabilitation and is a viable technique for suturing the corneal wound.

Technique of Selective Suture Removal

Suture patterns. The donor corneal button is sutured into the recipient with 8, 12, or 16 interrupted radial 10-0 nylon sutures. Twelve interrupted sutures allow adequate wound closure and sufficient choice of sutures for subsequent removal. A continuous 10-0 or 11-0 nylon suture is then placed in a single radial or "antitorque" bite between each of the interrupted sutures. Intraoperative keratometry and keratography may be used for decreasing astigmatism, with replacement of any tight sutures that are identified. All knots are buried in the recipient cornea.

Identification of tight sutures. Keratometry, photokeratoscopy, slitlamp examination, and manifest refraction aid in the identification of tight sutures. Keratometry provides quantitative input as to the magnitude and angle of corneal astigmatism. It is limited by its single ring, which is variably centered over the pupillary axis and may be discontinuous or unmeasurable.

Photokeratoscopy provides a photographic record of the contour of most of the corneal surface. It distinguishes steep and flat axes and the effects of individual sutures. Mires help predict the effect of interrupted suture removal. Very little has been written about the nuances of the use of photokeratoscopy in selective suture removal. Kozarsky and Waring[10] described qualitative patterns on the keratographs as an early guide to removal. Harris and colleagues[9] elaborated on the keratographic technique dividing the keratographs studied into six groups: (1) symmetric oval, (2) D-shaped oval, (3) focally indented, (4) mildly disrupted, (5) incomplete, and (6) uninterpretable. This excellent guide to selective suture removal is highly recommended for the novice embarking on this technique. Success is dependent on the surgeon's understanding of corneal topography and ability to identify the offending tight sutures.

On slitlamp examination, tight sutures can be identified by increased length, visible compression, Descemet's folds, and planar configuration of the suture. Manifest refraction is the final determinant in the need for intervention.

Criteria for suture removal. A tight suture is removed if (1) more than 3 D of astigmatism are present on keratometry readings and (2) there is no structural contraindication for interrupted suture removal, such as absence of the 11-0 running suture or wound abnormality.

Technique of suture removal. Topical anesthetic is instilled. At the slitlamp a bent 22-gage hypodermic needle cuts the suture, which is briskly pulled out with a pair of tying forceps. Topical antibiotic ointment is applied.

Timing of suture removal. Postoperatively, interrupted sutures may be removed as early as 3 weeks if a tight suture can be identified by use of a combination of keratometry, keratography, slitlamp examination, and manifest refraction. Epithelial irregularity may limit accuracy of tight suture identification immediately after surgery and delay removal of sutures. It is recommended to remove 1 or 2 interrupted sutures at a clinical visit. The optimal timing between clinical visits has not been established. Visual rehabilitation may be hastened with biweekly visits rather than monthly visits. Two weeks appears adequate time for the cornea to equilibrate to a new curvature after the removal of an interrupted suture. The changes in curvature is believed to be a two-phase response with an initial acute release of tension followed by a gradual redistribution of tension that changes corneal shape.

Advantages and Disadvantages of Selective Suture Removal. Both selective interrupted suture removal and the adjustable running suture techniques allow for the early modulation of the wound and rapid visual rehabilitation. Both methods attempt to set the wound in a more spherical configuration for the extended healing period. Van Meter and colleagues[15] compared the use of an adjustable single running suture with the use of the combined running and interrupted sutures. The adjustable suture group had reduced astigmatism compared to their combined suture group (1.5 D versus 3.2 D). When compared to other studies[1-8,14] on selective suture removal there is a much longer time to visual rehabilitation (9.6 months versus 4 to 5 months) and the residual astigmatism is in the high range (3.2 D compared to 1.5 to 3.5 D). Unfortunately, until all the interrupted and running sutures are removed in both groups, the final astigmatism cannot be compared.

Selective suture removal of interrupted sutures allows for adjustment of astigmatism because of wound healing many months after surgery. In the adjustable single continuous running suture method, the risk of breakage of the suture exists because of the biodegradation of the nylon suture.

Selective suture removal requires more frequent visits in the early postoperative period. However, the ability to dispense the optical correction in 3 to 4 months outweighs the disadvantage of multiple visits. Removal of any running suture can be associated with wide fluctuation in the amount of astigmatism. Subepithelial fibrosis and periodic breakage or loosening of sutures with secondary infection, inflammation, and vascularization are possible with any long-term retention of nylon sutures.

Recommendations. Despite problems associated with selective suture removal, it has been shown to reduce astigmatism to less than 3 D in two to three clinical visits after penetrating keratoplasty.

Current recommendations (Table 24-1) include use of combined single and 12 interrupted sutures, commencement of suture removal approximately 1

Table 24-1. Current Technique of Selective Suture Removal After Penetrating Keratoplasty

Sutures	12 interrupted 10-0
	12-bite running 11-0
Measurement of astigmatism	Keratograph
	Keratometry
	Refraction
Commence removal	1 month after operation
Number removed	1 or 2 sutures
Follow-up observation	Every 2 weeks
Expected stability	3 to 4 months

month after surgery, identification of tight sutures utilizing keratometry, keratographs, slitlamp examinations, and manifest refraction, and removal of one or two sutures in two or three visits with expected dispensing of optical correction at 3 to 4 months.

Summary. Many factors affect postkeratoplasty astigmatism including wound configuration, wound healing, and suture technique. Selective suture removal has been demonstrated to be useful in the modification of postkeratoplasty astigmatism. If tight sutures are identified and removed systematically in the early postoperative period, the visual rehabilitation period is significantly reduced. Despite its disadvantages, selective suture removal represents a technique that can be used until we develop better intraoperative methods to reduce postkeratoplasty astigmatism and have the ability to control wound healing.

REFERENCES

1. Binder PS: Selective suture removal can reduce postkeratoplasty astigmatism, *Ophthalmology* 92:1412-1416, 1985.
2. Binder PS: The effect of suture removal on postkeratoplasty astigmatism, *Am J Ophthalmol* 105:637-645, 1988.
3. Burk LL et al: Changes in astigmatism after removal of individual sutures in penetrating keratoplasty, *Invest Ophthalmol Vis Sci* 27(suppl):92, 1986.
4. Burk LL et al: The effect of selective suture removal on astigmatism following penetrating keratoplasty, *Ophthalmic Surg* 19:849-854, 1988.
5. Burk LL, Waring GO, Harris DJ Jr: Simultaneous and sequential selective suture removal to reduce astigmatism after penetrating keratoplasty, *Refract Corneal Surg* 6:179-187, 1990.
6. Cottingham AJ: New techniques for preventing high astigmatism in keratoplasty. In Boyd BF, editor: *Highlights of ophthalmology: silver anniversary*, vol 2, Panama, Republic of Panama: Highlights, 1979, pp 1182-1189.
7. Cottingham AJ: Residual astigmatism following keratoplasty, *Ophthalmology* 87(suppl):113-114, 1980.
8. Feldman ST, Brown SI: Reduction of astigmatism after keratoplasty, *Am J Ophthalmol* 103:477-478, 1987.
9. Harris DJ Jr et al: Late bacterial and fungal keratitis after corneal transplantation: spectrum of pathogens, graft survival, and visual prognosis, *Ophthalmology* 95:1450-1457, 1988.
10. Kozarsky AM, Waring GO: Photokeratoscopy in the management of astigmatism following keratoplasty, *Dev Ophthalmol* 11:91-98, 1985.
11. McNeill JI, Kaufman HE: A double running suture technique for keratoplasty: earlier visual rehabilitation, *Ophthalmic Surg* 8:58-61, 1977.
12. McNeill JI, Wessels IF: Adjustment of single continuous suture to control astigmatism after penetrating keratoplasty, *Refract Corneal Surg* 5:216-223, 1989.
13. Musch DC, Meyer RF, Sugar A: The effect of removing running sutures on astigmatism after penetrating keratoplasty, *Arch Ophthalmol* 106:488-492, 1988.
14. Stainer GA, Perl T, Binder PS: Controlled reduction of postkeratoplasty astigmatism, *Ophthalmology* 89:668-676, 1982.
15. Van Meter WS et al: Single continuous suture adjustment versus selective interrupted suture removal, *Ophthalmology* 98:177-183, 1991.

SURGICAL CORRECTION

PETER J. AGAPITOS
RICHARD L. LINDSTROM

Significant astigmatism may be induced after common surgical procedures including penetrating keratoplasty. In many cases the astigmatism may be minimized through appropriate incision and suturing techniques, but in some cases excessive astigmatism develops. Although the eye can often be visually rehabilitated through the use of spectacles or specialized contact lens fitting, some patients will require a surgical attempt to correct the high astigmatism.

In this chapter surgical techniques that have proved useful to us for the correction of high residual postoperative astigmatism after keratoplasty are described.

Surgical Approach to Postkeratoplasty Astigmatism. Before any surgical intervention in the postkeratoplasty patient, all sutures are removed and the stability of the refraction is observed for at least 1 month.

Astigmatism is evaluated using refraction, keratometry, and corneoscopy. Corneal topography is also routinely obtained by use of a corneal modeling system; however currently we do not use these data routinely in planning surgery. This sophisticated topographic method is being used by some investigators to plan incision location and extent, and the early results are encouraging.[3]

Our preferred approach to postkeratoplasty astigmatism involves various types of incisional techniques. It must be stressed that all incisions are performed at the graft-host interface or on the graft, so that the host tissues are not disturbed in case of the need for a regraft later on.

The initial approach to postkeratoplasty astigmatism that we advocate is intraincisional relaxing incisions with or without compression sutures. This technique can yield large astigmatic shifts and even in cases of high astigmatism we will always attempt this as a first procedure.

If relaxing incisions and compression sutures are not effective, one can utilize arcuate keratotomy on the graft at a 7 mm optical zone.

If a wound dehiscence is present or if there is a large area of the graft overriding onto the host (wound uplift), these are repaired. One does this by fracturing the wound, removing any epithelium, and simple resuturing, using interrupted sutures.

Wedge resections are reserved for extremely high cases of astigmatism.

Radial keratotomy can be performed for postkeratoplasty myopia in combination with intraincisional relaxing incisions, or arcuate keratotomy on the graft.[5] Once again it must be stressed that all incisions are made on the graft so as not to disturb the remaining host corneal tissues.

Relaxing Incisions. Most corneal surgeons have more experience with the relaxing incision technique for the reduction of postkeratoplasty astigmatism than any other. Several authors have reviewed their results utilizing this technique.[2,6-8,16-18] In the average patient a relaxing incision is capable of correcting 4 to 5 diopters of astigmatism with a range of 0 to 10 diopters. The technique has the advantage of being relatively simple to perform, requiring only an office procedure and topical anesthesia. In addition, the postoperative recovery period is relatively short and the improvement in refractive status can be rapid and dramatic.

The major disadvantages of this technique are significant undercorrections and overcorrections. Although these cases tend to undercorrect, the operation is relatively unpredictable: an identical operation in one patient may achieve a minimal effect with significant undercorrection, whereas another patient achieves a large effect with significant overcorrection. Additionally inadvertent perforations may occur, some of which may require suturing. Finally, some patients develop a prolonged instability of the corneal topography with fluctuating keratometry because the graft appears to migrate during healing.

Operative technique. The patient's refractive error is evaluated carefully preoperatively. All sutures are removed at least 1 month before any secondary surgical intervention. The relaxing incision technique flattens the steeper meridian and steepens the flatter meridian an equal amount. This means that the postoperative change in spherical equivalent is negligible. This operation therefore will not correct any residual hyperopia or myopia.

With refraction, keratometry, and corneoscopy each commonly gives the surgeon a different impression of the corneal topography. Since refraction is often quite difficult and inaccurate in keratoplasty patients, we tend to rely primarily on keratometry and corneoscopy in planning the operation. The corneoscopy picture will often graphically demonstrate areas where cicatricial wound healing has resulted in significant corneal distortion. In some cases this poor wound healing will be on only one side of the graft-host interface, and a single relaxing incision will be satisfactory. In most cases relaxing incisions must be performed on both sides of the graft-host interface in the axis of the steepest corneal meridian.

A minirelaxing incision can be performed at the slitlamp using a small needle or a 15-degree metal blade. This is done with topical anesthesia after instillation of an antibiotic drop, with or without a fine-wire speculum. A scratch incision to a depth of 50% to 75% can be made for 60 to 90 degrees on each side of the steep meridian. This can effectively reduce astigmatism by 4 to 5 diopters and can be repeated two or three times. It is well tolerated by patients already familiar with selective suture removal.

If a satisfactory result cannot be achieved with the minirelaxing incision approach, the patient is taken to the operating room where the procedure can be performed under an operating microscope using real-time monitoring with a quantitative surgical keratometer.

The eye is anesthetized with topical proparacaine hydrochloride. The periocular skin is prepped with a povidone-iodine solution. A sterile field is achieved with a plastic adhesive aperture drape, and the lids are separated with a fine-wire speculum. The patient is asked to fixate on the operating microscope light, and the keratometer mire is studied on the corneal surface. The axis of the steepest meridian is noted, and a mark is made with a blade in the epithelium on each side of the graft-host interface (Fig. 24-5, *A*). The appropriate incision size is approximately 60 to 90 degrees, or 15% to 25% of the circumference of the graft. The Katena 7 mm Lindstrom arcuate keratotomy marker can be used to demarcate the axis and arc of incision. The incision length and depth should vary, depending on the type of wound healing that has yielded the astigmatism. Utilization of intraoperative keratometry is especially useful during performance of the relaxing incision. The length and depth of the incisions can be graded according to the effect achieved during the surgical procedure.

The graft-host interface is carefully dissected in a graded fashion utilizing a microsharp metal blade

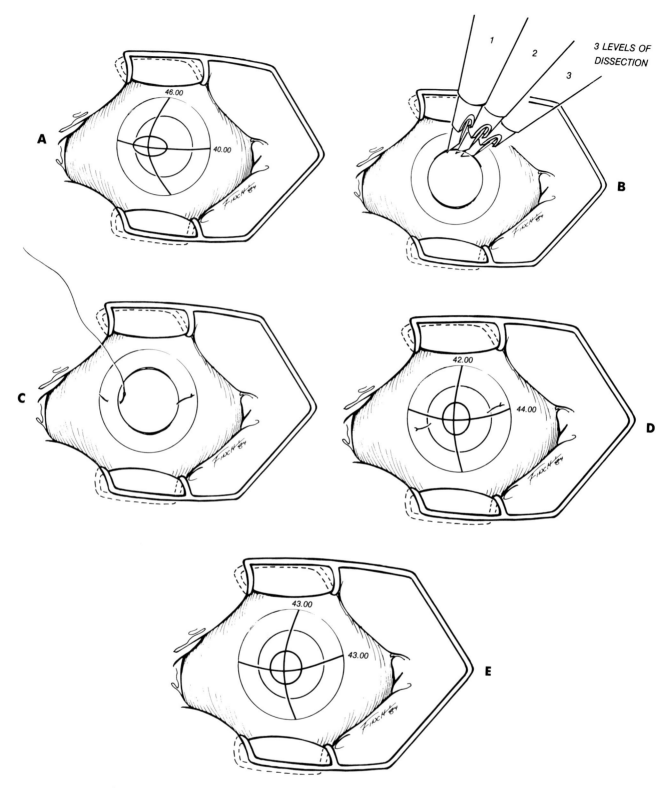

Fig. 24-5. Relaxing incision. **A,** Preoperative refraction: −3.00 +6.00 × 90 (spherical equivalent = plano). **B,** Incision in graft-host interface for 90 degrees. These incisions are perpendicular to graft at graft-host interface. **C,** Compression sutures are placed to increase wound gape. Two to six of these may be inserted. **D,** Adjust compression sutures to overcorrect ⅓ to ½. **E,** Final result—refraction: plano, 3 months postoperatively.

(Fig. 24-5, *B*). This technique allows the surgeon to scratch down gently into the incision while continuously observing the keratometer mire for correction of the astigmatism. Since wound healing is quite variable in postkeratoplasty patients, it is not unusual to enter areas of poor wound healing. In such cases the incision can be more carefully formed and adjusted by use of this technique. We have attempted to use preset diamond knives as those used in radial keratotomy; however, in many instances either perforations occurred or we were unable to maintain the incision in the graft-host interface because of poor visibility. In addition, the slow and careful deepening of the incision appears to be more controllable with the metal knife than with the nonguarded diamond knife. In some cases blunt dissection with the noncutting edge of the knife may be used. If perforation occurs with significant loss of chamber, suturing is necessary. Unfortunately, this suturing usually negates any effect of the operation. Occasionally early removal of the suture (4 to 6 weeks) will still allow for some effect.

Progressive deepening and lengthening of the incision is performed first on the one side and then on the other side until the keratometer mire is spherical. We used to attempt a mild overcorrection but now seek a spherical result on the table, as rare patients progress or regress in the postoperative period.

Compression sutures. If a satisfactory correction cannot be obtained by the simple relaxing incision technique, one to three 10-0 nylon compression sutures are placed on each side of the graft-host interface 90 degrees away from the relaxing incision (Fig 24-5, *C*). These sutures are tied with a simple slip knot and tightened under keratometric control until appropriate correction is achieved (Fig. 24-5, *D*). The knots are then cut short and buried.

After completion of surgery, the relaxing incisions are gently irrigated with a blunt cannula to remove any blood or debris. The globe is irrigated with topical gentamicin sulfate. In most cases a single drop of 0.25% scopolamine hydrochloride is placed on the eye for cycloplegia. The eye is covered with a patch and shield, and the patient is asked to return the following day for evaluation.

Postoperative course. Postoperatively the patient is treated with topical antibiotics four times daily for 1 week. Topical steroids are usually increased initially and then continued as appropriate for maintenance of graft clarity. Serial keratometry and refraction are performed, and when the eye is stable, optical correction is provided with glasses or a contact lens (Fig. 24-5, *E*).

If compression sutures have been utilized and overcorrection persists at 8 weeks, one or two of the sutures is removed. The patient is asked to return, and if overcorrection still persists, another one or two compression sutures is removed at 12 weeks. If an inadequate surgical correction is achieved, the operation may be repeated or an alternative procedure such as an astigmatic keratotomy or wedge resection may be considered.

Clinical results. In an early series at the University of Minnesota, 12 of 17 patients showed a mean reduction of 4.84 diopters of astigmatism by keratometry with a range from 1.75 to 10.50 diopters.[8] Sixteen of these 17 cases were relaxing incisions alone. Three patients had an increase of 3.42 diopters of astigmatism from preoperative levels with a range from 2.13 to 5.50 diopters as a result of overcorrection. One patient remained unchanged in the amount of residual astigmatism but was overcorrected as the axis shifted 90 degrees away.

Sugar and Kirk reported a mean reduction of cylinder of 7.50 diopters in 17 patients with a range from 2.50 to 11.50 diopters.[16] Krachmer and Fenzl found a mean of 4.25 diopters of improvement in 16 of their postkeratoplasty patients.[7] Troutman reported 8.38 diopters of improvement in four of his postkeratoplasty patients.[18]

Sugar measured a trend toward a more myopic spherical equivalent of 1.69 diopters with a range from 0.43 diopters of flattening to 5.50 diopters of steepening.[16] However, in the University of Minnesota experience, spherical equivalence was, in general, preserved after relaxing incisions. With exclusion of one patient with an eccentric graft, the mean ratio of flattening to steepening for 16 corneas was 0.975.[8] This implies that the relaxing incisions resulted in approximately the same amount of flattening in the steep meridian as steepening in the flat meridian. The mean change in spherical equivalent was +0.27 diopters (hyperopic shift). Six corneas were steeper after relaxing incisions, five were flatter, and five were essentially unchanged.

Three patients in the early Minnesota series required further surgery because of increased astigmatism after relaxing incisions. Two of these patients had wedge resections performed: one had an excellent result with 2.25 diopters of residual astigmatism and 20/25 vision; the other continued to have high astigmatism with unstable keratometry. A third patient with an overcorrection had compression sutures placed in the same axis as his relaxing incisions. These sutures decreased the total astigmatism from 11.37 to 1.25 diopters and achieved a best corrected visual acuity of 20/25.[8] One of the 17 patients sustained a perforation that required suturing. Three other patients had microperforations that did not require suturing.[8] In Sugar's series of 17 patients, one had a perforation at the time of the relaxing incision requiring suture repair. Another patient had a wound dehiscence 3 days after the relaxing incision, which also required suture repair.[16] These patients did not suffer any serious complication after being repaired.

Mandel and co-workers found that 21 patients who underwent relaxing incisions with compression sutures had a mean decrease of 6.56 diopters or 67%.[13] Additionally they found that in patients with greater than 8.5 diopters of astigmatism preoperatively, relaxing incisions with compression sutures yielded a 70% reduction in astigmatism compared to 39% for relaxing incisions alone.

We reported on 10 cases of relaxing incisions with compression sutures at the University of Minnesota.[1] The mean delta keratometry value was 6.9 diopters. Our analysis showed that most of these patients tended to undercorrection with only 1 overcorrection. The change in spherical eqivalent was a mean −1.50 diopter myopic shift.

Fronterre and Portesani,[4] reported on 100 cases and divided them into 3 groups based on preoperative astigmatism: *group 1:* 4 to 10 diopters; *group 2:* 10.5 to 15 diopters, and *group 3:* >15 diopters. Thirty-one patients had relaxing incisions alone, and 69 patients had relaxing incisions and compression sutures. Patients in group 3 had a two-stage procedure with repeat relaxing incisions and compression sutures. The mean reduction in astigmatism was 5.53 (77%), 9.68 (77%), and 14.87 (85%) diopters in groups 1, 2, and 3 respectively. Twenty-six of 69 patients with compression sutures had 1 to 5 sutures left in place. Group 1 had no change in spherical equivalent, with groups 2 and 3 having small hyperopic shifts.

Relaxing incisions with compression sutures appear to be useful in reducing even high levels of astigmatism and are relatively predictable.

Wedge Resections. The wedge resection technique for correction of postkeratoplasty astigmatism is appropriate for cases with relatively high levels of cylinder.[2,6-8,17]

Operative technique. The patient is evaluated preoperatively as described for the relaxing incision. The overall effect of the wedge resection is to steepen the flatter meridian approximately twice as much as it flattens the steeper meridian. This means that the average patient will have a slight increase in myopia or decrease in hyperopia after this surgical technique.

A wedge resection requires retrobulbar anesthesia because the dissection involved along with placement of the multiple sutures requires good akinesia. To begin with, the axis of the flattest meridian is located and verified, preferably under intraoperative surgical control with an operating keratometer (Fig. 24-6, *A*). In the wedge-resection technique a diamond micrometer radial keratotomy knife is useful. If a double-bladed knife as described by Troutman is available, it can be utilized.[17] In addition, intraoperative ultrasonic pachymetry is helpful.

Ultrasonic pachymetry is performed at the graft-host interface in the axis where the wedge resection is to be performed. It is usually impossible to obtain readings immediately over the scar; however, readings can commonly be obtained adjacent to the graft-host interface just onto the donor or recipient. After several corneal-thickness measurements are taken, the diamond knife is set at 100% of the thinnest reading. The blade setting is then checked with a coin gage or microscope. A 90-degree section of the keratoplasty wound is then incised with the diamond knife. An attempt is made to stay in the graft-host interface, but perfect accuracy is difficult. A wedge of recipient tissue is then excised with the diamond knife or with microscissors by use of a free-hand dissection (Fig. 24-6, *B*).

In the average case, resection of a tenth of a millimeter of tissue results in approximately 2 diopters of correction. This operation is usually reserved for patients with greater than 10 diopters of astigmatism and therefore resections of 0.5 to 1 mm of tissue are performed. A paracentesis is not usually necessary before resuturing of this wound. Five to seven deep, evenly spaced, interrupted 10-0 nylon sutures are placed (Fig. 24-6, *C*). Each of the sutures is placed with a slip knot, and under keratometric control the sutures are tightened until an overcorrection of one third to one half of the preoperative cylinder is achieved (Fig. 24-6, *D*). The sutures are then tied down with square knots, cut short, and buried.

Postoperative course. The immediate postoperative care is the same as that for relaxing incisions. The sutures are left in place for a minimum of 8 weeks. At 8 weeks a selective suture-removal technique in the axis of the steepest residual astigmatism is utilized, with one or two sutures being removed every 3 to 4 weeks. Once a satisfactory result is achieved the remaining sutures may be left in place (Fig. 24-6, *E*).

Clinical results. This technique is capable of correcting up to 20 diopters of astigmatism. We currently prefer to attempt to correct most cases with astigmatism less than 10 to 15 diopters by using re-

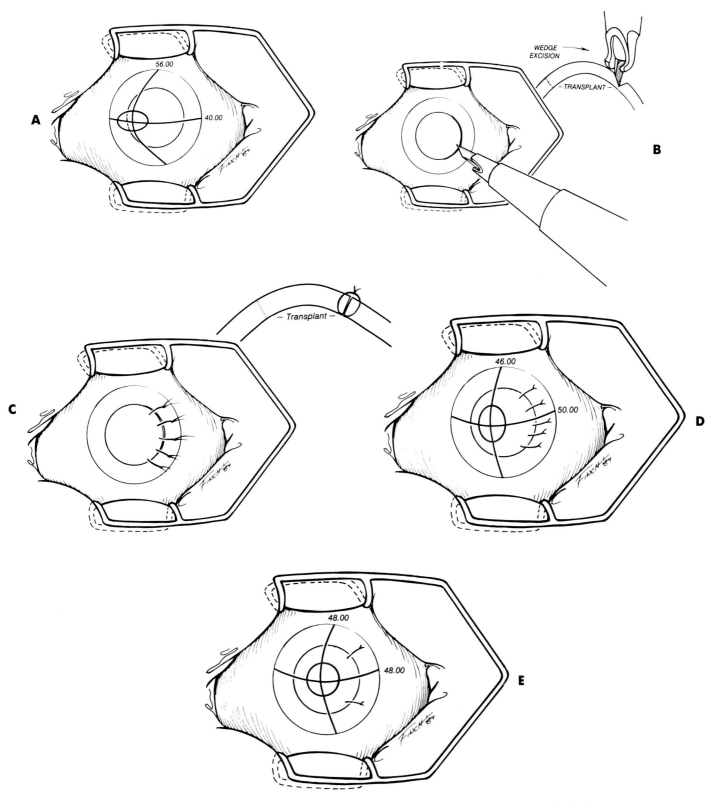

Fig. 24-6. Wedge resection. **A,** Preoperative refraction: −6.00 +12.00 × 90 (spherical equivalent = plano). **B,** Excise 0.6 mm of tissue from recipient cornea. **C,** Place 5 to 7 sutures (to Descemet's membrane). **D,** Adjust tension of sutures to overcorrect ⅓ to ½. **E,** Final result—refraction: −2.00 sph., 6 months postoperatively.

laxing incisions or astigmatic keratotomy before considering wedge resection. The wedge-resection approach requires a longer postoperative visual rehabilitation. The longer visual rehabilitation is needed because the multiple sutures induce significant irregular astigmatism, and wound healing must take place. Selective suture removal is needed to reduce the astigmatism before eventual visual rehabilitation. Nonetheless, the alternative to this procedure in patients with severe astigmatism may be consideration of repeat keratoplasty, and a wedge resection approach should always be attempted first.

Wound Revisions. In some cases where there is a donor override of the recipient (graft uplift), or a small wound dehiscence, simple wound revision may be utilized. Here the incision is debrided of any epithelium, simply dissected open, and resutured under keratometric control to achieve a spherical result.

The visual recovery is similar to that of wedge re-

sections because of multiple sutures. Selective suture removal can begin at 8 weeks.

Astigmatic Keratotomy. Astigmatism surgery is still evolving in technique, and further study is needed. Various different techniques have been used in the past and have been abandoned because of poor predictability. These include both intersecting and nonintersecting trapezoidal astigmatic keratotomy.[1]

Careful manifest refraction and keratometry are performed preoperatively. In most cases, the keratometric and refractive cylinder power and axis are compatible. In case of significant disparity, remeasurement and evaluation with more sophisticated methods of corneal topographic analysis, such as photokeratography, are performed. Surgery in postkeratoplasty astigmatism is based on the refractive cylinder and axis. A straight keratotomy at a 5 or 7 mm optical zone or an arcuate keratotomy at a 7 mm

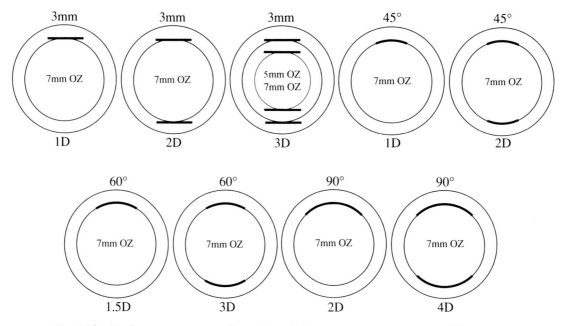

Fig. 24-7. Lindstrom nomogram for astigmatic keratotomy nomogram modifiers.
1. Optical zone: 7 mm for arcuate keratotomy, 7 and 5 mm for straight keratotomy.
2. Blade depth: 100% of thinnest paracentral pachymetry at zone mark in meridian of astigmatism.
3. Over/under 30 years of age: Increase or decrease efficacy 2% per year:
   Age 20 = 80% of effect at 30
   Age 55 = 150% of effect at 30
   Age 80 = 200% of effect at 30
4. Although mild overall corneal flattening may occur, assume a coupling ratio of 1:1.
5. Procedure may be combined with a 4-incision or 8-incision radial keratotomy, though radial and transverse incisions should not touch.
6. Assume a range of effect of ± 2.00 diopters when planning surgery.
Note that all incisions diagramed are for plus cylinder axis 90; 45, 60, and 90 degrees refer to length of arcuate incisions, not meridian of astigmatism. (From Lindstrom, R.L.: *Refract Corneal Surg* 6:441, 1990.)

optical zone are preferred. The nomogram utilized is depicted in Fig. 24-7. This nomogram, if adopted by others, needs to be adjusted to that particular surgeon's technique. The procedures are centered on the optical center as determined by fixation on the operating microscope light irrespective of graft centration. If the graft is decentered so that paired arcuate incisions cannot be placed at a 7 mm optical zone with both incisions on the graft, both incisions may be placed 0.5 to 1.0 mm interior to the graft-host interface as described by others.[12,14]

Operative Technique. The equipment utilized includes a Zeiss OPMI-6 operating microscope, Sinskey hook, and 0.12 colibrí corneal fixation forceps. Various zone markers are available. For arcuate

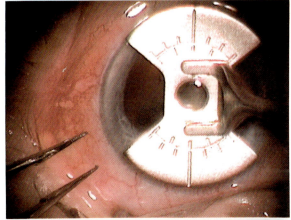

A

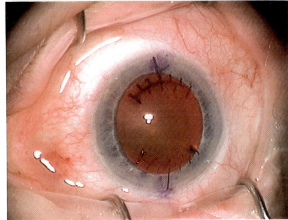

B

Fig. 24-8. A, Katena-Lindstrom arcuate marker is placed on cornea aligned with steeper meridian. This instrument marks two 90-degree incisions at a 7 mm optical zone. **B,** Cornea marked before astigmatic keratotomy. Perpendicular marks are centered at steep meridian. Internal notches demarcate 22.5 degrees of arc so that two of these segments give a 45-degree incision. External notches demarcate 15 degrees of arc so that four of these give a 60-degree incision and six of these give a 90-degree incision. (From Lindstrom, R.L.: *Refract Corneal Surg* 6:441, 1990.)

keratotomy, we currently utilize the Lindstrom arcuate marker (Katena K37996 7 mm) (Fig. 24-8). Several straight keratotomy markers are also available from various instrument manufacturers. As an alternative, 3, 5, and 7 mm round radial keratotomy optical zone markers and 8-, 12-, and 16-incision radial keratotomy incision markers may be used to demarcate incision location and length. A skin-marking pencil or stencil ink pad is used to clarify the marks. A high-quality vertical-blade (push) diamond micrometer knife is calibrated with a micronscope. An ultrasonic pachymeter is utilized to measure corneal thickness intraoperatively. A bottle of balanced salt solution and an irrigation cannula are utilized for wetting the cornea and irrigating the incision. Topical anesthesia is achieved with 0.5% proparacaine instilled every 5 minutes times 3. Peribulbar or retrobulbar anesthesia is not necessary. A surgical keratometer is useful for intraoperative monitoring, but the operations usually are not modified according to intraoperative keratometry. The patient is placed under the operating microscope and the eye adjusted to be perpendicular to the microscope. One marks the center of the pupil with a Sinskey hook by requesting that the patient fixate on the operating microscope light, which is turned down to a low level (Fig. 24-9). The zone for the keratotomies is then marked with a 7 mm round optical zone marker (Fig. 24-10). The steeper meridian is marked with a skin-marking pen with use of intraoperative keratometry or preoperative landmarks (Fig. 24-11).

To mark the length of a 3 mm straight relaxing keratotomy, a 3 mm circular zone marker is placed over the 7 mm zone mark (and also over the 5 mm

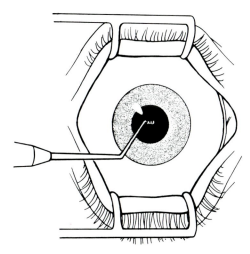

Fig. 24-9. Center of cornea is marked with a Sinskey hook. (From Lindstrom, R.L.: *Refract Corneal Surg* 6:441, 1990.)

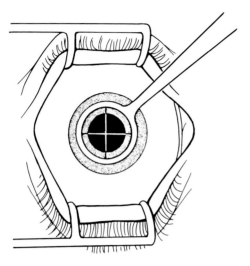

Fig. 24-10. Marking optical zone with a 7 mm zone marker. (From Lindstrom, R.L.: *Refract Corneal Surg* 6:441, 1990.)

zone if four cuts were planned) in the steeper meridian (Fig. 24-12). If an arcuate keratotomy is preferred, a 16-incision radial keratotomy marker can delineate an arc of 45 degrees (2 segments), a 12-incision radial keratotomy marker can delineate an arc of 60 degrees (2 segments), and an 8- or 16-ray marker for 90 degrees (2 or 4 segments respectively) (Fig. 24-13). The Lindstrom arcuate marker may also be used (Fig. 24-8). We do not utilize arcuate incisions of over 90 degrees, but others have reported success up to 120 degrees.[14]

The corneal thickness at the appropriate optical

zone in the steepest meridian is measured on one (for a single incision) or both sides of the cornea intraoperatively with ultrasonic pachymetry. A high-quality diamond knife (Magnum Diamond Lindstrom Lecut, Chiron Intraoptics, Irvine, California) is calibrated either preoperatively or intraoperatively with a Magnum Diamond Baribeau micronscope. Extreme care in knife selection, calibration, and maintenance is taken to assure reproducible cuts. The knife is set at 100% of the thinnest paracentral pachymetry. Secondary fixation is achieved with the corneal fixation forceps at the limbus.

The knife is set in the cornea, with a pause for the count of 1001, followed by slow guidance of the knife through the incision. A knife that allows the surgeon good visibility while pushing through the length of the keratotomy improves accuracy. All the incisions are made with the blade pushed forward (front cutting).

The incisions are irrigated with balanced salt solution. Several drops of gentamycin or tobramycin are placed on the eye. We do not routinely patch or use cycloplegia. If a significant perforation occurs, subconjunctival antibiotic, topical cycloplegia, and a pressure patch are utilized. The patient is seen 1 day, 1 week, 1 month, and 3 months postoperatively. Topical antibiotics are continued for 1 week.

Postoperative course. If significant undercorrection is observed, a topical steroid is used four times daily for 1 month in an attempt to delay wound healing and increase incision gape. If significant overcorrection is noted early, topical 5% sodium chloride drops four times daily are used for 1 month in an attempt to reduce corneal edema and wound

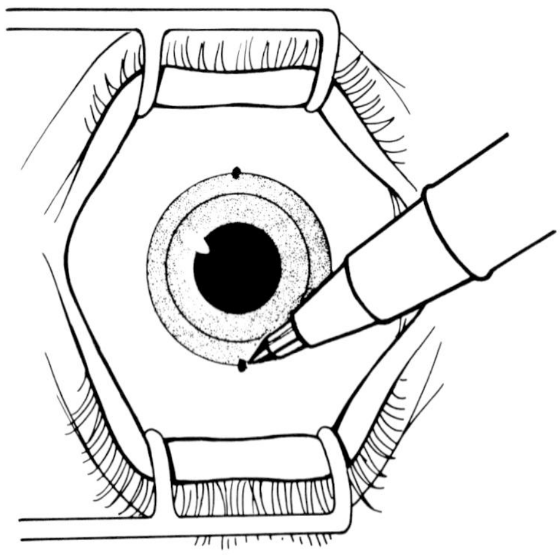

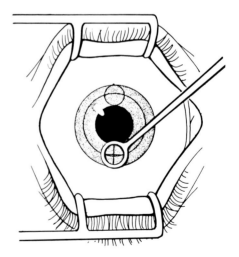

Fig. 24-11. Marking steeper meridian. (From Lindstrom, R.L.: *Refract Corneal Surg* 6:441, 1990.)

Fig. 24-12. Use of a 3 mm zone marker to delineate incision length for a straight incision. (From Lindstrom, R.L.: *Refract Corneal Surg* 6:441, 1990.)

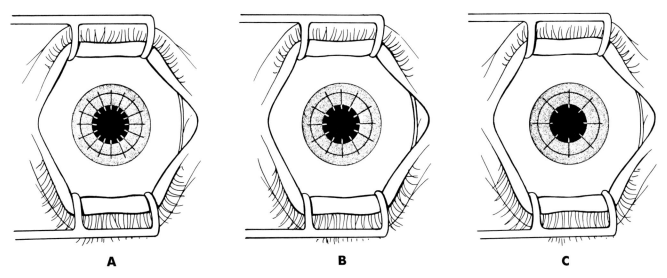

Fig. 24-13. A, Sixteen-cut radial keratotomy marker is useful to delineate 45-degree arcuate keratotomy (2 segments = 45 degrees). **B,** Twelve-cut radial keratotomy marker is useful to delineate 60-degree arcuate keratotomy (2 segments = 60 degrees). **C,** Eight-cut radial keratotomy is useful to delineate 90-degree keratotomy (2 segments = 90 degrees). (**A** to **C** from Lindstrom RL: *Refract Corneal Surg* 6:441, 1990.)

gape. If significant overcorrection persists, the epithelial plug is removed under topical anesthesia, and the incision is sutured back together with two or three 10-0 Mersilene sutures. Intraoperative control of suture tension with a surgical keratometer and the use of slip knots are employed. A spherical result to one-third overcorrection in the appropriate direction with the sutures is aimed for on the table, and selective suture removal beginning 8 weeks after suture placement is utilized if needed.[11]

Clinical results. Results with straight and arcuate keratotomy in the postkeratoplasty group are somewhat inconsistent with several overcorrections.[1,10] Intraincisional relaxing incisions with compression sutures are probably better and more predictable.

There are three series of arcuate keratotomy interior to the graft-host interface with compression sutures reported in the literature. McCartney and coworkers reported on 11 patients that had arcuate keratotomy with compression sutures. All incisions were made 0.5 mm internal to the graft-host interface. The amount of cylinder decrease was a mean of 8 diopters, correcting 68% of astigmatism.[14] A similar series by Lustbader and Lemp yielded similar results but corrected only 56% of preoperative astigmatism.[12] The series that corrected the most astigmatism was reported by Frangieh and co-workers,[3] giving an 81% reduction in preoperative astigmatism. The incision length and placement of compression sutures in this series was guided by corneal topographic analysis.[3]

Astigmatic keratotomy can certainly cause large shifts in corneal astigmatism. Current techniques have limited predictability. Each of the procedures described in this chapter is capable of correcting variable amounts of astigmatism in the postkeratoplasty patient. As more sophisticated methods develop, we should be able to improve on our results.

REFERENCES

1. Agapitos PJ, Lindstrom RL, Williams PA, Sanders DR: Analysis of astigmatic keratotomy, *J Cataract Refract Surg* 15:13-18, 1989.
2. Barner SS: Surgical treatment of corneal astigmatism, *Ophthalmic Surg* 7:43-48, 1976.
3. Frangieh GT, Kwitko S, McDonnell PJ: Prospective corneal topographic analysis in surgery for postkeratoplasty astigmatism, *Arch Ophthalmol* 109:506-510, 1991.
4. Fronterre A, Portesani GP: Relaxing incisions for postkeratoplasty astigmatism, *Cornea* 10:305-311, 1991.
5. Gothard TW, Agapitos PJ, Bowers RA, et al: Four incision radial keratotomy for high myopia post-penetrating keratoplasty, *Refract Corneal Surg* 1992. (Submitted.)
6. Krachmer JH, Ching SST: Relaxing corneal incisions for postkeratoplasty astigmatism, *Int Ophthalmol Clin* 23:153-157, 1983.
7. Krachmer JH, Fenzl RE: Surgical correction of high postkeratoplasty astigmatism, *Arch Ophthalmol* 98:1400-1402, 1980.
8. Lavery GW, Lindstrom RL, Hofer LA, Doughman DJ: The surgical management of corneal astigmatism after penetrating keratoplasty, *Ophthalmic Surg* 16:165-169, 1985.
9. Lindquist TD, Rubenstein JB, Lindstrom RL: Correction of

hyperopia following radial keratotomy: quantification in human cadaver eyes, *Ophthalmic Surg* 18:432-437, 1987.

10. Lindstrom RL: The surgical correction of astigmatism: a clinician's perspective, *Refract Corneal Surg* 6:441-454, 1990.

11. Lindstrom RL, Lindquist TD: Surgical correction of postoperative astigmatism, *Cornea* 7:139-148, 1988.

12. Lustbader JM, Lemp MA: The effect of relaxing incisions with multiple compression sutures on post-keratoplasty astigmatism, *Ophthalmic Surg* 21:416-419, 1990.

13. Mandel MR, Shapiro MB, Krachmer JH: Relaxing incisions with augmentation sutures for the correction of postkeratoplasty astigmatism, *Am J Ophthalmol* 103:441-447, 1987.

14. McCartney DL, Whitney CE, Stark WJ, et al: Refractive keratoplasty for disabling astigmatism after penetrating keratoplasty, *Arch Ophthalmol* 105:954-957, 1987.

15. Merlin U: Curved keratotomy procedure for congenital astigmatism, *J Refract Surg* 3:92-97, 1987.

16. Sugar J, Kirk AK: Relaxing keratotomy for post-keratoplasty high astigmatism, *Ophthalmic Surg* 14:156-158, 1983.

17. Troutman RC: Corneal wedge resections and relaxing incisions for postkeratoplasty astigmatism, *Int Ophthalmol Clin* 23:161, 1983.

18. Troutman RC, Swinger C: Relaxing incision for control of postoperative astigmatism following keratoplasty, *Ophthalmic Surg* 11:117-120, 1980.

Chapter 25

Contact Lens Fitting

FREDERICK S. BRIGHTBILL

Contact lenses fit after penetrating keratoplasty are usually provided either very early for therapeutic reasons, for example, a soft lens used to treat a persistent epithelial defect, or late after suture removal to correct residual refractive error, especially astigmatism.[1]

THERAPEUTIC FITTING

Rapid reepithelialization of the corneal graft is essential to reestablish a barrier to infection and to prevent subepithelial scarring. Medical treatment of epithelial defects seen on the first postoperative visit will usually result in complete healing, but frequent examinations are necessary to assure this. When the size of a defect fails to decrease or is persistent beyond 6 to 7 days, a soft bandage lens is chosen and is fitted over the graft.

Fitting Method. Any cosmetic daily or extended-wear soft contact lens with which one has experience can be fit for therapeutic reasons over a corneal transplant. Accuvue, CSI, and Softcon lenses are most often used in my practice. Centration with complete covering of the graft-host sutured junction, comfort, and slight movement on the blink are key signs to achieve satisfactory fitting. Patients are instructed that the initial 24 hours of lens wear may cause some discomfort and are asked to return the day after fitting and at 1 and 2 weeks. Treatment with an antibiotic, cycloplegic, and nonsuspension corticosteroid drop is given in the usual doses after keratoplasty.

When no underlying recipient cause exists for epithelial breakdown in the donor (such as exposure, dryness, or graft-host wound disparity), a therapeutic lens usually achieves healing in 1 to 2 weeks. Be-cause, in my opinion, prolonged wearing of bandage lenses may interfere with stromal wound healing, it is advisable to remove the soft lens at 2 to 3 weeks and observe carefully for a recurrence of the defect. Artificial tears such as Celluvisc, Cellufresh, 0.5% methylcellulose, or ocular lubricants such as Refresh PM, HypoTears, or Lacri-Lube should be used after lens removal to limit superficial punctate keratitis and to maintain wetting of the corneal graft surface.

Recently, corneal collagen shields have become popular devices advocated for a variety of corneal surface problems. Groden and White[6] studied the effect of the Bausch & Lomb 24-hour Bio-Cor collagen shield compared with Bausch & Lomb 04 plano bandage lenses in consecutive transplant patients with epithelial defects and found the therapeutic lens significantly more effective in achieving healing.

OPTICAL FITTING TO CORRECT REFRACTIVE ERROR

Clear corneal transplants are now obtainable for most recipient diseases using modern surgical and eye banking techniques. Other than homograft rejection, limiting post–suture removal graft astigmatism is the major problem faced by today's transplant surgeon.

Among the most significant factors in the determination of final transplant astigmatism are the recipient disease, graft centration, wound cut, suture placement, wound healing, and suture removal. Since no one technique has resolved this problem, the surgeon must be prepared to manage the frequent complications of both irregular and high corneal graft astigmatism.[2,5]

Unless a graft recipient wore spectacles preoperatively for correction of high astigmatism (some with keratoconus), patients are usually unable to tolerate more than 5.00 diopters of refractive cylinder in spectacles. Relaxing incisions and wedge resection procedures may be used in postgraft eyes with larger amounts of astigmatism. About 10% of grafts in my practice and in others[3] may require contact lens fitting postoperatively either because of (1) patient preference—usually keratoconus, (2) irregular astigmatism, (3) anisometropia, or (4) spectacle-intolerant high astigmatism.

Time of Fitting. Both rigid gas-permeable (RGP) and soft contact lenses can be fit on grafts with retained epithelialized sutures and buried knots (Fig. 25-1), but there is some inherent risk of suture erosion, inflammation, and possible rejection aggravated by contact lens movement and trauma. For these reasons, most transplant surgeons prefer to remove all graft sutures before fitting a contact lens. Since average healing times with nylon sutures vary between 4 and 12 months and since after suture removal K readings and refractive changes may occur for up to several months, recipients need to be forewarned that best vision may be delayed.

A review of our transplant data reveals that the overall average time of contact lens fitting after keratoplasty was 10 months. The earliest time of fit came at 6 months on a 30-year-old man and the latest was a 26-month fitting in a 70-year-old patient.

Contrary to common belief, contact lenses are well tolerated by grafts, and graft injury by them seldom occurs. In fact, transplanted corneas, despite requir-

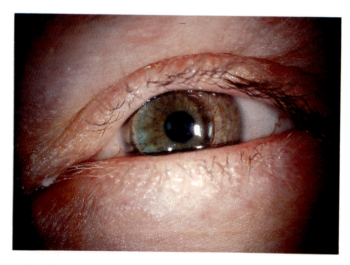

Fig. 25-1. RGP (rigid gas-permeable) lens fit 6 months after penetrating keratoplasty over retained 10-0 and 11-0 double running sutures. The lens diameter was 8.5 mm and the graft diameter 8.0 mm. K's were 44.50/44.25.

ing more time to fit, are often less likely to have problems than eyes of cosmetic patients.

Indications for Contact Lens Wear. Keratoconus graft recipients are by far our largest group of patients fit with RGP lenses. Many of these patients wore rigid lenses preoperatively to obtain adequate visual acuity, and most remain moderately myopic after penetrating keratoplasty, a condition enhanced by donor-to-recipient disparate buttons, which increases corneal steepness. Many patients require a contact lens in the opposite eye and choose a contact lens for either cosmetic value or of necessity because of postkeratoplasty anisometropia.

Postkeratoplasty unilateral aphakia is rarely encountered presently because of the availability of anterior or posterior intraocular lens insertion at the time of grafting. Elderly recipients generally find it impossible to insert and remove a contact lens, and extended aphakic lens wear may be complicated by frequent visits to the ophthalmologist for cleaning, lens loss, or infection.[9]

Factors in Grafted Eye Affecting Lens Fit. A poorly centered donor corneal button will limit a satisfactory contact lens fit in most cases (Fig. 25-2) and cause rapid aging of the technician and ophthalmologist. Decentered grafts may also be highly astigmatic. The tendency in recent years toward larger-diameter buttons (that is, 8.0 to 8.5 mm) surrounding, for example, the thinned cone in eyes with keratoconus has decreased the incidence of graft decentration.

Lid position and lid tension have long been known to adversely affect rigid contact lens centration, a fact observed in over 50% of our corneas. With rigid lens use, changing either the lens diameter or base curve or designing a toric lens has little effect on centration. Some effect, however, is achieved when one changes the lens edge, such as a lenticular to a single-cut design, a decrease in the anterior bevel, or the addition of prism ballast. Another alternative, if there is little or no astigmatism, is to select a large-diameter soft contact lens.

Astigmatic grafts frequently cause poor lens centration. Rigid lenses seldom center on highly astigmatic grafts, whereas soft lenses, which may center perfectly, usually provide suboptimal vision. Therefore, relaxing incisions and wedge-resection procedures are performed soon after suture removal to improve the prognosis for successful lens fitting by decreasing astigmatism by as much as 3 to 7 diopters. In fact, the need for a lens fit may be eliminated with these procedures when a significant astigmatic reduction makes spectacle correction acceptable.

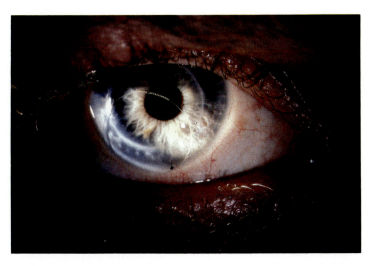

Fig. 25-2. Graft 8.5 mm was decentered inferiorly in eye with severe keratoconus causing final objective (keratometric) astigmatism of 12 D. All lenses fit in this eye rode inferiorly over lower limbus causing irritation and prismatic lens-edge distortion. Patient was unable to tolerate lens wear and underwent a wedge resection procedure.

Choosing the Lens

Rigid gas-permeable lenses

DESIGN. A thorough knowledge of the basic principles of contact lens design and modification based on fitting many cosmetic eyes is invaluable when one is selecting a contact lens for fitting a transplanted cornea.[11] We utilize a wide variety of lens designs, most often spherical, Soper, and prism ballast. Tricurve, back toric, bitoric, and aspheric designs are also used on both phakic and aphakic grafts.

MATERIALS. In the past 9 years, rigid lens materials have evolved to nearly exclusive use of oxygen-permeable materials. This has enabled grafts to be fit with tighter-fitting, larger diameter lenses, having less movement, which, even with some decentration, allow for adequate visual axis coverage and good acuity.

HARD VERSUS SOFT LENSES. Our bias is toward RGP lens fitting in grafts for these reasons:

1. The average refractive graft astigmatism requiring contact lens fitting is between 4 and 9 diopters. This precludes sharp visual acuity with most soft lenses.
2. Decreased corneal graft sensation allows for moderate comfort with RGP wear compared to the cosmetically fit eye.
3. Hard lenses are more durable and less likely to need replacement.
4. Small RGP contact lenses are less likely than larger-diameter soft contact lenses to stimulate existing corneal vessels and predispose to graft rejection.

MEASURING CORNEAL CURVATURE. A keratometer measures the central 3.16 mm of the cornea and will provide readings only for initial base curve selection for trial lens fitting. Manabe and associates[8] utilized photokeratoscopy to fit 30 post–suture removal eyes after keratoplasty with polymethylmethacrylate rigid lenses. They attributed their 90% success rate to being able to measure peripheral radii of curvature near the often irregular graft-host junction and to modify peripheral lens curvatures (often flatter than expected).

Without access to photokeratoscopy, a simple method to judge lens-corneal touch both centrally, midperipherally, and peripherally is to use trial lenses of known base, midperipheral, and peripheral curves, instill fluorescein, and observe with the slit-lamp areas of steep or flat fitting. The fitter then orders specific base and peripheral curves and reinserts the finished lens, restains for lens-corneal touch, and further modifies as needed. Often a blending of the intermediate or peripheral curve junction is necessary to avoid discomfort and to allow for tear exchange at the edge of the lens.

FITTING THE LENS. Fitting a contact lens on an eye after keratoplasty may best be summarized utilizing the *3T* technique: (1) *t*rial lenses, (2) *t*echnician, and (3) *t*ime. Graft fitting, like keratoconus fitting, can require the extensive use of numerous trial lenses and often more than one lens fabrication and trial in the eye before the best fit is achieved.

Lens selection. Measurements of corneal curvature

with the keratometer or corneoscope, or both, are useful only as starting points in the initial trial lens selection. Likewise, the unaided refraction is only helpful with regular astigmatism and when irregular astigmatism is present as a reference point for the final contact lens power. The suggested trial lens sets should include the following:

1. Spherical standard lenses
   a. Base-curve ranges (40 to 54 diopters with 0.50-diopter steps)
   b. Diameter (7.6 to 9.5 mm)
   c. Peripheral curves (standard + custom adjustment later)
2. Spherical variable (Soper, McGuire) lenses
   a. Base-curve ranges (39 to 52 diopters with 3-diopter steps)
   b. Diameter (7.5, 8.5, and 9.5 mm)
   c. Intermediate curves (43 and 45 diopters)
   d. Peripheral curves (standard + custom adjustment later)

Trial fitting. After the K readings or photokeratoscopy values and refraction are ascertained, the lid position and tension is evaluated and an initial lens is selected from the trial lens set. Topical anesthetic is instilled to decrease discomfort, blinking, and tearing, which may occur during a multiple lens trial. A large-diameter spherical base curve lens is selected. The base curve is chosen at about mid-K value, and the initial diameter selected is usually 9.5 mm. If a running nylon suture is still in place, a smaller diameter (7.6 to 8.2 mm) is the initial choice because these small lenses tend to position within the suture line. Initially, lens position, apical clearance, movement, and the peripheral curve are evaluated, followed by trial lenses of varying base curves and then varying lens diameters. It may be necessary to choose a lens by bracketing (for example, the best diameter may be judged to be between 8.8 and 9.5 mm, but no trial lens for that diameter is available and a 9.1 mm size is ordered). Finally, when a satisfactory trial lens is in place, a spherical over-refraction is done.

Other design variables that must be evaluated and specified by the fitter are the intermediate curve, anterior bevel, lenticular size, carrier power, ballast, and blends. When lens parameters are known and specified, subsequent adjustments based on fluorescein patterns are easily made.

Evaluation of Fit. A lens centered directly over the graft is in the ideal position, but with high or irregular astigmatism, a decentered graft, or a peripheral wound irregularity, perfect centration rarely occurs (less than 25% of eyes I fit) (Fig. 25-3). In difficult cases, even after many lens trials and modifications, the best lens fit may still have the patient apparently looking through the edge of the lens combined with a limbal override and a bizarre fluorescein pattern. If the visual acuity is good (20/15 to 20/25) and undistorted despite lens decentration, the contact is ordered and dispensed.

Although the patterns seldom resemble those of a cosmetic lens patient, one of the most useful tests for judging a lens fit is the evaluation of the lens-cornea relationship using topical fluorescein (Fig. 25-4). Ar-

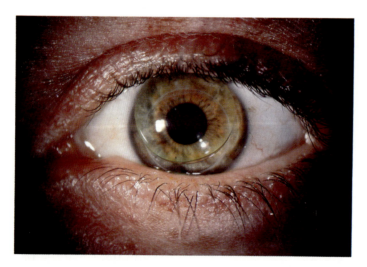

Fig. 25-3. RGP lens fit on grafted eye 6 weeks after suture removal. Notice that lens is decentered upward over superior wound but with good coverage of visual axis. Mild vertical or horizontal lens decentration over grafts is found in over 75% of cases we have fit and is generally well tolerated.

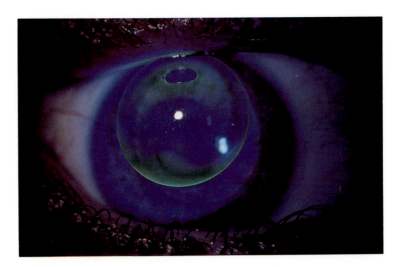

Fig. 25-4. Fluorescein tear film staining beneath lens fit on graft for keratoconus. Notice central nonstaining area of corneal touch over astigmatic graft axis and pooled dye superiorly and inferiorly, representing areas of nontouch. An air bubble is trapped beneath lens above superior wound. Peripheral curve clearance appears normal inferiorly between 4 and 8 but narrow from 3 to 9 above. RGP lenses have allowed us to fit larger diameter, tighter (that is, steeper) lenses with variable peripheral curve widths with excellent tolerance.

eas of paracentral lens-graft touch and strange astigmatic patterns invariably are seen. The object of fitting is to limit this touch and to design a peripheral curve that is at least 50% open so that adequate tear exchange can occur. The importance of retesting the ordered lens with fluorescein once it is returned from the lab and placed on the grafted eye cannot be overemphasized. Peripheral curve and edge modification in the office often ensures successful lens fitting.

Once the lens has been examined on the eye and found to be satisfactory, the patient is given thorough instruction in the cleaning and care of the lens and asked to practice insertion and removal of the lens under technician observation. Wearing schedules comparable to those in cosmetically fit eyes with all-day wear by 1 week are discussed. Patients are reassured regarding excessive lens movement, which may occasionally result in lens loss during the first week or two of wear. The usual course, however, is for rapid adaptation during ensuing weeks.

During the first visit at 1 week, I check for discomfort, lens retention (that is, displacement either off the cornea or falling out of the eye), and superficial punctate keratitis. Corneal edema is found only rarely in grafts fit with RGP lenses. At 1, 3, and 6 months I screen for evidence of inflammation (mild iritis, keratitic precipitates), progressive vascularization of the wound beneath the lens, and peripheral graft edema.

Complications. Superficial opacification of the graft epithelium has been a rare but notable occurrence (Fig. 25-5). This most likely results from secondary edema in corneas with recurrent erosion. Discomfort with rigid lens materials if not alleviated by lens modification may be improved by refitting with a soft contact lens, though visual acuity may be compromised. Chronic soft contact lens irritation may stimulate the ingrowth of preexisting corneal vessels, a dangerous sign that may lead to a homograft reaction.

Soft contact lenses. The indications for fitting soft contact lenses are as follows:
1. Aphakic grafts, particularly to aid with stereopsis with either daily or extended wear
2. Inability of the patient to handle or insert a hard contact lens
3. Corneal grafts with a low amount of astigmatism

Both spherical and toric soft contact lenses may be tried following suture removal after keratoplasty. In general, unless 2 diopters or less of regular keratometric astigmatism is present, visual acuity is usually less than ideal. Grafted eyes with higher astigmatism may achieve satisfactory vision with a toric soft lens (Fig. 25-6). Most toric soft lenses are available in

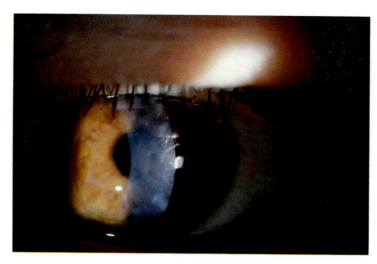

Fig. 25-5. Rare progressive subepithelial scarring centrally in keratoconus graft fit 1 year previously with PMMA lens. Majority of grafts tolerate lens application without complications.

0.75, 1.00, or 2.00 diopter minus cylinders powers. The Sunsoft Corporation (U.S.A. 1-800-648-2015) will provide toric soft contact lenses (methafilicon-A 55%) with cylindrical powers ranging in 0.25-diopter steps up to −7.0 diopters. These have been fit in several recent patients and are an additional tool in the arsenal sometimes needed to fit a grafted cornea.

The comfort achieved with soft lens wear certainly warrants soft lens trials. Over-refracting soft contact lenses on grafted eyes with hopes of providing resid-

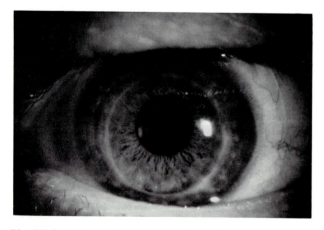

Fig. 25-6. Toric soft contact lens (Sunsoft) fit 8 months after penetrating keratoplasty for keratoconus. Manifest refraction: −4.50 +2.00 × 157, 20/50. K (keratometric) reading 44.00 − 47.37 × 114. Lens specifications: −2.75 −1.75 × 70, 8.9 base curve. Good centration, movement, and comfort in RGP-intolerant eye. Visual acuity, 20/25.

ual astigmatic correction in forward spectacles in my experience is generally unsatisfactory.

The SofPerm Lens (formerly Saturn lens). A unique soft/hard combination contact lens now in its second generation may occasionally be useful in some grafted eyes with astigmatism where base-curve measurements are flatter (less than 46 diopters) rather than steeper (Fig. 25-7). Initially reported by Hartstein,[7] the lens provides excellent optical correction and comfort. Manufactured from one solid button of silicone acrylate tertiary butylstyrene copolymer, the rigid optical center with a 6.5 mm diameter is blended after lathe cutting and hydrolyzation with a soft hydrophilic skirt of 13 mm diameter. A trial lens set is provided with base curves variable in 1 mm increments between 8.1 to 8.9 mm, and centration generally is excellent. Although less common in the second-generation design, the primary complication of the SofPerm lens fit is the tight-fitting lens with little-to-no movement and not infrequent problems with "steep lens syndrome" characterized by redness, keratitis, and corneal edema.

Rigid gas-permeable (RGP) scleral lenses. Schein and coauthors[10] describe their use of lathed fluorosilicone-acrylate copolymer high oxygen-permeable scleral lenses in seven postkeratoplasty eyes failing conventional lens treatment methods. An average follow-up time of 21 months in their population of between 29 and 55 years of age is noteworthy. Both anterior and posterior surfaces consist of three curves with the haptic portion resting on the sclera providing the base for the other two posterior secondary and posterior optic curves.

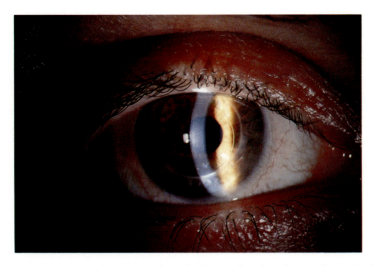

Fig. 25-7. Saturn "hard-soft" contact lens fit 9 months after keratoplasty for keratoconus. Despite objective graft astigmatism of 14 D, perfect centration was achieved with the following lens specifications: base curve, 7.20; power, −275; diameter, 13.0 mm. Residual astigmatism of 3.5 D was corrected in forward spectacles.

SUMMARY

Fitting a corneal graft with a contact lens is inherently challenging, particularly when a contact lens is the selected treatment for correction of astigmatism.

Skills in conventional rigid lens fitting are a necessary prerequisite as is a good supply of trial lenses. Additionally, a willingness to be creative and innovative in lens selection and persistent in lens modification increases the chance of a successful fit.

The expectation of what is a good fit on a graft cannot be based solely on criteria used for conventional contact lens fitting. Good visual acuity, lens stability, and patient comfort without any sign of superficial punctate keratitis or neovascularization may be present in a lens that looks like it doesn't fit.

Corneal surgeons will continue to strive for the ideal keratoplasty result, but until the time when low astigmatism is as predictable as graft clarity is now, a need will exist for postoperative visual correction with a contact lens.

ACKNOWLEDGMENT

The author wishes to thank Daniel J. Laux, B.S., C.O.T., for coauthorship of this chapter in the first edition.

REFERENCES

1. Beekhuis WH, van Rij G, Eggink FAGJ, et al: Contact lenses following keratoplasty, *CLAO J* 17:27, 1991.
2. Cohen EJ, Adams CP: Postkeratoplasty fitting for visual rehabilitation. In Dabezies OH, editor: *The CLAO guide to basic science and clinical practice*, New York, 1984, Grune & Stratton.
3. Cohen EJ, Genvert GI: Postkeratoplasty contact lens fitting, *Int Ophthalmol Clin* 26(1):119, 1986.
4. Davison JA, Bourne WM: Results of penetrating keratoplasty using a double running suture technique, *Arch Ophthalmol* 99:1541, 1981.
5. Genvert GJ et al: Fitting gas-permeable contact lenses after penetrating keratoplasty, *Am J Ophthalmol* 99:571, 1985.
6. Groden LR, White W: Porcine collagen corneal shield treatment of persistent epithelial defects following penetrating keratoplasty, *CLAO J* 16:95, 1990.
7. Hartstein J: Personal communication, St. Louis, 1985.
8. Manabe R, Matsuda M, Suda T: Photokeratoscopy in fitting contact lenses after penetrating keratoplasty, *Br J Ophthalmol* 70:55, 1986.
9. Mannis MJ, Matsumoto ER: Extended wear soft contact lenses after penetrating keratoplasty, *Arch Ophthalmol* 101:1225, 1983.
10. Schein OD, Rosenthal P, Ducharme C: A gas permeable scleral contact lens for visual rehabilitation, *Am J Ophthalmol* 109:318, 1990.
11. Soper JW, Girard LJ: Special designs and fitting techniques. In Girard LJ, editor: *Corneal contact lenses*, ed 2, St. Louis, 1970, Mosby–Year Book.

Chapter 26

Endothelial Cell Loss After Keratoplasty

ANN E. SCHWARTZ

WILLIAM M. BOURNE

Transplanted corneal endothelial cells remain viable as a chimera for years after successful penetrating keratoplasty.[4,10,34,64,93] Because the cornea is clear, it affords us the unique opportunity to observe these living human cells in vivo with the specular microscope. Because human endothelial cells divide or fuse only in exceptional circumstances,[44,45,92] cells that die or migrate are not replaced; such a cell loss is reflected by a decrease in the number of endothelial cells in the area in question. This chapter is a review of current knowledge about postoperative changes in donor and recipient endothelial cells and the use of preoperative and postoperative endothelial cell assay as a test of the efficacy of different methods of corneal preservation.

DONOR ENDOTHELIAL CELL SURVIVAL AFTER PENETRATING KERATOPLASTY

Many investigators have shown that a significant number of donor endothelial cells are lost in the weeks and months after penetrating keratoplasty.* Several studies have been carried out in a prospective manner, examining the donor endothelial cells both before and after transplantation.† Data on cell loss from various studies show that corneas lose an average of 17% to 39.8% at 1 year after keratoplasty.[47,84,90] However, these data are somewhat difficult to interpret as numerous other factors must be

taken into consideration, including type of operation and type of intraocular lens, if any. Recent data indicate that donor age, however, does not appear to affect postoperative cell loss for transplants done for a number of different conditions (Schwartz, unpublished data). This early cell loss must be attributed to the effects of both corneal preservation and transplantation. Some earlier studies demonstrated less than 10% cell loss postoperatively.[18,22]

Early endothelial cell loss can be influenced by both preservative and operative techniques. On average, all transplants lose a large number of central endothelial cells in the first several months postoperatively. Both prospective and retrospective large studies reported similar findings;[14,62] the central endothelial cell counts decreased by approximately 21% per year for 3 years after keratoplasty and then stabilized (Fig. 26-1), losing approximately only 0.5% per year as in normal aging.[21] A recent analysis of keratoplasties done for pseudophakic bullous keratopathy found an average of 22.6% to 27.4% cell loss in the first year after surgery, 31.7% to 38.6% after 2 years, and 52.4% to 54.1% after 5 years.[89] The percentage differences encompassed patients grouped by intraocular lens status. It is hypothesized that the majority of the endothelial cell damage (the true "loss") occurs intraoperatively.

Peripheral Cell Loss. The greatest degree of cell loss occurs from the peripheral graft and recipient near the wound. The remaining endothelial cells enlarge and migrate to cover these peripheral areas of cell loss (are "lost" from the central graft). Gradually

---

*References 1, 5-8, 13, 17, 20, 23, 25, 26, 31, 32, 36, 46, 51, 54, 55, 60, 62, 63, 68, 71-75, 77, 81, 82, 86, 87, 94, 96.
†References 2, 11, 12, 14, 18, 19, 22, 24, 29, 69, 70, 76, 91.

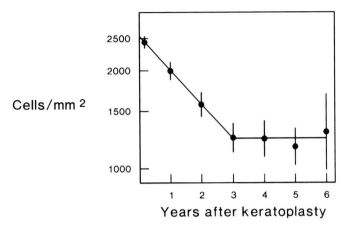

Fig. 26-1. Exponential decrease in central endothelial cell density of transplanted corneas over time after keratoplasty (semilog scale, mean ± SEM). Decrease in mean cell density is linear for 3 years and then minimal. Central cell loss during first 3 years is described by following equation:

$$\text{Central cell density} = 2522e^{-0.24t}$$

(From Bourne WM: *Cornea* 2[4]:289-294, 1983.)

a realignment of cells occurs and eliminates large discrepancies in mean cell size in different portions of the graft and recipient. This cell migration and realignment takes an average of 3 years after keratoplasty, after which cells are lost at a very slow rate, similar to that of normal corneas. This hypothesis is plausible because it requires severe (90%) cell loss from only the peripheral 1.5 mm of the graft and recipient.[20] This is consistent with the increased manipulation of the wound edge (cutting and suturing). Thus, when grafts are examined many years after keratoplasty, one would expect cell losses greater than 60% with no differences between central and peripheral counts. One study of 100 transplants at least 10 years postoperatively showed a mean endothelial cell density of 684 cells/mm². This would represent a 73% cell loss if one assumes a preoperative cell count of 2500 cells/mm². No difference between central and peripheral counts was found.[1]

The status of the recipient corneal endothelium after keratoplasty is less well known. One study found a decrease in recipient cell density in phakic eyes similar to that on the graft,[80] whereas two other investigations noted recipient cell counts much higher than those in the donor, even 12 years after keratoplasty.[68,77] The recipient corneal endothelium near the wound probably is considerably damaged during the keratoplasty procedure. No studies that have examined the peripheral recipient endothelium both before and after keratoplasty have yet been published.

Storage Method Versus Cell Loss. The method of corneal preservation and storage time can affect endothelial cell loss. McCarey-Kaufman (MK) medium was found to be clinically successful in the mid-1970s[57] and changed corneal storage methods. Corneas stored at 4° C in MK medium for 1 to 81 hours had the same mean endothelial cell loss (6%) 2 months after keratoplasty as the grafts using tissue stored in K-Sol medium for 1 to 13 days.[15,16] Cryopreservation of corneal tissue, a method rarely used in the United States today, yielded a mean cell loss of 23% over a 12-year period (from 2 to 14 years after transplantation) in a European study.[79] Organ-cultured donors preserved for up to 4 weeks showed a mean cell loss of 39.4% to 65% at the final postoperative evaluation (7.5 months to 5 years after keratoplasty).[3,52]

New corneal preservation media have been developed in an effort to increase donor cornea storage time while minimizing endothelial cell loss. In a study comparing corneas preserved in either K-Sol or CSM, the mean cell loss 12 months postoperatively was 27% ± 22% for corneas preserved in K-Sol and 17% ± 26% for those preserved in CSM solution. Thus the authors concluded that both chondroitin-based solutions were effective for corneal preservation.[49] Transferring corneas received in MK medium to K-Sol solution was shown to effectively increase storage time without a significant effect on endothelial cell density.[40] Also, the addition of 1% dextran to CSM solutions (DexSol) was found to significantly thin corneal tissue without adversely affecting endothelial cell density.[50] Perhaps one of the most exciting developments in recent years has been the addition of growth factors to corneal preservation media. Human epidermal growth factors (EGF) and human insulin were added to DexSol (CSM containing 2.5% chondroitin sulfate and 1% dextran[48]). Corneas stored in this solution were transplanted; their mates were stored in Dexsol and transplanted on the same day. The impetus for this study was both animal work and a pilot study that showed higher endothelial cell counts in corneas that had been exposed to EGF.[33,83] Results of this study are still pending.

Intraoperative Factors and Cell Loss. Operative techniques can also affect cell loss. One study showed a greater cell loss in phakic versus aphakic grafts;[24] this was attributed to contact between the graft endothelium and the iris during surgery and was eliminated by softening phakic eyes preoperatively.[12] The method of correcting aphakia at the time of keratoplasty can also affect cell loss.[47,78,84,89,90] Closed-loop anterior chamber lenses (AC IOL) are no longer used, but a retrospective study of these lenses inserted at the time of keratoplasty showed a 51.4% cell loss 3 years postoperatively.[90] Currently, most surgeons place either an open-loop AC IOL or a posterior chamber lens (PC IOL) sutured to the iris or the sclera in the region of the ciliary sulcus if capsular support is inadequate.* In one study, a 19% cell loss was found 1 year after keratoplasty with PC IOLs sutured to the iris.[84] Another group retrospectively analyzed open-loop AC IOLs versus iris-fixated sutured PC IOLs in eyes undergoing keratoplasty for aphakic or pseudophakic bullous keratopathy. The mean endothelial cell loss 1 year after keratoplasty did not significantly differ between the two groups (32% ± 26% for AC IOLs, 27% ± 26% for PC IOLs).[47] Similarly, one investigator reported 19.0% cell loss for iris-sutured PC IOLs and 16.5% cell loss for open-loop AC IOLs after 1 year.[89] It is not yet clear which of these methods is safest for the graft endothelium over a long period of time.

Other Factors Affecting the Endothelium. Trauma after keratoplasty can also be a source of cell loss. A case of two redundant graft wound dehiscences in the same eye was reported; the patient also had two graft-rejection episodes preceding the trauma. The endothelial cell density decreased 47%. More cell loss was attributed by the authors to the rejection episodes than to the trauma.[95]

Contact lens wear after keratoplasty may affect the endothelial cell density. A study comparing patients transplanted for keratoconus and then wearing poly(methyl methacrylate), or PMMA, contact lenses with similar patients who did not wear contact lenses showed a significantly lower endothelial cell density in the lens wearers than in the non–lens wearers.[53] Thus it appears that PMMA lenses may contribute to cell loss over time, probably by reducing the amount of oxygen reaching the epithelium. This leads to decreased pH and a buildup of lactate, which in turn may affect the endothelium. It is not clear if the same is true for rigid gas-permeable lenses or soft contact lenses.

Endothelial cells are also lost during immunologic graft rejection.[17,23,35,51,61,75] In one study, the central endothelial cells of 26 transplants were examined before and after an episode of endothelial rejection, with the mean cell loss over the interval being 28%.[14] A recent study compared mean cell loss before and after an episode of graft rejection in patients who had undergone keratoplasty for keratoconus with a control group transplanted for kera-

toconus who did not experience graft rejection. A decrease in endothelial cell density was observed that was of borderline significance, but those patients with severe graft rejection had much greater cell loss than controls (14.8% versus 6.5%) and than patients with mild graft reaction (1.8% cell density decrease).[58]

CLINICAL SPECULAR MICROSCOPY AS A SENSITIVE MEASURE OF ENDOTHELIAL CELL SURVIVAL

Basically the goal of corneal transplantation is to replace an abnormal central cornea with one that is as close to normal as possible. This entails transplanting as many viable donor endothelial cells as possible. The purpose of corneal preservation techniques is to maintain the donor corneas, especially the endothelial cells, in as viable and healthy a state as possible during the time between death of the donor and transplantation of the cornea, so that as many cells as possible will survive the trauma of the keratoplasty procedure. The ability to examine the central endothelial cells of donor corneas both before and after transplantation carries with it the opportunity to observe the combined effects of corneal preservation and transplantation on endothelial cell survival.

When corneas are excised from the donor eyes and placed in a medium for preservation, the endothelial cells can be observed if the corneas are stored in specialized viewing chambers[9,59] (Fig. 26-2). The central endothelial cells can be examined and photo-

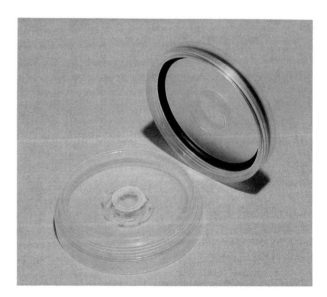

Fig. 26-2. Corneal storage chamber containing cornea in preservation medium. When lid is closed, corneal endothelium can be viewed from outside of container.

---

*References 27, 28, 30, 37-39, 41-43, 56, 65-67, 85, 88, 97.

graphed with an eye bank specular microscope through the window of the viewing chamber (Fig. 26-3). After keratoplasty, the transplanted endothelial cells can again be photographed with a clinical specular microscope. By comparing the two populations of endothelial cells one can estimate the operative cell loss—the proportion of cells that did not survive the preservation and transplantation process.

This assay of endothelial cell survival is a more sensitive measure of the efficacy of a method of corneal preservation than is the measurement used in the past—the clinical success rate (the proportion of clear, thin grafts several months after keratoplasty). Thus clinical studies have been able to demonstrate improved cell survival with modern corneal preservation techniques.* Similarly, the same system of specular microscopy can be used to assess the effects of numerous other variables on endothelial cell survival over time.

Increased endothelial cell survival in transplants is important for graft longevity. Despite excellent short-term clinical success rates, one would expect the corneas with fewer endothelial cells (more cell loss) to have less endothelial reserve to weather the effects of inflammation, healing, rejection, and aging. Their long-term survival would therefore be less than that of grafts with more endothelial cells (less cell loss).

Donor endothelial cells may also be assessed before and after corneal preservation (before transplantation). This assay measures cell survival of the preservation process itself but does not evaluate the ability of the preserved viable cells to withstand the trauma of transplantation. The best test of the efficacy of a method of corneal preservation, therefore, is to examine the central endothelium of the donor cornea before its preservation and after its transplantation; thus one can obtain an estimate of the cells that survived both the preservation and transplantation procedures. The techniques for performing these examinations are readily available, easy to perform, and not harmful to the donor cornea. All new methods of corneal preservation should be evaluated by endothelial specular microscopy.

---

*References 12, 14-19, 22-24, 33, 35, 47-49, 51-53, 58, 61, 75, 78, 83, 90, 95.

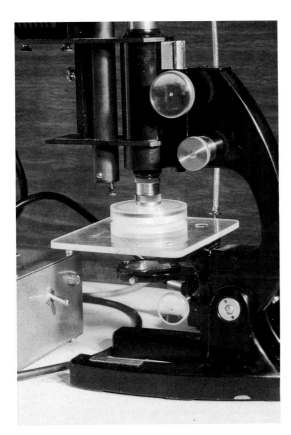

Fig. 26-3. Eye bank specular microscope with corneal storage chamber. Endothelium of donor cornea can be viewed and photographed from outside of container.

REFERENCES

1. Abbott RL, Fine M, Guillet E: Long term changes in corneal endothelium following penetrating keratoplasty: a specular microscopic study, *Ophthalmology* 90:676, 1983.
2. Abbott RL, Forster RK: Clinical specular microscopy and intraocular surgery, *Arch Ophthalmol* 97:1476, 1979.
3. Anderson J, Ehlers N: Corneal transplantation using 4-week banked donor material: long term results, *Acta Ophthalmol* 65:293, 1987.
4. Basu PK, Carré F: A study of cells in human corneal grafts: growth potential in vitro, cellular morphology, and fate of donor cells, *Can J Ophthalmol* 8:1, 1973.
5. Berry CC, Binder PS, Kahn M: Distribution of cell areas in normal and transplanted corneas, *Exp Eye Res* 31:623, 1980.
6. Bigar F: Specular microscopy of the corneal endothelium, *Dev Ophthalmol* 6:1, 1982.
7. Bigar R: Alte versus junge Spenderhornhäute, *Klin Monatsbl Augenheilkd* 184:344, 1984.
8. Bodereau X, Baikoff G, Quéré MA: Examen en microscopie spéculaire des greffes transparentes après kératites herpétiques graves, *Bull Soc Ophthalmol Fr* 82:965, 1982.
9. Bourne WM: Examination and photography of donor corneal endothelium, *Arch Ophthalmol* 94:1799, 1976.
10. Bourne WM: Penetrating keratoplasty with fresh and cryopreserved corneas: donor endothelial cell survival in primates, *Arch Ophthalmol* 96:1073, 1978.
11. Bourne WM: One-year observation of transplanted human corneal endothelium, *Ophthalmology* 87:673, 1980.
12. Bourne WM: Reduction of endothelial cell loss during phakic penetrating keratoplasty, *Am J Ophthalmol* 89:787, 1980.
13. Bourne WM: Chronic endothelial cell loss in transplanted corneas, *Cornea* 2:289, 1983.
14. Bourne WM: Morphologic and functional evaluation of the endothelium of transplanted human corneas, *Trans Am Ophthalmol Soc* 81:403, 1983.

15. Bourne WM: Endothelial cell survival on transplanted human corneas preserved at 4 C in 2.5% chondroitin sulfate for one to 13 days, *Am J Ophthalmol* 102:382, 1986.

16. Bourne WM: Results of transplantation of corneas preserved in 2.5% chondroitin sulfate, *Dev Ophthalmol* 14:106, 1987.

17. Bourne WM, Doughman DJ, Lindstrom RL: Organ-cultured corneal endothelium in vivo, *Arch Ophthalmol* 95:1818, 1977.

18. Bourne WM, Doughman DJ, Lindstrom RL: Decreased endothelial cell survival after transplantation of corneas preserved by three modifications of corneal organ culture technique, *Ophthalmology* 92:1538, 1985.

19. Bourne WM, Doughman DJ, Lindstrom RL, et al: Increased endothelial cell loss after transplantation of corneas preserved by a modified organ-culture technique, *Ophthalmology* 91:285, 1984.

20. Bourne WM, Kaufman HE: The endothelium of clear corneal transplants, *Arch Ophthalmol* 94:1730, 1976.

21. Bourne WM, Kaufman HE: Specular microscopy of human corneal endothelium in vivo, *Am J Ophthalmol* 81:319, 1976.

22. Bourne WM, Lindstrom RL, Doughman DJ: Endothelial cell survival on transplanted human corneas preserved by organ culture with a 1.35% chondroitin sulfate, *Am J Ophthalmol* 100:789, 1985.

23. Bourne WM, McCarey BE, Kaufman HE: Clinical specular microscopy, *Trans Acad Ophthalmol Otolaryngol* 81:743, 1976.

24. Bourne WM, O'Fallon WM: Endothelial cell loss during penetrating keratoplasty, *Am J Ophthalmol* 85:760, 1978.

25. Bron AJ, Brown NAP: Endothelium of the corneal graft, *Trans Ophthalmol Soc UK* 94:864, 1974.

26. Brooks AMV, Grant G, Gillies WE: Assessment of the corneal endothelium following keratoplasty, *Aust NZ J Ophthalmol* 17:379, 1989.

27. Busin M, Brauweiler P, Böker T, et al: Complications of sulcus-supported intraocular lenses with iris sutures, implanted during penetrating keratoplasty after intracapsular cataract extraction, *Ophthalmology* 97:401, 1990.

28. Cohen EJ, Brady SE, Leavitt K, et al: Pseudophakic bullous keratopathy, *Am J Ophthalmol* 106:264, 1988.

29. Culbertson WW, Abbott RL, Forster RK: Endothelial cell loss in penetrating keratoplasty, *Ophthalmology* 89:600, 1982.

30. Davis RM, Best D, Gilbert GE: Comparison of intraocular lens fixation techniques performed during penetrating keratoplasty, *Am J Ophthalmol* 111:743, 1991.

31. Doughman DJ: Prolonged donor cornea preservation in organ culture: long-term clinical evaluation, *Trans Am Ophthalmol Soc* 78:567, 1980.

32. Ehlers N, Olsen T: Long term results of corneal grafting in keratoconus, *Acta Ophthalmol* 61:918, 1983.

33. Fabricant RN, Salisbury JD, Berkowitz RA, et al: Regenerative effects of epidermal growth factor after penetrating keratoplasty in primates, *Arch Ophthalmol* 100:994, 1982.

34. Hanna C, Irwin ES: Fate of cells in the corneal graft, *Arch Ophthalmol* 68:810, 1962.

35. Hirst LW, Stark WJ: Clinical specular microscopy of corneal endothelial rejection, *Arch Ophthalmol* 101:1387, 1983.

36. Insler MS, Cooper HD, Caldwell DR: Analysis of corneal thickness and endothelial cell density in pseudophakic and aphakic patients undergoing penetrating keratoplasty, *Arch Ophthalmol* 103:390, 1985.

37. Insler MS, Kook MS, Kaufman HE: Penetrating keratoplasty for pseudophakic bullous keratopathy associated with semiflexible, closed-loop anterior chamber intraocular lenses, *Am J Ophthalmol* 107:252, 1989.

38. Johnson SM: Results of exchanging anterior chamber lenses with sulcus-fixated posterior chamber IOLs without capsular support in penetrating keratoplasty, *Ophthalmic Surg* 20:465, 1989.

39. Karnama Y, Khodadoust AA: Corneal endothelium in penetrating keratoplasty, *Am J Ophthalmol* 102:66, 1986.

40. Keates RH, Rabin B: Extending corneal storage with 2.5% chondroitin sulfate (K-Sol), *Ophthalmic Surg* 19:817, 1988.

41. Koch DD: The dilemma of pseudophakic bullous keratopathy, *Ophthalmic Surg* 20:463, 1989 (Editorial).

42. Koenig SB, McDermott ML, Hyndiuk RA: Penetrating keratoplasty and intraocular lens exchange for pseudophakic bullous keratopathy associated with a closed-loop anterior chamber intraocular lens, *Am J Ophthalmol* 108:43, 1989.

43. Kornmehl EW, Steinert RF, Odrich MG, et al: Penetrating keratoplasty for pseudophakic bullous keratopathy associated with closed-loop anterior chamber intraocular lenses, *Ophthalmology* 97:407, 1990.

44. Laing RA, Neubauer L, Leibowitz HM, et al: Coalescence of endothelial cells in the traumatized cornea. II. Clinical observations, *Arch Ophthalmol* 101:1712, 1983.

45. Laing RA, Neubauer L, Oak SS, et al: Evidence for mitosis in the adult corneal endothelium, *Ophthalmology* 91:1129, 1984.

46. Laing RA, Sandstrom M, Berrospi AR, et al: Morphological changes in corneal endothelial cells after penetrating keratoplasty, *Am J Ophthalmol* 82:459, 1976.

47. Lass JH, DeSantis DM, Reinhart WJ, et al: Clinical and morphometric results of penetrating keratoplasty with one-piece anterior chamber or suture-fixated posterior-chamber lenses in the absence of lens capsule, *Arch Ophthalmol* 108:1427, 1990.

48. Lass JH, Musch DC, Gordon JF, et al: Epidermal growth factor and insulin in use in corneal preservation: study design and objectives of a multi-center trial, *Refract Corneal Surg* 6:92, 1990.

49. Lass JH, Reinhart WJ, Bruner WE, et al: Comparison of corneal storage in K-Sol and chondroitin sulfate corneal storage medium in human corneal transplantation, *Ophthalmology* 96:688, 1989.

50. Lass JH, Reinhart WJ, Skelnik DL, et al: An in vitro and clinical comparison of corneal storage with chondroitin sulfate corneal storage medium with and without dextran, *Ophthalmology* 97:96, 1990.

51. Linn JG, Jr, Stuart JC, Warnicki JW, et al: Endothelial morphology in long-term keratoconus corneal transplants, *Ophthalmology* 88:761, 1981.

52. Lundh BL, Källmark B: Endothelial cell density after penetrating keratoplasty using long-time banked donor material after long distance transportation (Denmark-Sweden), *Acta Ophthalmol* 64:492, 1986.

53. Matsuda M, MacRae SM, Inaba M, et al: The effect of hard contact lens wear on the keratoconic corneal endothelium after penetrating keratoplasty, *Am J Ophthalmol* 107:246, 1989.

54. Matsuda M, Suda T, Manabe R: Long-term observations of the graft endothelium with different postoperative courses, *Jpn J Ophthalmol* 27:556, 1983.

55. Matsuda M, Suda T, Manabe M: Serial alterations in endothelial cell shape and pattern after intraocular surgery, *Am J Ophthalmol* 98:313, 1984.

56. Maus M, Sivalingam E: Alternate method for sulcus fixation of posterior chamber lenses in the absence of capsular support, *Ophthalmic Surg* 20:476, 1989.

57. McCarey BE, Kaufman HE: Improved corneal storage, *Invest Ophthalmol* 13:165, 1974.

58. Musch DC, Schwartz AE, Fitzgerald-Shelton K, et al: The effect of allograft rejection after penetrating keratoplasty on central endothelial cell density, *Am J Ophthalmol* 111:739, 1991.

59. Nesburn AB, Mandelbaum S, Willey DE, et al: A specular microscopic viewing system for donor corneas, *Ophthalmology* 90:686, 1983.

60. Neubauer L, Smith RS, Leibowitz HM, et al: Endothelial findings in cryopreserved corneal transplants, *Ann Ophthalmol* 16:980, 1984.

61. Olsen T: The specular microscopic appearance of corneal graft endothelium during an acute rejection episode: a case report, *Acta Ophthalmol* 57:882, 1979.

62. Olsen T: Post-operative changes in the endothelial cell density of corneal grafts, *Acta Ophthalmol* 59:863, 1981.

63. Olsen T, Ehlers N, Favini E: Long term results of corneal grafting in Fuchs' endothelial dystrophy, *Acta Ophthalmol* 62:445, 1984.

64. Polack FM: Four-year retention of ^{3}H thymidine by corneal endothelium, *Arch Ophthalmol* 75:659, 1966.

65. Polack FM: Results of keratoplasty for aphakic or pseudophakic corneal edema with intraocular lens implantation or exchange, *Cornea* 7:239, 1988.

66. Polack FM: Pseudophakic corneal edema. An 11-year study of its development, incidence, and treatment, *Cornea* 8:306, 1989.

67. Price FW Jr, Whitson WE: Visual results of suture-fixated posterior chamber lenses during penetrating keratoplasty, *Ophthalmology* 96:1234, 1989.

68. Rao GN, Aquavella JV: Peripheral recipient endothelium following corneal transplantation, *Ophthalmology* 88:50, 1981.

69. Rao GN, Waldon WR, Aquavella JV: Fate of endothelium in a corneal graft, *Ann Ophthalmol* 10:645, 1978.

70. Rao GN, Waldon WR, Aquavella JV: Morphology of graft endothelium and donor age, *Br J Ophthalmol* 64:523, 1980.

71. Rigal D, Roche C, Threil M, et al: Fate of the human corneal endothelium during perforating keratoplasty: study using specular microscopy (apropos of 45 cases), *Bull Soc Ophthalmol Fr* 83:731, 1983.

72. Ruben M, Colebrook E, Guillon M: Keratoconus, keratoplasty thickness, and endothelial morphology, *Br J Ophthalmol* 63:790, 1979.

73. Ruben M, Guillon M: Endothelial survival in transparent keratoplasty. In Trevor-Roper P, editor: *The cornea in health and disease*, Sixth Congr Eur Soc Ophthalmol, New York, 1981, Grune & Stratton, pp 591-596.

74. Ruusuvaara P: Effects of corneal preservation, donor age, cadaver time and postoperative period on the graft endothelium: a specular microscopic study, *Acta Ophthalmol* 57:868, 1979.

75. Ruusuvaara P: Histocompatibility and corneal graft endothelium, *Acta Ophthalmol* 57:868, 1979.

76. Ruusuvaara P: The fate of preserved and transplanted human corneal endothelium, *Acta Ophthalmol* 58:440, 1980.

77. Ruusuvaara P: Endothelial cell densities in donor and recipient tissue after keratoplasty, *Acta Ophthalmol* 88:50, 1981.

78. Ruusuvaara P, Setälä K: The triple procedure: penetrating keratoplasty, extracapsular cataract extraction and posterior chamber lens implantation: a clinical and specular microscopic study, *Acta Ophthalmol* 65:433, 1987.

79. Ruusuvaara P, Setälä K: Long term follow-up of cryopreserved corneal endothelium: a specular microscopic study, *Acta Ophthalmol* 66:687, 1988.

80. Saggau DD, Bourne WM, Ilstrup DM: Changes in recipient and donor corneal endothelium over time after keratoplasty, *Invest Ophthalmol Vis Sci* 26(suppl):146, 1985, ARVO abstracts.

81. Sato T: Studies on the endothelium of the corneal graft, *Jpn J Ophthalmol* 22:114, 1978.

82. Sawa M, Tanishima T: The morphometry of the human corneal endothelium and follow-up of postoperative changes, *Jpn J Ophthalmol* 23:337, 1979.

83. Skelnik DL, Pearlstein CS, Mindrup EA, et al: Corneal preservation at 4° with chondroitin sulfate containing medium supplemented with dextran and epidermal growth factor (EGF), *Invest Ophthalmol Vis Sci* 29(suppl):112, 1988.

84. Soong HK, Musch DC, Kowal V, et al: Implantation of posterior chamber intraocular lenses in the absence of lens capsule during penetrating keratoplasty, *Arch Ophthalmol* 107:660, 1989.

85. Speaker MG, Lugo M, Laibson PR, et al: Penetrating keratoplasty for pseudophakic bullous keratopathy: management of the intraocular lens, *Ophthalmology* 95:1260, 1988.

86. Sperling S, Olsen T, Ehlers N: Fresh and cultured corneal grafts compared by postoperative thickness and endothelial cell density, *Acta Ophthalmol* 59:566, 1981.

87. Stegmann R, Miller D: The protective function of sodium hyaluronate in corneal transplantation, *J Ocular Therap Surg* 1:28, 1981.

88. Stein RM, Laibson PR: Comparison of chondroitin sulfate to McCarey-Kaufman medium for corneal storage, *Am J Ophthalmol* 104:490, 1987.

89. Sugar A: An analysis of corneal endothelial and graft survival in pseudophakic bullous keratopathy, *Trans Am Ophthalmol Soc* 87:762, 1989.

90. Sugar A, Bhugra M, Felbeck P, et al: Follow-up of closed-loop anterior chamber intraocular lenses inserted at penetrating keratoplasty, *Trans Am Ophthalmol Soc* 88:255, 1990.

91. Sugar A, Meyer RF, Heidemann D, et al: Specular microscopic follow-up of corneal grafts for pseudophakic bullous keratopathy, *Ophthalmology* 92:325, 1985.

92. Treffers WF: Human corneal endothelial wound repair, in vitro and in vivo, *Ophthalmology* 89:605, 1982.

93. Van Rij G, Manschot WA, Renardel De Lavalette JGC, et al: Long-term survival of endothelial cells in a human corneal graft, *Am J Ophthalmol* 95:709, 1983 (Letter to the editor).

94. Waltman SR, Palmberg PF: Human penetrating keratoplasty using modified M-K medium, *Ophthalmic Surg* 9:48, 1978.

95. Watson AP, Simcock PR, Ridgway AEA: Endothelial cell loss due to repeated traumatic wound dehiscence after penetrating keratoplasty, *Cornea* 6:216, 1987.

96. Weekers JF, Malaise-Stals J: Etude à long terme de la densité cellulaire endothéliale après kératoplastie perforante, *J Fr Ophthalmol* 6:951, 1983.

97. Zaidman GW, Goldman S: A prospective study on the implantation of anterior chamber intraocular lenses during keratoplasty for pseudophakic and aphakic bullous keratopathy, *Ophthalmology* 97:757, 1990.

Part III

SPECIAL SITUATIONS IN KERATOPLASTY

Chapter 27

Chemical Burns

SHIGERU KINOSHITA

REIZO MANABE

Chemical and thermal burns are devastating ocular surface injuries that often occur bilaterally, resulting in permanent visual impairment. The surgical results obtained in the treatment of these injuries over the past few decades by use of techniques such as keratoplasty have not been encouraging.[6] Although there have been numerous reports regarding various aspects of the initial phase of chemical injury, for example, the collagenolytic activity in corneal ulceration,[2,3,24] information is relatively scarce concerning chemically injured cells at the late scarred phase of injury. This information is essential for understanding the postoperative complications of keratoplasty in burned eyes. With recent improvements in our understanding of the ocular surface epithelium[13,30] and underlying substrate[12,18] and new surgical approaches for chemical injuries[27,29] have been developed as a means of achieving a stabilized ocular surface and improved vision as well.

Chemical and thermal burns vary in their mechanism of injury, since alkali penetrates the eye very rapidly in contrast to acid or thermal burns, which tend toward rather superficial ocular surface destruction.[8,21] Special consideration of the chemical composition itself is important for medical management at the initial phase of chemical injury[22] but not for surgical management in the late scarred phase. Since the severity of an injury depends on the concentration of the chemical and the duration of chemical contact, a chemical or thermal agent can inflict injuries of any size and depth into the ocular surface. Thus the ocular manifestations of the burned cornea at the late scarred phase are rarely indicative of the injurious agent itself.

CLASSIFICATION OF SEVERITY

Initial Phase. Classification of severity in chemical injury was first proposed by Hughes,[9,10] mainly on the basis of the degree of corneal clouding and conjunctival blanching. This classification, however, indicates the extent of chemical penetration, rather than the extent of the damaged area; it divides injuries into three groups as follows:

Mild
  Erosion of corneal epithelium
  Faint haziness of cornea
  No blanching of conjunctiva or sclera
Moderately severe
  Corneal opacity blurring iris detail
  Minimal ischema of conjunctiva and sclera
Very severe
  Blurring of pupillary outline
  Blanching of conjunctiva and sclera

Severity here mainly reflects the type of chemical and its concentration, pH, and exposure time. Such a classification may be effective for prediction of the final visual acuity after medical treatment, however it does not always accurately reflect the relationship between degree of severity and final conjunctival invasion into the cornea, which seems the most important sequela to be dealt with in surgical manage-

Supported in part by Japanese Grant-in-Aid for Scientific Research 58570737.

309

ment. Ballen[1] and Roper-Hall[25] modified this classification to some extent, introducing the idea of area of chemical exposure and adding the category of total loss of corneal epithelium to group 3 (very severe) cases. Their modification has gained increasing importance in view of newer research discoveries.

Epithelial Injury. Recent laboratory experience in rabbits indicates that it may be of value to assess the area of ocular-surface epithelial defect after an injury. In fact, if the epithelial defect extends over the total surface of the cornea in a chemical injury, the conjunctival epithelium inevitably invades and covers the corneal surface. In cases of minimal inflammation, the regenerated epithelium of conjunctival origin covering the cornea gradually changes, histologically as well as biologically, and undergoes transdifferentiation into corneal epithelium.[26,30] Once a corneal wound or inflammatory response occurs, it seems that the transdifferentiated epithelium returns to the original characteristics of conjunctival epithelium, even as long as 6 months after the chemical injury.[20,31] A similar biologic progression can be assumed in humans. Thus, whether there is total loss of corneal epithelium in the initial phase of chemical injury is a key to predicting the final outcome of conjunctival invasion into the cornea. From this point of view, Thoft's classification[28] seems the more valuable; he distinguishes the following four grades on the basis of injured area.

Grade 1. Conjunctival hyperemia, with no more than diffuse superficial punctate keratitis

Grade 2. Conjunctival hyperemia, with partial corneal epithelial loss

Grade 3. Conjunctival hyperemia or areas of necrosis, with total corneal epithelial loss

Grade 4. More than 50% perilimbal conjunctival necrosis, with total corneal epithelial loss

Grades 1 and 2 possess a remnant of corneal epithelium after injury, resulting in corneal epithelial regeneration with minimal superficial vascularization, even given severe central scarring of the stroma and vascularization in the deep stromal layer. Since grades 3 and 4 show total loss of corneal epithelium and extensive conjunctival epithelial cell loss in combination with inflammatory response to chemical injury, the burned cornea eventually is covered by the well-vascularized conjunctival epithelium and subepithelial fibrous tissues. Thus Thoft's classification, based as it is upon the area of initial epithelial defect, shows closer relation to the degree of conjunctival invasion at the scarred phase than do other classifications based upon the depth of penetration.

In addition, although the total loss of corneal epithelium in grade 3 is a key point, completely different outcomes are sometimes seen: in one case minimal vascularization, whereas in another a fibrovascular corneal surface.[22] When total loss of corneal epithelium occurs, one must be sure to observe the limbal lesion, especially the palisades of Vogt.[7,17] Since laboratory work has shown that the limbal epithelium alone can resurface the totally denuded cornea with a regenerated epithelium quite similar to the corneal epithelium, with minimal invasion of the conjunctival epithelium and minimal superficial vascularization, the presence of the limbal epithelium is crucial.[15] Basal cells in the infolding of the palisades of Vogt often survive even in severe chemical injury because of less contact with chemicals. In clinical observation therefore total loss of corneal epithelium alone should be strictly distinguished from such loss together with complete disappearance of the limbal epithelium, that is, the palisades of Vogt. Thus a further subdivision may be needed in grade 3.

Scarred Phase. If the injured eye does not develop corneal perforation or corneal infection, the ocular surface will heal within a few years with corneal scarring and vascularization of varying degrees of severity. The final corneal opacity may be caused by scarring of the cornea itself, which is not a crucial consideration in penetrating keratoplasty, or by conjunctival invasion of the cornea, which is of crucial importance because of tendencies for postgraft persistent epithelial defects and corneal ulceration. These two different types of scarring are outlined below and illustrated in Figs. 27-1 to 27-3.

Scarring type A (Figs. 27-1, *left,* and 27-2)
   Corneal scarring
   Retention of most of corneal epithelium
Scarring type B (Figs. 27-1, *right,* and 27-3)
   Corneal scarring
   Conjunctival epithelial coverage
   Superficial vascularization
   Complete disappearance of palisades of Vogt

Although, preoperatively, the visual impairment and degree of corneal scarring are sometimes quite similar in types A and B, after keratoplasty both immunologic and cell biologic host responses are dramatically different in the two groups. Thus, even a case with severe corneal scarring from a chemical burn of type A would be a reasonable candidate for penetrating keratoplasty, resembling as it does the scarring caused by herpetic keratitis. On the other hand, in type B scarring the regenerated epithelium of conjunctival origin covers the scarred cornea, and even though the scar may be faint, long-term fol-

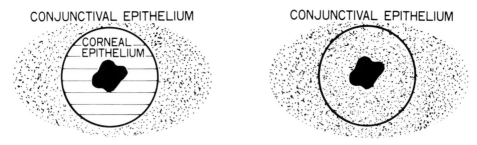

Fig. 27-1. Schema of two different types of scarring: *hatched,* corneal epithelium; *stippled,* conjunctival epithelium; *shaded,* scarring. *Left,* Scarring type A; *right,* scarring type B.

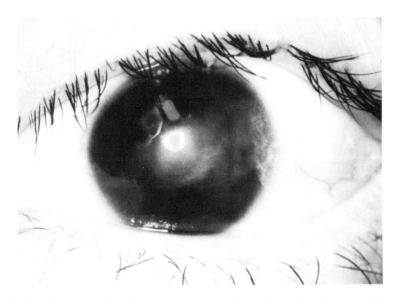

Fig. 27-2. Scarring type A. Observe corneal scarring with minimal superficial vascularization and minimal conjunctival invasion.

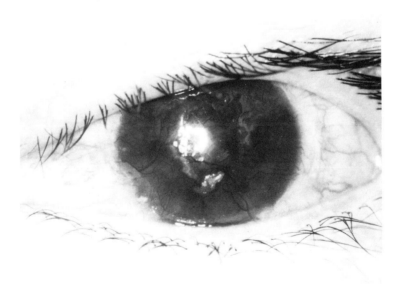

Fig. 27-3. Scarring type B. There is extensive vascularization and conjunctival invasion.

low-up study after keratoplasty often reveals a high incidence of epithelial problems resulting in graft failure. This is probably attributable to the fact that in type B the host corneal epithelium has been rejected or replaced over time[13] by conjuctival epithelium. Furthermore, transdifferentiated epithelium of conjunctival origin tends to revert to its original characteristics after surgical wounding.[31] Thus the surgeon must be especially careful in deciding to perform penetrating keratoplasty in cases of type B scarring.

SURGICAL MANAGEMENT

Keratoplasty. Since the process of wound healing after a chemical injury sometimes takes years, keratoplasty in cases of chemical or thermal burns should be postponed until the final scarring phase.[19] For acute corneal perforation, however, penetrating keratoplasty must be performed to preserve the integrity of the cornea and globe.

It has been suggested that when performing penetrating keratoplasty in chemical injury one should keep the donor corneal epithelium on the graft, especially in type B scarring.[4] In addition, should epi-

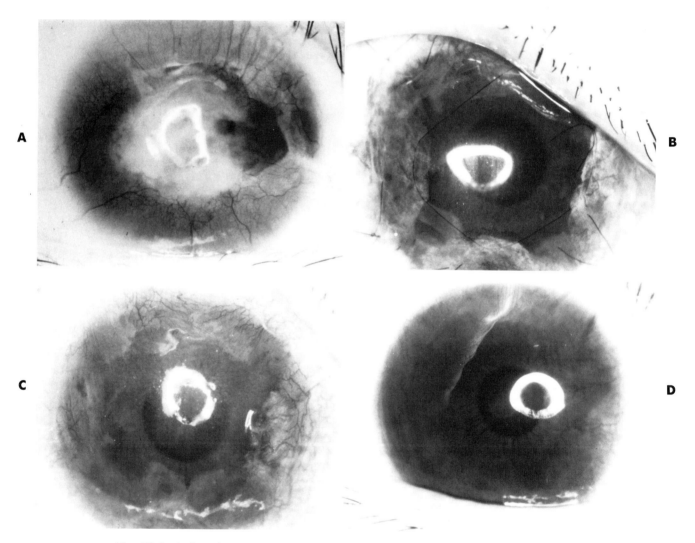

Fig. 27-4. A, Scarring type B in thermal burn before conjunctival transplantation. **B,** Same eye 7 days after conjunctival transplantation. Four pieces of free-flap conjunctiva are sutured onto limbal area with 10-0 nylon, with central portion of cornea becoming clear. **C,** One month after conjunctival transplantation. Notice thinning of free-flap conjunctiva and some haziness of corneal surface attributable to complete coverage by regenerated conjunctival epithelium. **D,** Seven years after conjunctival transplantation. Notice clear optic axis and superficial vascularization in peripheral cornea.

thelial disturbance of the graft occur because of entropion of the upper eyelid, trichiasis, or lagophthalmos resulting from chemical injury, the use of a soft contact lens may be necessary to preserve the epithelial layer on the graft.[4] It is difficult to expect excellent results from penetrating keratoplasty in type B scarring; however, some keratoplasties, if the donor epithelium is kept on the graft and a soft contact lens is continuously used, will yield somewhat better results, especially in cases where the histocompatibility antigen of the donor tissue is matched with that of the host.

Conjunctival Transplantation. In cases of type B scarring with minimal scarring of the deep stroma, (often in acid or mild thermal burns), conjunctival transplantation may be the surgery of choice, rather than keratoplasty (Fig. 27-4, *A*). The idea in this procedure is to replace scarred conjunctival epithelium with transdifferentiated epithelium of conjunctival origin, which migrates out from free-flap conjunctiva near the limbus, thereby achieving surface rehabilitation.[27] In fact, some cases of unilateral chemical injury, if operated at the scarred phase, have exhibited great visual improvement. The technique of surgery is as follows: After superficial keratectomy and extensive peritomy over 360 degrees, four pieces of free-flap conjunctiva obtained from the contralateral eye are sutured onto the limbal area with 10-0 nylon. Seven to 10 days postoperatively the keratectomized cornea is covered by regenerating epithelium from the free flaps, without much fibrovascular invasion (Fig. 27-4, *B*). The key point for success is to keep a large central portion of the cornea free from the conjunctiva. Conjunctiva transplanted near the limbus tends to thin at 1 to 2 months postoperatively; the cornea, including the free-flap conjunctiva, then becomes translucent (Fig. 27-4, *C*). The epithelium on the central portion of the cornea is believed to transdifferentiate into corneal epithelium, with superficial vascularization from the limbus being retained, resulting in an obscure borderline between cornea and conjunctiva even 7 years after operation (Fig. 27-4, *D*).

Since conjunctival transplantation cannot be used for chemical burns in both eyes, keratoepithelioplasty remains the surgery of choice in such cases.

Keratoepithelioplasty (Fig. 27-5). The surgical procedure of keratoepithelioplasty is similar to conjunctival transplantation. The primary difference is in the source of epithelial material: conjunctival transplantation uses autologous conjunctival epithelium, whereas keratoepithelioplasty uses allogeneic corneal epithelium. The original idea for this surgery, proposed by Thoft, is that donor corneal epithelium migrating

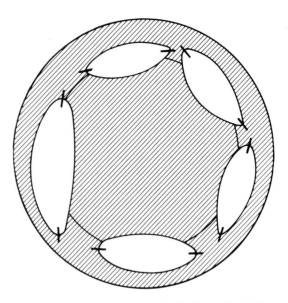

Fig. 27-5. Schema of keratoepithelioplasty: *hatched,* keratectomized and peritomized area: *open,* lenticules; *inner circle,* limbus.

from the peripheral cornea could be preserved permanently if the immunologic reaction were inhibited by topical use of steroid.[11,29]

In this surgical procedure, the severely vascularized cornea can be resurfaced by a relatively normal-looking epithelium. After peripheral placement of donor corneal lenticules the epithelium grows over the bare corneal surface, bringing about epithelial wound closure within 7 to 10 days as well as quieting of the eye (Fig. 27-6, *A* and *B*). At this time the donor corneal epithelium covers the cornea. One problem with Thoft's original idea is that donor corneal epithelium often encounters epithelial rejection and is subsequently replaced by host conjunctival epithelium (Fig. 27-6, *C*). A most interesting phenomenon occurs after such epithelial rejection, in that the eye remains silent afterward, with epithelium of host conjunctival origin covering the cornea (Fig. 27-6, *D*). Judging from these clinical observations, the donor lenticule in keratoepithelioplasty does not play a major role in the permanent supply of donor corneal epithelium though it may largely contribute to blocking subconjunctival fibrovascular tissue invasion at the limbal site.[14] There may also be involved other important biologic factors, such as corneal basement membrane deposition by donor corneal epithelium on the bare stroma.

Keratoepithelioplasty Combined with Keratoplasty (Fig. 27-7). As discussed above, the biologic purpose of keratoepithelioplasty is the blocking of conjunctival invasion and the providing of a tempo-

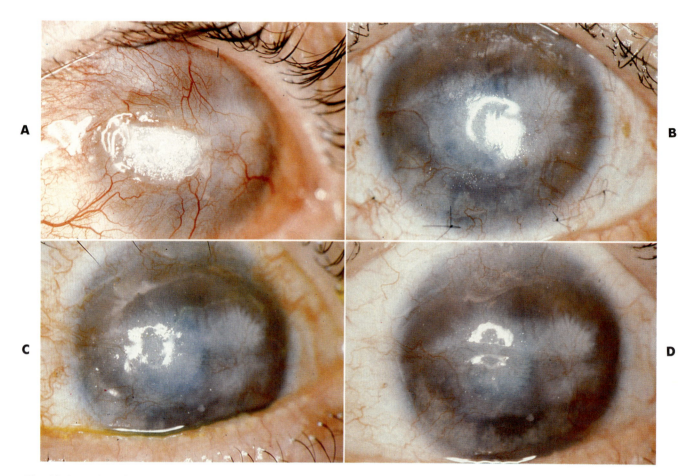

Fig. 27-6. A, Scarring type B from grade 3 alkali burn. Visual acuity is "hand movements." **B,** Same eye 1 month after keratoepithelioplasty. Notice relatively normal-looking corneal surface, deep stromal opacity, and some vessels, mainly in deep stroma. Postoperative visual acuity was 20/100. **C,** Epithelial rejection occurred 5 months after keratoepithelioplasty. Notice line produced by fluorescein staining. This rejection progressed toward central portion of cornea. **D,** Same eye 1 year after keratoepithelioplasty. Corneal epithelium is presumably replaced by host conjunctival epithelium. Eye looks the same as in **B.**

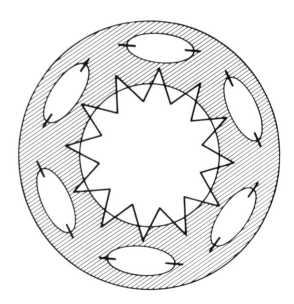

Fig. 27-7. Schema of keratoepithelioplasty combined with keratoplasty: *hatched,* keratoectomized and peritomized area; *open,* lenticules and graft.

rary source of epithelium; surgical results bear this out. In cases exhibiting extensive conjunctival invasion with descemetoceles after chemical injury, lamellar keratoplasty was performed with keratoepithelioplasty as a means of blocking conjunctival invasion (Fig. 27-8). With lamellar keratoplasty alone, epithelial defect or corneal ulceration frequently occurs at the wound edge as well as on the graft, but this occurs less often when the techniques are combined. Since after epithelial rejection the keratoepithelioplastied eye becomes silent, this procedure is ideal for reconstruction of the devastated cornea in chemical injury. It is also quite effective in Mooren's

ulcer,[16] probably for its blocking of perilimbal conjunctival invasion. Since relatively deep stromal opacity can be removed by means of lamellar keratoplasty, the combined procedure is the best choice for achievement of better vision with fewer postoperative complications.[23]

In the more severe chemical injuries that are often accompanied by secondary glaucoma, the corneal endothelium is sometimes destroyed. Penetrating keratoplasty with keratoepithelioplasty can be performed in such cases (Fig. 27-9, *A*). In penetrating keratoplasty, perilimbal subconjunctival tissue removal usually affords good results for the short term;[5]

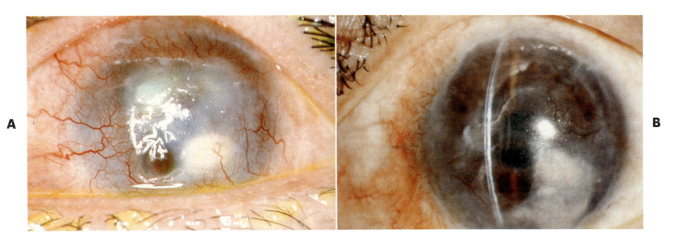

Fig. 27-8. A, Scarring type B with descemetocele in alkali burn. Visual acuity was "hand movements." **B,** One year after lamellar keratoplasty with keratoepithelioplasty. Corrected visual acuity, 20/60. Epithelium covering cornea is presumably of host conjunctival origin, since donor epithelial rejection occurred 2 months after this surgery.

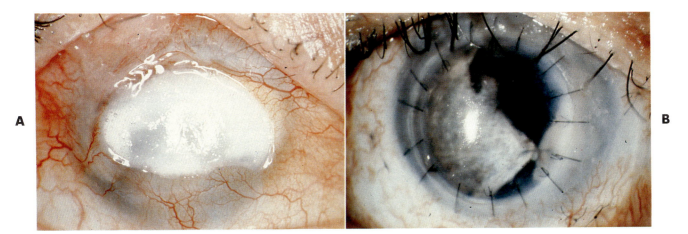

Fig. 27-9. A, Scarring type B from grade 4 alkali burn. **B,** Three months after penetrating keratoplasty with keratoepithelioplasty. Notice clear graft and several lenticules sutured onto sclera.

however, the placement of lenticules prevents conjunctival invasion into the wound edge and yields far better results, preventing neovascularization and corneal ulceration. As seen in Fig. 27-9, *B,* not only is the peripheral cornea white and silent, but the sclera is also. Since the donor cornea is placed upon the sclera, the graft can easily be sensitized by the host, resulting in the possibility of early immunologic reaction. Without keratoepithelioplasty, neovascularization easily reaches the wound edge, with the same results. In our clinical experience, curiously enough we have not seen early endothelial rejection, but rather less fibrovascular tissue reaction in the peripheral cornea and a stabilized ocular surface. Long-term follow-up study will reveal the true value of penetrating keratoplasty with keratoepithelioplasty. For grade 4 chemical injury the development of a new keratoprosthesis would offer greater hope.

REFERENCES

1. Ballen PH: Treatment of chemical burns of the eye, *Eye Ear Nose Throat Monthly* 43:57, 1964.
2. Berman MB, Leary R, Gage J: Evidence for a role of the plasminogen activator-plasmin system in corneal ulceration, *Invest Ophthalmol Vis Sci* 19:1204, 1980.
3. Berman MB, Manabe R: Corneal collagenase: evidence for zinc metalloenzymes, *Ann Ophthalmol* 5:1193, 1973.
4. Brown SI, Bloomfield SE, Pearce DB: A follow-up report on transplantation of the alkali-burned cornea, *Am J Ophthalmol* 77:538, 1974.
5. Brown SI, Tragakis MP, Pearce DB: Corneal transplantation for severe alkali burns, *Trans Am Acad Ophthalmol Otolaryngol* 76:1266, 1972.
6. Casey TA, Mayer DJ: Grafting in chemical burns. In *Corneal grafting: principles and practice,* Philadelphia, 1984, WB Saunders.
7. Davanger M, Evensen A: Role of the pericorneal papillary structure in renewal of corneal epithelium, *Nature* 229:560, 1971.
8. Grayson M: Acid and alkali injuries. In *Diseases of the cornea,* St. Louis, 1979, Mosby–Year Book.
9. Hughes WF: Alkali burns of the eye. 1. Review of the literature and summary of present knowledge, *Arch Ophthalmol* 35:423, 1946.
10. Hughes WF: Alkali burns of the eyes. 2. Clinical and pathological course, *Arch Ophthalmol* 36:189, 1946.
11. Kaufman HE: Keratoepithelioplasty for the replacement of damaged corneal epithelium, *Am J Ophthalmol* 97:100, 1984.
12. Kenyon KR et al: Regeneration of corneal epithelial basement membrane following thermal cauterization, *Invest Ophthalmol Vis Sci* 16:292, 1977.
13. Kinoshita S, Friend J, Thoft RA: Ocular surface epithelial regeneration and disease, *Int Ophthalmol Clin* 24:(2):169, Boston, 1984, Little, Brown.
14. Kinoshita S, Ohashi Y, Manabe R: Keratoepithelioplasty in chemical burn, *Jpn J Clin Ophthalmol.* (In press.)
15. Kinoshita S et al: Limbal epithelium in ocular surface wound healing, *Invest Ophthalmol Vis Sci* 23:73, 1982.
16. Kinoshita S et al: Keratoepithelioplasty in Mooren's ulcer. (In preparation.)
17. Kinoshita S et al: Palisades of Vogt in ocular surface disease, *Jpn J Clin Ophthalmol.* (In press.)
18. Khodadoust AA et al: Adhesion of regenerating corneal epithelium: the role of basement membrane, *Am J Ophthalmol* 65:339, 1968.
19. Kramer K: *Delay of keratoplasty to improve prognosis in alkali burns,* Presented to the Castroviejo Society, Las Vegas, 1982.
20. Liu SH et al: Secretory component of IgA: a marker for differentiation of ocular epithelium, *Invest Ophthalmol Vis Sci* 20:100, 1981.
21. McCulley JP: Chemical injuries. In Smolin G, Thoft RA, editors: *The cornea,* Boston, 1983, Little, Brown.
22. McCulley JP, Moore TE: Chemical injuries of the eye. In Leibowitz HM, editor: *Corneal disorders,* Philadelphia, 1984, WB Saunders.
23. Manabe R: *Therapeutic keratoplasty,* Presented to 39th Japanese Congress for Clinical Ophthalmology, Niigata, 1985.
24. Pfister RR et al: The efficacy of ascorbate treatment after severe experimental alkali burns depends upon the route of administration, *Invest Ophthalmol Vis Sci* 19:145, 1980.
25. Roper-Hall MJ: Thermal and chemical burns, *Trans Ophthalmol Soc UK* 85:631, 1965.
26. Shapiro MS, Friend J, Thoft RA: Corneal reepithelialization from the conjunctiva, *Invest Ophthalmol Vis Sci* 21:135, 1981.
27. Thoft RA: Conjunctival transplantation, *Arch Ophthalmol* 95:1425, 1977.
28. Thoft RA: Chemical and thermal injury, *Int Ophthalmol Clin* 19(2):243, Boston, 1979, Little, Brown.
29. Thoft RA: Keratoepithelioplasty, *Am J Ophthalmol* 97:1, 1984.
30. Thoft RA, Friend J: Biochemical transformation of regenerating ocular surface epithelium, *Invest Ophthalmol Vis Sci* 16:14, 1977.
31. Thoft RA, Friend J, Murphy HS: Ocular surface epithelium and corneal vascularization in rabbits. 1. The role of wounding, *Invest Ophthalmol Vis Sci* 18:85, 1979.

Chapter 28

Regrafting

JOHN D. GOTTSCH

MICHAEL E. SULEWSKI

WALTER J. STARK

The patient with apparent graft failure who is considered for a repeat corneal transplant requires a thorough examination to determine the cause of the graft failure, a prediction of the postregraft visual potential, and a rational surgical approach to maximize graft survival. To address these areas, this chapter focuses on the following subjects:

1. Work-up of the patient who presents with graft failure
2. Causes and relative risks of failed keratoplasties
3. Indications and contraindications for repeat penetrating keratoplasty
4. Update on recent efforts to decrease allograft rejection by HLA tissue typing
5. Surgical techniques that maximize the survival of the corneal regraft

DECREASED ACUITY AND THE POSTKERATOPLASTY PATIENT

The patient who complains of decreased visual acuity after penetrating keratoplasty needs to be evaluated promptly and thoroughly. Graft failure must be suspected, and if careful inspection of the cornea and anterior chamber reveals any inflammatory signs suggestive of rejection, appropriate therapy must be instituted immediately. Graft failure may not fully account for a drop in visual acuity, and other causes of decreased acuity, such as cataract, opacification of the posterior capsule in a pseudophakic eye, and retinal or optic nerve disease, must be excluded.

The contribution of stromal and epithelial edema during graft failure to the decrease in visual acuity can be predicted by an application of anhydrous glycerin and a hard contact lens over-refraction or potential acuity testing (PAM). Surprisingly good visual acuity may result if the corneal edema is a significant cause of the visual loss. Importantly, clearing of the edematous cornea will permit better visualization of ocular structures so that other possible causes of diminished acuity can be evaluated. Graft failure itself may only be one factor in causing reduced vision in eyes undergoing multiple surgery.[32] Eyes that have undergone multiple procedures are more likely to develop other problems such as cataract, raised intraocular pressure, retinal detachment, or cystoid macular edema.[38,55,28]

In those eyes with opaque corneas an estimation of macular function may be made with entoptic phenomenon and color-vision testing. An ultrasound evaluation is helpful to allow determination of the presence of a retinal detachment or a mass lesion.

CAUSES OF GRAFT FAILURE

Allograft Reaction. Maumenee[40] demonstrated that corneal graft failure could be caused by sensitization of the recipient to donor material. Later, Khodadoust and Silverstein[32,34] showed that the epithelium, stroma, and endothelium could each exhibit an immune reaction. The clinical manifestations and frequency of the different types of corneal rejections have been described[4,12,33,36] and include

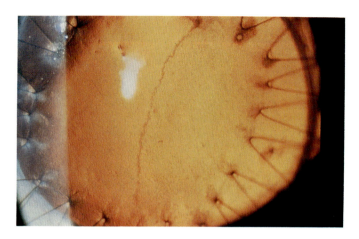

Fig. 28-1. Retroillumination of endothelial rejection line.

epithelial and endothelial rejection lines (Fig. 28-1), subepithelial infiltrates, keratic precipitates, and graft edema.

Since the introduction of microsurgical techniques and advances in corneal preservation, the allograft reaction has become the most common cause of graft failure.[5,6,30,60]

Predisposing Factors for Allograft Reaction

Vascularization. In vascularized recipient corneas (Fig. 28-2) rejection occurs in up to 65% of cases.[62] Khodadoust[30] studied the rejection rates of corneas with increasing recipient vascularization and found that rates were as high as 65% in densely vascularized corneas and the interval between the surgical procedure and allograft reaction was much shorter in the densely vascularized cornea. In a study of high-risk patients with vascularized recipient corneas, an immune event developed in 26% of cases.[60]

Graft failure from rejection occurred in 15% of these higher-risk cases.

Additionally, neovascularization of the graft-host interface or in the donor graft is associated with a significant increase in the risk of allograft reaction.[47]

Inflammation. Inflammatory conditions such as herpetic keratouveitis[18,21,49] or bacterial suppuration from a suture abscess (Fig. 28-3) may incite an allograft reaction. Ocular inflammation alone is believed to produce corneal opacification without the involvement of an allograft reaction.[50,51] Presumably endothelial dysfunction is induced in an eye with significant uveitis.

Regrafts. The prognosis for repeat keratoplasty (Fig. 28-4) has significantly improved with the recent advances in instrumentation, surgical technique, corneal preservation, and postoperative management. The success rate for clear regrafts has been re-

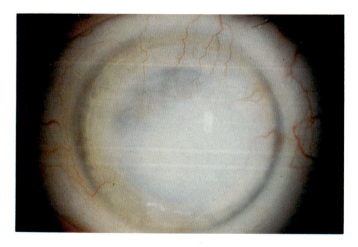

Fig. 28-2. Corneal opacification with vascularization after herpes zoster keratitis.

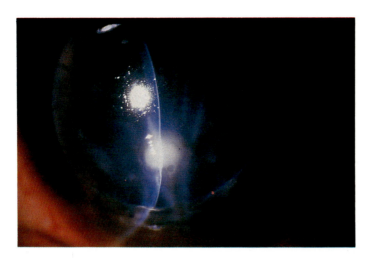

Fig. 28-3. Allograft reaction 1 week after presentation with suture abscess caused by *Streptococcus pneumoniae*.

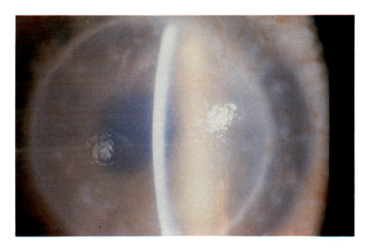

Fig. 28-4. Recurrent lattice dystrophy 5 years after keratoplasty.

ported to be 42% to 68% with follow-up observation ranging from 1 to 12 years.[6,14,20,35,38,55] Kirkness and co-workers[35] determined that allograft rejection was the most common cause of graft failure in repeat transplants but recurrence of the host disease and endothelial decompensation were also significant causes. However, in eyes with regrafts attributable to rejection episodes, the intervals between subsequent allograft reactions was significantly shortened.[31]

Other predisposing factors. Evidence has been produced that the presence of anterior synechiae,[5] bilateral grafts,[15] and younger age of the recipient[4] increases the risk for allograft rejection.

Glaucoma. Paton[48] reports ocular hypertension as a leading cause of graft failure. In Arentsen's[5] series, uncontrolled glaucoma accounted for 20% of all failed penetrating keratoplasties. The occurrence of glaucoma after aphakic keratoplasty is well documented,[29,43,44,66] and Olson and Kaufman[44] have suggested that an oversized graft in an aphakic eye may help prevent the development of elevated intraocular pressure. The incidence of postoperative glaucoma in repeat transplants was 47% in one series by Robinson,[55] whereas Kirkness and co-workers[35] reported an incidence of 38%. When the intraocular pressure is poorly controlled with all types of therapy, regrafting may be contraindicated.[55] In these very difficult cases one can attempt a combined keratoplasty and trabeculectomy.[27]

To reduce the probability of an unacceptably high rise in intraocular pressure postoperatively, it is imperative that the glaucoma be under good medical control before keratoplasty. Cyclocryotherapy[9,68] or filtering[23] procedures before or sometimes after keratoplasty may be necessary when medical therapy is inadequate to control intraocular pressure. The use of neodymium:YAG laser transscleral cyclodestruction of the ciliary body has been a promising procedure in difficult to control postkeratoplasty glaucoma patients.[13] Surgical techniques during keratoplasty that may aid in the prevention of postoperative glaucoma are as follows:

1. An oversized graft in aphakic or pseudophakic eyes
2. Lysis of previous anterior synechiae
3. A well-sutured wound to prevent a postoperative flat chamber and synechial formation
4. Simultaneous trabeculectomy in eyes with poorly controlled glaucoma

To achieve accurate postoperative monitoring of pressure, one may need to use a MacKay-Marg tonometer or a pneumotonometer. Cyclocryotherapy may be necessary after keratoplasty to control ocular tension if maximal medical therapy is unsuccessful[9] or if filtering surgery fails. The use of Molteno setons has been relatively successful in glaucomatous eyes refractory to other modes of therapy.[8,42]

Recurrent herpetic keratitis. The recurrence rate of herpetic keratitis (Fig. 28-5) after keratoplasty has been reported to be 15% to 47%.[18,19,21,49] The presence of preoperative inflammation does not seem to influence the graft survival rate or the incidence of recurrent herpes keratitis in the graft.[18] Grafts performed during active recrudescence may be complicated by defective wound healing, a flat anterior chamber, anterior synechiae, and glaucoma.[49]

The concomitant treatment of rejection episodes with intensive topical steroids and prophylactic topical antivirals has improved the results in herpetic keratoplasties.[18,19,53] One or more rejection episodes occur in about half of the grafts.[18] Ficker and co-workers[18] found that rejection episodes complicated 23% of herpes recurrences, an indication that these patients need careful follow-up study and the addition of sufficient topical steroids if uveitis is present. Herpes simplex keratitis recurrence accounted for 16% of all graft failures. In this study the major cause of failure overall was rejection, which was defined by the presence of anterior chamber inflammation and keratic precipitates limited to the donor corneal tissue. Previous studies[21,49] indicated that in those corneas with herpes recurrence from 50% to 60% will develop graft failure; however the combined use of steroids and antivirals has greatly reduced the failure rate. The long-term survival rate of herpes grafts was 70% in one series with a 10-year mean follow-up period. Subsequent regrafting decreases the overall survival rate, and the failure rate from rejection was greater for regrafts (69%) than for first grafts (40%).[18]

The patient with a penetrating keratoplasty for herpetic keratitis should be informed that any decreased vision, pain, photophobia, or redness may be recurrent herpetic disease or graft rejection and needs immediate attention. It may be difficult to distinguish an allograft reaction from recurrent herpetic keratouveitis.[60] Fine and Cignetti[21] indicate that many, large keratic precipitates in the presence of corneal edema that involve the donor and recipient cornea probably represents recurrent herpetic disease. Rose bengal should be topically applied to allow identification of active epithelial herpetic in-

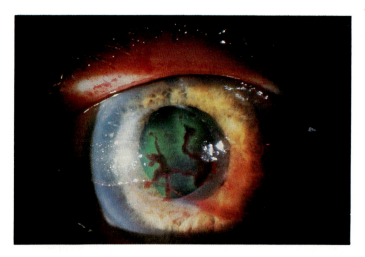

Fig. 28-5. Recurrent herpetic dendrite 20 years after keratoplasty.

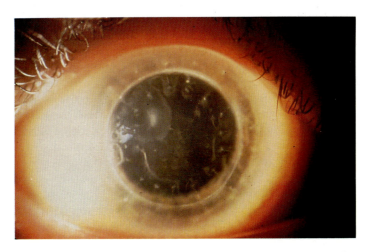

Fig. 28-6. Recurrent hereditary stromal dystrophy after keratoplasty.

volvement. Adjunctive therapy with orally administered acyclovir may benefit active herpetic keratouveitis, but evidence of its efficacy is inconclusive.

Interrupted sutures are recommended in highly vascularized recipient beds thereby allowing selected loose suture removal when necessary. There is an increased risk of bacterial infection associated with loose sutures.[18]

Graft failure. Primary graft failure is defined as corneal edema that is present from the time of keratoplasty, does not clear, and is unassociated with rejection or other secondary causes for graft failure. It is presumably attributable to a compromised or dysfunctional corneal endothelium. Primary graft failure has decreased to a minimal level with advances in surgical techniques, materials, and donor tissue preservation.

Primary graft failure has been reported as low as 4% in a series of failed corneal grafts.[5] In our most recent 1000 grafts, primary donor failure occurred in less than 1% of cases.

To ensure that the donor material is of adequate quality, slitlamp examination of the cornea and especially of the endothelium before surgery is essential.[26] The screening of donor endothelium by specular microscopy is performed by most eye banks today. Meticulous surgical technique must be utilized to protect the donor endothelium during keratoplasty.

Late graft failure seems to occur in corneal grafts in which a marginal endothelium proceeds to complete endothelial dysfunction. In the early postoperative period the graft is clear but may become edematous months to years later without any predisposing causes. The cause of continued endothelial cell loss may be the linear decrease in endothelial cell counts that has

been observed to occur after keratoplasty.[11,71] Other secondary causes include pseudophakic touch, vitreous touch, recurrent uveitis, glaucoma, and rejection. Even though there is a slow continuous cell loss over time, corneal grafts have a favorable prognosis for long-term clinical stability.[71] The remaining endothelium has a minimal functional reserve. Therefore corneal decompensation may occur if the endothelium is subjected to further trauma as in subsequent anterior segment surgery.[18,71]

Recurrent corneal dystrophy. The recurrence of hereditary stromal dystrophies (Fig. 28-6) after keratoplasty has been reported in Reis-Bücklers',[45] granular,[50,56] lattice,[31,37,41,53] and macular dystrophies.[54] Recurrences occur most commonly in grafts for lattice dystrophy, with 25% to 48% of grafts demonstrating recurrence within 25 years.[11,25,41] Regrafting may be necessary in 15% of patients in which primary corneal transplantation had been performed.[41] In our experience, recurrence of lattice dystrophy becomes evident in most cases within 5 years after surgery.

INDICATIONS FOR REGRAFTING

Primary Graft Failure. Corneal grafts that have gross stromal edema with large broad folds immediately after keratoplasty should be suspected of having endothelial decompensation. Intensive topical steroids may be of some benefit, but if no reversal is noticed within several days, irreversible graft failure is inevitable and regrafting within 2 weeks is recommended. Stromal edema may also be caused by ocular hypotony, which may clear when one discontinues ocular hypotensives and allows the intraocular pressure to increase.

Allograft Reaction. Despite the evidence that the risk for allograft reaction is increased with repeat keratoplasty,[31] HLA tissue typing may play a role in minimizing these risks.

Recurrence of Host Disease. Although many grafts with recurrent herpes keratitis remain clear, 23% to 30% will necessitate regrafting.[18,38] Recurrent corneal dystrophy, particularly lattice dystrophy, may reduce graft clarity.[41] A soft contact lens is usually of some benefit in reducing epithelial erosion symptoms; however, some patients will require a regraft. Recently, excimer laser phototherapeutic keratectomies have been performed on some recurrent anterior stromal dystrophies and have obviated the need for repeat keratoplasty.

CONTRAINDICATIONS FOR REGRAFTING

Uncontrolled Glaucoma. As discussed previously, an eye with increased intraocular pressure uncontrolled by medical or surgical therapy will certainly have difficulties after keratoplasty. The pressure should be in good control before surgery, with cyclocryotherapy, shunt, or filtering procedures utilized if necessary. In desperate situations, penetrating keratoplasty combined with a filtering procedure may be justified.

Inadequate Tear Function. Eyes with severe keratitis sicca or severe cicatrizing diseases should rarely be considered for keratoplasty. The postoperative prognosis for these eyes is extremely poor. If keratoplasty is attempted, a lateral and possibly medial tarsorrhaphy may be necessary to enhance the surface lubrication postoperatively.

Unsatisfactory Lid Margins. Trichiasis, chronic blepharitis, ectropion, entropion, extensive symblepharon, and scarred lid margins are relative contraindications for keratoplasty. These conditions should be corrected before one proceeds to keratoplasty.

HLA TISSUE TYPING AND CORNEAL GRAFTING

Studies of allograft reaction have centered on the two immune responses, humoral and cell medicated. Humoral immunity has been implicated in graft rejection when circulating antibodies to corneal endothelium were found.[1,10,17,39,61] Cell-mediated immune responses have been demonstrated by lymphocytes, which with the appropriate antigenic stimulus can produce the destruction of corneal cells. Natural killer cells, lymphocytes without a history of prior sensitization, have been shown to be spontaneously cytoxic to human corneal endothelium.[46]

The antigens that probably mediate the immunologic phenomenon of graft rejection in the corneas and in other organs as well are the human lymphocyte antigens (HLA). These are classified as class I (HLA-A and HLA-B loci) and class II (HLA-D and HLA-DR loci). In contrast to renal transplant studies, ABO antigens have not been shown to be important in corneal rejection.[2] Class I antigens have been considered important mediators of renal graft rejection, since they are believed to act primarily as targets for cytotoxic T cells or antibody, but recent studies have indicated that Class II antigens may be more important because they are believed to be responsible primarily for the recognition of foreign allografts.[60,64] Corneal epithelium and endothelium are known to express class I antigens, and dendritic (Langerhans') cells, which express class II antigens, are occasionally present in corneal epithelium.[57,63,69] It has been shown recently that class II antigens, not normally expressed on corneal cells, may be induced to do so on both corneal endothelial and stromal cells.[70]

The role of HLA in corneal graft rejection has been studied by utilization of two clinical approaches. The first is negative cross matching. Recipient serum is tested in vitro against donor lymphocytes, and if there is a reaction, the recipient may be preimmunized to the donor antigen. If there is no reaction (a negative cross match), there is no detectable preimmunization. The hypothesis that transplanting tissue to a high-risk recipient with a negative cross match might be more beneficial than one with a positive cross match has been tested in a nonrandomized, prospective trial.[62] The rates of rejection (26%) and graft failure (15%) were lower than the 60% to 70% reported in the literature.[7]

The second clinical approach has been direct HLA genotypic matching. Currently, the HLA A, B, and DR loci are used for matching. At least two A or B loci or two DR loci are matched before transplantation is used in our prospective, randomized clinical trial. Poor matching of these loci (that is, no match or one or two matches) has been shown to provide for a higher risk of rejection in renal transplantation than a higher degree of matching (that is, three or four loci matched).[59] For the cornea this question has been addressed indirectly,[58] retrospectively,[16] and in uncontrolled studies.[3,7,22,24,67] These results generally are consistent with renal studies, but some have shown opposite results.[3] The issue whether lymphocytotoxic antibodies play a role in this remains unanswered.

A prospective, randomized controlled clinical trial on cross-match testing and HLA matching for high-risk keratoplasty cases is in progress to determine if these clinical approaches have any value in reducing allograft reaction in high-risk patients.

SURGICAL CONSIDERATIONS

Fine[20] states that there are two principles to consider before regrafting:

1. The graft should be of appropriate size so that its margins lie in the most normal tissue, whether recipient or donor.
2. The graft margin should not be in proximity to the limbus.

We would add that the corneal surgeon should avoid successively increasing the donor size with each regraft. If the recipient bed includes a previous donor of excessive diameter and the tissue is of sufficient consistency, a penetrating keratoplasty may be performed within the boundaries of the original donor.

CONCLUSION

Repeat keratoplasty is now a relatively successful operation in eyes that once may have been believed to be inoperable. The improved success is related to better microsurgical techniques, advances in corneal preservation, and a more sophisticated understanding of the pathophysiology of corneal rejection and recurrent corneal disease. Progress in the medical management of allograft rejection and herpes simplex keratitis recurrence has helped enhance graft survival.

Currently, the Collaborative Corneal Transplantation Study (CCTS) is attempting to answer the question of whether tissue antigen cross matching enhances graft survival in high-risk keratoplasties. The Sandoz cyclosporin trial is underway to determine the efficacy of topical immunosuppressive therapy in reducing allograft rejection in the high-risk eyes. The results of these studies will, one would hope, pave new ground for further improvement in corneal transplantation.

REFERENCES

1. Alberth B, Leovey A, Balazs C: Anticorneal antibody examinations in human keratoplasty, *Albrecht von Graefes Arch Klin Exp Ophthalmol* 190:341, 1974.
2. Allansmith MR, Drell DW, Kajiyama G, Fine M: ABO blood groups and corneal transplantation, *Am J Ophthalmol* 79:493, 1975.
3. Allansmith MR, Fine M, Payne R: Histocompatibility typing and corneal transplantation, *Trans Am Acad Ophthalmol* 78:445, 1974.
4. Alldredge OC, Krachmer JH: Clinical types of corneal transplant rejection: their manifestations, frequency, preoperative correlate, and treatment, *Arch Ophthalmol* 99:599, 1981.
5. Arentsen JJ: Corneal transplant allograft reaction: possible predisposing factors, *Trans Am Ophthalmol Soc* 81:361, 1983.
6. Arentsen JJ, Morgan B, Green WR: Changing indications for keratoplasty, *Am J Ophthalmol* 81:313, 1976.
7. Batchelor JR, Casey TA, Gibbs DC, et al: HLA matching and corneal grafting, *Lancet* 2:551, 1976.
8. Beebe WE, Starita RJ, Fellman RL, et al: The use of Molteno implant and anterior chamber tube shunt to encircling band for the treatment of glaucoma in keratoplasty patients, *Ophthalmology* 97:1414, 1990.
9. Binder PS, Abel R, Kaufman HE: Cyclocryotherapy for glaucoma after penetrating keratoplasty, *Am J Ophthalmol* 79:489, 1975.
10. Binder PS, Chandler JW, Kaufman HE: In vitro demonstration of cytotoxic antibodies and their possible role in corneal graft rejections, *Invest Ophthalmol* 15:481, 1976.
11. Bourne WM: One-year observation of transplanted human corneal endothelium, *Ophthalmology* 87:673, 1980.
12. Chandler JW, Kaufman HE: Graft reactions after keratoplasty for keratoconus, *Am J Ophthalmol* 77:543, 1974.
13. Cohen EJ, Schwartz LW, Luskind RD, et al: Neodymium:YAG laser transcleral cyclophotocoagulation for glaucoma after penetrating keratoplasty, *Ophthalmol Surg* 20:713, 1989.
14. Cowden J, Morgan B, Green WR: Changing indications for keratoplasty, *Am J Ophthalmol* 78:523, 1974.
15. Donshil PC, Cavanaugh HD, Boruchoff SA, et al: Effect of bilateral and unilateral grafts on the incidence of rejections in keratoconus, *Am J Ophthalmol* 87:823, 1979.
16. Ehlers N, Kissmeyer-Nielsen F: Corneal transplantation and HLA histocompatibility, *Acta Ophthalmol* 57:738, 1979.
17. Ehlers N, Kissmeyer-Nielsen F: Corneal transplantation and rejection probably medicated by antibodies, *Acta Ophthalmol* 59:119, 1981.
18. Ficker LA, Kirkness CM, Rice NSC, et al: The changing management and improved prognosis for corneal grafting in herpes simplex keratitis, *Ophthalmology* 96:1587, 1989.
19. Ficker LA, Kirkness CM, Rice NSC, et al: Long term prognosis for corneal grafting in herpes simplex keratitis, *Eye* 2:400, 1988.
20. Fine M: Corneal regrafts: indications, techniques and results. In Barraquer JI et al, editors: *Symposium on medical and surgical diseases of the cornea*, St Louis, 1980, Mosby–Year Book.
21. Fine M, Cignetti FE: Penetrating keratoplasty in herpes simplex keratitis: recurrence in grafts, *Arch Ophthalmol* 95:613, 1977.
22. Foulks GN, Sanfilippo FP: Beneficial effects of histocompatibility in high risk corneal transplantation, *Am J Ophthalmol* 94:622, 1982.
23. Gilvarry AME, Kirkness CM, Steele ADMcG, et al: The management of post-keratoplasty glaucoma by trabeculectomy, *Eye* 3:713, 1989.
24. Foulks GN, Sanfilippo GP, Lo Cascio JA, et al: Histocompatibility testing for keratoplasty in high risk patients, *Ophthalmology* 90:239, 1983.
25. Herman SJ, Hughes WF: Recurrence of hereditary corneal dystrophy following keratoplasty, *Am J Ophthalmol* 73:689, 1973.
26. Hirst LW, Stark WJ: Donor corneal endothelium: slitlamp examination of buttons in storage medium, *Ophthalmic Surg* 9:51, 1978.
27. Insler MS, Cooper HD, Kastl PR, Caldwell DR: Penetrating keratoplasty with trabeculectomy, *Am J Ophthalmol* 100:593, 1985.
28. Insler MS, Pechous B: Visual results in repeat penetrating keratoplasty, *Am J Ophthalmol* 102:371, 1986.
29. Irvine AR, Kaufman HE: Intraocular pressure following penetrating keratoplasty, *Am J Ophthalmol* 68:835, 1969.
30. Khodadoust AA: The allograft rejection reaction: the leading cause of late failure of clinical corneal grafts. In Porter R,

Knight J, editors: *Corneal graft failure,* Ciba Found Symp 15:151, Amsterdam/New York, 1973, Elsevier Publishing Co./Associated Scientific Publishers.

31. Khodadoust AA, Abigadel A: The fate of corneal regrafts after previous rejection reactions. In Silverstein AM, O'Connor GR, editors: *Immunology and immunopathology of the eye,* New York, 1979, Masson.

32. Khodadoust AA, Silverstein AM: Transplantation and rejection of individual cell layers of the cornea, *Invest Ophthalmol* 8:180, 1969.

33. Khodadoust AA, Silverstein AM: Local graft versus host reactions within the anterior chamber of the eye: the formation of corneal endothelial pocks, *Invest Ophthalmol* 14:640, 1975.

34. Khodadoust AA, Silverstein AM: Induction of corneal graft rejection by passive cell transfer, *Invest Ophthalmol* 15:89, 1976.

35. Kirkness CM, Ezra E, Rice NJC, et al: The success and survival of repeat corneal grafts, *Eye* 4:58, 1990.

36. Krachmer JH, Alldredge OC: Subepithelial infiltrates: a probable sign of corneal transplant rejection, *Arch Ophthalmol* 96:2234, 1978.

37. Lanier JD, Fine M, Togni B: Lattice corneal dystrophy, *Arch Ophthalmol* 94:921, 1976.

38. MacEwen CJ, Khan ZUH, Anderson E, et al: Corneal regraft: indications and outcome, *Ophthalmol Surg* 19:706, 1988.

39. Manski W, Ehrlich G, Polack FM: Studies on the cytotoxic immune reaction. I. The action of antibodies on normal and regenerating corneal tissue, *J Immunol* 105:755, 1970.

40. Maumenee AE: The influence of donor-recipient sensitization on corneal grafts, *Am J Ophthalmol* 34:142, 1951.

41. Meisler DM, Fine M: Recurrence of the clinical signs of lattice corneal dystrophy (type I) in corneal transplants, *Am J Ophthalmol* 97:210, 1984.

42. McDonnell PJ, Robin JB, Schanelin DJ, et al: Molteno implant for control of glaucoma in eyes after penetrating keratoplasty, *Ophthalmology* 97:210, 1984.

43. Olson RJ: Aphakic keratoplasty: determining donor tissue size to avoid elevated intraocular pressure, *Arch Ophthalmol* 96:2274, 1978.

44. Olson RJ, Kaufman HE: A mathematical description of causative factors and prevention of elevated intraocular pressure after keratoplasty, *Invest Ophthalmol Vis Sci* 16:1085, 1977.

45. Olson RJ, Kaufman HE: Recurrence of Reis-Bücklers' corneal dystrophy in a graft, *Am J Ophthalmol* 85:349, 1978.

46. Opremeak EM, Whisler RL, Dangel ME: Natural killer cells against human corneal endothelium, *Am J Ophthalmol* 99:524, 1985.

47. Paque J, Poirer R: Corneal allograft reaction and its relationship to suture site neovascularization, *Ophthalmic Surg* 8:71, 1977.

48. Paton D: The principal problems of penetrating keratoplasty: graft failure and graft astigmatism. In Barraquer JI et al, editors: *Symposium on medical and surgical diseases of the cornea,* St. Louis, 1980, Mosby–Year Book.

49. Pfister RR, Richards JSF, Dohlman CH: Recurrence of herpetic keratitis in corneal grafts, *Am J Ophthalmol* 73:192, 1972.

50. Polack FM: The effect of ocular inflammation on corneal grafts, *Am J Ophthalmol* 60:259, 1965.

51. Polack FM: The pathologic anatomy of corneal graft rejection, *Surv Ophthalmol* 11:391, 1966.

52. Polack FM, Gonzales CE: The response of the lymphoid tissue to corneal heterografts, *Arch Ophthalmol* 80:321, 1968.

53. Rice NJC, Jones BR: Problems of corneal grafting in herpetic keratitis. In Porter R, Knight J, editors: *Corneal graft failure,* Ciba Found Symp 15:221, Amsterdam/New York, 1973, Elsevier Publishing Co./Associated Scientific Publishers.

54. Robin A, Green WR, Lapsa TP, et al: Recurrence of macular corneal dystrophy after lamellar keratoplasty, *Am J Ophthalmol* 84:457, 1977.

55. Robinson CH: Indications, complications and prognosis for repeat penetrating keratoplasty, *Ophthalmic Surg* 10:27, 1979.

56. Rodrigues MM, McGavic JS: Recurrent corneal granular dystrophy: a clinico-pathologic study, *Trans Am Ophthalmic Soc* 73:300, 1975.

57. Rodriques MM, Rowden G, Hackett J, et al: Langerhans cells in the normal conjunctiva and peripheral cornea of selected species *Invest Ophthalmol* 21:759, 1981.

58. Ruusuvaara P: Histocompatibility and corneal graft endothelium, *Acta Ophthalmol* 57:968, 1978.

59. Sanfilippo F, Vaughn WK, Spees EK, et al: Benefits of HLA-A and HLA-B matching on graft and patient outcome after cadaveric-donor renal transplantation, *N Engl J Med* 311:358, 1984.

60. Stark WJ: Transplantation immunology of penetrating keratoplasty, *Trans Am Ophthalmol Soc* 78:1079, 1980.

61. Stark WJ, Oplez G, Newsome D, et al: Sensitization to human lymphocyte antigens by corneal transplantation, *Invest Ophthalmol* 12:639, 1973.

62. Stark WJ, Taylor HR, Bias WB, et al: Histocompatibility (HLA) antigens and keratoplasty, *Am J Ophthalmol* 86:595, 1978.

63. Stigne LG, Kunihiko T, Katz SI: Origin and function of epidermal Langerhans cells, *Immunol Rev* 53:149, 1980.

64. Streilein JW, Bregslasser PR: Ia antigens and epidermal Langerhans cells, *Transplantation* 30:319, 1980.

65. Stuart JC, Mund ML: Recurrent granular corneal dystrophy, *Am J Ophthalmol* 79:18, 1975.

66. Thoft RA, Gordon SM, Dohlman CH: Glaucoma following keratoplasty, *Trans Am Acad Ophthalmol Otolaryngol* 78:352, 1974.

67. Völker-Dieben HJM, Kok-van Alphen CC, et al: Advances and disappointments: indications and restrictions regarding HLA-matched corneal grafts in high risk cases, *Doc Ophthalmol* 46:219, 1979.

68. West CE, Wood TO, Kaufman HE: Cyclocryotherapy for glaucoma pre- or postpenetrating keratoplasty, *Am J Ophthalmol* 76:485, 1973.

69. Whitset CF, Stulting RD: The distribution of HLA antigens on human corneal tissue, *Invest Ophthalmol* 25:519, 1984.

70. Young E, Stark WJ: Immunology of corneal allograft rejection: HLA-DR antigens on human corneal cells, *Invest Ophthalmol* 26:571, 1985.

71. Zacks CM, Abbott RL, Fine M: Long-term changes in corneal endothelium after keratoplasty, *Cornea* 9:92, 1990.

Chapter 29

Peripheral Corneal Disease

Terrien's marginal degeneration

MICHAEL S. INSLER

DELMAR R. CALDWELL

DAVID H. LEACH

Terrien's marginal degeneration, first described in 1881,[4] has a characteristically slow and chronically progressive course that extends over years and even decades. As the disease progresses, high corneal astigmatism and corneal ectasia, with the potential for rupture, become inevitable.[8] During the long-term course of this condition, the ophthalmologist may have to intervene surgically when the cornea is severely thinned, corneal astigmatism is great, and perforation either has or is likely to occur.

CLINICAL FINDINGS

Terrien's disease, or ectatic marginal degeneration, begins as a punctate infiltration of the anterior layers of the peripheral cornea with a clear limbal zone, resembling arcus senilis (Fig. 29-1). This degeneration is further characterized by the early development of a superficial vascularization extending from the limbal arcades. Because of thinning of the subepithelial tissue in the involved area, a depression in the anterior stromal surface results in a gutterlike furrow or trough usually located between the arcus and limbus but occasionally central to it. The epithelium, however, remains unaffected throughout the course of the disease. As the gutter deepens, the sharp edge between the periphery and the normal central cornea stands out as a white line (Fig. 29-2). As thinning continues, the superior cornea eventually begins to bulge, forming an ectasia. These ectatic areas may be localized or may involve the entire corneal periphery. Finally, rupture may occur, with aqueous loss and prolapse of iris, either spontaneously or after minor trauma.

Terrien's disease is uncommon. Men are affected more frequently than women. Most patients are over 40 years of age though the disorder has been observed in all age groups, including several children under 10 years. It is usually bilateral and limited to

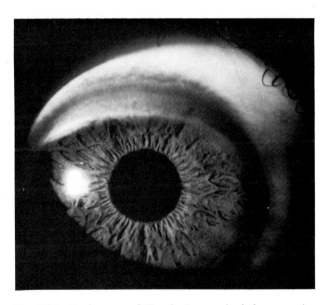

Fig. 29-1. Early case of Terrien's marginal degeneration with typical findings, including a clear limbal zone, resembling arcus senilis.

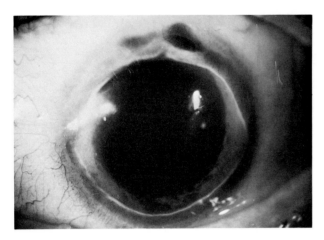

Fig. 29-2. As disease progresses, a depression in anterior stromal surface results in a furrow that can deepen and eventually form an ectasia.

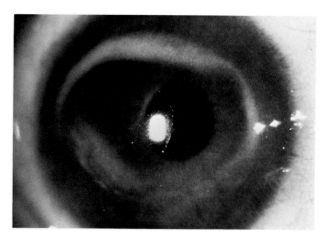

Fig. 29-3. Peripheral marginal corneal degeneration with superior and inferior involvement.

the upper portion of the cornea but is not always in the same stage of development in both eyes.

The cause of this condition is unknown; both inflammatory and degenerative causes have been proposed. The upper part of the cornea is usually affected first, but superior as well as inferior involvement with an ectasia above and a furrow below is not uncommon (Fig. 29-3). Peripheral involvement may spread circumferentially to involve the whole cornea. Atypical pterygium (pseudopterygium) in an unusual oblique axis has been described as an early presenting sign in Terrien's disease.[6] The earliest symptom may be a change in refraction; the shift follows the meridian of the furrow or ectasia and the cornea flattens in the vertical axis. The astigmatism thus produced is usually against the rule. This phenomenon can be shown with keratometry readings. It can be even more elegantly demonstrated with the use of computer-assisted corneal topographic analysis, which produces color-coded topographic maps that are easily interpreted clinically (Fig. 29-4).[11]

The process of peripheral corneal thinning is generally noninflammatory and painless. However, occasionally there are intermittent symptoms of inflammation resembling a mild conjunctivitis or episcleritis.[5] Similarly, several histopathologic studies of Terrien's have demonstrated both "quiescent" and "inflammatory" forms of the disorder.[7] There are no other significant ocular associations with Terrien's, except for corneal hydrops, which has been described in a series of patients.[10]

DIFFERENTIAL DIAGNOSIS

The differential diagnosis of Terrien's includes Mooren's ulcer and other progressive ectasias of the cornea, such as keratoconus, keratoglobus, and pellucid marginal degeneration. Mooren's ulcer (see p. 328) is a painful inflammatory autoimmune process in which the epithelium is lost. Although these ectasias are readily differentiated clinically, all are characterized by corneal thinning of unknown cause.

Keratoconus is the most common corneal thinning disorder and is characterized by slitlamp findings of central corneal thinning, vertical stress lines, Fleischer's ring, and breaks in Bowman's layer and Descemet's membrane with scarring or corneal hydrops. In keratoglobus, corneal thinning is quite diffuse and is greatest in the periphery, just the reverse of that seen in keratoconus. Eyes with pellucid degeneration have a narrow band of thinning in the lower half of the cornea with normal limbal, central, and superior corneal thickness. In contrast to Terrien's disease, vascularization, lipid deposition, and peripheral scarring are absent. It is reasonable to assume that cases of pellucid degeneration with or without keratoconus are a variant of keratoconus or a different manifestation of the same etiologic factor. Terrien's disease, under some circumstances, may also fall into this category.

We have measured differential corneal thinning in several patients with these disorders. One typical example is a 38-year-old man who presented to us with superior Terrien's marginal degeneration that was worse in the right eye (Fig. 29-5). Central keratometry readings were 35.25 diopters × 64.50 diopters, axis 164 degrees. The superior area of thinning showed a minimum thickness of 0.258 mm. The degree of astigmatism and corneal thinning precluded the use of spectacle or contact lens correction. When

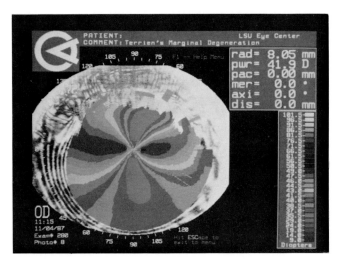

Fig. 29-4. Computer-assisted color-coded topographic map showing an advanced case of Terrien's disease with effectively 13 diopters of regular, against-the-rule astigmatism. (From Wilson SE, Lin DTC, Klyce SD, Insler MS: *Refract Corneal Surg* 6:15-20, 1990.)

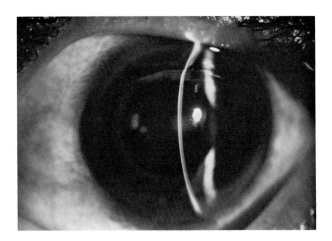

Fig. 29-5. Right eye of 38-year-old man with bilateral Terrien's marginal degeneration. Patient presented with 30 diopters of astigmatism and diffuse corneal thinning.

this stage is reached, surgical intervention is the only option for visually rehabilitating this type of patient.

SURGICAL TREATMENT

After a trial of spectacle and contact lens correction, other therapeutic measures used to correct corneal thinning disorders include the application of trichloroacetic acid, cautery, lamellar and penetrating keratoplasty, and excision of ectatic cornea, with or without conjunctival and scleral flaps.[1] However, medical therapy has not been shown to be effective in this condition. If thinning becomes severe and visual acuity is further compromised, surgical intervention becomes necessary (Fig. 29-6). In situations where there is impending or frank perforation, an annular or horseshoe-shaped lamellar graft appears to be the best method for treatment of Terrien's disease.[9] Inlay lamellar keratoplasty can be used to add corneal substance after a partial-thickness lamellar dissection is performed to remove recipient cornea. A recipient bed is fashioned and partial- or full-thickness donor cornea is used to restore corneal thickness and maintain the structural integrity of the globe (Fig. 29-7). Use of two trephines as markers for the dissection greatly facilitates the lamellar surgery in these instances.[2]

Because these techniques are difficult and the risk of perforation with flattening of the anterior chamber during the procedure is high, we have used an alternative approach to surgical treatment of Terrien's marginal degeneration.[3] With observation through an operating microscope, an incision is

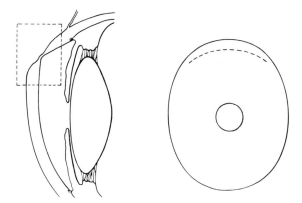

Fig. 29-6. Diagram of area of ectasia with resultant increased vertical diameter and flattened meridian.

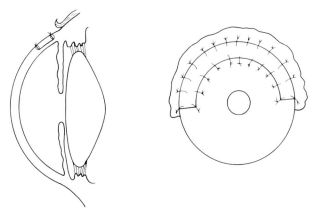

Fig. 29-7. Inlay lamellar keratoplasty after partial- or full-thickness donor tissue is sutured into position.

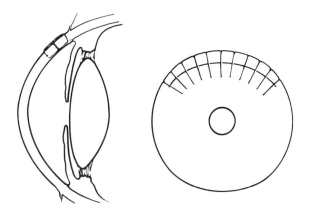

Fig. 29-8. Final placement of sutures and contour of cornea after dissection.

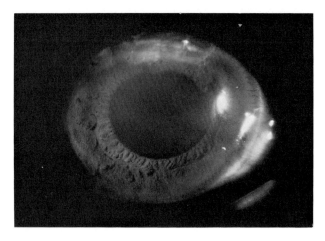

Fig. 29-9. Early postoperative photograph of resected superior cornea in eye with Terrien's marginal degeneration.

made into the stroma down to Descemet's membrane along the entire semicircular edge of the peripheral ectatic cornea using a razor blade knife or diamond knife set to a depth determined by preoperative pachymetry. A lamellar blunt dissection is performed with a dry field just to the level of Descemet's membrane along both sides of the incision, centrally as well as peripherally into the sclera. The dissection is continued until stroma of normal thickness is reached. The dissector is directed parallel to the bed of the stromal lamellae, rather than downward, so as to remain in the same plane and to prevent penetration into the anterior chamber.

At this stage, the wound edges of the undermined tissue are approximated; the goals are to restore normal stromal thickness, preserve the smooth corneal curvature, and avoid creating any stress lines. Interrupted 9-0 or 10-0 polypropylene sutures are

passed through the deep normal-thickness stroma 1 to 1.5 mm apart. The sutures are tied down and the knots are buried (Fig. 29-8). If necessary, an anterior chamber paracentesis may be created to help soften the eye while the wound is being closed. Postoperatively, the eye is treated with topical antibiotics, steroids, and mydriatic eyedrops (Fig. 29-9). The sutures are left in place indefinitely, and any remaining refractive error can be corrected with spectacles or contact lenses.

REFERENCES

1. Anderson FG: Repair of marginal furrow perforation, *Ophthalmic Surg* 8:25, 1977.
2. Brown AC, Rao GN, Aquavella JV: Peripheral corneal grafts in Terrien's marginal degeneration, *Ophthalmic Surg* 14:931, 1983.
3. Caldwell DR, Insler MS, Boutros G, Hawk T: Primary surgical repair of severe peripheral marginal ectasia in Terrien's marginal degeneration, *Am J Ophthalmol* 97:332-336, 1984.
4. Duke-Elder S, Leigh AG: Diseases of the outer eye: cornea and sclera. In Duke-Elder S, editor: *System of ophthalmology* 8(pt 2):909-914, St. Louis, 1965 (1976 reissue), Mosby–Year Book.
5. Etzine S, Friedmann A: Marginal dystrophy of the cornea with total ectasia, *Am J Ophthalmol* 55:150, 1963.
6. Goldman KN, Kaufman HE: Atypical pterygium: a clinical feature of Terrien's marginal degeneration, *Arch Ophthalmol* 96:1027, 1978.
7. Iwamoto T, DeVoe AG, Farris RL: Electron microscopy in cases of marginal degeneration of the cornea, *Invest Ophthalmol* 11:241-257, 1972.
8. Richards WW: Marginal degeneration of the cornea with perforation, *Arch Ophthalmol* 70:72, 1963.
9. Schanzlin DJ, Sarno EM, Robin JB: Crescentic lamellar keratoplasty in pellucid marginal degeneration, *Am J Ophthalmol* 96:253, 1983 (Letter).
10. Soong HK, Fitzgerald J, Boruchoff SA, et al: Corneal hydrops in Terrien's marginal degeneration, *Ophthalmology* 93:340-343, 1986.
11. Wilson SE, Lin DTC, Klyce SD, Insler MS: Terrien's marginal degeneration: corneal topography, *Refract Corneal Surg* 6:15-20, 1990.

Mooren's ulcer

GEORGE FRANGIEH

KENNETH R. KENYON

Mooren's ulcer is a peripheral ulcerative keratitis that begins as a sterile inflammatory infiltrate in the anterior stroma, destroys the epithelium overlying it, and then spreads circumlimbally or centripetally.[8] It is a diagnosis of exclusion and should be considered only when numerous other infectious and noninfectious, localized and systemic causes of peripheral corneal ulceration have been eliminated as possibilities. The differential diagnoses thus includes the collagen vascular disorders such as rheumatoid arthritis, systemic lupus erythematosus, Wegener's granulomatosis, and polyarteritis nodosa. The diagnosis of Mooren's ulcer can then be established only after thorough evaluation of all relevant data including a complete medical and ocular history, careful review of systems, and appropriate laboratory investigation.

Mooren's ulcer has been seen in all ages but usually occurs in males over 20 years of age. It is believed to be more common in Africa. Two types exist and differ according to age distribution and severity of clinical course.[6] One type occurs in older persons, with men more frequently involved and no racial predilection; it is unilateral in about 75% of cases and runs a slow and somewhat variable course with a fair prognosis. The second type occurs in young adults, especially common in black males in their thirties; it is bilateral in about 75% of cases and runs a progressive unrelenting course with a poor prognosis because one third of patients develop corneal perforations. The presence of many plasma cells in the conjunctiva, circulating antibodies against the conjunctiva and corneal epithelium, and the association of tissue-fixed immunoglobulins with complement in the conjunctival epithelium strongly indicates the disease is immunologic[4] (Fig. 29-10). Recently, macrophage inhibition factor to corneal tissue antigen has been demonstrated in the serum of patients with Mooren's ulcer.

The clinical signs and symptoms of Mooren's ulcer are typical. The eye is usually red and inflamed and may be excruciatingly painful to the extent that the patient may beg for enucleation. Clinically, the anterior stromal infiltrate with overlying epithelial defect adjacent to the limbus spreads circumlimbally or centripetally. No unaffected area remains between the ulcerative lesion and the limbus, unlike the peripheral ulcers associated with rheumatoid arthritis. Typically the ulceration process starts in the lateral and medial quadrants and features a gray and overhanging edge with involvement of the anterior one third to one half of the corneal stroma (Fig. 29-11). Some of the ulcerated areas appear active, whereas others seem to be healing. The disease normally runs a 3- to 12-month course and can occur in healed, scarred corneas.

The work-up of any suspected case of Mooren's ulcer should include a thorough medical examination and laboratory studies to rule out collagen-vascular diseases, malignancies, and leukemias. Stud-

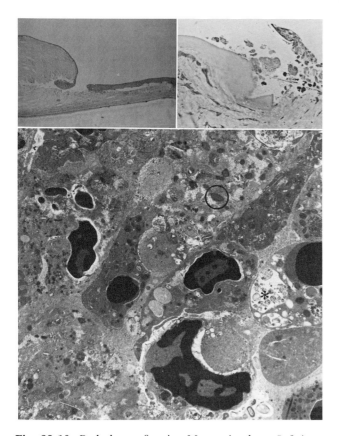

Fig. 29-10. Pathology of active Mooren's ulcer. *Left inset,* At low magnification, light microscopy of ulcerating interface compares normal thickness stroma at left with extremely thinned ulcerated stroma at right with typical overhanging stroma at margin of actively undermining ulceration. *Right inset,* Phase-contrast microscopy shows absence of epithelium, abrupt loss of Bowman's layer, and inflammatory cell accumulation (paraphenylenediamine, 500×). *Main figure,* Transmission electron microscopy of similar area reveals polymorphonuclear neutrophils actively involved in phagocytosis *(asterisk)* and degranulation *(circled)* (6500×).

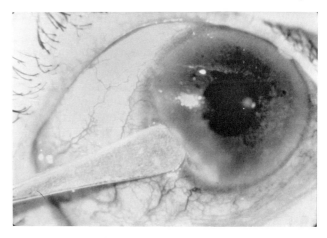

Fig. 29-11. Undermining of stroma at margin of active ulceration is demonstrated with advancement of spatula beneath overhanging anterior stroma.

ies should include complete and differential blood cell counts, platelet count, erythrocyte sedimentation rate, rheumatoid factor, chest x-ray examination, antinuclear antibodies, liver enzymes, VDRL (Venereal Disease Research Laboratory), fluorescent treponemal antibody absorption (FTA-ABS), blood urea nitrogen, serum protein electrophoresis, and urinalysis.

It is important to reiterate that many patients with active Mooren's ulcer have severe disabling ocular pain. Sulindac (Clinoril) is a new nonsteroid antiinflammatory drug that is an effective analgesic in Mooren's ulcer, affording more relief than other nonsteroidals or mild narcotic analgesic combinations in dosages up to 400 mg daily.

TREATMENT

A stepwise approach to the treatment of Mooren's ulcer is recommended. The goal of the treatment is to promote epithelialization of the ocular surface and to arrest the progression of the ulcerative process. Prophylactic topical antibiotics and cycloplegics are mandatory as is the specific treatment of concomitant ocular diseases. In cases also involving acne rosacea, for example, administration of systemic tetracycline may promote epithelial healing and may suppress the stromal inflammation and ulceration. In patients with moderate dry eyes, copious use of artificial tears and ointments may promote epithelial migration, and preparations that contain sensitizing preservatives like thimerosal should be avoided. Patients with severe dry eye conditions benefit from punctal occlusion by thermal or electrical cauterization. In patients with eyelid abnormalities, epithelial recovery is facilitated by correction of the anatomic disorder such as trichiasis, entropion, ectropion, or exposure.

Medical and Surgical Treatment of Active Mooren's Ulcer. The initial medical treatment should be initiated with topical corticosteroids, such as prednisolone acetate or prednisolone phosphate 1% hourly, as long as the infiltration and ulceration are not already so deep as to pose an immediate danger of perforation. If no epithelial healing occurs but ulceration does not progress within 2 to 3 days, the frequency of steroid application can be increased to every half an hour; if healing then occurs, topical steroid dosage can be slowly reduced over a period of several months. Aggressive pulse therapy with oral prednisone (60 to 100 mg daily) may be attempted if topical steroid therapy has not shown improvement after 7 to 10 days, or in cases where the infiltration is already deep and where intensive topical steroids in the face of an already thin cornea may

be worrisome. Since collagenolytic enzymes have been implicated in the stromal degradation of Mooren's ulcer, the use of inhibitors of these enzymes, predominantly metal-binding agents (such as 20% acetylcysteine, Mucomyst, or 0.2 M EDTA calcium) may be used in topical form and are relatively nontoxic. However their efficacy in humans has never been rigorously demonstrated. We do not recommend their use.

Conjunctival resection. If there is no response to topical medical therapy, the minor surgical procedure of conjunctival excision can readily be performed[1] (Fig. 29-12). Topical application of 0.5% proparacaine hydrochloride anesthetic will often suffice though some patients may require subconjunctival or retrobulbar anesthesia. With the aid of the operating microscope the conjunctiva should be incised so that the incision extends approximately 3 mm posterior to the corneoscleral limbus and parallel to the full extent of active ulceration. This conjunctiva is then dissected to the corneoscleral limbus and excised. The epithelium in the bed of the Mooren's ulcer may also be removed by simple débridement. Adjunctive cryotherapy, as recommended in the past, is seemingly unnecessary. Postoperatively a pressure dressing is used and topical corticosteroids and antibiotics should be continued. Conjunctival resection can be repeated if and as needed.

Immunosuppressives. If these therapies prove ineffective, immunosuppressive therapy[3] may be initiated after consultation with an internist or oncologist. Systemic cyclophosphamide (Cytoxan) at 100 mg per day and prednisone at 60 mg per day are our first-line drugs of choice. Alternatively methotrexate 10 to 30 mg per week and azathioprine 25 to 100 mg per day could be used and titrated to control the inflammation while not suppressing the white blood cell count below 3500/dl. Complete blood counts, urinalysis, hepatic and renal function tests, and other appropriate laboratory studies have to be conducted regularly for evaluation of the potentially adverse reactions of this chemotherapy. Such immunosuppression may need to be administered for many months up to 1 year and if recurrent inflammation occurs and before a significant beneficial response develops.

Perforation. If corneal perforation occurs and the size is less than 2 mm in diameter, the best treatment is the use of the tissue adhesive isobutyl cyanoacrylate (not FDA approved) (Fig. 29-13). Both experimental and clinical experience[2] confirm that the earlier application of tissue adhesive can substantially reduce the need for conjunctival flap, patch corneal

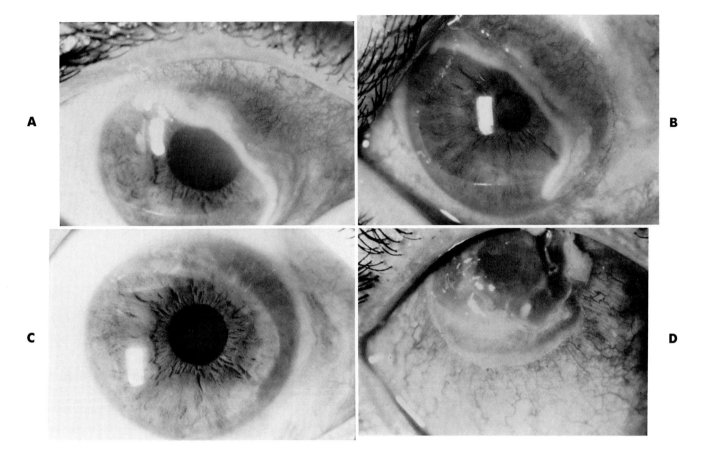

Fig. 29-12. A, 55-year-old white male with typical uniocular Mooren's ulcer that, **B,** progressed rapidly over 3-day interval, despite intensive topical corticosteroid therapy. Notice extensive stromal ulceration posterior to line of active stromal inflammatory infiltrate. Two days after conjunctival resection, **C,** intensity of inflammatory infiltrate has diminished. Four weeks later, **D,** entire inflammatory and ulcerative process has abated. Corneal and conjunctival epithelium is intact and corneal stroma is clear and free of inflammatory infiltrate in absence of topical steroid therapy.

graft, and other keratoplasty procedures. It is believed that the mechanism of action is through the exclusion of the inflammatory cells from the ulcerating stroma. Application of the cyanoacrylate glue involves instillation of local 0.5% proparacaine hydrochloride anesthesia while a lid speculum separates the lids. Small discs 2 to 4 mm in diameter may be cut from surgical drape material and are picked up by application of any ointment to the bare end of a cotton applicator; a small drop of adhesive glue is placed on the other side of the disc and held upright.

Alternatively a small polyethylene cannula or disposable needle (such as a half-inch no. 25 gage) may serve as an applicator. The area of perforation or ulceration is deepithelialized and dried with cellulose sponges; the adhesive in minimal amount is then applied to the area with gentle pressure. Because the adhesive rapidly polymerizes and substantially expands on contact with water, it must be applied carefully on a dry surface to minimize the formation of a large, rough, elevated mass. Once the adhesive has polymerized, a durable therapeutic soft contact lens is applied to provide comfort and to reduce the risk of glue dislodgment.

If the perforation is completely sealed, spontaneous deepening of the anterior chamber should then occur. If it is not sealed and the chamber does not reform, the adhesive can be removed and the procedure repeated. However in some cases of more extensive ulceration, a glued-on hard contact lens can protect the corneal stroma until reepithelialization

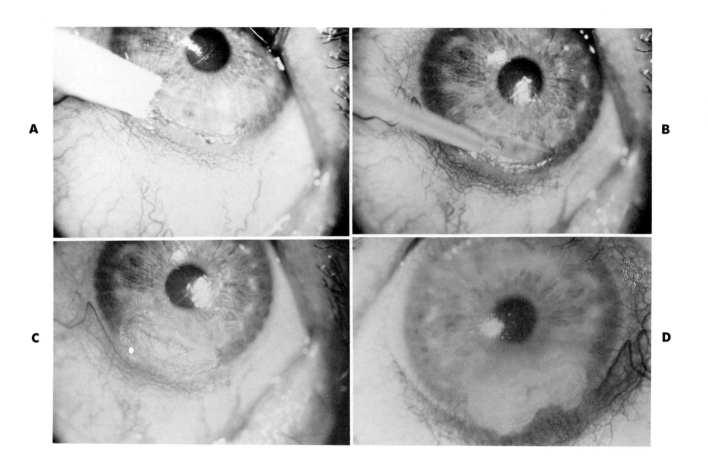

Fig. 29-13. Application of cyanoacrylate tissue adhesive in setting of extensive peripheral ulceration with small central perforation involves drying and débridement of ulcerated area with cellulose sponge, **A;** application of liquid cyanoacrylate adhesive by micropipette, **B;** and fitting of bandage soft contact lens, **C.** Four weeks later, **D,** ulcerative process has subsided and neovascularization has extended into stroma adjacent and beneath tissue adhesive to additionally inhibit stromal degradation.

occurs. Tissue adhesive can be left in place until it loosens or dislodges spontaneously after reepithelialization and neovascularization (Fig. 29-14). Prophylactic antibiotics and cycloplegics used with ocular lubricants and local steroids may reduce the inflammation and the discomfort.

Other surgical alternatives. If the ulceration is extensive and involves most of the cornea, the available surgical options are either a superficial keratectomy, complete or partial conjunctival flap, and lamellar or penetrating keratoplasty. Simple superficial keratec-

tomy to remove a central island of remaining anterior stroma is often followed by amelioration of the inflammatory process such that lamellar or penetrating keratoplasty can be subsequently performed.[7]

CONJUNCTIVAL FLAP. The conjunctival flap approach is especially useful for elderly debilitated patients where prolonged hospitalization and medical therapy may not be warranted. Although a conjunctival flap will not provide visual improvement, it will often provide comfort, reduce the ocular inflammation, and promote healing in these patients. If the

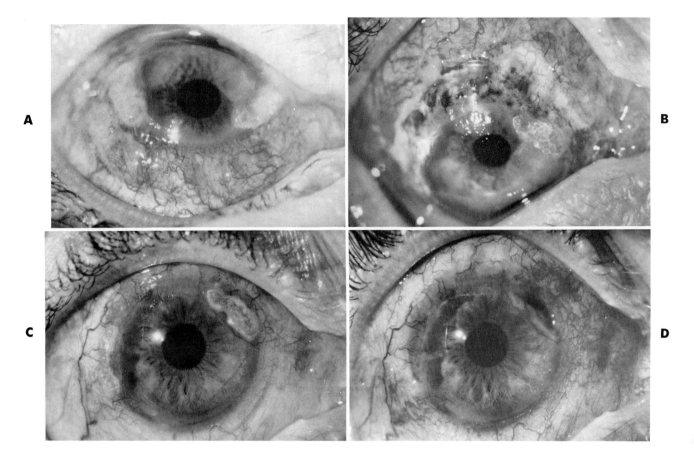

Fig. 29-14. Mooren's ulcer after cataract extraction displays intense conjunctival inflammation and peripheral stromal ulceration initially managed by tissue adhesive, **A,** with subsequent conjunctival resection and reinforcement of surgical incision dehiscence, **B.** Within 2 months, inflammation has subsided, **C,** and tissue adhesive can be safely removed from reinforced stroma without risk of reactive ulceration, **D.**

stromal ulceration is limited to the corneal periphery, a partial conjunctival flap may be mobilized to cover only the affected area. Such conjunctival advancement may temporarily succeed in halting the centripetal progression of the Mooren's ulceration while the patient is being immunosuppressed.

In 1958, Gundersen popularized the use of thin conjunctival flaps in the treatment of corneal ulcerations and thinning disorders of the cornea. Since then, many modifications have evolved. The following is a description of conjunctival flap as described by Gundersen.

Anesthesia may be local or retrobulbar, and after placement of the lid speculum, a 7-0 Vicryl (polyglactin 910) traction suture is placed through the peripheral cornea at the limbus from 11:30 to 12:30 o'clock allowing the surgeon to control the globe by rotating it downward and exposing the entire upper

bulbar conjunctiva. Subconjunctival injections of 2% lidocaine with epinephrine is used to baloon the upper bulbar conjunctiva. It is important not to puncture the portion of the conjunctiva that will be used to cover the cornea. The superior conjunctiva is then incised horizontally as far away from the limbus as possible in the upper conjunctival cul-de-sac. After the reflection of the bulbar conjunctiva on the supratarsal fold, the incision should be 30 to 35 mm long and should avoid underlying Tenon's fascia. A very thin flap of bulbar conjunctiva is dissected downward toward the limbus. Careful attention must be directed to prevent any "buttonholing" of the conjunctiva. When the limbus is reached, one frees the resultant flap by incising the limbus and completing a 360-degree conjunctival peritomy. At this stage, one should prepare the cornea by cleaning off any epithelium or necrotic material so that the conjunctiva-

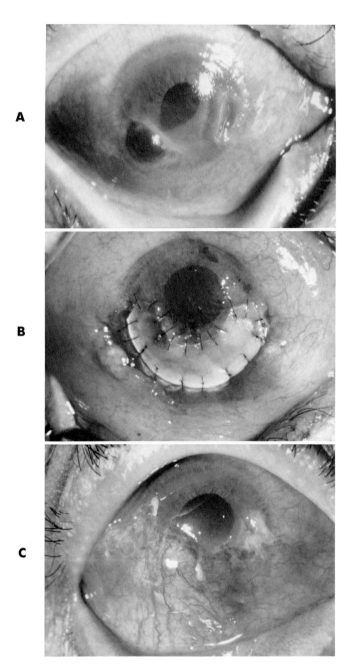

Fig. 29-15. Active ulceration with extensive peripheral stromal degradation and perforation with iris prolapse, **A,** is successfully managed by arcuate lamellar keratoplasty, **B,** and partial conjunctival flap, **C,** to provide tectonic support while systemic immunosuppression is accomplished.

val flap will adhere to the underlying stroma. The conjunctival flap may then be pulled down over the entire cornea and secured into position with 8-0 silk sutures placed in the superficial sclera just outside the limbus and also through the flap. The inferior conjunctiva can be secured to the conjunctival flap with interrupted 8-0 silk sutures. Similarly, the superior Tenon's capsule can be secured to the flap with interrupted 8-0 silk sutures. Cycloplegic agents and antibiotic ointments are instilled, and the sutures may be removed in 10 to 14 days.

KERATOPLASTY. The role of keratoplasty in the management of Mooren's ulcer is determined by the activity of the inflammatory and ulcerative process. In the acute phase of active ulceration, keratoplasty almost invariably only serves as a tectonic device to preserve the structural integrity of the anterior segment in situations of impending or actual perforation. Patch grafts or arcuate sectoral grafts of either full or partial thickness may also be required to reinforce a thinned or perforated area of usually peripheral cornea (Fig. 29-15). Concomitant conjunctival transplants from the other eye or keratoepithelioplasty[9] may also be used to reinforce the structural integrity of the globe. If the ulceration is extensive, large-diameter keratoplasty[5] even extending from limbus to limbus may be required. In the setting of acute inflammation, the prognosis for penetrating keratoplasty is poor, even if adjunctive immunosuppression is added. Immunologic rejection is almost inevitable, even if ulceration of the graft, dehiscence of the surgical wound, or secondary glaucoma can be avoided. Once the inflammatory phase is controlled keratoplasty can be repeated for visual restoration with a more favorable prognosis.

Case illustrations. To illustrate the stepwise approach to the management of Mooren's ulceration, two examples of different stages of the disease are presented.

Case 1 is a 55-year-old patient who presented with severe pain and decreased vision in the right eye (Fig. 29-16). Examination revealed peripheral corneal ulceration from 1 to 7 o'clock inferiorly with 50% thinning and a typical gray leading edge. Initial treatment should begin with prednisolone phosphate 1% topically applied every hour for 3 days. If no healing occurs within 3 days and no further ulceration occurs, the frequency can be increased to every half hour. If healing then occurs, the frequency can be reduced and the drops can be tapered slowly over a period of several months. Concomitant topical antibiotics should be used. Topical ocular lubricants and ointments can be used four or five times per day. If stromal ulceration progresses, a conjunctival resection is performed between 7 and 1 o'clock superiorly. Aggressive pulse therapy with orally administered prednisone 100 mg per day can be given for 1 to 2 weeks. If systemic steroid therapy is ineffective, immunosuppressive therapy can be started with cyclophosphamide 100 mg per day and prednisone 160 mg per day. Alternatively, one can use methotrexate or azathioprine depending on the response to the medication and the preference of the co-managing internist or oncologist.

If corneal perforation of less than 2 mm in diameter occurs, cyanoacrylate adhesive and a therapeutic soft contact lens should be used. If the ulceration is more than 2 mm in size, lamellar or penetrating keratoplasty and possibly a conjunctival flap are planned.

Case 2 shows advanced peripheral corneal ulceration in a 66 year old with perforation for at least 6 mm and iris prolapse (Fig. 29-17). In this patient, the options are quite limited. Topical steroids will hasten the ulcerative process and are contraindicated. Conjunctival resection alone will not suffice at this stage. A conjunctival flap over an area of perforation is not appropriate because it will result in fibrovascular ingrowth, prolonged hypotony, and loss of the eye. The preferred treatment is to start systemic immunosuppression with a combination of prednisone and cyclophosphamide followed by a limbus-to-limbus corneal transplant with conjunctival resection in the area of corneal ulceration. Recurrent ulceration of the graft leaves only two options: (1) conjunctival transplantation from the opposite eye or (2) a complete conjunctival flap. Once the systemic immunotherapy stabilizes the progressive immunologic destruction of the cornea, further visual rehabilitation may be attempted.

REFERENCES

1. Brown SI, Mondino BJ: Therapy of Mooren's ulcer, *Am J Ophthalmol* 98:1-6, 1984.
2. Fogle JA, Kenyon KR, Foster CS: Tissue adhesive arrests stromal melting in the human cornea, *Am J Ophthalmol* 89:795-802, 1980.
3. Foster CS: Systemic immunosuppressive therapy for progressive bilateral Mooren's ulcer, *Ophthalmology* 92:1436-1439, 1985.
4. Foster CS, Kenyon KR, Greiner J, et al: The immunopathology of Mooren's ulcer, *Am J Ophthalmol* 88:149-159, 1979.
5. Raizman MB, de la Maza MS, Foster CS: Tectonic keratoplasty for peripheral ulcerative keratitis, *Cornea* 10(4):312-316, 1991.
6. Schanzlin D: Mooren's ulceration. In Smolin G, Thoft R, editors: *The cornea: scientific foundations and clinical practice*, ed 2, Boston, 1983, Little, Brown.
7. Martin HF, Stark WJ, Maumenee AE: Treatment of Mooren's and Mooren's-like ulcer by lamellar keratectomy, *Ophthalmic Surg* 18:564-569, 1987.
8. Wood TO, Kaufman HE: Mooren's ulcer, *Am J Ophthalmol* 71:417-421, 1971.
9. Kinoshita S, Ohashi Y, Ohji M, Manabe R: Long-term results of keratoepithelioplasty in Mooren's ulcer, *Ophthalmology* 98:438-445, 1991.

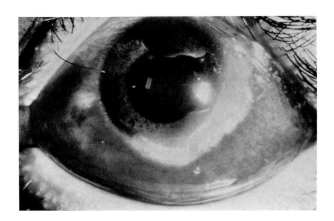

Fig. 29-16. Active Mooren's ulceration with peripheral stromal thinning from 1 to 7 o'clock without perforation.

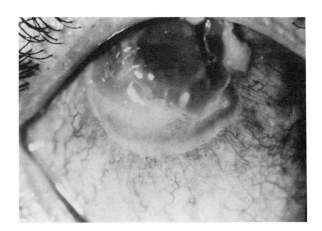

Fig. 29-17. Advanced Mooren's ulceration with extensive stromal ulceration and major perforation with iris prolapse.

Pterygium

MICHAEL S. INSLER

DELMAR R. CALDWELL

DAVID H. LEACH

A pterygium is caused by the fibrovascular overgrowth or extension of connective tissue from the bulbar conjunctiva onto the cornea. It generally occurs in the interpalpebral zone at the 3 and 9 o'clock positions adjacent to the limbus. Most commonly, the pterygium is located nasally, but it may occur temporally and, in some instances, in both clock-hour positions simultaneously (Fig. 29-18). Many cases are bilateral.

Fuchs's theory[6] that damaging external influences, such as sun glare, dust, wind, and heat, are responsible for the formation of a pterygium is supported by the fact that this disorder is observed more frequently in persons who work outdoors and that the incidence is higher in tropical and subtropical countries where prolonged exposure to intense solar radiation is common. The prevalence is higher in older people; the peak occurs in those 60 years of age or older. An increased tendency to develop pterygia has also been observed in the 40- to 49-year-old age group.[7]

There are a variety of theories concerning the origin and pathogenesis of pterygia.[16] Some investigators have proposed an inflammatory process with possible involvement of type 1 hypersensitivity in which stimulation by exogenous irritants such as pollens and dust particles containing antigenic material cause localized IgE production.[11] Others have cited

a primary degeneration of the cornea. Austin, Jakobiec, and Iwamoto suggested that elastodysplasia followed by elastodystrophy may be involved.[2]

The first visible sign of an impending pterygium is the presence of small grayish opacities near the limbus in Bowman's zone. These opacities always precede the apex of the pterygium in its progression toward the center of the cornea. In a fully developed pterygium, this grayish zone forms a flat rim around the apex (Figs. 29-19 and 29-20). The vessels of the pterygium tend to course horizontally toward this apex. In the growing pterygium, the base may become quite fleshy and vascularized. An iron line, called Stocker's line, may develop in the corneal epithelium at the leading edge of the pterygium.

Slitlamp examination is important in the evaluation of the rate of growth of a pterygium. Multiplication of the opacities preceding the apex and extension of vessels into this zone indicate a tendency toward rapid growth. Cessation of growth is characterized by decreased size and flattening, with attenuation of vascularity.

The ophthalmologist must be keenly aware of the fact that an atypical pterygium may be confused with an epibulbar tumor.[10] Most malignant lesions, including carcinoma in situ and invasive squamous carcinoma, are slow growing and advance from the limbus onto the cornea in a fashion similar to that of pterygia. Several factors account for the tendency of the limbal area to undergo degeneration and malignant transformation. The first is that the limbus represents a transitional zone where corneal epithelium changes into conjunctival epithelium. The second is

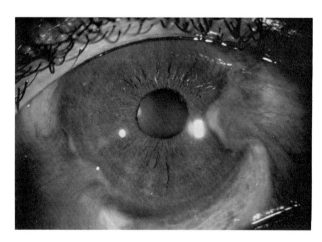

Fig. 29-18. Eye with temporal as well as nasal pterygia.

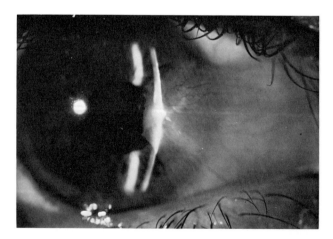

Fig. 29-19. Characteristic slitlamp changes of advancing pterygia include apex surrounded by flat gray rim and elevated fibrovascular overgrowth with radially oriented blood vessels.

that the interpalpebral portion of the limbus is continually exposed to environmental irritants as well as solar ultraviolet radiation.

Histologically, a pterygium shows elastotic degeneration in the substantia propria of the conjunctiva. A pinguecula shows the same changes without corneal involvement. The epithelium over the fibrovascular tissue may show dysplastic changes, such as hyperkeratosis, acanthosis, or dyskeratosis. Electron microscopic studies show the presence of active fibroblasts in the areas of tissue destruction, with Bowman's layer severely affected.[5]

TREATMENT

When the pterygium is confined to 1 to 2 mm of the peripheral cornea, there is little effect on vision and only a cosmetic concern; however, as the pterygium advances, it may induce irregular astigmatism and cause some decrease in visual acuity (Fig. 29-21). Additionally, the elevated area may disrupt the tear film, leading to an epithelial keratopathy with symptoms. Early treatment with lubricating drops and artificial tears may serve to prevent the progression of the keratopathy. When vision is affected or the symptoms become more bothersome, excision of the pterygium is indicated. Primary surgical resection using a bare scleral technique with meticulous conjunctival dissection is the initial surgical approach. Some authors have suggested transplanting the head of the pterygium during the resection by carrying it down into a conjunctival slit below and suturing it as a pedicle flap.[1]

Recurrence rates as high as 50% after primary ex-

cision have been reported. Recurrent pterygia are more difficult to control, and various adjunctive treatment modalities have been coupled with surgical excision in managing these cases.

Beta radiation has been used effectively to reduce the rate of recurrence of pterygium in many patients over the past several decades. Considerable variation in the rates of recurrence after treatment with strontium-90 radiation has been reported.[14] This procedure has an acceptable range of complications and results in a low recurrence rate when it is administered by an experienced radiation therapist and the calculations and calibrations are done precisely. The radiation treatments are best given early in the postoperative period, preferably within 48 hours of surgery. A total of 1800 to 2200 rad equivalent to beta radiation is usually administered.[3] Complications include cataract formation, corneal and scleral thinning and ulceration, and keratitis sicca.[13]

Another modality is the use of topical thiotepa solution diluted 1:1000. The drops are given immediately after surgery and continued for several weeks. Complications include allergic conjunctivitis, conjunctival hypertrophy, and depigmentation of the eyelid skin in darkly pigmented persons.[8]

A more recent approach to reducing the rate of recurrence of pterygium is the use of mitomycin-C, an antimetabolite-antineoplastic agent. A significant reduction in recurrences was shown with the application of a 0.4 mg/ml solution four times a day for 2 weeks after surgical excision.[12]

In severe cases of recurrence with some stromal thinning, lamellar keratoplasty may be used to rein-

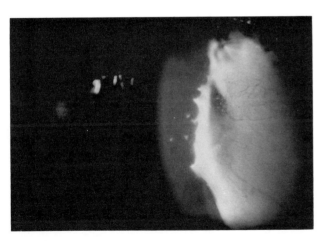

Fig. 29-20. Higher magnification showing grayish opacities preceding apex of pterygium. Opacities are commonly seen in association with Stocker's line, an iron line in corneal basilar epithelial cells sometimes seen at the leading edge of pterygia.

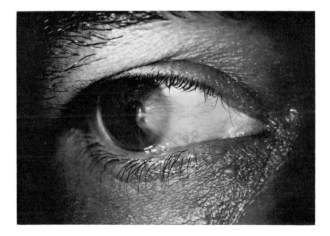

Fig. 29-21. Advanced pterygium encroaching on the visual axis may cause visual as well as symptomatic complaints because of scarring, increased astigmatism, and poor tear film apposition.

force the bed of the excised pterygium. More recently, free conjunctival grafts have been reported to have much promise in the prevention of recurrent pterygium.[9,15]

Finally, the argon laser can be used to prevent recurrences of pterygium.[4] The laser beam is applied most readily after the original surgical excision, when there is a smooth corneal surface remaining at the limbus. Laser burns (50 μm spot size) are made in the limbus in four parallel rows, with care taken to treat all neovascular fronds (Fig. 29-22). The patient is followed closely for signs of new fibrovascular formation, especially evidence of neovascular fronds. If any are found, laser treatment is repeated, with the setting adjusted to prevent conjunctival epithelial burn or shrinkage. This procedure can be repeated and has several advantages over repeated excision, beta radiation, or lamellar grafting.

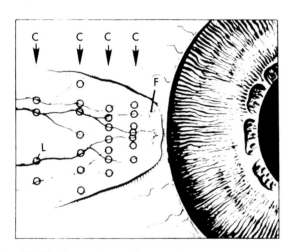

Fig. 29-22. Argon laser therapy for recurrent pterygia with four parallel rows of burns, including all neovascular fronds.

REFERENCES

1. Arruga H: *Ocular surgery,* ed 3, New York, 1962, McGraw-Hill, pp 321-333.
2. Austin P, Jakobiec FA, Iwamoto T.: Elastodysplasia and elastodystrophy as the pathologic bases of ocular pterygia and pinguecula, *Ophthalmology* 90:96-109, 1983.
3. Bahrassa F, Datta R: Postoperative beta radiation treatment of pterygium, *Int J Radiat Oncol Biol Phys* 9(5):679-684, 1983.
4. Boyd BF: *Highlights of ophthalmology, atlas and textbook of microsurgery and laser surgery,* 30th anniversary, 1:534-545, Panama, Republic of Panama, 1984, Highlights of Ophthalmology.
5. Cameron ME: Histology of pterygium: an electron microscopic study, *Br J Ophthalmol* 67:604-608, 1983.
6. Fuchs E: Ueber das Pterygium, *Arch Ophthalmol* 38:1, 1892.
7. Hilgers JH: Pterygium: its incidence, heredity, and etiology, *Am J Ophthalmol* 50:635-644, 1960.
8. Joselson GA, Muller P: Incidence of pterygium recurrence in patients treated with thio-tepa, *Am J Ophthalmol* 61:891-892, 1966.
9. Kenyon KR, Hettinger ME, Wagoner MD: Conjunctival autograft transplantation for advanced and recurrent pterygium, *Ophthalmology* 92:1461-1470, 1985.
10. Ni C, Searl SS, Kriegstein HJ, Wu BF: Epibulbar carcinoma, *Int Ophthalmol Clin* 22(3):1-33, 1982.
11. Pinkerton OD, Hokama Y, Shigemura LA: Immunologic basis for the pathogenesis of pterygium, *Am J Ophthalmol* 98:225-228, 1984.
12. Singh G, Wilson MR, Foster CS: Long-term follow-up study of mitomycin eye drops as adjunctive treatment of pterygia and its comparison with conjunctival autograft transplantation, *Cornea* 9:331-334, 1990.
13. Talbot AN: Complication for beta ray treatment of pterygia, *Trans Ophthalmol Soc NZ* 64(7):496, 1980.
14. Van Den Brenk H: Result of prophylactic postoperative irradiation in 1300 cases of pterygium, *Am J Roentgenol* 103(4):723-733, 1968.
15. Vastine DW, Stewart WB, Schwab IR: Reconstruction of the periocular mucous membranes by autologous conjunctival transplantation, *Ophthalmology* 89:1071-1081, 1982.
16. Wong WW: A hypothesis on the pathogenesis of pterygiums, *Ann Ophthalmol* 10:303, 1976.

Chapter 30

Corneal Thinning and Perforation

STEPHEN P. GINSBERG

FREDERICK S. BRIGHTBILL

Many ocular conditions predispose the cornea to thinning and possible perforation. These conditions range from chronic, indolent circumstances associated often with long-standing ocular or systemic problems to more acute and rapidly progressing processes. Common to them all are persistent corneal epithelial defects,[21,23,35,43] stromal dehydration with associated thinning, and often Descemet's membrane rupture and global collapse. Although the rapidity of the process varies from one condition to the next and the speed of the therapeutic response may often vary as well, the ultimate result of inadequately treated corneal thinning and perforation is devastating to the eye. The persistent loss of the integrity of the anterior chamber in an eye that is leaking aqueous through a corneal perforation can and probably will result in anterior synechia formation, absolute glaucoma, cataract formation, and possible endophthalmitis. Prompt measures to seal the perforation, even if only temporarily in preparation for a more definite treatment, must be instituted as quickly as possible.

FACTORS LEADING TO LOSS OF CORNEAL EPITHELIAL INTEGRITY

The factors that can lead to the loss of corneal epithelial integrity and subsequent potential for corneal perforation have been summarized by Doughman[23] (Fig. 30-1).

Infection. Although some bacterial organisms can enter the intact corneal epithelium, such as *Neisseria gonorrhoeae*, Koch-Weeks bacillus, and *Corynebacte-*

rium diphtheriae, most other bacteria, fungi, and viruses require a defect in the surface for entry.* Once established in the corneal stroma, these organisms create a necrotic process that can ultimately lead to loss of stromal mass with perforation. In addition to the destructive nature of the organism itself, the surrounding regenerating epithelial cells and the polymorphonuclear leukocytes called forth by the severe inflammatory reaction then liberate proteolytic enzymes, which further damage the collagen matrix and hasten the corneal dissolution. Herpes simplex corneal infections, both because of the often severe inflammation and the high frequency of recurrences, seem to be ideally suited for the creation of the string of events that may culminate in corneal perforation[13,17,44,65] (Fig. 30-2).

In herpes zoster ophthalmia (HZO), the corneal hypesthesia often seen may lead to a persistent epithelial defect and a subsequent corneal perforation from either the trophic (sterile) process or the active viral necrosis[52] or both.

Xerosis. Many systemic and local ocular conditions result in corneal desiccation caused by inadequate mucus and water components in the tear film. Diseases such as rheumatoid arthritis, erythema multiforme, epidermolysis bullosa, vitamin A and B complex deficiencies, and others are often associated with chronic epithelial abnormalities and persistent healing defects.† Inadequate corneal fibroplasia and

---

*References 13, 15, 17, 18, 24, 27, 29, 32, 42, 50, 62.
†References 6, 7, 12, 26, 32, 33, 36, 47, 50, 60, 69, 70.

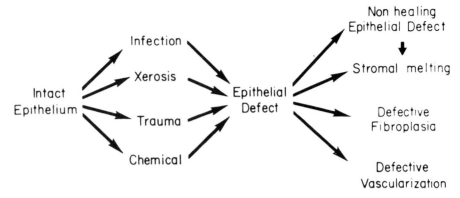

Fig. 30-1. Pathogenesis of corneal thinning and perforation (From Doughman D: *J Contin Educ Ophthalmol* 39:15, 1978.)

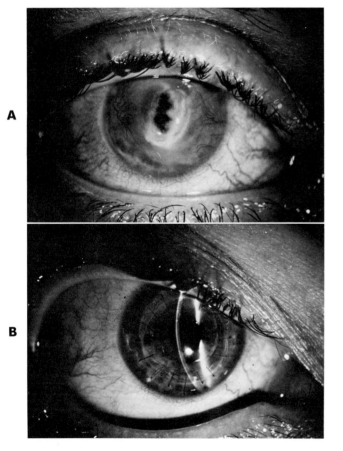

Fig. 30-2. A, Corneal perforation caused by stromal herpes simplex keratitis in 28-year-old woman. **B,** Same eye 6 months postoperatively. Eleven years later graft remains crystal clear, and vision is corrected to 20/20.

vascularization are also characteristic and retard corneal stromal healing. When combined with persistent epithelial defects, conditions are ripe for corneal perforation in these unfortunate patients.

Localized specific ocular diseases such as Mooren's corneal ulceration,[5,22,29] Terrien's marginal dystrophy, and severe cases of keratitis sicca[37] can, for reasons still unknown, lead to severe corneal stromal melting and perforation often in the corneal periphery.

The topical use of steroids for treating corneal disease, particularly when there is an epithelial defect, has led to melting of the corneal stroma and subsequent perforation.[44,65] The mechanism by which this occurs is as yet not fully understood, but corticosteroids probably act by perpetuating the lytic action of the proteolytic enzyme collagenase, produced by various corneal conditions, rather than by a direct alteration of the collagen molecule.[11] Conditions in which this may occur include corneal infections such as that by *Pseudomonas aeruginosa* and herpes simplex, neuroparalytic keratopathy, the ulcers of alkali-burned corneas, those of patients with rheumatoid arthritis and Stevens-Johnson syndrome, and in the corneal graft wounds of patients with collagen diseases, alkali burns, Stevens-Johnson syndrome, or ocular pemphigoid.

Trauma. Incidental corneal trauma such as an abrasion or, the more serious, penetrating or even perforating corneal laceration, can result in situations similar to those discussed and require the same vigorous therapeutic intervention.[2,16,25,35,43,60,67]

Superficial corneal abrasions, especially linear types such as a corneal scratch from the edge of a piece of paper or a baby's fingernail, can cause destruction of the hemidesmosome bonding of the basal epithelium to the underlying basement membrane. This can, in rare instances, lead to recurrent, nonhealing epithelial defects with ultimate stromal melting. The failure of prompt hemidesmosome reformation may be attributable to localized basement-membrane injury or can be associated with systemic conditions such as diabetes mellitus, severe malnutrition, and other metabolic derangements.[35,43,52,67]

Corneal ulcerations can also occur after cataract and intraocular lens surgery, especially if there is an associated dry eye condition.[52]

Chemical Injury. The classic chemical injury that frequently leads to persistent epithelial defects with associated stromal melting, defective fibroplasia, and vascularization is the alkali-burned cornea. The result of an increase in collagenase activity, the severe ischemia from the destructive effect of the burn on the limbal vessels, and the alteration in the fibroplastic response of these corneas often leads to corneal melting and perforation with perhaps the worst prognosis for treatment of all corneal perforations encountered so far.*

DIAGNOSIS

In the initial examination of the cornea the surgeon must decide (1) whether an epithelial defect is present, (2) the extent of stromal thinning, and (3) whether corneal perforation has occurred. When fluorescein pools over the thinned area rather than staining Bowman's membrane and the eye is not inflamed, the likely diagnosis is dellen—saucer-shaped excavations of dehydrated corneal stroma—rather than a more worrisome form of corneal thinning. Often the limbal area near the thinned portion is elevated causing problems with corneal wetting. The thinning may respond only to hydration and removal of the contiguous elevated area.[23]

If, in fact, a true epithelial defect is seen with associated stromal thinning and loss of tissue, one next needs to observe for white blood cell infiltration beneath the ulcer. When the involved tissue and surrounding area appear whitish gray or creamy yellow, one should assume the tissue is infected as well as edematous. Appropriate corneal scrapings should be obtained directly over and adjacent to the stromal infiltrate for Gram's, periodic acid–Schiff (PAS), or other fungal stains, and smears plated for bacterial (aerobic and anaerobic), viral, and fungal cultures.

When frank perforation is observed, one must determine the size of the opening. If the perforation site is large (over 2 mm), the treatment may be different from what it would be if it were small (less

than 2 mm). Preexisting conditions such as viral infections, corneal trauma with vegetable matter, prior topical use of steroid medication, generalized predisposing local or systemic problems, corneal exposure, or dry eye conditions, may indicate the source of the presenting problem.

The examination is completed when the visual acuity and intraocular pressure measurements are recorded. A careful examination is then made for evidence of anterior synechia formation or central iris adherence (leukoma), hypopyon or hyphema, cataract formation, or signs of an intraocular foreign body. Trauma associated with corneal perforation indicates the possibility of a penetrating foreign body, and orbital x-ray examination, ocular CAT scans and B-scan ultrasonography are then appropriate.

TREATMENT

The specific treatment of epithelial defects (ulcers) is dependent on the presence or absence of perforation, concomitant infection, size of the perforation, and possible association with an autoimmune disease process.

Epithelial defect with stromal *thinning* only:

1. Topical antibiotics even if there is no infiltrate present.[23]
2. With infiltration, specific antibacterial, antiviral, or antifungal treatment combined with frequent débridement, after initial scrapings for stains and cultures.
3. Corneal lubrication (artificial tears or bland ointment, or both) in case of dehydration (dellen) or associated corneal drying.
4. Avoid topical steroids to prevent stromal melting.
5. With or without collagenase inhibitors (acetylcysteine drops (Mucomyst) 10% to 20%, or EDTA).
6. Lid closure with tape, eye pad, or possible temporary tarsorrhaphy if exposure or corneal drying, or both, are present and nonresponsive to local lubrication measures including drops and ointments.
7. Extended-wear therapeutic standard soft lens fitting if this is preferable to point 6 (8.0 to 8.7 mm lenses are adequate for most cases).
8. Anterior stromal puncture (needle or laser) or epithelial débridement for resistant recurrent erosion syndrome epithelial defects.[31,48]
9. Conjunctival flap placement for unresponsive ulcers.

Noninfected epithelial defect with *corneal perforation:*

1. Antibiotic coverage with topical solutions.

---

*References 1, 3, 8-11, 14, 21, 39, 40, 49, 54, 55, 63.

2. Orally given carbonic anhydrase inhibitors (acetazolamide, Diamox) optional because decreased aqueous flow may help in sealing.
3. Topical collagenase inhibitors optional.
4. Short trial (6 to 8 hours) with pressure dressings if opening 1 mm or less in an attempt to reform anterior chamber and prevent anterior synechia formation until more definitive treatment is instituted.
5. Soft contact lens with pressure dressing if defect is 1 mm or less.
6. Tissue adhesive glue or fibrin sealant[45] with or without soft contact lens.
7. Partial conjunctival flap for small opening if glue is not successful or unavailable with the anterior chamber depth always being left observable.
8. "Blow-out" corneal patch graft if no reformation by other methods by 24 hours.

Noninfected marginal epithelial defect with extreme thinning or perforation, associated with autoimmune disease (such as Mooren's ulcer, Sjögren's syndrome, adult rheumatoid arthritis, polyarteritis nodosa, Wegener's granulomatosis, systemic lupus erythematosus):

1. Antibiotic coverage with topical solutions.
2. Topical corticosteroids for 1 to 3 days depending on response.
3. Conjunctival resection in quadrant of ulceration.[22]
4. Cytotoxic agents (cyclophosphamide or azathioprine, 50 to 100 mg per day, with dose adjustment depending on local and systemic effect).[22]
5. Tissue adhesive glue with or without soft contact lens for small (less than 2 mm) perforation.

6. Annular peripheral penetrating keratoplasty if ulcer inactive with extreme thinning or greater than 2 mm perforation.[22]
7. Autogenous periosteal graft in face of significant scleral thinning and failure of above methods to heal area.[19,52]

Infected epithelial defect with *2 mm OR LESS* corneal perforation:

1. Debride necrotic material.
2. Apply appropriate topical anti-infective agent or agents.
3. Subconjunctival antibiotics every other day, optional.
4. Carbonic anhydrase inhibitor (Diamox) optional.
5. Topical collagenase inhibitors, optional.
6. Avoid patching an infected eye.
7. After 24 to 48 hours of anti-infective therapy, a soft contact lens with or without a pressure dressing may be tried (allows observation and continued topical medication).
8. Tissue adhesive glue or fibrin sealant[45] with or without corneal patch and soft contact lens (Fig. 30-3).
9. Partial conjunctival flap after careful removal of all previously placed glue.
10. "Blow-out" corneal patch graft if no chamber reformation is effected by other methods within 24 hours (Fig. 30-4).

Infected epithelial defect with *3 mm OR MORE* corneal perforation:

1. Debride necrotic material.
2. Apply appropriate topical anti-infective agent or agents. Subconjunctival antibiotics optional.
3. Collagenase inhibitors optional.

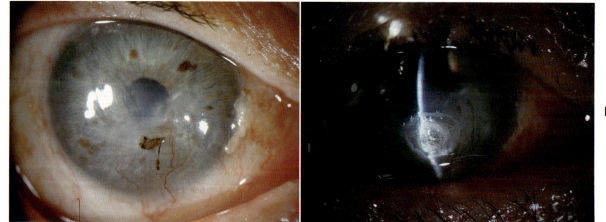

Fig. 30-3. A, Corneal perforation (beneath pigment) associated with herpes simplex keratitis. **B,** Corneal perforation in same eye 24 hours after sealing with cyanoacrylate tissue adhesive.

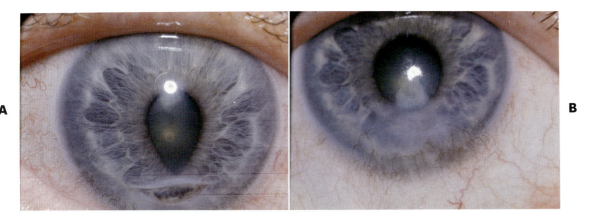

Fig. 30-4. A, Rheumatoid corneal melt with iris prolapse. Notice quiet, noninflamed nature of eye. **B,** Healed corneal patch graft in same patient.

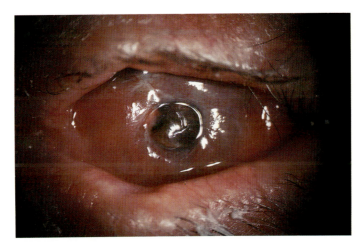

Fig. 30-5. Herpes simplex perforation through center of conjunctival flap. Total flap placement must be avoided in large corneal perforations (over 1 to 2 mm).

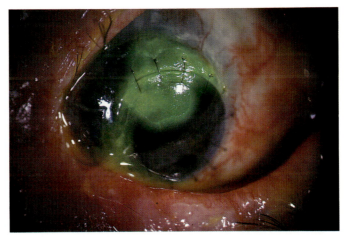

Fig. 30-6. Recurrence of epithelial herpes simplex infection in penetrating corneal graft. Many corneal grafts fail if done on inflamed or infected corneal ulcerations.

4. Avoid pressure bandage, soft contact lens, or conjunctival flap (Fig. 30-5).

5. Tissue adhesive glue or fibrin sealant[45] with or without corneal or scleral patch and with or without soft contact lens.

6. "Blow-out" patch graft if anterior chamber is not easily reformed after glue. Carefully remove all glue placed previously before positioning patch graft because glue-degradation products cause necrosis of overlying patch graft.

7. Avoid penetrating corneal graft in an inflamed, infected eye as initial therapy (Fig. 30-6). Spread of infection to donor graft along with failure is common. Use only as a last resort.[51]

SPECIFIC THERAPEUTIC MEASURES

Treatment of Recurrent Erosion By Anterior Stromal Puncture. Having observed that the so-called recurrent corneal erosion occurred more likely after incidental corneal trauma or even spontaneously as opposed to after embedded corneal foreign bodies or superficial lacerations, McLean[48] reasoned that the difference between these etiologic factors was the breaching of Bowman's membrane. On that assumption, he deduced in 1966, that a recreation of this Bowman's membrane disruption may be useful in treating nonresponsive corneal erosions. In a study reported in 1986, McLean and co-workers reviewed 21 eyes in 18 individuals that had nonhealing erosions by the conventional methods of ocular patching, lubrication, and soft lens wear. Using the anterior stromal needle puncture technique, all the 21 eyes treated (three requiring a second treatment) had remained healed during the follow-up period of 5 months to 12 years.

The technique described varies with each physician but generally consists in this sequence:

1. Topical anesthesia is required.

2. The area to be treated is left undisturbed and the loosened epithelium serves as the guide for the treatment locale.

3. With use of a 20-, 27-, or 30-gauge needle, approximately 15 to 25 punctures, spaced 0.5 to 1.0 mm apart, are created by penetrating Bowman's membrane with enough vertical pressure so as to enter the outer regions of the stroma.

4. Alternatively, the epithelium over the damaged area can be debrided by mechanical means (spatula or no. 15 Bard-Parker knife blade) or with use of the Nd:YAG laser. Set at energy levels between 1.8 and 2.2 mJ, rows of spots 0.20 to 0.25 mm apart are used to cover the area. The laser is focused just anterior to the basement membrane so that the induced shock wave hits the corneal surface and not the anterior stroma, thus limiting the size of the scar created and any potential visual effects.[31]

5. The treated eyes are given cycloplegia and antibiotics and are pressure patched until re-epithelialization has occurred.

6. Once the eye has become epithelialized, topical lubrication in the form of tears during the day and a bland ointment at bedtime should be continued at the discretion of the physician.

Glueing Technique for Corneal Perforation. Around 20 years ago, Refojo[59] reported the first successful closure of a small corneal perforation using a tissue adhesive. Since then multiple reports have appeared in the literature extolling the virtues of cyanoacrylate tissue adhesive as a first-line treatment to close leaking corneal wounds and to thereby restore temporarily or even permanently the integrity of the anterior chamber.[4,20,34,41,56-59,66,68] As a simple office procedure, the glueing of corneal wound leaks can restore a deep anterior chamber with normal intraocular pressure until a more definitive corneal procedure can be done.

By rapid polymerization of carbon molecules, the adhesive readily "set up" on contact with dry nonnecrotic tissue and bonds firmly with the cornea until the natural scarring process of the cornea can take over in from days to 1 or more weeks. Later on, the degradation of the polymer will occur with cleavage of its carbon-to-carbon backbone and release of formaldehyde and other products.[30,46] These toxic by-products have led to stringent criteria for the use of this product and the reluctance of the Food and Drug Administration to approve it for general use. In truth, however, there has not been good evidence to show any deleterious ocular effects from these toxic by-products and the inflammation observed with its use probably is more related to a foreign-body reaction.[34]

The degree of reaction to the glue is probably also related to the amount employed and the specific monomer utilized, with perhaps less reaction observed with the higher monomer.[34] The following three types of tissue adhesives have been used frequently: *n*-heptyl, octyl, and isobutyl cyanoacrylate monomers, with the last being the most popular (Bucrylate, from Ethicon Inc., Somerville, New Jersey, and Histoacryl, from Tri Hawk International, Montreal).

The actual technique for applying the glue (Fig. 30-7) varies among corneal surgeons,[34,41,53,56] but in general the following principles apply:

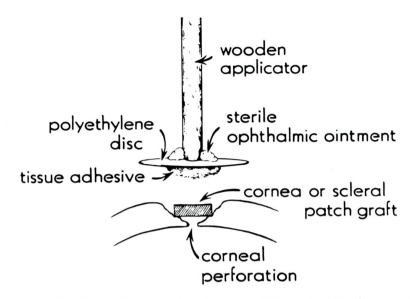

Fig. 30-7. Method for sealing corneal perforation utilizing a lamellar donor graft and cyanoacrylate tissue glue. (From Hyndiuk R, Hull D, and Kinyoun J: *Ophthalmic Surg* 5:50, 1974.)

1. Topical anesthesia is employed, with a lid speculum being optional but also useful.
2. All necrotic tissue and epithelium are removed around the perforation for at least 2 mm.
3. The area is thoroughly dried with cellulose sponges because the polymerization of the glue occurs more efficiently without moisture.
4. (Optional:) A lamellar piece of fresh or glycerin-preserved cornea or sclera is created and freehand cut to fill the defect.
5. A small polyethylene disc of a 3 to 4 mm diameter is cut and affixed to the blunt end of a wooden applicator stick with a small amount of sterile ophthalmic ointment.
6. A tiny drop of the cyanoacrylate glue is placed on the face of the disc, and the disc-glue combination is pressed onto the once-again dried perforation site and held in place for 1 to 2 minutes while polymerization occurs.
7. (Optional:) A soft contact lens is fitted over the corneal glue site with a small air bubble maintained to demonstrate vaulting. This contact lens acts to separate the lids from the often heaped-up and hardened glue that can appear around the edges of the disc, which is otherwise quite irritating to the eyelid.
8. If the chamber does not deepen, the area is not sealed, and the procedure can be repeated immediately.

9. If the glueing procedure is not successful and a lamellar patch graft with or without a partial conjunctival flap is contemplated, all the previously placed glue must be carefully removed just before placement of the patch graft. If this is not done, the underlying glue may cause considerable inflammation and necrosis of the

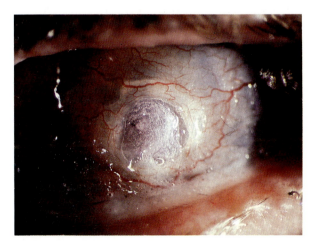

Fig. 30-8. Necrosis of conjunctival flap 3 weeks after placement over tissue adhesive used to seal perforation. Toxic breakdown products of glue cause severe necrosis of overlying tissue (conjunctival flap or corneal patch graft). All glue should be meticulously removed before placement of tissue over perforation site.

overlying tissue with continued leaking of the site[34] (Fig. 30-8).

Technique for Performing a Proper Conjunctival Flap. Since Trygve Gunderson's original description of his technique for creating a thin conjunctival flap over the cornea,[38] it has been utilized extensively to treat unresponsive corneal ulcers. Because the flap brings an immediate source of blood vessels and fibroblasts, rapid corneal healing and ocular comfort are achieved with the quieting of an inflamed eye. Later more definitive corneal surgery can be performed on a now normotensive, noninflamed eye.

The placement of a flap is indicated only after all medical therapeutic measures have been tried including patching, anti-infectives, and therapeutic soft lenses. It is particularly useful in treating nonhealing, infected corneal ulcers with corneal thinning. If perforation of the cornea has occurred, the application of a partial conjunctival flap remains controversial because wound leaking can persist under the flap surface and may be unrecognized by the physician, resulting in almost certain loss of the eye to absolute glaucoma or intraocular infection. This will certainly be the case if the entire cornea has been covered by the conjunctival tissue obscuring observation of the anterior chamber depth.

The actual technique for performing a flap has been described elsewhere,[53] but, subject to individual surgeon preference, the following general principles apply (Fig. 30-9).

1. Local anesthesia with lid and retrobulbar injections are utilized.
2. A lid speculum is applied.
3. All the corneal epithelium is removed as well as the necrotic tissue from the area about the perforation. This assures flap adherence.
4. Since the flap is easier to create from the superior bulbar area, the eye is rotated downward by either a traction suture placed in the cornea at a point below 12 o'clock or by means of a superior rectus bridle suture in the manner utilized in cataract operations.
5. A 360-degree conjunctival peritomy is cut as close to the limbus as possible with undermining of the inferior conjunctiva for a few millimeters. Smaller peritomies may be performed according to surgeon preference.
6. The conjunctival flap is meticulously dissected over the entire superior aspect of the globe. All underlying tissue is separated so that the flap is thin enough for one to see the shine on the dissecting scissors. A Max Fine stitch or Wescott scissors is ideal for this though the

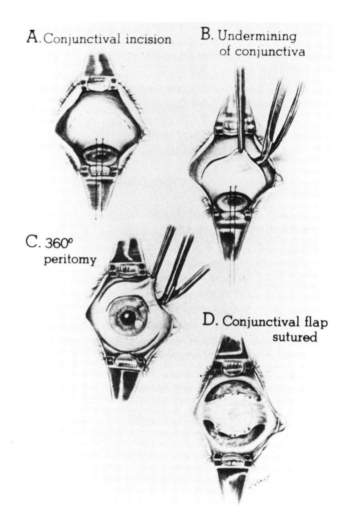

Fig. 30-9. Total conjunctival flap used primarily to cover areas of extreme corneal thinning without perforation. Partial flaps can be done to heal very small perforations as long as anterior chamber depth can be observed through areas of cornea not covered by flap. (From Raju VK: Corneal surgery. In Duane TD, Jaeger EA, editors: *Clinical ophthalmology*, vol 5, Philadelphia, 1984, Lippincott.)

points are quite sharp and extreme care must be taken to avoid flap perforation.

7. Once the flap is thinned and easily stretches over the entire cornea without excess tension, a relaxing incision is made in the area of the superior fornix. Any inadvertent "buttonholes" of the flap are repaired at once because these open sites will serve as areas for flap retraction and exposure of the underlying cornea.
8. The flap is smoothed down and closed over its entire open edge. This is done with interrupted 10-0 nylon sutures. The horizontal intact bridges are maintained to provide flap nutrition through its vascular supply.

9. Antibiotic and cycloplegic drops are applied and the sutures are removed in 2 to 3 weeks or longer. Gradual "whitening" and thinning of the flap occurs over the next few months, and often the flap becomes translucent enough to actually allow rough anterior segment inspection at a later date.

10. Subsequently vision can be restored by means of penetrating keratoplasty with no adverse effects created by the presence of a flap.

Technique for Lamellar "Blow-Out" Patch Grafting. If a corneal perforation of greater than a range of 2 to 3 mm is present, the site should be repaired with a small lamellar or full-thickness graft (Fig. 30-10). Penetrating keratoplasty is to be avoided because these grafts do poorly in inflamed, often infected, and hypotonous eyes.[51]

The technique itself varies, but general principles apply.[23,53]

Preparation of recipient perforation

1. Local anesthesia is preferred, but care must be taken to minimize ocular squeezing during the placement of the lid and retrobulbar block.

2. A lid speculum is placed.

3. The epithelium and necrotic tissue are carefully removed for 2 to 3 mm outside of the perforation site, and an application of cyanoacrylate glue can be made in the usual manner to seal the perforation (Fig. 30-10, *A*).

4. After the glue has been placed, a Haab knife paracentesis can be made and balanced saline solution or hyaluronate, or both, are injected into the anterior chamber to restore normal depth and pressure.

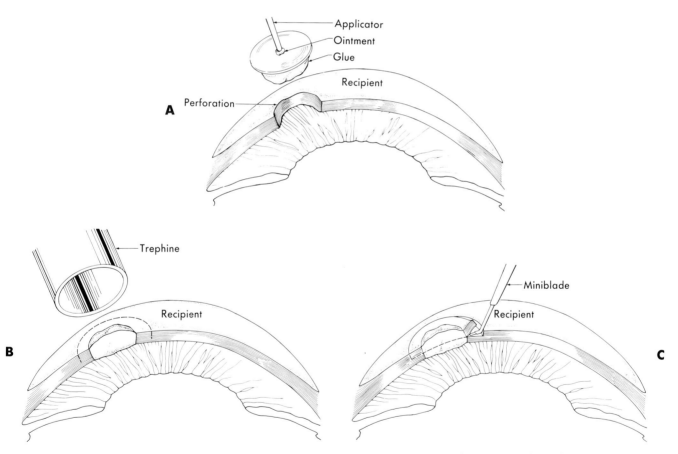

Fig. 30-10. Lamellar keratoplasty principles utilized in creating a "blow-out" patch graft for sealing a corneal perforation. **A,** Cyanoacrylate adhesive on rounded plastic drape before application over perforation site. Sodium hyaluronate can be used to push back adherent iris if necessary. **B,** Recipient perforation "plugged" with glue. Sizing trephine outlines one half to two thirds depth incision in normal cornea surrounding perforation. **C,** No. 6600 lamellar blade dissection inside trephine mark to create bed for "patch" graft. Notice perpendicular wall, which facilitates suturing of button into recipient bed.

Continued.

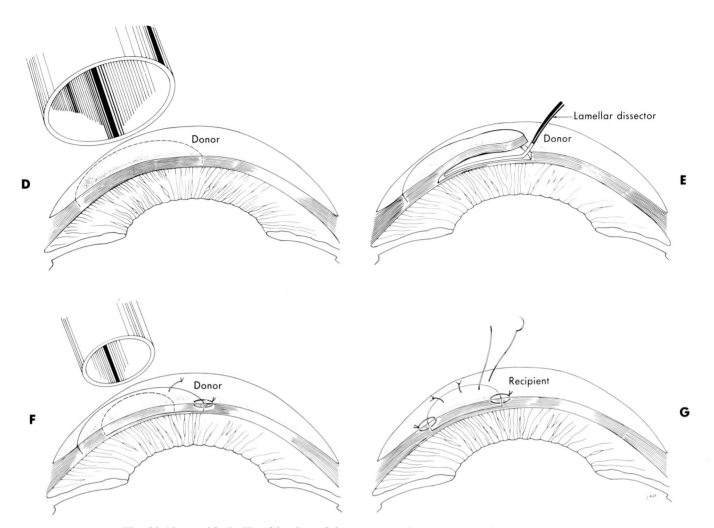

Fig. 30-10, cont'd. D, Trephination of donor cornea in same general area as recipient hole. Outlining incision 0.3 to 0.4 mm depth. In some cases full-thickness donor buttons trephined from anterior corneal surface are satisfactory and will ultimately thin down and conform to recipient bed thickness. **E,** One method for dissecting donor lamellar graft in deep stromal plane. **F,** After reanchoring of dissected lamellar button with suture, proper size trephine creates exact button desired. **G,** Donor cornea is sutured into perforation with 10-0 interrupted nylon. Knots should be trimmed short or buried.

5. Small "sizing" corneal trephines are gently placed over the perforation site so as to leave a small cuff of normal tissue about the central inflamed core (Fig. 30-10, *B*). Usually a 3 or 4 mm trephine will suffice.

6. A mark is made with a trephine, and the resulting circle is deepened with a razor blade or diamond knife to one half to two thirds the corneal depth (Fig. 30-10, *B*). The usual spinning trephination is more difficult because of the ocular hypotony.

7. The area of clear cornea inside the ring is dissected off to about one half the corneal depth

with a No. 6600 Beaver lamellar or comparable blade (Fig. 30-10, *C*).

Preparation of donor:

8. A donor whole eye, either fresh, frozen, or glycerin preserved, is inflated to normal, or just above normal, intraocular pressure and is placed in a donor eye holder. Kerato-Patch, available from American Medical Optics, (Irvine, California), provides a 10 mm, 0.3 mm thick, lathe-cut to plano, lamellar corneal button. Packaged as a freeze-dried tissue that requires rehydration with balanced salt solution—gentamicin (100 mg/ml), a 3 to 4 mm

patch can be fashioned with a Polack corneal punch or a freehand punch on a corneal well. The drawback is its high cost ($700 per button), but it is very useful in an emergency, and the tissue can probably remain stored in the operating room for a considerable time.

Technique for Creating a Lamellar Donor Button:

a. The epithelium of the donor is removed and a one-half corneal-depth trephination (0.3 to 0.4 mm) is made with a 6 to 8 mm Castroviejo corneal trephine (Fig. 30-10, *D*).

b. Using a lamellar dissector, a two-thirds corneal-depth incision is created over 80% of the button, with care being taken to allow a small area of nonseparated cornea to remain at the distal edge of the dissection so that the button created remains hinged along this remaining area (Fig. 30-10, *E*). The proximal edge of the button is sutured back to the edge of the adjoining corneal surface with 1 to 3 interrupted 10-0 nylon sutures

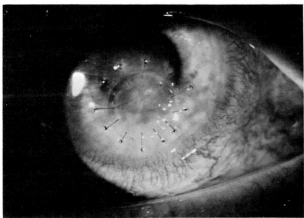
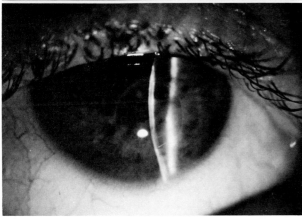

Fig. 30-11. A, Lamellar patch graft anchored with 10-0 interrupted nylon sutures for rheumatoid patient with corneal melt (early in postoperative course). **B,** Same eye after healing and suture removal.

(Fig. 30-10, *F*). The hinge on one side and the interrupted sutures on the opposite result in a firm seating of the lamellar button once again on its bed. This prevents graft rotation on subsequent trephination of the button to be used in creating the patch graft.

c. The appropriately sized trephine, determined on prior inspection of the recipient eye, is then used to create the exact-sized button for the patch graft (Fig. 30-10, *F*).

9. The donor button thus created is placed over the recipient site and affixed with either multiple interrupted sutures or a short running 10-0 nylon suture, or even by crossed figure-8 mattress sutures with buried knots (Figs. 30-10, *G*, and 30-11, *A*).

10. (Optional:) A soft contact lens may be used to promote re-epithelialization, and appropriate antibiotics and cycloplegic drops are administered.

11. Corneal sutures are removed 1 to 3 months after surgery (Fig. 30-11, *B*).

12. It should be pointed out, as well, that some surgeons prefer a full-thickness corneal button to use as the donor. In that case, it is appropriate simply to create a 3 to 4 mm full-thickness button with a corneal punch as described above.

REFERENCES

1. Abel R Jr et al: The results of penetrating keratoplasty after chemical burns, *Trans Am Acad Ophthalmol Otolaryngol* 74:584, 1975.
2. Adhikary HT, Taylor P, Fitzmaurice DJ: Prognosis of perforating eye injury, *Br J Ophthalmol* 60:737, 1976.
3. Ballen PH: Treatment of chemical burns of the eye, *Eye Ear Nose Throat Monthly* 43:57, 1964.
4. Boruchoff SA et al: Clinical applications of adhesives in corneal surgery, *Trans Am Acad Ophthalmol Otolaryngol* 73:499, 1969.
5. Brown SI: Mooren's ulcer: treatment by conjunctival incision, *Br J Ophthalmol* 59:675, 1975.
6. Brown SI, Grayson M: Marginal furrows: a characteristic corneal lesion of rheumatoid arthritis, *Arch Ophthalmol* 79:563, 1969.
7. Brown SI, Shahanian L: Diagnosis and treatment of ocular rosacea, *Ophthalmology* 85:779, 1978.
8. Brown SI, Tragakis MP, Pearce DB: Treatment of alkali-burned cornea, *Am J Ophthalmol* 74:316, 1972.
9. Brown SI, Wasserman HE, Dunn MW: Alkali burns of the cornea, *Arch Ophthalmol* 82:91, 1969.
10. Brown SI, Weller CA: Collagenase inhibitors in prevention of ulcers of alkali-burned corneas, *Arch Ophthalmol* 83:352, 1970.
11. Brown SI, Weller CA, Vidrich AM: Effect of corticosteroids on corneal collagenase of rabbits, *Am J Ophthalmol* 70:744, 1970.
12. Burgoon CF Jr, Collins JP: Ocular changes in skin disorders. In Harley R, editor: *Pediatric ophthalmology*, Philadelphia, 1975, WB Saunders.

13. Cavanaugh DH: Herpetic ocular disease: therapy of persistent epithelial defects, *Int Ophthalmol Clin* 15:67, 1975.

14. Chiang TS, Moorman CR, Thomas RP: Ocular hypertensive response following acid and alkali burns in rabbits, *Invest Ophthalmol* 10:270, 1971.

15. Christensen L, Beeman HW, Allen A: Cytomegalic inclusion disease, *Arch Ophthalmol* 57:90, 1957.

16. Cinotti A, Maltzman B: Prognosis and treatment of perforating ocular injuries: the John Luhr memorial lecture, *Ophthalmic Surg* 6:54, 1975.

17. Dawson C: Herpes virus infection of human mesodermal tissue (cornea) detected by electron microscopy, *Nature* 217:460, 1968.

18. Deckard PS, Bergstrom TJ: Rubeola keratitis, *Ophthalmology* 88:810, 1981.

19. Dingeldein SA et al: Mooren's ulcer treated with a periosteal graft, *Ann Ophthalmol* 22:56, 1990.

20. Dohlman CH, Boruchoff SA, Sullivan GC: A technique for the repair of perforated corneal ulcers, *Arch Ophthalmol* 77:519, 1967.

21. Dohlman CH et al: Artificial corneal epithelium in acute alkali burns, *Ann Ophthalmol* 3:357, 1969.

22. Donzis PB, Mondino BJ: Management of noninfectious corneal ulcers, *Surv Ophthalmol* 32:94, 1987.

23. Doughman DJ: Treatment of corneal thinning and perforation, *J Contin Educ Ophthalmol* 39(1):15, 1978.

24. Duke-Elder S: *System of ophthalmology*, vol 8: *Diseases of the outer eye*, St. Louis, 1965 (1976 reprint), Mosby–Year Book.

25. Eagling E: Perforating injuries to the eye, *Br J Ophthalmol* 60:732, 1976.

26. Forgacs J, Franceschetti A: Histologic aspect of corneal changes due to hereditary metabolic and cutaneous infection, *Am J Ophthalmol* 47:191, 1959.

27. Forster RK, Rebewll G: The diagnosis and management of keratomycoses. I. Causes and diagnosis, *Arch Ophthalmol* 93:975, 1975.

28. Forster RK, Rebell G: The diagnosis and management of keratomycoses. II. Medical and surgical management, *Arch Ophthalmol* 93:1134, 1975.

29. Francis E: Tularemia. In Christian HA: *Oxford loose-leaf medicine*, 1920-1942 (in 13 volumes with reprints to 1953), New York, Oxford University Press.

30. Gasset AR et al: Ocular tolerance to cyanoacrylate monomer tissue adhesive analogues, *Invest Ophthalmol* 9:3, 1970.

31. Geggel HS: Successful treatment of recurrent corneal erosion with Nd:YAG anterior stromal puncture, *Am J Ophthalmol* 110:404, 1990.

32. Giller H, Kaufman W: Ocular lesions in xeroderma pigmentosum, *Arch Ophthalmol* 62:130, 1959.

33. Ginsberg SP: Corneal problems in systemic disease. In Duane TD, Jaeger EA, editors: *Clinical ophthalmology*, vol 5, Philadelphia, 1984, Harper & Row.

34. Ginsberg SP, Polack FM: Cyanoacrylate tissue adhesive in ocular disease, *Ophthalmic Surg* 3:126, 1972.

35. Goldman JJ, Dohlman CH, Kravitt BA: The basement membranes of the human cornea in recurrent epithelial erosion syndrome, *Trans Am Acad Ophthalmol Otolaryngol* 73:471, 1969.

36. Granek H, Baden HP: Corneal involvement in epidermolysis bullosa simplex, *Arch Ophthalmol* 98:469, 1980.

37. Gudas PP et al: Corneal perforations in Sjögren syndrome, *Arch Ophthalmol* 90:470, 1973.

38. Gundersen T: Conjunctival flaps in the treatment of corneal disease with reference to a new technique of application, *Arch Ophthalmol* 60:880, 1958.

39. Hughes WF Jr: Alkali burns of the eye. I. Review of the literature and summary of present knowledge, *Arch Ophthalmol* 35:423, 1946.

40. Hughes WF Jr: Alkali burns of the eye. II. Clinical and pathological course, *Arch Ophthalmol* 36:189, 1946.

41. Hyndiuk RA, Hull DS, Kinyoun JL: Free tissue patch and cyanoacrylate in corneal perforations, *Ophthalmic Surg* 5:50, 1974.

42. Jones DB: Early diagnosis and therapy of bacterial corneal ulcers, *Int Ophthalmol Clin* 13:1, 1973.

43. Khodadoust AA et al: Adhesion of regenerating corneal epithelium the role of the basement membrane, *Am J Ophthalmol* 65:339, 1968.

44. Kibrick S et al: Local corticosteroid therapy and reactivation of herpes keratitis, *Arch Ophthalmol* 86:694, 1971.

45. Laqoutte FM, Gauthier L, Comte PRM: A fibrin sealant for perforated and pre-perforated corneal ulcers, *Br J Ophthalmol* 73:757, 1989.

46. Lehman RAW, West RL, Leonard F: Toxicity of alkyl 2-cyanoacrylates. II. Bacterial growth, *Arch Surg* 93:477, 1966.

47. Lockie GW, Hunder GG: Reiter's syndrome in children: a case report and review, *Arthritis Rheum* 14:767, 1971.

48. Mclean E, MacRae S, Rich LF: Recurrent erosion: treatment by anterior stromal puncture, *Ophthalmology* 93:784, 1986.

49. McLoughlin RS: Chemical burns of the human cornea, *Am J Ophthalmol* 29:1363, 1946.

50. Nataf R, Lepine P, Bonamour G: *Œil et virus*, Paris, 1960, Masson et Cie.

51. Nobe JR et al: Results of penetrating keratoplasty for the treatment of corneal perforations, *Arch Ophthalmol* 108:939, 1990.

52. Portnoy SL, Insler MS, Kaufman HE: Surgical management of corneal ulceration and perforation, *Surv Ophthalmol* 34:47, 1989.

53. Raju VK: Corneal surgery. In Duane TD, Jaeger EA, editors: *Clinical ophthalmology*, vol 5, Philadelphia, 1984, Harper & Row.

54. Ralph RA: Chemical burns of the eye. In Duane TD, Jaeger EA, editors: *Clinical ophthalmology*, vol 4, Philadelphia, 1984, Harper & Row.

55. Ralph RA, Slanskey HH: Therapy of chemical burns, *Int Ophthalmol Clin* 14:171, 1974.

56. Refojo MF: Adhesives in ophthalmology. In Polack FM, editor: *Corneal and external diseases of the eye*, Springfield, Ill, 1970, Charles C Thomas, Publisher.

57. Refojo MF, Dohlman CH: The tensile strength of adhesive joint between eye tissues and alloplastic materials, *Am J Ophthalmol* 68:248, 1969.

58. Refojo MF, Dohlman CH, Koliopoulos J: Adhesives in ophthalmology: a review, *Surv Ophthalmol* 15:217, 1971.

59. Refojo MF et al: Evaluation of adhesives for corneal surgery, *Arch Ophthalmol* 80:645, 1968.

60. Reinecke R, Beyer C: Lacerated corneas and prevention of synechiae, *Am J Ophthalmol* 61:131, 1966.

61. Roper-Hall MJ: Ocular aspects of rosacea, *Trans Ophthalmol Soc UK* 86:727, 1966.

62. Saxena RC, Gang KC: Ankyloblepharon following smallpox, *Am J Ophthalmol* 61:169, 1966.

63. Slanskey HH et al: Cysteine and acetylcysteine in the prevention of corneal ulcerations, *Ann Ophthalmol* 2:488, 1970.

64. Suan EP et al: Corneal perforation in patients with vitamin A deficiency in the United States, *Arch Ophthalmol* 108:350, 1990.

65. Takahashi GH, Leibowitz HM, Kibrick S: Topically applied steroids in active herpes simplex keratitis, *Arch Ophthalmol* 85:350, 1971.

66. Turss U, Turss R, Refojo MF: Removal of isobutyl cyanoacrylate adhesive from the cornea with acetone, *Am J Ophthalmol* 70:725, 1970.

67. Webster RG Jr: Corneal injuries. In Smolin G, Thoft RA, editors: *The cornea*, Boston, 1983, Little, Brown.

68. Webster RG Jr et al: The use of adhesives for the closure of corneal perforations: report of two cases, *Arch Ophthalmol* 80:705, 1968.

69. Wilson LA, Grayson M: Oculodermatologic disorders. In Wilson LA, editor: *External diseases of the eye*, Hagerstown, Md, 1979, Harper & Row.

70. Wilson W: Pellagra, beriberi, and vitamin deficiency. In Bruce A, editor: *Neurology*, Baltimore, 1955, Williams & Wilkins.

Chapter 31

Anterior Segment Reconstruction After Trauma

KENNETH R. KENYON

TOMY STARCK

PETER S. HERSH

A fundamental principle of management in ocular trauma is that definitive primary repair prevents secondary complications, thus minimizing the ocurrence of adverse sequelae. Such complications might include (1) corneal scarring, fibrovascular pannus, and astigmatism; (2) glaucoma secondary to peripheral anterior synechiae, pupillary block, or lens-induced inflammation; (3) vitreous incarceration within ocular wounds and associated chronic inflammation, cystoid macular edema, retinal detachment, and infection; (4) pupillary or cyclitic membranes; (5) conjunctival scarring and symblepharon; and (6) ocular surface epithelial damage with long-term consequences including persistent epithelial defects, and sterile stromal ulceration. This same principle can be extended to secondary reconstruction in which definitive anatomic restoration improves ultimate visual rehabilitation. Such reconstruction might include restoring the normal relationships of the lid, conjunctiva, and cornea; peeling or stripping organized corneal and iris membranes; removal of lens and vitreous remnants; and reconstruction of pupil and angle structures (goniosynechiolysis and iridoplasty).

Visual rehabilitation may additionally involve limbal autografting for definitive ocular surface stabilization and improved prognosis for subsequent penetrating keratoplasty, and clearing of any other anterior or posterior segment opacities. In this discussion, we suggest that by means of either single, combined, or staged reconstructive procedures, both anatomic and visual restorative goals can be definitively accomplished.

INSTRUMENTATION

In addition to standard ophthalmic microsurgical instrumentation, the anterior segment surgeon should be familiar with the following adjunctive measures that are invaluable in dealing surgically with the traumatized anterior segment:

1. Multifunctional aspiration, cutting, and sonication instruments. Such units as Ocutome II/Fragmatome II (Alcon Surgical Irvine, California) offer an atraumatic vitrectomy, aspiration or sonication of lens material, and removal of intraocular foreign bodies.
2. Motorized corneal trephines such as Mikro-Keratron (Geuder, Heidelberg, Germany) provide excellent visibility, control for perfect centration, and the ability to trephine safely even in the presence of corneal perforation or a flat anterior chamber.
3. Viscoelastic substances (Viscoat, Healon) are important adjuncts to reform the anterior chamber, replace vitreous, dissect iridocorneal adhesions, and protect the corneal endothelium.
4. Dry cellulose sponges (Weck-cel, Xomed-

Trease, Jacksonville, Florida) are excellent dissecting instruments to strip membranes from the surface of the cornea and iris. A disposable scarifier such as the Grieshaber 681.01 may be required for harvesting the tissue for the limbal autograft transplantation as well as for dissecting tenacious corneal pannus.

5. Cyanoacrylate tissue adhesive (Histocryl, Braun, Spangenberg, Germany) is useful both in the acute management of impending and actual corneal perforations and as a tool for tectonic support of the globe during various surgical procedures.

6. Suture materials such as 10-0 nylon, polypropylene (Propylene), or Mersilene in a round vascular needle (such as Ethicon BV100-4) are preferable to a spatula or cutting needle for iridoplasty and sulcus-fixated IOLs. We prefer 10-0 polypropylene for sutures that are placed under tension, as in the resuspension of dialyzed iris. If performed in a closed-eye situation, a long fine tapered needle (such as Ethicon CIF-4 or CTC-6) is useful to penetrate the sclera.

ANTERIOR SEGMENT RECONSTRUCTION TECHNIQUES—PREPARATORY AND ADJUNCTIVE PROCEDURES

Ocular Surface Stabilization. Appropriate preoperative preparation of the eye should always precede the definitive reconstructive effort in order to optimize the long-term prognosis. Ongoing abnormalities such as intraocular inflammation or increased intraocular pressure must be controlled, as well as anatomic restoration of the lids, and ocular adnexa before one performs definitive intraocular surgery. Furthermore, stabilization of the ocular surface is an important condition for the success of reconstructive penetrating or lamellar keratoplasty. Nonpreserved lubricants, soft contact lenses, patching, and tarsorrhaphy are all interventions that help to support, stabilize, and renew the ocular surface.[6] In cases of severe chronic damage to the ocular surface, pannus stripping with limbal autograft transplantation has widespread application for stable surface healing, decreased corneal vascularization, and improved prognosis for subsequent penetrating keratoplasty.[7] The success of this procedure relies on the availability of healthy limbal "stem" cells from the uninvolved eye (Fig. 31-1). When transplanted to the diseased corneal limbus, these cells transform, migrate, and adhere to the central stromal tissue, assuming biochemical and morphologic features of normal corneal epithelium.[16-18]

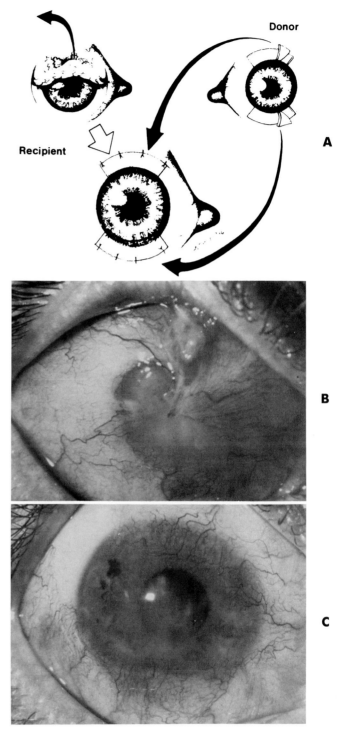

Fig. 31-1. A, Technique of limbal conjunctival transplantation for uniocular chemical burn. Notice transfer of free grafts of limbal conjunctiva from normal donor eye to recipient site, which has been prepared by peeling of corneal pannus. **B,** After chemical assault injury, vision is hand motions, and extensive symblepharon unites upper lid to scarred cornea. **C,** One year after limbal autograft transplantation, vision is 20/100 with a stable ocular surface and nebular stromal scar.

Superficial Keratectomy. If corneal surface irregularity and scarring are confined to a superficial fibrovascular pannus, only superficial keratectomy may be required to improve the vision, thus obviating penetrating keratoplasty. The procedure may be performed in the minor operating room under topical (proparacaine or cocaine) or local anesthesia. One removes the corneal epithelium overlying the involved area with a dry cellulose sponge and, if necessary, carefully scraping with a scarifier, avoiding sharp dissection. A distinct cleavage plane is typically present between pannus and relatively normal stroma. To identify this plane atraumatically, the tip of a dry cellulose sponge is insinuated beneath an edge of fibrovascular tissue (Fig. 31-2). The abnormal tissue is then peeled, or stripped, with use of dry sponges and fine tissue forceps. If sharp dissection with a scarifier or other blade is necessary to mobilize firmly adherent tissue, extreme caution should be exercised to remain parallel to the cleavage plane, thus avoiding further corneal scarring.

INTRAOCULAR TECHNIQUES

Penetrating Keratoplasty. Keratoplasty, though rarely indicated in primary repair after trauma, is a frequent concomitant of secondary reconstruction. Although the general surgical principles of penetrating keratoplasty apply in anterior segment reconstruction as well, additional specialized maneuvers and instrumentation are helpful.

Generally, a Flieringa ring is unnecessary because the principal meridians of cardinal suture placement may be delineated with an eight-blade radial keratotomy marker. The edges of the marker are first coated with a gentian violet tissue-marking pen to clarify the impressions made on the cornea. The eight cardinal suture meridians are then marked at the limbus with disposable cautery (Fig. 31-3). In this way, alignment of the donor tissue and proper suture placement are ensured even in the event of anterior segment and scleral distortion.

Fig. 31-2. Technique of superficial keratectomy. **A,** Dry cellulose sponge is used to remove overlying epithelium and to allow identification of cleavage plane beneath fibrovascular tissue. **B,** Pannus is stripped with a dry sponge and tissue forceps.

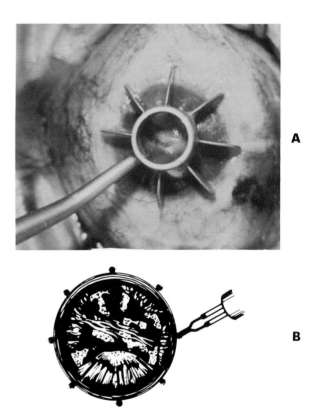

Fig. 31-3. A, An eight-blade radial keratotomy marker coated with gentian violet is used to delineate the meridians for placement of cardinal sutures. **B,** These meridians then are marked at the limbus with a disposable cautery.

If it is anticipated that a posterior chamber intraocular lens (IOL) will be sutured through the ciliary sulcus, conjunctival peritomy and scleral flaps are prepared in the appropriate meridians. These flaps are subsequently used to cover the anchoring polypropylene suture, thereby preventing erosion through the conjunctiva and potential microbial invasion of the globe. A scarifier blade is used to outline and dissect a rectangular or triangular half-thickness scleral flap approximately 3 mm at its base. The flap must span the limbus because the exit point of the suture from the ciliary sulcus should be no greater than 0.5 to 1 mm posterior to the limbus.

A donor cornea button is trephined 0.5 mm larger than the host bed. Such oversizing may aid in preventing peripheral anterior synechiae and glaucoma postoperatively.[5,20] For recipient trephination, an instrument allowing for good visualization and precise trephine placement should be used. Particularly valuable are motorized (Mikro-Keratron) and vacuum (Hessburg-Barron) trephines. More importantly, enhanced control makes trephination safer in the setting of a flat anterior chamber or corneal perforation. In such cases, a shallow trephination groove is made and deepened with a blade, and the corneal button is removed with Vannas or corneal

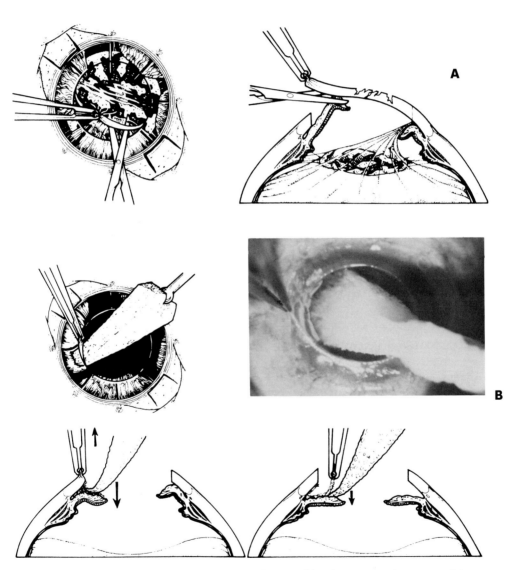

Fig. 31-4. A, Removal of recipient cornea. After trephination, cornea is separated from any posterior adhesions by blunt dissection with Vannas scissors or cellulose sponges. **B,** Technique of synechiolysis. Iridocorneal synechiae are broken with dry cellulose sponges while counter-traction with forceps is applied. Completion is achieved with removal of hyalinized membranes from anterior chamber.

scissors. If corneo-irido-lenticular adhesions are present, forceps, dry cellulose sponges, and Vannas scissors are used for careful separation, with particular care being taken to preserve any iris tissue that may be useful for a subsequent iridoplasty (Fig. 31-4).

Goniosynechiolysis. The presence of anterior synechiae after penetrating keratoplasty not only increases the risk of graft failure because of exposure of the donor endothelium to blood vessels or mechanical traction, but also has been associated with increased incidence of glaucoma after keratoplasty.[9,11,13,15,19] Although areas of trabecular meshwork that are uncovered by goniosynechiolysis may or may not resume a functional status, the method of lysing the anterior synechiae, peeling the organized fibrous membranes, and reestablishing a rigid iris diaphragm by iridoplasty appears to retard the formation and progression of anterior synechiae into areas of meshwork that are filtering.[1,2] Thus the lysis of iridocorneal synechiae constitutes a particularly important restorative maneuver not only to avoid secondary glaucoma and graft failure, but also to improve cosmesis and reduce glare. The major technique of synechiolysis is accomplished predominantly with blunt dissection with a dry cellulose sponge, which push the adherent iris posteriorly while supporting the keratoplasty wound margin anteriorly with forceps (Fig. 31-4). This anteroposterior dissection specifically avoids lateral sweeping with iris spatulas, vitreous sweeps, or other metallic instruments, which might induce bleeding. With a similar cellulose-sponge technique, fibrous or hyalinized membranes on the anterior iris surface can also be identified and peeled in much the same manner as corneal pannus (Fig. 31-4). When synechiae cannot be lysed despite meticulous effort, the iris may be cut radially on each side of the peripheral anterior synechiae and the included sector of iris excised.[2] This leaves a sector iris defect, which may be closed by iridoplasty techniques. More importantly, the risk of "zippering" new synechiae adjacent to the original peripheral anterior synechiae is reduced. If bleeding is encountered, viscoelastic should be placed into the anterior chamber to isolate the blood and prevent leakage posteriorly into the vitreous. Other methods of hemostasis include the direct application of epinephrine 1:10,000, thrombin-soaked cellulose sponges or Gel-foam (100 U/ml), or direct cauterization of the bleeding site with underwater microcautery.

Cataract Surgery. The state of the lens dictates the method by which it is managed surgically. If the lens is cataractous but the posterior capsule appears intact, a standard extracapsular cataract extraction is performed and a posterior chamber IOL may be placed. In many cases of eye trauma, the anterior and posterior capsules have been ruptured, the zonules have been disrupted, and the vitreous has been violated. In such cases, the lens material may be flocculent, and fibrotic incarcerated vitreous may be present. A lensectomy and anterior vitrectomy should be performed to prevent the well-recognized complications of chronic inflammation, cystoid macular edema, intraocular fibrosis, and retinal detachment.

Microvitrectomy suction and cutting instrumentation is used to perform the anterior vitrectomy traumatically and to lyse iridovitreal and other adhesions. When using an open-sky technique, infusion is not necessary. In some instances, cellulose sponges may be used to gently identify and isolate vitreous strands, which may then be excised with Vannas scissors. At the completion of the vitrectomy, the iris diaphragm should spontaneously fall back into its usual position.

The placement of an intraocular lens and selection of IOL type and implantation technique must be tailored to the individual case. The age, optical and physical status of the other eye, and architectural state of the injured eye will be factors in decisions regarding the advisability of IOL implantation. Some younger patients, for example, may be able to wear an aphakic contact lens, neutralizing the irregular astigmatism caused by a corneal scar and not requiring an IOL.[12] Other patients may require IOL insertion for optimal visual rehabilitation.

The potential benefits of a posterior chamber IOL include less compromise of the filtration angle and corneal endothelium. This, coupled with the recently successful implantation techniques of suturing the IOLs directly to the posterior surface of the iris or into the ciliary sulcus in the absence of posterior capsular support, makes this approach our preferred method.[3,10,14]

If sulcus fixation is desired, each haptic is secured respectively with one double-armed 10-0 polypropylene suture (Fig. 31-5). We prefer the Ethicon BV100-4 needle because of its sharpness and fine caliber, which prevent tissue trauma. A standard spatula needle (such as Ethicon TG160 or Alcon CU-5) may also be used. Occasionally, the longer Ethicon CIF-4 needle (generally most valuable for secondary posterior chamber IOL implantation without keratoplasty) may be used if the ciliary sulcus is difficult to reach with a short needle. The haptic may be secured by the suture either through a control hole at its tip or by a girth-hitch knot tied

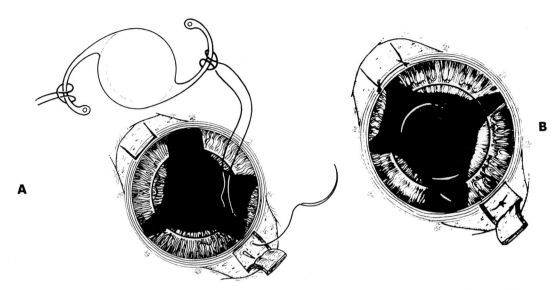

Fig. 31-5. Placement of sclera-sutured posterior chamber intraocular lens in absence of capsular support. **A,** Girth-hitch knot is used to secure IOL haptics with double-armed polypropylene sutures. Needles are brought under iris and through ciliary sulcus, exiting approximately 0.5 to 1 mm posterior to limbus. **B,** Sutures are tied in mattress fashion, and scleral flap is repositioned over knot and secured with sutures.

around the haptic itself.[18] The two sutures should be symmetrically positioned 180 degrees apart to ensure lens centration. The needles are then brought under the iris, through the ciliary sulcus, and out through the previously dissected scleral beds. The lens optic is positioned, the anchoring sutures are tied, and the scleral flaps are brought over the knot and secured.

Alternatively, the posterior chamber IOL may be sutured directly to the iris.[18] Two double-armed mattress sutures of 10-0 polypropylene on fine needles are placed through opposing positioning holes on the optic or around the optic-haptic junctions and brought up through the underside of the iris. The 2-inch Ethicon BV100-4 suture is specially tailored for this purpose. Each suture is tied over the iris, and the ends are trimmed close to the knot.

Although sutured posterior chamber IOLs have some theoretical advantages over anterior chamber designs, their long-term propriety is as yet unclear. If an anterior chamber IOL is chosen, a flexible uniplanar lens or a flexible tripod type with slightly angled haptics (such as Allergan AC21) may be preferred. If the latter is placed in a reversed position (haptics angled anteriorly) so that the optic is concave to the haptics, this configuration will mechanically push the angle open and displace the IOL optic posteriorly from the graft.

Iridoplasty. Some of the goals of iridoplasty have been reviewed in the previous discussion of goniosynechiolysis. Briefly, the restoration of a tight iris diaphragm and reconstruction of the pupil minimize the risk of further synechia formation and secondary closed angle glaucoma, improve the graft survival and cosmetic appearance, and prevent glare.

When iridoplasty is performed, simple interrupted sutures of 10-0 nylon, Prolene, or Mersilene are placed from iris edge to iris edge (Fig. 31-6). Polypropylene is preferred for sutures placed under tension, as in the resuspension of dialyzed iris (Fig. 31-7). Although polypropylene is also an excellent suture material for iris surgery in general, in more than 10 years of experience we have not encountered long-term degradation or separation of iris repair performed with nylon sutures. This is, of course, contrary to the fate of nylon used to fixate IOLs or corneal grafts. The suture needle should be passed completely through one edge of the iris, regrasped with the needle holder, and then passed through the other edge of the iris. This manuever prevents excessive traction and possible tearing of fragile iris tissue during the second needle pass. Any sector iridectomies created during goniosynechiolysis should be closed with interrupted sutures placed tangentially near the iris sphincter.

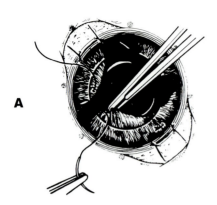

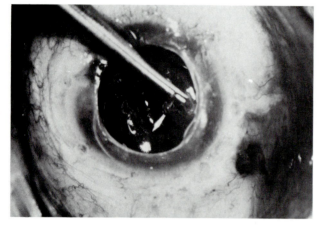

Fig. 31-6. Interrupted sutures of 10-0 nylon or polypropylene is used to perform iridoplasty.

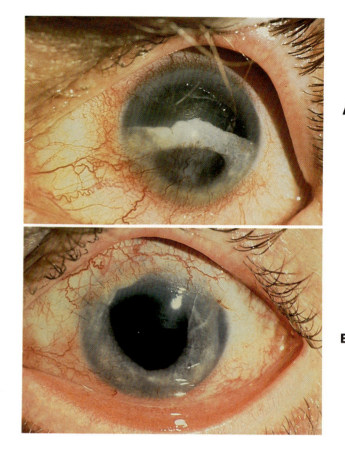

Fig. 31-7. A, After blunt trauma, fibrovascular pannus covers inferior cornea. An extensive iridodialysis, subluxated cataract, and vitreous herniated into anterior chamber are present. **B,** Six months after stripping of corneal pannus, suspension of iris, removal of cataract, and anterior vitrectomy, vision is improved to 20/80.

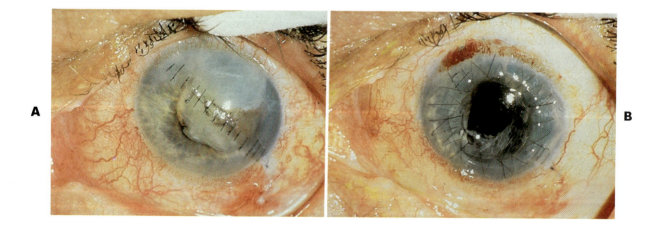

Fig. 31-8. A, Repaired corneal laceration with lens cortical material in anterior chamber and extensive iris loss. **B,** After penetrating keratoplasty, removal of lens remnants, anterior vitrectomy, iris reconstruction, and placement of anterior chamber intraocular lens, visual acuity is 20/70.

If an iridodialysis is present or only small amounts of iris remain, iris remnants and pedicle flaps may be anchored with one or more mattress sutures passed through the angle just anterior to the ciliary sulcus and secured through the limbus. Polypropylene suture material is preferred, with use of either a fine tapered needle or a longer needle (such as Ethicon CIF-4). A conjunctival peritomy and scleral flap should first be prepared as for sulcus-sutured posterior chamber IOLs to allow for easier needle penetration and for subsequent coverage and protection of the suture knot. At the completion of the procedure, the pupil should be central, the iris posterior, the angle open with a deep anterior chamber, and the vitreous behind the iris with a clear visual axis.

RESULTS OF ANTERIOR SEGMENT RECONSTRUCTION

We recently reviewed 39 consecutive cases of severe ocular trauma that had undergone penetrating keratoplasty and anterior segment reconstruction, and we evaluated visual outcome, graft survival, and secondary complications.[8] Postoperatively, 49% of eyes achieved >20/100 compared with 10% before surgery, and 72% improved at least two Snellen lines. With a mean follow-up period of 2 years, 80% of initial keratoplasties remained clear, and all four subsequently regrafted corneas maintained clarity, for an overall keratoplasty success rate of 90%. Preoperative anterior synechiae could be anatomically corrected at surgery in 80% of cases. We, as well as others,[4] found a high prevalence of postoperative glaucoma (46%). Such elevation of intraocular pressure postoperatively was predominantly restricted to those patients with preoperative glaucoma and persistent synechiae. Severe complications were rare. Thus, despite major trauma, both visual restoration and anatomic reconstruction were highly satisfactory (Fig. 31-8).

REFERENCES

1. Chandler PA, Simmons RJ: Anterior chamber deepening for gonioscopy at time of surgery, *Arch Ophthalmol* 74:177-190, 1965.
2. Cohen EJ, Kenyon KR, Dohlman CH: Iridoplasty for prevention of postkeratoplasty angle closure glaucoma, *Ophthalmic Surg* 13:994-996, 1982.
3. Cowden JW, Hu BV: A new surgical technique for posterior chamber lens fixation during penetrating keratoplasty in the absence of capsular or zonular support, *Cornea* 7:231-235, 1988.
4. Doren GS, Cohen EJ, Brady SE, et al: Penetrating keratoplasty after ocular trauma, *Am J Ophthalmol* 110:408-411, 1990.
5. Heidemann DG, Sugar A, Meyer RF, et al: Oversized donor grafts in penetrating keratoplasty, *Arch Ophthalmol* 103:1807-1811, 1985.
6. Kenyon KR: Decision-making in the therapy of external eye disease: non-infected corneal ulcers, *Ophthalmology* 89:44-51, 1982.
7. Kenyon KR, Tseng SCG: Limbal autograft transplantation for ocular surface disorders, *Ophthalmology* 96:709-723, 1989.
8. Kenyon KR, Starck T, Hersh PS: Penetrating keratoplasty and anterior segment reconstruction for severe ocular trauma, *Ophthalmology* 99:396-402, 1992.
9. Meyer RF, Musch DC: Assessment of success and complications of triple procedure surgery, *Am J Ophthalmol* 104: 233-240, 1978.
10. Price FW, Whitson WE: Visual results of sutured-fixated posterior chamber lenses during penetrating keratoplasty, *Ophthalmology* 96:1234-1240, 1989.
11. Rowsey JJ, Gaylor JR: Intraocular lens disasters: peripheral anterior synechiae, *Ophthalmology* 87:646-663, 1980.
12. Smiddy WE, et al: Contact lenses for visual rehabilitation after corneal laceration repair, *Ophthalmology* 96:293-298, 1989.
13. Smolin G, Biswell R: Corneal graft rejection associated with anterior iris adhesion: case report, *Ann Ophthalmol* 10:1603-1604, 1978.
14. Soong HK, Musch DC, Kowal V, et al: Implantation of posterior chamber intraocular lenses in the absence of lens capsule during penetrating keratoplasty, *Arch Ophthalmol* 107:660-665, 1989.
15. Tragakis MP, Brown SI: The significance of anterior synechiae after corneal transplantation, *Am J Ophthalmol* 74:532-533, 1972.
16. Tsai RJF, Sun TT, Tseng SCG: Comparison of limbal and conjunctival autograft transplantation in corneal surface reconstruction in rabbits, *Ophthalmology* 97:446-455, 1990.
17. Tseng SCG: Concept and application of limbal stem cells, *Eye* 3:141-157, 1989.
18. Tseng SCG, Chen JJY, Huang AJW, et al: Classification of conjunctival surgeries for corneal diseases based on stem cell concept, *Ophthalmol Clin North Am* 3(4):595-610, 1990.
19. Wilson SE, Kaufman HE: Graft failure after penetrating keratoplasty, *Surv Ophthalmol* 34:325-356, 1990.
20. Zimmerman TJ, Olson RJ, Waltman SR, et al: Transplant size and elevated intraocular pressure, *Arch Ophthalmol* 96:2231-2233, 1978.

Chapter 32

Lamellar Grafting

JUAN J. ARENTSEN

In the last three decades, with the availability of better donor material and surgical instrumentation and with the better understanding of the pathophysiology of corneal diseases that require corneal transplantation, the number of lamellar keratoplasties (LK) being performed has been dramatically reduced. Today the use of a lamellar keratoplasty is limited to a few conditions.

In 1976 we reported a series of 1057 keratoplasty buttons received by the pathology laboratory at the Wilmer Institute.[1] Whereas in the late 1950s 28.9% of all buttons were of the lamellar type, by the early 1970s this number had been reduced to 3.2% of all keratoplasties. Of the 128 lamellar keratoplasties in that series, most had been performed for conditions in which a penetrating keratoplasty (PKP) would be the first choice today (stromal scarring, viral infections, chemical burns, and different corneal dystrophies). Most current graduates of ophthalmology programs probably have never seen a lamellar keratoplasty during training.

In this chapter, I review only those situations in which lamellar keratoplasties are used frequently and with the "old-fashioned" techniques available to most ophthalmologists familiar with microsurgery.

INDICATIONS AND CONTRAINDICATIONS FOR LAMELLAR KERATOPLASTY

There are at least four indications for lamellar keratoplasties:[8]

Tectonic Lamellar Grafts. Tectonic grafts are the most common type and are used to restore the normal surface of the anterior segment by replacing localized or generalized areas of corneoscleral thinning. They are rarely used for visual purposes except for situations in which the normal corneal thickness needs to be restored in preparation for a penetrating keratoplasty. In many situations they are used to strengthen the cornea or sclera and to prevent rupture of the globe.

A tectonic graft can be employed after the removal of a recurrent pterygium involving the visual axis; in such cases a large graft is necessary to include this area[9] (Figs. 32-1 and 32-2). This technique is not indicated in primary or recurrent pterygia in which the visual axis is not involved; simpler techniques such as excision with or without a conjunctival transplant[14] or beta radiation can then be used.

Large descemetoceles without inflammation can also be managed with a lamellar keratotomy and keratoplasty. These, as any other LK should be handled with extreme care; if a perforation occurs during the procedure, it should be converted to a penetrating keratoplasty.

Marginal areas of thinning and ectasia can be reinforced with a lamellar graft.[8] This technique has been used in patients with Terrien's degeneration (Figs. 32-3 and 32-4) and in pellucid degeneration.[12] In both situations a crescentic lamellar graft including the thinned area not only will reinforce it, but also will increase the curvature of the cornea, partially or totally neutralizing the astigmatism and improving visual acuity. Both conditions should be operated upon only when inflammatory signs are not present and when a perforation is imminent.

Other less-understood situations such as "marginal ectasia," "furrow dystrophies," and noninflammatory keratomalacia can easily be managed with a lamellar graft when a perforation is a threat, after an appropriate lamellar bed has been created.

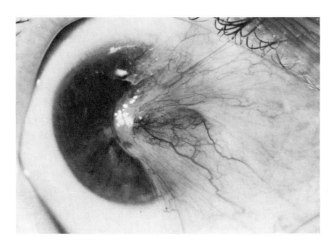

Fig. 32-1. Recurrent pterygium involving the visual axis after two previous excisions. Vision 6/60.

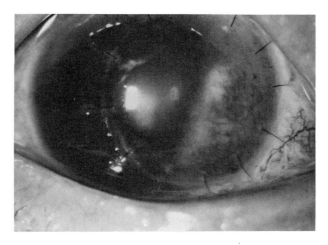

Fig. 32-2. Same patient 6 months after pterygium excision and lamellar keratoplasty. Despite deep peripheral scarring, visual axis is clear, with vision of 6/9.

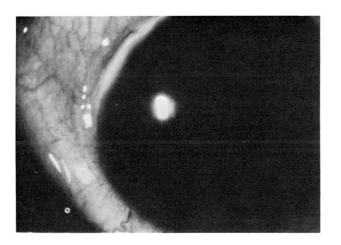

Fig. 32-3. Terrien's marginal degeneration with noticeable thinning.

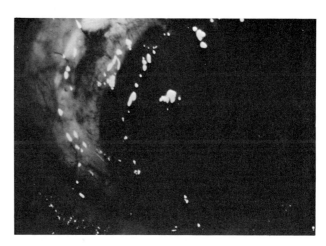

Fig. 32-4. Same eye after free-hand peripheral lamellar graft.

Finally, in the rare situation in which localized areas of very thin cornea are found before a penetrating keratoplasty, they can be "filled in" with a tectonic keratoplasty.

Optical Lamellar Grafts. Optical grafts are rarely used today since a penetrating keratoplasty has a better visual prognosis.[8] They have been used for superficial, noninflammatory, stable conditions of the anterior stroma when visual acuity is not of primary importance. Salzmann's nodular degeneration is a typical example. A lamellar keratoplasty for visual rehabilitation can also be the answer in young patients or those with mental retardation who have the potential of a more complicated and traumatic follow-up observation. Lamellar keratoplasties should be avoided in vascularized corneas where the possibility of vessel ingrowth into the graft or the donor-host interface and subsequent visual deterioration exists.

Therapeutic Lamellar Grafts. Therapeutic grafts may be necessary after a deep lamellar keratectomy when excess tissue has been removed. Again, this situation may arise after pterygium removal and in the management of certain tumors. This technique has been employed to restore the ocular surface and provide a clear cornea after the excision of benign corneal tumors such as dermoids.[15,16] The use of a lamellar keratoplasty to reinforce the area left after the removal of a malignant tumor is more questionable, since the strong possibility of a tumor recurrence exists.[13]

Cosmetic Lamellar Grafts. Cosmetic grafts are very rarely indicated and only in eyes with no visual potential. Many patients can be managed more easily today with cosmetic contact lenses if the corneal surface is regular and the tear supply is appropriate.

Lamellar keratoplasties should be avoided in any situation where a penetrating keratoplasty offers a better visual prognosis such as in the presence of vessels, especially if the vessels are deep and a PKP is being considered at a later date. (Vessels will grow into the PKP and will be closer to the endothelium, increasing the chances of an allograft reaction.)

In my experience, lamellar keratoplasties should not be performed in the presence of an active inflammatory disease, since it is practically impossible to remove all inflamed structures by lamellar dissection. This observation has been seen in lamellar keratoplasties in active and inactive herpetic keratitis. In cases of active keratitis the incidence of recurrence of the disease into the lamellar keratoplasty is extremely high, apart from other complications.[2,10] Fig. 32-5 shows this problem very clearly in a patient who had a stormy postoperative period after the lamellar keratoplasty for herpetic keratitis, with an eventual fungal superinfection and loss of useful vision.

Although lamellar keratoplasty has been recommended in the management of Mooren's ulcer and other marginal ulcerations associated with systemic diseases, my experience has been that sooner or later a lamellar graft will become involved in the ulcering process and become necrotic (Figs. 32-6 to 32-10.)[4,5] If a lamellar keratoplasty is absolutely necessary, the addition of a conjunctival flap offers a much better prognosis, probably by providing new healthy vessels for nourishment in that area.

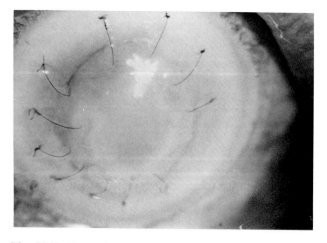

Fig. 32-5. Herpetic interstitial keratitis after lamellar graft for superficial active herpetic keratitis.

SURGICAL TECHNIQUES AND INSTRUMENTATION

As I mentioned previously, I am reviewing only those techniques and instruments that are available to most microsurgeons. Other instruments and techniques (cryolathes, epikeratophakia, refractive surgery with lasers, and so on) are discussed elsewhere.

General Considerations. Most lamellar transplants, with the exception of those in children, can be performed under local anesthesia on an outpatient basis.

If the possibility exists that the keratectomy to remove the altered tissue will extend deep, it is advisable to have preserved full-thickness corneal tissue in case the procedure has to be converted into a penetrating keratoplasty. When the anterior chamber is accidentally penetrated, and if a relatively large segment of cornea is missing, it is then advisable to perform a penetrating keratoplasty. Otherwise aqueous will move into the stroma through the gap and result in persistent corneal edema and sometimes a cystic formation.

A lamellar keratoplasty and the removal of the lamellar graft from the donor eye can be performed basically with the help of the disposable trephines (Storz no. E-3096 or 171), with a Troutman and adjustable handle (Weck no. 1737) and a flat spatula-shaped knife. The Martinez knife (Storz no. E-3001) has been the most satisfying one in my cases (provided that the knife is kept sharp at all times).

Several aspects of lamellar keratoplasty should be taken into account before one starts the procedure:[8]
1. Donor corneas do not need to be fresh, since their endothelium is not a concern as in penetrating keratoplasty. Two- or 3-day-old whole eyes are acceptable. Glycerin-preserved or lyophilized tissue can also be used.
2. In general, the graft should be slightly larger than the recipient bed. Exceptions are peripheral grafts in conditions of marginal thinning with large astigmatism in which a slightly smaller graft would help reduce the astigmatism by steeping the meridian.
3. The grafts should be of uniform thickness and slightly thicker than the recipient bed. (The initial swelling of the donor cornea will rapidly disappear, and if the donor button is too thin, this area may be depressed postoperatively.)
4. The margin of the graft ideally should exactly match that of the recipient's bed.
5. If the graft includes the limbus, I personally prefer to match a donor corneoscleral segment with the area removed from the recipient. If only cornea is used, there may be some protru-

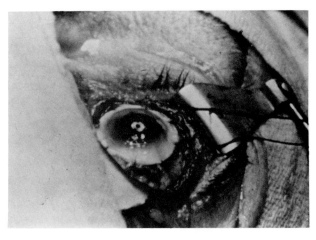

Fig. 32-6. Peripheral corneal ulceration after cataract extraction, repaired with total lamellar graft. (Courtesy John H King, MD, Washington, DC.)

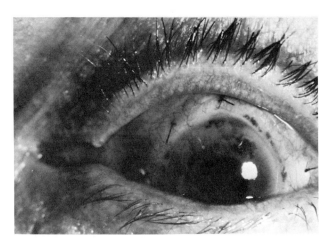

Fig. 32-7. Postoperative aspect of total lamellar keratoplasty in same case as in Fig. 32-6.

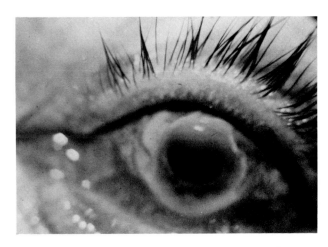

Fig. 32-8. Same case as in Fig. 32-6, 4 months after surgery, with recurrence of peripheral ulceration.

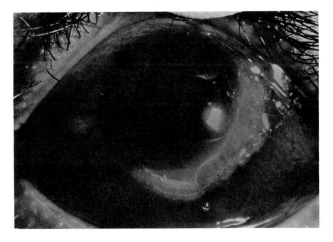

Fig. 32-9. Mooren's ulcer in 36-year-old patient.

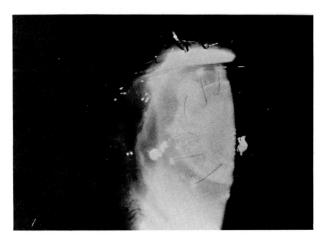

Fig. 32-10. Same patient as in Fig. 32-9, with melting of peripheral corneal graft a month after surgery.

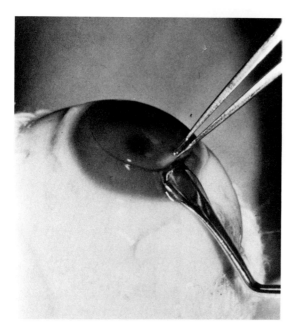

Fig. 32-11. Beginning of dissection of lamellar graft from donor eye, using Martinez knife after a 0.3 mm deep trephine mark has been placed.

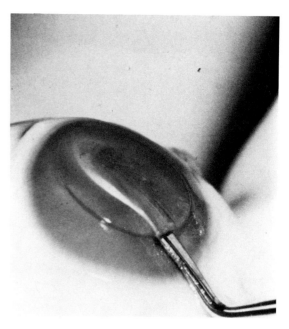

Fig. 32-12. Martinez knife has been advanced to center of donor cornea, and now peripheral dissection is started, toward trephine mark.

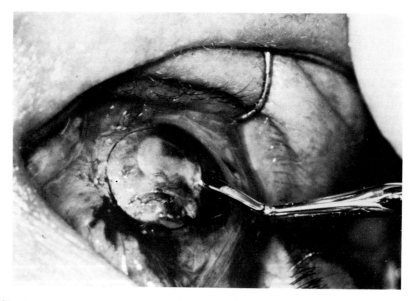

Fig. 32-13. Similar to Fig. 32-12, Martinez knife is being used to dissect plane in recipient eye of patient with recurrent pterygium.

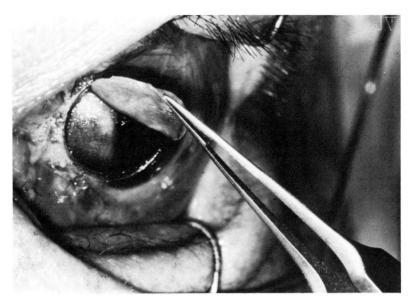

Fig. 32-14. Recipient lamellar button is being lifted, showing corneal bed (same patient as in Figs. 32-1 and 32-2).

sion at the limbus because of the smaller radius of curvature of the cornea compared to that of the limbus and sclera. This is not a major problem, however.

Removal of Donor Tissue. Removal of the donor lamellar graft can be accomplished in two ways:

1. A perpendicular cut is made at the limbus of the donor to a depth of 0.3 to 0.4 mm. Then the Martinez spatula is placed in the incision in such a way that it is parallel to the surface of the cornea and with its end very slightly directed upwards. This way an interlamellar plane is easily formed. The spatula is gently pushed and rotated as it advances toward the center of the cornea. The same type of motion is continued toward the limbus in its whole circumference. Once the entire cornea has been dissected, different-size trephines can be used to remove a lamellar graft of the appropriate size.

2. The donor lamellar graft can be removed with the same technique as is used in a keratectomy in the recipient eye. A trephine of the desired diameter with an adjustable blade set at the necessary depth is used to penetrate the cornea. The Martinez knife is introduced into the groove, and the lamellar resection is carried out in the same way (Figs. 32-11 to 32-14).

For peripheral grafts, use of a trephine that encompasses the opacity to be removed offers a better

possibility of a more precise procedure, rather than cutting by freehand.

After removal of a total lamellar graft from the donor, the graft can be cut into any desired shape to match the recipient keratectomy. These grafts can be central, total, peripheral, or annular (Figs. 32-15 to 32-18).[3]

Although it is much easier to remove a lamellar graft from a whole donor eye, an artificial anterior chamber is available (Ophthalmic Specialties, P.O. Box 27, St. Gabriel, CA 91778), in which tissue culture-preserved corneas can be affixed to allow removal of anterior lamellar sections with a microkeratome.[6] It is becoming evident that in the very near future frozen or lyophilized lamellar corneal tissue of known thickness will become available to the ophthalmic surgeon. These will allow the surgeon to save time and avoid the possibilities of contamination from whole eyes.[11]

COMPLICATIONS OF LAMELLAR GRAFTS

Complications are rare when candidates for lamellar keratoplasty have been properly selected. As mentioned earlier the intraoperative perforation of the cornea with aqueous leakage or a flat anterior chamber is relatively common and it is mandatory in such cases to proceed with a penetrating keratoplasty.

A uniform depth and margin can be removed with little difficulty from a nonvascularized and

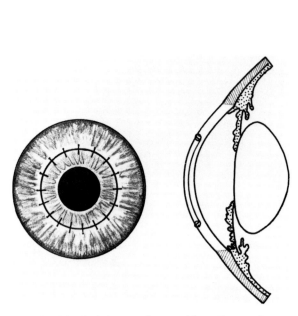

Fig. 32-15. Schema of central lamellar graft.

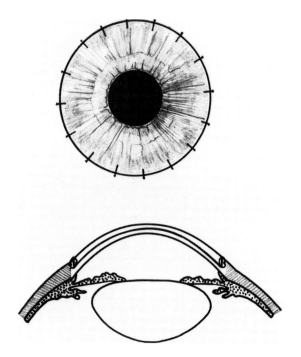

Fig. 32-16. Schema of total lamellar graft.

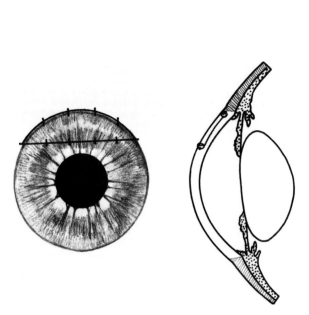

Fig. 32-17. Schema of peripheral lamellar graft.

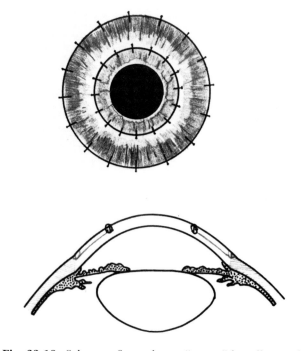

Fig. 32-18. Schema of annular or "crown" lamellar graft.

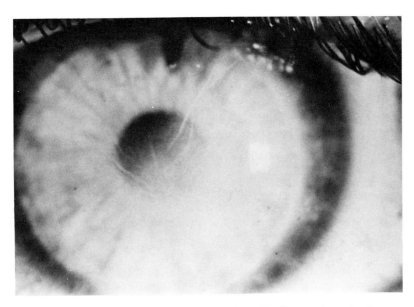

Fig. 32-19. Stromal allograft reaction of large lamellar keratoplasty for keratoconus.

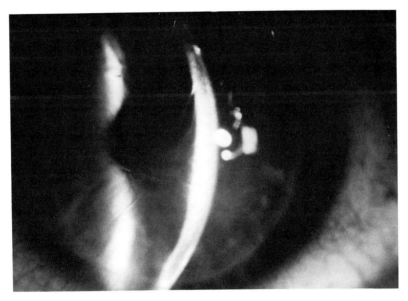

Fig. 32-20. Slitlamp view of same case as in Fig. 32-19.

lightly scarred cornea. However, keratectomies in heavily scarred vascularized corneas are difficult and many times result in residual scarring and irregular surfaces and margins.

Just as in penetrating keratoplasties, an allograft reaction can occur (Figs. 32-19 and 32-20). If a reaction is not properly treated, it may result in a failed graft.[7]

An irregular interface and lipid deposition is more often seen in vascularized corneas and will contribute to decreased visual acuity. Because of this, central lamellar grafts have gradually been replaced by penetrating keratoplasty.

Other problems that can be encountered postoperatively are epithelial defects, melting of the graft, or superinfection, especially in cases in which the lamellar graft has been done on a cornea that is still actively inflamed.

REFERENCES

1. Arentsen JJ, Morgan B, Green WR: Changing indications for keratoplasty, *Am J Ophthalmol* 81:313-318, 1978.
2. Beekhuis WH, Renardel de Lavalette JGC, van Rij G, Schaap GJ: Therapeutic keratoplasty for active herpetic corneal disease: viral culture and prognosis, *Doc Ophthalmol* 55:31-35, 1983.
3. Buxton JN: Lamellar keratoplasty: indications. In King JH, McTigue JW, editors: *The Cornea World Congress,* London, 1965, Butterworth & Co.
4. Christiensen JM, Arentsen JJ: Surgical therapy of Mooren's ulcer, *Ophthalmology* 7:1507-1509, 1975.
5. King JH: Destructive marginal corneal ulceration: a saga of surgical treatment, *Trans Am Ophthalmol Soc* 63:311-316, 1965.
6. Maguen E, Villaseñor RA, Ward DE, et al: A modified artificial anterior chamber for use in refractive keratoplasty, *Am J Ophthalmol* 89:742-744, 1980.
7. Maumenee AE: Clinical patterns of corneal graft failures. In Porter R, Knight J editors: *Corneal graft failures,* Ciba Found Symp 15:5-15, Amsterdam/New York, 1973, Elsevier Publishing Co./Associated Scientific Publishers.
8. Paton D: Lamellar keratoplasty. In *Symposium on medical and surgical disease of the cornea,* Transactions of the New Orleans Academy of Ophthalmology, St. Louis, 1980, Mosby–Year Book.
9. Pearlman G, Susal AL, Hushaw J, et al: Recurrent pterygium and treatment with lamellar keratoplasty with presentation of a technique to limit recurrences, *Ann Ophthalmol* 2:763-771, 1970.
10. Poliquen Y, Petroutsos G, Goichot EL, et al: Eléments du pronostic des kératoplasties sur kératites herpétiques, *J Fr Ophthalmol* 4(12):825-827, 1981.
11. Rich LF: A technique for preparing corneal lamellar donor tissue using simplified keratomileusis, *Ophthalmic Surg* 11:606-608, 1980.
12. Schanzlin DJ, Sarno EM, Robin JB: Crescentic lamellar keratoplasty for pellucid marginal degeneration, *Ophthalmology* 96:253-254, 1983.
13. Stucchi CA, Bianchi G, Lo Votrico A: Mélano-sarcome cornéoscléral: kératoplastie, *Klin Monatsbl Augenheilkd* 176:637-639, 1980.
14. Thoft RA: Indications for conjunctival transplantation, *Ophthalmology* 89:335-339, 1982.
15. Topilow HW, Cykiert RC, Goldman K, et al: Bilateral corneal dermis-like choristomas, *Arch Ophthalmol* 99:1387-1391, 1981.
16. Zeidman GW, Johnson B, Brown SI: Corneal transplant in an infant with corneal dermoid, *Am J Ophthalmol* 93:78-83, 1982.

Chapter 33

KERATOPROSTHESIS

FRANK M. POLACK

Blind eyes caused by corneal disease not amenable to transplantation can be rehabilitated with an artificial cornea, or keratoprosthesis. This procedure has been tried for many years with varying degrees of success. Several factors that influence long-term good results include:

- Biocompatibility of material and mechanical design of the implant
- Patient selection and preparation of recipient eye
- Operative technique.

HISTORY

In the United States, pioneering work was done since 1955 by William Stone,[16] later by Cardona,[6,7] Castroviejo and DeVoe,[8,9] and also Girard.[11] In England, Choyce used an acrylic prosthesis,[10] and, in Spain, Barraquer[2] used various types of prosthetic implants of the Cardona design. All these implants consisted of an optical cylinder made of methyl methacrylate and a supporting flange made of various materials (methacrylate, polytef (Teflon), Dacron mesh, polycarbon, and so forth). Strampelli used a very successful but technically difficult procedure called osteo-odontokeratoprosthesis.[17] It consisted of an optical acrylic cylinder inlaid in a sliver of maxillary bone. An acrylic lens with a platinum supporting flange was used in Odessa at the Filatov Institute, and, in Mexico, Alamillo[1] used a similar implant with success. In 1977 we developed a two-piece implant made of aluminum oxide (corundum) following a Cardona design.[13,15] This material has been used with success in bone and dental implants.[12] Corneal prosthesis using glass-ceramic have been tried in Germany and Switzerland.[4,5,14]

SELECTION OF PATIENTS

In my experience, keratoprosthesis have not been successful in patients with ocular pemphigoid, extremely dry eyes, or severely scarred conjunctiva, which required that the implant be placed through the lids. It is contraindicated in patients with diabetes and advanced glaucoma. Good candidates for prosthesis are patients with vision of hand motion or light perception with fair projection and vision of colored lights. Best results have been obtained in cases where the cornea was not receptive for additional corneal transplants because of severe scarring and vascularization (usually from chemical burns). Enough normal conjunctival tissue is needed to produce a flap to cover the cornea and the prosthesis. The eye should have a minimum amount of tears to keep the conjunctiva smooth and glistening. Preparatory surgery to improve the condition of the eye may include plastic work on the eyelids to correct an entropion or ectropion, grafting of conjunctiva from the other eye or buccal mucosa to reform fornices, cataract extraction, and control of glaucoma with diathermy or YAG laser.

OPERATIVE TECHNIQUE

We use instruments for corneal transplantation and plastic lid work. The techniques require the grafting of either fascia lata or periosteum. The fascia lata can be obtained through a direct approach from the side of the quadriceps, and the periosteum is acquired from the upper third of the tibial surface (3 × 3 cm). Instruments required for this procedure include scalpel, Stevens scissors, skin retractors, Freie periosteal elevator, 4-0 catgut and 5-0 nylon.

Periosteal Removal. About 5 ml of 1% or 2% lidocaine with epinephrine is infiltrated along the anterior crest of the tibia in its upper third. The skin is then prepped and draped. An incision is made with the scalpel on the skin over the crest of the tibia, deep to the bone for an extension of about 15 cm. The skin is then retracted, and blunt dissection is made with the scissors to separate the subcutaneous fat from the surface of the periosteum. About 4 × 4 cm of periosteal tissue is then isolated from the fat and connective tissue, which is elevated from the bony surface with the periosteal elevator and removed with scissors. This tissue is saved in a Petri dish over a moist gauze. The subcutaneous tissue is approximated with 4-0 catgut suture, and the skin is closed with interrupted or continuous 5-0 nylon suture. A compressive dressing is then applied to the leg.

Extremely thin corneas will require a full-thickness total corneal graft. A cryogenic unit for intracapsular cataract extraction may be required, and a vitrectomy instrument should be available. Fine hemorrhages are controlled with a solution of 0.002% epinephrine.

Trephines. Ten or 11 mm trephines are used in cases where the corneas must be replaced. A 3 mm trephine is needed for the optical portion of the keratoprosthesis.

Sutures. Use 8-0 black silk for keratoplasty, 6-0 black silk (Ethicon TG-140-8) to secure a Flieringa ring, 5-0 catgut to fix the periosteal donor tissue, and 5-0 nylon for skin closure when required. The footplate of the keratoprosthesis is sutured to the cornea with a special-order Ethicon 8-0 Prolene on a TG-140-8 needle.

Ceramic Keratoprosthesis. The prosthesis is made of a special type of ceramic formed almost exclusively of AL203. The substance is obtained in a powder form called corundum. These crystals measure about 0.001 mm and after melting they form a polycrystalline opaque material (used for the flange) or a crystalline material with a refractive index of 1.767. It has an structure similar to ruby or sapphire and must be cut with diamond tools. The implant consists of a flange of 8 mm in diameter with a central threaded perforation and several holes for sutures. The optical element is 3 mm in diameter and 10 mm long. It has 60-diopter power (Fig. 33-1).

Prosthesis Implantation. The surgical technique, with small modifications, are those of Castroviejo, Cardona, and DeVoe.[9] Cases with scarred conjunctiva require previous conjunctivoplasty or buccal mucosa graft. The prosthesis can be sutured to the cornea only if it has normal thickness. After insert-

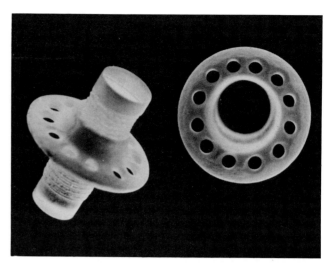

Fig. 33-1. Ceramic keratoprosthesis, which consists of an optical cylinder 10 mm long and 3 mm in diameter. It is threaded into an 8 mm–diameter supporting plate.

ing a lid speculum or traction sutures to the lid borders, a 360-degree peritomy of conjunctiva and Tenon's capsule is done. The dissection is followed toward the fornices. Bleeding is controlled with diluted epinephrine (1:20,000) drops and cautery. A single Flieringa ring (18 to 20 mm) is sutured to the sclera with 6-0 silk sutures immediately in front of the rectus muscles. The corneal limbus, or the corneal center, may need identification and should be marked for future reference. A corneal transplant (11 mm in diameter) is done at this point if it is required. (In this case, the 3 mm trephination is done from the endothelial side in the center of the cornea before the graft is sutured in place). Lens extraction and total iris excision are done before vitrectomy. If the eye is aphakic, a large and wide basal iridectomy is done through a limbal incision. Vitrectomy can be performed through this incision or through the 3 mm opening in the center of the cornea (Fig 33-2, *A*).

The plate of the keratoprosthesis is placed over the cornea and the central opening is aligned with the 3 mm trephination marking, and then two or three preplaced 8-0 polypropylene sutures are passed through the cornea and through the perforations in the prosthesis plate (Fig. 33-2, *B*). At this time the 3 mm perforation is completed with a razor-blade knife and Vannas scissors. The optical portion of the prosthesis is assembled, with about 4 mm of the optical portion being left to protrude in front of the retaining plate. The optical cylinder is introduced into the eye. The preplaced sutures are

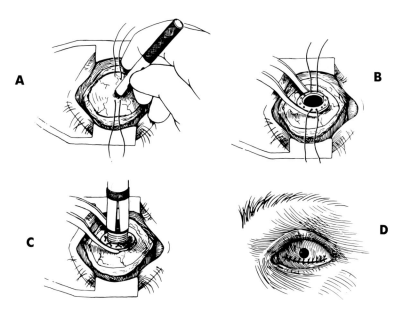

Fig. 33-2. Transcorneal technique (Cardona). **A,** Central area of cornea has been identified and a partial 3 mm trephination is performed. Two 8-0 polypropylene preplaced sutures are placed near limbus. **B,** Corneal button is removed, and ring of prosthesis is secured with two sutures (the Flieringa ring is not shown). **C,** Prosthesis is assembled and additional sutures are placed. Periosteum is applied over prosthesis. Conjunctiva and Tenon's fascia are brought over optical cylinder. **D,** Conjunctiva is opened 1 or 2 weeks later. (From Polack FM: *Cornea* 2:189, 1983.)

tied, and additional sutures are applied (Fig. 33-2, *C*). The knots are buried under the prosthesis.

Balanced salt solution is injected into the globe through a small keratotomy, or between sutures if a graft was used, to give the eye normal pressure. Fluorescein solution may be used to check for fast leaky spots.

The periosteum, which had been preserved in a petri dish with balanced salt solution, is placed over the prosthesis and trimmed if necessary. A small slit is made in its central portion so that the optical cylinder can be pushed through it, and it is then sutured to the sclera with 5-0 catgut or 7-0 Vicryl (polyglactin 910). The conjunctiva and Tenon's capsule are sutured over the prosthesis with 8-0 silk, and the sutures should be kept away from the optical lens (Fig. 33-2, *D*). Sliding flaps may be required so that healthy and thick conjunctiva can be placed over the implant.

POSTOPERATIVE TREATMENT

The conjunctiva over the implant is not opened for at least 3 weeks. It will then retract and adhere to the sides of the optical implant. Topical steroids and antibiotics are used daily for 3 to 4 weeks. Conjunctival sutures are removed in 4 weeks. Also at this time, vision can be corrected with glasses if necessary.

COMPLICATIONS OF KERATOPROSTHESIS

Extrusion of the implant and intraocular infection are the most common and serious problems to all corneal prostheses. In part, the problem of extrusion or dislocation of the implant is caused by degenerative structural or inflammatory changes in the recipient cornea. It is also caused by lack of incorporation of the prosthesis to the surrounding tissues (adhesion) and in part attributable to shearing forces caused by eye movements and lid rubbing against the optical lens. As mentioned before, patient selection, biocompatibility of the prosthesis material, and good design will minimize these problems.

Thinning and retraction of the conjunctiva surrounding the implant is often seen and requires grafting of new conjunctival tissue. Fixation of the supporting flange depends on the sutures and the condition of the recipient cornea. If a corneal graft was done to receive the prosthesis, one should keep in mind that rejection usually occurs, and this may cause loosening of the retaining sutures. In these

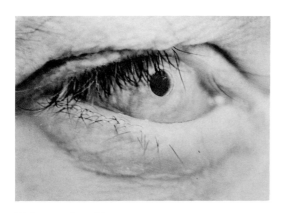

Fig. 33-3. Results of keratoprosthesis in eye with a chemical burn.

cases (usually corneal grafts of large size), patients are kept on topical steroids for long periods of time (1 to 2 years).

The optical cylinder has a large portion protruding from the back of the cornea to prevent retrocorneal membrane growth. If this occurs however, YAG laser lysis of the membrane can be performed.[3]

RESULTS

In general, visual results depend on the status of the retina, and stability of the implant depends on the structural condition of the anterior segment of the eye. In the absence of retinal disease or glaucoma some cases have obtained visual acuities near 20/20 (Fig. 33-3). The procedure of implantation through the lids for cases of pemphigoid or severe scarring of the conjunctiva has been abandoned several years ago because of the high incidence of infections and extrusions.

The ceramic prosthesis shows excellent biocompatibility when placed through the cornea and conjunctiva. Some cases retain good vision for 7 to 8 years. Permanent stability however has not been obtained. The periosteal subconjunctival graft is usu-

ally reabsorbed centrally and leaves the prosthesis solely covered by conjunctiva. After 2 to 3 years there has been a need to reoperate to cover a portion of the implant with new conjunctiva because of the retraction of this tissue. The results are shown in Table 33-1.

SUMMARY

A ceramic keratoprosthesis with the design of Cardona has been used with good results for the past 10 years. Patients have been selected on the basis of having enough conjunctival tissue to cover the implant, absence of glaucoma and dry eye, vision of light perception or better. Patients require frequent follow-up observation to prevent complications.

REFERENCES

1. Alamillo M, Alamillo R: Implantation of an artificial cornea, *Am J Ophthalmol* 56:937-941, 1963.
2. Barraquer J: Inclusion de prótesis ópticas corneanas, córneas acrílicas o queratoprótesis, *Ann Inst Barraquer* 1:243-347, 1960.
3. Bath PE, McCord RC, Cox KC: Nd:YAG laser discission of retroprosthetic membrane: a preliminary report, *Cornea* 2:225, 1983.
4. Bigar F, Frahenmann A, Landolt E, et al: *Die Gewebeverträglichkeit bioaktiver Glaskeramik in der Hornhaut und Bindehaut,* Bericht über die Kunststoffimplantat in der Ophthalmologie, Munich, 1977, Bergmann Verlag.
5. Blencke A, Hagen P, Bromer H, et al: Untersuchungen über die Verwendbarkeit von Glaskeramiken zur Osteo-Odonto-Keratoplastik, *Ophthalmologica* (Basel) 176:105-112, 1978.
6. Cardona H: Keratoprosthesis: acrylic optical cylinder with supporting intralamellar plate, *Am J Ophthalmol* 54:284-294, 1962.
7. Cardona H: Keratoprosthesis Round Table. In Corneal and external disease of the eye, Polack FM, editor: Springfield, Ill, 1970, Charles C Thomas, Publisher.
8. Cardona H, Castroviejo R, DeVoe AG: Advances in prosthokeratoplasty. In Casey TA, editor: *Corneal grafting,* London, 1972, Butterworth, p 313.
9. Castroviejo R, Cardona H, DeVoe AG: Present status of prosthokeratoplasty, *Am J Ophthalmol* 69:613-625, 1069.
10. Choyce DP: The treatment of bullous keratopathy with acrylic inlays: experience with Choyce two-piece acrylic kera-

Table 33-1. Vision: Clinical Results

Number	Age	Diagnosis	Before	After	Years After Operation
1	50	Corneal scar	LP	HM	8
2	38	Alkaline burn	HM	20/200	5
3	37	Alkaline burn	LP	20/50	7
4	40	Alkaline burn	HM	20/30	6
5	35	Alkaline burn	LP	HM	6
6	42	Alkaline burn	LP	20/50	2
7	38	Alkaline burn	LP	20/40	2
8	27	Heat	LP	20/200	1
9	21	Alkaline burn	LP	20/30	1

LP, light perception; *HM*, hand movement.

toprosthesis. In Rycroft PV, editor: *Corneo-plastic surgery, Proc II International Corneo-Plastic Conf,* London, 1967, Pergamon Press, p 399.

11. Girard LJ, Moore CD, Soper JW, et al: Prostheto-sclerokeratoplasty implantation of a keratoprosthesis using full thickness onlay sclera and sliding conjunctival flap, *Trans Am Acad Ophthalmol* 73:936-961, 1969.

12. Heimke G, Griss P: Ceramic implant material, *Med Biol Eng Comput* 18:503, 1980.

13. Heimke G, Polack FM: Keramische Keratoprosthesen, *Proc German Congress Ophthalmol* (Heidelberg), Munich, 1977, Bergmann Verlag, pp 28-35.

14. Hoffman F, Harnisch JP, Strunz V, et al: Osteo-Keramo-Keratoprothese: eine Modifikation der Osteo-Odonto-Keratoprothese nach Strampelli, *Klin Monatsbl Augenheilkd* 173:747-755, 1978.

15. Polack FM, Heimke G: Ceramic keratoprosthesis, *Ophthalmology* (AAO) 87:693, 1980.

16. Stone W Jr: Study of patency of openings in corneas anterior to intralamellar plastic artificial discs, *Am J Ophthalmol* 39:185, 1955.

17. Strampelli B: *Osteo-odontocheratoprotesi,* Ospedali Riuniti di Roma Reporte Oculistico, Rome 1963, Ospedale di S Giovanni, pp 1039-1044.

Chapter 34

Penetrating Keratoplasty in Children

R. DOYLE STULTING

At one time, corneal transplantation in children was considered doomed to failure and even contraindicated.[3,16,23] More recently, limited success has been reported,[1,4,6,8,15,19-21,25] but the prognosis for pediatric keratoplasty is clearly not so good as that for an adult (Table 34-1). Several factors account for the poorer prognosis for keratoplasty in children. The surgery itself is technically more difficult because the infant cornea and sclera are less rigid, the iris is more adherent, and the vitreous is more tenacious than in adults. The eye is smaller and tends to collapse at the time of surgery. In phakic eyes there may be spontaneous extrusion of the lens.

Postoperative care in children is more difficult than that in adults. An adequate examination often requires general anesthesia. Healing of the child's eye is rapid, and so sutures loosen quickly. The problems of postoperative care are compounded because children are unable to communicate their symptoms to the physician, delaying care. The child's eye is capable of mounting a fulminating, intense inflammatory response to the grafted tissue. Thus rejection episodes are very difficult to detect and treat before they become irreversible. Although technical success in pediatric keratoplasty has now been reported, visual results have been disappointing because failure to place a focused image on the retina during the early years of life leads to irreversible amblyopia. The lack of predictable refractive results after keratoplasty is a major contributing factor.

We reviewed our experience with 152 penetrating keratoplasties in 107 eyes of 91 children, analyzing results and identifying variables that influence the surgical outcome.[22] We summarize here these results and offer recommendations for the management of children with corneal opacities.

METHODS

Patients. One hundred eleven eyes of 95 children less than 15 years of age underwent penetrating keratoplasty utilizing allogeneic tissue for visual rehabilitation at Emory University (Atlanta, Georgia) between March 1977 and June 1982. Four cases could not be analyzed because of incomplete or unobtainable records. The remaining 152 penetrating keratoplasties in 107 eyes of 91 patients were reviewed retrospectively in July 1983. An attempt was made to locate and obtain information on patients who had not been examined within the 6 months before review.

Donor Corneas. The time of donor death, time of enucleation, and the time that the cornea was placed in storage medium were available in 145 cases. One hundred forty-two donor corneas were stored in TC-199 with dextran and antibiotics (McCarey-Kaufman [MK] medium), and three whole eyes were stored in moist chambers before utilization. The mean length of time from donor death to transplantation was 48.8 hours (range 2 to 122 hours).

Surgical Technique. Surgery was performed under an operating microscope with the patient under general anesthesia. Surgical technique varied, depending on the preference of the four surgeons involved and the complexity of the case. Preoperative intravenously administered mannitol and ocular massage were used in some cases. The lids were retracted with sutures, a lid speculum, or a Goldmann-McNeill blepharostat. Single or double scleral rings were used in some cases. The donor corneal buttons

Table 34-1.   Summary of Selected Reports of Penetrating Keratoplasty in Children

| | | Number of Eyes that Maintained a Clear Graft After Penetrating Keratoplasty | | |
| | | | Acquired | |
Author, Year	Follow-up Years Mean (range)	Congenital	Nontraumatic	Traumatic
Picetti,[19] 1966	2 (1-14)	100% (3/3)	84% (21/25)	83% (5/6)
Stone,[21] 1976	14 months	67% (2/3)	—	—
Waring,[25] 1977	3 (2-5)	11% (1/9)	83% (10/12)	100% (2/2)
Beauchamp,* 1978	4 (3 months to 26 years)	50% (9/18)	63% (22/25)	48% (10/21)
Gordon,[8] 1979		75% (3/4)	71% (5/7)	50% (1/2)
Schanzlin,[20] 1980	4 (1-10)	60% (9/15)	—	—
Cowden,[4] 1990	(1-10)	56% (14/25)	50% (8/16)	56% (9/16)
Legeais,[15] 1990	2.1	38% (6/16)	79% (69/87)	71% (17/24)
Erlich,[6] 1991	1.7 (3 months-9 years)	29% (7/24)	40% (2/5)†	71% (12/17)
TOTAL		49% (33/68)	81% (127/156)	64% (35/55)

Modified from Stulting RD et al: *Ophthalmology* 91:1222, 1984.
*Series includes 23 patients 15 to 19 years of age at the time of surgery.
†Herpes simplex keratitis only.

were cut manually with a disposable trephine from the epithelial side on a cutting block. The donor cornea was sutured to the recipient cornea with a single running 10-0 nylon suture in 139 cases, an interrupted 10-0 nylon sutures in 10 cases, and a combination of running and interrupted sutures in 2 cases. In one case, the suturing technique could not be determined. Operative procedures performed in addition to penetrating keratoplasty included iridoplasty, iridectomy, synechiolysis, lensectomy, membranectomy, vitrectomy, and repair of retinal detachment.

Postoperative Care. Topical antibiotics were begun during the early postoperative period and continued for as long as 6 months postoperatively. Topical cycloplegics, subconjunctival antibiotics, and subconjunctival steroids were also used in some cases. Eyes were patched for 5 to 14 days after surgery.

The postoperative steroid regimen included topical prednisolone acetate 1% or dexamethasone phosphate 0.1% hourly for 1 or 2 days, with a reduction in dosage to 5 times a day by about the third postoperative day. By 6 months, steroid therapy had been discontinued in most phakic eyes and decreased to 1 drop daily in most aphakic eyes.

Postoperative examinations were performed at intervals varying from daily to monthly during the first year. Uncooperative children (generally those less than 4 years of age) were examined under insufflation anesthesia. In young children, visual acuity was estimated by fixation patterns or graded opticonystagmus (Catford scanner). In older children who were cooperative, Allen picture cards, an HOTV chart, the illiterate E chart, or a Snellen

Table 34-2.   Indications for Penetrating Keratoplasty

Diagnosis	Number of Eyes
Congenital	
Peters' anomaly	27
Glaucoma with corneal edema	6
Posterior polymorphous dystrophy	5
Multiple anterior segment anomalies	4
Sclerocornea	3
Acquired, nontraumatic	
Herpes simplex keratitis	16
Bacterial keratitis	4
Stevens-Johnson syndrome	3
Keratoconus	2
Neurotrophic keratitis	2
Interstitial keratitis	1
Fungal keratitis	2
Exposure keratopathy (coloboma of upper lid)	1
Acquired, traumatic	
Corneal or corneoscleral laceration	23
Blood stain	4
Nonpenetrating injury with scar	4
TOTAL	107

From Stulting RD et al: *Ophthalmology* 91:1222, 1984.

chart was used. A clear graft was defined as one with compact central stroma without epithelial or stromal edema that allowed a clear view of iris detail through a slitlamp. Probable graft rejection was defined as a sudden loss of graft clarity associated with inflammation in a previously clear graft 2 or more weeks postoperatively when no other cause for loss of clarity could be found. Definite graft rejection was defined as the presence of an endothelial or epithelial rejection line. Optical correction and occlusion therapy for amblyopia were initiated at a time determined on an individual-case basis by the attending physician.

Statistical Analysis. Data were analyzed by the Kaplan-Meier method of survival analysis utilizing the Breslow and Mantel-Cox tests for significance or by Cox regression analysis of right-censored survival data.[5,11,14] The association between candidate predictive factors and final visual acuity was evaluated by one-way analysis of variance.

RESULTS

Indications for penetrating keratoplasty in the series is shown in Table 34-2. For the purposes of analysis, these have been divided into congenital, acquired nontraumatic, and acquired traumatic corneal opacities. Additional data on the population examined are shown in Table 34-3. The average follow-up observation for all eyes was 30 months, with a follow-up period of less than 1 year in only four first grafts. Thus survival data are not biased by a large number of successful grafts followed for only a short period of time.

First graft survival analysis for the three major diagnostic groupings is shown in Fig. 34-1. Although the probability of survival differs somewhat for the three groups with grafts for congenital opacities having the worst prognosis, these differences are not statistically significant. Because the three diagnostic categories compared in Fig. 34-1 are heterogeneous

Table 34-3. Summary of Clinical Data

Variable	Congenital	Acquired Nontraumatic	Traumatic	Total
Grafts	72	42	38	152
Patients	33	28	30	91
Eyes	45	31	31	107
Patients with bilateral disease	21	5	2	28
Patients with unilateral disease	12	23	28	63
Patients with bilateral grafts	12	3	1	16
Patients with unilateral grafts	21	25	29	75
Right eye	23	14	16	53
Left eye	22	17	15	54
Eyes with one graft	29	24	23	76
Eyes with two grafts	4	3	8	15
Eyes with three grafts	8	3	0	11
Eyes with four grafts	4	1	0	5
Patients with previous failed grafts performed elsewhere	3	1	1	5
Grafts performed elsewhere	5	1	1	7
Age at onset of opacity				
Mean	0	49 mo.	79 mo.	—
Median	0	40 mo.	65 mo.	—
Range	0	2-144 mo.	3-175 mo.	—
Age at first Emory surgery				
Mean	30 mo.	97 mo.	98 mo.	—
Median	15 mo.	100 mo.	94 mo.	—
Range	1-144 mo.	31-171 mo.	17-176 mo.	—
Patients <6 months of age at surgery	12	0	0	12
Time from onset of opacity to surgery (mean)	30 mo.	48 mo.	20 mo.	—
Follow-up per eye				
Mean	34 mo.	24 mo.	30 mo.	—
Range*	2-75 mo.	3-66 mo.	1-68 mo.	—
Eyes with clear grafts at time of review	31 (68%)	23 (74%)	23 (74%)	77(71%)

From Stulting RD et al: *Ophthalmology* 91:1222, 1984.
*The fate of all first grafts at 6 months postoperatively is known, since only opaque grafts were lost to follow-up study during this period. Between 6 months and 1 year postoperatively, only four successful first grafts were lost to follow-up study.

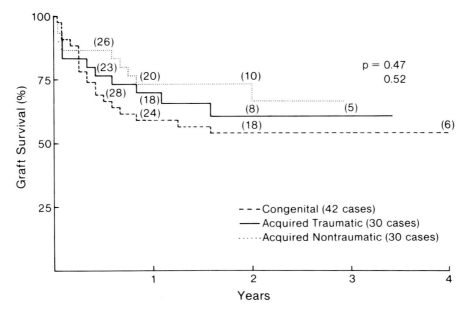

Fig. 34-1. Penetrating keratoplasty in children—first graft survival by diagnostic group. Survival analysis was performed by Kaplan-Meier method. Breslow and Mantel-Cox tests showed no significant difference in graft survival among the three groups (p = 0.47 and 0.52 respectively). *Figures in parentheses,* Number of patients remaining under observation. (Total number of eyes shown in this figure for each group is less than total number of eyes shown in Table 34-3, line 2, because five eyes received their first graft elsewhere and follow-up data were not available.) (From Stulting RD et al: *Ophthalmology* 91:1222, 1984.)

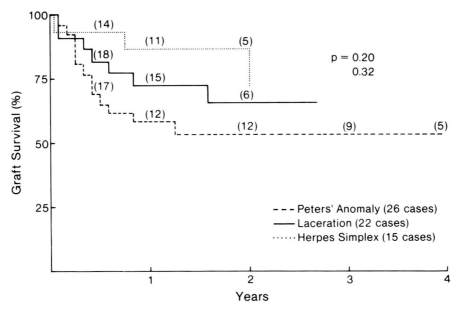

Fig. 34-2. Penetrating keratoplasty in children—first graft survival by diagnosis. Survival analysis was performed by the Kaplan-Meier method. Breslow and Mantel-Cox tests showed no significant difference in graft survival among the three groups (p = 0.20 and 0.32 respectively). *Figures in parentheses,* Number of patients remaining under observation. (From Stulting RD et al: *Ophthalmology* 91:1222, 1984.)

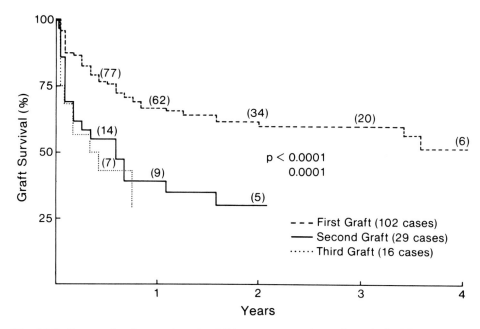

Fig. 34-3. Penetrating keratoplasty in children—comparison of survival of first, second, and third grafts. Survival analysis was performed by the Kaplan-Meier method. Breslow and Mantel-Cox tests showed a significant difference in survival of first grafts compared to second or third grafts ($p < 0.0001$) but not for second grafts compared to third grafts. *Figures in parentheses,* Number of patients remaining under observation. (From Stulting RD et al: *Ophthalmology* 91:1222, 1984.)

(Table 34-2), graft survival was also analyzed for the three most common diagnoses (Fig. 34-2). Grafts for herpes simplex had the best prognosis and grafts for Peters' anomaly, the worst. Again, these differences did not reach statistical significance. Overall, graft survival was better in older patients than in younger patients, but the correlation between patient age and graft survival failed to reach statistical significance in this series ($p = 0.12$).

As can be seen (Fig. 34-3), first grafts were much more likely to remain clear than second or third grafts. Only 5 fourth grafts were available for analysis. Four of these remained clear at 1, 2, 17, and 33 months postoperatively.

In most cases, transplanted corneas failed by gradual loss of clarity without inflammation or signs of rejection (Table 34-4). It is suspected that some of these failures might have been attributable to immunologic graft rejection that was unrecognized because of difficulty in examining and communicating with these patients.

Several preoperative and intraoperative variables were analyzed to determine whether they might have influenced graft survival (Table 34-5). Of those variables examined, the presence of deep or superficial vascularization was most closely correlated with decreased graft survival. Intraoperative lensectomy and vitrectomy were also associated with poor graft survival. Whether these procedures by themselves are responsible for a poor prognosis or eyes requiring lensectomy or vitrectomy are inherently less likely to do well after keratoplasty cannot be determined from the data.

The final postoperative vision was improved compared to the preoperative vision in 71% of patients with acquired traumatic or nontraumatic opacities (Figs. 34-4 and 34-5). In contrast, only 50% of patients with congenital corneal opacities showed an improvement in vision (Fig. 34-6). Of those patients with congenital corneal opacities and unknown preoperative vision, the best postoperative vision achieved was 20/80. Only eyes with posterior polymorphous dystrophy achieved a final visual acuity better than 20/100. In these cases, corneal opacities were present at birth but gradually became more dense during the first few months or years of life, leading to surgical intervention. Thus visual deprivation was not so severe as in eyes with other diagnoses.

In addition to loss of graft clarity, irreversible amblyopia, strabismus, nystagmus, and glaucoma accounted for failure to achieve good postoperative vi-

Table 34-4. Reasons for Failure of Grafts After Penetrating Keratoplasty in Children

| | Number of Grafts | | | |
| | Congenital | Acquired | | |
Reason for Failure	*Congenital*	*Nontraumatic*	*Traumatic*	*Total*
Unknown	18	10	7	35
Sterile ulcer	6	2	3	11
Homograft reaction (probable or definite)	3	3	2	8
Retrocorneal fibrous membrane	6	0	0	6
Bacterial keratitis	5	0	1	6
Phthisis	2	0	2	4
Herpes simplex keratitis	0	2	0	2
Endophthalmitis	1	1	0	2
Trauma	0	1	0	1
TOTAL	41	19	15	75

From Stulting RD et al: *Ophthalmology* 91:1222, 1984.

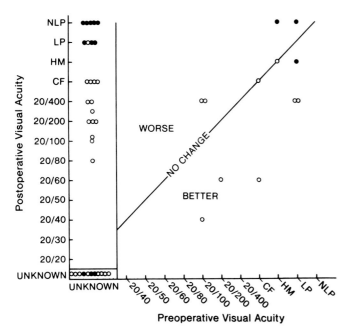

Fig. 34-4. Final visual acuity after keratoplasty for congenital corneal opacities. Preoperative visual acuities were the most recently obtained prior to initial keratoplasty. Postoperative acuities were the most recently obtained. In some cases, additional surgical procedures were performed between time of initial keratoplasty and final postoperative acuity. *Open circles,* Clear grafts; *closed circles,* failed grafts; *circles to right of diagonal line,* patients with final visual acuity better than preoperative visual acuity; *circles to left of diagonal line,* patients with final visual acuity worse than preoperative visual acuity. (From Stulting RD et al: *Ophthalmology* 91:1222, 1984.)

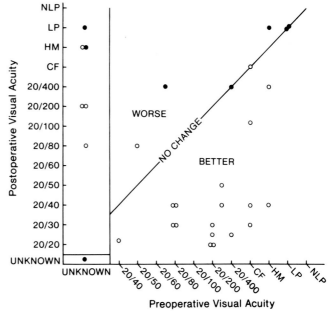

Fig. 34-5. Final visual acuity after keratoplasty for acquired, nontraumatic corneal opacities. Preoperative visual acuities were the most recently obtained before initial keratoplasty. Postoperative acuities were the most recently obtained. In some cases, additional surgical procedures were performed between time of initial keratoplasty and final postoperative acuity. *Open circles,* Clear grafts; *closed circles,* failed grafts; *circles to right of diagonal line,* patients with final visual acuity better than preoperative visual acuity; *circles to left of diagonal line,* patients with final visual acuity worse than preoperative visual acuity. (From Stulting RD et al: *Ophthalmology* 91:1222, 1984.)

Table 34-5. Factors Examined for Effect on Graft Survival

Preoperative Variables	p Value*
Epithelial defect	0.01
Pupillary membrane	0.05
Tear/surface abnormality	0.05
Vascularization†	0.0001
Age of recipient at surgery	ns
Aphakia	ns
Fibrous proliferation in anterior chamber	ns
Glaucoma	ns
Inflammation‡	ns
Anterior synechiae	ns
Thinning of cornea	ns
Intraoperative Variables	
Lensectomy	0.005
Vitrectomy	0.002

From Stulting RD et al: *Ophthalmology* 91:1222, 1984.
*Obtained by Breslow and Mantel-Cox tests for significance, or by Cox regression analysis of right-censored survival data. No correction has been made for the number of variables (13) examined. *ns*, Not significant; $p < 0.05$.
†Deep or superficial, as determined by clinical observation and microscopic examination of pathologic specimens. When analyzed independently, both deep and superficial vascularization were significantly associated with decreased graft survival.
‡Presence of inflammation clinically or a leukocyte infiltrate in the histologic section.

Table 34-6. Factors Examined for Effect on Final Visual Acuity

Preoperative Variables*	p Value†
Age of recipient at onset of opacity	0.03
Aphakia	0.03
Edema of cornea	0.04
Glaucoma	0.05
Anterior synechiae	0.02
Time from onset of opacity to surgery	ns
Epithelial defect	ns
Fibrous proliferation in anterior chamber	ns
Inflammation‡	ns
Pupillary membrane	ns
Tear/surface abnormality	ns
Thinning of cornea	ns
Vascularization§	ns
Intraoperative Variables	
Vitrectomy	0.003
Lensectomy	ns
Postoperative Variables	
Aphakia	0.0002

From Stulting RD et al: *Ophthalmology* 91:1222, 1984.
*Preoperative and operative variables were obtained for the initial keratoplasty. Final visual acuity was the most recent obtained, even though additional surgical procedures might have been performed since the initial keratoplasty.
†p values were obtained by χ^2 analysis of contingency tables. *ns*, Not significant; $p < 0.05$. No correction was made for the number of variables examined (16).
‡Presence of inflammation clinically or a leukocyte infiltrate in the histologic section.
§Neither deep nor superficial vascularization was significantly correlated with final acuity.

sion. Factors that are associated with poor postoperative visual acuity are shown in Table 34-6.

DISCUSSION

Adult versus Pediatric Grafts. Although the prognosis in pediatric keratoplasty is not so good as that in adult keratoplasty, our data and the data of others[1,4,6,8,15,19,21,25] indicate that success can be achieved in these patients (Table 34-1 and Fig. 34-7). The prognosis for graft clarity is poorer in children with congenital corneal opacities than it is in children with acquired opacities, but statistical significance was not reached in our series. Similarly, grafts tended to remain clear longer in older children than in younger children, but statistical significance was not reached. We suspect that a larger series might demonstrate statistical significance in both of these comparisons.

In the pediatric age group, first grafts have a better prognosis than subsequent grafts (Fig. 34-3). One cannot determine from the available data whether failure of a previous graft by itself is a poor prognostic indicator or the subset of patients requiring multiple grafts simply represents a selected group with a poor prognosis from the outset. Perhaps both factors play a role.

There are several reasons that might explain why penetrating keratoplasty has a poorer prognosis in children than in adults. The surgical procedure itself is technically more complex. Postoperative follow-up observation is difficult because children are often uncooperative and cannot be examined adequately without general anesthesia. Healing, vascularization, and probably rejection also occur more rapidly in children than in adults.

The infant eye is smaller than that of the adult, but it is the decreased rigidity and increased elasticity of the infant cornea and sclera that make transplantation technically much more difficult than in the adult eye. In phakic eyes, it is imperative that the intraocular pressure be reduced by preoperative massage, intravenous mannitol, and pharmacologic paralysis of extraocular muscles. Supplemental preoperative retrobulbar anesthesia should be avoided because of the small volume of the orbit. A Goldmann-McNeill blepharostat or lid sutures are valuable in reducing pressure on the globe intraoperatively. Despite these precautions, the lens and iris invariably move forward as soon as the eye is opened, and spontaneous extrusion of the lens may be unavoidable. In phakic eyes, visualization and division of iridocorneal adhesions are difficult and often best

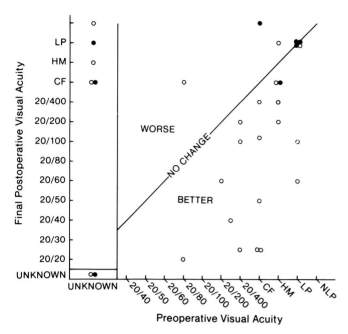

Fig. 34-6. Final visual acuity after keratoplasty for acquired, traumatic corneal opacities. Preoperative visual acuities were most recently obtained before initial keratoplasty. Postoperative acuities were most recently obtained. In some cases, additional surgical procedures were performed between time of initial keratoplasty and final postoperative acuity. *Open circles,* clear grafts; *closed circles,* failed grafts; *circles to right of diagonal line,* patients with final visual acuity better than preoperative visual acuity; *circles to left of diagonal line,* patients with final visual acuity worse than preoperative visual acuity. (From Stulting RD et al: *Ophthalmology* 91:1222, 1984.)

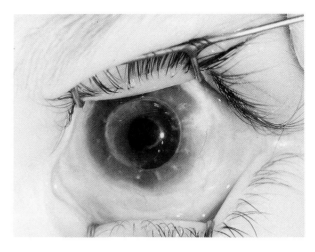

Fig. 34-7. Clear corneal graft in 5-year-old patient with congenital glaucoma 2 years after surgery for irreversible corneal edema that followed several surgical procedures to lower the intraocular pressure.

performed after closure of the wound. A viscoelastic substance is useful in coating the lens to protect the corneal endothelium from damage during synechiolysis. After synechiolysis, one must obtain adequate hemostasis by intraocular diathermy or by waiting for spontaneous clotting. A fibrin clot that remains in the anterior chamber may lead to the reformation of synechiae postoperatively. Tissue plasminogen activator can be used intraoperatively to remove fibrin.

Suture and Donor Tissue. A running 10-0 nylon suture should be used in most cases for closure. This facilitates rapid wound closure, minimizing the time of contact between the lens, iris, and grafted corneal endothelium, reducing the likelihood that iris will adhere to the peripheral cornea or surgical wound because of fibrin. Postoperatively, a single running suture is much easier to remove. The selective removal of interrupted sutures or adjustment of a single-running suture for control of astigmatism is not practical in infants and very small children with symmetrically vascularized corneas, since sutures loosen

quickly and typically must be removed early in the postoperative period.

A running suture should not be used for corneas with asymmetric vascularization. Rapid healing and wound contraction in vascularized areas could cause exposure of a portion of a running suture while the wound has not healed elsewhere. In such cases of asymmetric vascularization, interrupted 10-0 nylon should be used.

Since there is no correlation between donor age and graft survival and since adult donor tissue is easier to handle, adult donor tissue is probably preferable in pediatric keratoplasty unless the recipient is aphakic. In aphakic eyes, the use of infant tissue has the advantage of increasing the corneal curvature to compensate for the loss of the crystalline lens.[12,18,28]

Because of the increased elasticity of the infant cornea and sclera, it is recommended that donor tissue be sized 0.5 to 1 mm larger than the recipient opening, particularly in aphakic eyes. Donor diameters of 5.5 to 7 mm are recommended for infants. The use of oversized donor buttons is particularly important when the recipient tissue is thin. Watertight closure is more easily achieved when the incision in the recipient is angled so as to leave a posterior ledge.

Postoperative Care. The postoperative care of young, uncooperative children is difficult. They may traumatize their eyes by rubbing them or may injure them while at play. Arm restraints may be necessary in some cases. Parents often find it difficult to administer medications and comply with occlusion therapy, and careful instruction may be required to assure compliance with the physician's instructions. Some children are irritated more by a patch than they are by the unpatched eye. In these cases, it may be better to leave the eye unpatched.

It is important to provide pleasant conditions in the office or hospital and to assure the child's comfort whenever possible so that he or she will be more likely to cooperate with the examiner. Examination of small children should be performed without touching the child, if possible. Infants less than 1 year of age can usually be examined without anesthesia using the portable slitlamp. They are often more cooperative if they can be examined while feeding. Those over 4 years of age are often cooperative for slitlamp examination, and those over 7 years of age may even allow suture removal in the office. Between 1 and 4 years of age, however, children are usually not cooperative for slitlamp examination and cannot be effectively restrained. In this age range, an examination under anesthesia is required for adequate evaluation of the cornea.

Rapid Healing Rate. The infant cornea heals much faster than the adult cornea, particularly when there is vascularization. Healing and contraction of the operative scar causes loosening of the suture, which collects mucus, irritates the lids, stimulates vascularization, increases the risk of infectious keratitis, and places the transplanted cornea in danger of rejection (Fig. 34-8). Parents of children with corneal transplants should be taught to recognize loose sutures. Loose sutures should be removed immediately, and routine suture removal may be performed 4 to 6 weeks postoperatively in children less than 1 year of age.[1,2,20,26]

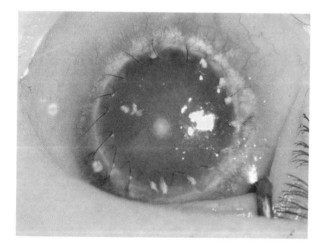

Fig. 34-8. Loose sutures collecting mucus and a failed graft in a 2-year-old 3 weeks after keratoplasty for Peters' anomaly.

Frequent Follow-up Observation. Young children are often unable to report symptoms involving postoperative complications: pain, decreased vision, and photophobia. It is therefore important that they be examined frequently, perhaps every 1 or 2 days during the first 2 weeks after surgery and every 1 or 2 weeks during the first postoperative year when most failures occur. It is imperative to train the parents to observe the graft when they are instilling medicines and even give them a penlight to help them see. They should promptly report loss of graft clarity, redness of the eye, or the appearance of mucus at the suture line. Suspicion should also be aroused when a child with a corneal transplant becomes irritable, doesn't sleep, rubs his eye, refuses to open the operated eye, tries to avoid bright lights, or ambulates poorly.

Rejection. In this series, allograft rejection accounted for only 11% of graft failures (Table 34-4). In the congenital opacity group, 6 times more grafts failed for unknown reasons than failed from rejection. We suspect that many of the failures that occurred for unknown reasons were actually failures from rejection. One possible explanation for this large number of unexplained graft failures is that the children were not examined during the acute rejection episode. Another possible explanation is that the classical signs of rejection (rejection lines and keratic precipitates in association with graft edema) are not seen as commonly in children as they are in adults. In support of this latter hypothesis is my observation that endothelial rejection lines are extremely rare in infants.

Glaucoma. The management of glaucoma is often quite difficult in children, and uncontrolled glaucoma may lead to graft failure or irreversible optic nerve damage. Intraocular pressure should be measured by applanation and confirmed by another method (such as pneumotonometer). Until recently, the only effective means of controlling glaucoma in these patients has been cyclocryopexy, which exposes the patient to the risk of irreversible hypotony. The Molteno implant now appears to be safer and more effective for the control of glaucoma in pediatric eyes.[17]

Visual Results. The final visual acuities obtained in our series of children undergoing keratoplasty for congenital corneal opacities were disappointing (Fig. 34-4). Although poor visual results in pediatric keratoplasty are partly attributable to loss of graft clarity and noncorneal ocular abnormalities, amblyopia is a significant factor limiting postoperative acuity. Postoperative aphakia and a young age at the onset of opacity are correlated with poor visual acuity (Table

34-6), as would be expected if irreversible amblyopia played a role in limiting postoperative acuity. It is well known that visual deprivation during the early months of life produces severe, irreversible damage to the developing central visual system.[9,10,27] Asymmetric visual deprivation, such as that created by unilateral corneal opacities or high anisometropia (monocular aphakia), is especially damaging because of binocular competition. The importance of a sharp retinal image during the first few months of life is emphasized by the relatively good postoperative acuities achieved in children with posterior polymorphous dystrophy. In these cases, the retinal image was less distorted during the first few months than in children with dense corneal opacities at birth (such as Peters' anomaly).

The average age at the time of surgery in the congenital opacity group is 30 months, and so it is not surprising that irreversible amblyopia would be a major factor in limiting postoperative acuity in our series (Table 34-3). For optimal visual results, the graft must not only be successful, but must also be performed at an early age, perhaps as early as 2 weeks, with immediate optical correction and appropriate amblyopia therapy.

Even though the final visual acuities obtained after penetrating keratoplasty for congenital corneal opacities have been disappointing, several points should be emphasized. First, many of these eyes were severely damaged, with coexisting noncorneal ocular disease and vascularization of the cornea significantly reducing the prognosis for successful keratoplasty and recovery of vision. Many of these children underwent surgery because the eye would have no chance at all of providing useful vision without any surgical intervention. Secondly, even a cloudy graft often provides better vision than the densely opaque cornea that the patient had preoperatively. There is often a noticeable postoperative improvement in the behavior of, communication with, and ambulation of children with bilateral corneal opacities despite the fact that they have a cloudy graft or a measured visual acuity of 20/200 or less. Finally, it should be recognized that the visual results shown in Figs. 34-4 to 34-6 might be somewhat misleading, since some of the patients with poor acuities were awaiting regraft, optimal optical correction, or additional improvement from amblyopia therapy at the time of review.

Since publication of our original report, the visual acuities of some of the subjects have progressively improved. For example, one of the oldest subjects with bilateral Peters' anomaly who was born March 3, 1977, underwent penetrating keratoplasty at 4 months (OD) and 13 months (OS) of age, followed by cataract extraction at 2 years (OD) and 4½ years (OS) of age. When last examined on November 18, 1991, at 14½ years of age, his acuities were 20/40 OD and 20/100 OS with spectacle correction. Thus it is possible to obtain reading vision with penetrating keratoplasty for Peters' anomaly.

Indications for penetrating keratoplasty in children are similar to those in an adult, but the decision to proceed with surgery must be tempered by the extreme difficulty of the surgical procedure, problems with follow-up observation, severity of associated ocular anomalies with trauma, and the likelihood that amblyopia will limit visual rehabilitation.

Bilateral Disease. Our present philosophy is to operate as soon as possible on both eyes of infants with dense corneal opacities to provide the maximal opportunity for development of the visual pathways. "Saving" one eye for surgery later (when the prognosis for graft clarity may be better) assures that irreversible amblyopia will severely limit visual acuity. It is also difficult to predict which eye will have the better prognosis for early surgery. Another reason for operating on both eyes is that when a graft fails, useful vision in the opposite eye may be important in the psychosocial development of the child.

In the presence of corneal vascularization or previous corneal graft rejection, the use of histocompatible donor tissue of immunosuppression with cyclosporin A may improve the prognosis for graft survival.[7,24]

Informed Consent. Decisions regarding keratoplasty in a child with one normal eye and one eye with a corneal opacity must be made circumspectly. Is the potential visual result worth the time, effort, and money to be invested? What is the probability that the graft will remain clear for the long term? What is the likelihood that amblyopia can be treated and reversed? What is the likely outcome if nothing is done?

Undertaking the care of a child with a corneal opacity is a long-term commitment on the part of both parents and physician, particularly if the opacities are congenital. The prognosis for success must be discussed realistically and openly with the parents before a decision is made to proceed with surgical intervention. Obtaining informed consent for keratoplasty from the parent of a child with congenital corneal opacities means telling them that the likelihood of first graft survival is about 50%, that further surgical intervention may be necessary, that postoperative care will be difficult and will require a major commitment of time on their part, and that the expected visual outcome after the exercise is only about 20/400. In older children with acquired corneal opacities, one can be more optimistic about the visual prognosis (Figs. 34-5 and 34-6).

The child's socioeconomic environment must be considered when the probability of surgical success is estimated. Who will be home to give the child his medications? How will he get to and from the doctor? Assuring an optimal milieu for good postoperative care often means assembling a team of personnel including social workers, philanthropic institutions, relatives, and other physicians when the resources of the immediate family and corneal surgeon are inadequate[13,26] (Fig. 34-9).

The emotional reaction of parents to their child's ocular abnormalities must be recognized and dealt with appropriately by the ophthalmologist. There are often unjustified feelings of guilt that the physician must help the parents to recognize and resolve. (I must have done something wrong during pregnancy. I should have prevented my child from getting herpes. If I had taken better care of the transplant, it would not have failed.) The parents invariably want to "do anything" to help the child and tend not to hear discussions of possible surgical complications or the merits of no surgical intervention at all, and so these negative points must be emphasized repeatedly. A counselor or psychiatrist might be needed to help the family cope with their emotional problems.

It is easy for parents to form the impression that "everything will be all right" if surgery is "successful." Thus, the likely appearance of the eye and the expected postoperative vision should be realistically and carefully explained. One helpful technique is to use trial lenses to reduce the parents' vision so that they can understand what the child might see after "successful" surgery and to show them pictures of an eye with a graft in place.

Five eyes in this series became phthisical after penetrating keratoplasty or subsequent surgical procedures, and an additional eye developed an inoperable retinal detachment, for an overall severe complication rate of 5.6%. Thus enthusiasm for penetrating keratoplasty in children should be tempered not only by technical surgical difficulties and difficult postoperative care, but also by the real possibility that eyes can be lost from surgical intervention. This, too, is a fact that should be shared with the parents of such children.

ACKNOWLEDGMENT

I am grateful to Dr. George O. Waring, III, for discussion and review of the manuscript.

REFERENCES

1. Beauchamp GR: Pediatric keratoplasty: problems in management, *J Pediatr Ophthalmol Strabismus* 16:388-394, 1978.
2. Brown SI: Corneal transplantation of the infant cornea, *Trans Am Acad Ophthalmol Otolaryngol* 78:461-466, 1974.
3. Castroviejo R: Selection of patients for keratoplasty, *Surv Ophthalmol* 3:1-12, 1958.
4. Cowden JW: Penetrating keratoplasty in infants and children, *Ophthalmol* 97:324-328, 1990.
5. Cutler SJ, Ederer F: Maximum utilization of the life table method in analyzing survival, *J Chron Dis* 8:699-712, 1958.
6. Erlich CM, Rootman DS, Morin JD: Corneal transplantation in infants, children, and young adults: experience of the Toronto Hospital for Sick Children, 1979-1988, *Can J Ophthalmol* 26:206-210, 1991.
7. Foulks GN, Sanfilippo F: Beneficial effects of histocompatibility in high risk corneal transplantation, *Am J Ophthalmol* 94:622-629, 1982.
8. Gordon YJ, Mokete M: Penetrating keratoplasty in children, *J Pediatr Ophthalmol Strabismus* 16:297-300, 1979.
9. Hubel DH: Exploration of the primary visual cortex, *Nature* 299:515-524, 1982.
10. Jampolsky A: Unequal visual inputs and strabismus management: a comparison of human and animal strabismus. In *Transactions of the New Orleans Academy of Ophthalmology Symposium on Strabismus*, St. Louis, 1978, Mosby−Year Book.
11. Kaplan EL, Meier P: Nonparametric estimation from incomplete observations, *J Am Statistical Assoc* 53:457-481, 1958.
12. Koenig S, Graul E, Kaufman HE: Ocular refraction after penetrating keratoplasty with infant donor corneas, *Am J Ophthalmol* 94:534-539, 1982.
13. Laibson PR, Waring GO: Diseases of the cornea. In Harley RD, editor: *Pediatric ophthalmology*, ed 2, Philadelphia, 1983, WB Saunders.
14. Lee ET: *Statistical methods for survival data analysis*, Belmont, Calif, 1980, Lifetime Learning Publication, pp 75-128, 306-317.

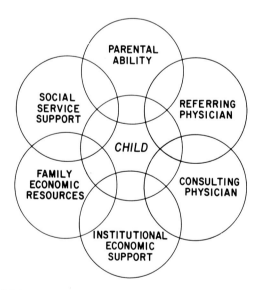

Fig. 34-9. Venn diagram illustrating complex support network often required to provide optimal postoperative care to child after keratoplasty. (From Waring GO, Laibson PR: Keratoplasty in children. In Kwitko ML editor: *Surgery of the infant eye*, New York, 1979, Appleton-Century-Crofts.)

15. Legeais JM, Jobin D, Pouliquen Y: Kératoplasties chez l'enfant, *J Fr Ophtalmol* 13:116-120, 1990.
16. Leigh AG: Corneal grafting, *Br J Clin Pract* 5:329-332, 1958.
17. Lynch MG, Brown RH, Stulting RD, Drews-Botsch C: The Molteno implant for pediatric glaucoma, *Ophthalmology*. (Submitted.)
18. Pfister RR, Breaud S: Aphakiac refractive penetrating keratoplasty using newborn donor corneas: a preliminary report on an alternative approach to refractive correction, *Ophthalmology* 90:1207-1212, 1983.
19. Picetti B, Fine M: Keratoplasty in children, *Am J Ophthalmol* 61:782-789, 1966.
20. Schanzlin DJ, Goldberg DB, Brown SI: Transplantation of congenitally opaque corneas, *Ophthalmology* 87:1253-1264, 1980.
21. Stone DL, Kenyon KR, Green WR, Ryan SJ: Congenital central corneal leukoma (Peters' anomaly), *Am J Ophthalmol* 81:173-193, 1976.
22. Stulting RD, Sumers KD, Cavanagh HD, et al: Penetrating keratoplasty in children, *Ophthalmology* 91:1222-1230, 1984.
23. Thomas JWT: On advising a corneal graft, *Br Med J* 1:880-882, 1956.
24. Völker-Dieben HJM: *The effect of immunological and nonimmunological factors on corneal graft survival,* The Hague and Boston, 1984, Dr W Junk bv Publishers.
25. Waring GO, Laibson PR: Keratoplasty in infants and children, *Trans Am Acad Ophthalmol Otolaryngol* 83:283-296, 1977.
26. Waring GO, Laibson PR: Keratoplasty in children. In Kwitko ML, editor: *Surgery of the infant eye,* New York, 1979, Appleton-Century-Crofts.
27. Wiesel TN: Postnatal development of the visual cortex and the influence of environment, *Nature* 299:583-591, 1982.
28. Wood TO, Nissenkorn I: Infant donor corneas for penetrating keratoplasty, *Ophthalmic Surg* 12:500-502, 1981.

Part IV

REFRACTIVE CORNEAL SURGERY

Chapter 35

CLASSIFICATION AND TERMINOLOGY

GEORGE O. WARING, III

Most specialized fields develop their own technical terminology and jargon. Corneal surgery is no exception. The penchant for professional shorthand has produced jargon such as "keratorefractive" surgery, a Greek-Latin hybrid that flows easily from the tongue and pen of those enamored by neologisms. Some surgeons have become "keratotomists," and their patients are "keratotomized." Words have been invented, such as "lenticle," instead of the correct term, lenticule—the piece of tissue or synthetic material used to change corneal shape. Commercial trademarked terms have appeared; the donor lenticule used in epikeratoplasty has been dubbed Kerato-Lens™. Eponyms abound. Common use of some colloquial terms has fixed them in our vocabulary. For example, some say "myopic keratomileusis" (Is the keratomileusis myopic?), instead of the more precise designation, keratomileusis for myopia. Thus far we have been spared "myopic radial keratotomy."

To clarify the language we use in this rapidly changing area of ophthalmology, I propose a classification of refractive corneal surgery, which I hope is broad enough to include all corneal procedures that have a major refractive component, systematic enough to organize our present knowledge, flexible enough to accommodate new developments, and precise enough to decrease the proliferation of jingly keratospeak.

REFRACTIVE SURGERY

Refractive surgery is any operation intended to alter the refractive state of the eye.[1] Thus radial keratotomy, cataract extraction with implantation of an intraocular lens, and scleral reinforcement to treat degenerative myopia are all forms of refractive surgery. Refractive corneal surgery refers to operations on the cornea, which are intended to alter the refractive state of the eye. This type of surgery is popularly referred to as refractive keratoplasty, an appropriate term, since keratoplasty means "molding the cornea."

CLASSIFICATION OF REFRACTIVE CORNEAL SURGERY

The classification I propose (Table 35-1) is based on surgical technique. It describes basic techniques that can be applied to many refractive errors, such as keratomileusis for both myopia and hyperopia. It accommodates new techniques that are modifications of previously used ones, such as epikeratoplasty as a modification of keratomileusis. It requires only one description of a technical procedure that is used in different refractive operations, such as the use of a microkeratome in keratomileusis, keratophakia, and keratokyphosis.[14]

This classification specifies first the surgical technique and then the refractive disorder being treated, for example, keratomileusis for myopia. Of course, precision demands appropriate modifiers, such as alloplastic keratophakia for aphakia using a hydrogel lenticule or "aphakic hydrogel intracorneal lens (ICL)," which unfortunately makes the terminology more cumbersome.

This study was supported by National Eye Institute Grant No. EY-03761.

Table 35-1. Classification of Refractive Surgery 1991

Type of Refractive Surgery	Surgical Technique	Variations of Surgical Technique	Refractive Error Treated	Comment
Lamellar	Keratomileusis (carving corneal disc)	Barraquer cryolathe	Myopia, hyperopia aphakia	Secured with or without sutures Manual or computerized
		BKS nonfreeze microkeratome with suction mold	Myopia, hyperopia, aphakia	
		Excimer laser (argon fluoride gas, 193 nm)	Myopia	FDA trial in USA
	Keratomileusis in situ (carving corneal bed)	Microkeratome (plano excision)	Myopia	Multiple techniques evolving
		Keratokyphosis (refractive mold in microkeratome)	Myopia	In laboratory development
		Excimer laser (ArF gas, 193 nm)	Myopia	FDA trial in USA
	Lamellar keratotomy	Single deep microkeratome pass	Hyperopia	Early clinical trials
	Epikerato-plasty	Human donor, cryolathe (lyophilized, commercially available), circular keratotomy	Aphakia Keratoconus	If IOL contraindicted If PK contraindicted
		BKS nonfreeze and suction mold,	Myopia	FDA core study
		Synthetic (such as collagen; coated hydrogel)	None	In laboratory development
	Intracorneal lens (keratophakia)	Hydrogel	Aphakia, myopia	FDA trial in USA
		Fresnel intracorneal lens, hydrogel	Aphakia, myopia	In laboratory development
		High index of refraction (such as fenestrated polysulfone)		In laboratory development
		Intracorneal ring (PMMA, hydrogel)	Myopia, hyperopia	FDA trial in USA
		Gel injection adjustable keratoplasty (GIAK)	Myopia	In laboratory development
		Human donor, cryolathe	Aphakia, hyperopia	Not in clinical use
		Autokeratophakia, corneal flap		Under development in Russian Federation
	Lamellar keratoplasty	Central	Astigmatism and myopia from keratoconus	
		Crescentic	Astigmatism from marginal thinning (such as Terrien's)	
Refractive keratotomy	Radial	Single nomogram	Myopia	
		Staged with repeated adjustments		

From Waring GO: *Arch Ophthalmol* 103:1472-1477, 1985.
ArF, Argon fluoride; *BKS,* Barraquer-Krumeich-Swinger; *FDA,* Food and Drug Administration; *IOL,* intraocular lens; *PMMA,* poly(methyl methacrylate); *PK,* penetrating keratoplasty; *RK,* radial keratotomy; *YAG,* yttrium-aluminum-garnet laser.

Table 35-1. Classification of Refractive Surgery 1991—cont'd

Type of Refractive Surgery	Surgical Technique	Variations of Surgical Technique	Refractive Error Treated	Comment
	Transverse	Straight or arcuate (T cuts)	Astigmatism naturally occurring postoperatively	
		Isolated incisions Combined with radial Between radial Interrupted transverse Interrupted radial Trapezoidal (Ruiz, semiradial)		Used infrequently
	Modification of penetrating keratoplasty		Astigmatism	Staged under keratoscopic or keratometric control
		Wound revision Incision in wound or donor (relaxing incision)		
		Suture adjustment (removal or cutting of interrupted, distribution of tension on running)		Acts like keratotomy
	Circumferential	Hexagonal nonconnected with transverse (T-hex)	Hyperopia	Multiple techniques evolving
		Circular partial thickness trephination with running suture	Astigmatism	Early clinical trials evolving
Laser	Excimer laser (ArF gas, 193 nm)	Photorefractive keratectomy (PRK) (central sculpting; sculpting; large area ablation)	Myopia	FDA trial in USA
		Therapeutic PRK	Postoperative myopia (as after RK, PK)	FDA trial in USA
		Linear keratectomy (radial, transverse)	Myopia, astigmatism	Not in clinical use
	Intrastromal, solid-state laser	"Central intrastromal photokeratectomy"; picosecond YAG 1053 nm	Myopia	In laboratory development
		"Intrastromal photorefractive keratectomy, laser plasma-wave keratectomy"; nanosecond YAG 1064 nm		
Keratectomy, manual	Crescentic wedge	Wedge resection after penetrating keratoplasty	Astigmatism	
		Wound repair during or after cataract extraction		
	Crescentic lamellar	Corneal tuck or flap for Terrien's pellucid degeneration	Astigmatism	

Continued.

Table 35-1. Classification of Refractive Surgery 1991—cont'd

Type of Refractive Surgery	Surgical Technique	Variations of Surgical Technique	Refractive Error Treated	Comment
Thermokerato-plasty	Holmium:YAG laser	Peripheral, intrastro-mal radial pattern	Hyperopia	FDA trial in USA
		Flat meridian	Astigmatism	
	Stromal thermo-coagualation	Hot needle, peripheral radial pattern	Hyperopia	Early clinical evalua-tion
		Arcuate in one merid-ian	Astigmatism	
	Central surface coagu-lation	Thermophore	Keratoconus	Seldom used clinically
Penetrating kera-toplasty and cataract surgery (refractive as-pects)	Incisions	Uniform and small	Astigmatism	
	Wound closure	Sutures uniform	Astigmatism	
	Astigmatism reduction	Suture adjustment		
		Transverse keratotomy		
		Wound revision		
Phakic IOL	IOL calculations	Monofocal		Minimal spherical ametropia
		Multifocal		
	Clear lens extraction	With or without IOL	High myopia	Risk of retinal detach-ment
	Anterior chamber	Multiflex	Myopia	FDA trial in USA: Eu-rope
	Iris fixated	Spider claw		Japan, Europe
	Posterior chamber	Silicone		Russian Federation
Posterior scleral support	Multiple techniques (X, Y, I shapes)	Sclera, fascia lata, car-tilage, synthetics	Pathologic myopia with staphyloma	Retard progression of staphyloma

The classification includes corneal, scleral, and in-traocular lens surgery.

Lamellar Refractive Keratoplasty. Lamellar re-fractive keratoplasty involves the placement of a lenticule on or within the cornea to alter its refrac-tive power, usually by changing its anterior curva-ture. There are four lamellar refractive keratoplasty techniques:

1. *Keratomileusis* (Fig. 35-1) is the removal of an an-terior disc of corneal tissue, which is then carved on its posterior stromal surface to change its radius of curvature, using a cryolathe, a planar microkera-tome technique, or an excimer laser. Alternatively, tissue can be removed from the bed of the resection. The disc is then sutured back in place onto the cor-nea.

2. *Epikeratoplasty* (Fig. 35-2), in which a lenticule with power is fashioned from a human donor cornea (by either a cryolathe or a nonfreeze technique) or a synthetic lenticule, such as one made from collagen, is manufactured with power (currently an experi-mental technique in animals), and the lenticule is at-tached to the deepithelialized surface of Bowman's layer. Currently, the most commonly used attach-ment technique is a circular, undermined keratot-omy with running or interrupted sutures. In the fu-ture tissue adhesives might be used.

3. *Intracorneal lens (or keratophakia, lens in the cor-nea).* Classically, a human donor[25] lenticule was fash-ioned on a cryolathe, but currently a synthetic plastic lenticule is placed within the corneal stroma (Fig. 35-3), with use of either a hydrogel lenticule placed beneath a corneal disc removed with a microkera-tome or a fenestrated lenticule of high index of refrac-tion placed in a lamellar pocket incision (experimen-tal technique in laboratory animals). A new technique being developed in laboratory animals is to place an intracorneal ring in a lamellar circular dissection in the peripheral cornea, with use of the volume of the ring to change the curvature of the central cornea.

4. *Lamellar keratoplasty[19] or epikeratoplasty in which the lenticule has no refractive power* is used to diminish the myopia and irregular astigmatism of keratoco-nus (Fig. 35-4) or of some corneal thinning disor-ders.[20]

New techniques will have new appellations, such as those that use a mold to shape the corneal bed or the lenticule as they are cut with a microkeratome, including keratokyphosis[14] ('a protrusion of the cor-nea').

Keratotomy. Keratotomy ('cutting the cornea') involves making a partial-thickness incision into the cornea to flatten it and reduce its refractive power in that meridian. The term "refractive keratotomy" designates all such incisions. A description of the pattern of the incisions usually modifies the term,[10] such as radial[32] (Fig. 35-5), transverse incisions across the steep corneal meridian (T-cuts), and trapezoidal-Ruiz incisions (transverse incisions between two semiradial ones) (Fig. 35-6). In general, four to eight radial incisions are used to decrease myopia, often in a sequential or staged manner to approximate the desired final correction. Transverse incisions may be either straight or arcuate and are used along or in combination with radial incisions to reduce astigmatism. Arcuate transverse incisions are used after penetrating keratoplasty in the donor or

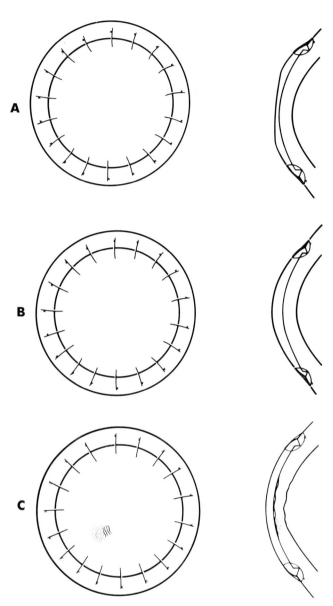

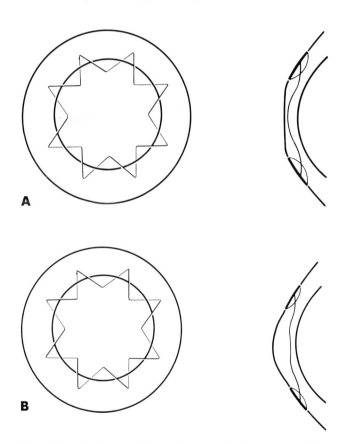

Fig. 35-1. A, Keratomileusis for myopia involves excision of a lamellar disc of patient's cornea with a microkeratome, carving of disc on a cryolathe or die to form a concave lenticule, and suturing the lenticule back onto cornea. This flattens central corneal curvature and decreases refractive power. **B** Keratomileusis for aphakia involves a similar process using a convex lenticule that steepens corneal curvature and increases refractive power. (From Waring GO: *Arch Ophthalmol* 103:1472-1477, 1985.)

Fig. 35-2. A, Epikeratoplasty for myopia involves removal of a lamellar disc from a donor cornea, carving it on a cryolathe or die to form a concave lenticule, placing it on surface of deepithelialized recipient cornea, and suturing it into a peripheral circumferential groove or incision. This flattens the central corneal curvature and decreases refractive power. **B,** Epikeratoplasty for aphakia involves a similar process using a convex donor lenticule that steepens corneal curvature, increasing refractive power. **C,** Epikeratoplasty for keratoconus employs a donor lenticule without power to flatten cornea and diminish myopia and irregular astigmatism. (From Waring GO: *Arch Ophthalmol* 103:1472-1477, 1985.)

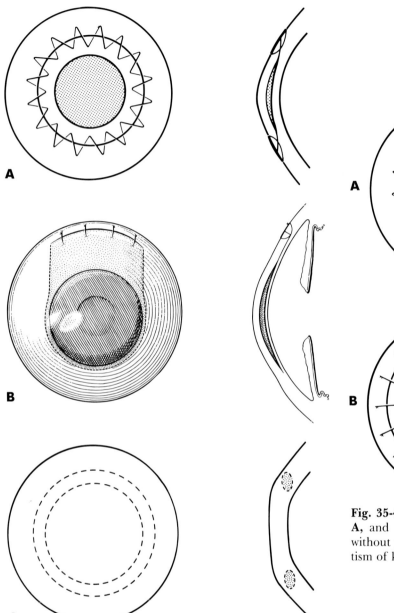

Fig. 35-3. Keratophakia involves placement of a lenticule within corneal stroma to change refraction of cornea. **A,** If lenticule is designed to change curvature of anterior surface of cornea, excision of a lamellar disc of cornea with a microkeratome is necessary. Then lenticule of a human donor cornea or hydrogel material is placed in lamellar bed, and disc of recipient cornea is resutured into its original position. **B,** If donor lenticule has a different index of refraction, thereby changing refraction of cornea, it can be placed in a deep lamellar pocket. **C,** Developing technology involves use of intracorneal rings placed in peripheral cornea, reducing hazard of placing a lenticule in visual axis. (**A** and **B** from Waring GO: *Arch Ophthalmol* 103: 1472-1477, 1985.)

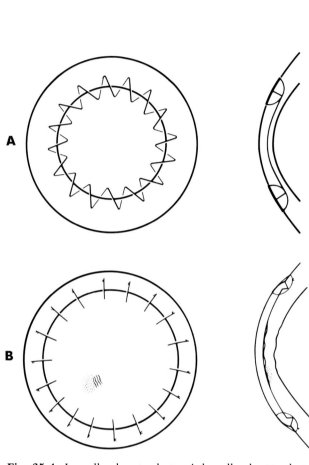

Fig. 35-4. Lamellar keratoplasty. A lamellar keratoplasty, **A,** and epikeratoplasty, **B,** can employ donor lenticules without power to diminish myopia and irregular astigmatism of keratoconus.

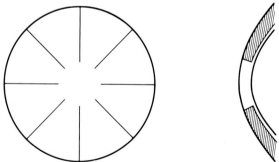

Fig. 35-5. Radial keratotomy for myopia. Equally spaced radial incisions made deeply into corneal stroma flatten central cornea and decrease its refractive power, reducing refractive error in myopia.

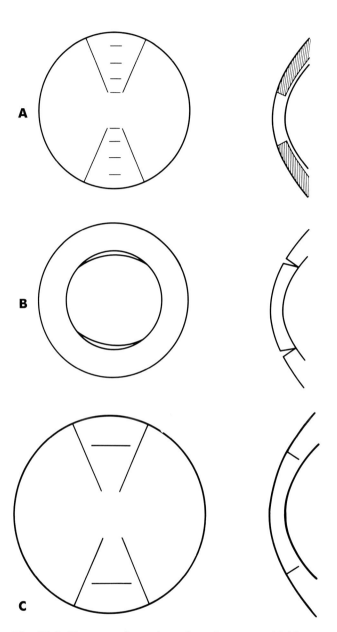

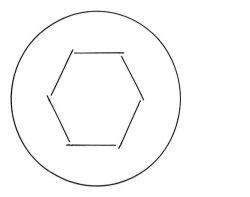

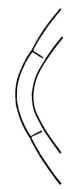

Fig. 35-7. Circumferential keratotomy (hexagonal keratotomy) for management of hyperopia is undergoing trial-and-error refinement.

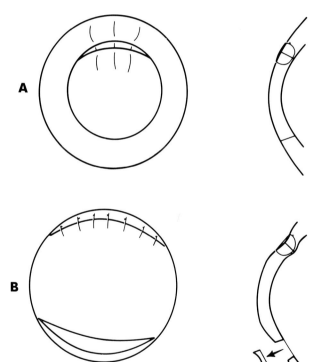

Fig. 35-6. Keratomy for astigmatism. **A,** Trapezoidal keratotomy consists in two semiradial incisions and four non-connecting transverse incisions that flatten corneal curvature and decrease its refractive power in axis of surgery. **B,** Arcuate keratotomy (relaxing incision) consists in deep incisions into healed scar in steepest axis that flatten that axis and reduce astigmatism after penetrating keratoplasty. **C,** Keratotomy for astigmatism involves transverse incisions made in steep meridian that do not intersect other incisions. The incisions flatten steep meridian and steepen flat meridian.

Fig. 35-8. Keratectomy for astigmatism. A crescentic wedge resection, **A,** can reduce astigmatism after a penetrating keratoplasty by removal of a piece of tissue from corneal scar in flat axis and resuturing wound together, which steepens that axis and increases refractive power of cornea. A crescentic lamellar keratectomy, **B,** can help manage thinning disorders of peripheral cornea by strengthening thin areas and by steepening flat axis of central cornea.

in the wound to decrease astigmatism (relaxing incisions)[10,24] (Fig. 35-6).

Keratotomies to treat hyperopia by creating a circular keratotomy either partial thickness with a trephine or the making of nonconnected hexagonal incisions around a 7 mm zone without the addition of transverse incision outside the apices (hexagonal keratotomy, T-hex procedure) are under development (Fig. 35-7).

Keratectomy. Keratectomy designates excision of a piece of cornea, used in this context to change the refraction of the cornea. There are three basic types of keratectomy: (1) keratectomy with an excimer laser (discussed below), (2) wedge-shaped keratectomy (wedge resection) to decrease astigmatism after penetrating keratoplasty[15] or cataract surgery, and (3) a lamellar crescentic keratectomy for Terrien's marginal degeneration or pellucid degeneration[5] (Fig. 35-8). Revising and resuturing a slipped or separated corneal or limbal wound acts like a keratectomy because it steepens the cornea in the meridian of surgery.[6,28]

Laser Refractive Corneal Surgery.[31] Because the field of laser corneal surgery is expanding rapidly, I present here more detail concerning the classification and terminology used in laser corneal surgery (Fig. 35-9).

Fundamental to all designations is the fact that the pulsed laser light removes tissue from the cornea. Therefore a cut made with the laser is an excision—a keratectomy—that leaves a defect, not an incision—a keratotomy—that leaves only a dehiscence. A term such as "excimer laser radial keratotomy" is inaccurate. The fundamental effect of a pulsed excimer laser on tissue is a photochemical one, the breaking of molecular bonds with tissue fragments flying from the surface at supersonic speeds. This process has been designated photoablative decomposition—photoablation for short. This process contrasts with the more familiar photocoagulation of an argon laser and photodisruption of an Nd:YAG laser emitting at 1064 nm.

The use of other types of lasers in corneal surgery complicates the terminology. For example, a frequency-doubled Nd:YAG or an Nd:YLF (yttrium-lithium-fluoride) laser produces photodisruption by shock waves, not photoablation. So, intrastromal sur-

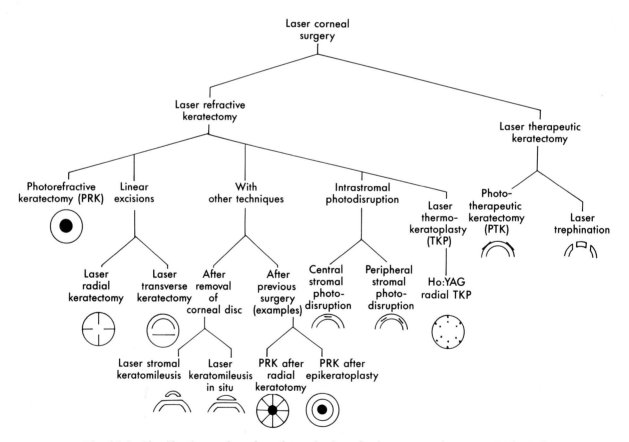

Fig. 35-9. Classification and preferred terminology for laser corneal surgery. (Adapted from Waring GO: *Refract Corneal Surg* 6:318-320, 1990.)

gery done with this type of laser is called intrastromal photodisruption, not intrastromal ablation.

The generic term "laser corneal surgery" can easily be modified to the terms "laser refractive corneal surgery" or "laser therapeutic corneal surgery," in order to designate the two major categories. Since lasers remove tissue, the term "keratectomy" is used in the proposed terminology; this should be strictly adhered to regarding usage of such terms as "laser refractive keratectomy" and "laser therapeutic keratectomy."

There are four types of laser refractive keratectomy: (1) removal of a graded amount of tissue from the anterior central cornea, (2) the creation of linear excisions in a radial or transverse pattern, (3) removal of stroma after a microkeratome disc resection (laser keratomileusis), and (4) intrastromal photodisruption.

The term "photorefractive keratectomy" (PRK) has come to mean the central removal of a specific profile of Bowman's layer and anterior stroma to change the anterior curvature of the cornea. This is a good example of how the usage of language determines its meaning because, strictly speaking, the term "photorefractive keratectomy" refers to all types of laser refractive corneal surgery. Nevertheless, photorefractive keratectomy (PRK) has become the preferred term for what is otherwise called "laser anterior keratomileusis," "large area ablation," and "reprofiling or sculpting of the cornea" (Fig. 35-10).

Designations of other refractive surgery techniques that involve the laser simply borrow preexisting terms and add the prefix "laser" or "excimer laser" to designate this new method of surgery, such as "excimer laser keratomileusis" (usage analogous to cryolathe keratomileusis and nonfreeze keratomileusis) and "excimer laser keratomileusis in situ"—both designating the removal of stromal tissue with a laser after a lamellar disc of cornea has already been removed with a microkeratome.

Using a laser to make a linear cut is analogous to making cuts with a diamond knife, except that the cuts are excisions rather than incisions of tissue. The laser actually creates a groove or trough in the tissue and does not merely sever the tissue; the proper term is "laser radial or transverse keratectomy." Removing stromal tissues without disrupting the surfaces of the cornea requires a nonultraviolet laser that is not absorbed by the cornea but that can focus energy within the stroma, such as an Nd:YLF. This creates an intrastromal cavity by photodisruption. Whether this technique can create a predictable refractive change in the cornea remains to be determined.

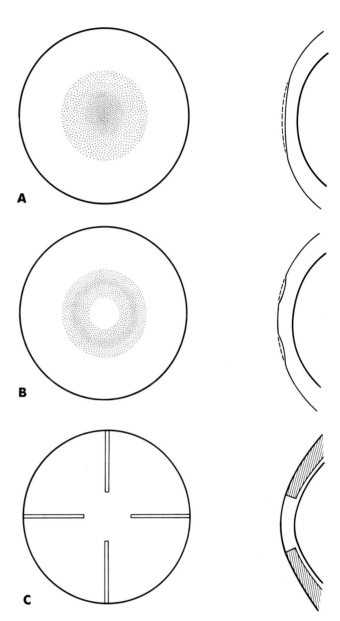

Fig. 35-10. Laser refractive keratectomy involves use of ultraviolet excimer or other type of laser to remove tissue from cornea. One technique is anterior keratomileusis (large-area ablation corneal etching or reprofiling), in which center of cornea is carved, **A,** to increase its minus power to treat myopia or, **B,** to increase its plus power to treat hyperopia. **C,** Another technique is excision of fine radial grooves (radial keratectomy), which function in the same way as radial keratotomy. Transverse excisions also can be made to correct astigmatism.

Another surgical use of the laser is to refine the result of a previous refractive surgical procedure; I suggest simply using the term "photorefractive keratectomy" (PRK) in conjunction with the original procedure: for example, PRK after radial keratotomy. If the modification is done on a synthetic epikeratoplasty, a new acronym such as LASE (laser adjustable synthetic epikeratophakia) may emerge (Fig. 35-11).

Using the laser to create a lenticule of corneal tissue, in the same way that a microkeratome or a manual lamellar dissection does, involves a lamellar cut tangent to the apex of the cornea, and can therefore be called a "lamellar resection" or "tangential resection." This is distinguished from a "tangential ablation," in which the laser coming from the side ablates the tissue from the central anterior surface of the cornea, rather than the usual en face technique.

Laser therapeutic keratectomy comes in two varieties. The first involves the removal of a superficial corneal opacity or irregularity. Some have termed this "superficial keratectomy," which is an accurate but inadequate term because the term also includes photorefractive keratectomy, which is a type of superficial keratectomy. Again, usage dictates meaning, and the term "phototherapeutic keratectomy"

(PTK) generally means the removal of anterior diseased layers of the cornea.

There is a second type of laser therapeutic keratectomy, laser trephination—using the laser to make circular or elliptical incisions for penetrating or lamellar keratoplasty.

I have not mentioned some terms for procedures that are not yet in use, such as making a circular oblique keratectomy as the bed for the wing of an epikeratoplasty, where the laser cut substitutes for the vertical trephination and lateral undermining. As new uses for the laser develop, there will certainly be new terms to describe them, such as "laser intrastromal thermokeratoplasty."

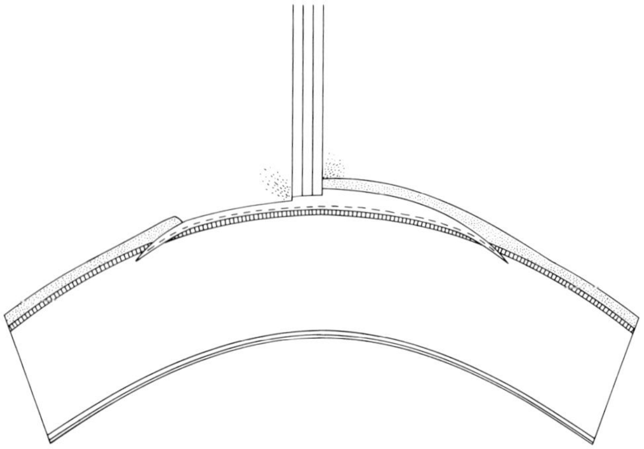

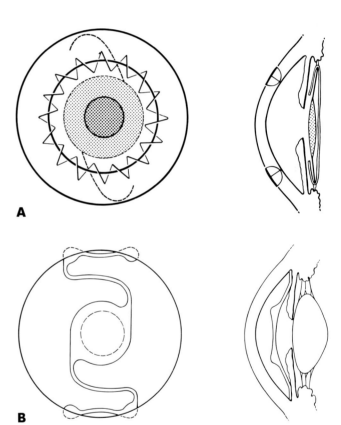

Fig. 35-12. A, In penetrating keratoplasty, residual astigmatism can be diminished by careful attention to wound configuration, suture pattern, and trephination. In eyes that contain an intraocular lens, spherical power of corneal graft should correlate appropriately with that of intraocular lens and with axial length of globe to achieve desired final refraction. **B,** Placement of a vaulted, open-loop anterior chamber intraocular lens into a phakic eye to correct myopia raises questions about long-term development of damage to angle with glaucoma, endothelial damage with rubbing of eye, and possible cataract formation in clear crystalline lens. (From Waring GO: *Arch Ophthalmol* 103:1472-1477, 1985.)

Fig. 35-11. Laser-adjustable synthetic epikeratoplasty. A synthetic epikeratoplasty lenticule (clear in this figure) has been placed onto surface of Bowman's layer and into a peripheral circular keratotomy. Epithelium has grown over epikeratoplasty lenticule. If curvature of lenticule is not that desired, a laser is used to recarve lenticule into new shape. This has advantage of repeated adjustability, absence of wound healing, since lenticule contains no cells, and potential replaceability, since lenticule can be removed and replaced. (From Waring GO: *Arch Ophthalmol* 103: 1472-1477, 1985.)

Penetrating Keratoplasty. The major reason for doing a penetrating keratoplasty is to replace the central portion of a scarred or distorted cornea by clear regular donor tissue. Between 1940 and 1980, the major clinical challenge was to maintain a clear graft. However, now that grafts remain clear in approximately 85% of cases,[4,29] control of the refractive effect of the donor has become increasingly important, especially when an intraocular lens is used, as in a combined penetrating keratoplasty, cataract extraction, and intraocular lens insertion (triple procedure, Fig. 35-12). The surgeon not only must control factors that affect the spherical power of the graft (such as wound configuration, suture pattern, donor size), but also must select an intraocular lens power that appropriately matches the final refractive power of the graft and the axial length of the globe.[7]

Control of astigmatism during and after penetrating keratoplasty is an important refractive component. Creating the most uniform wound configuration and suture placement will help diminish astigmatism. Adjustment of sutures after surgery can do the same, either by selective removal of interrupted sutures in the steep semimeridian or by adjustment of the tension on a running suture to distribute it more evenly and create a more spherical cornea.[12,15,16]

Thermokeratoplasty. There are four general categories of applying heat to the cornea to change its curvature: (1) Actual coagulation of the corneal surface with a hot cautery tip, as may be done to flatten a keratoconus cornea during surgery;[13] (2) use of temperature-controlled flat probe to heat the anterior cornea and shrink the collagen to flatten the cornea in keratoconus, a procedure now abandoned[11] (Fig. 35-13, A); (3) intrastromal thermal coagulation using a hot-tipped probe that penetrates deeply into the stroma and shrinks the collagen, with this being done in a radial fashion in the peripheral cornea in order to steepen the central cornea and treat hyperopia (Fig. 35-13, B); (4) laser thermokeratoplasty, which can be done using a holmium:YAG laser to create focal spots of intrastromal thermal coagulation. The spots contract the stromal collagen, flattening the peripheral cornea and steepening the central cornea to treat hyperopia. If done in only one meridian, the intrastromal burns can steepen the flat meridian to treat astigmatism.[21]

Other Classification Systems. There are other approaches to the classification of refractive corneal surgery. One is to use the ametropia being treated[22]—myopia, hyperopia, aphakia, or astigmatism—as the basis, but this requires repeated description of similar surgical techniques for each refractive error, such as keratomileusis for myopia and for aphakia. A more

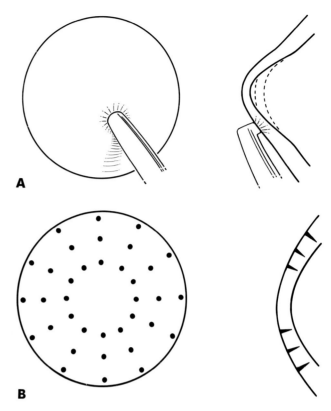

Fig. 35-13. In thermokeratoplasty, controlled application of heat into stroma can shrink and scar stromal collagen. **A,** Central-surface thermokeratoplasty involves application of heat to surface to shrink underlying collagen and reduce ectasia of cornea in keratoconus. **B,** Radial intrastromal thermokeratoplasty shrinks peripheral and paracentral stromal collagen, producing a central steepening of cornea to treat hyperopia. (From Waring GO: *Arch Ophthalmol* 103:1472-1477, 1985.)

abstract classification is based on the type of alteration of the cornea[1] resection of tissue (for example, keratomileusis, wedge resection), relaxation of the tissue (for example, radial keratotomy, suture removal), addition of tissue (for example, keratophakia, epikeratoplasty), substitution of tissue (for example, penetrating keratoplasty, keratomileusis using a donor cornea), retraction of tissue (for example, thermokeratoplasty), and compression of tissue (for example, tight sutures, epikeratoplasty for keratoconus). One may also classify refractive corneal surgery in bioengineering terms: changes in corneal volume, thickness, surface area,[27] and, in the future, even stress-strain forces. Meanwhile, a classification based on surgical technique (Table 35-1) will enhance communication and understanding among those interested in refractive surgery.

TERMINOLOGY USED IN TRANSPLANTATION

The fields of genetics, tissue transplantation, and refractive corneal surgery share a common language that seems to remain in flux, creating confusion about words that contain the Greek prefixes auto-, iso-, syn-, allo-, homo-, xeno-, and hetero-. Consensus among the three fields is emerging[2,22] for the usage outlined in Table 35-2.

An autograft involves tissue from the host, as in keratomileusis. An allograft involves tissue from a donor of the same species who has a different genetic makeup, as in a penetrating keratoplasty, epikeratoplasty, and both keratophakia and keratomileusis using a human donor cornea. The term "alloplastic" refers to use of synthetic donor material as in keratophakia using a hydrogel lenticule. Unfortunately, there is confusion here, since an allograft with donor tissue is sometimes colloquially referred to as an "alloplasty." In a xenograft, the donor tissue comes from a species different from the host. No xenografts give good clinical results in human corneal surgery.

TERMINOLOGY FOR CORNEAL TOPOGRAPHY

To best understand the results of refractive corneal surgical procedures, one must apply methods of measuring the change in the shape of the cornea. The most current method is videokeratography, a technique that has allowed us to better define the terminology and concepts underlying the measurement of corneal curvature and shape.

In an attempt to improve communication in the field of corneal topography and measurement, I propose here some terminology usage that I hope will become conventional.[30] The terms presented here refer to the corneal surface, its topography, and related items and do not cover corneal optics. See Table 35-2.

Measurement of Corneal Curvature and Shape

Corneal light reflection. The image formed by light reflected from the convex anterior corneal surface is first called the Purkinje image, the corneal light reflex, or the corneal light reflection. This virtual, erect image is viewed during keratometry and keratoscopy and is located approximately 4 mm posterior to the surface of the cornea at the level of the anterior lens capsule. Because the reflected image size is determined by the curvature of the cornea (the greater the curvature, the smaller the image), it can be used to quantify corneal curvature and power.

Keratometer (ophthalmometer). This is a good example of how colloquial usage can set linguistic standards. "Keratometer" is the trade name of Bausch & Lomb, but like Xerox and Kleenex, the commercial term has taken on a generic use. The original designation by von Helmholtz (1853) for an instrument that measures the central corneal curvature was

Table 35-2. Types of Grafts Used in Refractive Corneal Surgery

Type of Graft	Synonym	Source of Tissue	Genetic Identity of Donor	Examples from Human Corneal Surgery
Autograft (G. *autos*, self)	Autoplastic procedure	Host	Identical (autogeneic)	Keratomileusis Penetrating keratoplasty donor from opposite eye
Isograft (G. *isos*, equal)	None	Monozygotic twin	Near identical isogeneic, syngeneic	Penetrating keratoplasty donor from identical twin
Allograft (G. *allos*, another—in the sense of another person)	Homograft (G. *homos*, same—in the sense of same species) Homoplastic procedure	Another member of same species	Dissimilar (allogeneic homogeneic	Keratomileusis or keratophakia with human donor Epikeratoplasty Penetrating keratoplasty Lamellar keratoplasty
Alloplastic (G. *allos*, another—in the sense of another material)	Synthetic or inert implant, Intracorneal lens	Nonbiologic material	None	Keratophakia with plastic implant
Xenograft (G. *xenos*, foreign)	Heterograft (G. *heteros*, different)	Member of different species	Very dissimilar (xenogeneic, heterogeneic)	None

G., Word of Greek origin.

"ophthalmometer," a term still used outside the United States.[8]

Keratometry (ophthalmometry). A keratometer measures corneal curvature in designated meridians by reflection of a mire from small areas along an annulus 3 to 4 mm in diameter, centered around the apex of the cornea.[8,23] Keratometry done outside the central cornea must be designated as paracentral or peripheral, using instruments such as the topogometer or American Optical keratometer, neither of which is currently marketed.

Radius of curvature and refractive power of the cornea. The radius of curvature of the anterior and posterior corneal surfaces affects its refractive power (Fig. 35-14). A shorter radius of curvature creates a steeper arc and a greater refractive power. Conversely, a longer radius of curvature creates a flatter arc and less refractive power. All keratometers and keratoscopes measure the size of the image reflected from the anterior surface of the cornea and calculate the radius of curvature of the anterior surface and the refractive power of the whole cornea, using 1.3375 as the "keratometric" index of refraction for the cornea instead of the true index of 1.376.[8,23]

Keratoscope. An instrument that presents a series of mires, most commonly rings, to the corneal surface is a keratoscope. Keratoscopes fitted with a still film camera are called photokeratoscopes; those fitted with a video camera are called videokeratoscopes. The term "corneoscope" is the trade name used by the Kera Corporation.

Keratoscopy. Direct observation of the images of mires reflected from the surface of the cornea is keratoscopy, in the same sense that examination of the ocular fundus with an ophthalmoscope is ophthalmoscopy.

Keratography. The term "keratography" denotes a record or portrayal of the cornea in the same sense that angiography records the pattern of vessels. Currently, there are two methods of recording pictures (keratographs) of the mires reflected from the corneal surface: (1) With photographic film, one uses a

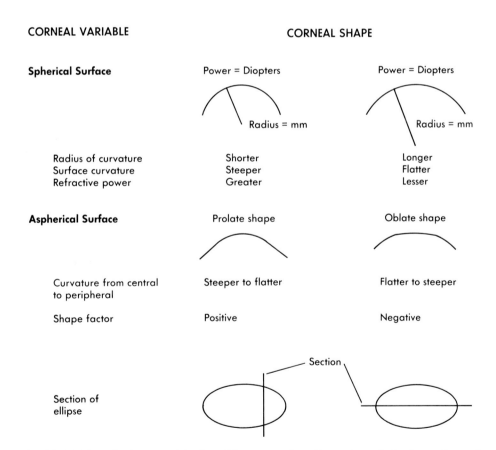

CORNEAL VARIABLE

CORNEAL SHAPE

Spherical Surface

	Power = Diopters	Power = Diopters
Radius = mm	Radius = mm
Radius of curvature	Shorter	Longer
Surface curvature	Steeper	Flatter
Refractive power	Greater	Lesser

Aspherical Surface

	Prolate shape	Oblate shape
Curvature from central to peripheral	Steeper to flatter	Flatter to steeper
Shape factor	Positive	Negative

Section of ellipse

Fig. 35-14. Terminology used in describing corneal configurations. *Left column,* Corneal variables described; *right columns,* terminology descriptive of topography of both spherical corneas and aspherical corneas. (From Waring GO: *Refract Corneal Surg* 5:360-367, 1989.)

photokeratoscope to produce a photokeratograph, a process called "photokeratography" (in the same sense that one uses a photomicroscope to take a photomicrograph). (2) With video recording, one uses a videokeratoscope to produce a videokeratograph, a process called "videokeratography."

A keratograph can be interpreted qualitatively or quantitatively. A qualitative interpretation is done by visual inspection of the shape and spacing of the mires and has practical value in the diagnosing of corneal disorders such as keratoconus or in the adjustment of sutures after penetrating keratoplasty. Quantitative keratography is done by the assignment of numerical coordinate values to points on the mires and the mathematical description of the curves that the points form. Complex formulas and algorithms are required for accurate quantitation of its topography. Quantitative is usually done with the assistance of a computer that uses image analysis programs and is located in a separate instrument (as in the Kera and Nidek systems—both photokeratoscopes) or in the keratoscope itself (as in the Computed Anatomy, Visio, and KeraView systems—all computer-assisted videokeratoscopes).

Topography. Topography refers to the shape of surfaces, whether they be the surface of the earth or the surface of the cornea. The most common representation is a topographic map on which the relative elevations of the surface are delimited by contour lines.

Topographic displays. The mires used to study corneal shape have many configurations: circles, arcs, parallel lines, interference fringes, steps. Those most commonly used are circular rings. The concentric ring mires are commonly called Placido* rings, but strictly speaking, that designation should describe only Placido's flat disc with the equally spaced circular black rings. Modern keratoscope rings are designed differently. By convention, the rings are numbered from innermost to outermost. This can be confusing, because a specific ring (such as ring 3) in different instruments may cover a different location on different corneas. Therefore it is important to designate the diameter of a projected ring and indicate the area on the cornea that it covers.

There are four basic methods of displaying corneal topographic information: (1) the keratograph, (2) representation of the radius of curvature or dioptric power at various locations on the surface of the cornea, either in a fixed pattern on a "face plate" or at any location identified by a cursor in a computer-assisted videokeratoscope, (3) graphic three-

dimensional figures often with exaggerations to show changes in curvature, and (4) color-coded maps using colors to designate areas of uniform radius of curvature and refractive power. The most widely used system of color coding[17] is reds and oranges to indicate steeper areas with greater refractive power and greens and blues to indicate flatter areas with less refractive power (LSU Topography System, Computed Anatomy Corneal Modeling System). A quantitative scale indicates the values corresponding to each color.

Shape of the Anterior Cornea

Corneal asphericity. The anterior corneal surface is asymmetrically aspheric; that is, the radius of curvature changes from the center to the limbus and does so at a different rate along different semimeridians. Some day our simplified conception of the cornea as a spherocylindrical lens may be replaced by more accurate "shape factors," mathematical indices or ray-tracing diagrams.[9]

A useful simplification to understand the topography of the cornea is to consider the corneal curvature as a section of an ellipse. In most normal corneas, the central zone is steeper than the paracentral and peripheral zones, a configuration referred to as having a positive shape factor (positive because the radius of curvature becomes larger from the center to the periphery) and a prolate shape (the shape of a section across the steep end of an ellipse). The opposite topographic pattern rarely occurs in normal eyes but appears commonly after radial keratotomy: the central zone is flatter than the paracentral and peripheral zones, a configuration referred to as having a negative shape factor and an oblate shape (because it resembles a section across the flatter side of an ellipse) (Fig. 35-14).

Surface zones of the cornea. A similar oversimplification takes place when the cornea is divided into surface zones (such as "optical zone," "apical zone"). None of these areas is discrete, because the cornea forms continuous curves. Nevertheless, for practical optical and anatomic purposes, we can divide the surface of the cornea into two overall regions: the central optical zone and the remainder of the cornea (sometimes called the "periphery").[18] The optical zone forms the foveal image through the entrance pupil of the eye; its size, shape, and curvature vary among individuals. The rest of the cornea serves as a refracting surface for peripheral vision and for the foveal image when the pupil is widely dilated, as a mechanical structure, and as a source of cells during normal turnover and repair.

Conventionally, four concentric anatomic zones are recognized (Fig. 35-15): central optical zone,

---

*Accent always on first syllable.

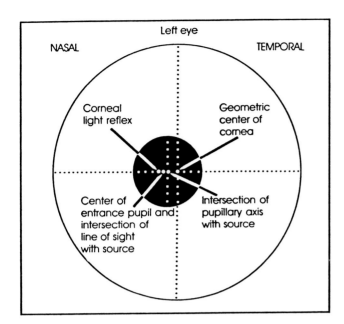

Fig. 35-15. Intersection of various axes with cornea. (Redrawn from Waring GO: *Refract Corneal Surg* 5:364, 1989.)

paracentral intermediate zone, peripheral transitional zone, and limbal zone (Fig. 35-16).

Central zone. The central zone is approximately 4 mm in diameter and has been called the apical zone, the corneal cap, the optical zone, the central spherical zone—all terms intended to designate this region of the cornea as the more spherical, symmetric, and optically important. Now that corneal topography is requiring more careful definitions, we must distinguish among four designations: (1) the anatomic central zone, which is 3 to 4 mm in diameter; (2) the functional optical zone, which is the area that overlies the entrance pupil; (3) the "spherical" central part of the cornea, which is present in a minority of normal corneas; and (4) the apex of the cornea, which is the highest spot on the cornea (as discussed subsequently).

The center of the optical zone can be defined in one of five ways, depending on the optical circumstances: (1) the anatomic center of the cornea equidistant from the limbus; (2) the optical axis, which connects the center of curvature of the cornea and centers of curvature of the crystalline lens; (3) the pupillary axis which connects the center of the entrance pupil and the center of curvature of the cornea; (4) the line of sight which connects the fixation point with the center of the entrance pupil; and (5) the visual axis which passes from the center of the foveola through the nodal points of the eye (Fig. 35-16). Detailed discussion of these often confusing axes can be found in most standard ophthalmic and

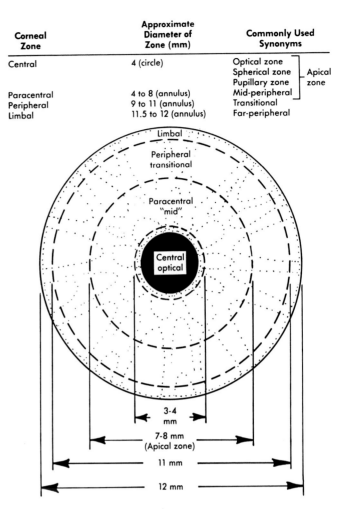

Corneal Zone	Approximate Diameter of Zone (mm)	Commonly Used Synonyms	
Central	4 (circle)	Optical zone Spherical zone Pupillary zone	Apical zone
Paracentral	4 to 8 (annulus)	Mid-peripheral	
Peripheral	9 to 11 (annulus)	Transitional	
Limbal	11.5 to 12 (annulus)	Far-peripheral	

Fig. 35-16. Terminology for describing *anatomic* (not optical) topographic regions (zones) of cornea, including circular central zone and three concentric annular zones. (From Waring GO: *Refract Corneal Surg* 5:360-367, 1989.)

physiologic optics textbooks. For practical purposes, the center of the optical zone should be considered the intersection of the pupillary axis with the cornea because the entrance pupil determines the image-forming bundle of rays that reach the fovea.

The term "optical zone" is used with four different meanings in the context of refractive surgery. The first meaning is that just defined, the central more spherical portion of the normal cornea overlying the entrance pupil. The second meaning refers to the portion of a keratomileusis lenticule, epikeratoplasty lenticule, or excimer laser surface ablation that creates the major refractive change; in this context, it is possible to decenter the "optical zone." The third meaning is the central uncut clear zone in radial keratotomy; the term optical zone (OZ) is so engrained in the radial keratotomy literature that it is not likely to disappear, even though the preferred designation is "clear zone." The fourth meaning is the diameter of any circular mark on the cornea, such as a "7 mm optical zone" used for placement of transverse incisions; in this context, "optical zone" is truly a misnomer and should be replaced by the simple designation "zone" or "zone mark," as in "the transverse incisions were placed at the 7 mm zone."

Paracentral zone. The paracentral zone is an annulus approximately 4 to 7 mm in diameter and has been called the "mid-", "intermediate" or "midperipheral" cornea. The term "midperipheral" is a misnomer because this zone does not occupy the middle of the periphery; a transverse incision made at the 6 mm zone is not "midperipheral" because it is still within the central anatomic half of the cornea. The central and paracentral zones together compose what contact lens fitters call the apical zone.

Peripheral zone. The peripheral zone is an annulus from approximately 7 to 11 mm in diameter. This is the area in which the normal cornea flattens the most and becomes more aspheric. For this reason it has been called the "transitional zone."

Limbal zone. The limbal zone is the rim of cornea approximately 0.5 mm wide that abuts the sclera.

Apex of the cornea. The apex of the cornea is the high spot of the cornea, the location of the greatest sagittal height on the surface. It is from this point that the corneal light reflection emanates, and therefore it is the point around which the keratoscopy rings center. The apex or high point of the normal cornea is close to the optical axis. However, in pathologic states such as keratoconus and after corneal surgery, the apex may be so displaced that the keratoscopy rings no longer center around any clearly identifiable point or axis on the cornea or over the entrance pupil. Thus the patient may be looking through an area of the cornea eccentric to that in the center of the keratography mires.

Directions on the Cornea: Meridians, Semimeridians, and Axes. Locations on the surface of the cornea are designated along meridians, lines that span the diameter of the cornea from one point on the limbus to the opposite point. Meridians are designated from 0 to 180 degrees, proceeding counterclockwise starting at 3 o'clock for both the right and left eyes (Fig. 35-17).

The term "axis" designates the direction in a cylindrical lens along which there is no power; it is parallel to the focal line. Because clinicians align the axes of cylindrical lenses with meridians on the cornea, it is common practice to substitute the term "axis" for "meridian" when referring to directions on the cornea. Thus clinicians commonly refer to the steep

"axis" of a cornea when they mean steep "meridian," a habit that is unlikely to change. When a clinician says that a correcting cylindrical lens is placed at a certain axis, he is simply using a short way of saying that the axis of the cylinder is placed along a certain corneal meridian; this short method is used so commonly as to be acceptable. However, when clinicians refer to the "steep axis" or the "flat axis" of the cornea, the term "axis" is used incorrectly; the term "meridian" should be used when referring to the direction of corneal refractive power.

Designating meridians as 0 to 180 degrees is conventional, but, unlike geographers, ophthalmologists have no north-south longitude lines to indicate a point along a meridian. Thus, if one refers to removing a tight corneal suture in the 90 degree meridian, it is not clear whether the activity occurs in the 12 o'clock direction or in the 6 o'clock direction. Therefore directions from the center of the cornea are designated as semimeridians and are located around the 360 degree circumference of the cornea measured in degrees, such as "the 225 degree semimeridian" (The term "semimeridian" is preferred, since both components are derived from Latin. The term "hemi-meridian" is a Greek-Latin hybrid, which etymologic purists eschew.) Another convention is to consider the cornea as the face of a clock so that 7:30 o'clock indicates the 225 degree semimeridian. This clock-hour system is too crude for refractive surgery, which requires more accuracy.

A specific point on the surface of the cornea is designated by an indication of its location in millimeters from the center of the cornea along a semimeridian. For example, at 3 mm from the center along the 225 degree semimeridian the corneal power may be 41.00 diopters (D). The location of a transverse incision could be accurately described as follows: it was placed 3 mm from the center at the 6 mm zone perpendicular to the 225-degree semimeridian (in current jargon, "A T cut was made at the 6 mm optical zone at 7:30.").

Refraction and Astigmatism. Finally, I include some meat-and-potatoes terminology commonly used in the correction of refractive errors. Definitions and details are contained in standard textbooks.

Refraction of the eye. Clinical refraction is the measurement of the spherocylindrical lens required to correct an ametropia.

Cylinder axis. The axis of a cylindrical lens lies along the direction that produces no refractive power. The axis of a plus cylinder lens that corrects corneal astigmatism is oriented along the steepest corneal meridian; the axis of a minus cylinder is aligned with the flattest meridian.

Direction of Refractive Power on the Cornea:
Meridians and Axes from 0° to 180°

Meridian: Arc across the cornea from limbus to
            limbus along which corneal power is
            measured
Axis: Orientation of cylindrical lens where
            there is no refractive power

Examples of three power meridians or cylindrical axes:

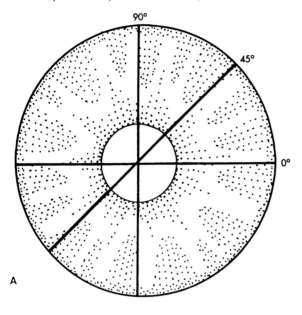

Locations on the Cornea: Semimeridians from
0° to 360° or from 1:00 O'Clock to 12 O'Clock
Plus Distance from Center of Cornea

Examples of point locations on three semimeridians

Point **A** is located on the 0°, or 3:00 o'clock, semimeridian
at 2 mm from the center. This is on the 4-mm
diameter zone mark.

Point **B** is located on the 90°, or 12:00 o'clock, semimeridian
at 3.5 mm from the center. This is on the 7-mm
diameter zone mark.

Point **C** is located on the 215° semimeridian at 5 mm
from the center. This is on the 10-mm diameter zone
mark.

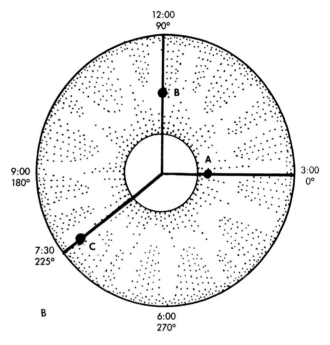

Fig. 35-17. Directions and locations on cornea **A,** Terminology describing meridional
directions on surface of cornea and axes of correcting cylindrical lenses. **B,** Locations of
specific points on cornea are described in terms of semimeridian along which point lies
and distance from geometric center of cornea. (From Waring GO: *Refract Corneal Surg*
5:360-367, 1989.)

Astigmatism. (Greek: *a-,* privative + *stigma,* 'a
puncture, spot') The optical condition under which
an eye cannot bring an image to a focal point because the refractive power varies in different meridians. Naturally occurring astigmatism is sometimes
mislabeled "congenital" astigmatism, an error because it is not always present at birth.

Regular astigmatism. A deviation of the ocular refraction or the corneal surface from spherical, such
that the radius of curvature changes gradually from
one meridian to the next.

Irregular astigmatism. Variation in corneal curvature such that the amounts or orientations of the
greatest and least curvatures vary across the refractive aperture. This cannot be completely corrected
by a cylindrical spectacle lens.

Net change in astigmatism. The total change in
astigmatism between two refractions or two keratometric measurements, regardless of the change in
the axis of the correcting cylinder.

Total induced astigmatism. The difference in the
amount of astigmatism at the preoperative axis and
the amount of astigmatism at the postoperative axis,
as calculated by vector analysis.

ACKNOWLEDGMENTS

This chapter is a modification of three previous publications on "Keratospeak" from Waring GO: Making sense of keratospeak: a classification of refractive corneal surgery, *Arch Ophthalmol* 103:1472-1477, 1985; Waring GO: Making sense of keratospeak II: conventional terminology for corneal topography, *Refract Corneal Surg* 5:363-367, 1989; and Waring GO: Classification and terminology of laser corneal surgery: making sense of keratospeak III, *Refract Corneal Surg* 6:318-320, 1990.

Appropriate acknowledgements of other contributors are made in the original publications.

REFERENCES

1. Barraquer JI: Basis of refractive keratoplasty, *Arch Soc Am Oftalmol Optom* 6:21-68, 1967.
2. Bellanti JA: *Immunology II*, Philadelphia, 1978, WB Saunders, p 82.
3. Binder PS: Refractive surgery: its current status and its future, *CLAO* 11:358-375, 1985.
4. Bourne WM: Current techniques for improved visual results after penetrating keratoplasty, *Opthalmic Surg* 12:321-327, 1981.
5. Caldwell DR, Insler MS, Boutros G, Hawk T: Primary surgical repair of severe peripheral marginal ectasia in Terrien's marginal degeneration, *Am J Ophthalmol* 97:332-336, 1984.
6. Cravy TV: Modification of postcataract astigmatism by wound revision. In Binder PS, editor: *Refractive corneal surgery: the correction of astigmatism*, Boston, 1983, Little, Brown, vol 23, pp 111-126.
7. Crawford GJ, Van Meter WS, Waring GO, et al: Prediction of intraocular lens power in the triple procedure, *Ophthalmology* 91(suppl):88, 1984.
8. Dabezies OH, Holladay JT: Measurement of corneal curvature: Keratometer (ophthalmometer). In Dabezies OH, editors: *Contact lenses: the CLAO guide to basic science and clinical practice*, Orlando, Fla, 1984, Grune & Stratton, 17.1-17.27.
9. Dingeldein SA, Klyce SD, Wilson SE: Quantitative descriptors of corneal shape derived from computer-assisted analysis of photokeratographs, *Refract Corneal Surg* 5:372-378, 1989.
10. Franks JB, Binder PS: Keratotomy procedures for the correction of astigmatism, *J Refract Surg* 1:11-17, 1985.
11. Gassett AR, Kaufman HE: Thermokeratoplasty in the treatment of keratoconus, *Am J Ophthalmol* 79:226-232, 1975.
12. Harris DJ, Waring GO, Burk LL: Keratography as a guide to selective suture removal for the reduction of astigmatism after penetrating keratoplasty, *Ophthalmology* 96:1597-1607, 1989.
13. Hatch JL: Thermal wedge with penetrating keratoplasty to reduce high corneal cylinder, *Am J Ophthalmol* 90:137-141, 1980.
14. Hoffmann F, Jessen K, Pahlitzsch T, Buchen R: Hypermetropic and myopic keratokyphosis: a new method of refractive keratoplasty. I. Effect of a synthetic lens on intraocular pressure, *Cornea* 1:137-141, 1982.
15. Krachmer JH, Fenzl RE: Surgical correction of high post-keratoplasty astigmatism: relaxing incisions versus wedge resection, *Arch Ophthalmol* 98:1400, 1980.
16. McNeill JI, Wessels, IF: Adjustment of single continuous suture to control astigmatism after penetrating keratoplasty, *Refract Corneal Surg* 5:216-223, 1989.
17. Maguire LJ, Singer DE, Klyce SD: Graphic presentation of computer-analyzed keratoscope photographs, *Arch Ophthalmol* 105:223-230, 1987.
18. Miller D, Carter J: A proposed new division of corneal functions. In Cavanagh HD. *The Cornea*, Transactions of the World Congress on the Cornea III, New York, 1980, Raven Press.
19. Richard JM, Paton D, Gasset AR: A comparison of penetrating keratoplasty and lamellar keratoplasty in the surgical management of keratoconus *Am J Ophthalmol* 86:807-811, 1978.
20. Schanzlin DJ, Sarno EM, Robin JB: Crescentic lamellar keratoplasty for pellucid marginal degeneration, *Am J Ophthalmol* 96:253-254, 1983.
21. Seiler T, Matallana M, Bende T: Laser thermokeratoplasty by means of a pulsed holmium:YAG laser for hyperopic correction, *Refract Corneal Surg* 6:335-339, 1990.
22. Stites DP, Stobo JD, Fudenberg HH, Wells JV: *Basic and clinical immunology*, ed 5, Los Altos, Calif, 1984, Lange Medical, pp 763-773.
23. Stone J: Keratometry. In Ruben M: *Contact lens practice: visual, therapeutic and prosthetic*, Baltimore, Md, 1975, Williams & Wilkins, pp 104-129.
24. Sugar J, Kirk AK: Relaxing keratotomy for postkeratoplasty high astigmatism, *Ophthalmic Surg* 14:156, 1983.
25. Taylor DM, Stern AL, Romanchok KG, Keilson LR: Keratophakia: clinical evaluation, *Ophthalmology* 88:1141, 1981.
26. Troutman RC: Microsurgical control of corneal astigmatism in cataract and keratoplasty, *Trans Am Acad Ophthalmol Otolaryngol* 77:563, 1973.
27. Troutman RC, Gaster RN, Swinger C: Refractive keratoplasty. In *Symposium on Medical and Surgical Disease of the Cornea*, Transactions of the New Orleans Academy of Ophthalmology, St. Louis, 1980, Mosby–Year Book.
28. van Rij G, Waring GO: Changes in corneal curvature induced by sutures and incisions, *Am J Ophthalmol* 98:773-783, 1984.
29. Völker-Dieben HJ, Kok-van Alphen CC, Lansbergen Q, Persijn G: Different influences on corneal graft survival in 539 transplants, *Acta Ophthalmol* 60:190-202, 1982.
30. Waring GO: Making sense of keratospeak II: proposed conventional terminology for corneal topography, *Refract Corneal Surg* 5:362-367, 1989.
31. Waring GO: Classification and terminology of laser corneal surgery: making sense of keratospeak III, *Refract Corneal Surg* 6:318-320, 1990.
32. Waring GO, Moffitt SD, Gelender H, et al: Rationale for and design on the National Eye Institute Prospective Evaluation of Radial Keratotomy (PERK) Study, *Ophthalmology* 90:40-58, 1983.

Chapter 36

Synthetic Keratophakia

Synthetic lamellar refractive keratoplasty

BERNARD E. McCAREY

Refractive keratoplasty procedures[1] are an attempt to alter corneal power either by (1) changing the anterior corneal curvature without an implant, as with radial keratotomy or photorefractive keratoplasty, (2) changing the anterior curvature with an implant, as with a hydrogel intracorneal lens or intrastromal corneal ring implant, or (3) changing the refractive power of the cornea without altering the anterior curvature, as with a high refractive index inclusion or a Fresnel optic lens.

The hydrogel polymers used for intracorneal implants have a high water content (generally 70% water by weight) and a refractive index approximating corneal stroma. The hydrophobic polymer has a refractive index significantly greater than stroma has and is designed to minimize the nutritional barrier effect by the addition of fenestration that is, penetrating holes perpendicular to the lens surface. The greater the refractive index difference between implant and stroma, the greater is the refractive alteration per the lens thickness. The intrastromal corneal ring implant has unique requirements, which are discussed later. Factors to be considered with intracorneal implant procedures include toxicity of the material, biocompatibility with the physiologic processes within the corneal tissue, anatomic relationships, and the refractive index of the material.

BIOCOMPATIBILITY

Material biocompatibility is related to chemical and physical properties of the material. Chemically pure polymers rarely demonstrate chemical toxicity. A pure polymer will not have residual monomers within its matrix. The surface charge of an implant may create a nontoxic problem to the tissue. A positive or negative surface charge can result in specific attraction to keratocytes,[22] proteins, and so on. This surface adsorption may coat the material, reduce its permeability, or create light-scatter problems. Toxicity may occur postoperatively from in situ solute uptake in hydrogel materials. The hydrogel may absorb toxic solutes, such as benzalkonium chloride, or excessive concentrations of a drug, directly from fluid within the stroma and indirectly from the tear film. Most importantly, the implant must not be soluble or break down in the stromal environment.

Long-term biocompatibility has been demonstrated in the monkey eye by Parks and co-workers.[18] After 8 postoperative years, the corneal morphology demonstrated normal stroma and keratocytes anterior to the implant and normal endothelium posterior to the implant. The morphologic abnormalities were limited to a reduction in the number of cells in the epithelial layer anterior to the central zone of the aphakic implant and the presence of an incomplete thin layer of keratocytes adjacent to the implant.

MATERIAL CHARACTERISTICS

There are numerous physical properties of implant materials that are important. The implant material must not be porous to the stromal tissue be-

This work was supported in part by an Allergan Medical Optics Grant, NIH Grant EY-03696, a departmental grant from Research to Prevent Blindness, Inc., New York, and in part by NIH Grant RR-00165 from the Division of Research Resources to Yerkes Primate Research Center. The Yerkes Center is fully accredited by the American Association for Accreditation of Laboratory Animal Care.

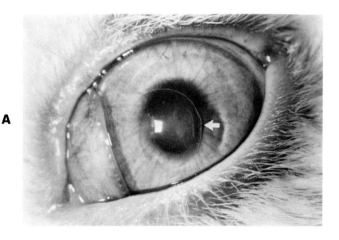

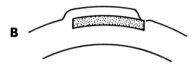

Fig. 36-1. Thinning of corneal stroma often developed anterior to edge of a thick-edged hydrogel intracorneal lens. **A,** Thinning was slow to develop, taking, on average, 4 months before implant was exposed in rabbit cornea. Arrow, Stromal erosion. (From McCarey BE, Andrews DM: *Invest Ophthalmol Vis Sci* 21:107, 1981.) **B,** Cross-sectional diagram illustrates thick-edged implant and its relationship to erosion.

cause the keratocytes migrating into the material may cause scarring and loss of transparency. The intrastromal corneal ring implant has a unique set of requirements and is discussed on p. 411. The following discussion is for an implant that is a solid disc.

Implant permeability, diameter, and design are important parameters. The net flux of glucose and water across the disc-designed implant is important in the maintenance of normal corneal nutrition.[10] A steady supply of nutrients can be maintained with increasing implant diameter by an increase in the implant permeability or a decrease in implant thickness. A thick-edge implant can actually erode through the tissue. McCarey and Andrews[14] demonstrated that even a 70% water-content hydrogel with an abrupt edge design can cause the stromal collagen to break down resulting in surface exposure of the implant. A lesser thick edge can create a gap in the stroma, which is filled with scar tissue, resulting in light scatter (Fig. 36-1). Implant rigidity is important, since an inflexible lens may have the potential of creating endothelial damage with blinking or rubbing of the eye.

EFFECT ON CORNEAL NUTRITION

The influence of the synthetic polymer intracorneal disc-designed implant on the nutritional aspects of corneal function is one of the most important factors to the success of this refractive procedure. The cornea receives its necessary glucose[10] and water[2,7] from the aqueous humor. Some water is lost by evaporation from the corneal surface resulting in a need for a constant supply of water entering into the tissue (Fig. 36-2). The cornea receives some of its nutritional needs from the limbal blood supply, but because the geometric shape of the cornea is comparable to a flat disc and the stromal diffusion rate for glucose is equal in all directions in the stroma, this nutritional supply is significant only to the peripheral corneal tissue.

In 1969, David Maurice[17] presented a theoretical analysis on the influence of an intracorneal impermeable implant on the glucose supply to the corneal epithelium. He assumed an aqueous glucose supply of 90 mg% and a uniform corneal glucose consumption of 50 g/cm^2 per hour. These calculations can be adjusted for a permeable implant when one adds the amount of glucose that can flow across the implant. The algorithm illustrates that with an impermeable 4 mm diameter implant located as deep as possible in the cornea, the glucose supply to the epithelium anterior to the implant will be approximately zero, that is, depleted. A glucose-permeable implant, such as that made from Lidofilcon-A, similarly implanted within the tissue will result in a slight amount of reserve glucose anterior to that implant. Surprisingly, based on David Maurice's calculations, the permeable Sauflon implant results in a theoretical anterior stromal starvation of glucose when the implant is at 50% depth. This theoretical analysis demonstrates the tenuous nutritional balance created by an intracorneal implant.

McCarey and Schmidt (1990)[16] expanded this analytical approach into a three-dimensional electrical resistance network to define the distribution of glucose in the stroma around or through the implant. The model is in agreement with Maurice (1969) that a 4 mm diameter impermeable implant would reduce the glucose in the central epithelium to approximately zero. There were only minor advantages to locating the implant at less than maximum depth in the stroma. Six millimeters is a practical implant diameter to provide an optical zone of greater than 5 mm for the patient. Fig. 36-3 demonstrates the effect of implant depth and glucose available to the epithelium. A interesting finding from the model is that a semipermeable implant can permit

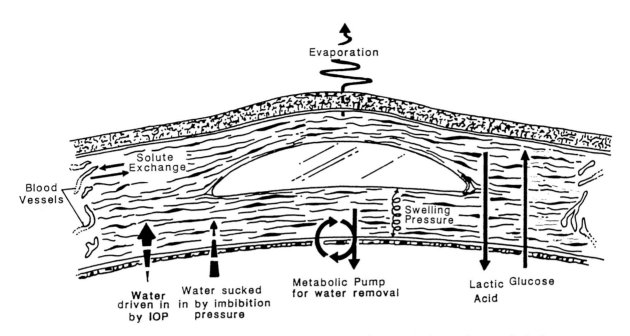

Fig. 36-2. Cornea is free of blood vessels; therefore it must obtain nutrients and eliminate waste products by diffusion across the posterior corneal surface and limbal blood vessels. Stromal hydration is controlled passively by water evaporation from tear film and a metabolic pump located in endothelium. An implant within the stroma may become a barrier to these processes. (From McCarey BE: *Int Ophthalmol Clin* 31:87-99, 1991.)

greater epithelial glucose availability when implanted immediately below the epithelium than deep within the stroma.

A hydrogel polymer will have pore dimensions ranging from the 0.4 to 6 nm.[19] The high-water-content (60% to 80%) hydrogels were measured to have pore dimensions of 0.6 to 2.2 nm. The pores will exclude stromal cells, collagen, and proteoglycans. The hydrogel, even while imbedded within the stroma, could be predicted to contain water and electrolytes. A theoretical hydrogel with 100% water would have a glucose-diffusion coefficient equal to an aqueous solution, that is, 6.73×10^{-6} cm^2/sec.[21] A 70% water-content hydrogel has a glucose diffusion coefficient of 1.09×10^{-6} cm^2/sec.[11] This is less than the diffusion coefficient for stroma, that is, 2.47×10^{-6} cm^2/sec.[16] The stroma contains 78% water by weight, that is, dry weight per wet weight. The ground substance between the collagen fibrils, where solute diffusion occurs, contains 98% water by weight. It would be difficult to design a hydrogel to have 98% water content and good mechanical properties; thus it would be difficult to design a hydrogel to have a glucose-diffusion coefficient equivalent to stroma.

One is led to ask, What hydrogel diffusion coeffi-

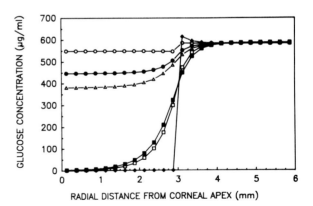

Fig. 36-3. Depth at which intracorneal lens is implanted can alter glucose epithelial cell availability and is dependent on intracorneal lens glucose permeability. The 6 mm diameter implants are at minimum, middle, and maximum depth with corneal stroma. Locations of hydrogel with 70% water content are at a minimum (○), middle (●), and maximum (△) depth. Water-impermeable intracorneal lenses are at minimum (◆), middle (□), and maximum (■) depth. (From McCarey BE, Schmidt FH: *Curr Eye Res* 9:1025, 1990.)

cient will provide safe nutritional availability to the anterior stroma? A comparable question may also be asked for impermeable material with fenestrations, that is, pores. What percent surface opening, that is, pore size multiplied by the number of pores, will provide safe nutritional availability to the anterior stroma? These questions cannot be answered until we know the minimum nutrient needs of the cornea to maintain normal cell biology. The answer to this question is still unknown.

SURGICAL TECHNIQUE AND OPTICAL PRINCIPLES

As stated in the opening paragraph, there are three procedures to alter the corneal refractive power. A discussion of each will give insight as to the technical feasibility of the variety of refractive surgical techniques. The implant design greatly influences the surgical technique to be selected. The three surgical approaches are (1) the freehand pocket incision, (2) a lamellar keratectomy with a microkeratome incision, and (3) peripheral tunneling for the ring implant.

Anterior Corneal Curvature Change Without an Implant. Radial keratotomy is a unique surgical technique when compared to the other refractive keratoplasty procedures discussed in this chapter. It creates an alteration in the optical zone by weakening the corneal shell biomechanics and therefore destabilizing the peripheral architecture. Photorefractive keratectomy (PRK) excimer beam delivery technique may vary, but the objective is to use laser ablation to alter the curvature of the patient's cornea within a specific optical zone for the desired

effect. In Fig. 36-4, a 5 mm optical zone is altered from a base corneal power of 45 diopters, that is, 7.5 mm anterior corneal radius calculated with a Bausch & Lomb keratometer with a refractive index of 1.3375, by 5-diopter steps within +20 to −20 diopters range. This causes a corneal radius of curvature change of 5.19 to 13.5 mm. The relationship between corneal power and anterior cornea radius is sensitive. Interestingly, flattening the cornea 10 diopters causes a 2.14 mm increase in anterior curvature, but steepening the cornea 10 diopters causes a 1.36 mm reduction in anterior curvature. Myopic corrections require greater alteration in anterior corneal curvature per diopter of correction, but the hyperopic (aphakic) correction will require greater precision in alteration of corneal curvature per diopter of correction.

Anterior Corneal Curvature Change With an Implant. The two techniques within this category are the use of hydrogel intracorneal lenses in conjunction with a microkeratome dissection and the use of an intracorneal rigid peripheral ring implant.

Hydrogel intracorneal lens. A lamellar keratectomy with microkeratome incision creates different biomechanical conditions from that with a pocket incision. The entire anterior segment of the cornea is removed, the implant is placed on the lamellar bed, and the corneal disc is contoured over the implant and sutured into position. In this way, an anterior curvature change is produced. Since the arc length of the cornea is constant, the cornea disc edge will be at a new position (Fig. 36-5). For a 15-diopter, 6 mm diameter implant made of a hydrogel with a refractive index of 1.402, the cornea disc edge will be displaced centrally by 0.03 mm, that is, 0.06 mm per diameter.

The implant refractive index selection will have important consequences on the implant design and surgical approach. If the implant material is a hydrogel, there will be a direct relationship between the water content of the hydrogel and the refractive index (Fig. 36-6). At zero water content, the refractive index relevant to the material selected will steadily increase with respect to the density of the material. The influence of the implant's refractive index and geometric shape can be determined with first-order optics (Fig. 36-7). The algorithm is used to calculate the back vertex power of each of the three segments of the cornea/implant complex, that is, stroma anterior to the implant, the implant, and the stroma posterior to the implant. One may calculate each of the back vertex powers assuming that they are immersed in air. Their addition will approximate the postoperative cornea refractive

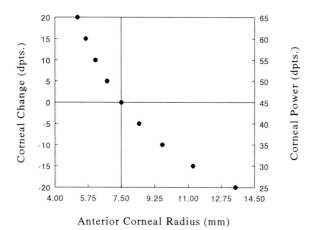

Fig. 36-4. Altering anterior corneal radius over a 5 mm optical zone. Bausch & Lomb keratometer value (1.3375) was used to define these relationships from an initial corneal power of 45 diopters.

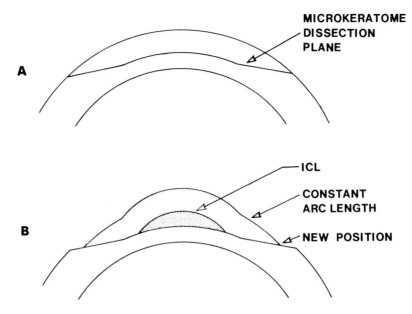

Fig. 36-5. A, Lamellar keratectomy with a microkeratome will result in an incision parallel to corneal surface. **B,** Implant alters corneal anterior curvature while repositioning corneal disc edges.

power. The principles are the same for either the freehand pocket incision or the lamellar keratectomy. The trick is to determine the radius of curvature for each of the surfaces that are illustrated in Fig. 36-7. One of the factors of the lamellar keratectomy incision technique is the depth of the implant within the stroma. The deeper the implant is placed within the cornea, the less is the effect on the anterior radius of curvature. The maximum surface

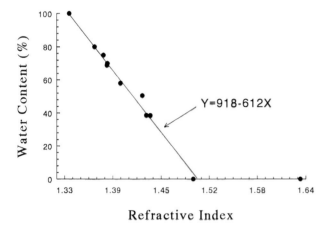

Fig. 36-6. Hydrogel materials have a linear relationship between the material's water content and refractive index. Hydrophobic materials can have large refractive indexes depending on density of material. Equation defines linear regression line for hydrogel materials.

powers of the implant-stroma interfaces is about a diopter, which is relatively insignificant.

The optical calculations are based on:

$$D = \frac{n_{to} - n_{from}}{r}$$

where D is the dioptric anterior surface power of the implant; n_{to} is the refractive index of the substance that the light is traveling to, that is, the implant; n_{from} is the refractive index of the substance the light is traveling from, that is, the stroma; and r is the radius of the anterior surface of the implant in meters. Since the refractive index is in the numerator, it has a direct influence on the dioptric power. The theoretical corneal power change can be calculated by use of these optical principles and factors such as depth of implant and surgical incision. With a microkeratome incision the refractive index of the implant will have minimal influence on the corneal power change. In Fig. 36-8 implants with refractive indexes of 1.633 and 1.402 illustrate this point. The relationship is quite different with the pocket incision. The implant in a pocket incision results in the cornea bulging posteriorly with the anterior corneal curvature unaltered. In this case, there is an advantage by increasing the refractive index of the implant material (Fig. 36-9).

Intrastromal corneal ring. The surgical technique utilizes a unique corkscrew-like dissector that theo-

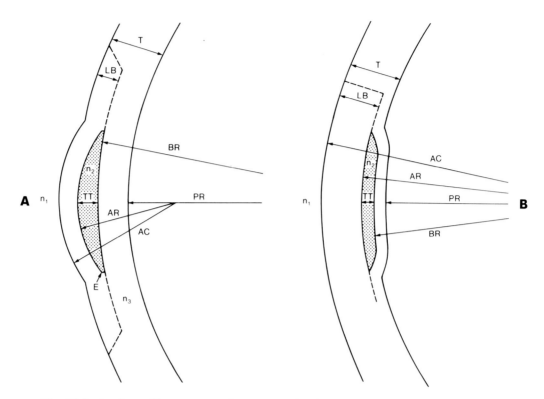

Fig. 36-7. Implant affect on corneal power can be determined by first-order optics. **A,** Intracorneal implant creates an anterior corneal radius change when used with a microkeratome incision. **B,** Same implant within a pocket incision will result in a posterior corneal bulging.

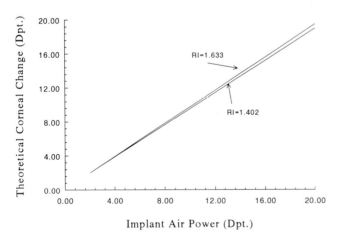

Fig. 36-8. With use of first-order optics, theoretical change in corneal power after intracorneal lens implantation with a microkeratome incision technique was determined with implants of various dioptric powers and two refractive indexes. Influence of refractive index on outcome is minimal.

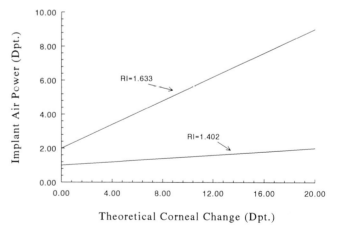

Fig. 36-9. With use of first-order optics, theoretical change in corneal power after intracorneal lens implantation with a pocket incision technique was determined with implants of various dioptric powers. High refractive index implants demonstrate greater effectiveness, that is, greater corneal power change, than low refractive index materials do.

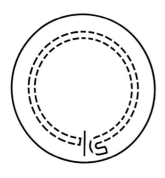

Fig. 36-10. Diagram representing intrastromal corneal ring (ICR) in peripheral corneal stroma. ICR is inserted through a single peripheral radial incision. (From Fleming JF et al: *CLAO J* 15:146, 1989.)

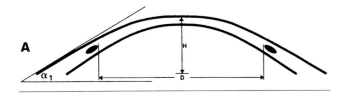

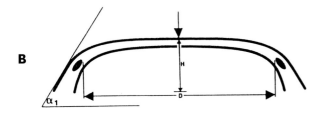

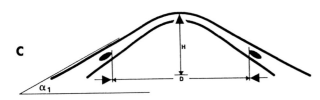

Fig. 36-11. A, Corneal configuration after intrastromal corneal ring insertion but before expansion or constriction. Corneal sagittal height (H), relaxed intrastromal ring diameter (D), and peripheral corneal angle (α) are represented. **B,** Corneal configuration after intrastromal corneal ring expansion. D is increased, H is decreased, α is increased, and central curvature is flattened. **C,** Corneal configuration after intrastromal corneal ring construction. D is decreased, H is increased, α is decreased, and central curvature is steepened. (From Fleming JF: *CLAO J* 15:146, 1989.)

retically separates without cutting the collagen lamellae in the peripheral cornea (Fig. 36-10).[8] A peripheral tunnel will disrupt a minimum number of collagen lamellae and thus cause minimal disruption of the shell biomechanical properties of the cornea. This assumption is probably not achieved, yet the surgical technique is the least invasive of all refractive surgical procedures and it does not violate the corneal tissue within the optical zone.

An intrastromal corneal ring (ICR) is designed to create tension laterally within collagen lamellae such that the diameter of the ICR is reduced or increased (Fig. 36-11) from the relaxed insertion dimensions, resulting in a corresponding steepening or flattening of the central cornea. Fleming and co-workers (1989)[8] described the algorithm used to model the influence of the ICR diameter change on the corneal curvature. The relationship must include the initial ICR diameter, initial corneal curvature, and the change in ICR diameter. For example, with a ICR diameter of 6 mm and initial corneal curvature of 7.67 mm (44 diopters), a 0.2 mm constriction of the ICR diameter results in an 8-diopter steepening of the cornea (6.49 mm, or 52.00 diopters). A 0.2 mm expansion of the ICR diameter results in an 10-diopter flattening of the cornea (9.93 mm or 34 diopters) (Fig. 36-12).

By increasing the initial diameter of the ICR, one notes that the relationship between the change in ICR diameter and change in anterior corneal curvature becomes less sensitive; a 0.2 mm constriction results in a 4-diopter change, and a 0.2 mm expansion

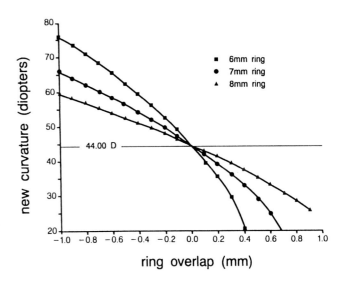

Fig. 36-12. Predicted changes in corneal curvature with intrastromal corneal ring procedure (44.00 D preoperative curvature). (From Fleming JF: *CLAO J* 15:146, 1989.)

results in a 3-diopter change. The human cornea diameter is 10.6 mm vertical and 11.7 mm horizontal.[9] Placement of the 8 mm diameter ICR would result in a 1.3 mm margin of tissue between the limbus and ICR. Surgical centering and precise ICR diameter control (0.5 diopters per 33 μm) will be necessary.

Corneal Power Change without Altering Anterior Corneal Curvature. With a freehand pocket incision a 75-degree arc of collagen fibers running from limbus to limbus is cut to open the pocket. The remaining 285-degree arc of fibers remain intact. The forces generated in the cornea by an implant within a pocket incision are similar to forces generated by edema of the stroma. The scleral shell and cornea will not change in circumference; that is, the anterior corneal arc length does not enlarge with corneal edema or the presence of the implant. The posterior surface (the endothelium) of the cornea will move posteriorly, displacing aqueous humor without a change in the anterior corneal curvature. This will occur regardless of the implant rigidity.

Performing a refractive keratoplasty procedure without relying on a precise alteration of anterior corneal radius and resulting corneal remodeling would greatly simplify the task. This has been accomplished with intracular lens implants in the aphakic eye and in the phakic eye in limited myopic trials. The implant creates the desired refractive alteration, rather than the need for a surgical alteration of the corneal topography. A high-refractive-index polymer lens placed within a intrastromal dissection has been performed by Choyce[3,5] and investigated in the laboratory by Climenhaga et al.,[6] Rodrigues et al.,[20] McCarey et al.,[15] and Lindstrom et al.[12] The data support the concept that an impermeable intrastromal lens will result in anterior-stroma nutrition deficits.

Surgidev Corporation (Goleta, California) has designed a high-refractive-index material with numerous 10 μm fenestrations that permit a glucose flux sufficient to support tissue nutrition anterior to the implant. Animal studies are being performed by Lindstrom, Lane and Associates (Minneapolis). Some of the advantages of the hydrogel implant, such as being impervious to tissue growth and soft and pliable, are lost with a fenestrated rigid polymer. It is also unknown if the fenestrations will mimic a fiber-optic bundle, causing unwanted light scatter. The advantages of the refractive surgery implant are sufficient to warrant further investigation.

An intrastromal lens (ISL) implant has been designed by Optical Radiation Corporation (Azusa, California).[13] Two hydrogel polymers of sufficiently

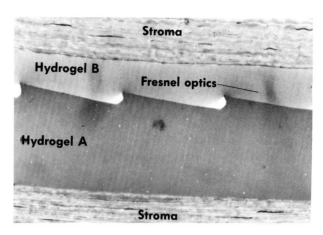

Fig. 36-13. Fresnel hydrogel intracorneal lens within the stroma of a rabbit cornea. Fresnel optics is the interface between two hydrogel layers. (From McCarey BE: *Refract Corneal Surg* 6:40, 1990.)

different refractive indexes have been bonded together such that the interface is a refracting surface with a Fresnel optic design of a unit dioptric power (Fig. 36-13). The implant design permits a thin, unit-thickness hydrogel to have an extensive range of dioptric powers. Therefore the implant mechanical stress on the stroma does not vary with implant dioptric power because the implant cross-sectional profile does not vary. This could be an exciting concept if it can provide good optical resolution and minimal image contrast loss.

In summary, the principles of refractive keratoplasty with intracorneal implants made of synthetic materials have been presented. The theoretical principles indicate excellent possibilities for this approach.

REFERENCES

1. Barraquer JI: Modification of refraction by means of intracorneal inclusions, *Int Ophthalmol Clin* 6(1):53-78, 1966.
2. Brown SI, Mishima S: The effect of intralamellar water impermeable membranes on corneal hydration, *Arch Ophthalmol* 76:702-708, 1966.
3. Choyce DP: The present status of intra-cameral and intracorneal implants, *Can J Ophthalmol* 3:295-311, 1968.
4. Choyce DP: *Semi-rigid corneal inlays used in the management of albinism, aniridia, and ametropia*, 24th Congress of Ophthalmology, Philadelphia, 1983, Lippincott.
5. Choyce DP: The correction of refractive errors with polysulfone corneal inlays: a new frontier to be explored, *Trans Ophthalmol Soc UK* 104:332, 1985.
6. Climenhaga H, Macdonald JM, McCarey BE, Waring GO: Effect of diameter and depth on the response to solid polysulfone intracorneal lenses in cats, *Arch Ophthalmol* 106:818-824, 1988.
7. Dohlman CH, Brown SI: Treatment of corneal edema with a

buried implant, *Trans Am Acad Ophthalmol Otolaryngol* 70:267-280, 1966.

8. Fleming JF, Wan WL, Schanzlin DJ: The theory of corneal curvature change with the intrastromal corneal ring, *CLAO J* 15:146-150, 1989.

9. Hogan MJ, Alvarado JA, Weddell JE: The cornea. In Hogan MJ, Alvarado JA, Weddell JE, editors: *Histology of the human eye*, Philadelphia, 1971, WB Saunders.

10. Knowles WF: Effect of intralamellar plastic membranes on corneal physiology, *Am J Ophthalmol* 51:1146-1156, 1961.

11. Lane SS, McCarey BE, Lindstrom RL: Alloplastic corneal lenses. In Schwab IR, editor: *Contemporary Issues in Ophthalmology*, New York, 1987, Churchill Livingstone.

12. Lindstrom RL, Lane SS, Cameron JD, et al: Intracorneal lenses. In Caldwell DR, editor: *Cataracts*, Transactions of the New Orleans Academy of Ophthalmology, New York, 1988, Raven Press.

13. McCarey BE: Current status of refractive surgery with synthetic intracorneal lenses: Barraquer lecture, *Refract Corneal Surg* 6:40-46, 1990.

14. McCarey BE, Andrews DM: Refractive keratoplasty with intrastromal hydrogel lenticular implants, *Invest Ophthalmol Vis Sci* 21:107-115, 1981.

15. McCarey BE, Lane SS, Lindstrom RL: Alloplastic corneal lenses, *Int Ophthalmol Clin* 28(2):155-164, 1988.

16. McCarey BE, Schmidt FH: Model glucose distribution in the cornea, *Curr Eye Res* 9:1025-1039, 1990.

17. Maurice DM: Nutritional aspects of corneal grafts and prosthesis. In Raycroft PV, editor: *Corneo-plastic surgery*, Proceedings of the Second International Corneo-Plastic Conference, London, 1967, New York, 1969, Pergamon Press.

18. Parks RA, McCarey BE: Hydrogel keratophakia: Long term morphology in the monkey model, *CLAO J* 17(3):316-222.

19. Refojo MF: Permeation of water through some hydrogels, *J Appl Polymer Sci* 9:3417-3426, 1965.

20. Rodrigues MM, McCarey BE, Waring GO III, et al: Lipid deposits posterior to impermeable intracorneal lenses in rhesus monkeys: clinical, histochemical, and ultrastructural studies, *Refract Corneal Surg* 6:32-37, 1990.

21. Weast RC, editor: *CRC handbook of chemistry and physics*, ed 58, Cleveland, 1977-1978, CRC Press, p F-62.

22. Zavala EY, Nayak S, Deg JK, Binder PS: Keratocyte attachment to hydrogel materials, *Curr Eye Res* 3(10):1253-1262, 1984.

Polysulfone intracorneal lenses

STEPHEN S. LANE
RICHARD L. LINDSTROM

Keratorefractive surgical techniques have been under investigation as an alternative to spectacle or contact lens correction of refractive errors for several decades. Fyodorov refined techniques previously described by Sato and popularized radial keratotomy. Although serious eye-threatening complications are rare in radial keratotomy, fluctuation of vision is frequent, and predictability is poor in the higher myopic range, making it a suitable procedure

This work has been supported in part by Surgidev Corporation, Goleta, California.

for only relatively small degrees of myopia. Barraquer pioneered the development of keratophakia and keratomileusis. Although efficacious, these techniques are technically complex and require expensive sophisticated instrumentation. Based on Barraquer's work, Werblin and Kaufman developed epikeratoplasty, which, although technically simpler, is quite unpredictable, requires months for full visual rehabilitation, and demands a normal anterior surface for its maintenance.

In an attempt to overcome some of these problems, attention has turned to the use of alloplastic materials as intrastromal lenses.

Early work has shown that rigid, impermeable plastic membranes of appropriate size as well as larger more permeable lenses such as hydrogel lenses can be well tolerated over a significant period of time.[3,5,6,10,15,16,21,23] Previously, McCarey, Lane, and Lindstrom[17] categorized alloplastic materials according to their refractive indexes (Table 36-1). Materials with refractive indexes approximating corneal stroma (1.38 to 1.40) affect refraction only when used in combination with a 360-degree lamellar keratectomy using a microkeratome dissection. In this way, the anterior corneal curvature is altered, accomplishing a change in refraction. Materials with a higher refractive index (greater than 1.45) are effective in a freehand intralamellar pocket dissection. With the use of a lens of appropriate power, the native refractive error is corrected with no alteration of the anterior corneal curvature but rather by the inherent power of the lens itself.

PHYSIOLOGY

Physiologically the diameter of an impermeable inlay should not exceed 5.0 mm.[8,11,15] Maurice[15] calculated that the concentration of glucose above the center of an impermeable membrane would fall to zero in rabbits as the diameter of the membrane approached 4 mm. He concluded, however, that based on the experience of Knowles[11] and Dohlman and Brown[8] 5.0 mm was the maximum diameter for impermeable discs that could be safely implanted in humans. Although smaller lenses would allow nutrients to reach the anterior stroma and epithelium more easily, they would likely be poorly tolerated because of the monocular diplopia that would occur from poor centration on the visual axis in different lighting situations. In addition, Maurice concluded that an impermeable barrier within the stroma is more deleterious to the anterior corneal layers the more anteriorly it is placed. Because the nutrition of the epithelium is largely derived from the aqueous, the closer an impermeable barrier is to the epithe-

Table 36-1. Hydrogel Contact Lens Refractive Index Versus Water Content

Brand	Polymer	Water Content (%)	Refractive Index (hydrated)
Sauflon PW	Lidofilcon B	79	1.3686
Sauflon 70	Lidofilcon A	70	1.3853
Permalens	Perfilcon	68.9	1.3845
Hydrocurve II	Bufilcon A	50.5	1.43
Bausch & Lomb	Polymacon	38.6	1.435
CSI	Crofilcon A	38.5	1.44
Vistacon	Etafilcon A	58	1.402
Vistacon	Etafilcon A	70	1.385
Vistacon	Etafilcon A	75	1.380
Polysulfone	—	0	1.633
Polycon II	Silafocon A	0	1.495
Cornea	—	78	1.376
Aqueous	—	100	1.336

lium, the greater is the decline in the nutrient supply reaching the superficial layers. This has been supported by Werblin and co-workers[24] experimentally and Choyce[7] clinically.

LENS MATERIALS

In 1949, Barraquer[1] originated the idea of placing intracorneal lenses of *flint glass* (6 mm in diameter) in rabbits and cats. Tolerance of these lenses was poor, with eventual extrusion in all eyes. Despite later modifications of the radius curvature and diameter (5 mm), and a change in material (*Plexiglas,* that is, poly[methyl methacrylate]), loss of transparency with vascularization and extrusion of lenses occurred in all cases.

With the development of new polymers, Belau,[2] Choyce,[5,7] Knowles,[11] and others[2,9,19,22] searched for the ideal intracorneal lens material (see Box). Knowles investigated three polymers (*polyethylene, polyvinylidine,* and *polypropylene*) in 1961.[11] Corneal

---

Materials used for Alloplastic Intracorneal Lenses

Flint glass
Poly(methyl methacrylate), or Plexiglas
Celloidin
Glyceryl methacrylate
Polyvinylidine
Polypropylene
Silicone elastomer (Silastic)
Hydroxyethyl methacrylate
Polysulfone

---

changes anterior to the lenses occurred in all rabbit eyes regardless of the material or depth of placement. Most of these eyes developed a dimple or crater in the epithelial surface with microscopic degeneration and disappearance of the substantia propria. Little or no inflammation was observed. As mentioned earlier, results in monkey eyes were more favorable, especially when smaller-diameter lenses were used. Knowles suggested that the degeneration of the stroma and epithelium anterior to the intracorneal lenses was caused not only by interference with diffusion, but also by selective desiccation at the corneal epithelium anterior to the lens. The favorable results noted in primate eyes were hypothesized to be secondary to rapid, spontaneous blinking, which maintained a tear film that prevented desiccation. This was later confirmed by Brown and Mishima[4] who found that the amount of corneal thinning that occurred anterior to a *Silastic (silicone elastomer) intralamellar membrane* was dependent on evaporation of the precorneal tear film, tear film tonicity, and the blink epithelial rate. Turss and co-workers,[22] however, were unable to maintain epithelial integrity after placement of an intracorneal lens despite performing a prophylactic tarsorrhaphy. They believe that the forward diffusion of nutrients derived from the aqueous maintains epithelial integrity. Corneal thinning then was secondary solely to inadequate diffusion of metabolites across the lens membrane rather than a local drying effect.

Dohlman and colleagues[9] were the first to look at the intracorneal inclusion of a hydrophilic polymer—*glyceryl methacrylate* (GMA). Intracorneal lenses in rabbits, 4.0 mm in diameter and with a thickness varying from 0.25 to 0.57 mm, were noted to ex-

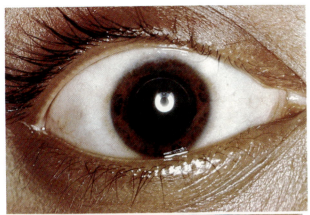

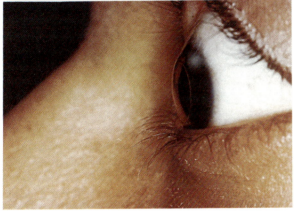

Fig. 36-14. Twenty-year-old patient 30 months postoperatively. Preoperative refraction, −16.00 +4.00 × 130; postoperative refraction, −3.00 +1.00 × 135.

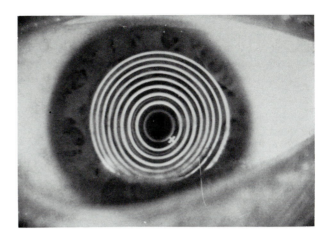

Fig. 36-15. Corneoscopic view of eye of patient in Fig. 36-14.

trude without evidence of inflammation or toxicity. The authors believed that this was related to the water permeability of GMA and not to the toxicity of the lens material. Mester[18] and associates were the first to report the use of hydrophilic polymers specifically for alloplastic keratophakia. The implantation of 4.0 mm discs of hydroxyethyl methacrylate (thickness 0.2 mm) was well tolerated by 40 rabbits during a period of up to 18 months. In addition, reproducible changes in refraction were obtained using 0.2 mm hydroxyethyl methacrylate lenses. More recently, McCarey and Andrews[16] have demonstrated that high-water-content hydrogels are biologically compatible in rabbits. Binder[3] has shown these same materials to be compatible in nonhuman primates. However, in contrast to the work of McCarey and his co-authors, Samples and co-workers[20] found activated keratocytes, phagocytic keratocytes, macrophages, and newly formed collagen at the edges of the implanted lenses. Yet at 23 months postoperatively, all baboons maintained clear corneas.

Recently McDonald, Nordan, and Price have successfully implanted hydrogel lenses manufactured by American Medical Optics into human sighted eyes. Although the results are preliminary, the procedure appears to be well tolerated and efficacious.

Attracted by the high refractive index (1.633) and superior optical quality of *polysulfone*, Choyce pioneered the use of this material as an intracorneal lens for the correction of refractive errors in 1981. An independent retrospective review of his patients was reported and showed the procedure to be efficacious[12,13,17] (Figs. 36-14 and 36-15). A protocol was subsequently established to prospectively study the safety and efficacy of the procedure in a laboratory cat and monkey model. Results of this multicenter study showed 70% of the cat corneas ($n = 24$) remained clear; however, complications including interface opacification (Fig. 36-16), interface refractile particles (Fig. 36-17), epithelial dimple formation, irregular astigmatism, anterior corneal necrosis, vascularization (Fig. 36-18), and lens extrusion were encountered[13,17] (Table 36-2). Because of these complications, the reversibility of polysulfone corneal lenses was also investigated. Three months after removal of the lens, the opacification noted preoperatively was reversed.[17] In the baboon model ($n = 8$), the majority of the procedures were considered failures since they were complicated by lens extrusion, anterior stromal necrosis, interface opacification, and anterior corneal edema with vascularization. All the monkeys tested ($n = 4$) tolerated the lens well without complications. When specimens with nebular opacities and refractile particles were examined histologically, multiple discrete oil-red-O−positive deposits were noted at the same corneal depth as the

Table 36-2.   Complications of Polysulfone Intraocular Lenses*

Complication	Minus Lenses (n = 6)	Plus Lenses (n = 7)	Total (n = 23)
Interface opacity (slitlamp)	94% (15)	100% (7)	96% (22)
Interface opacity (visually significant)	12.5% (2)	71% (5)	30% (7)
Refractile particles	67% (10)	57% (4)	61% (14)
Epithelial dimple	6% (1)	29% (2)	13% (3)
Irregular astigmatism	6% (1)	14% (1)	9% (2)
Anterior corneal necrosis	12.5% (2)	0% (0)	9% (2)
Vascularization	19% (3)	14% (1)	61% (4)
Lens extrusion	6% (1)	29% (2)	13% (3)

*The number of cases is shown in parentheses.

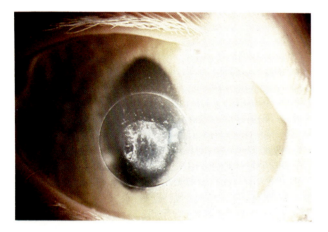

Fig. 36-16. Visually significant nebular opacity. Posterior pole landmarks were not visualized through this opacity with a direct ophthalmoscope.

opacities seen clinically.[17] We believe that these lipid deposits originated from keratocytes that were composed secondary to inadequate nutrition anterior to the nonpermeable intracorneal lens.

FENESTRATED INTRACORNEAL LENSES

To investigate the above-mentioned hypothesis, we surgically implanted 5 mm fenestrated polysulfone lenses (35 μm fenestrations) encompassing 20% of the surface area of the lens within the corneal stroma in one eye of each of six cats. A nonfenestrated, otherwise identical, 5 mm polysulfone lens was placed at the same corneal depth in the other eye. One hundred percent of the eyes that received a fenestrated lens maintained ophthalmoscopically clear central media at 1 year with no evidence of any central interface nebular opacities. Thirty-three percent (2) of the fenestrated lens eyes did, however, show peripheral nebular opacification in some areas over the nonfenestrated portion of the lens. One eye was particularly interesting because within the area of peripheral nebular opacification were multiple

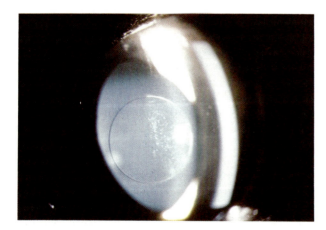

Fig. 36-17. Refractile particles, not visually significant in this case.

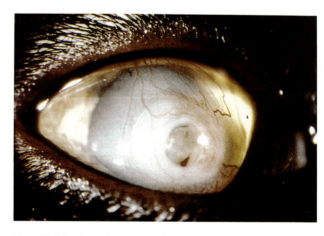

Fig. 36-18. Anterior corneal necrosis and vascularization in presence of a polysulfone lens.

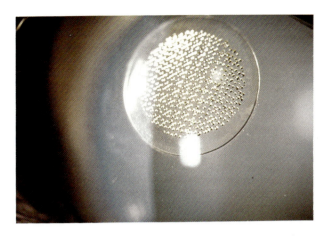

Fig. 36-19. Peripheral opacification at lens-cornea interface in fenestrated lens eye. Notice Swiss-cheese appearance over far peripheral fenestrations.

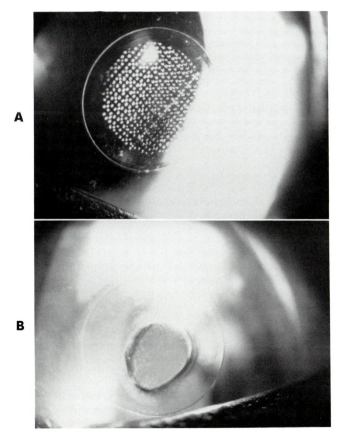

Fig. 36-20. A, Fenestrated polysulfone lens in right cornea of cat with no evidence of interface opacification at 1 year. **B,** Nonfenestrated polysulfone lens in left cornea of same cat with significant central opacities at lens-cornea interface and a large central aseptic melt (1 year).

clear areas directly overlying open fenestrations of the peripheral lens (Fig. 36-19). This supports the hypothesis of nutritional stress as the cause for the nebular opacification. The clear stromal areas overlying the fenestrations represent adequately nourished cornea surrounded by opaque cornea, which is inadequately nourished.

In contrast to the fenestrated lens eyes, no nonfenestrated lens eyes achieved ophthalmoscopically clear media at 1 year, with all the eyes showing some degree of interface change (Fig. 36-20). Complications seen in the nonfenestrated lens eyes included nebular interface opacities (100%), refractile particles (100%), anterior thinning (50%), extrusion of lens (33%), vascularization (33%), and anterior corneal necrosis (17%). These percentages correlate quite closely with those from previous studies,[13] and these complications were not noted in the fenestrated lens group (Table 36-3).

Histopathologic evaluation of these fenestrated specimens reveals the presence of normal keratocytes and stroma within the fenestrations. (Figs. 36-21 and 36-22). Examination of the endothelium and epithelium was normal with no central epithelium thinning or peripheral epithelial thickening (Fig. 36-23).

Although this study indicated increased safety with the fenestrations, the lenses, unfortunately, proved to be optically unsatisfactory. Ophthalmoscopic examination through the fenestrated lenses utilizing a direct ophthalmoscope revealed a poor view of retinal structures. Confirmation of this was achieved when ophthalmoscopic photographs of the cat's posterior pole were taken with the fenestrated lens in situ. Photographic details of posterior pole anatomy was poor because of optical distortion caused by the fenestrated lenses.

A second generation of fenestrated polysulfone lenses was developed in 1989. In an attempt to im-

Table 36-3. Complications of Fenestrated and Nonfenestrated Intracorneal Lens Implantation in Six Cats 1 Year Postoperatively

Complications	Fenestrated Eyes % (number)	Nonfenestrated Eyes % (number)
Nebular opacities	33 (2)*	100 (6)
Refractile particles	0	100 (6)
Anterior thinning	0	50 (3)
Extrusion	0	33 (2)
Necrosis	0	17 (1)
Vascularization	0	33 (2)

*Peripheral opacification only over nonfenestrated portion of the lens.

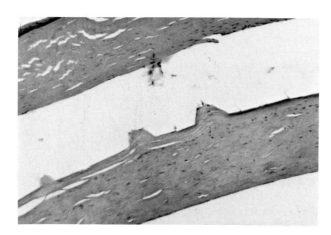

Fig. 36-21. Histologic section of interlamellar pocket after removal of a fenestrated lens. Notice normal keratocytes within pegs of corneal stroma that grew through the fenestrations. (10×.)

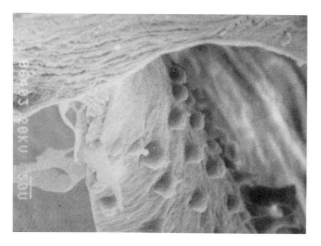

Fig. 36-22. Scanning electron micrograph demonstrating corneal stromal pegs and smooth interlamellar pocket. (22×.)

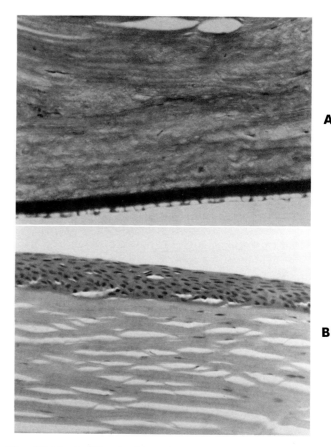

Fig. 36-23. **A,** Histologic section of cat cornea at 1 year showing normal endothelium in fenestrated lens eye. (10×.) **B,** Histologic section of cat cornea at 1 year showing normal epithelium in fenestrated lens eye. (10×.)

prove the optical resolution, microfenestrated lenses were manufactured with fenestration diameters less than 10 μm. The fenestration size and percentage of open area have been investigated, and several of these lenses have been placed in laboratory animal models. Postoperative examinations including tests of optical quality have been performed and have given us clues as to the optimal fenestration size and percentage of open area. Results from this pilot series have been encouraging. Lenses manufactured with fenestrations several micrometers or less in diameter can give optical qualities equivalent to standard intraocular lenses, including optical resolution

(Fig. 36-24). Based upon results gleaned from this preliminary pilot series and optical bench studies, a large controlled study in laboratory cats and monkeys is underway to evaluate safety and efficacy. Special emphasis will be placed on obtaining information regarding the optical resolving power of these lenses in situ, and examination techniques including photographic analysis will be utilized.

Fenestrations that allow nutrients to pass from the aqueous through the lens to the anterior cornea greatly improve the safety margin of polysulfone as an intracorneal lens material.[14] Additionally, microfenestrations, although allowing the same movement of nutrients across the membrane, appear to give satisfactory optical lens quality. Unfortunately, the process in manufacturing microfenestrated polysulfone lenses is complex. Consequently, other microfenestrated high-refractive-index alloplastics are also being investigated as possible alternatives to polysulfone. The ideal material, one of high refrac-

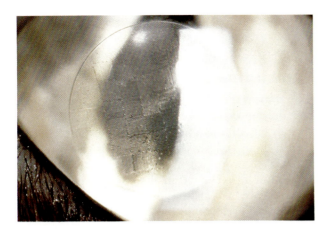

Fig. 36-24. Clear microfenestrated intracorneal lens in cat model.

tive index to allow surgical placement within a lamellar pocket and of suitable permeability to sustain the nutritional requirements of the cornea, remains elusive to investigators. Only with continued active investigation in the laboratory and in animal models can suitable alternatives to the ideal material be realized.

REFERENCES

1. Barraquer JI: Modification of refraction by means of intracorneal inclusions, *Int Ophthalmol Clin* 6:53-78, 1966.
2. Belau PG, Dyer JA, Ogli KN, et al: Correction of ametropia with intracorneal lenses, *Arch Ophthalmol* 72:541-547, 1962.
3. Binder PS, Deg JK, Zavala EY, Grossman KR: Hydrogel keratophakia in non-human primates, *Curr Eye Res* 1(9):535-542, 1981/1982.
4. Brown SI, Mishima S: Effect of intralamellar water impermeable membranes on corneal hydration, *Arch Ophthalmol* 76:702-708, 1966.
5. Choyce DP: The present status of intracameral and intra-corneal implants, *Can J Ophthalmol* 3:295-311, 1968.
6. Choyce DP: Semi-rigid corneal inlays used in the management of albinism, aniridia, and ametropia. In Henkind P, editor: *XXIV International Congress of Ophthalmology*, Philadelphia, 1983, JB Lippincott.
7. Choyce DP: *The correction of refractive errors with polysulfone corneal inlays*, Presented at the Oxford Ophthalmological Congress, July 3, 1984.
8. Dohlman CH, Brown S: Treatment of corneal edema with a buried implant, *Trans Am Acad Ophthalmol Otolaryngol* 70:267-279, 1966.
9. Dohlman CH, Refojo MF, Rose J: Synthetic polymers in corneal surgery: I. Glyceryl methacrylate, *Arch Ophthalmol* 77:252-257, 1967.
10. Gillette TE, Udell IJ, Abelson MB: Hydrogel keratophakia. In Schachar RA, Levy NS, Schachar L, editor: *Keratorefraction*, Proc Keratorefractive Society Meeting, Denison, Texas, 1980, LAL Publishing, pp 127-139.
11. Knowles WF: Effect of intralamellar plastic membranes on corneal physiology, *Am J Ophthalmol* 51:1146-1156, 1961.
12. Lane SS, Lindstrom RL: Polysulfone intraocular lenses. In Brightbill FS editor: *Corneal surgery*, St. Louis, 1986, Mosby–Year Book.
13. Lane SS, Lindstrom RL, Cameron JD, et al: Polysulfone corneal lenses, *J Cataract Refract Surg* 12:(1)50-60, 1986.
14. Lane SS, Lindstrom RL, Mindrup EA, Cameron JD: One year follow-up on fenestrated intracorneal lenses: complications, reversibility, and histopathology, *Invest Ophthalmol* 29(suppl):311, 1988.
15. Maurice DM: Nutritional aspects of corneal grafts and prosthesis. In Raycroft PV, editor: *Corneo-plastic surgery*, Proc Second International Corneo-Plastic Conference, London, 1967, New York, 1969, Pergamon Press, pp 197-207.
16. McCarey BE, Andres DM: Refractive keratoplasty with intrastromal hydrogel lenticular implants, *Invest Ophthalmol Vis Sci* 21:107-115, 1981.
17. McCarey BE, Lane SS, Lindstrom RL: Alloplastic corneal lenses, *Int Ophthalmol Clin* 28:155, 1988.
18. Mester U, Heimig D, Dardenne MU: Measurement and calculation of refraction in experimental keratophakia with hydrophilic lenses, *Ophthalmic Res* 8:111-116, 1976.
19. Pollack IP: Water movement in rabbit corneas containing a plastic intralamellar disk, *Am J Ophthalmol* 60:481-487, 1965.
20. Samples JR, Binder PS, Zavala EY, et al: Morphology of hydrogel implants used for refractive keratoplasty, *Invest Ophthalmol Vis Sci* 25(7):843-850, 1984.
21. Sendele DD, Abelson MB, Kenyon KR, Hanninen LA: Intracorneal implantation, *Arch Ophthalmol* 101:940-944, 1983.
22. Turss R, Friend J, Dohlman CH: Effect of a corneal fluid barrier on the nutrition of the epithelium, *Exp Eye Res* 9:254-259, 1970.
23. Werblin TP, Blaydes JE, Fryczkowski A, Peiffer R: Refractive corneal surgery: the use of implantable alloplastic lens material, *Aust J Ophthalmol* 11:325-331, 1983.
24. Werblin TP, Blaydes JE, Fryczkowski A, Peiffer RL: Stability of hydrogel intracorneal implants in non-human primates, *CLAO J* 9(2):157-161, 1983.

Evaluation of published results

THEODORE P. WERBLIN

Synthetic keratophakia has several theoretical advantages over conventional refractive surgery. Because synthetic material rather than corneal tissue is used, the lens required at the time of surgery can be manufactured in limitless quantity to precise specifications. In contrast, procedures using lathed corneal lenses require, in some cases, donor corneal tissue, and the precision of the lathing process cannot be verified before clinical usage. Additionally, synthetic lenses do not require any internal healing or repopulation by stromal keratocytes. The cornea, during the surgical procedure, is minimally affected; thus healing is quite rapid.

HISTORY OF DEVELOPMENT

The work of José Barraquer[1] forms the basis for most corneal refractive procedures that alter the anterior corneal curvature. He began his work with impermeable plastics as inlays in the cornea over three decades ago but had problems with melting and necrosis of the anterior corneal cap and abandoned this as a clinical entity. Several investigators in the 1960s using impermeable substances as inlays for other than refractive reasons (such as bullous keratopathy) participated in studies and again observed eventual necrosis and dissolution of the anterior cornea. McCarey[7] really set the stage for the current work in hydrogel implant surgery. He demonstrated biocompatibility with the high-water-content hydrogel implants used by many current investigators. Several years later, Binder[3] and Werblin[8] used hyperopic implants in various animal models, confirming their biocompatibility and observing that significant hyperopic refractive changes (such as increased anterior corneal curvature) could be achieved with these materials.

Choyce[5] began work quite some time ago with another synthetic material, polysulfone. In contrast to hydrogels, these materials affect the refractive properties of the cornea, not by changing its shape but by altering its refractive index. Unlike the hydrogels, polysulfone material is water impermeable and similar to material originally used by Barraquer.

Several years ago, Binder[2] investigated myopic hydrogel implants but was unable to achieve satisfactory myopic corrections with his technique. His demonstration of the reversibility of the hydrogel implant procedure[4] was one of the major reasons why

hydrogels seem to be a more desirable medium. More recent success has been achieved by Werblin[9] with specially designed myopic hydrogel implants.

ANIMAL MODEL

The appearance of a myopic hydrogel implant in a female rhesus monkey 2 weeks after surgery is shown in Fig. 36-25. The cornea appears quite clear, and at 6 months, little change in clarity is seen (Fig. 36-26). Observation for up to 18 months in these animals shows little change in the corneal appearance. Biomicroscopy reveals the implant material to be an optically void area within the cornea. In Fig. 36-27, a hyperopic corneal implant is shown, with the central portion of the lens being thick as opposed to its thin periphery. Myopic implants, oppositely, are thin centrally and thickest just inside the peripheral edge (Fig. 36-26). The obvious flattening of the anterior corneal surface achieved with this type of myopic hydrogel inlay is evident in Fig. 36-26.

MEASUREMENT OF REFRACTIVE CHANGE

How best to measure or quantitate the refractive change that occurs after hydrogel inlay surgery in nonhuman studies remains controversial. The corneoscope provides a picture of the topography of the cornea that may be too simplified to allow one to predict what is happening refractively. The keratometer gives us information that is somewhat removed from the central visual axis and also may be

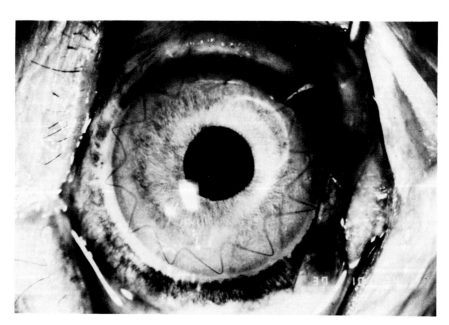

Fig. 36-25. Nonhuman primate cornea with myopic hydrogel implant in place for 2 weeks. 10-0 nylon suture is seen securing anterior corneal cap.

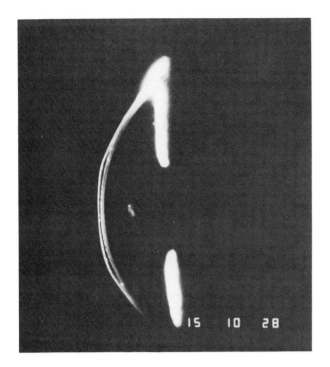

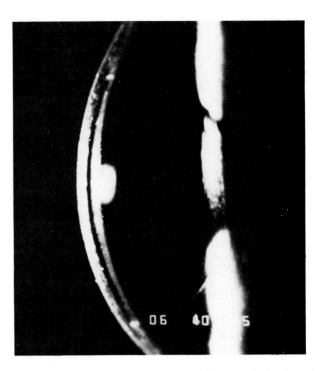

Fig. 36-26. Slitlamp appearance of myopic hydrogel implant. Lens appears as an optically void area within stroma. Edge of myopic lens is thick in contrast to thin central area.

Fig. 36-27. Slitlamp appearance of hyperopic hydrogel implant. Lens appears as an optically void area within stroma. Edge of hyperopic lens is thin compared to its center.

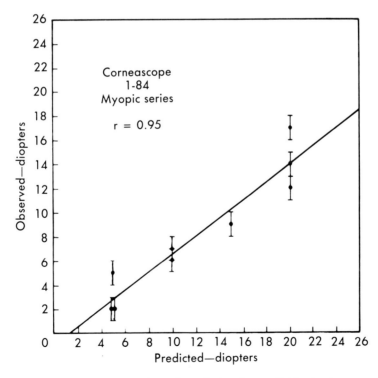

Fig. 36-28. Plot of myopic hydrogel implant design "power" (abscissa) versus observed (ordinate) central ring corneoscopic topography (in diopters). Implants of −5 D, −10 D, −15 D, and −20 D were used for this study. Each point represents measurements on different eyes.

Table 36-4. Relative Power per Corneoscopic Ring

Animal Number	Power	Ring				
		First	Second	Third	Fourth	Fifth
884K	−20	−17.5	−12.5	−9.3	−4.0	−2.8
432K	−15	−10.5	−12.2	−7.0	−3.0	−3.0
437K	− 5	− 0.7	− 0.5	−2.0	−1.0	+0.7

inaccurate in terms of predicting what effect has been achieved optically.

In myopic implants, when one compares the central ring to the successive peripheral rings on the corneoscope (Table 36-4), significant flattening is seen only within the first and second corneoscopic rings. There is a rapid dropoff in the effect on the cornea beyond that. Fig. 36-28 demonstrates the central corneoscopic ring flattening achieved with several different myopic implants (−5.00, −10.00,

−15.00, and −20.00 diopter implants). Several different animal eyes were measured at each of these points. Although the amount of flattening achieved at each of these points was not exactly what was predicted, each given implant design produced the same amount of flattening. The early myopic implants showed definite central flattening but also some irregularity in the appearance of the corneal surface (Fig. 36-29). However, recent advances in the design of these implants have demonstrated a

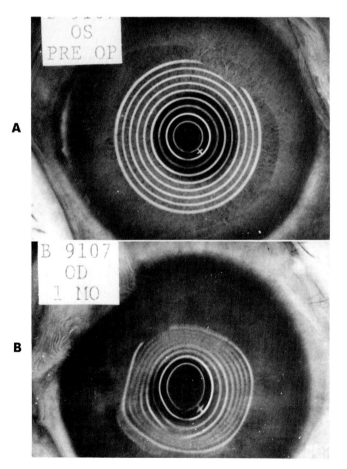

Fig. 36-29. Corneoscopic analysis of myopic hydrogel implant. Preoperative appearance, **A,** and postoperative appearance, **B,** are shown. Dramatic central flattening is evident postoperatively.

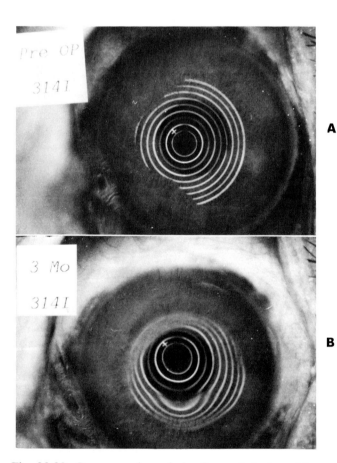

Fig. 36-30. Corneoscopic analysis of myopic hydrogel implant. Preoperative appearance, **A,** and postoperative appearance, **B,** are shown. Symmetric central corneal flattening is demonstrated with this myopic lens design.

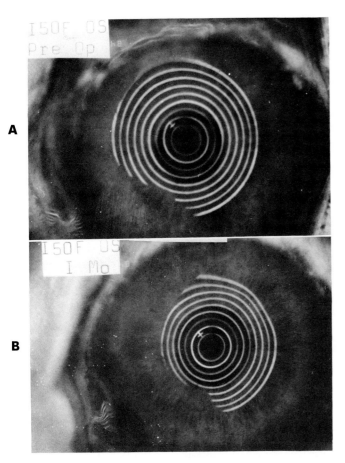

A

B

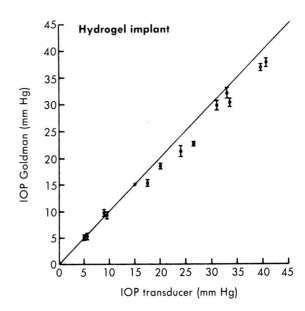

Fig. 36-32. Plot of actual intraocular pressure (IOP) (abscissa) versus observed IOP (ordinate) in eye with a myopic hydrogel implant. Goldman tonometer was used to measure IOP over a 0 to 40 mm Hg range.

Fig. 36-31. Corneoscopic analysis of hyperopic hydrogel implant. Preoperative appearance, **A,** and postoperative appearance, **B,** are shown. Symmetric central steepening is demonstrated.

fairly even, symmetric flattening of the central cornea (Fig. 36-30). With the hyperopic implants it has been easy to demonstrate a very even and symmetric pattern with steepening of the central cornea (Fig. 36-31).

STABILITY

It has been shown that the anterior corneal curvature stabilizes between 2 and 4 weeks postoperatively in the hyperopic implants. Similarly, the position of the implant, the thickness of the cornea in front of the implant, the thickness of the implant itself, and the thickness of the posterior corneal stroma are constant. Thus the implant does not appear to show any migration or progressive dissolution of the anterior corneal cap as a function of time.

INTRAOCULAR PRESSURE MEASUREMENT

Recent studies in primate eyes have demonstrated the accuracy of intraocular pressure measurements

using Goldmann and pneumotonometry in eyes with hydrogel implants. Cannulation of the anterior chamber was performed with balanced salt solution infusion to regulate intraocular pressure while another needle was connected to a pressure transducer. Data generated over a wide range of intraocular pressures showed that routine forms of tonometry could be easily and accurately performed with the hydrogel implants in place (Fig. 36-32). This contrasts with the usage of polysulfone implants, which are more rigid than hydrogel implants and may hamper accurate measurement of intraocular pressure.

COMPLICATIONS

Historically, there have been several problems with hydrogel implantation, largely attributable to variable manufacturing standards, that have now been resolved. Early in the study of hydrogels, we demonstrated the deleterious effects of chemical contaminants on the surface of the hydrogel. Abnormal keratocytes (Fig. 36-33) were demonstrated both in front of and behind the implant, positions that make it unlikely that nutrient flow factors were causative. In addition, thickened implant edges have caused anterior corneal necrosis 6 to 8 months after apparently successful surgery (Fig. 36-34).

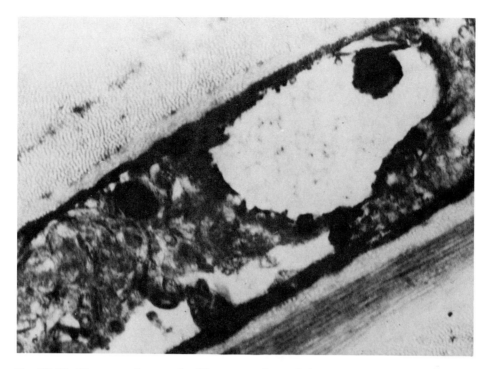

Fig. 36-33. Electron micrograph of keratocyte located deep to hydrogel implant, demonstrating pronounced vascularization and dense body formation.

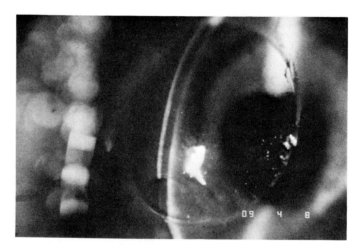

Fig. 36-34. Slitlamp appearance of poorly designed hydrogel implant with thick edges. Lower edge of lens is shown eroding through anterior cornea, having been in place for 8 months.

HYDROGEL VERSUS POLYSULFONE MATERIAL

A large impermeable barrier placed within the corneal stroma will lead to aseptic necrosis of the anterior corneal surface. Polysulfone implants are impermeable to water and nutrients, and to succeed physiologically, they must (1) be positioned very deep within the cornea close to Descemet's membrane, (2) be made in small diameters, thereby making the impermeable barrier less effective for the anterior cornea (Fig. 36-35), or (3) be perforated to allow nutrients to pass through the implant (Fig. 36-36). The polysulfone implant planted deep within the cornea does not achieve its refractive effect by modifying the corneal curva-

IMPERMEABLE LENS

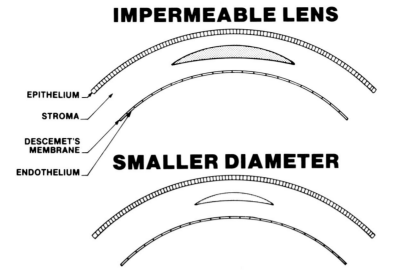

EPITHELIUM

STROMA

DESCEMET'S MEMBRANE

ENDOTHELIUM

SMALLER DIAMETER

Fig. 36-35. Diagram of small-diameter polysulfone implant within corneal stroma. The larger the lens diameter, the greater the tendency to prevent nutrient flow to anterior corneal layers.

IMPERMEABLE LENS

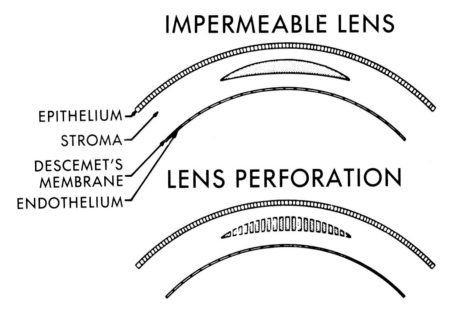

EPITHELIUM

STROMA

DESCEMET'S MEMBRANE

ENDOTHELIUM

LENS PERFORATION

Fig. 36-36. Diagram of perforated polysulfone implant within corneal stroma. Perforation allows nutrient flow to anterior cornea and allows usage of a larger-diameter implant without compromising nutrient supply.

ture but instead by changing the refractive index of the cornea. In contrast, the hydrogel, to have any effect, must be planted anteriorly enough so as to change the anterior radius of curvature of the cornea (Fig. 36-37).

The long-term stability of corneal inlays is an important consideration. Up to now most solid polysulfone lenses used in animal models have induced significant pathologic changes in the corneal stroma an-

terior to the implant.[6] In contrast hydrogel lenses in animal model systems have demonstrated good long-term tolerances with almost a decade of stability noted in some cases.[10]

Histopathologic data, again from nonhuman primate modeling systems, have demonstrated little reactivity to the implanted hydrogel material. Slight thinning of the epithelium overlying the implant is seen in most cases. The implant cavity shows some

POLYSULFONE

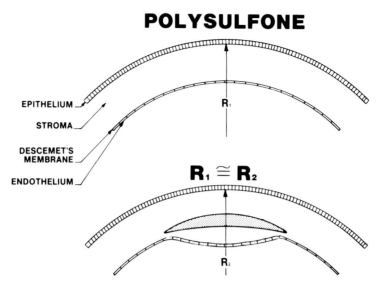

Fig. 36-37. Diagram of deeply placed polysulfone implant having no effect on anterior corneal shape in contrast to hydrogels, whose effect is largely dependent on altering anterior corneal surface.

minimal collagen deposition around the implant with very little cellular section.[10]

Clinical Studies. Having demonstrated a reasonable degree of safety and efficiency in modeling systems, the Food and Drug Administration beginning in 1988 has allowed limited clinical testing of hydrogels within and without the United States. A summary of the existing clinical data are presented here though very little has been published up to now.

Both hyperopic and myopic hydrogel inlays have been tested in human subjects. In one study of hyperopic hydrogel inlays, about 30 patients have been implanted. Patients enrolled in the study were contact lens intolerant and poor candidates for intraocular procedures because of preexisting disorder. Twenty patients have been followed for at least 1 year, and the accuracy of the refractive result was ±1.5 diopters (standard deviation). Lens exchange, to improve accuracy, has not been routinely performed up to now. By 2 months postoperatively most patients achieved their maximal dioptric correction and remained stable through at least 6 months. Data on 16 patients at 6 months indicated an average induced cylinder of about 1 diopter (scalar analysis). Recovery of best corrected vision was relatively slow, but at 1 year patients generally seemed to approach preoperative acuity levels whereas at 6 months patients were about two lenses below postoperative correction. Generally there was good tolerance of the implant material though several intraoperative and postoperative complications

occurred. These included irregular microkeratome sections, epithelial ingrowth and implant migration.

Data surrounding myopic inlays is even more limited. The first myopic hydrogel inlays in humans were implanted by Dr. José Barraquer in Bogotá, Columbia. Because both data and follow-up period are limited, a few case summaries illustrate the best and worst results up to now. One patient, R.M., had preoperative best corrected vision of 20/30 with a refraction of −9.50 D. A −10 D lens was implanted, and at 6 months the corrected acuity was 20/45, uncorrected acuity 20/150, and residual refraction of −2.0 −2.0 × 60°. At 2 years the corrected acuity was 20/25 and the uncorrected acuity was 20/60 with a residual refraction of −1.5 −2.0 × 30°. Another patient, M.M., had a preoperative best corrected acuity of 20/50 with a refraction of −13.0 −1.0 × 20°. A −13 D lens was implanted, and at 6 months the corrected acuity was 20/50, uncorrected acuity was 20/200, and residual refraction was −4.0 −2.0 × 45°. At 2 years the residual refraction had decreased to −6.5 −2.0 × 70°, with corrected acuity of 20/25 and uncorrected acuity of finger counting. In the first case, there was noted a good refractive result, which appeared to be stable, whereas in the second case, the refractive result was initially much less than adequate, but in addition a significant loss of effect was seen over time. Lens replacements to correct for residual refractive errors have not been performed but should improve accuracy considerably. In Dr. Barraquer's hands, no intraoperative complications occurred, but in the limited experience in the United States, some microkeratome-related problems were encountered. Some long-term changes have been noted in the interface in some cases, particularly those of Dr. Barraquer. These interface deposits did not appear to significantly affect acuity.

SUMMARY

Synthetic keratophakia using hydrogel inlays remain a feasible alternative for treating both aphakia and high myopia. Early human clinical testing of these inlays has demonstrated some limited success. However the ultimate success of this concept will require longer periods of clinical follow-up observation as well as additional efforts in redesign of the microkeratome. Finally, the ultimate goal of a highly accurate procedure will be achieved only with lens exchange for which these procedures are exquisitely suited.

ACKNOWLEDGMENT

I wish to acknowledge the assistance of Anil Patel, Ph.D., of Alcon Laboratories, Inc., Fort Worth, Texas, and Patty Knight, Ph.D., and Blake Storje, both of Allergan Medical Optics, Santa Ana, California, for their assistance in furnishing data from the human clinical studies cited in the text.

REFERENCES

1. Barraquer JI: *Queratoplastia refractiva*, Barcelona, 1949, Instituto Barraquer, vol 2, chapter 10, pp 1-21.
2. Binder PS: Hydrogel implants for the correction of myopia, *Curr Eye Res* 2:7, 1982-1983.
3. Binder PS, Deg JK, Zavala EY, Grossman KR: Hydrogel keratophakia in non-human primates, *Curr Eye Res* 1:535-542, 1981-1982.
4. Binder PS, Zavala EY, Deg JK: Hydrogel refractive keratoplasty: lens removal and exchanges, *Cornea* 2(2):119-125, 1983.
5. Choyce DP: Semi-rigid corneal inlays used in the management of albinism, aniridia, and ametropia. In Henkind P, editor: *Acta XXIV International Congress of Ophthalmology*, New York, 1982, Lippincott, pp 1230-1234.
6. Climenhaga H, Macdonald J, McCarey BE, Waring GO: Effect of diameter and depth on the response to solid polysulfone intracorneal lenses in cats, *Arch Ophthalmol* 106:818-824, 1988.
7. McCarey BE, Andrews DM: Refractive keratoplasty with intrastromal hydrogel lenticular implants, *Invest Ophthalmol* 21:107-115, 1981.
8. Werblin TP, Blaydes JE, Fryczkowski AW, Peiffer RL: Stability of hydrogel intracorneal implants in non-human primates, *CLAO J* 9(2):157-161, 1983.
9. Werblin TP, Blaydes JE, Fryczkowski AW, Peiffer RL: Alloplastic implant in non-human primates. III. Myopic correction: preliminary report, *Ann Ophthalmol* 16(12):1127-1130, 1984.
10. Werblin TP, Peiffer RL, Binder PS, McCarey BE, Patel AS: *Eight years experience with Permalens[R] intracorneal lenses in non-human primates.* (In preparation.)

Chapter 37

Myopic Keratomileusis

Theory, case selection, and major variables in success or failure

KEVIN H. CHARLTON

Keratomileusis and keratophakia are modified lamellar keratoplasties used for the correction of large ametropias. Keratomileusis involves a lamellar resection on the patient's cornea with a modification of the resected cornea on a cryolathe to produce an alteration of the anterior corneal curvature (Fig. 37-1). The advantage of keratomileusis is that it is an autoplastic procedure not relying upon the need for a donor cornea. It can correct a high range of myopia from −6.00 to −18.00, or hyperopia from +5.00 to +11.00.

Keratophakia also involves a lamellar resection of the patient's cornea. However, a donor cornea modified on the cryolathe is inserted at the lamellar interface to cause an increase in the anterior corneal curvature when the resected lamellar corneal tissue is resutured to the cornea (Fig. 37-2). Keratophakia may correct from +11.00 to +18.00 diopters of hyperopia.

HISTORY

We are all indebted to the ingenuity and perseverance of Dr. José Barraquer of Bogotá, Colombia, for the development of keratomileusis and keratophakia. Dr. Barraquer began in 1949 experimenting in the techniques of lamellar keratoplasty for the correction of refractive errors. His work led to the development of the microkeratome to make the lamellar corneal resection needed for the surgery, and the cryolathe to freeze and carve the resected lamellar cornea. Keratophakia was first performed on humans by Dr. Barraquer in 1963 and keratomileusis for myopia in 1964. Recent advances include

but are not limited to new computer programs to make the necessary calculations to modify the resected cornea.

THEORY

The refractive changes produced by keratomileusis and keratophakia are caused by alteration of the anterior corneal curvature. Theoretically the calculations are based upon the following equation:

$$R_f = [(n' - n) \div (D_i + D_c)]\, 1000$$

The equations are based upon the patient's initial diopter power of corneal surface (D_i), the index of refraction for corneal stroma 1.376 (n'), the index of refraction of air (n), the diopter power of refractive error (D_c), and the final radius of curvature (R_f) needed to produce the desired effect. Furthermore, these calculations are modified by the incremental changes produced by expansion of the cornea and contraction of the cryolathe during freezing.[2]

The theoretical calculations have tended to produce undercorrections in the clinical setting. To compensate for this in keratomileusis for myopia, the patient's diopter power of myopia is measured at a vertex of 12 mm and that value is used in the calculations instead of the value of myopia converted at the corneal plane.[6] For example, for −12.00 diopters of myopia at 12 mm vertex, the amount of dioptric power at the cornea is −10.37. The −12.00 diopter number is used in the calculations to produce the needed overcorrection for clinical results.

In patients with astigmatic refractive errors, the refraction at the 12 mm vertex is converted into minus cylinder form, and the spherical portion of the refraction is then used for the calculations.[4] For example, −7.00 −2.00 × axis. The −7.00 is used in the calculations. An ideal result after surgery would

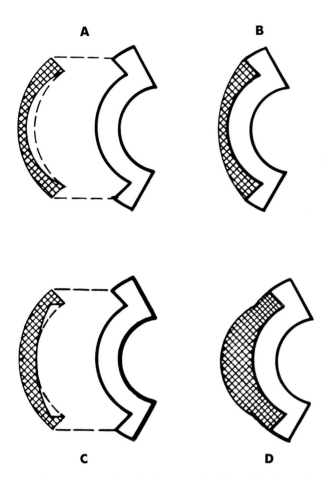

Fig. 37-1. Keratomileusis for myopia, **A** and **B.** Lamellar disc is carved for minus correction, **A,** and flattens corneal curvature, **B.** Keratomileusis for hypermetropia, **C** and **D.** Lamellar corneal disc is carved for plus correction, **C,** and steepens curvature, **D.**

then be plano −2.00 × axis. The astigmatic refractive error could then be managed postoperatively if the keratotomy incisions are relaxed.

Dr. Barraquer recommends the average keratometric reading used for the theoretical calculations. Keratometers differ in calibration based upon the index of refraction of the corneal tissue. It is necessary to convert the keratometric readings to those compatible with Dr. Barraquer's calculations based upon a corneal index refraction of 1.376.[6]

A simplified way of conceptualizing the surgery is as follows. The microkeratome produces a lamellar resection of anterior cornea creating a disc composed of parallel faces approximately 7 to 8 mm in diameter and 0.25 to 0.40 mm in thickness. The anterior surface of this disc is composed of epithelium and Bowman's layer. The posterior surface is corneal stroma. One then modifies this disc by carving the stromal surface to create a lens. A minus power lens is made for the correction of myopia, the shape being thin in the center and thicker on the edges. For hyperopia the corneal stroma is carved as a plus lens, being thicker in the center and thinned at the edges. In keratophakia a donor cornea is carved as a plus lens and inserted at the lamellar interface produced by the keratectomy.

KEYS TO SUCCESS

Successful surgery is based on good case selection, adequate preparation, good surgical technique, and proper postoperative care.

Case Selection. Keratomileusis for myopia can generally correct between −6.00 and −18.00 diopters of myopia. We are limited in the amount of correction possible by the initial radius of curvature of the patient's cornea. In general a final radius of curvature after surgery needs to be greater than 33.00

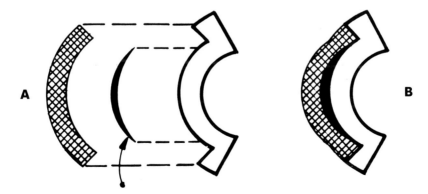

Fig. 37-2. Keratophakia. **A,** Donor cornea carved to plus lens. **B,** Intracorneal lens steepens cornea.

diopters[2] to be stable and provide good visual acuity. Thus a patient with a 43.00 diopter initial radius curvature of the cornea can be flattened to 33.00 diopters, and a correction of 10 diopters at the corneal plane (−11.50 diopters at 12 mm) would be all that would be possible in that patient.

Keratomileusis for hyperopia can correct between +5.00 and 11.00 diopters of hyperopia. Keratophakia is necessary for greater hyperopic corrections from +11.00 to +18.00.

Again we are limited by the final radius of curvature postoperatively. Corneas steeper than 57.00 diopters[2] tend to have poor vision.

Keratomileusis for hypermetropia and keratophakia are alternatives to intraocular lens implantation in those patients who are contact lens intolerant and are not intraocular lens candidates.[6]

In the correction of aphakia it is doubtful that keratophakia or hypermetropic keratomileusis will be widely used, since intraocular lenses provide a fast safe alternative.

Contraindications. Keratoconus and irregular scarred corneas are contraindications to surgery. Corneas of abnormal size or shape may not be compatible with the necessary suction rings and microkeratome to perform an adequate keratectomy. Preoperative corneal curvatures flatter than 39 diopters or steeper than 48 diopters should be avoided.[4] Corneas thinner than 0.48 mm may not provide enough tissue for correction and stability postoperatively. The surgery is therefore usually limited to older children or adults. Keratoconjunctivitis sicca, amblyopia, and glaucoma are relative contraindications, depending on their severity.

Myopic macular degeneration is not a contraindication, since many patients improve vision because of reduction of minification by myopic lenses.[6]

Preparation. Since the microkeratome and cryolathe are difficult procedures, different from regular ophthalmic techniques, training should include a practical hands-on course with the opportunity to perform practice surgery and lathing in the laboratory under supervision of experienced surgeons. After the practical course the surgeon is encouraged to practice regularly and become familiar with the multiple steps necessary to perform successful surgery. An ophthalmic technician knowledgeable in the technique is useful to supervise the rest of the operating room crew during the surgery. For a surgeon's initial cases it is recommended an experienced keratomileusis surgeon be present in the operating room for support.

Surgical Technique. Surgery may be performed on an outpatient using either local or general anesthesia. Retrobulbar injection of Marcaine (bupivacaine hydrochloride) and lidocaine (Xylocaine) will greatly decrease the incidence of postoperative pain and have the beneficial effect of 2 to 4 mm of proptosis that aids in exposure making the microkeratome resection easier. The eye is draped with plastic drapes, since they are lint free. Care must be taken to allow adequate exposure so that the microkeratome does not get caught on the eyelid speculum or drapes.

The keys to a good keratectomy are adequate and stable suction, good centration, and a slow, steady forward movement of the microkeratome.

Centration. One accomplishes centration by marking the visual axis similar to radial keratotomy. Furthermore, a reference mark is made in the corneal epithelium from the center out to the periphery using a series of minute epithelial scratches so that the orientation of the resected cornea can be resutured exactly. These reference marks should be a series of small microabrasions and not a continuous line to avoid having the epithelium slough off after freezing. The suction ring is then centered around the marked visual axis.

Suction. Loss of suction during the keratotomy may result in an irregular or inadequate keratectomy, or even perforation of the anterior chamber.

To avoid this, the section ring needs to be adequately adapted to the globe such that it does not lose suction during the keratectomy. To ensure adequate adaption and suction, two tests are performed before the keratotomy.

The suction applied to the eye by the suction rings raises the intraocular pressure to a range of 60 to 85 mm Hg. The pressure is needed to ensure a good keratectomy. However, the measured pressure of 60 mm Hg does not ensure adequate adaptation of the suction ring. The applanation lens, which measures the diameter of cornea presented to the microkeratome to be resected, applanates the cornea similar to the microkeratome. Listening to the suction apparatus for breaks in suction when the lens is applanated is useful in the determination of an adequate adaptation of the suction ring. A second test involves the positioning of the microkeratome. The microkeratome is positioned in the dovetail groove of the suction ring and pushed forward. The cornea is applanated before one cuts with the microkeratome blade. Because of the design of the microkeratome, approximately one half of the cornea is applanated before the oscillating blade of the microkeratome comes into contact with the cornea. At this point, observation to detect breaks in suction during this initial applanation will allow the surgeon to abort before turning on the keratome and cutting the cornea. Once adequate suction is established the keratectomy may be accomplished consistently.

Chemosis. Conjunctival chemosis may interfere with proper adaptation of the suction ring. If this is the case, a 360-degree limbal peritomy will ensure adequate fixation of the suction ring. Good hemostasis is necessary.

Microkeratome. The microkeratome needs to be properly assembled, and an adequate plate chosen for the depth of the incision desired. The microkeratome is checked before use to determine that the oscillating blade moves freely. The microkeratome should also be placed in the selected suction ring and moved across to make sure that there are no hangups in the suction ring to be used during surgery. For new microkeratomes the depth of cut should be measured by use of human cadaver eyes or PK20 rubber.[4]

Once committed, one pushes forward the microkeratome in a slow, smooth motion. When the keratectomy is completed, both the suction and the microkeratome are turned off at the same time by release of the foot pedals. The exposed lamellar cornea is then protected with a protective shield.

Lathing. After measurement and emersion in cryoprotectants, the resected lamellar cornea is then placed on the Delrin base of the cryolathe. Before this, the Delrin base has been precarved, and the lathe is visually checked to make sure that the tool has adequate clearance from the Delrin base based upon the calculator-generated lathe settings for the amount of myopia and the thickness of the resected cornea. Doing so ensures that a perforation of the lenticule will not occur unless the lenticule is detached. It is useful to have a Delrin base of similar diameter to that of the resected corneal tissue. If a small cornea is placed on a large Delrin base, it is difficult to center; whereas, if the Delrin base and the resected cornea are of very similar sizes, centering is much easier. Care must be taken to allow no air bubbles between the cornea and the Delrin base. After the cornea is placed on the Delrin base, centered, and checked for air bubbles, the excess fluid is drained with a sponge. Murocel sponges are useful, since they have less fibrous material than other types. It is important that the carbon dioxide pressure in the tanks be greater than 800 mm Hg or inadequate freezing and adherence of the cornea to the Delrin base may occur and the cornea may become dislocated. An electronic digital displacement gage is useful since it enables you to control visually the end point to the depth of the carving. Before use of the digital gage, this end point was controlled by a manual stop, which could be passed by excessive pressure.

Removal of particles and inclusions. Proper preparation of the resected corneal bed is necessary to ensure the absence of interface particulate matter and epithelial inclusions. The bed is carefully irrigated with saline solution, preferably filtered, and some surgeons utilize a mohair brush to brush the bed to relieve particulate matter. Studies by Krumeich[4] and Barraquer[2] have shown a lesser incidence of epithelial inclusions and interface particles during their later cases than in their earlier cases. The plastic drapes, the absence of gloves, and careful irrigation ensure that few if any particles will be present at the interface.

Suture. A running antitorque suture is used to secure the graft.

Postoperative Care. Healing the corneal epithelium is the main concern during the immediate postoperative period because the lamellar epithelium is freeze damaged and sloughs off. Tarsorrhaphy sutures, patching, and occasionally bandage contact lenses are used to provide reepithelialization along with topical antibiotics. Complete healing of the epithelium is usually present by 3 to 5 days. Any enlarging epithelial inclusions observed in the graft periphery need removal by lifting of the graft and scraping. If epithelial inclusions occur within the visual axis, early intervention is recommended,[5] since it may be possible to lift the resected cornea, scrape, and then resuture. In general these complications occur in the first few weeks of surgery and are readily apparent. Extensive scarring or epithelialization of the interface may be treated with a repeat keratectomy and donor cornea.

Residual refractive errors, that is, astigmatism or myopia, can be managed by radial keratotomy or Ruiz astigmatic keratotomy relaxing incisions. It is best to delay this until 1 year after surgery for stabilization of the cornea to occur.

NEW ADVANCES

New advances in keratomileusis technique involve an automated microkeratome, resection of stroma with the microkeratome (keratomileusis in situ), and keratomileusis in combination with excimer laser stromal ablation.

The new self-propelled microkeratome works on the same principle as the original microkeratome. However, it has been modified with gears and a track to propel the microkeratome across the cornea at a constant speed, thus eliminating the surgeon's influence on the microkeratome resection.

Keratomileusis in situ utilizes the microkeratome

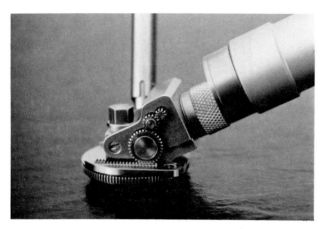

Fig. 37-3. Automatic corneal shaper. (Courtesy Steinway Instrument Company, San Diego, Calif.)

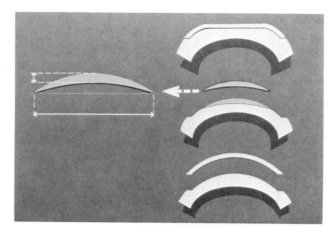

Fig. 37-5. Keratomileusis in situ with resection of midstromal tissue by second pass of microkeratome.

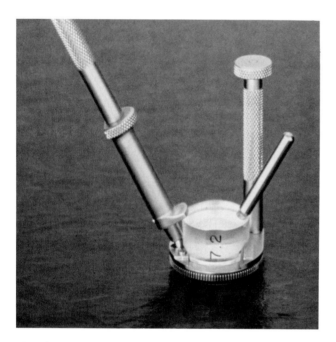

Fig. 37-4. Adjustable fixation ring. (Courtesy Steinway Instrument Company, San Diego, Calif.)

to resect corneal stroma instead of lathing on the cryolathe. A microkeratome resection (Fig. 37-3) is used to remove the corneal cap in the standard manner. Next, a different set of fixation rings or adjustable fixation rings (Fig. 37-4) are used to guide the microkeratome for a second pass over the cornea resecting the middle layer of stroma. The diameter and depth of this second resection determines the refractive correction (Fig. 37-5). The resected cap is then sutured in place, and the resected material

from the second pass of the microkeratome is then discarded.

Most recently investigations have begun into the combination of keratomileusis with the excimer laser.[3] A microkeratome resection is made in the standard manner, and then the excimer laser is used to remove stromal tissue to obtain the refractive correction. The resected cap is then sutured in place. This technique avoids the ablation of Bowman's membrane with the excimer laser and the corneal haziness that occurs when ablating the front surface of the cornea.

REFERENCES

1. Barraquer JI: Calculations for refractive keratoplasty, *Arch Soc Am Oftalmol Optom* 8:103-164, 1970.
2. Barraquer JI: Keratomileusis for myopia and aphakia, *Ophthalmology* 88:701-708, 1981.
3. Brint SF: U.S. trial of excimer MKM, *Ocular Surgery News* 9(15):1, 1991.
4. Krumeich JH: Indication, techniques and complications of myopic keratomileusis, *Int Ophthalmol Clin* 23(3):75-91, 1983.
5. Nordan LT: Personal communication, La Jolla, Calif, 1985.
6. Swinger CA, Barker BA: Prospective evaluation of myopic keratomileusis, *Ophthalmology* 91:785-792, 1984.
7. Troutman RC: Indications, techniques, and complications of keratophakia, *Int Ophthalmol Clin* 23(3):11-23, 1983.
8. Villaseñor, RA: Introduction to and historical overview of surgical procedures for the correction of refractive errors, *Int Ophthalmol Clin* 23(3):1-9, 1983.

Improvements in technique, technology, and instrumentation

RICHARD A. VILLASEÑOR

CASIMIR A. SWINGER

Myopic keratomileusis (MKM) is a form of lamellar refractive keratoplasty that flattens the corneal

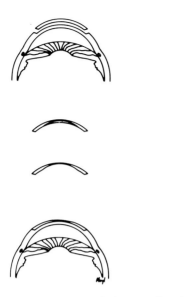

Fig. 37-6. Lamellar resection; myopic keratomileusis lenticule before and after being lathed, with resultant flattened cornea.

curvature and reduces moderate to high myopic refractive errors (Fig. 37-6). Although surgeons have been performing this surgery since 1963,[3] world experience has been relatively small. We review the literature on MKM in the next section, p. 440.

BARRAQUER'S EARLY RESEARCH

Barraquer's earliest attempts to correct refractive errors surgically have previously been described by Villaseñor.[14] In 1949 he resected a peripheral ring of corneal tissue, made a freehand lamellar dissection of the remaining central cornea, and resutured it onto the lamellar bed under tension to flatten its anterior contour.

In 1958, he attempted to freeze a rabbit cornea in situ before reshaping it. However, the low temperature resulted in irreversible damage to the iris and clear crystalline lens. He next prepared lenticules from donor eyes by performing a freehand lamellar dissection, lathing the disc on an ordinary watchmaker's lathe, and sewing the lenticule onto a lamellar recipient bed, dissected freehand, on the patient's eye. In 1964, Barraquer first utilized a microkeratome on a patient's cornea and modified the disc on a prototype of the current cryolathe. This first autoplastic lenticule was then sewn onto its original bed.

Since then, Barraquer has successfully performed hundreds of cases of MKM with good results. Similar results have subsequently been reported by various investigators.

EARLY AMERICAN EXPERIENCE

We began performing MKM in 1980 and have continuously performed the surgery since that time. Beginning a new and complicated procedure like MKM in a country far from its developer, we found that there were inevitable complications reflected in the initial series. The complication rate was high, with three central perforations of the disc during lathing and two cases of irregular astigmatism. In addition, three eyes had epithelial cells in the interface that were located out of the visual axis and did not affect the visual acuity. Endothelial cell counts on six patients revealed a mean cell loss of 13.6%.

IMPROVEMENTS IN TECHNIQUE

Microcomputer Programs. Early calculator programs utilized the programmable Texas Instrument 59 with printer. The programs were initially written by Barraquer and required the following data input:
1. Mean corneal radius of curvature (mm)
2. Desired refractive correction (diopters, D)
3. Thickness of resected corneal disc (mm)
4. Thickness of corneal disc after freezing (mm)

The computer then generated the lathe settings, after which the surgeon "set up" the lathe and modified the tissue. There was one datum that was time consuming to obtain, was often inaccurate, and resulted in a prolonged freezing time. This was the thickness of the frozen lamellar disc. After the microkeratome section, the resected tissue was measured, placed on the cryolathe, and frozen. Freezing resulted in an increase in corneal thickness, which must be taken into account mathematically. The method of measuring this increment during surgery was difficult and gave variable results.

Unpublished data have indicated that the freezing increment may not have changed considerably during autoplastic surgery. This led to abandonment of measuring the freezing increment during surgery and assumption of a fixed value (1.0908) close in value to the coefficient of expansion of water. Elimination of this step now enables the microcomputer to generate the lathe settings before placement of the cornea on the cryolathe. Adequate tool clearance can be microscopically verified before lathing, which eliminates setup errors and greatly reduces the chances of perforation. In addition, the freezing time is now significantly reduced to approximately 60 to 90 seconds. Our research has shown that reducing the freezing time increases the number of viable keratocytes and epithelial cells.[9] The clinical significance of these findings has yet to be documented.

Further recent improvements include factors taking into consideration the patient's age, resected disc diameter, resected disc thickness, and optic zone diameter, all determined by multivariate analysis.[1,5] Most surgeons now use a personal computer during surgery.

Modification of Cryolathe. Early models of the cryolathe utilized mechanical micrometer heads to set the cutting radius and displacement. The divisions of the micrometers were small and difficult to read and occasionally resulted in lathing errors (Fig. 37-7). These mechanical micrometer heads have been replaced by electronic displacement indicators with light-emitting diode readouts that read to 1 μm (Fig. 37-8).

The cutting tool of the cryolathe has also been modified. The previous tool was pointed with a 0.1 mm curvature at its cutting tip (Fig. 37-9). Even with high-speed rotation, a uniform, smooth cut was sometimes difficult to obtain, especially in hyperopia. The tool has been changed to a 5.0 mm semioval configuration (Fig. 37-10) that provides a much smoother transition at the periphery of the optic zone, allowing for better wound coaptation.

Other improvements include rust-resistant metal surfaces, a rechargeable battery for the microkeratome, and a new heat exchanger to prevent the escape of carbon dioxide gas from the freezing circuit. Previously, gas could sometimes pass through the Delrin base, causing dislodgment of the lamellar disc.

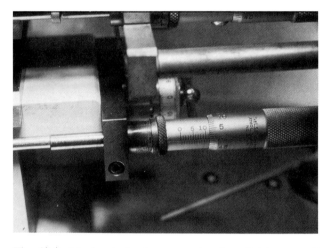

Fig. 37-7. Mechanical micrometer heads—divisions small and difficult to read.

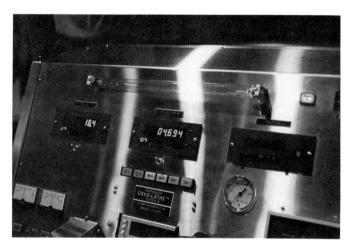

Fig. 37-8. Electronic displacement indicators with light-emitting diode readouts.

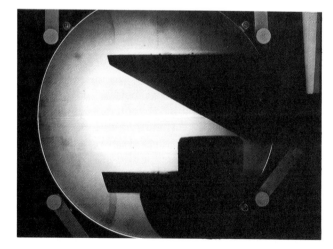

Fig. 37-9. Tool 0.1 mm visualized on shadowgraph from top and side.

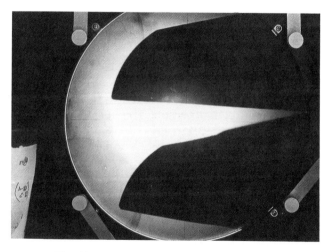

Fig. 37-10. Semioval configuration 5 mm.

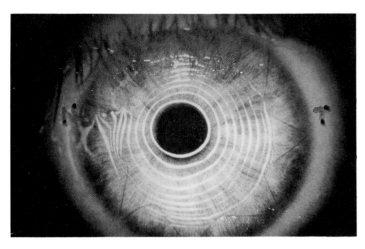

Fig. 37-11. Center ring photokeratoscope is displaced nasally corresponding to visual axis. MKM sutures visible.

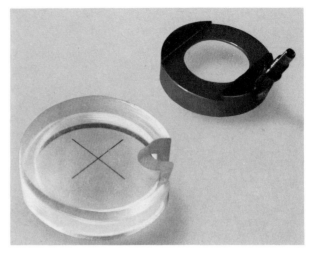

Fig. 37-12. Cross hairs of applanation lens are aligned with visual axis before microkeratome section.

Microkeratome Section. The diameter of the microkeratome section in myopic keratomileusis typically measures 7.00 to 7.50 mm. It is critical that this section be aligned as closely as possible to the visual axis of the eye, which is usually located slightly nasal to the anatomic center of the cornea (Fig. 37-11). The pneumatic suction ring, when applied to the eye, usually centers itself with the anatomic center of the cornea. Grasping the sclera with forceps when the pneumatic ring is applied allows the surgeon to decenter it slightly nasally before doing the microkeratome section. An epithelial reference mark made with a blunt instrument on the visual axis, similar to that made during radial keratotomy surgery, is useful in centering the pneumatic ring. One of us (C.A.S.) has developed an applanation lens with cross hairs (Fig. 37-12) that greatly facilitates the alignment of the microkeratome section with the previously marked visual axis.[10]

Should the microkeratome resection still be decentered, we have achieved good results by centering the visual axis mark on the disc with the center of rotation of the lathe or the center of the BKS die (p. 438). This ensures that the optic zone created will be concentric with the visual axis, even though it may be decentered within the lenticule.

Automated Microkeratome. Luis Ruiz and Jörg Draeger have each developed automated microkeratomes that standardize the passage of the microkeratome during the resection. Initial experience has shown smooth and regular resections, though in one instance with the Ruiz unit the passage halted during the keratectomy and needed to be completed manually. Another major advantage of these instruments is that the diameter of the resection can be varied without a change in the suction rings, which increases safety.

Partial Conjunctival Peritomy. One of the complications sometimes encountered by the novice refractive surgeon is a break in suction during the microkeratome section. This usually results in a small corneal section, necessitating suturing of the small, irregular corneal piece onto its bed and cessation of surgery. The surgeon must allow several months of healing before repeating the surgery. Interruption of suction can occur because of excessive upward traction on the suction ring by the surgeon or obstruction of the suction port by the perilimbal conjunctiva. A small 3 mm peritomy, corresponding to the proposed site of placement of the suction port, greatly reduces the chances of this complication, in cases where newer models of the suction ring or microkeratome are not employed.

Suction Ring Manifold. Another attempt to reduce the incidence of aborted resections has been the development of newer suction rings having a manifold with many ports to deliver the suction, rather than a single port. This distributes the suction through a more or less continuous channel, thereby increasing safety because one or several ports may become occluded and still allow a satisfactory keratectomy.

Interface Hygeine. Epithelial cells are frequently observed in the interface after keratomileusis and keratophakia (Fig. 37-13). They may be deposited there either by the blade of the microkeratome or by later peripheral epithelial cell ingrowth because of poor wound coaptation. The latter cause is fre-

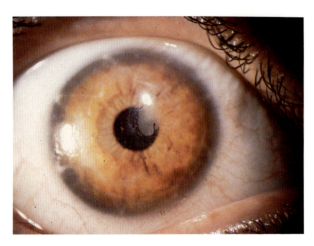

Fig. 37-13. Epithelialization of interface after MKM procedure.

quently overcome as the surgeon becomes more skilled. The epithelial cells that are deposited in the interface during the surgical procedure must be removed by careful irrigation with filtered saline. There is a tendency in the surgeon's initial cases to minimize this important step. Time must be taken for cleansing of the interface to remove epithelial cells or foreign bodies. All accomplished refractive surgeons notice a dramatic reduction in the incidence of this complication as they become more comfortable with this procedure and have more time to direct their attention toward this important step.

Cryopreserving Solution. Before freezing, the corneal tissue is placed in a cryopreserving solution for 1 minute. Initially, this solution consisted of glycerol (8%), DMSO (dimethyl sulfoxide) (4%), and Fast green dye (0.25%) in distilled water. Research has indicated that DMSO may be toxic to the corneal endothelium and possibly the keratocytes, and it has recently been eliminated from the solution. In addition, many surgeons make the solution up in a buffered media.

CURRENT DEVELOPMENTS AND TRENDS

Homoplastic Surgery. Despite the improved surgical techniques discussed in this chapter, myopic keratomileusis remains extremely demanding with little margin for error. There are currently less than 15 refractive surgeons in the United States performing MKM on a regular basis. This is surprising, since approximately 350 surgeons have taken a complete lathing course. Some have purchased a cryolathe only to have subsequently abandoned the technique.

We have observed that homoplastic MKM has produced accuracy comparable to autoplastic MKM. A lenticule made specifically for the individual patient can be manufactured in the laboratory and shipped to the surgical site. Lenticules may be made using the cryolathe, BKS device, or excimer laser. This would enable the surgeon to electively schedule homoplastic MKM cases and eliminate the need to purchase costly equipment other than the microkeratome.

In addition, we have found other advantages to homoplastic MKM. These include greater safety, since the patient's original cap may be stored and replaced should it be determined after surgery that the microkeratome resection was irregular. This allows restoration of the original cornea. Also, we have been able to obtain greater corrections with the technique while maintaining a relatively normal final corneal thickness and good optic zone diameter, which enhances stability.

Combined Surgery. Even though the accuracy of MKM is satisfactory, some patients may still have less than desirable unaided acuity after surgery. This is especially so because some surgeons have taken the approach of slightly undercorrecting patients, to avoid cases of hyperopia. In such cases the residual refractive error can be corrected by subsequent radial or transverse keratotomy, 6 to 12 months later, to achieve a result close to emmetropia.

Nonfreeze Keratomileusis. Another advancement is a new instrument (BKS, Barraquer-Krumeich-Swinger device) developed by Swinger and Krumeich that allows the preparation of lenticules without freezing (Fig. 37-14), thereby eliminating cryodamage to the corneal tissue.[12] In addition to being less expensive than a cryolathe, this device provides several potential advantages such as rapid visual rehabilitation, reduction of subjective symptoms, portability, complete sterilizability, and a technically simplified surgical procedure. This instrument is capable of preparing lenticules for use in keratophakia, myopic keratomileusis, hyperopic keratomileusis, and epikeratophakia.

Keratomileusis in Situ. A modification of the original keratomileusis procedure has been developed by Ruiz. The procedure is a nonfreeze operation that eliminates the cryolathe and BKS device. A shallow microkeratome resection is performed on the patient's eye, and the resected tissue is set aside in a container. The ring of the microkeratome, being adjustable, is then set to provide a resection of much smaller diameter (3 to 5 mm). A second microkeratome resection is then performed within the confines of the first to remove a positive meniscus lens. The originally resected cap is then replaced, effecting a flattening of the cornea.

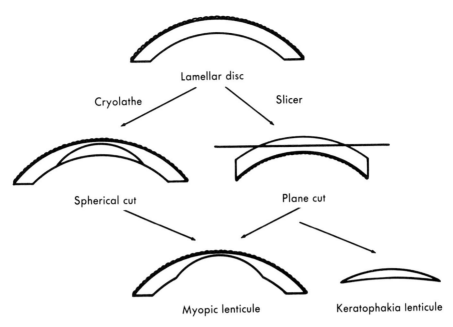

Fig. 37-14. Comparison of myopic lenticule produced by cryolathe versus nonfreezing technique. Cryolathe makes a spherical cut, whereas nonfreeze technique obtains same result when a planar cut is made. Resected area is destroyed by cryolathe but is spared by planar cut, producing a keratophakia lenticule.

This procedure requires great technical skill and is relatively irreversible should the second resection not be centered on the visual axis. Centration is thus very critical to avoid subjective symptoms. There have not been, unfortunately, any controlled studies reported in the literature, though several reports at symposiums have described good results.

Excimer Laser Keratomileusis. There is increasing use of the 193 nm excimer laser in corneal surgery. It is inevitable that this technology will be employed to replace MKM in some way or be used with it to produce the tissue-modification step. Just recently, a small study in the United States has begun using an excimer laser to replace the cryolathe and BKS as the modification device. Otherwise, the operation is the same. An early report at a symposium described promise for this approach.

CONCLUSIONS

The future of refractive surgery is most promising. Although most myopes may be surgically corrected with radial keratotomy, the moderate to high myope will require lamellar refractive surgery, unless a new laser technique is developed. The advances in technique discussed in this chapter will allow the surgeon who chooses to perform myopic keratomileusis a greater margin of safety and predictability for the patient. The use of homoplastic lenticules prepared in a central laboratory and the advent of the excimer laser promise to further simplify the technique and to make it a practical procedure for the general ophthalmologist in the future.

REFERENCES
1. Barraquer C, Gutierrez AM, Espinosa A: Myopic keratomileusis: short-term results, *Refract Corneal Surg* 5:307, 1989.
2. Barraquer JI: Method for cutting lamellar grafts in frozen cornea: new orientations for refractive surgery, *Oftalmol Optom* 1:1-271, 1958.
3. Barraquer JI: Autokératoplastie avec surfaçage pour la correction de la myopie (quératomileusis): technique et résultats, *Ann Oculiste* 198:401-425, 1965.
4. Barraquer JI: Keratomileusis for the correction of myopia, *Arch Soc Am Oftalmol Optom* 16:221, 1982.
5. Barraquer JI, Viteri E: Results of myopic keratomileusis, *J Refract Surg* 3:98, 1987.
6. Binder P: Refractive keratoplasty: tissue dyes and cryoprotective solutions, *Arch Ophthalmol* 101:1591-1596, 1983.
7. Maxwell WA: Myopic keratomileusis: initial results and myopic keratomileusis combined with other procedures, *J Cataract Refract Surg* 13:518, 1987.
8. Nordan LT: Myopic keratomileusis. In *Current status of refractive surgery*, San Diego, 1983, Steinway Instrument Company.
9. Schanzlin DJ, Jester JV, Pacheco LF, Villaseñor RA: Effects of keratorefractive cryo-techniques on the cornea: in vivo studies, *Invest Ophthalmol Vis Sci* 22(suppl):201, 1982, ARVO abstracts.
10. Swinger CA: Myopic keratomileusis. In Sanders D, Hofmann R, editors: *Refractive surgery*, ed 2, Thorofare, NJ, 1985, Slack Inc.

11. Swinger CA, Barker BA: Prospective evaluation of myopic keratomileusis, *Ophthalmology* 91:785-792, 1984.
12. Swinger CA, Krumeich J, Cassiday D: Planar lamellar refractive keratoplasty, *J Refract Surg* 2:17, 1986.
13. Villaseñor RA: *Recent improvements and results of myopic keratomileusis,* Presented at the International Society of Refractive Keratoplasty Symposium, Chicago, 1982.
14. Villaseñor RA: Homoplastic myopic keratomileusis. In Sanders D, Hofmann R, editors: *Refractive surgery,* ed 2, Thorofare, NJ, 1985, Slack Inc.

Evaluation of published results

CASIMIR A. SWINGER
RICHARD A. VILLASEÑOR

Myopic keratomileusis (MKM) is a form of lamellar refractive keratoplasty developed by José I. Barraquer of Bogotá, Colombia. The first clinical results with MKM were described by him in 1964.[3] The technique was performed by Barraquer alone until taken up by Ainslie in the early 1970s.[1] It was introduced into the United States in 1980.[16]

Myopic keratomileusis was developed as an autoplastic procedure and has been applied primarily to congenital myopia. The technique can also be performed on patients who have undergone prior surgery, such as radial keratotomy.[17] Also, MKM may be performed as a homoplastic procedure whereby a donor refractive lenticule replaces the resected anterior lamellae of the patient. The use of homoplastic MKM to obtain further myopic correction in patients who have previously undergone radial keratotomy has been described by Swinger.[17]

Clinical reports on MKM have been limited primarily to the correction of congenital myopia with autoplastic MKM.[1-16,18,19,21] This chapter is a review of these studies, which are tabulated in Table 37-1.

OPTIC CORRECTION

Refractive change after myopic keratomileusis can be determined by refraction, keratometry, or computerized topography. It has been documented that there is a poor correlation between the changes determined by keratometry and corneoscopy with those determined by refraction.[9] Therefore, since a change in the refraction is the goal of MKM, it is perhaps best that refraction be used to describe and analyze surgical results.

As in radial keratotomy, younger patients appear to obtain less correction than older patients do, averaging 0.50 D per decade.[7] Also, as with radial keratotomy, flatter corneas may achieve greater correction for the same procedure.[2]

High corrections are obtainable with MKM. In two series, for example, corrections of greater than 20 D

Table 37-1. Clinical Studies of Myopic Keratomileusis

Investigator	Year	Number of Cases
Barraquer	1964	12
Ainslie	1976	47
Barraquer	1981	72
Swinger, Barraquer	1981	85
Barraquer	1982	33
Barraquer	1983	23
Krumeich	1983	151
Swinger, Barker	1984	42
Swinger, Barker	1985	3
Swinger, Villaseñor	1985	10
Maxwell, Nordan	1986	23
Nordan, Fallor	1986	74
Polit	1986	147
Barraquer, Viteri	1987	74
Maxwell	1987	58
Barraquer, Gutierrez	1989	97
Neumann, McCarty	1989	4
Colin, Mimouni	1990	26

were reported.[10,16] Although very high corrections can be obtained, they necessarily result in excessive thinning of the central cornea in the majority of cases, unless the surgeon feels comfortable with the procedure and accepts a smaller optical zone. Therefore most surgeons presently limit the maximal dioptric correction requested to approximately 15 D and reserve homoplastic MKM for larger corrections. That MKM can provide high correction is also indicated by the mean refractive changes in these two series based on subjective testing, which were 13.58 D and 11.96 D respectively.[10,16]

Several studies have documented a significant underestimation of the refractive change when determined by keratometry. For example, the refractive and keratometric (here in parentheses) changes induced by MKM in several series were 5.92 D (4.09 D), 10.04 D (4.89 D), and 11.96 D (7.05 D) respectively.[8,10,12]

Barraquer claims there is an upper limit (10.06 mm) to which the corneal radius of curvature, measured by keratometry, can be flattened by MKM and remain stable, features implying an upper limit to the amount of optic correction possible.[4] However, two studies have documented radii flatter than this value, with values of 10.38 and 11.25 mm being reported.[6,16] Establishing an upper limit for corneal flattening with respect to radius of curvature and predicting the amount of correction obtainable in a given case on the basis of the initial radius of curvature and the theoretical upper limit are perhaps best avoided because there are examples of very high refractive corrections that have much lower changes when measured by keratometry. This further establishes the danger when one employs keratometry in assessing or predicting surgical results. In one series, for example, the maximal change determined by refraction was 23.25 D, whereas the maximal change determined by keratometry was only 12.31 D.[16] These considerations become especially important in a research setting on animals.

There is only one reported case of a patient whose myopia was worsened after MKM.[19] In this case, which was 7 years after surgery, the myopia was 1.87 D more than the preoperative value. Although such a finding may well be attributable to axial elongation, the patient also had excessive tissue resection that left the final corneal thickness less than desired, resulting in ectasia and corneal steepening. It has been recommended that the final corneal thickness not be left thinner than 0.30 mm and that corneas thinner than 0.50 mm not undergo autoplastic surgery.

Homoplastic MKM can provide greater optic correction than autoplastic MKM, and corrections of up to 25 D have been obtained.[20] The reason why greater correction is possible with homoplastic MKM is that the total thickness of the donor cornea is available for the production of the lenticule, whereas in autoplastic MKM only approximately 0.20 mm is available. Thus, regardless of the amount of optic correction, the final corneal thickness after homoplastic MKM can be left relatively normal.

ACCURACY

As with all refractive surgical techniques accuracy has been a concern. Because keratometry produces underestimates of the refractive correction, the percentage corrections obtained in different series may vary, depending on what modality of measurement was utilized in the calculations. In a prospective study, the mean percentage correction determined by refraction was 94.1%, with a range of 22% to 148%, a standard deviation of 24%, and a correlation coefficient of 0.43.[16] When determined by keratometry, the mean percentage was 67.2% with a range of 2.4% to 145%, a standard deviation of 33%, and a correlation coefficient of 0.11.[16] However, as previously mentioned, keratometry is not a useful modality for determination of the refractive change after MKM. In another study, 93.9% of the desired refractive correction was obtained with a standard deviation of 28.3%.[10] The mean follow-up observation was 10 months in the first series and 17 months in the second series.

In series with long follow-up times, the final optic result may be in greater part determined by stability or progressive myopia than by accuracy. For example, one study with a 5.5-year follow-up time found a mean percentage correction of 51.3%, based on refraction, with a standard deviation of 27.8%.[19] In another study, with a mean follow-up time of 6.1 years, the mean correction was 57.8%.[4] The standard deviations, which range anywhere from 20% to 30% in the literature, reflect significant inaccuracy.

It must be emphasized that the data reported above are for the early series of only several investigators. However, recent modifications in the computer program and surgical technique have given rise to greater accuracy.[2] In one study, for example, 57% of eyes were within 1 diopter of emmetropia and 87% within 2 diopters.[12]

ASTIGMATISM

Myopic keratomileusis induces minimal regular astigmatism, and in a prospective study there was no increase in the mean refractive cylinder and a maximal increase of 2 D with a maximal decrease of 3 D.[9] When the mean cylinder was measured by keratometry, there was a mean increase of 0.50 D with a maximum of 4.5 D. In a retrospective study of 97 eyes, the refractive cylinder increased by 0.53 D.[2] In another retrospective series there was a mean increase of 0.77 D, determined by refraction, with a maximum of 3.25 D, and there was an increase of 0.69 D, when determined by keratometry, with a maximum of 5.5 D.[19] In a study of long-term results with a mean follow-up time of 9.3 years there was no significant increase when determined by refraction and a maximal increase and decrease of 2 D respectively.[6] The axis changed by more than 10 degrees in half the patients and by greater than 20 degrees in over a third of the patients.

In a prospective study of 50 consecutive cases of autoplastic MKM, a keratometric, suture-induced astigmatism of 0.89 D was found, and the final surgically induced astigmatism was increased by 0.41 D.[18] However, there was no increase when determined by refraction. The vector-corrected astigmatism was also calculated and showed a surgically induced astigmatism of 2.17 D when determined by keratometry and 1.67 D when determined by refraction.

In addition to regular astigmatism, irregular astigmatism is also induced by MKM, as it is by other lamellar refractive techniques. It is of greater importance than regular astigmatism because it can reduce the best-corrected acuity. In one study 9% of eyes had a reduction in best-corrected acuity because of irregular astigmatism.[14] In another study it was determined that the majority of patients who had undergone MKM had some recognizable irregularity on the corneoscope photograph, regardless of how slight.[18] In no case, however, did this irregular astigmatism lead to a reduction in the best-corrected acuity. However, this possibility always exists, and it is not yet known whether minor alterations, unaccompanied by decreases in acuity, can cause poor contrast sensitivity or subjective symptoms.

VISUAL RESULTS

Although there have been several studies of MKM, the reported visual results have usually not provided good documentation of the effects of such surgery on the visual acuity. Few studies have provided both the individual's preoperative and postoperative best-corrected acuities. Another shortcoming has been that authors have averaged the denominators of Snellen visual acuities. Because Snellen visual acuities are not numeric interval data, such averages are relatively meaningless. Nevertheless, most investigators at one time or another have presented data in this way to give some indication of the results of surgery, and these are considered in this chapter for lack of better data.

In a prospective study, none of 19 patients with a minimum of 1 year of follow-up observation had a reduction in spectacle acuity.[16] This proves that the lamellar keratectomy across the visual axis does not, in itself, reduce the best-corrected vision. In addition, 63% of patients in this series had an improved spectacle acuity, averaging 1.5 lines with a maximum of 5 lines. In a retrospective series it was found that the spectacle acuity was increased in 67.1% with a maximal increase of 6 lines, whereas it was decreased in 8.2% with a maximal decrease of 4 lines.[19] In another series it was found that the best-corrected acuity was increased in 15% of patients and decreased in 6%.[10] It is obvious therefore that MKM has the potential to increase and decrease the best-corrected visual acuity. The major cause of decreased best-corrected acuity is irregular astigmatism, and the major reason for an improvement in spectacle acuity is reduction of image minification by elimination of the highly myopic spectacles.

Although averaging the denominators of Snellen visual acuities is inappropriate, several series have shown improvements in the spectacle acuity from mean preoperative to mean postoperative acuities of 20/49 to 20/33,[6] 20/57 to 20/48,[10] and 20/94 to 20/49.[16] Barraquer states that visual improvement is greater in patients with poorer preoperative vision. For example, he has provided data on patients whose preoperative acuity was worse or better than 20/50 before surgery. In the former the mean visual acuity improved from 20/100 to 20/39, whereas in the latter it remained relatively constant (20/29 to 20/28) and did not improve.[6] Experience has also shown that the visual improvement is maintained over the long term, even though the myopia may return or the results may be unstable.

With respect to uncorrected acuity, in one series 85% of eyes achieved an uncorrected acuity of 20/50.[12]

VISUAL REHABILITATION

Visual rehabilitation after MKM is rapid when compared with hyperopic lamellar techniques. In a prospective study the mean reduction in acuity 1 week after surgery was 2.3 lines for spectacle acuity.[16] In our experience,[16] patients will be within 2 or 3 lines of the preoperative acuity by 3 to 4 weeks after surgery, regardless of the preoperative vision. To reach the final acuity, 20/15 or 20/20, for example, it may, however, take anywhere from 3 to 12 months.

In another study in which Snellen acuities were averaged, a mean preoperative acuity of 20/57 was reduced to 20/66 at 8 weeks and improved to 20/55 at 6 months and 20/48 at 1 year after surgery.[10] In a series by Barraquer with a mean preoperative acuity of 20/49, the mean postoperative acuity was 20/47 at 1 month and 20/33 at 1 year.[6]

STABILITY

Until now there has been no satisfactory prospective evaluation of the stability of the correction after MKM. Although studies have reported data on stability, they have been unaccompanied by measurements of axial length, which is a critical factor in the assessment of stability. Previously, it was believed that keratometry could accurately describe the change in corneal power after MKM and that refraction was related to both keratometry and axial length. Studies have described stability in terms of keratometric stability, whereas attributing increase in myopia over time to corneal steepening, axial elongation, or both. However, based on recent evidence that keratometry cannot accurately be used to describe the change in corneal curvature after MKM, previous studies of stability are open to question.[9]

In a prospective evaluation it was found that MKM was unstable for up to 6 months after surgery because shifts in the refraction, both in the myopic and hyperopic directions, were observed.[16] Recent changes in the configuration of the cutting process and the computer programs have eliminated some of this early instability.

In another study it was found that the refractive correction obtained was unstable for as long as 18 months after surgery but appeared stable thereafter. In this study it was found that there was a mean loss of refractive correction of 1.17 D during the interval from 2 weeks to 6 months after surgery, a mean loss of 0.45 D between 6 months and 1 year, and an additional mean loss of 0.45 D between 12 and 17 months after surgery.[7] These measurements were based on refraction.

In a study with a mean follow-up time of 5.5 years it was found that the mean loss of correction, based on refraction, was 0.30 D per year, with a very large standard deviation of ±0.54 D per year.[19] When keratometry alone was evaluated, a mean decay of 0.09 D per year was found. Barraquer has stated that there is a mean loss of correction of 15.42% during the first year because of a reduction in edema of the lenticule.[6] In a study that had a mean follow-up time of 9.3 years and a maximal follow-up time of 21 years, he found a mean loss of correction of 1.43 D between the first and twelfth months and a further loss of 1.87 D between 1 and 9.3 years. However, in the unoperated fellow eye there was a mean increase in myopia of 1.42 D between 1 and 9.3 years. It appears, therefore, that the actual loss of correction attributable to steepening of the corneal curvature is very small after the first year.

In a study by Barraquer it was determined that stability is greatest in cases where the resection thickness is less than 0.30 mm, the resection diameter not greater than 7.00 mm, and the optic zone diameter less than 5.5 mm.

COMPLICATIONS

Following is a list of previously reported complications of myopic keratomileusis:

Operative Complications
Microkeratome
Thin lamellar section
Thick lamellar section
Irregular lamellar section
Perforation into anterior chamber
Cryolathe/BKS
Perforation of corneal disc
Dislodgment of corneal disc from device
Postoperative optical complications
Undercorrection
Overcorrection
Regular astigmatism
Irregular astigmatism
Postoperative corneal complications
Delayed epithelialization
Epitheliitis
Filamentary keratitis
Necrosis of Bowman's membrane

Epithelialization of interface
Amorphous deposits in interface
Foreign bodies in interface
Interface opacification
Hudson-Stähli line
Peripheral scarring
Ectasia
Endothelial cell loss

Operative complications can arise from the use of the microkeratome, the cryolathe, or the BKS device. In some instances, the thickness of the microkeratome resection can be thinner or thicker than the proposed resection. If the resection is too thin, an undercorrection may result, unless the surgeon resorts to homoplastic surgery or accepts a small optical zone. A thicker resection is of no consequence, unless the surgeon has inappropriately requested a thickness that leaves the posterior layer too thin. In a prospective series a thin resection (0.03 mm or less than the desired thickness) or a thick resection (0.03 mm or greater than the proposed thickness) was obtained in 3 of 42 cases.[16] There were no irregular microkeratome resections.

In another series, however, it was reported that the incidence of irregular keratectomy was 11% for the first 63 cases and 1.8% for the last 54 cases.[10] However, it was not stated how irregular a resection needed to be before being considered such.

Perforation into the anterior chamber has also occurred.[2] Such a complication is attributable to failure to place the base plate of the microkeratome, and it can result in damage to the lens.

Damage to the corneal disc during modification on the cryolathe/BKS appears to occur in most series, and the incidence of this complication is about 1%. Recent modifications in the technique should keep this complication to a minimum. If it occurs, the surgeon must complete the procedure with donor tissue.

Although a large number of postoperative complications, both optical and corneal, have been reported, the majority do not necessitate further surgery and are not deleterious to vision. Small undercorrections or overcorrections and minimal amounts of astigmatism, both regular and irregular, are of little consequence, and can be corrected by a keratotomy procedure.

The major complication that requires reoperation is epithelium in the interface that is either central and occludes the visual axis or is paracentral and causes irregular astigmatism. Such epithelium is easily removed by débridement. The incidence in a prospective series of cases that required reoperation for this complication was slightly greater than 2%.[16]

The most feared complication of MKM seen with any degree of frequency is irregular astigmatism. Although occurring in up to 10% of cases, it is not easily treated.[14] If attributable to a complication in the preparation of the lenticule, it is easily corrected by replacement of the lenticule. However, if it is attributable to an irregular keratectomy, replacement of the lenticule may or may not alleviate the situation. In this case, the surgeon must wait for the lenticule to heal to the bed and reoperate upon the patient, performing a keratectomy deeper than the initial one. The cornea is then reconstructed accordingly. In some cases, penetrating keratoplasty may be required.

Until now, there has been no adequate study of endothelial cell loss after MKM. In one study of six patients there was a mean cell loss of 13.6%, with a maximum of 26%.[13]

SUMMARY

Myopic keratomileusis has been shown to be able to correct high myopic refractive errors. Presently, the accuracy of the technique appears to be sufficient to provide the majority of patients with good uncorrected vision and the attainment of their goal. In some cases, further surgery such as radial or transverse keratotomy may be used to bring the patient close to emmetropia. In addition, it has been well documented that MKM can provide an improvement in the best-corrected spectacle acuity. In this sense, MKM is visually rehabilitative and not cosmetic surgery. In some instances, this visual improvement can be dramatic and equal to 5 lines or more. Astigmatism usually is minimal, though irregular astigmatism can be produced and, if severe, can result in visual loss. Although it may take up to a year for the refractive correction to fully stabilize, the long-term stability of MKM appears satisfactory though further studies are necessary.[22]

The complication rates should be relatively low because one is performing surgery on an eye for optical reasons. The reported complication rates do not appear excessively high, though the technique is difficult and may result in significant complications in untrained hands. Further studies are necessary for full documentation of the safety and efficacy of MKM.

REFERENCES

1. Ainslie D: The surgical correction of refractive errors by keratomileusis and keratophakia, *Ann Ophthalmol* 8:349, 1976.
2. Barraquer C, Gutierrez AM, Espinosa A: Myopic keratomileusis: short-term results, *Refract Corneal Surg* 5:307, 1989.
3. Barraquer JI: Queratomileusis para la corrección de la miopía, *Arch Soc Am Oftalmol Optom* 5:25, 1964.
4. Barraquer JI: Keratomileusis for myopia and aphakia, *Ophthalmology* 88:701, 1981.
5. Barraquer JI: Keratomileusis for the correction of myopia, *Arch Soc Am Oftalmol Optom* 16:221, 1982.
6. Barraquer JI: Long term results of myopic keratomileusis—1982, *Arch Soc Am Oftalmol Optom* 19:37, 1983.
7. Barraquer JI, Viteri E: Results of myopic keratomileusis, *J Refract Surg* 3:98, 1987.
8. Colin J, Mimouni F, Robinet A, et al: The surgical treatment of high myopia: comparison of epikeratoplasty, keratomileusis and minus power anterior chamber lenses, *Refract Corneal Surg* 6:245, 1990.
9. Kornmehl EW, Swinger CA, Pugh W, et al: Corneascope evaluation of myopic keratomileusis, *Invest Ophthalmol Vis Sci* 26(suppl):283, 1985, ARVO abstracts.
10. Krumeich JH: Indications, techniques, and complications of myopic keratomileusis, *Int Ophthalmol Clin* 23:75, 1983.
11. Maxwell WA: Myopic keratomileusis: initial results and myopic keratomileusis combined with other procedures, *J Cataract Refract Surg* 13:518, 1987.
12. Maxwell WA, Nordan LT: Myopic keratomileusis: early experience, *J Refract Surg* 1:124, 1986.
13. Neumann AC, McCarty G, Sanders DR: Delayed regression of effect in myopic epikeratophakia vs myopic keratomileusis for high myopic, *Refract Corneal Surg* 5:161, 1989.
14. Nordan LT, Fallor MK: Myopic keratomileusis: 74 consecutive non-amblyopic cases with one year follow-up, *J Refract Surg* 2:124, 1986.
15. Polit F: Keratomileusis for myopia: initial experience in Saudi Arabia, *Arch Soc Am Oftalmol Optom* 20:195, 1986.
16. Swinger CA, Barker BA: Prospective evaluation of myopic keratomileusis, *Ophthalmology* 91:785, 1984.
17. Swinger CA, Barker BA: Myopic keratomileusis following radial keratotomy, *J Refract Surg* 1:53, 1985.
18. Swinger CA, Barker BA, Forman JS: Myopic keratomileusis: postoperative astigmatism. (Submitted for publication.)
19. Swinger CA, Barraquer JI: Keratophakia and keratomileusis: clinical results, *Ophthalmology* 88:709, 1981.
20. Swinger CA, Villaseñor RA: Homoplastic keratomileusis for the correction of myopia, *J Refract Surg* 1:219, 1985.
21. Tucker DN, Barraquer JI: Refractive keratoplasty: clinical results in sixty-seven cases, *Ann Ophthalmol* 5:335, 1973.
22. Villaseñor RA: Unpublished results, 1985, Mission Hills (Los Angeles), California.

Chapter 38

Epikeratophakia

Theory, case selection, and variables in success or failure

MARGUERITE B. McDONALD

KEITH S. MORGAN

HERBERT E. KAUFMAN

DAVID H. LEACH

PRINCIPLES OF LAMELLAR KERATOREFRACTIVE SURGERY

The development of epikeratophakia was based on the principles of refractive surgery, first elucidated by José I. Barraquer, of Bogotá, Colombia.[2] Barraquer realized that the surgical modification of the shape of the anterior surface of the cornea could provide a permanent refractive correction, and he developed two procedures, keratophakia and keratomileusis, both of which accomplish this goal. To this end, he invented the microkeratome, an instrument that involves suction rings and raising the intraocular pressure so that one can remove a corneal lamella of precise thickness and diameter. He also developed the cryolathe, a modified contact lens lathe, that freezes the corneal lamella and shapes it to the required dioptric power, based on a series of complex computer calculations, also originated by Barraquer.

In his first procedure, keratophakia, the cryolathe was used to shape a piece of donor corneal tissue, which was then sandwiched between the patient's corneal lamella and the bare stromal bed (Fig. 38-1). In the second procedure, keratomileusis, the patient's corneal lamella was removed, frozen, shaped, and replaced in the stromal bed (Fig. 38-1). Keratomileusis is also done with use of the donor lamella, in which case it is called "homoplastic keratomileusis."

In the late 1970s, Barraquer demonstrated the elegance of these procedures to a number of American surgeons, and it was obvious that in his experienced hands, good visual results could be obtained. It also seemed clear, however, that the learning curve associated with the microkeratome conferred some stress on the surgeon and some risk to the patient. Additionally, the esoteric complexities associated with machining the tissue lenticules on the cryolathe seemed to preclude a widespread acceptance of these procedures among general ophthalmic surgeons.

The idea behind the development of epikeratophakia was to simplify the surgery--make the procedure easy to learn and easy to perform—and to minimize the risk to the patient while achieving the same permanent visual correction. The first problem was the cryolathe (Fig. 38-2). Having each surgeon shape each tissue lens for each patient would be comparable to requiring each surgeon to manufacture individual intraocular lenses or contact lenses. To eliminate this sort of cottage industry, donor tissue lenses for refractive surgery would have to be shaped by and supplied from a central source. This, in turn, meant finding a way to preserve the shaped donor tissue for storage and shipping.

The current state-of-the-art technology in shaping donor tissue lenses requires that the tissue be frozen on the cryolathe before it is carved, and it might seem natural to preserve the shaped tissue by freezing as well. However, we have considerable experience with cryopreservation of tissue for penetrating keratoplasty, and the subtleties of this method have

This work was supported in part by PHS grants EY-03635, EY-02580, and EY-02377 from the National Eye Institute, National Institutes of Health, Bethesda, Maryland, and an unrestricted grant from Research to Prevent Blindness, Inc., New York City.

Keratophakia

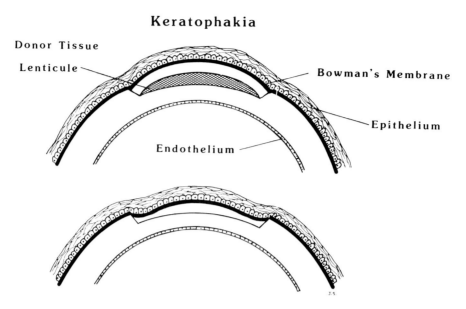

Keratomileusis

Fig. 38-1. *Keratophakia.* This procedure, developed by Barraquer, involves removal of a corneal lamella with microkeratome. A stromal lenticule, *hatched area,* is lathed from donor tissue and placed in dissected stromal bed. Patient's lamella is sutured over lenticule, providing a host-donor-host sandwich. Because cryolathe shapes donor lenticule by grinding on both sides, there is no donor Bowman's membrane. Patient's Bowman's membrane, which forms the anterior surface of corneal lamella, is covered with epithelium. Increased curvature results in desired hyperopic correction. Keratophakia can be used to correct aphakic vision and hyperopic errors in phakic patients. It cannot be used to correct myopia.

Keratomileusis. This procedure, also developed by Barraquer, involves removal of a corneal lamella with microkeratome, freezing and shaping tissue on cryolathe, and replacing it in stromal bed. A more recent adaptation of keratomileusis uses a preshaped donor tissue lamella instead of patient's own tissue. Again, result is a single Bowman's membrane covered with epithelium. With changes in shape of lathed tissue, keratomileusis can be used to correct both hyperopic and myopic errors.

proved it to be unsuitable for the storage of tissue for refractive surgery. The absence of living cells in the shaped tissue is not the problem: the living keratocytes in the donor tissue are killed during the shaping on the cryolathe, even before storage.[25] It has also been shown that this tissue is repopulated with living cells from the host cornea within a matter of weeks. The problem is that the arrangement of the collagen matrix and the basement membrane must remain intact, so that the tissue lens can recover within a reasonable period of time after being placed on the eye. If ice crystals are permitted to grow in the tissue and the stromal matrix is disrupted, the tissue remains cloudy for a long period of time and optical function is compromised. Our previous work has shown that cryopreserved corneal tissue can be kept only at the very lowest of temperatures, that is, −270° C, the temperature of liquid nitrogen. Above that temperature, the frozen tissue

degenerates. Even at −70° C, the temperature of dry ice, ice crystals grow, and the network of collagen fibrils is damaged. Early studies of Barraquer procedures in this country have shown that significantly poorer visual results are obtained with frozen tissue.[3]

Therefore a method of preserving the shaped tissue was needed. We studied fresh, frozen, and lyophilized (freeze-dried) tissue on nonhuman primate eyes, in terms of clarity and stability, and found that although the frozen tissue was less satisfactory the lyophilized tissue was equal in quality to the fresh tissue. In this procedure the graft is punched out, frozen, and shaped on the cryolathe and then lyophilized (Fig. 38-3) and stored under vacuum in a small vial. At the time of surgery, the donor tissue lens is rehydrated in balanced salt solution containing gentamicin for approximately 20 minutes (Fig. 38-3) while the patient is being draped.

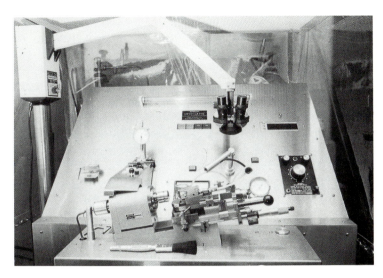

Fig. 38-2. Cryolathe is a modified Levin lathe that is cooled with carbon dioxide. Carbon dioxide tanks are connected by tubing to both headstock, where tissue is placed, and tool, which holds blade that shapes tissue. A microscope suspended from wall by an articulated arm is used to observe lathing process. For each piece of tissue, an optical zone and sometimes a wing and multiple blends, as well as a finishing cut, are made. Three to 5 minutes are needed to enter patient's measurements into computer and generate radius displacement and angle setting, followed by about 5 minutes to cool lathe with carbon dioxide, another 3 to 5 minutes to lathe tissue, and about 25 minutes for cryolathe to warm up to room temperature. This sequence is repeated for each lenticule that is produced. A major problem with cryolathe is that metal parts contract during cooling, which introduces significant but unpredictable errors in lathing; even minute contractions can result in serious dioptric errors in power of finished lenticule.

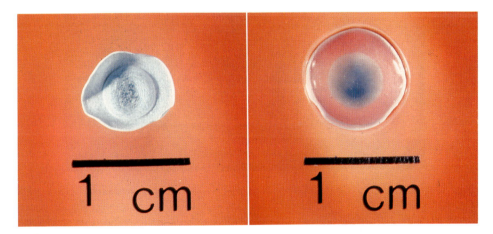

Fig. 38-3. For improvement of visualization during lathing, donor tissue is colored with an innocuous tissue dye called Fast Green. After tissue is shaped on cryolathe, it is preserved for storage and shipping by lyophilization and sealed in a small vial under vacuum. Lyophilized tissue lens is opaque and green in color. Before surgery, tissue lens is rehydrated for 20 minutes in balanced salt solution with antibiotics. Dye begins to dissipate during this time, and tissue becomes more transparent. Tissue lens is still faintly green, particularly in thickest areas, when it is placed on eye, but by end of surgery, green color is barely discernible. No dye remains visible by first postoperative day. *Left,* Lyophilized tissue lens; *Right,* Rehydrated tissue lens. This is an aphakic epikeratophakia lens; so thickest area is central optical zone, which still retains some of the green tissue dye.

To obtain the appropriate tissue lens, the surgeon makes a few common refractive measurements on the patient (keratometry readings combined with the spherical equivalent of the spectacle correction corrected to the corneal plane), and a lens is ordered. With the development of adequate storage procedures, the responsibility for the tedious and complicated preparation of the tissue has been shifted to a central facility where quality control can be maintained by well-trained technical personnel.

More recently, other investigators have used epikeratophakia tissue lenses for myopia prepared from unfrozen tissue. The donor tissue is fresh (usually less than 1 week) and is stored in McCarey-Kaufman (MK) medium. The tissue lens is shaped to the required specifications with the use of the BKS (Barraquer-Krumeich-Swinger) 1000 refractive set, which includes various dyes, fixation rings for the donor tissue lamella, and a microkeratome. Results have been encouraging and, in some series, comparable to the results with lyophilized tissue.[7]

The second problem to be overcome was the need for the microkeratome (Fig. 38-4). Although frequent use of this instrument certainly enhances the surgeon's skill, there still exists a risk of entering the anterior chamber or producing irregular cuts that result in high astigmatism. The lamellar dissection of the cornea with the microkeratome is an invasion of the optical zone. Our idea was that eliminating this lamellar dissection would not only increase the safety of the procedure, but also make it reversible. If for any reason the tissue lens was not satisfactory, it could be removed, and the cornea would revert essentially to its preoperative state within a few days. To this end, we found that we could remove the epithelium from the patient's cornea and attach the donor tissue lens directly onto the anterior corneal surface, directly apposed to the bare Bowman's membrane.

To provide a site for stroma-to-stroma contact between the tissue lens and the recipient cornea, one must make a defect in Bowman's membrane. Some surgeons still create an annular keratectomy in the

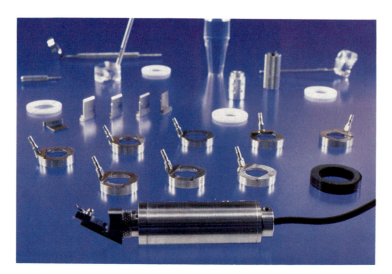

Fig. 38-4. Microkeratome has many small pieces that must be assembled correctly to prevent complications in removal of corneal lamella. It is not uncommon for infrequent users to neglect to insert footplate into bottom of instrument. Footplate serves as a guard to maintain appropriate distance between blade and applanated corneal surface, and its absence permits blade to enter anterior chamber, possibly hitting iris and lens. Microkeratome is designed to pass through a track in top of suction ring, which sits at limbus and helps blade to pass evenly over surface of cornea. Depending on height of suction ring, various amounts of corneal tissue are presented for excision. A very tall suction ring allows only a small amount of cornea to protrude above surface, and therefore a very small amount will be resected; a very low suction ring, only 1 or 2 mm tall, allows most of cornea to protrude above surface for resection. Suction ring drives intraocular pressure up to 65 mm Hg. This is required for a good cut, but surgeon must move quickly because such high pressure does not allow any arterial blood to circulate in eye, or to optic nerve head, and can cause blindness if maintained for more than a few minutes.

peripheral cornea, outside the optical zone, into which the edge of the tissue lens is placed and sutured. Most surgeons, however, use an annular keratectomy only in keratoconus cases. In other cases, a lamellar dissection is usually performed to provide the stroma-stroma interface. The circular trephine incision is extended peripherally at its base, and the edge of an oversized tissue lens is tucked into the dissection bed and sutured into position.

It is through this area of contact that the matrix of the tissue lens is repopulated with living cells from the patient's cornea. It is also only in this circular groove that healing between the tissue lens and cornea takes place; there is no scarring between the posterior stromal surface of the tissue lens and the anterior surface of the cornea in the optical zone. Therefore removal of the tissue lens involves only the separation of the circular scar, after which the tissue lens can be peeled from the cornea. The cor-

neal surface usually reepithelializes within 4 to 5 days. If desired, the epikeratophakia procedure can be repeated, either immediately if the eye is quiet, or within a few weeks. Epikeratophakia tissue lenses have been removed from human eyes as long as 2 years after attachment, and no permanent damage to the host cornea, scarring across the host Bowman's membrane, or loss of visual acuity has been seen.

CASE SELECTION

Epikeratophakia was originally developed for the correction of monocular aphakia.* The tissue lens for the correction of aphakia is shaped to be thicker centrally over the optical zone and thinner peripherally in the wing area (Fig. 38-5). This increases the anterior curvature of the cornea and provides the necessary hyperopic correction. The first patients to

---

*References 4, 8-13, 28, 29, 31-33.

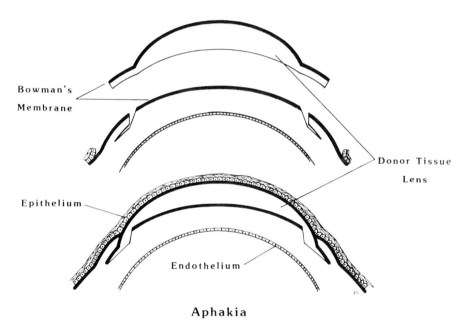

Aphakia

Fig. 38-5. Epikeratophakia for correction of aphakia. Donor tissue lens is ground only from endothelial side, so that anterior surface, including Bowman's membrane, remains intact. Epithelium is removed from patient's cornea, and peripheral trephination and dissection are completed. Posterior stromal surface of tissue lens is apposed to bare Bowman's membrane of patient's cornea, and wing of tissue lens is tucked and sutured into peripheral keratectomy. Result is a cornea nearly doubled in thickness, with two Bowman's membranes. Up to now, we have achieved increases in anterior curvature to correct as much as 34 D of hyperopia. The patient's epithelium grows over anterior surface of tissue lens, and patient's stromal keratocytes migrate through peripheral interruption of host Bowman's to populate stroma of tissue lens. No scarring occurs across stroma-host Bowman's interface. Tissue lens is permanently attached to patient's cornea only in area of keratectomy. Therefore one can easily remove graft, should it be necessary, in physician's office by opening scar and peeling graft off cornea. Within a few days, host cornea is re-covered with epithelium and, except for a small circular scar well out of visual axis, is essentially restored to its preoperative state.

receive these lenses were unilaterally aphakic adults who were contact lens–intolerant and unable to wear aphakic spectacles because of the image disparity and were not candidates for secondary intraocular lens implantation. These were patients who had no acceptable alternative for restoration of visual function in an otherwise sound eye. The second group of patients to receive epikeratophakia tissue lenses were children with unilateral aphakia resulting from congenital or traumatic cataract.[1,16-23] Such children who were, for one reason or another, unable to use contact lenses also had little prospect for visual rehabilitation, even if the cataract was successfully removed.

The epikeratophakia procedure was adapted to a third group, patients with keratoconus.[6,14] In this case the tissue lens was plano, that is, of equal thickness throughout (Fig. 38-6) and by itself conferred

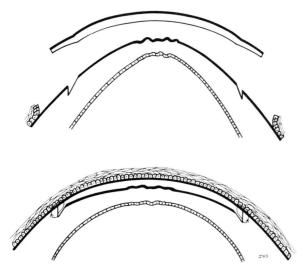

Fig. 38-6. Onlay epikeratophakia graft for treatment of keratoconus. For this procedure, donor tissue is of uniform thickness (0.3 mm), with a wing 0.75 mm across and 0.13 mm thick. A 10.0 mm epikeratophakia tissue lens is sutured tightly across thinned and ectatic cornea into a 9.0 mm bed. Some surgeons perform an annular keratectomy; others prefer to undermine and perform a lamellar dissection in the recipient bed. In either case, the results provide reinforcement and flattening of the irregular protrusion, so that the patient can resume daily wear of hard contact lenses comfortably. Although there is no optical power shaped into donor tissue, change in corneal contour results in a decrease in myopia of about 5 D. In immediate postoperative period, folds are visible in both Bowman's layer and Descemet's membrane, beneath graft. These folds apparently do not interfere with vision, however, and generally resolve by about 6 weeks after surgery, except in rare cases.

no additional optical power. The fourth and most recent group of patients to benefit from the development of epikeratophakia comprised patients with high myopia, many of whom were unable to be corrected even with a combination of spectacles and contact lenses.[5,9,12,15,26,27,30] For myopic patients, the tissue lens is shaped to be thinner centrally, with a thicker shoulder area and a thin wing (Fig. 38-7). When draped over the cornea, this tissue lens flattens the anterior curvature and can correct, theoretically, as much as 80 diopters of myopia, far beyond the actual myopic optical error in any human eye.

Indications for Aphakic Epikeratophakia in Adults. The majority of adult patients who have a cataract removed receive an intraocular lens simultaneously. However, there are some patients for whom epikeratophakia, as an extraocular procedure, may be somewhat safer than an intraocular lens. These include eyes at risk for endothelial damage and corneal decompensation, as well as eyes with disorganized anterior chambers, possibly lacking the necessary iris or angle to support the secondary implant. Other candidates include aphakic patients without an intact posterior capsule and adults with recurrent uveitis, glaucoma, marginal endothelial cell counts, cornea guttata, or vitreous in the anterior chamber, as well as patients with poorly controlled diabetes, who may require panretinal photocoagulation or vitrectomy. There may also be patients whose occupations make refractive surgery preferable to contact lens correction: those working in dusty or dirty environments and those who must pass vision screening without prosthetic correction.

Indications for Epikeratophakia in Pediatric Patients. Pediatric patients who are young enough to benefit from amblyopia therapy are candidates for epikeratophakia. Children with traumatic cataracts can receive epikeratophakia tissue lenses in a combined procedure with cataract extraction.[23] In cases of traumatic cataract and corneal laceration, epikeratophakia can provide a faster visual recovery than penetrating keratoplasty can; the sutures are generally removed within 2 to 3 weeks, and amblyopia therapy is begun 1 week later. Preoperative astigmatism caused by scarring is reduced 10% to 20%, and the epikeratophakia tissue lens provides a splinting effect on the lacerated cornea.[17]

For children with congenital cataracts, we have found that the correction provided by the epikeratophakia tissue lens is inadequate up to about 1 year of age for reasons that are not entirely clear.[1] As a result and because of the rapidly changing dioptric needs of these very steep and rapidly growing eyes, we now recommended that early cataract extraction

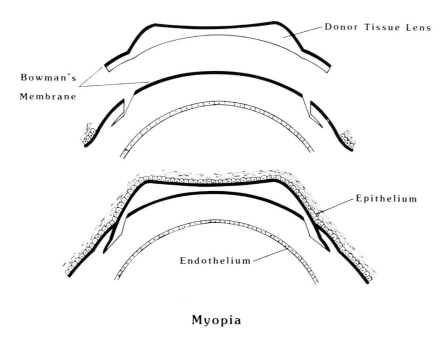

Myopia

Fig. 38-7. Epikeratophakia for myopia. Donor tissue lens is shaped to be thinner centrally, with a thicker shoulder and thin wing. This results in a net flattening of anterior corneal curvature. Potential myopic correction available with these tissue lenses exceeds 50 D, beyond what is obtainable through any other refractive surgical procedure or combination of procedures. This drawing exaggerates thickness of shoulders for illustrative purposes. Although this exaggeration appears to show a resulting concavity at surface of tissue lens, in reality final anterior curvature is still somewhat convex, albeit flatter than patient's cornea was preoperatively.

be followed by contact lens correction and that epikeratophakia be considered as a secondary procedure when the child is approximately 1 year old. This is generally the time when the use of contact lenses becomes increasingly difficult because the child is able to manipulate the eye and lens. This is also the time when the refractive needs of the eye stabilize, and the accuracy of correction provided by epikeratophakia at this age is excellent.

Epikeratophakia has also been used to correct aphakia in a few children with bilaterally symmetrical congenital cataracts.[16] There is some additional risk, compared to contact lens or spectacle correction, but with carefully selected patients and assiduous follow-up observation the risk may be acceptable. The parents are freed from the problems associated with contact lenses and spectacles, and the benefit to the child of a permanent and maintenance-free correction may be both visual and psychologic.

Indications for Epikeratophakia for Keratoconus.
Patients with mild to moderate keratoconus and no central scarring are ideal candidates for epikeratophakia. These patients are generally losing their ability to wear hard contact lenses on a full-time basis or are totally unable to wear contact lenses; however, they must be able to demonstrate 20/40 or better best-corrected visual acuity with a hard contact lens placed on the eye for a few minutes for diagnostic purposes.

The extraocular nature of the epikeratophakia procedure, with the partial-thickness graft laid on the anterior surface of the cornea, appears to preclude the possibility of an immune reaction. For this reason, patients with keratoconus who have rejected a penetrating keratoplasty graft in the first eye are good candidates for epikeratophakia for keratoconus in the second eye. In such a patient the contraindication of central scarring can be overcome by a surgical maneuver known as "reefing sutures." These 10-0 nylon sutures are placed into two adjacent quadrants 90 degrees from one another and are used to pull the central scar out of the visual axis just before the epikeratphakia tissue lens is attached. The reefing sutures are removed at 3 weeks, when the scar has settled into its new position.

Patients with Down's syndrome are good candidates for epikeratophakia for keratoconus unless they have a hydrops scar that is very dense and centrally located. Reefing sutures can also be used in these cases to reposition a small to moderately large central scar. Epikeratophakia confers better vision and less discomfort, with a shorter postoperative course and earlier return of vision, than penetrating keratoplasty and is therefore perhaps preferable to penetrating keratoplasty in patients with other physical disabilities and in children and teen-agers.

For keratoconus, the plano donor tissue is sutured tightly across the cone, flattening the protruding cornea and providing tectonic support to the thinned and ectatic tissue. Although the graft is not shaped to provide an optical correction, compression of the cone does reduce myopia by about 5 diopters.

Indications for Epikeratophakia for Correction of Myopia. Nationally, most surgeons select spectacle- and contact lens-intolerant patients with 10 or more diopters of myopia that has been stable for at least 1 year to be corrected with epikeratophakia; occasionally selected cases with as few as 6 diopters of myopia have undergone this procedure.

Patients with high myopia have generally been unable to achieve satisfactory corrections with any combination of optical aids. Patients with lesser amounts of myopia who have not attempted contact lens wear in the recent past should be encouraged to try some of the newer lenses before refractive surgery is contemplated. More than 2 diopters of preexisting astigmatism can be compensated for by a modified surgical protocol involving a controlled postoperative wound dehiscence in the steepest quadrant. Toric epikeratophakia tissue lenses, which have been tested at the Louisiana State University Eye Center, show promise for the correction of astigmatism. Children with unilateral high myopia, who are at risk for developing anisometropic amblyopia, are also potential candidates for epikeratophakia.

MAJOR VARIABLES IN SUCCESS OR FAILURE

The two major variables in success or failure of epikeratophakia are careful patient selection and close, careful, and consistent early postoperative care. The success of the surgery and the survival of the graft depend on the selection of patients with a suitable physical ocular environment, followed by alert conscientious postoperative observation and immediate intervention in case of trouble.

Contraindications. Severe or uncontrolled blepharitis, dry eyes, or lagophthalmos will predispose the epikeratophakia tissue lens to failure. Because these conditions also make contact lens wear difficult or impossible, the refractive surgeon is likely to see a

number of such patients presenting as candidates. However, these conditions must be treated successfully before surgery can be undertaken, and the patients must be made aware that chronic treatment of these conditions will be necessary to guarantee the survival of the refractive graft. It is essential that the surgeon be assured that the patient is both compliant and reliable; we suggest that compliance with therapy for severe blepharitis or dry eyes be monitored for at least 2 months before surgery is scheduled, in order that the problem be brought under control and the reliability of the patient be established. Severe lagophthalmos must be treated surgically to restore normal lid function.

In keratoconus patients, hydrops scars within 1 mm of the visual axis may be moved into the optical zone when the epikeratophakia tissue lens flattens the cone. In myopic patients, the presence of large posterior staphylomas, progressive myopic macular degeneration, previous rhegmatogenous retinal detachment with poor macular function, and any unstable or progressive posterior pole disorder are relative contraindications; the more severe these conditions, the less likely it is that good vision will result, and the surgeon must make a judgment as to whether the patient will obtain sufficient improvement to justify the risk.

Postoperative Care. Here the personality of the surgeon becomes a major factor. Epikeratophakia patients must be monitored closely by a physician who is familiar with the earliest signs of trouble. Therefore it is not a good idea to schedule the surgery immediately before the physician is planning to go on vacation because follow-up care cannot be delegated. Furthermore, because this is still a relatively new procedure, it is important that the surgeon be in close touch with the medical monitoring system and be willing to ask for advice or assistance if there is the slightest doubt as to the best course of action.

After surgery, the first week to 10 days of postoperative care are critical to ensure that the patient's epithelium covers the graft surface. Any hint of a persistent epithelial defect during this period must be treated aggressively and immediately. If the eye is patched, a bandage lens is tried; an eye that already has a bandage lens in place is patched. If no improvement is seen after 3 or 4 days, a "bow-tie" tarsorrhaphy with interrupted 5-0 Dermalon (monofilament nylon) sutures is performed, so that the tarsorrhaphy can be opened, the eye examined every 7 days for 3 weeks, and the sutures retied without the somewhat painful tarsorrhaphy procedure being repeated.

At the Louisiana State University Eye Center, a

temporary tarsorrhaphy is performed routinely at the end of the procedure. This protective measure has been shown to promote rapid reepithelialization uniformly and more reliably than other methods; Furthermore, it is more convenient for the patient, who need not return for follow-up observation for 10 to 14 days. If the epithelial defect has not diminished in size halfway through the course, the graft is removed. Over the longer postoperative period, loose or vascularized sutures must be removed promptly, and the eye pressure patched for 24 hours or until the epithelial defects have disappeared.

Because epikeratophakia is reversible, it is not a complicated procedure to remove the graft and repeat the surgery in a couple of weeks when the eye is quiet. Persistent epithelial defects or potentially damaging infections should lead to immediate consideration of graft removal, before any permanent damage is done to the host cornea. The epikeratophakia graft is much more easily removed and replaced than a penetrating keratoplasty, and the surgeon needs to overcome a natural reluctance to consider a graft "lost" and must suppress the inclination to continue to treat in a deteriorating situation.

Special Considerations for Pediatric Epikeratophakia. The major variable in the success of pediatric epikeratophakia is patient selection. Since the visual success of this procedure in most cases of unilateral aphakia depends on the determination of the parents in meeting the requirements of the amblyopia therapy, the evaluation of the suitability of a given child for this surgery includes not only the age and condition of the child, but also the likelihood that successful surgery will be followed by conscientious attention to the occlusion schedule over the next months or years. Therefore the surgeon must attempt to determine first whether the child meets the criteria for potential success, as described below, and then whether the parents are sufficiently concerned and motivated to follow through over the long-term rehabilitative course.

Children with traumatic cataracts and corneal lacerations are perhaps the best candidates for epikeratophakia. In these cases, the graft not only corrects the optical problems, but also lends support to the scarred and irregular cornea, allowing the sutures to be removed earlier and the eye to be rehabilitated more rapidly. Our experience is that children with traumatic cataracts can undergo a surprisingly long period of deprivation. Unfortunately in most of these children, the period of deprivation is prolonged as a result of repeated attempts at contact lens fitting in patients who are ultimately conceded to be totally noncompliant. Even so, we have found that almost 60% of children who have had an injury at 2½ years of age and who have had no formed vision to the eye for 10 months achieved 20/80 or better acuity with an epikeratophakia graft and intense patching.[17,23]

Analysis of the visual acuity results from children who have had epikeratophakia surgery for unilateral congenital cataracts revealed few cases of visual acuity results better than 20/200 when the children had the cataract in place for 1 year.[24] In contrast, some very good visual results were seen where children had cataracts removed and contact lenses prescribed within the first year of life and then underwent epikeratophakia when contact lens compliance became a problem. We have also seen excellent acuities after cataract extraction and refractive surgery in children with progressing incomplete congenital cataracts. Our experience has been that most ophthalmologists are reluctant to remove partial cataracts because of the problems associated with contact lens compliance. Our success rate, predictability, and visual acuity results for epikeratophakia in children over 1 year of age are so good that we suggest considering surgery when there is documented progression of vision loss despite conservative measures such as patching, spectacle overcorrection, and dilatation.

We have encountered a variety of problems in dealing with neonates and epikeratophakia. First, it is difficult to compute accurately the power required by means of traditional intraocular lens formulas, using A-scan ultrasonography and keratometry, because these formulas do not accurately predict the powers required in short eyes. The powers achieved in these very young children were generally less than the predicted powers.[1] Also, since the grafts tend to retain their shape as the eye grows and the growing eyes become myopic over a period of time, if the correction is accurate at 3 months of age, the child will be very myopic at 6 years of age and may need to have the graft replaced. We now circumvent all these problems in neonates with dense unilateral congenital cataracts by fitting them with an extended-wear contact lenses, which usually work well for the better part of the first year of life. Beyond this point and when contact lens problems occur, epikeratophakia can be performed with the expectation of a high rate of surgical success and a resulting correction that should be appropriate for the life of the child. As the epikeratophakia procedure evolves, it may become feasible to accurately correct optical errors in newborns very quickly and to achieve a better visual acuity than is possible with a contact lens, which is often decentered in these infant eyes. Such early surgery would, however, require changing the power at a later date as the eye becomes myopic with growth. However, the relative ease with which these grafts can be removed and replaced makes this prospect worth considering, compared to the problems associated with prosthetic correction of unilateral aphakia in a young child over the 7- or 8-year course of amblyopia therapy.

REFERENCES

1. Arffa RC, Marvelli TL, Morgan KS: Keratometric and refractive results of pediatric epikeratophakia, *Arch Ophthalmol* 103:1656, 1985.
2. Barraquer JI: Keratomileusis and keratophakia. In Rycroft PV, editor: *Corneoplastic surgery:* Proc Second International Corneo-Plastic Conference, New York, 1969, Pergamon Press.
3. Friedlander MH et al: Clinical results of keratophakia and keratomileusis, *Ophthalmology* 88:716, 1981.
4. Kaufman HE: The correction of aphakia, *Am J Ophthalmol* 89:1, 1980.
5. Kaufman HE, McDonald MB: Refractive surgery for aphakia and myopia, *Trans Ophthalmol Soc UK* 104(1):43, 1984.
6. Kaufman HE, Werblin TP: Epikeratophakia for the treatment of keratoconus, *Am J Ophthalmol* 93(3):342, 1982.
7. Krumeich JH, Swinger CA: Nonfreeze epikeratophakia for the correction of myopia, *Am J Ophthalmol* 103:397-403, 1987.
8. McDonald MB: The current state of epikeratophakia. In Jakobiec FA, Sigleman J, editors: *Advanced techniques in ocular surgery*, New York, 1984, WB Saunders.
9. McDonald MB, Kaufman HE: *Refractive corneal surgery.* Module 11: *Focal points*, 1984: clinical modules for ophthalmologists, San Francisco, 1984, American Academy of Ophthalmology, pp 1-12.
10. McDonald MB, Kaufman HE: Refractive keratoplasty. In Steele AD, McG, Drews RC, editors: *Cataract surgery* (Butterworths International Medical Reviews: Ophthalmology 2), Sevenoaks, Kent, Eng, 1984, Butterworth & Co., Publishers.
11. McDonald MB, Kaufman HE: Refractive surgery for visual rehabilitation of aphakia. In Ginsberg SP, editor: *Cataract and intraocular lens surgery: a compendium of modern theories and techniques*, Birmingham, Alabama, 1984, Aesculapius Publishing, vol 2, pp 622-632.
12. McDonald MB, Kaufman HE: Epikeratophakia for aphakia, myopia, and keratoconus in the adult patient. Chapter 21 in Sanders DR, Hofmann RF, Salz JJ, editors: *Refractive corneal surgery*, Thorofare, NJ, 1985, Slack Inc.
13. McDonald MB et al: Epikeratophakia: the surgical correction of aphakia, update: 1982, *Ophthalmology* 90(6):668, 1983.
14. McDonald MB et al: Onlay lamellar keratoplasty for the treatment of keratoconus, *Br J Ophthalmol* 67:615, 1983.
15. McDonald MB et al: Epikeratophakia for myopia correction, *Ophthalmology* 92:1417, 1985.
16. Morgan KS, Arffa RC, Marvelli TL: Epikeratophakia in the pediatric patient. Chapter 22 in Sanders DR, Hofmann RF, Salz JJ, editors: *Refractive corneal surgery*, Thorofare, NJ, 1985, Slack Inc.
17. Morgan KS, Stephenson GS: Epikeratophakia in children with corneal lacerations, *J Pediatr Ophthalmol Strabismus* 22(3):105, 1985.
18. Morgan KS et al: The use of epikeratophakia grafts in pediatric monocular aphakia, *J Pediatr Ophthalmol Strabismus* 18(6):23, 1981.
19. Morgan KS et al: Epikeratophakia in the pediatric patient: a case report, *J Ocular Ther Surg*, pp 198, May/June 1982.
20. Morgan KS et al: Preliminary visual results of pediatric epikeratophakia, *Arch Ophthalmol* 101:1540, 1983.
21. Morgan KS et al: Epikeratophakia in children, *Ophthalmology* 91:780, 1984.
22. Morgan KS et al: Pediatric epikeratophakia. In Reinecke RD, editor: *Strabismus II*, Proc Fourth meeting of the International Strabismological Association, Oct 25-29, Asilomar, Calif, New York, 1984, Grune & Stratton.
23. Morgan KS et al: Epikeratophakia in children with traumatic cataracts, *J Pediatr Ophthalmol Strabismus* 23(3):423, 1986.
24. Morgan KS et al: Five year follow-up of epikeratophakia in children, *Ophthalmology* 93(4):423, 1986.
25. Rich LF et al: Keratocyte survival in keratophakia lenticules, *Arch Ophthalmol* 99:677, 1981.
26. Suarez E et al: Efficacy of surgical modifications in myopic epikeratophakia, *J Refract Surg* 1(4):156, 1985.
27. Suarez E et al: Suarez spreader for epikeratophakia, *J Refract Surg* 1(4):180, 1985.
28. Werblin TP, Kaufman HE: Epikeratophakia: the surgical correction of aphakia. II. Preliminary studies in a non-human primate model, *Curr Eye Res* 1(3):131, 1981.
29. Werblin TP, Klyce SD: Epikeratophakia: the surgical correction of aphakia. I. Lathing of corneal tissue, *Curr Eye Res* 1(3):123, 1981.
30. Werblin TP, Klyce SD: Epikeratophakia: the surgical correction of myopia. I. Lathing of corneal tissue, *Curr Eye Res* 1(10):591, 1981-1982.
31. Werblin TP et al: Epikeratophakia: the surgical correction of aphakia. III. Preliminary results of a prospective clinical trial, *Arch Ophthalmol* 99:1957, 1981.
32. Werblin TP et al: A prospective study of the use of hyperopic epikeratophakia grafts for the correction of aphakia in adults, *Ophthalmology* 88(11):1137, 1981.
33. Werblin TP et al: Epikeratophakia: the surgical correction of aphakia, update 1981, *Ophthalmology* 89(6):916, 1982.

Surgical technique and improvements in technology and instrumentation

DANIEL S. DURRIE

Epikeratophakia is a form of optical onlay lamellar keratoplasty that changes the topography of the anterior corneal surface resulting in alteration of the refracting power of the cornea. This procedure has been the focus of a national prospective study to evaluate its use in the treatment of adult[2,5,10,11,13-15] and pediatric[6-8] aphakia, keratoconus,[3] and high myopia.[4,12] The purpose of this chapter is to describe the surgical technique and instrumentation used for this procedure.

The tissue that I have used in the present study is processed human cornea in a lyophilized (freeze-dried) state. Information regarding tissue ordering and postoperative management is also included in this chapter.

MATERIALS AND SUPPLIES

The corneal tissue used for this procedure is obtained by a commercial processing center from existing eye banks throughout the country. It is handled using standard eye-banking techniques. Viable endothelium is not needed in this type of corneal grafting. Therefore this procedure does not compete for tissue that is needed for penetrating keratoplasty.

One of the major advantages of using precarved tissue from a central source is that the complicated cryolathing process and associated calculations do not need to be performed by the operating surgeon. The only information that needs to be provided by the surgeon is the spherical equivalent of the patient's refraction at the corneal plane and the average central keratometer readings. All other calculations needed to design the lens are performed by the technicians processing the tissue.

The spherical equivalent is usually calculated from the patient's manifest refraction. If a refraction cannot be obtained as from an uncooperative child, the corneal plane power can be calculated by use of the SRK formula:[9]

$$P_{cl} = 85.8 - 1.87L - 0.67K$$

P_{cl}, Expected contact lens power in diopters; L, axial length in millimeters; K, averaged keratometry in diopters.

The tissue is custom lathed for each patient based on the above parameters and is usually delivered to the surgeon within 10 days.

Instrumentation and supplies for the procedure are quite simple. A basic ophthalmic instruments set is used along with the following additional items:

Hessburg-Barron vacuum trephine
Infant feeding tube or 14 g intercath
Cannula for irrigation and suction
Storz clear plastic shield (for child)

OPTICAL CENTERING

In all corneal refractive surgery procedures it is of paramount importance that the surgery is well centered on the patient's optical axis. The technique used to locate the optical axis depends on the type of patient. In high myopia, the patient can usually fixate on the filament in the microscope and the standard radial keratotomy technique for the PERK (Prospective Evaluation of Radial Keratotomy) Study can be used. Aphakic patients usually cannot fixate well on the microscope filament, and therefore this technique may sometimes be unreliable. In these patients, as well as pediatric patients, the topographic center of the cornea can be measured by calipers.

The optical center is usually located 1 mm nasal of the topographic center of the cornea.

After the optical center of the cornea is located, a small scratch is made in the epithelium with a needle to mark the site for later reference (Fig. 38-8, *A*).

In patients with keratoconus, it is important that the onlay graft cover as much of the cone as possible. The size of the cone can usually be easily found by analysis of the preoperative keratoscopic photograph (Fig. 38-9). The extent of ring distortion can be used to measure the size and location of the cone. The mark on the epithelium should be placed so that the lenticule will cover as much of the cone as possible. In greatly decentered cones the geographic center of the cornea is usually preferred over decentration of the graft.

Centering the graft around the optical axis is most important in myopic patients because the postoperative shape of the patient's cornea is very flat centrally and steepens very rapidly around the midperiphery (Fig. 38-10). If the surgery is off center, the patient may have glare problems when the pupil dilates.

EPITHELIAL REMOVAL

Careful and complete removal of the central epithelium is most important in prevention of the regrowth of epithelial cell rests between the recipient cornea and the onlay graft. This is performed by a combination of mechanical and chemical débridement. A 3 mm area of central epithelium is temporarily left on the cornea at this time, and this area includes the optical centering mark to be used for centering the trephine. The midperipheral epithelium is removed by scraping with a blunt spatula (Fig. 38-8, *C*). Care must be taken not to damage Bowman's layer during this maneuver to avoid any scarring between the recipient cornea and the graft in this area. One must remember that the goal is to have only adherence between the graft and the recipient cornea in the periphery so that the lenticule can be removed in the future if necessary.

After mechanical débridement, the cornea is carefully irrigated to remove any debris and residual epithelial cells (Fig. 38-8, *D*). This is done with a combination of irrigation through an infant feeding tube (or a 14 g intercath cannula) and suction in the fornix to remove excess fluid and debris. During the irrigation, the end of the feeding tube can also be used to scrub the surface of Bowman's layer to loosen any remaining epithelial cells. This irrigation step is repeated several times during the procedure to ensure that no particles remain to be trapped between the lenticule and the recipient cornea.

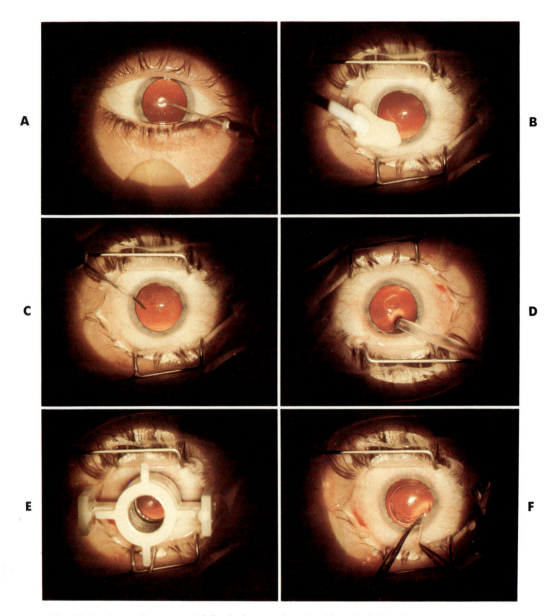

Fig. 38-8. Operative steps. **A,** Optical centering. **B,** Chemical débridement. **C,** Mechanical débridement. **D,** Meticulous cleansing. **E,** Vacuum trephine. **F,** Annular keratectomy.

ANNULAR KERATOTOMY

The next part of the procedure is the annular keratotomy. This not only is the site of adhesion between the two corneas, but also allows for migration of host keratocytes into the graft. If the keratotomy is not performed properly, the suturing can be very difficult with resulting astigmatism. This step is done in two stages. First, a vertical cut is obtained with trephine and then the edges are undermined toward the periphery. The trephine is carefully positioned around the previously marked optical center.

The diameter of the trephine and the size of the lenticule used are listed in Table 38-1. It should be noted that the lenticule for aphakia and myopia are oversized by 1.5 mm and only 1.0 mm in keratoconus.

The trephine cut is most accurately made with a Hessburg-Barron suction trephine (Fig. 38-8, *E*). This device creates a vertical keratotomy of consistent depth. The desired depth of 0.25 mm is obtained by advancement of the blade 2½ one-fourth turns once the blade has engaged the cornea. Care

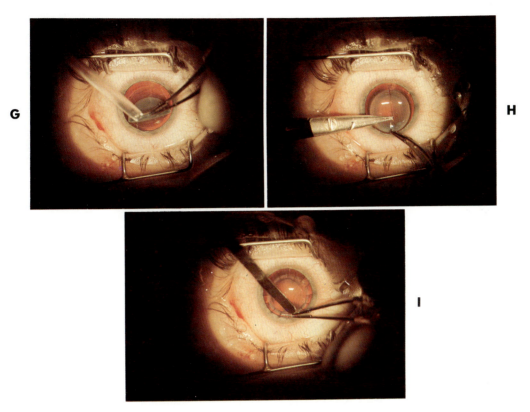

Fig. 38-8, cont'd. Operative steps. **G,** Lenticule application. **H,** Suturing. **I,** Edge tucking.

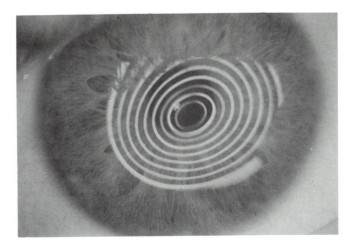

Fig. 38-9. Preoperative keratoscope photograph in patient with keratoconus.

Table 38-1. Lens and Trephine Diameters in Millimeters

| | For Aphakia | | For Myopia | For Keratoconus |
	Adult	Pediatric		
Lens diameter	8.5	8.5	8.5	9.5
Trephine diameter	7.0	7.0	7.0	8.5

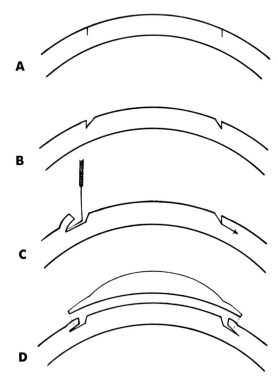

Fig. 38-11. Annular keratectomy technique steps for adult aphakia. **A,** Trephine keratotomy, 0.3 mm deep. **B,** Annular keratectomy, 0.3 mm deep and 0.5 mm wide. **C,** Spreading technique, 1 mm undermined. **D,** Lens edges designed to fit keratectomy.

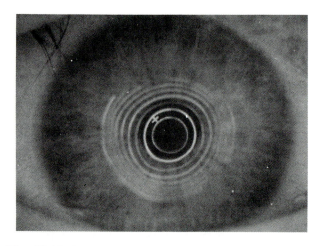

Fig. 38-10. Postoperative keratoscope photograph in patient with high myopia.

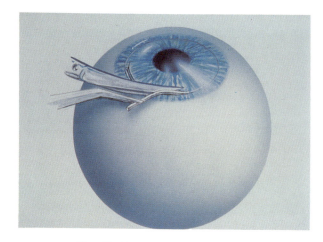

Fig. 38-12. Annular keratectomy.

must be taken not to break the suction during the keratotomy or an irregular cut will result. After the suction is released and the trephine has been removed, the depth of the cut is checked to confirm that it is 0.25 mm deep and consistent in all areas.

In aphakic and myopic procedures the additional preparation of the annular keratotomy is necessary because of the diameter difference between the lenticule and the keratectomy. The keratotomy bed is concentrically undermined 1 mm toward the periphery by use of a Suarez spreader or comparable instrument to allow the edge of the oversized graft to fit down in the keratotomy without buckling (Fig. 38-11).

In keratoconus an annular keratectomy is performed to allow for a larger area of adhesion between the lenticule and the stroma.

A wedge of anterior corneal stroma is then removed from the inner aspect of the trephine cut with a Vannas scissors being held at a 45-degree angle (Figs. 38-8, *F,* and 38-12). The resulting V-shaped groove should be 0.3 mm deep and 0.5 mm wide. The central epithelium is then removed and irrigated in accord with the previously described techniques. After all epithelium is removed and irrigated and just before the lenticule is sutured in place, a small amount of absolute alcohol is placed on the de-epithelialized surface to further prevent the possibility of epithelial inclusion cysts. This is best performed with a blunted Weck-cel sponge, and I first dip the sponge in the absolute alcohol and then squeeze all I possibly can out of the sponge so that it is barely moist and use this to paint the surface. As soon as the alcohol is applied, it is irrigated vigorously to make sure there are no residual toxic effects (Fig. 38-8, *B*).

SUTURING

The lenticule is sutured in place with use of 10-0 nylon in an interrupted fashion (Fig. 38-8, *H*). Sixteen sutures are used in myopia, adult aphakia, and pediatric aphakia, and 24 sutures are used in keratoconus. Ideally, the suture bites should extend from 0.5 mm on the donor side to 1 mm on the recipient side. The needle should be passed full thickness through the wing of the graft, completely into the recess of the annular keratotomy, and out the recipient corneal surface. This will bury the wing in the annular keratotomy and prevent dehiscence of the keratectomy, which might cause postoperative astigmatism during the healing process.

It is important not only to center the trephine on the optical center, but also to center the lenticule in the recipient bed during the suturing process. When one is placing the first four sutures, care must be taken to make sure that there is an equal amount of corneal tissue between each suture bite or the tissue will buckle, leading to an astigmatic result. The sutures should be cut short and the knots rotated. It is important that the knots be left just under the surface on the recipient side so that the sutures can be removed easily without excess pulling on the graft-host interface.

Next, the edges of the graft are tucked down into the keratectomy between each pair of sutures to prevent graft override, which would interfere with reepithelialization (Fig. 38-8, *I*).

In keratoconus, the suture technique is slightly different. Because the purpose of this procedure is to force the cone posteriorly, these sutures are under more tension and need to be carefully tightened. It is helpful to have the assistant place pressure on the center of the graft to press the cone posteriorly during the suturing. These suture bites should be slightly longer, 1.0 mm on both the host and recipient side for greater strength.

POSTOPERATIVE CARE

A bandage contact lens may be applied at the end of the procedure if desired, but this has not been found to be necessary for reepithelialization. Subconjunctival antibiotics and steroids are used as well as topical antibiotics at the end of the procedure.

The postoperative recovery occurs in three stages. The first stage is graft epithelialization. This usually takes place in 2 to 4 days in uncomplicated cases. It is very important to treat persistent epithelial defects aggressively or graft scarring or melting can occur. If lubrication or patching is not successful after 10 days, a temporary lateral lid adhesion should be done. The second stage of healing is an adhesion between the graft and host in the area of the annular keratotomy. In pediatric patients, this usually takes 1 week, whereas adults generally require approximately 2 weeks. After this adhesion occurs, the sutures can be removed. In keratoconus, the sutures remain in for 3 months because of the greater amount of tension on the graft edges in these cases. Topical steroids should be used very carefully in the early healing stages to avoid slowing the reepithelialization and healing. The third phase of the healing process is the repopulation of the graft with host keratocytes, which is believed to require between 4 and 6 months.[1,16]

It is important in the postoperative period to remember that, since this tissue contains no living cells, it is very susceptible to melting and infection if not handled properly. The graft should be considered "dead" tissue, and the role of the surgeon is to bring it back to "life" during the first 6 months of the healing process.

As with all corneal graft patients, there is a large variation in the healing rate of individual patients, and the surgeon should use discretion in early removal of loose sutures and the use of anti-inflammatory agents for vascularization of sutures.

FUTURE IMPROVEMENTS

Future advancements in this technique will simplify the procedure and also speed the patient's recovery and return of visual acuity. Advances will occur in the areas of instrumentation, tissue processing, improved lenticule designs, and substances aimed at improving tissue healing.

Further future advancements in corneal topography analysis will make possible better analysis of the patient's preoperative corneal shape, which should translate into a better "custom" fit of the lenticule to the corneal surface, allowing better predictability of the patient's postoperative refraction.

Improved methods of tissue processing and storage not only will improve the shelf life of the tissue, but should also increase the rate at which the tissue clears and result in more rapid return of good visual acuity.

With better instruments to perform the keratotomy and improved edge design of the graft, the

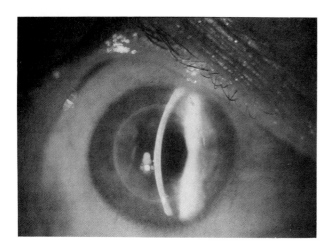

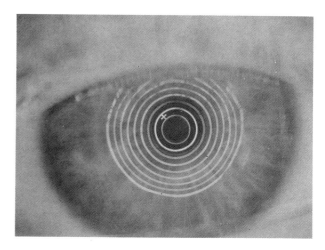

Fig. 38-13. Postoperative adult aphakia patient showing a clear onlay graft.

Fig. 38-14. Postoperative keratoscopic photograph of adult aphakia patient with minimal regular and irregular astigmatism.

length of time needed for epithelialization and adhesion at the keratectomy site should decrease.

Tissue adhesives and tissue-growth enhancers, which promote rapid wound healing, will simplify the procedure and shorten recovery.

CONCLUSION

Epikeratophakia is a simple ophthalmic surgical technique that uses basic surgical instruments. It is within the capabilities of most ophthalmic surgeons. One must remember that this procedure changes not only the structure of the cornea, but also its optical power. Care must be taken to obtain a symmetric keratotomy, good optical centering, a clean graft interface, and a well-tucked graft edges in order to result in not only a clear graft (Fig. 38-13), but also a symmetric optical surface (Fig. 38-14).

REFERENCES

1. Googe JM et al: The histology of epikeratophakia grafts, *Invest Ophthalmol Vis Sci* 20:8, 1981.
2. Kaufman HE: The correction of aphakia, Thirty-sixth Edward Jackson Memorial Lecture, *Am J Ophthalmol* 89:1, 1980.
3. Kaufman HE, Werblin TP: Epikeratophakia for the treatment of keratoconus, *Am J Ophthalmol* 93:342, 1982.
4. Keates RH, Kelley CG: Epikeratophakia for myopia: preliminary considerations, *J Refract Surg* 1:25, March-April 1985.
5. McDonald MB: Epikeratophakia: the surgical correction of aphakia, *Ophthalmology* 90:668, June 1983.
6. Morgan KS: The use of epikeratophakia grafts in pediatric monocular aphakia, *J Pediatr Ophthalmol Strabismus* 18:23, 1981.
7. Morgan KS et al: Surgical and visual results of pediatric epikeratophakia, *Metab Pediatr Syst Ophthalmol* 7:45, 1983.
8. Morgan KS et al: Epikeratophakia in children, *Ophthalmology* 91:780, July 1984.
9. Retzlaff J, Sanders D, Kraff M: Manual of implant power calculations, New York, Feb 1982, Sonometrics Systems, Inc.
10. Werblin TP, Kaufman HE: Epikeratophakia: the surgical correction of aphakia. II. Preliminary results in a non-human primate model, *Curr Eye Res* 1:31, Nov 1981.
11. Werblin TP, Klyce SD: Epikeratophakia: the surgical correction of aphakia. I. Lathing of corneal tissue, *Curr Eye Res* 1:123, Nov 1981.
12. Werblin TP, Klyce SD: Epikeratophakia: the surgical correction of myopia. I. Lathing of corneal tissue, *Curr Eye Res* 1(10):591, 1981-1982.
13. Werblin TP et al: Epikeratophakia: the surgical correction of aphakia, *Arch Ophthalmol* 99:957, Nov 1981.
14. Werblin TP et al: A prospective study of the use of hyperopic epikeratophakia grafts for the correction of aphakia in adults, *Ophthalmology* 88:1137, Nov 1981.
15. Werblin TP et al: Epikeratophakia: the surgical correction of aphakia, *Ophthalmology* 89:916, Aug 1982.
16. Yamaguchi T: Histological study of epikeratophakia in primates, *Ophthalmic Surg* 15:230, March 1984.

Chapter 39

Radial Keratotomy

Theory, case selection, and variables in success or failure

SID MANDELBAUM

MICHAEL J. LYNN

Myopia is the refractive state in which the refractive power of the eye is too great for its axial length, resulting in images being focused anterior to the retina rather than directly on it.[23] Since in the average eye more than 70% of the refractive power is attributable to the cornea,[12] alterations in corneal curvature can significantly affect the eye's refractive state. Radial keratotomy is one of several surgical procedures for flattening central corneal curvature, thus decreasing the eye's refractive power to better match its axial length.

Whereas other surgical keratorefractive procedures (keratomileusis, epikeratoplasty, photorefractive keratectomy using the excimer laser) correct myopia by altering anterior corneal curvature in the visual axis, radial keratotomy depends on the effect of adjacent incisions to alter central corneal curvature. Fyodorov postulated that radial keratotomy worked because a circular ligament present in the corneal periphery was incised.[6,7] No such structure has been generally recognized histologically, however. Knauss and associates constructed a synthetic model of the anterior segment of the eye and measured changes in curvature resulting from radial incisions.[13] Scha-

char, Black, and Huang derived a mathematical model for the cornea from which they predicted the anterior curvature after radial incisions.[31] The agreement between predicted curvature using these two models and actual measurements obtained in eye-bank eyes indicates that the curvature changes resulting from radial keratotomy may be explained mechanically, without the necessity of postulating a corneal circular ligament. The deep radial incisions weaken the paracentral and peripheral cornea, allowing the normal intraocular pressure to bulge the peripheral cornea outward. Since the cornea remains relatively fixed at the limbus, this peripheral bulge results in central corneal flattening.

The amount of central flattening depends on the interaction between the surgery performed (the number of incisions and their length and depth) and the response of the individual eye to these incisions. This chapter reviews the major surgical parameters and patient variables that have been proposed to influence the outcome of radial keratotomy.

SURGICAL VARIABLES

The effect of variations in the surgical technique has been evaluated by mathematical modeling, in eye-bank eyes, and in animal and patient eyes that have undergone radial keratotomy. Surgical variables that have been examined include the number of incisions, size of the central uncut optical zone, and incision depth and whether the incision extends beyond the limbus.

Incision Number. Fyodorov and Durnev reported that the optimum number of radial incisions was 16 and that a greater number of incisions did not increase the effect of the procedure.[6] Analysis of change of corneal curvature after radial keratotomy in eye-bank eyes indicated that 8 incisions produced

From the Prospective Evaluation of Radial Keratotomy (PERK) Clinical Center at the Bascom Palmer Eye Institute, University of Florida, and the Biostatistical Coordinating Center at Emory University, Atlanta, Georgia.
Supported by National Institutes of Health grants EY-03764 (University of Miami) and EY-03752 (Emory Statistical Center).

85% of the flattening of 16 incisions.[10] Based on their mathematical model, Schachar and associates similarly theorized that 8 incisions should produce about 91% of the flattening as 16.[31] When 8- and 16-incision radial keratotomies were compared in owl monkey eyes, there was no significant difference in corneal flattening that occurred with the greater number of incisions.[9,32] Preliminary results in patients undergoing radial keratotomy confirmed this.[19,22]

Since substantial corneal flattening was predicted[31] and noted experimentally[10,28] after four radial corneal incisions, some surgeons began to evaluate this approach clinically.[1] Experience has shown four-incision radial keratotomy to be effective, especially in lower degrees of myopia.

Incision Depth. Deep incisions are believed by most to be a major variable in attaining significant corneal flattening.[8] Intuitively, the deeper the incisions, the more the peripheral cornea is weakened, the more it can flex forward, and the greater the resultant flattening of the central cornea. A statistical analysis of radial keratotomy in cadaver eyes confirmed this intuitive concept, with the finding that depth of incision was the single best predictor of the amount of central corneal flattening attained.[10]

The importance of incision depth has been more difficult to establish in the clinical setting. Deitz found that incision depth (measured at 3 months with the Haag-Streit optical pachymeter) explained approximately 16% of the variability in outcome of radial keratotomy.[5] Using an average incision depth of 90%, Deitz achieved an average refractive change of 5.0 diopters at 1 year.[5] Nirankari, with an average incision depth of 50%, reported an average decrease in refractive myopia of 2.7 diopters.[19] Because of differences in surgical technique and data collection, these two series are not directly comparable; however, the difference in refractive effect may at least be partially related to differences in incision depth. In the series of patients reported from UCLA, refractive change after radial keratotomy was found to be greater for those eyes that sustained a microperforation, also indicating that deeper incisions may result in a greater effect.[8]

In the PERK Study, an ultrasonic pachymeter was used to intraoperatively measure corneal thickness at the edge of the central uncut zone at the 3, 6, 9, and 12 o'clock meridians. The micrometer diamond knife was then set to 100% of the thinnest of these four readings. This blade setting was used for all eight incisions. At follow-up examinations, attained incision depth was estimated by use of the slitlamp to estimate the depth of the scar in the central, middle,

and peripheral portions of each incision.[37] The estimate of depth of each portion of the eight cuts were averaged. The correlation noted between this average depth of incision and refractive change in the 413 eyes studied was 0.2.[16] Patients with shallow incisions generally did not have as great a change in refraction as those with deeper incisions, who had a wide range in refraction achieved.[16]

In cadaver-eye studies, incision depth can be accurately determined by histologic examination; such is not the situation clinically. The difficulty in establishing the role of incision depth in clinical series relates at least in part to difficulties in determining the actual incision depth in patients who have undergone radial keratotomy. It is not known how well the slit-lamp estimation of the depth of the scar resulting from a radial keratotomy incision correlates with the actual depth of the cut at surgery, or how reproducibly this can be estimated.

Even if incision depth could be measured accurately, the incisions themselves cannot be performed in an absolutely reproducible manner. Early cadaver-eye studies indicated a variation in incision depth of between 30% to 100% of corneal thickness when incisions were performed with metal blades and thickness was measured with optical pachymetry.[10,26] Although the use of ultrasonic pachymetry and the diamond micrometer knife has improved the reproducibility of performing incisions, there is still variability in incision depth. In a more recent cadaver study using these instruments, an average incision depth of 84% was achieved, but the depth of cuts still ranged from 61% to 98% of corneal thickness.[27] A histologic analysis of corneal cuts performed by one surgeon in eye-bank eyes with diamond knives confirmed significant differences in depth along single incisions.[33]

Factors that may account for this variation include differences in the configuration of the knife blade and foot processes and the difficulty in maintaining the blade precisely perpendicular to the cornea at all times. A small tilt to the side will result in obliquity of the cut and a shallower depth attained. Tilting in the forward-backward direction also affects depth as does the direction of the cut (toward the center or toward the limbus). Variation in pressure exerted on the knife and the speed with which the cut is made are also probably important. Variation in pressure exerted on the fixating forceps affects how much and how evenly the cornea domes upward and hence the depth of the cut. Anatomic considerations such as the prominence of the brow, the bridge of the nose, the eyelid position, and the amount the globe is displaced posteriorly when pressure is exerted on the eye make it more difficult to achieve consistent depth in some incision positions and in some patients. These difficulties in uniformly and reproducibly making incisions undoubtedly account for some of the variability seen in the outcome of radial keratotomy.

Diameter of Central Clear (Uncut) Zone. Fyodorov first suggested the concept of varying the central clear zone as a means of adjusting the effect of radial keratotomy.[6,7] In eye-bank eyes, Rowsey[20] and Salz[25,28] have observed that leaving a smaller central uncut zone results in more corneal flattening than a larger zone does. Similar conclusions have been reached in several clinical series of radial keratotomy.[5,21] Most clinical studies have incorporated multiple surgical variables, however, making analysis of the effect of clear zone more difficult.

Within the PERK Study, the sole surgical variable was the clear zone size.[36] The clear zone was assigned based on the spherical equivalent of baseline cycloplegic refraction: a 4.0 mm clear zone was used for -2.00 to -3.12, a 3.5 mm zone for -3.25 to -4.37, and a 3.0 mm zone for -4.50 to -8.00.[36] Baseline refractions were such that the patients were roughly equally divided into the three clear-zone groups.[37]

At 1 year postoperatively, PERK patients who underwent radial keratotomy with a 4.0 mm clear zone had an average of 2.73 diopters of refractive change. Patients with a 3.5 mm clear zone had about ¾ diopter more change (3.41 diopters), whereas patients in the smallest 3.0 mm group had an average of 4.49 diopters of refractive change.[16] On the average, then, the smaller the central uncut zone, the greater the effect of the procedure. A wide range of refractive change, at least 5 diopters, was noted within each group, and considerable overlap occurred between the three clear-zone groups.[16]

Termination Point of Incision. Although Fyodorov originally recommended extending incisions past the limbus, experimental radial keratotomy performed in cadaver eyes indicated that this may result in less effect than incisions that do not extend through the limbus.[10,26] When this variable was examined in patients, a similar decrease in effect was observed.[21] In cadaver eyes, some incisions through the limbus were found to have inadvertently damaged the trabecular meshwork.[26] Clinically, incisions through the limbus have resulted in superficial scarring and neovascularization.[14] It is therefore logical to recommend that radial keratotomy incisions stop just within the limbus both to maximize refractive effect and minimize structural ocular damage.

PATIENT CHARACTERISTICS AS VARIABLES

Besides the variables in surgical technique, variations posed by individual patient characteristics must also be considered in the outcome of the procedure. Factors that might influence outcome include age, sex, baseline refraction, preoperative corneal curvature, intraocular pressure, corneal diameter and thickness, and ocular rigidity.

Age. It has been noted that older patients obtain more effect from the same surgical procedure than younger patients do.[5,21,29] To test this, the PERK Study patients were divided into the following three age ranges: 20-29, 30-39, 40-58. On the average, older patients were found to have a greater change in refraction than younger patients have, with about ¾ diopter more effect in each successively older age group.[16] There was, however, considerable overlap between the three age ranges.

Sex. Slightly greater effect of radial keratotomy has been noted in males than in females.[5,29] In the PERK Study, males over 40 years of age had more effect from the procedure than females did, again with considerable variation.[16]

Baseline Refraction. At 1 year postoperatively, there was a tendency for PERK patients with greater baseline myopia to have a greater change in refraction from radial keratotomy, with a correlation coefficient of -0.56.[16] Recall that incorporated in these changes are different clear zones for different baseline refractions. For any given refractive error, however, the amount of change was quite variable.

Corneal Curvature. The effect of baseline keratometry as a predictor of outcome of radial keratotomy has been examined in eye-bank eyes with contradictory results. In one analysis, preoperative keratometry readings were not found to be helpful,[26] whereas in another study, preoperative corneal curvature did appear to contribute to the outcome.[10] Some of the predictive nomograms offered for radial keratotomy indicate that steeper corneas may have a greater response to the same surgery than flatter ones do.[30] In other clinical series, however, preoperative central keratometry has been found to have either little or no effect on outcome.[21] A preliminary attempt to utilize more complex corneal shape factors obtained from corneoscope photographs rather than from standard central keratometry did not improve prediction of refractive change.[11]

PERK Study data comparing preoperative keratometry and change in refraction did not show any effect of preoperative keratometry readings on the amount of correction obtained.[16] Although intuitively one might expect that the steeper the cornea is initially, the more it can flatten as a result of the surgery, this concept is *not* borne out by PERK Study results at 1 year.

Intraocular Pressure. Intraocular pressure has been suggested in various nomograms as a factor that should be taken into account in determining operative parameters,[17,30] on the theory that greater intraocular pressure will result in greater effect. PERK data indicate only a very weak relationship between intraocular pressure and change in refraction at 1 year (correlation = 0.19).[16]

Corneal Diameter and Corneal Thickness. No significant effect of either corneal diameter or corneal thickness on outcome of radial keratotomy could be demonstrated in the PERK Study.[16]

Ocular Rigidity. Ocular rigidity was included in Fyodorov's original formula as a determinant of the outcome of radial keratotomy.[6] In the PERK Study, ocular rigidity was determined by the method of Friedenwald[17] incorporating applanation tonometry (measured with a Goldmann tonometer) and Schiøtz tonometry. As determined in this fashion, ocular rigidity did not demonstrably affect the outcome of radial keratotomy in PERK Study patients.[16]

REGRESSION ANALYSIS VARIABLES

Before discussing the results of regression analyses on the PERK data, we present the following example, which illustrates a potential problem with the way regression analysis is typically used with radial keratotomy data. The computer was used to generate an imaginary set of data on 100 patients consisting of random values for baseline and follow-up refraction with no correlation between them. These imaginary data are plotted in Fig. 39-1, *A*, with a regression line shown and an R^2 value of 0.002. Besides R^2, another expression that can be calculated for variability is the mean squared error, or MSE, which is a measure of the variability of data around the regression line. The MSE for these data is 2.48.

Using the same set of imaginary noncorrelated data, the change in refraction is plotted against the baseline refraction in Fig. 39-1, *B*. The pattern of data and slope of the regression line certainly seems seems to indicate some relationship. The R^2 value has improved to 0.45. Notice that the MSE is unchanged by this manipulation of data. In this example, the use of the change in refraction as the outcome measure and the baseline refraction as the explanatory variable results in an inflated R^2 value. For this reason, R^2 should not be used as the sole measure of variability or of precision in the regression model.[18]

Using the best subset selection method[18] applied to the PERK data in an attempt to explain the variability in outcome, a regression analysis model including baseline refraction, age, and depth of incision gave the best fit, as follows: Change in refraction = $-1.69 - 0.48$ (baseline refraction) $+0.05$ (age) $+0.02$ (depth of incision). The R^2 value for this model is 0.45, and the MSE is 1.04. Using the MSE, one can calculate a more clinically meaningful measure of the variability associated with the model, called the "prediction interval."[18] The prediction interval is the range in which the outcome for a new patient can be expected to fall. The more variability is unexplained by the model, the wider the prediction interval will be.

As an example, consider a patient whose baseline refraction is -6.00 diopters, whose age is 33, and where the achieved depth of the incisions is 85%. Using the regression equation above, one finds the predicted value for the final refraction is -1.28. Using our MSE to calculate the 95% prediction interval, we can say with 95% confidence that we expect the patient's refraction after surgery to fall between -3.30 and $+0.74$ diopters. The amount of variability unexplained in this regression model results in a prediction interval about 4.00 diopters wide.

The regression equation presented above indicates that the average response is affected by several factors, most notably the baseline refraction, which incorporates different clear-zone sizes, age, and depth of incision. The response of an individual patient is highly variable, however, and the precision with which we can predict individual patient response based on these data is ±2.00 diopters.

Although we are unable to clearly isolate the contribution of many of the individual patient characteristics noted above, they and perhaps others must interact in some way to determine the refractive outcome. One lesson being learned from radial keratotomy reoperations is that some corneas will flatten only a certain amount, no matter how many deep incisions are performed, even if done as separate procedures.[34] This indicates that an individual eye will perhaps allow only a maximum amount of corneal flattening. Unfortunately, in some patients, this amount is insufficient to fully correct the existing myopia. Currently, we are unable to predict the maximum flattening that an individual cornea is capable of achieving.

One final patient variable whose contribution is uncertain but probably important is the rate of corneal wound healing. Although refraction seems stable in some patients by 3 months postoperatively, in others it is changing for several years after radial

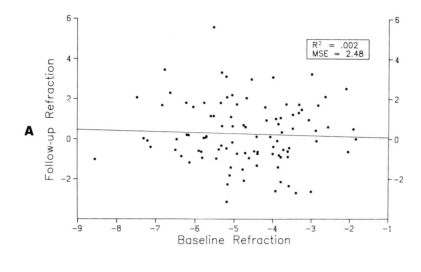

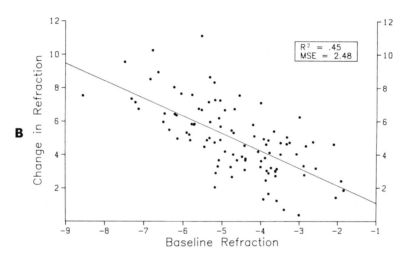

Fig. 39-1. A, Plot of 100 random, computer-generated pairs of numbers representing baseline refraction and follow-up refraction. These *imaginary* numbers do not represent actual data. **B,** Same set of imaginary noncorrelated data as in **A,** replotted as *change* in refraction versus baseline refraction. Notice that data now *appear* to be correlated and that R^2 has increased from 0.002 to 0.45. Mean squared error (MSE), however, remains constant at 2.48.

keratotomy. A subgroup of patients has been observed to have a continued decrease in myopia for years after surgery,[4,5] an indication that the incisions in these patients may not have completely healed. Waring and Steinberg have called our attention to featherlike stromal projections perpendicular to the incisions that appear several months after radial keratotomy (Fig. 39-2) and variably disappear over several years.[35] Their significance is uncertain, but they are another indication that in some cases these wounds are still undergoing remodeling for at least 3 years after radial keratotomy.

PATIENT SELECTION

Favorable publicity, media advertisements that focus on the positive aspect of discarding glasses, and the scientific aura surrounding medicine may create unrealistically high expectations in some if not most patients seeking radial keratotomy. Since radial keratotomy is an elective procedure that permanently alters an anatomically normal and crucial organ, it is particularly important that the patient be carefully informed of the risks and the desired benefits of the procedure as well. Only then can the patient realistically decide if he or she is willing to un-

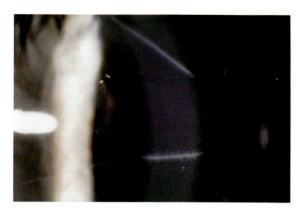

Fig. 39-2. Slitlamp photograph showing featherlike intrastromal projections perpendicular to a radial keratotomy scar 12 months after procedure.

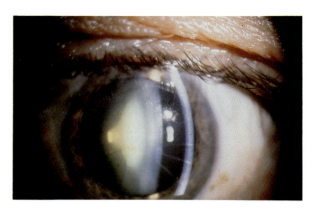

Fig. 39-3. Slitlamp photograph of 57-year-old male about 18 months after radial keratotomy showing radial corneal scars and nuclear sclerosis. Historically, patient was experiencing increasing myopia before procedure was performed, a probable indication of developing nuclear sclerosis preoperatively.

dergo the procedure. In counseling the patient preoperatively, the surgeon should consider the factors outlined below.

Baseline Refractive Error. Most studies have demonstrated that the majority of patients whose preoperative refraction is between −2.00 and −4.50 diopters will achieve an uncorrected acuity of 20/40 or better postoperatively. Even within this group, however, the outcome for an individual patient cannot be precisely predicted at the present time; some patients obtain much more or much less correction than desired. More myopic patients are less likely to achieve useful, uncorrected acuity. Prospective patients should understand that radial keratotomy may induce astigmatism even if not previously present and that procedures designed to correct astigmatism are also unpredictable at the present time.

Stability of Preoperative Refraction. Records of previous refractions should be obtained to verify that the refraction is stable. Progressive myopia in a younger patient may indicate pathologic rather than simple myopia. Keratometric readings that have become steeper over time should alert the ophthalmologist to the possibility of early, as yet unrecognized, keratoconus. In older patients, progressive myopia may be the first indication of an accelerating phase of nuclear sclerosis, the biomicroscopic signs of which may be slight. The patient in Fig. 39-3 was referred about 18 months after radial keratotomy. By history, he was already experiencing increasing myopia at the time the procedure was performed. It would seem to be in the best interests of both the patient and surgeon to avoid radial keratotomy in situations such as this.

Age. Radial keratotomy should not be performed until the refractive error stabilizes, the patient has

had the opportunity to try the wide variety of contact lenses available, and he or she is sufficiently mature to provide informed consent. These requirements are not yet met in most patients until their early twenties. Although all patients need to be informed of the effects of a reduction of myopia on presbyopia, this is particularly relevant to patients 40 years of age or older who, if they are fully corrected or overcorrected may experience symptoms of presbyopia immediately after surgery. The concept of presbyopia is difficult for most patients who have not previously required reading glasses to grasp; the decrease in unaided near vision should be demonstrated with appropriate trial lenses. Depending on the baseline refractive error, age, and occupation the surgeon and patient may plan on performing radial keratotomy on only one eye, resulting in monovision—one eye corrected for distance whereas the other remains uncorrected to provide best unaided near-range acuity.

Occupation. Although available data indicate that most patients who undergo radial keratotomy do not do so for job-related reasons,[2] occupation must be considered in patient counseling. The need for near- and intermediate-range vision in the patient's work should be assessed, particularly in light of the patient's age. Although glare usually resolves over several months, some patients remain symptomatic for much longer postoperatively; this may be particularly troublesome with jobs, especially any involving night driving. In experimental animals, globe rupture occurs with lesser force after radial keratotomy than in unoperated eyes,[15,24] patients in occupations at risk for blunt ocular trauma (such as security personnel) must particularly be apprised of this fact. Some patients require 20/20 uncorrected acuity to apply for or to function successfully in specific jobs. The likelihood of achieving this level of vision must be realistically discussed with the patient preoperatively; the patient should have plans for alternative employment if the required level of vision is not achieved.

Other Ocular Abnormalities. In selection of patients for radial keratotomy, significant ocular pathologic conditions should be ruled out. In particular, ocular surfacing disorders and anterior basement membrane dystrophies may be aggravated by this procedure. Reactivation of herpes simplex keratitis may be precipitated by radial keratotomy as by other forms of corneal trauma. Patients with less than 20/20 best-corrected acuity preoperatively are not likely to achieve a significant improvement in their best-corrected vision as a result of radial keratotomy.

■　■　■

In addition to counseling based on these considerations, informed consent for radial keratotomy should include a discussion of other available options for improving acuity (particularly the many available contact lenses), currently known complications of the procedure (including the potential of blindness if infectious endophthalmitis or keratitis were to develop), and the uncertainty of long-term effects of the procedure on the eye. It is critical to stress realistic expectations based on the likelihood that a person's specific visual goals can be met, given their particular refractive error. One approach is a discussion of a person's odds of achieving certain levels of vision, based on existing data. Demonstration of these approximate levels of vision with trial lenses as suggested by Deitz[3] may be helpful. It is of paramount importance that the patient understand our current inability to predict precise outcome in an individual case.

Thorough patient education, careful selection, and obtainment of truly informed consent are critically important to achieving patient satisfaction after radial keratotomy.

REFERENCES

1. Bonham RD, Hays JC, Rowsey JJ: Efficacy of four incision radial keratotomy, *Invest Ophthalmol Vis Sci* 26(suppl):202, 1985, ARVO abstracts.
2. Bourque LB et al: Psychosocial characteristics of candidates for the prospective evaluation of radial keratotomy (PERK) Study, *Arch Ophthalmol* 102:1187, 1984.
3. Deitz MR: Patient selection and counseling. In Sanders DR, Hofmann RF, editors: *Refractive surgery: a text of radial keratotomy*, Thorofare, NJ, 1984, Slack Inc.
4. Deitz MR, Sanders DR: Progressive hyperopia with long-term follow-up of radial keratotomy, *Arch Ophthalmol* 103:782, 1985.
5. Deitz MR, Sanders DR, Marks RG: Radial keratotomy: an overview of the Kansas City study, *Ophthalmology* 91:467, 1984.
6. Fyodorov S: Surgical correction of myopia and astigmatism. In Schachar RA, Levy NS, Schachar L, editors: *Keratorefraction*, Proc Keratorefractive Society Meeting, Denison, Texas, 1980, LAL Publishing Co.
7. Fyodorov SN, Durnev VV: Operation of dosaged dissection of corneal circular ligament in cases of myopia of mild degree, *Ann Ophthalmol* 11:1885, 1979.
8. Hoffer KJ et al: Three years experience with radial keratotomy: the UCLA study, *Ophthalmology* 90:627, 1983.
9. Jester JV et al: Radial keratotomy in non-human primate eyes, *Am J Ophthalmol* 92:153, 1981.
10. Jester JV et al: A statistical analysis of radial keratotomy in human cadaver eyes, *Am J Ophthalmol* 92:172, 1981.
11. Justin N, Asbell PA, Klyce SD: The role of corneal shape in radial keratotomy, *Invest Ophthalmol Vis Sci* 26(suppl):149, 1985.
12. Katz M: The human eyes as an optical system. In Duane TD, Jaeger EA, editors: *Clinical ophthalmology*, Philadelphia, 1982, Harper & Row, Publishers, vol 1.
13. Knauss WG et al: Curvature changes induced by radial keratotomy in Solithane model of eye, *Invest Ophthalmol Vis Sci* 20(suppl):69, 1981, ARVO abstracts.
14. Kremer FB, Marks RG: Radial keratotomy:prospective evaluation of safety and efficacy, *Ophthalmol Surg* 14:925, 1983.
15. Larson BC et al: Quantitated trauma following radial keratotomy in rabbits, *Ophthalmology* 90:660, 1983.
16. Lynn M et al: Factors affecting the outcome of radial keratotomy in the PERK study, *Invest Ophthalmol Vis Sci* 26(suppl):203, 1985, ARVO abstracts.
17. Moses RA: Intraocular pressure. In Moses RA, editor: *Adler's physiology of the eye:clinical application*, St. Louis, 1981, Mosby–Year Book.
18. Neter J, Wasserman W, Kutner M: *Applied linear statistical models*, Homewood, III, 1985, Richard D Irwin, Inc., pp 99, 246, 421-429.
19. Nirankari VS et al: Ongoing prospective clinical study of radial keratotomy, *Ophthalmology* 90:637, 1983.
20. Rowsey JJ: Ten caveats in keratorefractive surgery, *Ophthalmology* 90:148, 1983.
21. Rowsey JJ, Balyeat HD: Preliminary results and complications of radial keratotomy, *Am J Ophthalmol* 93:437, 1982.
22. Rowsey JJ et al: Predicting the results of radial keratotomy, *Ophthalmology* 90:642, 1983.
23. Rubin ML: *Optics for clinicians*, Gainesville, Florida, 1977, Triad Scientific Publishers, p 131.
24. Rylander HG, Welch AJ, Fremming B: The effect of radial keratotomy in the rupture strength of pig eyes, *Ophthalmic Surg* 14:744, 1983.
25. Salz JJ: Pathophysiology of radial keratotomy incisions. In Sanders DR, Hofmann RF, editors: *Refractive surgery: a text of radial keratotomy*, Thorofare, NJ, 1984, Slack Inc.
26. Salz J et al: Radial keratotomy in fresh human cadaver eyes, *Ophthalmology* 88:742, 1981.
27. Salz JJ et al: Analysis of incision depth following experimental radial keratotomy, *Ophthalmology* 90:655, 1983.
28. Salz JJ et al: A study of optical zone size and incision redeepening in experimental radial keratotomy, *Arch Ophthalmol* 103:590, 1985.
29. Sanders DR, Deitz MR: Factors affecting predictability of ra-

dial keratotomy. In Sanders DR, Hofmann RF, editors: *Refractive surgery: text of radial keratotomy*, Thorofare, NJ, 1984, Slack Inc.

30. Sanders D et al: Determination of operative parameters. In Sanders DR, Hofmann RF, editors: *Refractive surgery: a text of radial keratotomy*, Thorofare, NJ, 1984, Slack Inc.
31. Schachar RA, Black TD, Huang T: A physicist view of radial keratotomy with practical surgical implications. In Schachar RA, Levy NS, Schachar L, editors: *Keratorefraction*, Denison, Texas, 1980, LAL Publishing.
32. Steel D, et al: Modification of corneal curvature following radial keratotomy in primates, *Ophthalmology* 88:747, 1981.
33. Unterman SR, Rowsey JJ: Diamond knife corneal incisions, *Ophthalmic Surg* 15:199, 1984.
34. Villaseñor RA, Cox KO: Radial keratotomy: reoperations, *J Refract Surg* 1:34, 1985.
35. Waring GO III, Steinberg EB, Wilson LA: Slitlamp microscopic appearance of corneal wound healing after radial keratotomy, *Am J Ophthalmol* 100:218, 1985.
36. Waring GO III et al: Rationale for and design of the National Eye Institute prospective evaluation of radial keratotomy (PERK) study, *Ophthalmology* 90:40, 1983.
37. Waring GO III et al: Results of the prospective evaluation of radial keratotomy (PERK) study one year after surgery, *Ophthalmology* 92:177, 1985.

Surgical technique and improvements in technology and instrumentation

MICHAEL R. DEITZ

The surgical technique of radial keratotomy (RK) can be broken down into four main steps as follows:
1. Locating the visual axis at the point where it intersects the cornea and adjusting this center point for any eccentricity of the pupil.
2. Calculating the appropriate size of the optical zone and imprinting it on the corneal surface.
3. Measuring the exact corneal thickness and precisely setting the diamond knife to achieve the correct depth of cut.
4. Actually making each of the radial cuts in a consistent manner.

The surgery usually requires less than 10 minutes, and it appears to be quite simple. However, this is very deceptive because each step requires a considerable degree of precision to achieve good predictability and reasonably consistent results. It is easy to underestimate the skill and knowledge required for effective elimination of myopia with radial keratotomy.

CONSIDERATIONS

Radial keratotomy has become simpler and more accurate as better instrumentation has been developed, but basically the technique differs little from that advocated by Fyodorov in the mid-1970s and by Bores in the United States since 1978. However, the exquisitely sharp diamond blades (Fig. 39-4, *B*) set in handles with consistently reproducible micrometer settings (Fig. 39-5) have made the surgery more precise and convenient than it was originally.

These developments along with surgery formulas based on regression analysis have significantly improved predictability. Blade setting based on accurate ultrasonic pachymetry has been another major improvement (Fig. 39-6).

FOUR PRINCIPLE VARIABLES THAT CONTROL OUTCOME OF SURGERY

Size of Optical Zone. The size of the clear zone, or uncut window in the center of the cornea corresponding to the pupil, has traditionally been the most important factor in controlling the amount of myopic correction. The smaller the optical zone (OZ), the greater is the effect of the surgery: 3 mm or slightly smaller gives the greatest effect; 5 mm gives 1 diopter or less. The size of the OZ is chosen by the use of a regression formula or nomogram.

Depth of the Incision. The second factor in determining the refractive change is the depth of the cut. Normal procedure is to maintain a uniform depth of cut, as much as is possible from one cut to the next and from one case to the next. Eighty-five percent to 90% is preferred. Less than 85% does not weaken the cornea enough and thus gives too little effect. Also there appears to be more regression of effect and unpredictability with "shallow" cuts. Optimally deep cuts, 85% to 90%, allow a somewhat larger OZ to be used with reduced star pattern and glare. Cuts deeper than 90% can weaken the cornea unduly resulting in more risk of over-correction and increased fluctuation of vision. Successful myopic correction in the range of 9 to 10 diopters can be achieved but usually requires depths of 93% to 95% (the actual depth of all the cuts averaged together). This implies that a few of the radials will appear to touch Descemet's membrane. A disproportionate number of such cases of radial keratotomy with deep cuts show late increasing hyperopia termed "progressive hyperopic shift" (PHS).

Number of Cuts. Historically nearly all radial keratotomy done in 1979 and most of 1980 had 16 cuts as per the Russian influence. However, 8 cuts became standard within another year, and many milder myopes having RK surgery today require only 4 cuts. Cadaver data and mathematical models based on elastic spheres show that 4 cuts will give 55% to 60% of the maximum effect that can be ob-

A   **B**   **C**

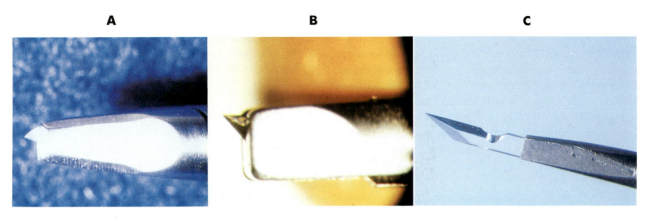

Fig. 39-4. **A,** Steel blade, **B,** Double-cut diamond blade. **C,** Sapphire blade.

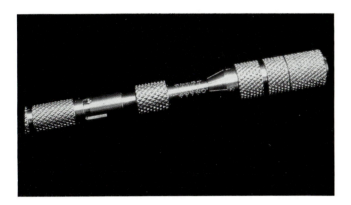

Fig. 39-5. Micrometer adjustment on knife handle.

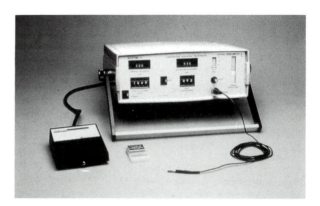

Fig. 39-6. Ultrasonic pachymeter—corneometer II.

tained by surgery; 8 cuts give 88% to 90%; 16 cuts give 98%. Only in the mathematical model can any more be achieved by use of 24 or 32 cuts. Actually, healing of this excessive trauma can cause more regression, and thus less effect than 8 or 16 cuts.

Two schools of thought have evolved on correcting milder myopes. Those advocating 4 cuts, usually with a 3.0 to 3.5 mm OZ cite the advantage of less trauma and fewer over-corrections although redeepening procedures may be necessary. Those advocating 8 cuts note that they can use larger optical zones, 4.0 to 4.5, and have fewer reoperations. This difference of opinion, along with the debate as to what order or sequence the cuts should be made, seems to be two areas where personal preference is the *main* determinant, with the pros and cons of each advocated technique balancing out the other.

Direction of Cut (Centripetal or Centrifugal). A moment's thought reveals that the radial cuts can be made either *inward* (toward the center or OZ, the so-called Russian technique) or *outward* (from the OZ to

the limbus, the so-called American technique). Both work. However, significant differences are inherent. Excursions into the optical zone are almost impossible when one is cutting outward from the OZ to the limbus. Therefore it is safer and easier for most beginners. The cuts are easier to keep straight; however depth control is more difficult. This is because the cutting edge of the blade is 45 to 60 degrees from the perpendicular to the direction of the cut. This results in a downward vector forcing tissue down away from the tip, into the anterior chamber like someone standing on a trampoline. The upward or outward force of the intraocular pressure, particularly as created by the fixation forceps or fixation ring, is the principal force to counteract this downward vector. By somewhat increasing the pressure of the fixation device as one proceeds through the radial cut one can compensate a bit for the increasing thickness of the peripheral cornea. This reduces the need for zone cutting with blade advancement.

Cutting from the limbus to the OZ results in a

more uniform depth of cut. Diamond blade settings are usually *no greater* than the thinnest paracentral pachymetry reading because you *get* what you *set*. On the other hand, outward-cutting surgeons set their blade extension to greater amounts than the pachymetric reading to get equally deep cuts. (I use 108% of paracentral or 104% of central pachymetry.)

It is often surprising to surgeons learning radial keratotomy that settings of the cutting blade in excess of paracentral pachymetry are frequently used. For example, for a cornea whose paracentral thickness measurement is 0.54 mm (540 μm) the blade setting for many surgeons would be 0.575 mm. Apparently the blade does not cut as deeply as it is set.

OTHER FACTORS

Age has a very significant effect on the amount of correction achieved by a given amount of surgery. Since age cannot be changed, it *must* be adjusted for by the surgical formula or nomogram to be used. Younger people get less effect, older people more effect. Patients 70 years and older get about the same effect as cadaver eyes, and 30 year olds get only half as much effect from the same amount of surgery.

Sex, intraocular pressure (IOP), and keratometric findings have been suggested as determinate of outcome, but they appear to be of much less significance, and although included in some formulas and nomograms, they are not found in others. Probably variations in surgical technique are of greater importance, and often mask these effects. Of the three, only IOP has been of real significance in the formula based on my Kansas City Study, the DRS (Deitz-Raanan-Sanders) formula.

To document the role of IOP one must take exceptionally careful applanation readings until the lowest stable pressure reading is obtained. Many of these patients have never, or rarely, had a pressure check, and they are a bit tense or apprehensive. The initial reading will often be 18 or 19 mm Hg. However, as the patient is urged to relax and becomes accustomed to the technique, the pressures frequently stabilize at 10 to 12 mm Hg.

The temptation of most examiners is to stop applanation as soon as a "normal" or nonglaucomatous reading is obtained. However, that may not be the patient's true IOP. One must remember that it will be the true, every-day IOP that will be causing the peripheral cornea (weakened by the radial cuts) to bulge and thus force the central cornea to flatten. In the final analysis it is the IOP that makes radial keratotomy work initially, and it is the IOP that helps prevent the natural tendency of all scar tissue to contract, from causing excess regression. If the IOP is carefully measured and followed serially, it has a significant effect on the outcome of radial keratotomy.

For example, in a recent case of a 54-year-old male with −5.00 diopters of myopia and keratometry of 43.00 diopters the OZ to be used for 10 mm Hg was 3.14 mm; for 14 mm Hg it was 3.42 mm; and for 18 mm Hg it was 3.70 mm. This shows a significant 0.56 mm difference in the procedure to be performed if there was an 8 mm difference in IOP.

This explains why a marijuana user with an IOP of 5 or 6 mm Hg may not achieve significant improvement in myopia with radial keratotomy, and some patients with borderline ocular hypertension can easily be overcorrected.

PROCEDURE—ANESTHESIA

In its simplest form, radial keratotomy can be performed with only topical anesthesia. Multiple doses of 0.5% tetracaine or proparacaine anesthetic drops are used. The corneal tissues are very easily anesthetized, but deep anesthesia of the episcleral tissue is necessary so that fixation forceps can be used to grasp the eye just beyond the limbus. Many surgeons using topical anesthesia recommend the use of diazepam (Valium), 5 to 10 mg by mouth, 30 to 60 minutes preoperatively.

The use of a retrobulbar block immobilizes the eye and helps to create a mild proptosis with slightly increased intraocular pressure. Most surgeons believe that the rare instance of optic nerve damage and permanent visual loss does not justify a retrobulbar block.

Although more than 80% of radial keratotomies being performed in the United States today involve only the use of topical anesthesia, a retrobulbar block will be required if a fixation ring (Thornton) or suction device is used. For a reasonably calm patient who has a normal degree of self-control, topical anesthesia is simpler, safer and quite satisfactory. However, for extremely nervous patients concerned that they might move during the actual surgery, general anesthesia may be utilized, if available at the surgery site.

SURGERY

Locating and Marking the Visual Axis. Although finding and marking the center is relatively easy for an experienced operator, it can be one of the most frustrating tasks for the beginning surgeon until a consistent and accurate system is worked out. The dot itself may be made with a disposable 25-gage needle on a 2½ ml syringe (Fig. 39-7). Blunter markers can be used including a fine irrigator, or a

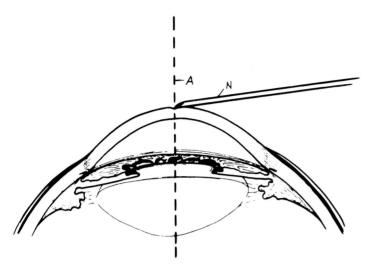

Fig. 39-7. Placing dot on cornea with a 25-gage needle.

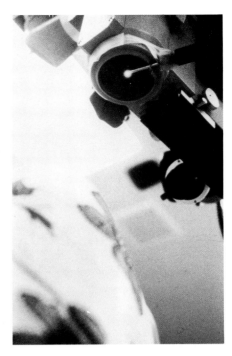

Fig. 39-8. Fiberoptic transilluminator used as a centering device.

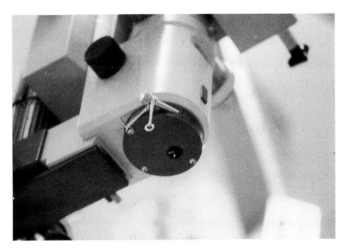

Fig. 39-9. Jed Med centering device developed for Dr. Robert Osher, Cincinnati, Ohio.

fine-tipped dye-containing marker that is disposable. Although retrobulbar and general anesthesia are not commonly utilized, it should be noted that they cannot be performed until the center mark is placed, and this requires the patient to be awake and cooperative. For the usual topical procedure, multiple drops are necessary for good episcleral anesthesia and more should be used at this point.

Numerous methods are available for finding and marking the center of the optical zone. The center is the intersection of the visual axis and the corneal surface.

The most accurate method employs a fiberoptic device (Fig. 39-8) that is not so dazzlingly bright as to cause the patient to fixate parafoveally. The patient is instructed to look right at the tip of the fiber optic light, which is pinhead in size. The physician, fixating binocularly, can make a dot on the cornea exactly where the reflection of the light appears. If the light or dot is placed in the center of the objective-lens cover glass, the surgeon must exercise good stereopsis to place the mark correctly. Alternately the surgeon can purposely mark both with his right eye and then with his left eye. Two dots on the cornea about 0.3 mm apart will delineate the visual axis. If the fiberoptic dot is in line with the left objective lens and the surgeon's right eye is obscured, as in the Osher/Jed Med device (Fig. 39-9), there should be no error in alignment. However, the mark must be made without benefit of stereopsis. The surgeon can partially compensate for the loss of stereopsis by focusing sharply on the cornea and then moving the focus *slightly* above the corneal plane. As the marking tip is lowered toward the cornea, it will come

into sharp focus a moment before contact is made, thus warning the surgeon that touch is imminent.

If the dazzling glare of the operating microscope light can be tolerated by the patient, the reflex can be seen on the cornea and the dot placed in correct location to its position. In a Zeiss OpMi-6 the mark is made at the lower edge of the reflex near the end opposite to the eye the surgeon is fixing with. Thus,

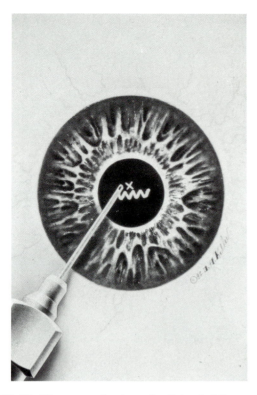

Fig. 39-10. Filament reflection of a Zeiss OpMi scope and desired placement of visual axis dot.

if the surgeon is using his right eye, the mark will be near the left end of the filament image and at its lower edge (Fig. 39-10).

If any attempts to correct astigmatism are contemplated, it is necessary to note some distinct anatomic spot (as a pigment spot or identifiable blood vessel) or make some reference mark on the patient's eye to delineate the 90- or 180-degree meridians. This must be done while the patient is sitting up, since significant torsional movements of the eye occur when the patient is lying down. The baseline reference must be indentifiable after the prep and draping are done. A mark on the cornea at the 6 o'clock position just below the pupil has been very useful to me (Fig. 39-11). If some anatomic landmark is found, it should be put on a diagram or the surgeon will find it impossible to align the protractor and thus establish the major axis of astigmatism during the surgery.

Routine Prep and Drape. A routine prep and drape should be done at this point. Care should be taken not to permit foreign substances, soaps, or disinfectants to get into the eye or on the cornea.

Fixation. Although the surgery can be performed with a simple conjunctival forceps, bipronged fixation with a Kremer spanning forceps (Fig. 39-12) or Bores' limbal forceps is superior. Bipronged fixation is a necessity for oblique or transverse cuts.

Optical Zone. The choice of clear or optical zone size will be determined by (1) the degree of myopia and (2) the planned depth of cut. Empiric formulas appear to improve predictability and greatly ease the burden of choosing the optic zone size for the beginning surgeon. They reflect not some theoretical mathematics, but simply what has happened to a group of patients who previously have undergone radial keratotomy. Although prospective studies have shown they work well for the surgeon from whose cases they were derived, little has been published to prospectively test these by other surgeons.

After good fixation is achieved and the cornea is dried with a Merocel sponge, the center mark

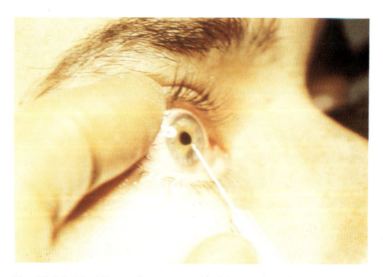

Fig. 39-11. Meridian reference mark with patient in sitting position.

should be clearly visible and the appropriate optical zone marker applied to the cornea concentrically around the dot delineating the visual axis (Fig. 39-13). Numerous devices are available for making this mark. The trephine should not be so sharp as to damage Bowman's membrane and leave a scar, but, on the other hand, its edge must be thin enough to leave a clearly defined mark. I prefer a low-profile marker with an outside bevel. Both the deeper trephines and trephines with an inside bevel are also usable but not ideal. This is because it is harder to sight down the inner surface for placement of the trephine. Cross hairs may seem useful, but many experienced surgeons prefer a marker without cross hairs, which introduce an element of parallax. Direct sighting through the inside surface of the trephine and making the dot absolutely central to the edge or rim give the best centering.

The microscope is zoomed *down* from the high magnification used for blade setting to low magnification for the optical zone marking. It is possible to mark multiple zones at this time. Care should be made not to put so many marks on as to cause confusion.

If cutting from the limbus to the clear zone is contemplated, the "cookie-cutter" imprinting device should be used to delineate the specific cuts. Otherwise, the tendency is to slightly torque these cuts unless a guideline is available for the direct observation of the cutting edge of the blade to follow. Cuts made from the clear zone to the limbus do not require this. Actually, the knife tends to obscure them for most of the cut, but they can help to mark where the radial cut is to be located at the start.

Depth Setting. Corneal thickness should be ascertained in the office or intraoperatively in the operat-

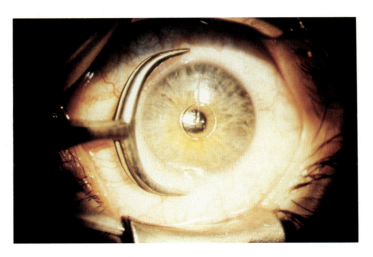

Fig. 39-12. Fixation device. Kremer's forceps at 5:30 and 12:30 position.

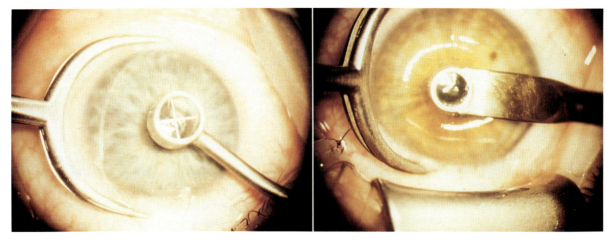

Fig. 39-13. Optical zone marker in position.

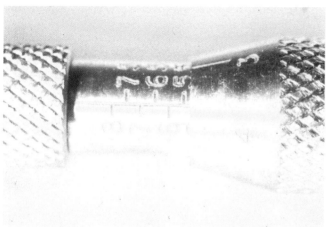

Fig. 39-14. Micrometer setting at 0.536 mm.

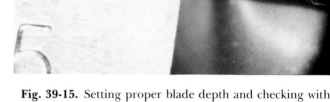

Fig. 39-15. Setting proper blade depth and checking with a Bores gage block.

ing room using ultrasonic pachymetry. Optical pachymetry is less reproducible and, except in experienced and skilled hands, has fallen into disuse. Using the pachymetry measurements, the surgeon chooses a blade setting that will, in his experience, give the desired depth of cut.

Until uniform, standardized, accurate gage blocks and knives are used universally, the beginning surgeon may have problems. I use a depth setting of 108% of *paracentral* ultrasonic pachymetry, or 104% of *central* ultrasonic pachymetry. But unless your gage block is carefully calibrated against my block, this number is almost meaningless, since differences of 25 μm are commonplace between different gage blocks. The cutting instrument (blade and footplate design), the gage block, the pachymeter, and the surgeon's technique form an interrelated complex that must be adjusted (titrated) to achieve the desired depth of cut.

Intraoperative pachymetry can be utilized to obtain necessary measurements, or the pachymetric readings can be measured in the office and the chosen depth settings calculated ahead of time.

Blade Setting. Knife-blade settings should be done with the maximum achievable accuracy. This requires the use of the *highest* power of the operating microscope and an appropriate gage block. Some micrometer knives have very accurate settings (Fig. 39-14), whereas others are found to be significantly off, in some cases by as much as 0.1 mm or 100 μm. Since the uncut lamella is usually no more than 50 μm, every attempt should be made to keep accuracy to within 10 μm for consistent results.

Care in using the gage block is essential, since any cutting instrument will be destroyed by the *slightest*

contact of the cutting edge against the block. This step must be practiced carefully. Care must be utilized to ensure that the knife is in exactly the same plane as the gage block. This must be judged by the surgeon if a hand-held block is utilized. If a cradle type of device is used, it will be achieved automatically. The whole apparatus or system must be absolutely perpendicular to the line of sight from the surgeon's eye through the microscope to the instrument. This usually requires closing one eye and looking for the reflex of the fiberoptic light off the surface of the block (Fig. 39-15). Then one should determine that the tip of the knife is at the appropriate setting. If blade setting is done intraoperatively, care must be taken to ascertain that the cornea does not dry during the setting procedure. Either an assistant should systematically check the corneal hydration and replenish it with balanced salt solution, or the eyelid speculum should be removed and the eye closed until the blade setting and confirmation have been achieved.

Newer instrumentation such as the Micron-Scope II (Fig. 39-16) eliminates parallax errors by using a coplanar alignment and can reproducibly measure blade extension within micrometers. The Micron-Scope features 100% magnification and retroillumination, which can pinpoint imperfections in blade quality such as chips or broken points, blade or footplate malalignments, and improper cleaning, which may not be evident under the maximum 25+ power of the operating microscope. The Micron-Scope is often used to check the calibrations of the micrometer handles of diamond knives before surgery. Since the blade is not placed near a hard surface during measurement, as with coin or block gages, there is

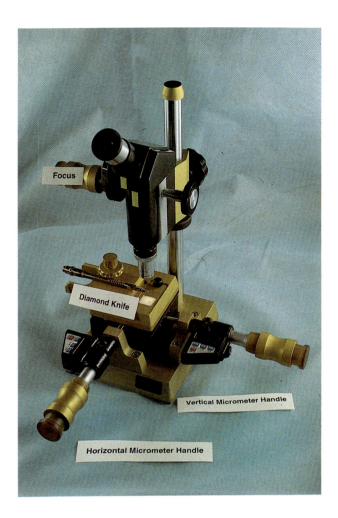

Fig 39-16. Micron-Scope II (Chiron Intraoptics, Irvine, California). Diamond knife tip beneath microscope objective lens can be inspected for damage and depth setting checked within several micrometers. (Photograph and comments courtesy C. Joseph Anderson, M.D., Madison Wisconsin.)

little risk of damage by touch to the fragile gem blade or its footplate.

Care of Gem Blades. The care of a gem blade knife requires the most exquisite, meticulous, and cautious technique. The knife should not be extended until one is ready to set the blade and confirm it with the gage block, or Micron-Scope II. It should be especially clean, since any loose dirt on the surface will be carried into the very first cut. Even more important, hardened debris must be removed because it will cause the knife to cut poorly, with increased drag, and may result in chattered or shallow incisions.

Drying. After the eyelid speculum is inserted and a final cleansing irrigation is applied, the cornea is dried with a Merocel sponge. Merocel is a man-made polymer sponge. It has been found to leave far less lint on the cornea than cellulose sponges do. Drying is done with a blotting, up-and-down motion, *not* a wiping motion. Wiping will cause more epithelial damage and more postoperative discomfort. The cul-de-sacs are carefully dried also.

Fixation. The fixation device is applied to the limbus. I prefer the spanning fixation device of Kremer and apply it at the 12:30 and 5:30 positions. Thus it is neither in line with nor interfering with either 6 o'clock or 12 o'clock cuts. If incisions at an oblique meridian are to be used for astigmatism correction, the fixation should be adjusted to a position where it will not interfere with them.

Immediately upon drying of the cornea, the center dot and meridian mark should be readily visible. The timing of the procedure should be started at precisely the point when the cornea is dried. Any delays in the procedure must be evaluated as to whether the cornea should be rehydrated or a decrease in depth cut should be attempted. Corneal thickness may decrease as much as 10% in 10 minutes if the microscope light is hot, the room air very dry, or the patient has prominent bulging eyes. Thus perforations can easily occur if adjustments are not made for significant delays.

Surgery: Incising the Cornea. The actual cutting is accomplished by gentle plunging of the diamond knife into the cornea at the edge of the clear zone and cutting to but not through the limbus. Some nicking of the upper limbal arcades may be necessary to maintain the same length of cut above as has been used below and temporally. *The blade should pause momentarily after the plunge into the cornea is made* to allow the knife to completely set itself and before the forward motion of the knife is begun. The actual cut should proceed in a very slow, methodical fashion, and the knife must be kept perpendicular to the cornea in both lateral and vertical directions (Fig. 39-17). Slow cutting is important for at least three reasons: (1) the cuts are more uniformly deep, (2) the cut can be stopped should a perforation occur and it can be kept to a minute microsize instead of being extended into a large macroperforation, and (3) the cuts can be more accurately and evenly placed. Since the thinnest portion of the cornea usually is the infratemporal quadrant, some surgeons prefer to perform this cut early before the cornea has undergone any drying. On the other hand, others state that it should be done last when a perforation will be of less consequence. Normally the rate of change may be slower than 10% in 10 minutes, but one needs to watch the duration of the procedure, since corneal thinning readily allows a microperfora-

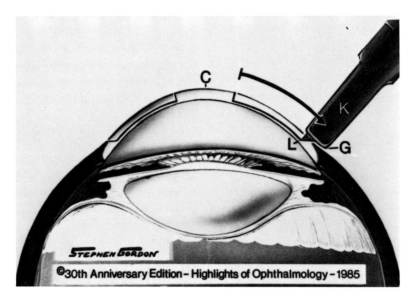

Fig. 39-17. Diagram of incision showing perpendicularity to tangent at surface of cornea at point of contact.

tion. The order in which radial keratotomy incisions are made appears to be totally at the surgeon's discretion. There is an advocate for every possible sequence of doing the cuts.

My preference is to make the infratemporal cut early before the cornea has had a chance to dry. Most surgeons agree that the cut at 12 o'clock, that is, the No. 16 radial, is the most difficult. For right-handed surgeons, the 1:30 cut is the next most difficult. *Conscious awareness of the pressure with the fixation forceps is essential.* It is used to increase intraocular pressure, particularly as the periphery of the cut is approached. This appears to allow a slightly deeper cut in the thicker peripheral cornea. Doing this can save the extra trauma of recutting (often referred to as redeepening). Once all eight radials have been placed any additional cuts can be performed. I do no zone cutting, or redeepening, but this would be the appropriate time for the zone measurement and any further increase in blade setting to be done.

When the formula or nomogram indicates that the degree of myopia requires an optical zone significantly smaller than 3 mm, I prefer recutting the radial cuts with the same blade setting, that is, no blade advancement, for their entire length. Accomplish it by gently slipping the knife into the original cut, at the edge of the clear zone, and cutting again to but not through the limbus. There must be *no* downward pressure. No resetting or extension of the blade is done. Recutting or redeepening is when most perforations occur; therefore its use must be undertaken cautiously.

Depth Check. The next step is to make some attempt to check the depth of the cut. Although most experienced surgeons eventually abandon the use of the depth gage, the beginning surgeon may find it more useful. The hockey-stick depth gage (Fig. 39-18) can be slipped into the wound, with its lower surface bearing on the bottom of the recently made cut (Fig. 39-19). It should be done very gently. The top edge of the hockey-stick blade should be noted. If it actually protrudes up out of the cornea and thus is above the corneal epithelium, the incision is less than 50% to 60% deep. If it is flush with the cornea, the depth of the cut will more likely be appropriate. If it appears to plunge into the cornea and no irrigation has been carried out, the cut is very deep. It is important not to press down, especially with the more pointed "dip-stick" variety of depth gage. Remember there is a possibility of perforation with a depth gage if Descemet's membrane has been partially severed.

Irrigation. The radials are next flushed with balanced salt solution. Great care should be taken not to allow the irrigating needle to damage the deepest portion of the cuts (Fig. 39-20). The uncut lamellae may be very thin and Descemet's membrane may be partially incised. Any pressure at all may cause a perforation and leakage. Each radial cut is flushed out one or two times.

Postoperative Dressing. Although some surgeons omit bandaging the eye, most believe that a *light* pressure bandage (such as two pads) is desirable, at least for a few hours. Most agree that an antibiotic eyedrop and possibly a mydriatic drop (cyclopento-

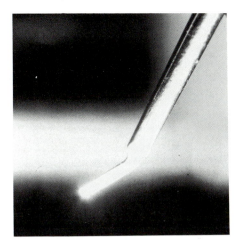

Fig. 39-18. Hockey-stick depth gage.

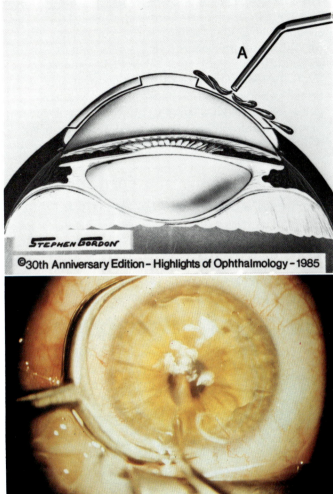

©30th Anniversary Edition - Highlights of Ophthalmology - 1985

STEPHEN GORDON

Fig. 39-20. Irrigation of wound with balanced salt solution.

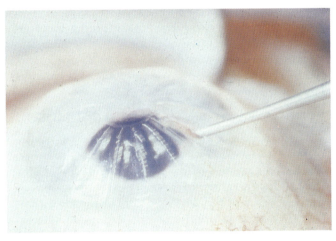

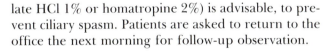

Fig. 39-19. Hockey-stick depth gage in radial cut.

late HCl 1% or homatropine 2%) is advisable, to prevent ciliary spasm. Patients are asked to return to the office the next morning for follow-up observation.

SUMMARY

The simplicity of radial keratotomy and the apparent ease with which large amounts of myopia can be reduced to near emmetropia has prompted a major revision in our attitude about the advisability of refractive surgery. Although skepticism may be waning, extreme caution and meticulous precision are important if the distress of serious complications such as infection, overcorrection, and irregular corneal scarring are to be kept to a minimum.

RADIAL KERATOTOMY VERSUS PHOTOREFRACTIVE KERATECTOMY (RK vs PRK)

There is no question after 18 months to 2 years of experience with the excimer laser (VISX 2020), that PRK can correct myopia with results roughly comparable to RK for 1- to 6-diopter myopes. Of the 120 photorefractive procedures we have done up to now at the Eye Foundation of Kansas City, 21 were in the original IIA phase of this FDA-monitored study. We have 18 months of follow-up study on 18 of them, and most are stable at 6, 12, and 18 months, within 20/40 or better uncorrected acuity in 75% and with 1 diopter of emmetropia in 62%. The 25 patients in phase IIB are at this time 10 months after the operation and appear to be following a pattern similar to that in phase IIA. These data compare favorably with our early RK results and the PERK study. If refinements in technique improve the predictability, it should match or possibly exceed the results of a carefully optimized mature RK series, that is, 20/40 or better in 90+% of cases. Since PRK removes only 5% to 10% of the anterior corneal tissue, it may well be more stable over time and certainly weakens the globe less than RK. However, currently it is more painful and slower to achieve good vision than RK. Truly "the jury is still out."

Factors affecting the corneal surgeon's decision to perform radial keratotomy

R. BRUCE GRENE

SCIENTIFIC FACTORS: ANALYSIS OF SURGICAL RESULTS

The objective assessment of surgical results is the most commonly discussed basis for exclusion of radial keratotomy (RK) from one's ophthalmic practice. Although there are legitimate concerns regarding the safety, stability, and accuracy of radial keratotomy, objective analysis of published data is only a small component of the decision-making process.[1,2,4,5,7] Few areas of ophthalmology have provoked such intense emotion as radial keratotomy has. One's scientific assessment of the published results is often an objective justification for behavior motivated by the subjective nonmedical factors discussed below. Familiarity with the numerous published series on radial keratotomy is necessary but insufficient to make a decision whether to perform radial keratotomy.

PHILOSOPHICAL FACTORS: THE EVOLVING PARADIGM OF SURGICAL INDICATIONS

The complex set of beliefs and values that guide our view of "appropriate surgery" is constantly evolving.[3,8] Thoft has described four general categories of surgical indications: (1) emergent life or death circumstances, (2) potentially life-threatening circumstances, (3) restoration of function, and (4) improved cosmetic status.[6] As ophthalmologists, we generally work within the third arena—restoration of function.

Historically, those in ophthalmology have spent the bulk of their existence striving to prevent blindness. Recently, with the advent of the intraocular lens, our goal has become the optimization of best corrected vision. Today, the standard of visual function has moved us further from our historical battle with blinding pathoses. Refractive surgery and radial keratotomy are based upon the belief that best uncorrected vision is the legitimate goal of both patients and ophthalmic surgeons.

The corneal surgeon must move from the comfort of performing penetrating keratoplasty for advanced keratoconus (pathosis that is causing functional blindness and for which no alternative exists) to performing radial keratotomy (surgery in the absence of any pathosis for which nonsurgical alternatives exist that provide a best corrected vision of 20/20).

This philosophical leap is difficult for many surgeons. Failure to examine one's beliefs carefully may lead to an ambivalent and ineffective foray into refractive surgery. This prevalent practice pattern is characterized by numerous instructional courses, minimal or absent marketing efforts, and extremely restrictive surgical indications. The resultant radial keratotomy "practice" rarely exceeds one or two cases per month. The surgeon considering incorporation of radial keratotomy into his or her practice must be comfortable with the basic philosophical tenet of refractive surgery: optimization of a patient's best uncorrected visual acuity.

ETHICAL FACTORS: PATIENT ACQUISITION

The scientific and philosophical issues raised by refractive surgery and radial keratotomy should be carefully examined before we move on to consider the factors encountered in the competitive arena of contemporary ophthalmology. One of the most challenging factors facing the prospective radial keratotomy surgeon is the ethical dilemma of patient acquisition. In the absence of injury or disease, few myopic men and women seek care from cornea and external disease specialists. Simply alerting one's existing referral base to the availability of radial keratotomy surgery is likely, at best, to result in an occasional endorsement. The successful creation of a radial keratotomy practice is based upon direct advertisement to the public. This effort can take the form of low-key marketing of newsletters or seminars. The other end of the spectrum is aggressive promotion by television and radio featuring implied guarantees of excellent vision without correction. Generally, the more modest the advertising "campaign" the more comfortable is the corneal surgeon beginning radial keratotomy. Unfortunately, the more aggressive the campaign, both in scope and implied benefits, the more effective for patient acquisition. The adage "no ad, no RK" creates another challenge to be resolved in considering the initiation of radial keratotomy in a corneal practice.

POLITICAL FACTORS: THE SPECTER OF COLLEGIAL RESPONSE

To have a low-profile radial keratotomy practice is possible, but like a low-volume "heavy metal" rock concert, infrequent and ineffective. Significant surgical volume is needed to justify both the expense of equipment and the time and effort required to learn the procedure. As with all complex surgical procedures, the comfort and skill of the surgeon is dependent on frequent, regular surgery. To accomplish this generally requires a visible public identity as a radial keratotomy surgeon. This identity and the advertising required to create and sustain it may lead to alienation of one's colleagues. The fear that "I'll lose my graft referrals" may be justified in some circumstances.

An ironic twist in negative collegial response is occurring with increasing frequency. The judgmental disdain for refractive surgery and its practitioners is being replaced by growing interest in alternatives to Medicare-reimbursed procedures. In some circumstances, the corneal surgeon may be encouraged to avoid radial keratotomy because of his colleagues' interest in entering the refractive surgical arena themselves.

ECONOMIC FACTORS: OPPORTUNITY VERSUS OPPORTUNITY COST

The factors preventing corneal surgeons from successfully integrating radial keratotomy into their practice are complex. Those practices that do succeed are generally driven by a more simple factor—economics. Refractive surgery is an extremely promising business area of ophthalmology, and radial keratotomy remains the heart of refractive surgery.

The traditional corneal transplant practice is built on the shoulders of external disease. From a purely economic perspective, the transplant surgeon earns his or her living providing time-consuming, low-paying office care to identify transplant candidates. These candidates require a time-consuming, low-paying surgical procedure and postoperative care when compared to both cataract surgery and radial keratotomy.

This gloomy, present-day view of the "business" of corneal and external disease faces a future with dramatic reductions in reimbursement, rising instrument and labor costs, and increasing competition from fellowship-trained and general ophthalmologists. On the other hand, refractive surgery is exempt from the radical regulatory and reimbursement constraints of our current government. Increased public acceptance and promising technology may create dramatic increases in the number of men and women seeking correction of their refractive error.

A corneal surgeon should not ignore the scientific, philosophical, ethical, and political ramifications of his decision. However, should these factors lead to a decision to not perform radial keratotomy, he must acknowledge the economic impact of that decision.

Although the opportunity is great, the opportunity cost of developing a strong refractive surgical practice is significant. The development of the technical skills required, analysis of equipment purchases, and development of advertising programs require tremendous time and energy. Of equal importance is the retraining of technicians, surgical assistants, receptionists, and billing and insurance staff. The refractive surgical practice is fundamentally different from the cornea and external disease practice, and this change in identity should not be underestimated. To "do a few RKs" is a straightforward task. To build a refractive surgery practice is no less complex and time consuming than the fellowship and early practice challenges of building a cornea and external disease practice. If all the previously discussed concerns have been satisfied, one must still ask whether he or she wants to make such a major career change.

CONCLUSION

The combination of changes negatively impinging on the cornea specialty and the promise of refractive surgery force the surgeon to make a difficult decision. Only by exploring the factors discussed above can one identify his or her own best direction. Regardless of one's decision, for all of us the future appears to bear little resemblance to the past.

REFERENCES

1. Arrowsmith RN, Marks RG: Visual, refractive and keratometric results of radial keratotomy: five-year follow-up, *Arch Ophthalmol* 107:506-511, 1989.
2. Deitz MR, Sanders DR, Raanan MG: A consecutive series (1982-1985) of radial keratotomies performed with the diamond blade, *Am J Ophthalmol* 103:417-422, 1987.
3. Grene RB: [Forward]. In Nordan LT, Maxwell WA, Davison JA, editors: *The surgical rehabilitation of vision*, New York, 1991, Gower Medical Publishing.
4. Salz JJ et al: Ten years experience with a conservative approach to radial keratotomy, *Refract Corneal Surg* 7:12-22, 1991.
5. Sawelson H, Marks RG: Five-year results of radial keratotomy, *Refract Corneal Surg* 5:8-20, 1989.
6. Thoft RA: Symposium of Radial Keratotomy, *J Refract Surg* 3(5):198-199, 1987.
7. Waring GO et al: Results of the prospective evaluation of radial keratotomy (PERK) study five years after surgery, *Ophthalmology* 98(8):1164-1176, 1991.
8. Weinstein GW: The buccaneer eye surgeon, *Ophthalmol Surg* 11:831, 1980 [Editorial].

Chapter 40

Laser Corneal Surgery: Fundamentals and Background

GEORGE O. WARING, III

THEO SEILER

All types of refractive keratotomy share one weakness—the inability to predict accurately the outcome of surgery for an individual patient. This defect results from variability in technique among surgeons and from variability in corneal biomechanical properties and wound healing among patients.

The development of pulsed lasers, particularly the argon fluoride (193 nm) excimer laser, offers a potential solution to the first of these two problems because these lasers can create accurate and precise excisions of corneal tissue to an exact length and depth with minimal disruption of the remaining tissue. In addition, this minimal tissue disruption and the smooth edges may allow more uniform stromal wound healing. Laser surgery can also make cuts in almost any conceivable configuration, without touching the cornea. Using computers to control these lasers may create robotic refractive surgery, removing the art from the procedure and allowing the surgeon to perform the exact desired operation in case after case.[1,17,18,27]

Since 1983, when excimer lasers were first sug-

gested as instruments for refractive surgery, researchers in numerous laboratories around the world have raced to define the conditions that might make this technology a clinical reality. Depending on one's perspective, progress has moved either rapidly—approximately five systems of varying sophistication are available for laboratory and clinical experimentation, or slowly—many fundamental technical and biologic questions about the process remain unanswered.

Of the three types of excimer laser corneal surgery—photorefractive keratectomy (laser keratomileusis, surface area ablation), linear laser keratectomy, and laser therapeutic keratectomy—we discuss only the first two.

Table 40-1 presents a proposal for conventional terminology for laser corneal surgery.

PRINCIPLES OF LASERS

To understand the use of lasers in photorefractive keratectomy, it is helpful to review briefly the basic principles of lasers at a level suitable for ophthalmic clinicians. Details are presented in textbooks.[39,43] We use the argon fluoride excimer laser to illustrate these principles.[14,18,30,31,39] Light has both wave-like and particle-like properties. Wave-like properties explain optical phenomena such as refraction and interference; particle-like properties explain how tissues acquire and release energy—the absorption and emission of light by atoms and molecules.

This chapter is modified from a thesis previously published in the *Transactions of the American Ophthalmological Society* (Waring GO: Development of a system for excimer laser corneal surgery, *Trans Am Ophthalmol Soc* 87:854-983, 1989) and has been published in a modified form by Seiler T, Fantes FE, Waring GO III, Hanna K: "Laser Corneal Surgery," a chapter in Waring GO III: *Refractive keratotomy for myopia and astigmatism*, St. Louis, 1992, Mosby–Year Book, Inc.)

Table 40-1. Proposed Terminology for Laser Corneal Surgery

Type of procedure	Preferred term	Colloquial alternatives
I. General term	Laser corneal surgery	Laser keratoplasty Laser ablation of the cornea Laser keratectomy
II. Refractive A. Removal of central Bowman's layer and anterior stroma	Laser refractive keratectomy Photorefractive keratectomy (PRK)	Laser anterior keratomileusis Large area ablation Reprofiling Sculpting En face ablation Tangential ablation
B. Linear keratectomy	Laser radial keratectomy Laser transverse keratectomy (straight, arcuate)	Laser RK

C. In conjunction with other techniques
    1. After removal of anterior lamellar disc (microkeratome)
    2. After previous refractive surgery
	Laser stromal keratomileusis
	Laser keratomileusis in situ
	
	For example, PRK after radial keratotomy
	For example, PRK after epikeratoplasty
		Ablation of disc
		Ablation of bed
		
		Laser-adjustable synthetic epikeratoplasty (LASE)

D. Intrastromal laser surgery	Intrastromal photodisruption Intrastromal thermokeratoplasty	Intrastromal keratomileusis Intrastromal linear keratectomy Intrastromal radial keratectomy, transverse keratectomy

III. Therapeutic
  A. Removal of superficial corneal opacity
  B. Trephination
	Laser therapeutic keratectomy
	Phototherapeutic keratectomy (PTK)
	Laser circular or elliptical keratectomy
		Surface smoothing
		Superficial therapeutic keratectomy
		Laser penetrating keratoplasty
		Laser lamellar keratoplasty

IV. Removal of lamellar disc (replaces microkeratome)	Laser lamellar resection	Tangential lamellar resection

From Waring GO: *Refract Corneal Surg* 6:318-320, 1990.
Type of laser to be specified (for example, excimer, argon fluoride.)

Therefore we use the terms "wave" and "photon" interchangeably, depending on the phenomena we want to explain.

The electromagnetic spectrum is composed of a broad range of wavelengths, from long radio waves to short gamma waves. Our interest is in the optical wavelengths in the invisible ultraviolet range (approximately 100 to 300 nm). Each wavelength of the electromagnetic spectrum interacts with the cornea in a specific way. The cornea absorbs well the ultraviolet and infrared radiation and transmits effectively the radiation between 300 and 1300 nm. Numerous wavelengths have been tested for photorefractive keratectomy: 193, 248, 2900, and 10,600 nm.

Specific Characteristics of Laser Light as Applied to Corneal Surgery

Monochromaticity. Light of a single wavelength forms a specific color in the visible spectrum and a specific invisible "color" outside that spectrum. Absolute monochromaticity is an unobtainable goal—even our best laser light is a mixture of some wavelengths. It is this characteristic that determines the amount of laser energy absorbed or transmitted by the cornea.

Directionality. Laser light is essentially collimated light that has a very small divergence, or spread, as it leaves the laser cavity. This characteristic allows laser light to be directed at a very small spot a relatively long distance from the laser itself and is the characteristic that allows laser light transmission through the delivery system to the eye. The directionality is measured by the full-angle beam divergence in radians. The typical laser beam increases in size for every meter of travel.

Brightness. The intense brightness of the laser light is an expression of the energy contained in the laser beam; because the energy is concentrated in a single wave train moving in one direction, the energies are extraordinarily high. This energy absorbed in the cornea is responsible for the ablation of tissue. The radiant energy is measured in joules; the radiant exposure of the tissue is measured in joules/cm^2; the radiant power is measured in watts; the irradiance is measured in watts/cm^2.

Coherence. Coherence occurs when the light waves in the laser are in phase and there is a predictable and constant correlation between the peak and the trough of the waves. The great regularity of coherence depends on the laser's monochromaticity and directionality and is measured by interferometry. Coherence is not a very important characteristic in the use of lasers for corneal or ophthalmic surgery, in which the major emphasis is on absorption of specific wavelengths and the energy of the beam. Coherence becomes important, however, in the use of lasers for communication, holography, and measurement. The coherence of an excimer laser beam is generally poor.

Mode structure. The distribution of energy in the laser beam is characterized as the mode of the beam, the energy distribution across the beam being called the "transverse mode" and that along the beam being called the "longitudinal mode." The mode structure of the laser is important in determining its potential uses on the basis of the divergence and coherence of the beam. The transverse mode—more specifically, the transverse electromagnetic mode (TEM)—can have many patterns and configurations. When there is more power in the center of the beam than at the edge of the beam, the mode is designated "TEM$_{00}$." If there is less power in the center and the distribution is bimodal, the designation is "TEM$_{01}$." Depending on the resonant properties in the laser cavity, laser beams can acquire many different mode structures (multimode). Excimer lasers produce a multimode beam that is more difficult to render homogeneous than are the beams of solid state or dye lasers. A homogeneous beam is an advantage in creating a smooth surface after photoablation.

Creation of Laser Light. To create laser light, three basic conditions must exist (Fig. 40-1). First, there must be an active medium—a collection of atoms, molecules, or ions that emit radiation in the optical part of the electromagnetic spectrum. The medium can be (1) a gas such as krypton, carbon dioxide, or those in an excimer, for example, argon fluoride; (2) a solid such as neodymium-doped yttrium-aluminum-garnet (YAG) crystal; or (3) a liquid, such as a dye laser. Second, there must be a source of energy for the laser, a pump that can cause a population of atoms to undergo the transition from their ground state to the higher energy level—a population inversion. The pumping may be achieved with an electrical discharge, as in an argon or excimer laser; by a flash lamp, as in a Nd:YAG laser; or by an optical source, as in dye lasers. The third necessary element is the optical resonator that allows the emitted light beam to feed back by being reflected between two mirrors, stimulating other atoms to a higher energy level in the process, thereby amplifying the light and creating a much more powerful

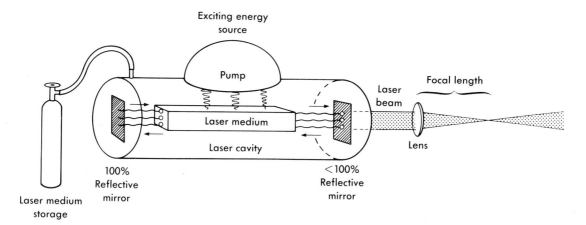

Fig. 40-1. Basic configuration of excimer laser demonstrates active laser medium as gas in storage tank and in laser cavity. Excited energy is pumped from a source illustrated as a bank of electrical capacitors whose discharge can create a population inversion in laser medium. Laser cavity has mirrors at each end to amplify laser beam before it is emitted through a delivery system containing lenses. (From Waring GO: *Trans Am Ophthalmol Soc* 87:854-983, 1989.)

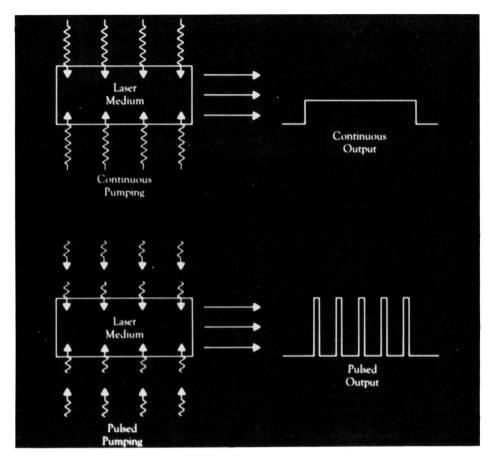

Fig. 40-2. Pattern of emission of laser light can be either a continuous wave from continuous pumping of the laser medium or individual pulses from intermittent pumping of laser medium. (From Waring GO: *Trans Am Ophthalmol Soc* 87:854-983, 1989.)

beam. The number of feedback or resonating cycles varies greatly among lasers, from many in the argon to few in an excimer.

Emission of Laser Light. Laser light is emitted either continuously or in pulses (Fig. 40-2). With continuous wave (CW) lasers, a constant pumping of the laser medium leads to a stationary emission of light, as in the familiar argon laser. With pulsed lasers, excitation of the laser medium is achieved by single events, such as the flash from a flash lamp or an electrical discharge, leading to a single short emission of light—the laser pulse. This is familiar in the pulsed Nd:YAG laser. The power of a pulsed laser is on the order of 1000 to 1,000,000 times higher than that of a continuous-wave laser. Only pulsed lasers are useful in refractive corneal surgery. The power emitted from a pulsed laser can be increased by decreasing the pulse length, for example by Q-switching or mode locking.

INTERACTION OF LASER LIGHT WITH THE CORNEA

There are four interactions that laser light may have with the cornea: transmission, scattering, reflection, and absorption (Fig. 40-3). Which of these four interactions occurs depends on the laser characteristics and the tissue characteristics, and most importantly, the amount of light energy that is absorbed by the molecules in the tissue—the chromophores.

Transmission of laser light through the normal human cornea generally occurs between wavelengths of 300 and 1600 nm.[18] Thus lasers such as the argon and the Nd:YAG pass through the cornea without difficulty. Laser light can also be scattered by the tissue, thus decreasing the efficiency of the laser. Reflection of the laser beam seldom occurs from the cornea.

The most important interaction is absorption of the laser energy by the cornea.

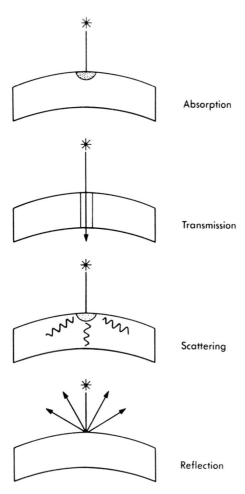

Fig. 40-3. Four types of interaction of laser light with cornea. (From Waring GO: *Trans Am Ophthalmol Soc* 87:854-983, 1989.)

Table 40-2. Absorption bands for components of cornea

Cornea component	Absorption wavelength (nm)	Location of major concentration	Optimal radiation
Protein	<220	Stroma	Ultraviolet
GAG	<200	Stroma	Ultraviolet
Collagen	<250	Stroma	Ultraviolet
Nucleic acid	<260	Epithelium	Ultraviolet
Ascorbic acid	<250	Epithelium	Ultraviolet
Water	2900	Stroma	Infrared
	10,000		
	<170		

Table 40-3. Lasers potentially usable for corneal surgery

Laser	Wavelength (nm)	Pulse duration (nsec)	Penetration depth (μm)
Excimer (ArF)	193	10-20	2
Excimer (KrF)	248	10-20	10
Excimer (XeCl)	308	10-20	300
Fifth harmonic Nd:YAG	213	10	2
Holmium:YAG	2060	20000	400
Hydrogen fluoride	2870-2910	50	1.5
Er:YAG	2940	20000	0.75
Er:YSGG	2790	20000	1.5
CO₂ TEA (transversely excited atmospheric pressure)	10,600		

Absorption of Laser Light by the Cornea. The higher the absorption, the more "opaque" the cornea to a given wavelength and the easier the process of surface ablation. Therefore the key to understanding the appropriate selection of lasers for keratectomy lies in the absorption spectrum of the corneal tissues (Figs. 40-4 and 40-5; Table 40-2).[4,27] The highest absorption in the cornea is by macromolecules, in the far ultraviolet region at wavelengths less than 300 nm, and by water, in both the middle infrared region near 3000 and 6000 nm and the far infrared region above 10,000 nm.

A good way to conceive of absorption is in terms of the penetration depth of the laser light: the greater the absorption, the less the penetration of a better potential for surface ablation and a decreased chance of thermal damage. Table 40-3 lists the penetration depths of lasers that have been used for keratectomy and demonstrates that the argon fluo-

ride excimer laser and the fifth harmonic Nd:YAG ultraviolet lasers have the smallest penetration depth and therefore are best suited for corneal surgery. The hydrogen fluoride and erbium-doped YAG (Er:YAG) are also well absorbed. Wavelengths absorbed by nucleic acids, such as the 248 nm excimer, may be mutagenic and therefore not appropriate for clinical use.

When laser light is absorbed by the cornea, there are three types of effects that can occur: (1) photothermal, (2) photodisruption, and (3) photochemical.

Photothermal effects. Photothermal effects occur when the energy absorbed by photons produces molecular vibration. This vibration produces heat and increases the temperature enough to break weaker bonds, such as hydrogen bonds, producing protein denaturation.

There are two types of thermal effects: photocoagulation and photovaporization. Photocoagulation

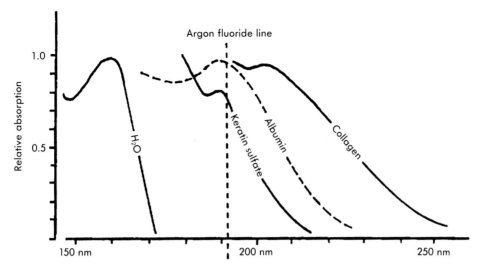

Fig. 40-4. Absorption spectrum for molecules in cornea. The *x*-axis indicates wavelength in nanometers. The *y*-axis indicates relative absorption. *Wavy dotted line,* Reference point for albumin; *vertical dotted line,* argon fluoride at 193 nm, where there is a relatively high absorption for collagen and keratin sulfate.

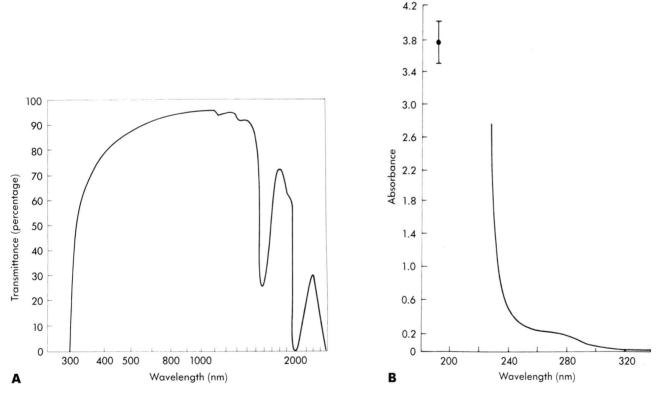

Fig. 40-5. Transmission and absorption of light by cornea. **A,** Transmission of light through human cornea. **B,** Plot of absorbance versus wavelength in far ultraviolet spectrum for a 32 μm thick section of bovine cornea. The point at 193 nm represents average of laser transmission measurements made on eight different 32 μm thick samples. Error bar indicates one standard deviation. (**A** from Boettner EA: *Invest Ophthalmol Vis Sci* 1:776-783, 1962; **B** from Puliafito CA et al: *Ophthalmology* 92:741-748, 1985.)

is the most common use of CW lasers in ophthalmology, such as argon and krypton laser photocoagulation of the retina and choroid. The laser needs to elevate temperature only 10 to 20 Celsius degrees to coagulate the tissue. Variables set by the surgeon are power, duration of exposure, and spot size. The holmium laser is used to coagulate corneal tissue during thermokeratoplasty.[48]

In photovaporization, very high radiant densities are used and tissue temperature rapidly reaches the boiling point of water, where both coagulation and excision of tissue occur. Photovaporization is the mechanism for keratectomy by the infrared lasers, such as HF and CO_2. The higher the irradiances, the greater the amount of tissue removed and the less the coagulation. For example, a CO_2 laser can ablate corneal tissue with less thermal damage if a pulsed laser rather than a continuous-wave laser is used.

Photodisruption effects. Photodisruption by means of ionization occurs at a very high irradiance, with pulse durations shorter than 20 nanoseconds. The high-energy density tears electrons from their atomic orbitals and disintegrates the tissue into a collection of ions and electrons and electrons called "plasma," a gas with the electrical properties of a metal. The effect produces mechanical shock waves. This is the mechanism used by the Nd:YAG laser and the pulsed dye laser.

Photochemical effects. Photochemical effects usually occur at shorter wavelengths, with low to moderate radiant exposures. There are two basic types of photochemical reactions: photoradiation and photoablation. Photoradiation is used in photoradiation therapy (PRT), in which a hematoporphyrin derivative is selectively taken up by active tumor cells and the laser radiation produces an excited state of the porphyrin, which triggers chemical reactions that destroy the cell.

The process most commonly used in refractive corneal surgery is ablative photodecomposition (photoablation for short) and is accomplished with ultraviolet and infrared radiation. The ultraviolet photons are almost completely absorbed by the surface of the cornea. They also have an extremely high photon energy (6.4 electron volts at 193 nm), an energy that is in excess of the intermolecular bond energy of approximately 3.5 eV. Thus the absorption of this energy at the surface breaks up the molecules with such energy that the fragments leave the surface at supersonic velocities of 1000 to 3000 m/sec. Thus the excess energy is carried off, and there is minimal thermal damage in the residual tissue.*

---

*References 8, 16, 18, 22, 32, 35, 41, 44, 50, 53, 54, 56, 59.

LASERS USED FOR CORNEAL SURGERY

As laser refractive corneal surgery continues to develop and expand, an increasing number of lasers are being used for the process (see Table 40-3). Presently, numerous types of lasers are under active investigation.

Excimer Lasers. Excimer lasers are discussed in detail in this chapter and are briefly defined here. In an excimer laser, the active medium is most commonly the excited combination of an excited rare gas atom (such as argon or krypton) combined with a diatomic halogen molecule (such as fluorine or chlorine). The laser is pumped by a high-voltage electrical discharge across the laser cavity and is emitted with megawatt intensity of ultraviolet light in the range of 190 to 350 nm, which is absorbed by the macromolecules (proteins, nucleic acids, proteoglycans) in the cornea. Excimer lasers have the potential advantage of precisely removing very small amounts of tissue with each pulse, leaving behind minimal thermal or acoustic damage.

Excimer lasers were first developed in 1975.[44,58] Extensive research on the excimer-polymer interactions was performed by Srinivasan, Sutcliffe, Dyer, and others,[8,22,52,55] who demonstrated that because the ultraviolet wavelengths were useful for etching silicones and other polymers,[50] they might be used for manufacturing microcircuits. Reed and co-workers were the first to use the excimer laser on the cornea, and they demonstrated that the corneal epithelium is very sensitive to the wavelengths of krypton fluoride at 248 nm.

Their first application for refractive corneal surgery occurred when R. Srinivasan, IBM Research Center, Yorktown, N.Y., and Stephen Trokel, Columbia University, N.Y., reasoned that if excimer lasers could be used to etch and carve polymers, they might be used also to etch and carve the cornea. This resulted in their 1983 publication demonstrating exquisite linear excisions in the cornea and suggesting the use of these lasers for refractive corneal surgery (Fig. 40-6)

Carbon Dioxide Laser. In a carbon dioxide laser the lasing medium is a mixture of nitrogen, helium, and carbon dioxide. Pumping is usually accomplished by a high-voltage electric current that excites the nitrogen atoms, whose electrons are rapidly transferred to the carbon dioxide atoms. The excited carbon dioxide atoms decay, emitting infrared light, most commonly at a wavelength of 10,600 nm. This is amplified within the resonance cavity at high efficiency and can produce tremendous amounts of output power. Thermal interaction relies on water content to determine the effect produced by the

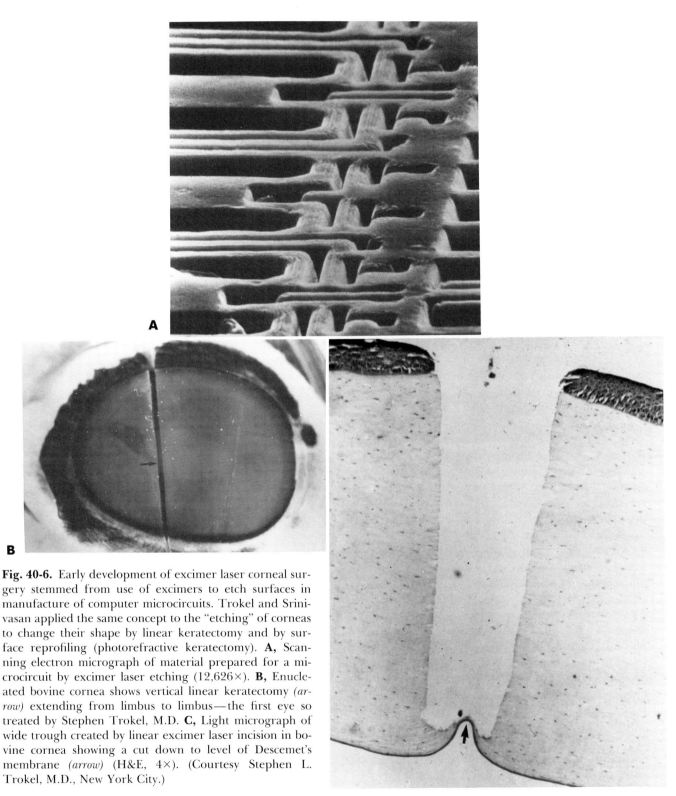

Fig. 40-6. Early development of excimer laser surgery stemmed from use of excimers to etch surfaces in manufacture of computer microcircuits. Trokel and Srinivasan applied the same concept to the "etching" of corneas to change their shape by linear keratectomy and by surface reprofiling (photorefractive keratectomy). **A,** Scanning electron micrograph of material prepared for a microcircuit by excimer laser etching (12,626×). **B,** Enucleated bovine cornea shows vertical linear keratectomy *(arrow)* extending from limbus to limbus—the first eye so treated by Stephen Trokel, M.D. **C,** Light micrograph of wide trough created by linear excimer laser incision in bovine cornea showing a cut down to level of Descemet's membrane *(arrow)* (H&E, 4×). (Courtesy Stephen L. Trokel, M.D., New York City.)

CO_2 laser. The intracellular and extracellular water undergoes an abrupt phase change, creating steam and vaporizing the tissue. The dispersed energy can be absorbed by the tissue adjacent to the ablation, resulting in coagulation and carbonization of the remaining tissue. However, reducing the exposure time can minimize the thermal effect.

The features of the pulsed CO_2 laser that make it particularly suitable for corneal surgery are (1) CO_2 laser energy is strongly absorbed by water molecules and (2) the marginal pulse duration for neglecting thermal dissipation from the volume in which CO_2 light has penetrated is about 10^{-3} second. Because the cornea is composed of 78% water, the corneal endothelium, as well as other portions of the eye, is protected from thermal damage from transmitted energy delivered with short exposure times. The thermal relaxation time of biologic tissue is different from that of water. However, with a pulse width shorter than 200 μsec, it should be possible to vaporize tissue without creating thermal damage to adjacent areas. A large amount of power will need to be delivered during the short-pulse duration, creating high-power densities. The poor hemostatic ability of the laser used in this fashion may be of concern in other tissues, but in an avascular tissue like the cornea, this is not relevant.

The first laser incisions in the cornea were made with a continuous-wave carbon dioxide laser by Fine and colleagues in 1967.[9,10] The deep penetration of about 25 μm caused large zones of thermal damage adjacent to the incision, resulting in inflammation and corneal scarring, with a need for penetrating keratoplasty. Beckman and colleagues[5] used a pulsed carbon dioxide laser, reducing thermal damage to the cornea but still leaving enough damage to render its use impractical for corneal surgery. Keates and colleagues[15] used a pulsed carbon dioxide laser and a specially designed delivery system to create a narrow cut into the cornea. The edges of the excised tissue were ragged compared with those achieved with an excimer laser. We have used a pulsed TEA (transversely excited atmospheric pressure) carbon dioxide laser for experimental corneal surgery.

Hydrogen Fluoride Lasers. The lasing medium in a hydrogen fluoride laser consists of hydrogen and sulfur hexafluoride gases. The laser is pumped by an electrical discharge into vibrationally excited hydrogen fluoride molecules that have a number of emission lines, ranging from 2740 to 2960 nm. These wavelengths can be amplified in the stable resonator cavity and are emitted to be absorbed by the water in the cornea, with a penetration depth on the order of 1 μm.

Two groups have reported on the use of hydrogen fluoride lasers for surgery. Seller and colleagues[47] observed that the excisions of tissue made with the laser created more thermal damage and a more irregular margin than those made with an argon fluoride (193 nm) excimer laser. However, with more careful design of the delivery system and more careful focusing of the laser, sharp-edged excisions with minimal remote thermal damage can be achieved.

Loertscher and co-workers[26,29] have used the hydrogen fluoride laser to perform laser circular trephinations using an axicon lens delivery system (see Fig. 40-21) with a narrowly focused beam. Trephinations performed in eye bank eyes demonstrated a perfectly vertical incision with reasonably smooth edges but not as smooth as those obtained with an argon fluoride excimer.

The experiments performed by these two groups have produced somewhat contradictory results. Seiler and co-workers[47] used lower radiant exposures of 100 mJ/cm^2, whereas Loertscher and co-workers[28] operated with higher fluences between 700 and 2300 mJ/cm^2, identifying an ablation threshold of 400 mJ/cm^2 and an optimal radiant exposure to minimize thermal damage of 4 mJ/cm^2. Both groups have found thermal damage extending 10 to 30 μm laterally from the excision.

The advantages of a hydrogen fluoride laser are the simplicity of the laser itself and the greater possibility of creating delivery systems using fiberoptics.

Erbium:YAG Laser. Very similar to the Nd:YAG laser, the Er:YAG type of solid-state laser uses a YAG crystal doped with erbium ions as a lasing medium. The emitted wavelength is 2.94 μm (2940 nm), near the maximal absorption of water. Commercial devices include a Q-switched mode that is able to create pulses with an energy of 100 mJ and a maximum pulse duration of 280 nsec and a non–Q switched mode with a pulse diameter at about 150 μsec. Only repetition rates of less than 10 Hz are available.

The advantages of this laser include its small size, its easy technical handling, and its transmission through optical fibers, making both direct application to the cornea and intraocular surgery possible. Manufacturing difficulties include the need for special optical elements that contain no absorbed water.

Bende and colleagues[6] used an Er:YAG laser for corneal surgery. They found an ablation threshold of about 13 mJ/cm^2. Thermal damage extended up to 25 μm into the tissue adjacent to the excisions. This damage was larger compared to those around excimer laser keratotomies, but did not have a significantly different healing rate in rabbit eyes.

Pulsed Holmium:YAG Laser. Seiler and colleagues[48] used a pulsed holmium:YAG laser emitting at a wavelength of 2.06 μm (2060 nm) to make focal thermokeratoplasty burns within the stroma, in an attempt to correct hyperopia by shrinking a paracentral ring of cornea and steepening the central cornea. The laser light was guided by a quartz fiber and focused by means of a handpiece. The beam was focused about 400 μm in front of the handpiece. The pulse duration was approximately 200 msec. The output energy was maximally 35 mJ per pulse at a repetition rate of 4 Hz. The fluence at the cornea ranged from 10 to 28 mJ/cm^2. For every coagulation, 30 pulses were applied. The studies were carried out in human cadaver eyes, demonstrating that a total energy delivered to the cornea of 15 to 20 mJ produced the maximal amount of correction. The smaller the diameter of the clear zone along which the burns were made, the greater was the change in refraction. Histologically the coagulation formed a conical illusion, wider near the surface and tapered to approximately 50 μm in front of Descemet's membrane. In a series of four blind human eyes, corrections of approximately 3.00 to 5.00 D were achieved, with the values present at 1 month persisting to approximately 9 months.

Dye Lasers. In general, lasers that emit visible light are not used for corneal surgery because they are not absorbed by the cornea. However, if a sufficiently high energy density can be applied in a short enough pulse, a keratectomy can be achieved by tissue disruption or ionization.

In a dye laser, an organic dye dissolved in a solvent is irradiated with a strong light source, such as an argon laser, which causes the dye to fluoresce over a broad spectrum of colors. A specific wavelength can be made to lase when a birefringent crystal is inserted into the laser cavity. By turning this crystal one can find an appropriate angle that will transmit only a narrow wavelength of light, allowing the operator to turn the crystal and dial the desired wavelength.

Troutman and colleagues[60] have used a pulsed dye laser to perform intrastromal keratectomies by focusing the laser in the center of the stroma. The rationale behind this approach to laser refractive surgery is to preserve an intact Bowman's layer and anterior corneal stroma so that the all-important anterior corneal surface is essentially undisturbed. The dye laser emitted a wavelength of 595 nm (yellow), which allowed the investigators to obtain radiances of up to 10^{15} watts/cm^2 when in focus, using picosecond pulses. Histologic examination of animal and human eye bank eyes showed creation of space within the stroma, with damage to the adjacent tissue extending 20 to 40 μm from the wound.

For such an approach to be successful, it must not only produce negligible stromal scarring and opacification from the intrastromal ablation, but must also change the anterior corneal curvature. Because Bowman's layer and the anterior cornea may be reasonably rigid compared with Descemet's membrane and the posterior cornea, and because there is a pressure differential across the cornea from the posterior side (the intraocular pressure exceeding atmospheric pressure), it seems more likely that the posterior layers of the cornea will collapse forward, leaving the anterior layers in their preoperative configuration, with minimal change in refraction. It seems that this approach will have more impact in linear excisions than in the central surface type of excisions.

SYSTEMS TO COUPLE LASER AND EYE

Because laser corneal refractive procedures must be performed with micrometer accuracy, the demands for stability of the eye are greater than those required during other ophthalmic laser procedures. For example, during argon laser photocoagulation of the retina or Nd:YAG photodisruption of the posterior lens capsule, the eye can move between laser shots because the interaction between the laser and a single spot on the tissue is brief and because the location of the laser shot needs to be controlled only within tenths of a millimeter. In photorefractive keratectomy, even though interaction between the laser and the tissue lasts only nanoseconds, the train of pulses must be delivered to the same or exactly adjacent areas of the cornea during the entire 20-second to 8-minute procedure. The eye must therefore be kept in a fixed position with respect to the laser, using a coupling system.

Position of the Patient. The first element in coupling is to have the patient comfortably in a stable position in front of the delivery system. Early attempts to accomplish this with the patient in a seated position before a slitlamp apparatus achieved less control, and so most systems now allow the patient to lie on a bed with the head stabilized beneath the overhanging delivery system.

Observation of the Cornea. The surgeon should have visual control through an operation microscope of the ablation process to monitor its progress, viewing coaxially with the laser beam path.

Aiming the Laser. Because the lasers used for photorefractive keratectomy have wavelengths outside the visible spectrum, an auxiliary aiming laser that is coaxial to the ablating laser is required to align and aim the laser. Helium-neon lasers or laser diodes are the standard for this. In automated systems, this is used only for initial alignment, but in manually controlled systems, it is used to align each location.

Stabilization of the Eye. Eye movements during ablation create two problems. The first is ablation of undesired areas of the cornea so that linear ablations become wide, V-shaped troughs and areal ablations have more irregular margins and surfaces. The second is inaccurate optical correction caused by aberrant pulses that deviate from the calculated amount of tissue ablation and disrupt the desired new corneal profile. The exact amount of eye movement allowable during ablation is unknown. Microsaccades that move the eye only a few micrometers may not be enough to disrupt the overall pattern of ablation, and the small movements may have an overall smoothing effect because they are somewhat random.

Manual stabilization. Early attempts at excimer laser corneal surgery used manual stabilization of the eye and manually directed micromanipulators to aim the beam while the patient fixated on a target. This can be adequate for therapeutic purposes, such as ablating the bed of an excised pterygium, but the level of control is far from that required for refractive purposes.

Contact lens mask. By having slits in a contact lens applied directly to the cornea, ablations remain in the same position. If the eye moves, the contact lens moves and the ablated area remains located beneath the opening in the mask (see Fig. 40-18).

Fixation rings. The eye can be stabilized by a mechanical device. The simplest of these is a Thornton compression ring, as used in radial keratotomy. A suction ring, such as a Barraquer or Gelender suction ring, may also be used to stabilize the eye. The Meditec system uses a mask containing radial or transverse slits held within a circular suction ring. Hanna and Parel have designed a conical suction ring that adheres to the limbus and contains ports for blowing humidified nitrogen over the surface and for aspirating air and debris from over the surface (Fig. 40-7).

Each of these devices can be held manually or can be attached mechanically to the end of the delivery system to help keep the eye properly aligned. The mechanism of attachment to the delivery system should have some flexibility to allow observation and manipulation of the position of the eye before ablation and to take up any compressive force that might be applied when the delivery system or the patient's head is moved up and down during surgery.

Eye-tracking systems. The most elegant type of coupling system is an optical tracking system. Com-

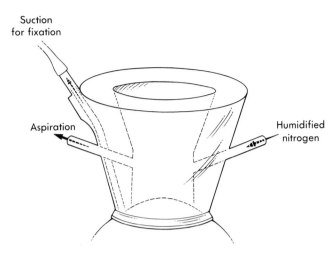

Fig. 40-7. Drawing of suction cone coupling and surface conditioning system. Suction cone adheres to conjunctival limbus and can be connected mechanically to end of delivery system. Ablated debris and air are aspirated from surface of cornea as humidified nitrogen is blown across surface. (From Waring GO: *Trans Am Ophthalmol Soc* 87:854-983, 1989.)

plex systems of eye tracking have been designed for research and military purposes and are just now being applied to laser corneal surgery. Tracking the eye in an *x-y* direction parallel to the corneal surface can be done by use of infrared lights or other methods of creating two serial images on the ocular surface or at the pupil; these images are detected, their position is related to computers, and the resulting electrical signal is used to move mirror or lenses in the delivery system so that the laser beam will always hit the desired area of the cornea. The passive tracker could control firing of the laser so that it is fired only when the eye was in an acceptable position. Confocal microscopy can be used to track the eye in the *z*-plane, perpendicular to the corneal surface. Such an eye-tracking system has been integrated with a picosecond Nd:YLF laser system by Intelligent Surgical Lasers, San Diego, California.

Environment Over Area of Ablation. Even the most homogeneous and perfectly shaped laser beam that emerges from the delivery system must still traverse the distance between the condensing lens and the surface of the tissue. Things can happen here to disrupt the beam and make it less effective.

Tissue fragments ejected from the surface may interfere with successive pulses. Even though the fragments of tissue clear the area before the next nanosecond pulse arrives, the cumulative effect of this debris falling back onto the surface of the cornea or accumulating in the trough of a linear ablation may create an irregular surface and may absorb some of the energy, disrupting the exact calculations for the amount of tissue ablated. One can decrease this problem in part by blowing or sucking gas across the surface of the cornea so that the effluent is removed and does not accumulate in the area of ablation (Fig. 40-7).

Ultraviolet excimer laser light is absorbed to some degree by particles in room air, and it is an advantage to remove this air from the delivery system and corneal surface and replace it with an inert gas such as nitrogen. However, blowing nitrogen gas across the surface will dehydrate and thin the cornea, disrupting the calculated tissue ablation. Therefore the area over the surface could be humidified, using very small water particles that will not absorb the laser beam.

Fluid on the corneal surface, whether from tears or irrigation, will also absorb the laser photons, so the surface must be kept dry during photoablation. This can be accomplished by use of an eyelid speculum to prevent blinking, by mechanical drying, and by use of grooves in a contact lens mask to wick away surface liquid.

EXCIMER LASERS

Physics of Excimer Lasers

Lasing medium. Two gases in the laser resonating chamber, an inert gas (such as argon) and a diatomic halide gas (such as fluorine), left by themselves do not interact, but under the impact of the energy from a high-powered electrical discharge, the electrons are moved to a higher energy state and the atoms become excited and form unstable molecules such as argon fluoride. When the molecules decay, they emit highly energetic photons of ultraviolet light.[14]

Within the excimer laser cavity are three gases. The first is a buffer gas, which simply mediates the transfer of energy. It is helium or neon and fills 88% to 99% of the cavity. The rare gas (argon, krypton, or xenon) constitutes 0.5% to 12% of the mixture. The halogen (fluorine or chlorine) contributes approximately 0.5% of the mixture. The combination of the rare gas and halogen gas produces photons of a specific wavelength (see Table 40-3). Modulation of the buffer gas and the addition of other gases, such as neon, affect the quality of the laser beam.

Electrical pumping. Pumping of the laser is produced by an electrical discharge, up to 5% of it being converted into laser energy. Electron beam pumping is achieved with a series of high-voltage potentials that accelerate electrons to high energies that are transmitted to the laser cavity at beam currents on the order of 100 kiloamperes. Lasing action is obtained parallel to the electrodes, perpendicular to the electric discharge path. With multiple uses, the gases deteriorate and need to be refilled frequently to maintain the high energy and the quality of the laser beam.

Optics and resonator cavity. If the gain produced by the population inversion is so large that lasing occurs without feedback between the mirrors, the laser is termed "superradiant." Excimer lasers are almost superradiant but still have a resonator configuration. The back mirror of the laser resonator cavity is completely reflective, and the front mirror has a reflectivity of about 4%, which is quite enough because of the high gain of the laser. The partial transmission of the front mirror allows the laser beam to escape in nanosecond pulses. The shape of the emergent beam is determined by stable or unstable configuration of the mirrors of the resonator cavity, as described earlier.

Effect of excimer laser on materials and tissue. The mechanism of ablative photodecomposition achieved by this laser is illustrated in Fig. 40-8. Puliafito and colleagues[40,41] used high-speed photography to chronicle the ejection of fragments from the surface (Fig. 40-9).

Excimer laser variables. Many variables control the effect of an excimer laser on the cornea; the variables in the laser include wavelength, pulse duration, pulse energy, radiant exposure (fluence), and peak power. The variables the surgeon can easily change include the pulse repetition rate, beam configuration, and the total number of pulses. The interaction between the laser and the tissue is determined by the depth of penetration of a pulse, the depth of ablation achieved by a single pulse, and the depth of the total excision of tissue. Table 40-4 lists the typical values for these variables.

Wavelength. Many ultraviolet wavelengths can be generated by excimer lasers (see Table 40-3); laboratory experiments and histopathologic studies have demonstrated that the argon fluoride laser emitting at 193 nm creates the most regular margin of excision with the least damage to residual tissue.[20,21,35,41,59] Presumably, the reason is that the shorter wavelengths have the higher photon energies and small penetration depths and achieve a more purely photochemical process of ablative pho-

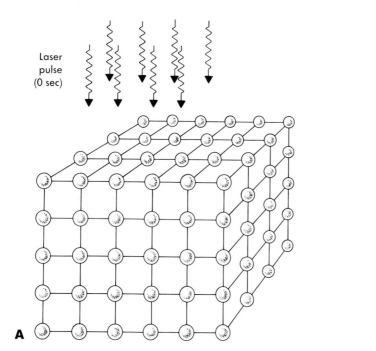

Laser
pulse
(0 sec)

A

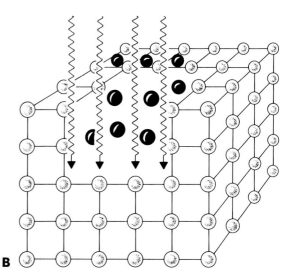

Ablative photodecomposition
(1 picosec)

B

Ejection of tissue fragments
(4 picosec)

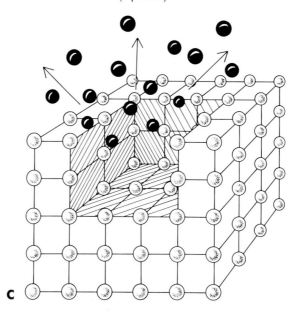

C

Fig. 40-8
For legend see opposite page.

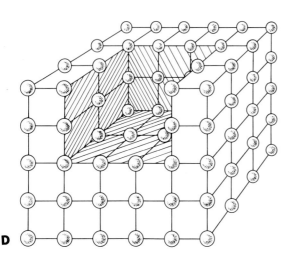

Termination of laser pulse and
tissue ablation (15 nanosec)

D

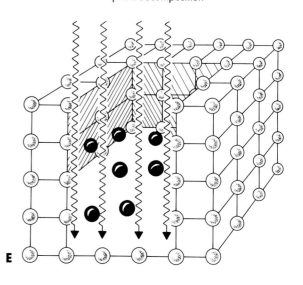

Repeated laser pulse and
photodecomposition

E

Table 40-4. Variables of Pulsed Lasers Used for Keratectomy

Variable	Dimension	Typical Values
Variables in the laser		
Wavelength	nm	200 (UV)
		3000 (IR)
		10,000 (IR)
Pulse duration	nsec	10-50
Pulse energy	mJ	200-250
Fluence or radiant energy density	mJ/cm^2	100-300
Peak power	Watts	10^8
Beam profile and spatial regularity	Percent deviation from mean	±5% to 10%
Variables adjusted by the surgeon		
Repetition rate	Hz	5-50
Total number of pulses	n	50-5000
Laser-tissue interactions		
Penetration depth	μm	1-5
Ablation depth	μm/pulse	0.1-0.5 for UV
		0.1-5.0 for IR
Excision depth	μm	20-400

Fig. 40-8. Model for ablative photodecomposition of cornea by argon fluoride (193 nm) laser ultraviolet radiation. **A,** Highly energetic (approximately 6.4 eV) ultraviolet photons head toward organic material, with intermolecular bond strength of approximately 3.5 eV. **B,** Photos break the intermolecular bonds, creating smaller molecular species, such as ^{2}H, CO, CH$_3$, H$_2$. Entire laser pulse is absorbed in approximately 0.1 to 0.5 μm of material. **C,** Because of excess energy from the photons and concentration of this energy in thin layers of material at surface, there is an intense buildup of energy and pressure that ejects the fragments off the surface at speeds approximating 1500 meters per second. The fragments leave the tissue perpendicularly and clear the surface in times of picoseconds to a few nanoseconds. **D,** Laser pulse terminates at approximately 15 nanoseconds, leaving the surface clear of effluent and allowing time for dissipation of any thermal energy that may have accumulated. **E,** Repeated laser pulses ablate successive layers of the material, requiring that the fragments travel farther to clear the surface and allowing fragments to fall back into ablated area, possibly interfering with successive pulses if they are fired at a rapid rate. (Modified from Garrison BJ and Srinivasan R: *Appl Phys Lett* 44:849-851, 1984.)

todecomposition near the surface whereas the longer wavelengths of krypton fluoride (248 nm) and xenon chloride (308 nm) have more energy dissipated in the adjacent tissue, causing thermal damage.

Specifically, Puliafito and colleagues[41] compared in human and bovine corneas the quality of the ablation achieved with argon fluoride at 193 nm and krypton fluoride at 248 nm. They found a better quality of ablation with the 193 nm laser. The zone of condensation and thermal damage was 0.1 to 0.3 μm thick with 193 nm, but it extended 2.5μm for the 248 nm. The 248 nm wavelength also created more disorganization of the residual stromal tissue. They concluded that the 193 nm excision was similar to the incision made with the diamond knife and that this was the preferred wavelength. Similar findings resulted from studies of Krueger[20] using 193 nm, 248 nm, and xenon chloride laser emitting at 308 nm. The walls of the remaining tissue at 193 nm showed only a thin layer of condensed tissue at the surface, but at 248 nm the residual tissue was irregular and vacuolated, and at 308 nm there was a wide area of cornea necrosis and coagulation, suggestive of thermal damage. Similar findings were reported by Peyman and colleagues[42] using 308 nm excimer wavelength. Indeed, the 308 nm wavelength may pass through the cornea and damage intraocular structures. Marshall and colleagues[35] demonstrated that 193 nm could create a smooth ablation surface in contrast to 248 nm, where edges and surface of

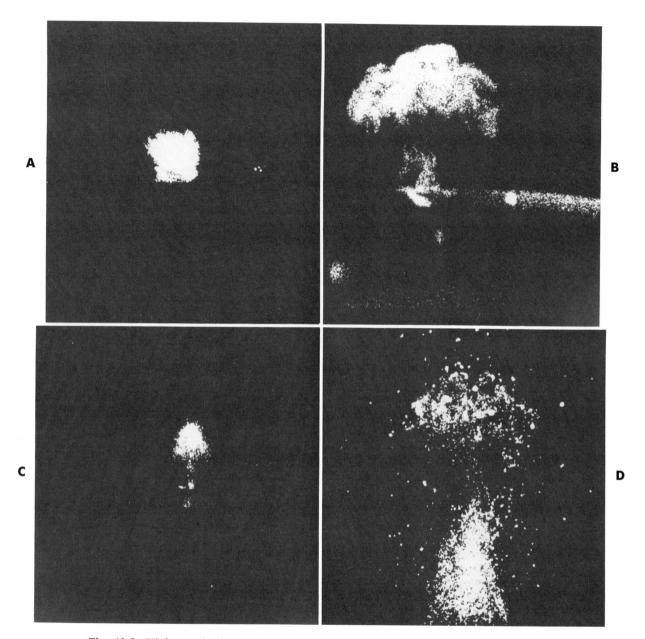

Fig. 40-9. High-speed photography of excimer laser ablation plume from cornea. Ablated fragments of tissue are leaving surface in a vertical direction at speeds of approximately 2000 meters per second. **A,** Plume from 193 nm laser approximately 5 msec after ablation shows cloud of tissue fragments immediately above surface. **B,** Plume from 193 nm laser approximately 50 msec after ablation resembles a nuclear mushroom cloud, with fragments expanding away from surface. **C,** Plume from 248 nm laser approximately 5 msec after ablation shows fragments farther from surface with expansion into a larger cloud than that seen with 193 nm. **D,** Plume from 248 nm laser approximately 150 msec after ablation shows tissue fragments leaving central cloud. Ablations with 193 nm laser were performed at 900 mJ/cm². Ablations with 248 nm laser were performed at 500 mJ/cm². (From Waring GO: *Trans Am Ophthalmol Soc* 87:854-983, 1989.)

the ablated zone were rougher with a 2 to 3 μm wide area of disruption of residual stromal tissue.

Thus the experience of all researchers seems consistent at this point: 193 nm argon fluoride lasers produce the most acceptable wounds in the cornea. As mentioned earlier, the proteins and proteoglycans of the cornea have a peak absorption at 190 nm, making the argon fluoride laser ideal. Collagen and nucleic acids have absorption at slightly higher wavelengths of 240 to 250 nm.

However, these wavelengths and their high energies impose limitations on the design of laser delivery systems. For example, excimer lasers cannot be transmitted through fiberoptic bundles, and they may damage lenses and mirrors that do not have special nonabsorbing coatings.

Pulse duration. The duration of a single excimer laser pulse depends on the short lifetime of the excited molecules—10 to 20 nanoseconds. The longer the wavelength, the shorter the pulse required to enhance the ablative action and minimize thermal effects. For example, at the 248 nm wavelength, a pulse duration as low as 300 femtoseconds can be achieved to improve the uniformity of the remaining surface.

Pulse energy. Interestingly, the total energy delivered in a single excimer laser pulse is not very great, usually a few hundred millijoules. However, because the pulses are of such short duration, a high power is achieved, more than 10 million watts. This power may produce some plasma along with the ejected tissue fragments but is far below the threshold for optical breakdown. There must be a uniform energy in each pulse so that the total ablation of the tissue can be calculated and a uniform surface can result. Using a 193 nm excimer, the fluctuation of pulse energy is on the order of 5% to 10%,[14] a level too high to obtain refractive corrections of ±0.25 D accuracy. However, when a pulse train of about 1000 pulses is used, this fluctuation averages out to less than ±0.3%.

Radiant exposure (fluence). Radiant exposure, or fluence, is a measure of the energy flux per unit area at the surface of the material ablated. It is usually expressed as millijoules per square centimeter (mJ/cm^2). An ablation curve plots the amount of tissue removed and the cornea experiences only surface photochemical changes. Tissue removal begins at the ablation threshold, which is approximately 50 mJ/cm^2 for 193

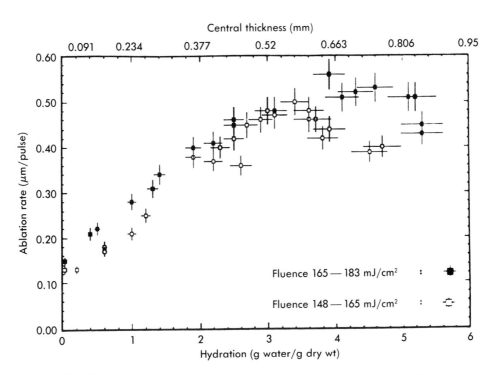

Fig. 40-10. Effective corneal hydration on ablation rate demonstrates that a pronounced effect is present below normal corneal thickness. In range of normal corneal thickness from approximately 0.50 to 0.60, ablation rate is reasonably constant. However, swollen corneas demonstrate some fall off the ablation rate, which can substantially alter number of pulses needed to remove a specific amount of tissue to effect a given refractive change. (From Waring GO: *Trans Am Ophthalmol Soc* 87:854-983, 1989.)

nm in the cornea. The curve rises slowly as the radiant exposure increases, until it reaches a level-off point, at which point it flattens at approximately 600 mJ/cm^2. After this point, increasing fluences are not associated with increased tissue ablation.[3,21,35,40,51] The ablation threshold and the inflection on the curve vary with corneas from different species.[3,34]

The rate of tissue ablation and consequently the location of the inflection point on the ablation curve vary with the hydration and thickness of the cornea (Fig. 40-10). This can be important in calculating the number of pulses used for a given refractive procedure in individuals with corneas of varying thickness and may have its greatest effect if excimer lasers are used in a therapeutic setting, such as the treatment of corneal infections or of superficial opacities, such as band keratopathy. Thus, in calibrating a laser on corneal tissue to determine its rate of ablation and the number of pulses necessary for a surgical procedure, one must dehydrate the cornea to a normal thickness.

As the radiant exposure increases, an optimal fluence is reached where, for a minimum exposure, tissue is most effectively removed. The exact location of this point is not known, though most studies have been done between 150 and 250 mJ/cm^2.[3,20,45,56] This is in the middle of the steepest part of the curve, but the value has been commonly derived from experiments on enucleated eyes, which may have been swollen. At this fluence, the laser ablates approximately 0.45 μm of tissue per pulse. It is difficult to work on this ascending part of the ablation curve at values of approximately 200 mJ/cm^2 because small differences in the energy density will create significant differences in the amount of tissue removed. Therefore, the beam must have a homogeneous energy profile and there must be uniform energy delivered from pulse to pulse. Variations in these factors will produce a rougher surface. On the other hand, working at higher fluences of 600 mJ/cm^2 or above may obviate this problem because in this flat part of the curve, the same amount of tissue is removed regardless of the energy density, and so the technical demand for a homogeneous beam and a uniform pulse is not as great as those at lower fluences[18,38] (Fig. 40-11).

The fact that the amount of tissue removed can be precisely determined for a single pulse at a given fluence is the basis for the exquisite accuracy and precision promised by excimer lasers for photorefractive keratectomy. However, accuracy may change under different surface conditions, such as humidity, or different degrees of corneal hydration—losing, therefore, the precision in excision depth.

Homogeneity of the laser beam and uniformity of the ablated surface. Beam uniformity is important because the energy profile of the beam is projected onto the surface of the cornea, leaving its "fingerprint" (Fig. 40-11). For example, if the beam has more energy concentrated in the center, the ablated area will have a central depression, whereas a beam with more energy concentrated at the periphery will create a doughnut configuration in the tissue. Because one of the goals of photorefractive keratectomy is to create as smooth a surface as possible, it is desirable to have as homogeneous a beam as possible. The laser beam at 193 nm is not homogeneous when it emerges from the resonating cavity, since its energy density is greater in the center. The beam does not have a defined mode structure and is therefore characterized only as a profile of energy density transversely and longitudinally. The beam profiles can change between pulses and have a tendency to become less uniform as the gases in the active medium become degraded.

There are few commercially available instruments to measure the energy distribution in the excimer laser beam. This is an extremely important variable, however, because the contour of the beam is imprinted on the tissue and the more irregular the beam, the more irregular the surface of the ablated cornea. Increasingly, manufacturers of delivery systems for excimer lasers are including methods to present a profile of the beam homogeneity to the user.

Another way to visualize the creation of a smooth surface is to use an immersion fluid to create a smooth surface.[7] The beam will remove from an irregular surface an equal amount of tissue over the exposed surface so that the high points and low points will be ablated at the same rate and the original surface contour will persist (Fig. 40-12). The fluid protects the low points of the surface from photoablation, which takes place only at the tissue elevated from the "sea," or fluid level. Thus a leveling process starts during photoablation leading to a smooth surface. Seiler and colleagues have used this method since 1986 to smooth the corneal surface after pterygium surgery, putting methyl cellulose on the surface to fill in the depressions and then ablating the entire surface with a 193 nm excimer laser beam.

Pulse repetition rate. The rate of delivery of the laser pulses to the cornea is measured as the number of pulses per second, expressed in hertz (Hz). Ideally, laser corneal surgery should be completed as rapidly as possible to decrease the chances of patient movement. Therefore a higher repetition rate is most desirable. There are definite limitations, how-

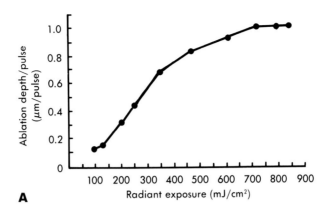

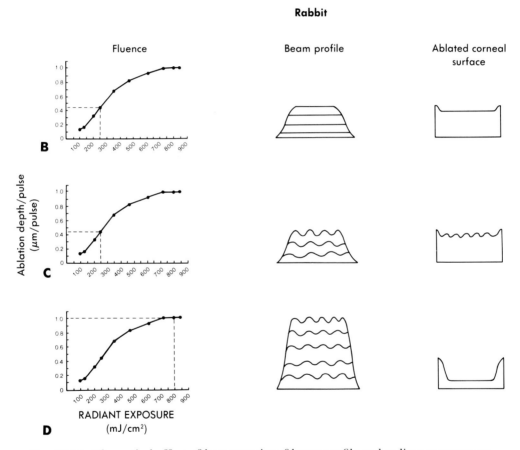

Fig. 40-11. Theoretical effect of homogeneity of beam profile and radiant exposure on rabbit cornea. **A,** Ablative curve for 193 nm excimer laser ablation of cornea in living rabbits with epithelium intact. Ablation threshold could not be determined in this system, but there was a gradual increase in ablation depth per pulse with increasing radiant exposure up to approximately 700 mJ/cm², where a plateau occurred. **B,** A homogeneous beam profile at a fluence of 250 mJ/cm² will give a smooth ablated corneal surface. **C,** An inhomogeneous beam with variable pulse energy at 250 mJ/cm² will give an irregular surface because the ablation depth per pulse is greatly influenced by radiant exposure. **D,** Working higher fluences on order of 700 to 800 mJ/cm² creates a smooth surface despite inhomogeneities and variable pulse energy because amount of tissue removed with each pulse does not depend on radiant exposure at this level. (From Fantes FE, Waring GO: *Lasers Surg Med* 9:533-542, 1989.)

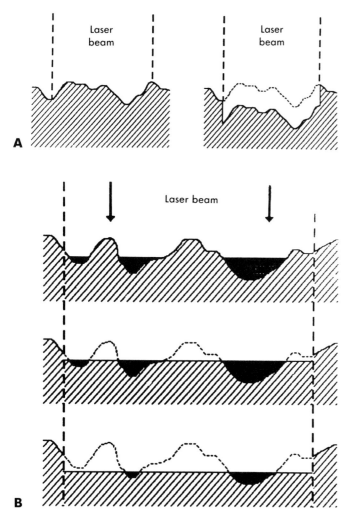

Fig. 40-12. Effect of surface contour on pattern of ablation with a homogeneous excimer laser beam. **A,** As laser beam encounters an irregular surface, it ablates an equal amount of tissue from the high points and low points of surface so that original contour of surface remains. **B,** By application of a fluid to surface to fill in depressions, the elevations will be preferentially ablated, and as fluid is also ablated and removed from surface, it is possible to convert an irregular surface to a smooth one. Seiler and colleagues have used this method to smooth the corneal surface after pterygium surgery, putting methyl cellulose on the surface to fill in depressions and then ablating entire surface with a 193 nm excimer laser beam.

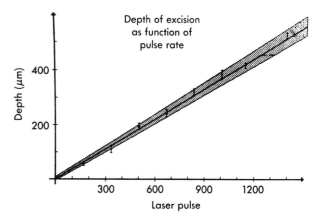

Fig. 40-13. Graph demonstrates that depth of excision of corneal tissue in microns is proportionate to number of 193 nm excimer laser pulses. *y*-Axis indicates depth in micrometers; *x*-axis indicates number of laser pulses. Points with error bars indicate actual data from human eye bank eyes. *Line,* Best-fit curve: *shaded area,* zone encompassing one standard deviation around line of best fit. (From Seiler T, Wollensak J: *Ophthalmologica* 192:65-70, 1986.)

ever, to the use of higher repetition rates (>60 Hz) with excimer lasers because the rapid sequence of pulses creates a thermal effect in the tissue and damages the optical components of the delivery system. In addition, the consistency of the pulse energy and beam profile may decline at higher rates.[49]

Currently, repetition rates from 5 to 15 Hz are being used,[11,12,35,37,41,59] the most common being around 10 Hz.

Number of pulses. The most important factor the surgeon controls is the number of pulses because this determines the amount of tissue removed. Potentially, this allows the surgeon to make a radial or transverse linear excision of an exact known depth, uniform from end to end, or perform photorefractive keratectomy by ablating a profile on the cornea of exact contour. The surgeon would compute the overall excision depth before surgery by multiplying the ablation depth per pulse times the total number of pulses. For example, if the surgeon wants to excise 100 μm of the cornea at 0.45 μm per pulse, a value of 222 pulses (100 × 0.45) would be entered into the operation terminal of the laser before surgery (Fig. 40-13). In another example, limiting excision depth to 40 μm during photorefractive keratectomy (ablation rate 0.3) means that only 40 ÷ 0.3 = 133 pulses may be applied. This limits too the number of steps of the iris diaphragm.

The simplicity of these data is confounded by several problems. First, the consistency of the pulse energy and the spatial uniformity of the beam profile vary 5% to 10%, creating some inherent irregularity of the surface. Second, different tissues are ablated at different rates; the epithelium faster than Bowman's membrane for example. This would have been taken into consideration in preoperative calculations for the amount of tissue removed. Third, laser keratomileusis requires removal of different amounts of tissue in different areas of the cornea to create a new optical profile, and this presents a chal-

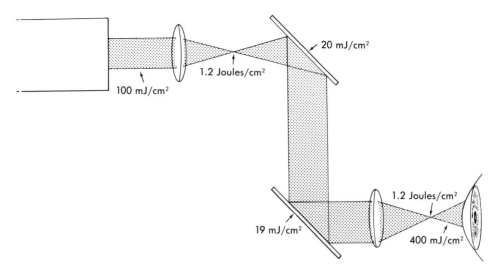

Fig. 40-14. General depiction of elements of excimer laser delivery system. Cylindric and spheric lenses can shape the beam, and mirrors can direct the beam. In general, optical elements should be placed at a distance from focal point where energy density is high to decrease damage caused by laser beam. Not depicted are other elements of a delivery system, such as mask to shape beam, prisms or mirrors that homogenize beam, and detectors that measure beam. (From Waring GO: *Trans Am Ophthalmol Soc* 87:854-983, 1989.)

lenge in the design of the delivery system. Fourth, changes in conditions during the surgery, such as movement of the eye, variation in corneal thickness from changes in hydration, and contamination of the surface with fluid, make the exact determination of the amount of tissue removed more difficult.

Excimer Laser Delivery Systems. Between the time the laser beam emerges from the resonating cavity and the time it strikes the surface of the cornea, it must be directed, homogenized, and shaped by a delivery system. In general, the delivery systems required for excimer lasers are more complex than those needed for the more familiar continuous-wave argon or pulsed Nd:YAG lasers. This requires a combination of lenses, mirrors, masks, homogenizers, motors, computers, and detectors—all assembled in a clinically useful device that must be simple to use, versatile, and able to withstand the impact of the excimer beam itself (Fig. 40-14).[12,57] Numerous experimental and commercial delivery systems are in development (Fig. 40-15).

Optical elements. The high-energy excimer laser will easily damage conventional lenses, mirrors, and prisms, even if made of quartz. To solve this problem, the optics should be coated with magnesium fluoride or calcium fluoride because of their strong ionic bond. In addition, the beam can be optically expanded so that the energy density is less at the optical interface, and then it is refocused by an objec-

tive lens at the end of the system. At every optical interface, some of the energy is lost, and so the more complex the delivery system and the less efficient its components, the more powerful is the laser required to deliver a beam of useful energy to the cornea, especially if there is a need to work at higher fluences along the upper part of the ablation curve.

Control of beam uniformity. The energy profile of the beam as it is emitted from the laser must be maintained or improved as it travels through the delivery system to present the best possible quality beam to the tissue. All optical elements must have smooth, nondegraded surfaces so that they do not disrupt the beam. Masking the peripheral part of the beam and using only its more homogeneous central part will enhance uniformity (Fig. 40-16). Using rotating prisms or lenses and spatial beam integrators can make the beam more homogeneous.

The beam homogenization is important because areas of higher and lower energy within the beam (hot spots and cold spots) will produce an irregular surface on the cornea. If portions of the beam are folded back into the beam by prisms, the hot spots and cold spots cancel each other out, producing a more homogeneous beam.

Shaping the beam for refractive ablation. The shape of the ablated area on the cornea is determined by the shape of the beam that strikes the cornea. The ideal shape is selected based on the

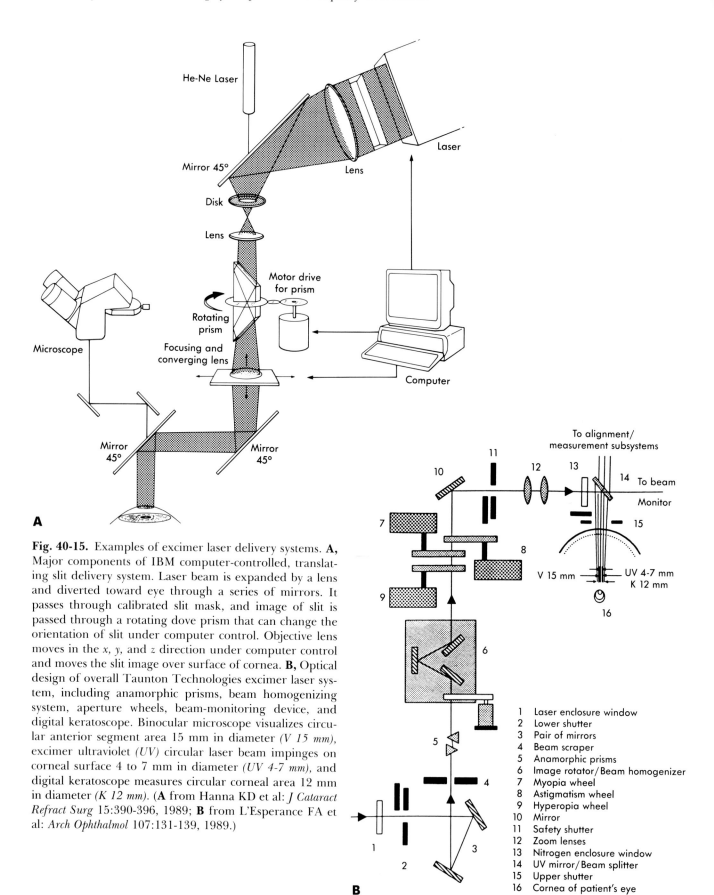

Fig. 40-15. Examples of excimer laser delivery systems. **A,** Major components of IBM computer-controlled, translating slit delivery system. Laser beam is expanded by a lens and diverted toward eye through a series of mirrors. It passes through calibrated slit mask, and image of slit is passed through a rotating dove prism that can change the orientation of slit under computer control. Objective lens moves in the *x, y,* and *z* direction under computer control and moves the slit image over surface of cornea. **B,** Optical design of overall Taunton Technologies excimer laser system, including anamorphic prisms, beam homogenizing system, aperture wheels, beam-monitoring device, and digital keratoscope. Binocular microscope visualizes circular anterior segment area 15 mm in diameter *(V 15 mm),* excimer ultraviolet *(UV)* circular laser beam impinges on corneal surface 4 to 7 mm in diameter *(UV 4-7 mm),* and digital keratoscope measures circular corneal area 12 mm in diameter *(K 12 mm).* (**A** from Hanna KD et al: *J Cataract Refract Surg* 15:390-396, 1989; **B** from L'Esperance FA et al: *Arch Ophthalmol* 107:131-139, 1989.)

1 Laser enclosure window
2 Lower shutter
3 Pair of mirrors
4 Beam scraper
5 Anamorphic prisms
6 Image rotator/Beam homogenizer
7 Myopia wheel
8 Astigmatism wheel
9 Hyperopia wheel
10 Mirror
11 Safety shutter
12 Zoom lenses
13 Nitrogen enclosure window
14 UV mirror/Beam splitter
15 Upper shutter
16 Cornea of patient's eye

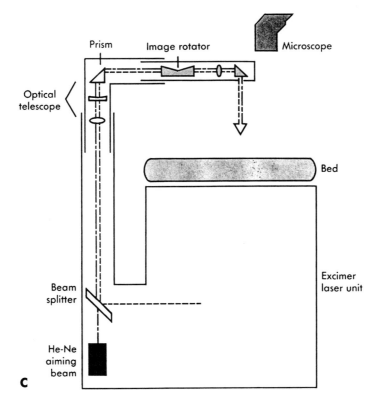

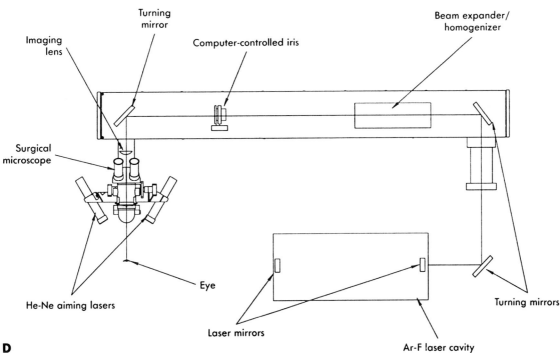

Fig. 40-15, cont'd. C, A basic design of Meditec excimer laser system. System consists of excimer laser unit and helium-neon laser aiming beam located in bed beneath patient. Delivery system consists of a beam splitter and optical telescope that transmits laser beam to image rotator, which orients beam on eye. A final focusing lens and prism transmit image to eye, as viewed by an operation microscope. **D,** Summit Technology UV 200 Optical Delivery System. Excimer laser resonating cavity is shown below with its two mirrors. Beam enters optical "rail" that is filled with nitrogen to decrease interaction of beam with air. Rectangular shape of beam is made square by beam expander, and computer-controlled iris determines diameter of circle of beam that impinges on cornea. Helium-neon aiming lasers are used to focus instrument before corneal ablation, which is observed through surgical microscope. (**C,** Courtesy Aesculap-Meditech, Heroldsberg, Germany; **D,** courtesy Summit Technology, Watertown, Mass.)

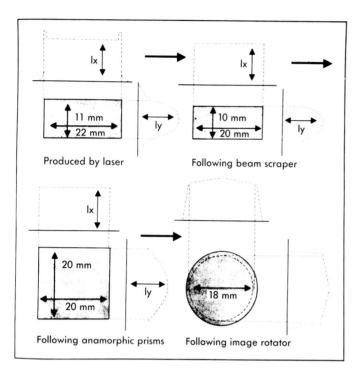

Fig. 40-16. Cross section of excimer laser beam intensity distribution as it emerges from laser *(top left)* and after edges of beam are scraped away *(top right)*, which may contain irregular and high-intensity energy areas. Anamorphic prisms convert rectangular beam into square beam *(bottom left)*, which is then homogenized by image rotator into axisymmetric intensity distribution *(bottom right)*. (From L'Esperance FA et al: *Arch Ophthalmol* 107:131-139, 1989.)

ametropia to be corrected and the refractive surgical technique used.[61] A linear slit is used for radial and transverse linear keratectomy.

Two methods are available to shape the beam: masks and lenses. The principle of using a mask is to create an aperture that will ablate a desired configuration and profile on the cornea (Fig. 40-17). Lenses project a beam of desired configuration on the cornea.

Any moving mask system, whether slit diaphragm or disc, will require control of the rate of movement to govern the number of pulses that strike the cornea in a given area and to ensure an accurate ablation profile. This requires accurate mathematic calculations that take into account the configuration of the aperture in the mask, the rate of movement of the aperture over the surface of the cornea, the repetition rate of the laser, and the ablation per pulse.

STATIONARY SLIT MASKS. The simplest method of shaping the beam is a rectangular narrow slit to make a linear radial keratectomy to correct myopia

or a linear transverse or arcuate excision to correct astigmatism. If enough energy is available, four or eight radial slits could be irradiated at the same time to make simultaneous radial excisions, but this would waste a lot of energy impacting the areas between the slits in the mask. Therefore a cylindrical lens can be used to shape the beam into a narrow rectangle that is then imaged onto one slit aperture in the mask, so that each of the four or eight slits is irradiated in turn.

Seiler and colleagues[45] have used a PMMA contact lens with slits cut in it as a mask placed directly on the surface of the cornea, the slits being oriented in the desired direction of ablation. Two important modifications of the contact lens allow use with the excimer laser. The first is coating the anterior surface with a metal foil film that blocks the transmission of the beam in all areas except the slit. The second is to carve out a recess on the back of the lens in the area of the slit that pulls fluid and tears away from the slit area by surface tension, decreasing the amount of fluid present to absorb and quench the laser beam (Fig. 40-18). This method has been used particularly in making transverse incisions for the correction of astigmatism, as described later.

A slit mask can also be incorporated into a suction ring and suspended over the surface of the cornea, as done in the Meditec.

MOVING SLIT. For photorefractive keratectomy a slit image can move over the surface of the cornea, either rotating around the center or translating across the surface. The rotating slit is not ideal because the center ablation is not always smooth, and it is difficult to keep the eye aligned exactly in the center during ablation. The shape of the slit can be designed to correct a variety of ametropias. A slit wider near its central portion would ablate more tissue from the central cornea; one wider near its outer portion would ablate more of the paracentral cornea and correct hyperopia. One could correct astigmatism by varying the rate of movement of the slit so that one meridian was exposed to more pulses than another or by passing the slit more frequently over one meridian than the other. A moving slit system has been described by Hanna and colleagues[11-13] in the IBM system (see Fig. 40-14, *A*). Its disadvantages include long operation time (up to 8 minutes) and absolute stabilization of the eye.

DIAPHRAGM MASK. For myopic photorefractive keratectomy a circular mask can be used. Obviously, if a simple disc-shaped mask is used, a circular depression with steep edges will appear without useful refractive effect. However, if a slowly constricting or dilating diaphragm is used to ablate a fixed circular

Excimer Laser Mask Systems

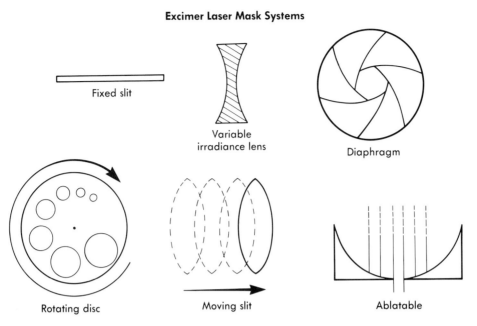

Fig. 40-17. Types of masks to shape excimer laser beam. Slit mask makes an elongated beam for radial or transverse keratectomy. A variable irradiance lens can distribute energy over corneal surface in desired patterns. Diaphragm can expand or contract for myopic correction. Disc with multiple apertures rotates to create successively smaller or larger ablation zones. Movable slit that is wider in the middle creates myopic correction. Ablatable mask is shape of desired tissue to be removed; as mask ablates, beam passes through to ablate tissue.

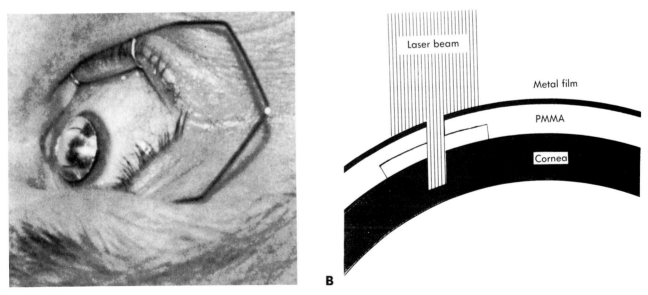

Fig. 40-18. Contact lens mask for transverse linear keratectomy. **A,** Foil-coated contact lens is placed on surface of patient's cornea, and rectangular laser beam is aligned with slit aperture in mask. Slit is 0.12 mm wide and 3.5 to 5.0 mm long. **B,** Drawing of modifications of PMMA contact lens shows surface coat of metal film that blocks part of laser beam, with slit in contact lens allowing transmission of laser beam and groove in back of contact lens to pull fluid away from corneal surface in area of slit by surface tension.

area of the central cornea (for example, 5 mm in diameter), the outer portion of the ablation will be shallower than the continuously exposed inner portion. The profile of this ablation is controlled by the rate of movement of the diaphragm and the number of pulses delivered. This creates a minus lens effect on the surface of the cornea to treat myopia. The diaphragm can be controlled mechanically and linked to a feedback system for fine control. This approach has been used in the VISX and Summit excimer laser systems.[37]

Advantages of the diaphragm are its relative simplicity and ease of centration. Another advantage is the rapid rate at which an area ablation can be accomplished—less than 30 seconds. Disadvantages include the limitation of treating only myopia. In addition, the central cornea is exposed to all pulses, possibly elevating the temperature there and requiring that the ejected fragments be removed from the surface by suction or blowing air. The diaphragm steps are etched on the corneal surface, creating some irregularity; the more the steps, the smoother is the surface (Fig. 40-19).

MULTIPLE DISC MASKS. Another type of mask delivery system uses different-sized apertures in a single circular disc. A sequence of circular apertures, from large (7 mm diameter) down to small (1 mm diameter) can be used to make a series of progressively constricting, stepped excisions of tissue by first exposing the large mask, then the next smallest, and so on. This creates a negative lens effect to correct myopia (Fig. 40-20). A similar approach can be used to correct hyperopia, using a translucent glass to mask the central unablated zone. A sequence of slits of different orientation could be used to create linear keratectomies. This system is used by Taunton Technologies (Monroe, Connecticut).[23,24]

OPTICAL SHAPING OF BEAM. Several optical methods can shape the beam. Spherical lenses that focus graded amounts of the laser beam across the optical zone can be fashioned to correct myopia and hyperopia, an approach currently under development in the Russian Federation. A cylindric lens in the delivery system creates a linear beam configuration that ablates radial or transverse linear keratectomies in the cornea. This is one of the earliest methods used to test the different effect of wavelengths of excimer lasers.[41] A properly graded cylindric lens probably can create an astigmatic correction.

Spherical lenses that transmit different amounts of energy in different areas of the lens can be used to modify the energy distribution over the surface of the cornea. This variable irradiance through an optical system can be achieved by a gas cell filter or by use of lenses that absorb ultraviolet radiation selectively. Thus a lens thinner in the middle and thicker in the periphery will transmit more laser energy in the central portion than the periphery, creating a myopic correction on the cornea.

An axicon lens can be used to create a circular pattern. The axicon lenses are coin-shaped, and refract the laser light from the original central axis out to the edge of the ring-shaped lens, projecting a circle onto the cornea. This system has been used by

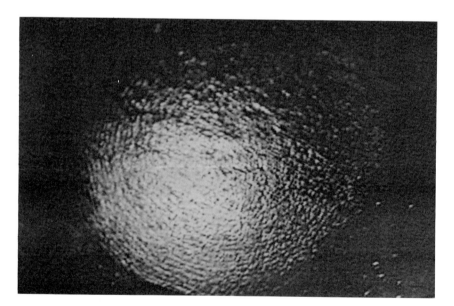

Fig. 40-19. Photograph of surface of rabbit eye after ablation using a dilating diaphragm shows multiple small concentric ridges indicating steps as diaphragm opens.

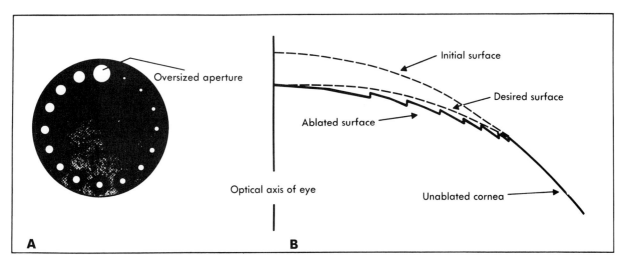

Fig. 40-20. Taunton laser mask system. **A,** Aperture wheel that allows laser beam to ablate central cornea more deeply than peripheral cornea to flatten anterior surface curvature and increase anterior corneal surface radius of curvature, thereby reducing myopia. **B,** Exaggerated representation of stepped profile ablation of cornea to reduce myopia. (From L'Esperance FA et al: *Arch Ophthalmol* 107:131-139, 1989.)

Loertscher and colleagues[26-29] for circular corneal trephination (Fig. 40-21). This system could be modified to create two parallel surfaces that would image two transverse slits simultaneously for the correction of astigmatism.

Properly coated optical systems transmit more energy than masks that block considerable areas of the laser. If the beam is optically shaped to conform to the size of the mask aperture, less energy is wasted on the edge of the mask.

Delivery of the beam to the eye. Final focusing lenses are necessary to collect the expanded, homogenized, and shaped beam for delivery to the eye. The energy density at the surface of the cornea will be determined largely by the distance between the focal point of the objective lens and the corneal surface.

The excimer laser beam may be aimed parallel rather than perpendicular to the corneal surface to fashion a tangential cut and to excise a lenticule.[10] The tangential method may create clearer corneas with less damage to the endothelium in rabbit eyes.

Measuring the beam. All the processes that modify the beam affect its energy profile. The surgeon needs the confidence that the pulse impinging on the cornea meets the calculated specifications. This requires detectors built into the system that can measure the final pulse energy, homogeneity, and shape (Fig. 40-22). Ideally, this detecting system would be linked to a computer-controlled feedback mechanism that could modulate both the output from the

laser and the beam management in the delivery system to ensure that each pulse meets exact specifications.

EXCIMER LASER INTERACTIONS WITH THE CORNEA

Ablative Photodecomposition. The atomic and molecular events that occur when a pulse of excimer laser light strikes the cornea and the effects of different wavelengths of excimer lasers on the cornea are discussed in the preceding sections. The essential feature of this process is the ability of an argon fluoride (193 nm) excimer laser to remove a few molecular layers or portions of a single cell with each pulse, the total amount of tissue removed being determined by the pulse energy, the number of pulses, and the radiant exposure at the surface of the cornea.

Ablation of Corneal Epithelium and Stroma. Different corneal tissues ablate at different rates, and so the amount of tissue removed with each pulse varies. This is important in calculating the rate and amount of tissue removal to create an exact refractive change. Topical medications, both in the tears and absorbed into the stroma, theoretically can act as a dopant and change the ablation rates of corneal tissue. We have investigated the ablation rate of gels doped with cocaine, oxybuprocaine, proxymetacaine, and pilocarpine and found no change in ablation rates, though with fluorescein the ablation rate decreased from 0.30 to 0.18 µm/pulse.[19]

The corneal epithelium is an inhomogeneous structure and ablates at a faster rate than the corneal stroma. In a human donor eye model, the epithelium ablated at a rate of 0.68 ± 0.15 μm/pulse, whereas the stroma ablated at a rate of 0.55 ± 0.1 μm/pulse.[46] Within the epithelium the nuclei are more resistant than the cytoplasm to ablation (Fig. 40-23). The irregular ablation of the multilayered epithelium could created an irregular surface on the stroma, and so the epithelium is simply mechanically scraped off before the ablation and calculations do not have to take the effect of the epithelium into account.

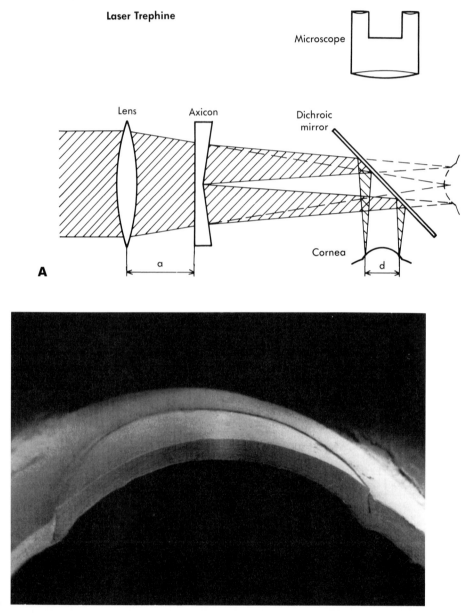

Fig. 40-21. Axicon lens used for circular trephination with a hydrogen fluoride laser. **A,** Optical setup for use of an axicon lens creates a circular pattern for corneal trephination. Diameter of annulus, *d*, can be varied by adjustment of distance between axicon and lens, *a*. Cornea is observed with a microscope. **B,** Scanning electron microscopic cross-sectional view of an eye bank cornea after trephination shows asymmetric depths, approximately 90% of corneal thickness at 11 o'clock and 50% at 5 o'clock. Walls of trephination are parallel. (From Loertscher H, Mandelbaum S, Parel J-M, and Parrish RK: *Am J Ophthalmol* 104:471-475, 1987.)

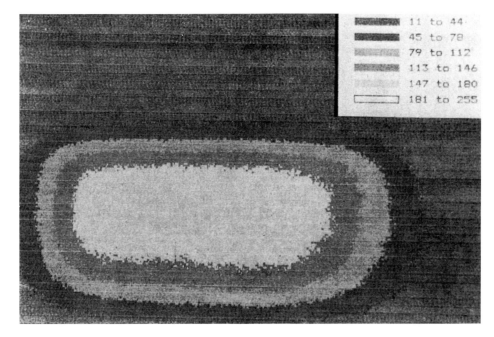

Fig. 40-22. Profile of laser beam energy emerging from laser shows greater concentration of energy in center and less at periphery of rectangular beam, as indicated in gray scale of photograph (mJ/cm^2). (Courtesy Questek, Inc., Billerica, Mass.)

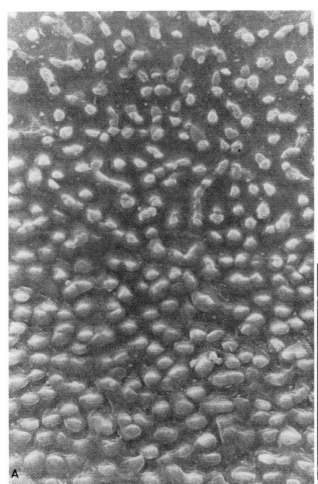

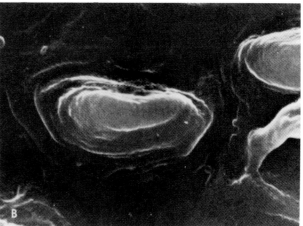

Fig. 40-23. Scanning electron micrographs of ablated corneal epithelium in a human eye bank eye. **A,** Photograph at junction of more sparsely spaced polygonal cells *(above)* and more compact basal cells *(below)* demonstrates nuclei protruding from surface of surrounding cytoplasm (500×). **B,** Higher power view demonstrates single nucleus with sloping ablated margins rising above cytoplasm (20,000×). (Courtesy Gilles Renard, M.D., Paris.)

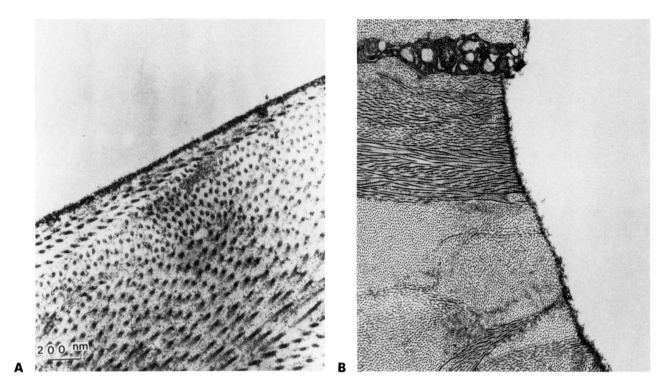

Fig. 40-24. Effect of different radiant exposures on surface of ablated area in human corneal stroma as examined by transmission electron microscopy. **A,** Exposure at 205 mJ/cm². **B,** Exposure at 205 mJ/cm². Higher magnification reveals residual surface condensate approximately 0.04 μm thick with essentially no disruption of underlying collagen stromal architecture (9100×).

Bowman's layer ablates slower than the stroma. In a human donor eye model, the ablation rate was 0.38 ± 0.05 μm/pulse compared with the stromal rate of 0.55 ± 0.1 μm/pulse at a radiant exposure of 2.5 mJ/cm².[46] This difference in ablation rate by a factor of 1.45 between stroma and Bowman's layer may create a difference in the calculations for photorefractive keratectomy.

Electron microscopic studies of the surfaces and edges of corneal stroma ablated at 193 nm, emphasizes three important findings (Fig 40-24). First, the surface is generally smooth but contains focal irregularities that result from inhomogeneities of the beam and surface irregularities of the tissue that are carried forward as "shadows" during the ablation process. The second observation is the frequent appearance on transmission electronmicroscopy of a layer of condensed material on the surface, sometimes called "pseudomembrane." This tissue is approximately 0.02 to 0.05 μm thick and has a very smooth surface. Its composition is unknown. Presumedly it results from thermal effects at the surface. This condensed matter is less permeable to wa-

ter than normal stroma and can decrease stromal swelling. It may also provide a smooth surface over which epithelial cells can migrate, with the usual layer of fibronectin appearing in front of them. The third finding of electronmicroscopic studies is the general lack of disruption of remaining tissue. Beneath the pseudomembrane, a layer of slightly condensed and disrupted tissue, approximately 1 μm thick, is present in some areas, but beyond that disruption the tissue retains its normal ultrastructural configuration.

The clinical meaning of these three observations is being determined by continued investigation. One of the tacit assumptions of excimer laser corneal surgery is that a generally smooth surface, with minimal underlying tissue disruption, will allow rapid normal epithelial wound healing and will stimulate little or no stromal fibrosis and scarring. Unfortunately, biologic reality is not so simple; clinical and histopathologic reports in monkeys and human beings demonstrate a wide spectrum of tissue responses after excimer laser corneal surgery, especially photorefractive keratectomy. Epithelial hyperplasia and subepithelial scaring have occurred frequently, but technical refinements may be able to reduce their frequency and severity.[24,32]

Thermal Effects. The cornea is a temperature-sensitive tissue, and corneal collagen extracts denature at approximately 40° C.

The time for heat diffusion in the cornea is on the order of 1 second, and so heat accumulates when repetition rates higher than 1Hz are used. To shorten the time required for a surgical procedure, repetition rates of 5 to 20 Hz are commonly used, and so temperature increases adjacent to the area of ablation do occur. The gaseous mixture formed by the ablation process has a temperature of more than 1000° C, but most of this heat is dissipated as the fragments are ejected from the surface. The highest residual temperature is at the boundaries of the ablated tissue, and it declines logarithmically as the dis-

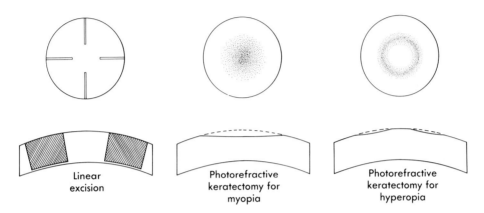

Linear
excision

Photorefractive
keratectomy for
myopia

Photorefractive
keratectomy for
hyperopia

Fig. 40-25. Two basic types of laser keratectomy. Linear excesions can be done radially for myopia, transversely for astigmatism, or circularly for corneal trephination. Photorefractive keratectomy (anterior keratomileusis) can be done to correct myopia, hyperopia, and, potentially, astigmatism. (From Waring GO: *Trans Am Ophthalmol Soc* 87:854-983, 1989.)

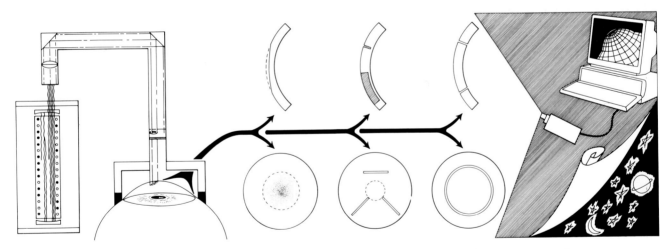

Fig. 40-26. Scope of laser corneal surgery is illustrated by composite montage, read from left to right. Appropriate laser passes through an effective delivery system that is coupled to eye. Interaction of laser with corneal tissue sets stage for wound healing. Patterns include photorefractive keratectomy (surface-area ablation) for all ametropias, transverse linear keratectomy for astigmatism, radial keratectomy for myopia, and circular trephination for corneal transplantation. Measurement of topography and thickness of cornea allows computation of effect of refractive surgery and, with biomechanical data, computer simulation of surgery. The future is bright but, like the exploration of space, fraught with technical challenges and the unknown. (From Waring GO: *Trans Am Ophthalmol Soc* 87:854-983, 1989.)

tance from the edge decreases. Seiler has measured a maximal temperature rise in the corneal tissue of 11 Celsius degrees adjacent to the trough, with a half value distance of 650 μm. This the temperature at the edge of the ablation rises to approximately 45° C and, at a distance of 650 μm, it rises to approximately 40° C. On this basis, one would expect collagen denaturation, but the only evidence of thermal damage is the surface condensate (pseudomembrane) and slight disruption of tissue at a distance of 1 μm. Thus clinical experience demonstrates that most of the heat energy is dissipated into the air, away from the tissues.

Mutagenesis Induced by Excimer Lasers. Ultraviolet light is absorbed by DNA and therefore may have a mutagenic and carcinogenic effect on the rapidly multiplying corneal epithelium. The less active stromal fibroblasts are at less risk. It is well known that excimer laser radiation between 248 and 308 nm is mutagenic. The best experimental evidence shows that 193 nm radiation is not mutagenic.[36]

Excimer Laser Keratectomy. Two basic types of corneal laser surgery have been described (Fig. 40-25): linear excisions, either radial to correct myopia, transverse to correct astigmatism,[2,12,37,45,57] or curcular trephination for corneal transplantation.[26] Photorefractive keratectomy (anterior keratomileusis, large-area ablation) can be done to correct myopia, hyperopia, and astigmatism,[38] and superficial keratectomy can be done to remove corneal scars and to smooth an irregular corneal surface.[26]

The scope of laser corneal surgery is illustrated in the montage of Fig. 40-26, which emphasizes the technical demands of the laser, the delivery system, and the coupling system as well as the variety of types of surgery that can be done with the laser. Whether the excimer laser itself will remain the primary surgical tool or other, less cumbersome, less expensive, and more user-friendly lasers will be developed requires future research. Measurement of the topography and optics of the cornea after photorefractive keratectomy is an essential feature of the study of this new technology, which is certainly opening windows to the future.

REFERENCES

1. Absten GT, Joffe SN: *Lasers in medicine,* New York, 1985, Chapman Co.
2. Aron-Rosa DS, Boerner CF, Bath P, et al: Corneal wound healing after laser keratotomy in a human eye, *Am J Ophthalmol* 103:444-464, 1987.
3. Aron-Rosa DS, Boulnoy JL, Carre F, et al: Excimer laser surgery of the cornea: qualitative and quantitative aspects of photoablation according to the energy density, *J Cataract Refract Surg* 12:27-33, 1986.
4. Beaver GH, Holiday ER: Ultraviolet absorption spectrum of protein and aminoacids, *Adv Protein Chem* 7:319-386, 1952.
5. Beckman H, Rota A, Barraco R: Limbectomies, keratectomies, and keratotomies performed with a rapid-pulse carbon dioxide laser, *Am J Ophthalmol* 71:1277-1283, 1971.
6. Bende T, Kriegerowski M, Seiler T: Photoablation in different ocular tissues performed with an erbium:YAG laser, *Laser Light Ophthalmol* 2:263-269, 1989.
7. Berlin M, Bende T, Seiler T: Corneal resurfacing by excimer laser photocoagulation, *Invest Ophthalmol Vis Sci* 29(suppl):310, 1988.
8. Dyer PE, Srinivasan R: Nanosecond photoacoustic studies on ultraviolet laser ablation of organic polymers, *Appl Phys Lett* 48:445-447, 1986.
9. Fine BS, Fine S, Peacock GR, et al: Preliminary observations on ocular effects of high power, continuous CO₂ laser irradiation, *Am J Ophthalmol* 2:209-222, 1967.
10. Fouraker BD, Holme RJ, Schanzlin DJ: A comparison of en face and tangential wide-area excimer surface ablation in the rabbit, *Invest Ophthalmol Vis Sci* 31(suppl):476, 1990.
11. Hanna K, Chastang JC, Pouliquen Y, et al: A rotating slit delivery system for excimer laser refractive keratoplasty, *Am J Ophthalmol* 103:474, 1987.
12. Hanna K, Chastang JC, Pouliquen Y, et al: Excimer laser keratectomy for myopia with a rotating slit delivery system, *Arch Ophthalmol* 106:245-250, 1988.
13. Hanna KD, Chastang JC, Asfar L, et al: Scanning slit delivery system, *J Cataract Refract Surg* 15:390-396, 1989.
14. Hecht J: Excimer laser update, *Lasers Applications* 12:43-48, 1983.
15. Keates RH, Pedrotti L, Welchel H, et al: Carbon dioxide laser beam control for corneal surgery, *Ophthalmic Surg* 12:117-122, 1981.
16. Keyes T, Clarke RH: Theory of photoablation and its implication for laser phototherapy, *J Chem Phys* 89:4194-4196, 1985.
17. Koch JW, Lang GK, Naumann GOH: Endothelial reaction to perforating and non-perforating excimer laser excisions in rabbits, *Refract Corneal Surg* 7(3):214-222, 1991.
18. Krauss JM, Puliafito CA, Steinert R: Laser interactions with the cornea, *Surv Ophthalmol* 31:37-53, 1986.
19. Kriegerowski M, Bende T, Seiler T: Do eye drops influence ablation rate during laser keratomileusis? *Invest Ophthalmol Vis Sci* 31:478, 1990.
20. Krueger RR, Trokel SL: Quantitation of corneal ablation by ultraviolet laser light, *Arch Ophthalmol* 103:1741-1742, 1985.
21. Krueger RR, Trokel SS, Shubert H: Interaction of UV light with the cornea, *Invest Ophthalmol Vis Sci* 26:1455-1464, 1985.
22. Lazare S, Srinivasan R: Surface properties of polyethylene terephthalate films modified by far-ultraviolet radiation at 193 nm (laser) and 185 nm (low intensity), *J Phys Chem* 90:2124-2132, 1986.
23. L'Esperance FA, Taylor DM, Warner JW: Human excimer laser keratectomy: short-term histopathology, *J Refract Surg* 4:118-124, 1988.
24. L'Esperance FA, Warner JW, Telfair WB, et al: Excimer laser instrumentation and technique for human corneal surgery, *Arch Ophthalmol* 107:131-141, 1989.
25. Lieurance RC, Patel AC, Wan WL, et al: Excimer laser cut lenticules for epikeratophakia, *Am J Ophthalmol* 103:475-476, 1987.
26. Loertscher H, Mandelbaum S, Parel JM, et al: Noncontact trephination of the cornea using a pulsed hydrogen fluoride laser, *Am J Ophthalmol* 104:471-475, 1987.
27. Loertscher H, Mandelbaum S, Parrish RK, et al: Preliminary

report on corneal incisions created by a hydrogen fluoride laser, *Am J Ophthalmol* 102:217-221, 1986.

28. Loertscher H, Parel JM, Parrish RK, et al: Effect of selected beam parameters on corneal incisions produced with a hydrogen fluoride laser, *Am J Ophthalmol.* (In press.)

29. Loertscher H, Parel JM, Parrish RK, et al: Laser trephination of the cornea, *Am J Ophthalmol.* (In press.)

30. Mainster MA: Ophthalmic applications of infrared laser—thermal considerations, *Invest Ophthalmol Vis Sci* 18:414-420, 1979.

31. March WF: *Ophthalmic lasers,* Thorofare, NJ, 1984, Slack, Inc.

32. Marshall J, Trokel SL, Rothery S, Krueger RR: Long-term healing of the central cornea after photorefractive keratectomy using an excimer laser, *Ophthalmology* 95:1411-1421, 1988.

33. Marshall J, Trokel S, Rothery S, et al: An ultrastructural study of corneal incisions induced by an excimer laser at 193 nm, *Ophthalmology* 92:749-758, 1985.

34. Marshall J, Trokel S, Rothery S, et al: A comparative study of corneal incisions induced by diamond and steel knives and two ultraviolet radiations from an excimer laser, *Br J Ophthalmol* 70:482-501, 1986.

35. Marshall J, Trokel S, Rothery S, et al: Photoablative reprofiling of the cornea using an excimer laser: photorefractive keratotomy, *Lasers Ophthalmol* 1:21-48, 1986.

36. Matchette LS, Waynant RW, Royston D, et al: Induction of lambda prophage near the site of focused UV laser radiation, *Photochem Photobiol* 49:161-167, 1989.

37. McDonald MB, Beuerman R, Falzoni W, et al: Refractive surgery with excimer laser, *Am J Ophthalmol* 103:469, 1987.

38. Munnerlyn R, Kooms SJ, Marshall J: Photorefractive keratectomy: a technique for laser refractive surgery, *J Cataract Refract Surg* 14:46-52, 1988.

39. O'Shea DC, Callen WR, Rhodes WT: *Introduction to lasers and their applications,* Reading, Mass, 1977, Addison-Wesley Publishing.

40. Puliafito CA, Wong K, Steinert RF: Quantitative and ultrastructural studies of excimer laser ablation of the cornea at 193 and 248 nanometers, *Lasers Surg Med* 7:155-159, 1987.

41. Puliafito CA, Steiner RF, Deutsch TF, et al: Excimer laser ablation of the cornea and lens, *Ophthalmology* 92:741-748, 1985.

42. Reed RD, Taboada J, Midsell JW: Response of the corneal epithelium to krypton fluoride excimer laser, *Health Phys* 40:677-683, 1981.

43. Scientific American Readings: *Lasers and light,* San Francisco, 1969, WH Freeman.

44. Searles SK, Hart GA: Stimulated emission at 281 nm XC, *Br Appl Phys Lett* 27:243-245, 1975.

45. Seiler T, Berlin M, Bende T, et al: Transverse keratectomy: laboratory and clinical experience, *Ophthalmology.* (In press.)

46. Seiler T, Kriegerowski M, Schnoy N, Bende T: Ablation rate of human corneal epithelium and Bowman's layer with the excimer laser (193 nm), *Refract Corneal Surg* 6:99-102, 1990.

47. Seiler T, Marshall J, Rothery S, et al: The potential of an infrared hydrogen fluoride laser or corneal surgery, *Lasers Ophthalmol* 1:49-60, 1986.

48. Seiler T, Matallana M, Bende T: Laser thermokeratoplasty by means of a pulsed holmium:YAG laser for hyperopic correction, *Refract Corneal Surg* 6:335-339, 1990.

49. Seiler T, Wollensak J: In vivo experiments with excimer lasers—technical parameters and healing processes, *Ophthalmologica* 192:65-70, 1986.

50. Srinivasan R: Ablation of polymers and biological tissue by ultraviolet lasers, *Science* 234:559-565, 1986.

51. Srinivasan R, Dyer PE, Braren B: Far-ultraviolet laser ablation of the cornea: photoacoustic studies, *Lasers Surg Med* 6:514-519, 1987.

52. Srinivasan R, Braren B, Dreyfus RW, et al: Mechanism of ultraviolet laser ablation of polymethylmethacrylate at 193 and 248 nm: laser-induced fluorescence analysis, chemical analysis, and doping studies, *J Opt Soc Am* 3:785-791, 1986.

53. Srinivasan R, Braren B, Seeger DE, et al: Photochemical cleavage of a polymeric solid: details of the ultraviolet laser ablation of poly(methyl methacrylate) at 193 nm and 248 nm, *Macromolecules* 19:916-920, 1986.

54. Sutcliffe E, Srinivasan R: Dynamics of UV laser ablation of organic polymer surfaces, *J Appl Phys* 60:3315-3322, 1986.

55. Sutcliffe E, Srinivasan R: Dynamics of the ultraviolet laser ablation of corneal tissue, *Am J Ophthalmol* 103:470-471, 1987.

56. Sutcliffe E, Srinivasan R: Time-dependent analysis of he UV laser ablation of corneal tissue, *Lasers Ophthalmol* 2:1201-1208, 1987.

57. Tenner A, Neuhann T, Schroder E, et al: Excimer laser radial keratotomy in the living human eye: a preliminary report, *J Refract Surg* 4:5-8, 1988.

58. Trokel SL: Development of the excimer laser in ophthalmology—a personal perspective, *Refract Corneal Surg* 6:357-362, 1990.

59. Trokel SL, Srinivasan R, Braren BA: Excimer laser surgery of the cornea, *Am J Ophthalmol* 96:710-715, 1983.

60. Troutman RC, Veronneau-Troutman S, Jakobiec FA, et al: A new laser for collagen wounding in cornea and strabismus surgery: a preliminary report, *Trans Am Ophthalmol Soc* 84:117-332, 1986.

61. Waring GO: Development and evaluation of refractive surgical procedures. Part 1. Five stages in the continuum of development. *J Refract Surg* 3:142-157, 1987.

Chapter 41

Human Application

Excimer laser photorefractive keratectomy: theory, case selection, and variables

ROGER F. STEINERT

The excimer laser can directly reprofile the optical zone of the cornea in vivo. Except for microscopic acoustic transients, the impact of the laser beam does not distort the cornea. Excimer laser photorefractive keratectomy therefore does not require artificial means for stabilization of the cornea during the procedure, in contrast to procedures, such as surgical keratomileusis, that require freezing of the cornea to stiffen it for lathing and the use of a suction ring to create high intraocular pressure during corneal lamellar splitting. In addition, because the ultraviolet radiation energy etches the corneal stroma with submicrometer accuracy, the excimer laser–ablated surface is smoother than that obtainable by any known surgical technique, including the use of gemstone blades. These two basic properties (nondistortion and smoothness) are the foundation of excimer laser–refractive surgical techniques. In this chapter, I explore the principal photorefractive techniques under active investigation and the variables identified thus far that influence the outcome.

CORNEAL WOUND HEALING RESPONSE TO EXCIMER LASER ABLATION

Chapter 40 details the preclinical experimental studies performed on excimer laser ablation of the cornea. In summary, the 193 nm radiation from the argon-fluorine (argon fluoride, ArF) excimer laser etches the cornea with submicrometer accuracy.[11,13,14,24,29,40] The stroma exhibits preservation of normal morphology and absence of thermal in-jury within less than 0.5 μm of the ablation zone. In contrast, at 248 nm, krypton-fluorine excimer laser ablation results in several micrometers of adjacent thermal disruption of the normal collagen architecture.[29] An incision with the ArF excimer compares favorably to a diamond-knife incision.[11,29] In addition to the absence of thermal injury, the excimer beam can split epithelial cells and the cell nucleus, preserving a normal-appearing cellular remnant and deposition of an electron-dense layer that Marshall and co-workers termed a "pseudomembrane."[11,24]

The precision of excimer laser ablation at 193 nm and the resultant smooth surface that can be obtained through large-area ablation of the corneal surface is theorized to be a key element in minimizing the corneal wound-healing response after ablation. The cornea does mount a wound-healing response, however, that directly affects the optical performance of the cornea. Histopathologic studies of the rabbit, monkey, and blind human eye ablation zones have consistently shown both new collagen deposition and epithelial hyperplasia* in the bed of the ablation.

In investigations in our laboratory by Carmen Puliafito, Deborah Malley, Eric Mandel, Ronald Krueger, and myself, the monkey wound-healing response has been studied in detail with correlation of light microscopy and immunohistochemistry to pachymetric and keratometric changes.[13,22] Acutely, after ablation, the wounded area exhibits deposition of laminin and fibronectin. Beginning after the first week and peaking at about 1 month, new collagen deposition occurs (Fig. 41-1). A major component is type III collagen. Type III collagen is absent in the normal developed corneal stroma but occurs after

---

References 1, 4-7, 10, 16, 22-25, 29, 34, 35, 41.

512

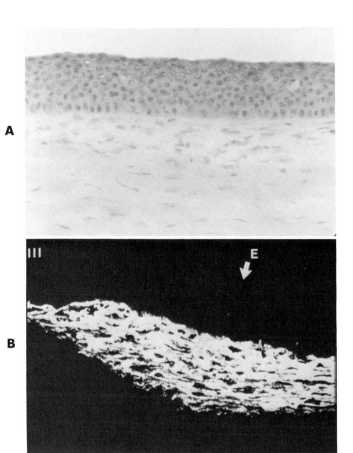

Fig. 41-1. An approximately 80 μm deep ablation was performed 1 month earlier in this monkey cornea. **A,** Light microscopy discloses epithelial hyperplasia and a different staining pattern of underlying collagen. An increased density in keratocytes in bed of ablation is noted. **B,** Immunohistochemical staining for type III collagen discloses intense staining of bed of ablation. Underlying normal stroma does not stain. Epithelial surface is indicated by *E.* (From Malley DS et al: *Arch Ophthalmol* 108:1316-1322, 1990.)

injury. Normal keratin sulfate is present in the non-treated stroma but absent in the area of newly deposited collagen. These pathologic changes correlate in time with partial regression of the initial induced corneal thinning and flattening as documented by pachymetry and keratometry. Biomicroscopy frequently reveals some degree of anterior stromal corneal haze in the bed of the ablation, again peaking 1 to 2 months after the ablation.

Overlying the new collagen, the epithelium is clinically stable, having reepithelialized within several days. On histopathology, the epithelium is orderly but hyperplastic, with 10 or more cell layers. The hyperplasia is most noticeable at the periphery of the ablation zone but typically present centrally as well.

Tuft, Marshall, and co-workers[41] and Goodman and co-workers similarly demonstrated new collagen deposition in the ablation bed of their primates. They utilized the dye DTAF (dichlorotriazinyl amino fluorescein) to label the host stroma immediately after ablation. In studies pursuing the factors responsible for the new collagen formation, they performed partial-thickness trephinations of small stromal buttons and then thinned the button from either its posterior or its anterior surface. The button was then replaced, simulating a disc ablation contour. They found that with retention of Bowman's layer (when the button was thinned from the posterior side) epithelial hyperplasia occurred but with no new collagen deposition. When Bowman's layer and the anterior stroma were excised, however, both new collagen deposition and overlying epithelial hyperplasia occurred in the button.

In the first published series of excimer ablation performed in blind human eyes treated before enucleation, Taylor and co-workers showed histopathologic evidence of epithelial hyperplasia over the ablation zone.[37] The underlying stroma showed disorganization. The number of keratocytes were increased, and the keratocyte microstructure indicated high metabolic activity. These findings were consistent with a corneal wound healing response similar to that demonstrated in the animal studies.

These preclinical studies identified therefore the anatomic basis for instability and partial regression of the optical effect achieved by the initial ablation. Haze in the ablation zone (Fig. 41-2) is also presumably related to new collagen deposition, with disorganization of the collagen fine structure and lack of the normal proteoglycans in the interfibrillar spaces.[17] The haze is maximal 1 to 2 months after ablation in humans and then typically improves in subsequent months, disappearing completely in some cases. One hypothesis is that the improvement in haze reflects remodeling of the initially deposited collagen and production of proteoglycans.

Laboratory studies thus far indicate that mutagenic and carcinogenic potential of 193 nm light is low.[8,12,27,39]

Overall human results, though parallel to animal studies, are generally better, with less haze and less regression.[15,18-21,23,31,33,37,38,43] The human cornea possibly mounts a less vigorous wound-healing response. The improved results may also result from the sophistication of the commercially produced ophthalmic excimer lasers. Current-generation clinical ophthalmic lasers achieve a more spatially homogenous beam profile, resulting in a smoother ablation bed.

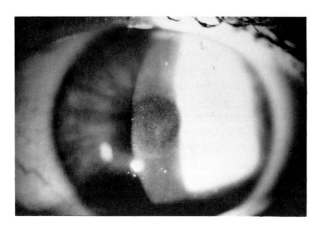

Fig. 41-2. Slitlamp photograph demonstrates maximum amount of anterior stromal reticular haze usually seen in ablation zone 1 to 2 months after myopic photorefractive keratectomy. Patient had no visual symptoms from his haze.

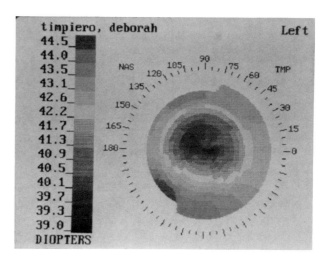

Fig. 41-3. Computer-assisted topographic analysis 6 months after myopic photorefractive keratectomy. Central flattening is demonstrated.

SPHERICAL MYOPIA

The refractive application of excimer laser large-area ablation under the most active clinical investigation is photorefractive keratectomy (PRK) for spherical myopia. A more accurate term for this procedure is "laser anterior myopic keratomileusis." The nonspecific term, PRK, is widely used to designate the myopic procedure, however.

Large-area ablation for myopia is a natural application for the excimer laser ablation technique. The central cornea is flattened relative to its original curvature (Fig. 41-4, *A*), with progressively less flattening toward the periphery of the optical zone (Fig. 41-3).

The laser beam is manipulated to achieve central corneal flattening through one of several techniques. The most common is through the use of a diaphragm. By changing the size of the aperture over the course of the exposure, the maximum laser ablation is in the central cornea with progressively less exposure toward the periphery. One commercial laser permits choosing between decreasing the aperture with progressive pulses or increasing the size of the diaphragm with successive pulses. It is not known whether these opposite approaches translate into clinically important differences. In principle, particularly in a system that is dependent on patient fixation during the exposure, starting with a small aperture that progressively increases achieves the critical central correction during the beginning of the exposure, and instability in fixation later in the exposure is less critical. In either case, the smoothest contour is achieved if the diaphragm changes size

with each pulse. In that manner, the "step" created with each laser pulse is limited to the ablation depth of a single pulse, typically about 25 μm.

One commercial laser achieves a similar effect through a rotary wheel with apertures of progressively increasing size.[15] Under investigation in Europe but not currently available in the United States are excimer laser systems that sweep the central cornea with slits of excimer pulses that summate into the desired overall corneal flattening pattern.[9,30]

Entering into current investigation is the use of an ablatable mask. The mask consists of a polymer that is ablated with successive excimer laser pulses. By placing the mask in the laser beam path, a myopic mask that is thinnest at the center and progressively thicker toward the edges should achieve the same overall contour as the previously mentioned mechanical systems. The excimer beam will ablate and penetrate the center first. Successive pulses will ablate the peripheral mask. In that manner, the central cornea will receive the most ablation, and myopic correction will be achieved.

Munnerlyn and co-authors derived the theoretical equations for the amount of stroma that must be ablated to achieve a given optical correction.[26] Reduced to a simple yet fairly accurate approximation,

$$t = \frac{S_2 D}{3}$$

where *t* is the maximal (central) depth of stromal ablation, *S* is the diameter of the optical zone, and *D* is the dioptric correction desired.

The depth of ablation is therefore highly dependent on the size of the optical zone. For example, to correct a 4-diopter myope with a 6 mm optical zone, 48 μm of stroma would have to be ablated. Bowman's layer is generally believed to be 10 to 15 μm in depth. To limit the ablation to the acellular Bowman's layer, one would have to reduce the optical zone to 3.4 mm to achieve a 4-diopter flattening with only 15 μm of ablation.

It is evident therefore that correction of moderate myopia will require ablation of the anterior stroma. To minimize halos and edge glare yet not perform deep ablation, most clinical investigations are employing optical zones of 5 ±0.5 mm.

Published series from Seiler[31,33] and McDonald,[18,19,43] as well as early experience by other investigators in the United States, uniformly indicates a great decrease in the stability and predictability of the refractive change for corrections exceeding 5 to 6 diopters. Below this level, human myopic corrections are generally hyperopic initially and then predictably regress toward emmetropia over several months. After approximately 2 to 4 months the corrections largely become stabilized. Typically over 90% of patients will achieve 20/40 or better uncorrected acuity and be within 1 diopter of emmetropia.

In contrast, in corrections exceeding 5 to 6 diopters, the incidence of eventual undercorrection because of regression dramatically increases. Regression is not uniform; this variability makes it impossible to compensate through initial overcorrection. Neither is the regression clearly correlated with increased haze, though some patients experience both simultaneously.

Pharmacologic modulation of the corneal response to myopic PRK has centered on topical steroid therapy thus far. Most investigators employ topical steroids intensively for the first 3 to 4 months after PRK. For example, dexamethasone 0.1% or prednisolone acetate 1% is applied from 4 times daily up to every 2 hours for the first month and then gradually tapered down and discontinued by the fourth month. The rate of tapering depends on the rate of regression and the refractive status of the patient. Steroids can, of course, reduce any inflammatory response in the ablated cornea and reduce new collagen formation. No published study has randomized patients between treatment and non-treatment or between different intensities of steroid treatment.

Other agents may be more effective than corticosteroids at modulating the corneal wound-healing response. Talamo and colleagues have shown some potentiation of effect by combining steroid and mitomycin, an antimetabolite.[36] Subsequent follow-up studies in our laboratory have indicated, however, that mitomycin may have unacceptable corneal toxicity. Presumably other agents will be developed to assist the surgeon in postoperative pharmacologic modulation of the refractive outcome.

In corneal surgical procedures such as penetrating keratoplasty and radial and astigmatic keratotomy, other variables in wound healing have become well known. In particular, elderly patients have slower and less intense wound healing than younger patients, and female patients may exhibit a greater effect in linear refractive keratotomies than males. Paradoxically, initially flatter corneas achieve a greater average effect from radial keratotomy than steeper corneas. Similar variables may effect the outcome after excimer laser PRK, but they have yet to be systematically studied in adequate numbers.

Presence of ocular pathoses that may affect reepithelialization is a relative contraindication. Lid structural abnormalities and lagophthalmos may lead to persistent epithelial defects. Keratitis sicca will cause postoperative punctate keratitis and occasionally persistent epithelial defects with secondary ulceration. Anticipation of healing difficulties in a patient with mild tear insufficiency facilitates prophylactic treatment, ranging from artificial tear substitutes to punctal occlusion. Blepharitis and meibomitis, even when well tolerated preoperatively, can lead to punctate keratitis and occasionally more severe reepithelialization difficulties. Relative or total corneal anesthesia strongly predisposes to postoperative difficulties with reepithelialization. Patients with underlying collagen-vascular disease, such as rheumatoid arthritis, may have keratitis sicca. They are also strongly predisposed to sterile stromal ulceration. It is important for all the above conditions to be recognized and treated preoperatively if possible. Proceeding with PRK in the face of these disorders risks prolonged healing at best and an increased risk of stromal scarring and ulceration with permanent loss of best corrected acuity.

ASTIGMATISM

Clinical investigation of excimer laser large-area ablation to correct astigmatism is beginning. The goal is the creation of a toric contour in the visual axis.

Two basic strategies are coming into clinical investigation. In one, the laser beam is directed through a slit-moving aperture[21] (Fig. 41-4, *B*). The parallel blades of the aperture expand with each successive pulse. In one meridian the entire optical zone is ex-

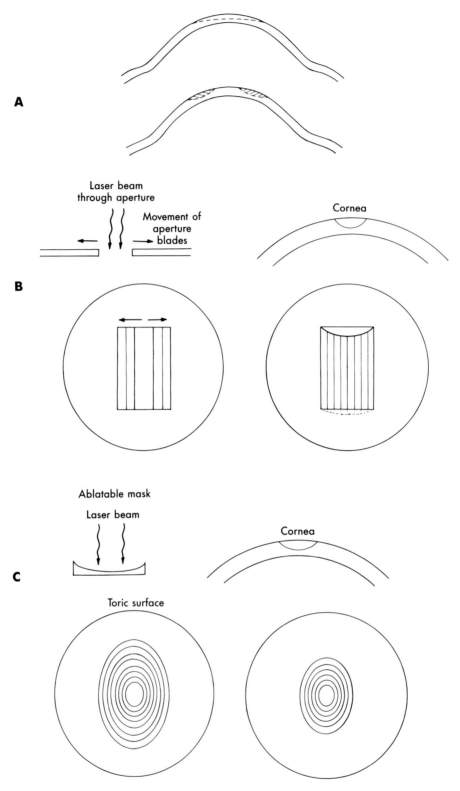

Fig. 41-4. A, Schematic exaggerated representations of new profiles achieved in myopic photorefractive keratectomy and hyperopic correction by ablation of midperiphery. **B,** Schema of ablation for correction of astigmatism, using method of an expanding slit aperture. **C,** Schema of ablation through an erodable mask to achieve a toric contour.

posed to each pulse. In the other meridian the ablation becomes progressively shallower moving to the periphery. The initial ablation contour, at the completion of treatment, is therefore a true cylinder with sharply truncated ends. Clinical experience with this approach is quite preliminary. Extensive remodeling appears to occur at the two truncated ends along the axis of the ablated cylinder. As a result, there is a net hyperoptic shift. The procedure is therefore suitable for compound myopic astigmatism but inadvisable for patients with minimal spherical equivalent myopia or with overall hyperopia.

The second approach employs the erodable (ablatable) mask in the beam path (Fig. 41-4, *C*). The mask consists of a polymer that is progressively ablated with successive excimer laser pulses. The mask has an optical zone contour similar to that of a toric hard contact lens. The excimer laser beam will penetrate through the mask initially at its thinnest areas, and the later pulses will progressively ablate the thicker areas of the mask. In theory, the mask can precisely and smoothly control the energy delivery to the cornea and achieve a contour compensating for astigmatism, myopia, or both. Unpublished early results in Europe by Theo Seiler are promising, but no data have yet been published, and investigation in the United States is just beginning.

HYPEROPIA

Large-area ablation for the correction of hyperopia must involve removal of tissue in the midperiphery relative to the center, achieving an overall steepening of the optical zone. The contour must then return to the existing peripheral corneal contour. This approach is illustrated in Fig. 41-4, *A*.

Clinical experience with this approach is extremely limited and anecdotal. The preclinical studies of large-area ablation would indicate, however, that the attempted hyperopic correction will be prone to regression because of epithelial hyperplasia as well as new collagen formation. In the correction of myopia, the new contour follows the original corneal contour with a flattening of the central zone. In contrast, the hyperopic correction is biphasic, requiring both relative flattening of the more peripheral treated zone and relative steepening of the more central zone as one approaches the visual axis. In principle, this change in contour may be particularly prone to "filling-in" by regenerating epithelium and new collagen formation.

REFERENCES

1. Aron-Rosa D, Boerner C, Bath P, et al: Corneal wound healing after excimer laser keratotomy in a human eye, *Am J Ophthalmol* 103:454-464, 1987.
2. Bende T, Seiler T, Wollensak J: Side effects in excimer corneal surgery: corneal thermal gradients, *Albrecht von Graefes Arch Clin Exp Ophthalmol* 226:227-280, 1988.
3. Dehm E, Puliafito C, Adler C, Steinert R: Corneal endothelial injury in rabbits following excimer laser ablation at 193 and 248 nm, *Arch Ophthalmol* 104:1364-1368, 1986.
4. DelPero R, Gigstad J, Roberts A, et al: A refractive and histopathologic study of excimer laser keratectomy in primates, *Am J Ophthalmol* 109:419-429, 1990.
5. Fantes F, Hanna K, Waring G, et al: Wound healing after excimer laser keratomileusis (photorefractive keratectomy) in monkeys, *Arch Ophthalmol* 108:665-675, 1990.
6. Gaster R, Binder P, Coalwell K, et al: Corneal surface ablation by 193 nm excimer laser and wound healing in rabbits, *Invest Ophthalmol* 30:90-98, 1989.
7. Goodman GL, Trokel SL, Stark WJ, et al: Corneal healing following laser refractive keratectomy, *Arch Ophthalmol* 107:1799-1803, 1989.
8. Green H, Boll J, Parrish J, et al: Cytotoxicity and mutagenicity of low intensity 248 and 193 nm excimer laser radiation in mammalian cells, *Cancer Res* 47:410-413, 1987.
9. Hanna K, Chastang J, Pouliquen Y, et al: A rotating slit delivery system for excimer laser refractive keratoplasty, *Am J Ophthalmol* 103:474, 1987.
10. Hanna K, Pouliquen Y, Savoldelli M, et al: Corneal wound healing in monkeys 18 months after excimer laser photorefractive keratectomy, *Refract Corneal Surg* 6:340-345, 1990.
11. Kerr-Muir M, Trokel S, Marshall J, Rothery S: Ultrastructural comparison of conventional surgical and argon fluoride excimer laser keratectomy, *Am J Ophthalmol* 103:448-453, 1987.
12. Kochevar I: Review: cytoxicity and mutagenicity of excimer laser radiation, *Lasers Surg Med* 9:440-444, 1989.
13. Krauss J, Puliafito C, Steinert R: Laser interactions with the cornea, *Surv Ophthalmol* 31:37-53, 1986.
14. Krueger R, Trokel S, Schubert H: Interaction of ultraviolet laser light with the cornea, *Invest Ophthalmol Vis Sci* 26:1455-1464, 1985.
15. L'Esperance F, Warner J, Telfair W, Yoder P, Martin C: Excimer laser instrumentation and technique for human corneal surgery, *Arch Ophthalmol* 197:131-139, 1989.
16. L'Esperance F, Taylor D, Warner J: Human excimer laser keratectomy: short term histopathology, *J Refract Surg* 4:118-124, 1988.
17. Lohmann C, Gartry D, Kerr-Muir M, et al: "Haze" in photorefractive keratectomy: its origins and consequences, *Lasers and Light in Ophthalmology* 4:15-34, 1991.
18. McDonald MB, Frantz JM, Klyce SD, et al: Central photorefractive keratectomy for myopia, *Arch Ophthalmol* 108:799-808, 1990.
19. McDonald MB, Liv JC, Byrd TJ, et al: Central photorefractive keratectomy for myopia: partially sighted and normally sighted eyes, *Ophthalmology* 98:1327-1337, 1991.
20. McDonnell PJ, Garbus JJ, Salz JJ: Excimer laser myopic photorefractive keratectomy after undercorrected radial keratotomy, *Refract Corneal Surg* 7:146-150, 1991.
21. McDonnell PJ, Moreira H, Garbus J, et al: Photorefractive keratectomy to create toric ablations for correction of astigmatism, *Arch Ophthalmol* 109:710-713, 1991.
22. Malley DS, Steinert RF, Puliafito CA, Dobi ET: Immunofluorescence study of corneal wound healing after excimer laser anterior keratectomy in the monkey eye, *Arch Ophthalmol* 108:1316-1322, 1990.
23. Marshall J, Trokel S, Rothery S, Krueger R: Long-term heal-

ing of the central cornea after photorefractive keratectomy using an excimer laser, *Ophthalmology* 95:1411-1421, 1988.

24. Marshall J, Trokel S, Rothery S, Krueger R: Photoablative reprofiling of the cornea using an excimer laser: photorefractive keratectomy, *Lasers in Ophthalmology* 1:21-48, 1986.
25. Marshall J, Trokel S, Rothery S, Schubert H: An ultrastructural study of corneal incisions induced by an excimer laser at 193 nm, *Ophthalmology* 92(6):749-757, 1985.
26. Munnerlyn C, Koons S, Marshall J: Photorefractive keratectomy: a technique for laser refractive surgery, *J Cataract Refract Surg* 14:46-52, 1988.
27. Nuss R, Puliafito C, Dehm E: Unscheduled DNA synthesis following excimer laser ablation of the cornea in vivo, *Invest Ophthalmol Vis Sci* 28:287-294, 1987.
28. Puliafito C, Wong K, Steinert R: Quantitative and ultrastructural studies of excimer laser ablation of the cornea at 193 and 248 nanometers, *Lasers Surg Med* 7:155-159, 1987.
29. Puliafito C, Steinert R, Deutsch T, et al: Excimer laser ablation of the cornea and lens, *Ophthalmology* 92:741-748, 1985.
30. Schröder E, Dardenne M, Neuhann T, Tenner A: An ophthalmic excimer laser for corneal surgery, *Am J Ophthalmol* 103:472-473, 1987.
31. Seiler T, Wollensak J: Myopic photorefractive keratectomy (PRK) with the excimer laser: one year followup, *Ophthalmology* 98:1156-1163, 1991.
32. Seiler T, Kriegerowski M, Schnoy N, Bende T: Ablation rate of human corneal epithelium and Bowman's layer with excimer laser (193 nm), *Refract Corneal Surg* 6:99-102, 1990.
33. Seiler T, Kahle G, Kriegerowski M, Bende T: Myopic excimer laser (193 nm) keratomileusis in sighted and blind human eyes, *Refract Corneal Surg* 6:165-173, 1990.
34. Steinert RF, Puliafito CA: Lasers in corneal surgery, *Ophthalmol Clin North Am* 2:611-623, 1989.
35. Sundar Raj N, Geiss MJ III, Fantes F, et al: Healing of excimer laser ablated monkey corneas: an immunolohistochemical evaluation, *Arch Ophthalmol* 108:1604-1610, 1990.
36. Talamo JH, Gollamudi S, Green WR: Modulation of corneal wound healing after excimer laser keratomileusis using topical mitomycin C and steroids, *Arch Ophthalmol* 109:1141-1145, 1991.
37. Taylor DM, L'Esperance FA Jr, DelPero RA, et al: Human excimer laser lamellar keratectomy: a clinical study, *Ophthalmology* 96:654-664, 1989.
38. Tenner A, Neuhann T, Schröder E, Salz J, Maguen E: Excimer laser radial keratotomy in the living human eye: a preliminary report, *Refract Surg* 4:5-8, 1988.
39. Trentacoste J, Thompson K, Parrish R, et al: Mutagenic potential for a 193 nm excimer laser in fibroblasts in tissue culture, *Ophthalmology* 94:125-129, 1987.
40. Trokel S, Srinivasan R, Braren B: Excimer laser surgery in the cornea, *Am J Ophthalmol* 96:710-715, 1983.
41. Tuft S, Marshall J, Rothery S: Stromal remodelling following photorefractive keratectomy, *Lasers in Ophthalmology* 1:177-183, 1987.
42. Waring GO III: Development of a system for excimer laser corneal surgery, *Trans Am Ophthalmol Soc* 87:854-983, 1989.
43. Wilson SE, Klyce SD, McDonald MB, et al: Changes in corneal topography after excimer laser photorefractive keratectomy for myopia, *Ophthalmology* 98:1338-1347, 1991.

Use of the 193 nm excimer laser for photorefractive and phototherapeutic keratectomy

NEAL A. SHER

JANET DEMARCHI

RICHARD L. LINDSTROM

The 193 nm excimer laser, by virtue of its ability to remove corneal tissue in a precise and incremental manner, can be used for both therapeutic scar removal and for refractive surgery. When used to ablate the cornea and remove opacities, the procedure is called "phototherapeutic keratectomy" (PTK). The same excimer laser can also be used to ablate small amounts of corneal tissue in a preprogrammed manner to alter the curvature of the cornea and reduce or eliminate myopia, hyperopia or astigmatism in a procedure called "photorefractive keratectomy" (PRK).

Several excimer laser systems have been developed and are being tested in this country and abroad. In the United States, clinical investigations have been underway for several years on three different laser systems including the Taunton Technologies (Monroe, Connecticut), VISX Co. (Sunnyvale, California), and Summit Technologies (Watertown, Massachusetts). In 1990, Taunton Technologies and VISX Company merged but parallel investigations on both laser systems are continuing. This chapter details some of our data and observations from the experience with the Taunton excimer laser system on over 100 patients at the Phillips Eye Institute in Minneapolis, Minnesota, and several other investigative sites using the same laser.

INSTRUMENTATION

The Taunton Technologies excimer laser had its genesis in the early work of Francis L'Esperance[5,6,16] as well as the work of Trokel and Srinivasan.[5,17] Our initial phase II and IIA studies utilized the Model LV 2000, which was replaced in 1991 with the Model LV 2015 (Fig. 41-5). Both models use a mixture of argon-fluorine (argon fluoride) gas to produce a 193 nm wavelength output at 10 Hz, which was adjusted to deliver a fluence at the eye of 100 to 120 mJ/cm^2 with a maximum beam diameter of 6.0 mm. The entire laser system has a computer control module with an interactive menu, real-time monitoring of procedure parameters, and an integrated digital keratoscope. During surgery, the patient is supine, and with a head-restraint system and three-axis

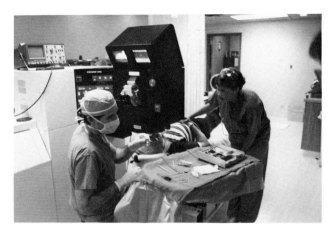

Fig. 41-5. Taunton Technologies Model 2015 Excimer Laser System. Patient is being positioned under laser before a procedure. Control console not visible in this photograph.

alignment, the eye is positioned by viewing through the integrated binocular surgical microscope as well as two video monitors. A technician runs the laser from a free-standing computer console, and the surgeon sits at the operating microscope in the usual surgical configuration.

SURGICAL PROCEDURE

These studies were carried out under the guidelines of the United States Food and Drug Administration under an Investigational Device Exemption.[2] The basic surgical technique for both PTK and PRK was similar and fully described by use elsewhere.[12,13,21] Our initial patients, in phase II and IIA, had peribulbar or retrobulbar anesthesia. This was later found unnecessary and in subsequent patients topical 0.5% proparacaine only was used. The eye was positioned by our viewing through an integrated binocular surgical microscope, and the patient was asked to fixate on an internal fixation target within the laser coaxial to a point midway between the two objective lenses of the operating microscope. The epithelium was then gently marked with a Sinskey hook over the center of the entrance pupil as suggested by Uozato and Guyton.[19] A 7.0 mm trephine, premarked with blue dye, was centered on the epithelial impression to demarcate the ablation zone. In PRK, the epithelium was always removed using a Tooke knife. In PTK, the epithelium was frequently left intact, especially in more recent cases because of modulating effect of the epithelium in smoothing irregular astigmatism. The eye was usually fixated with a 0.12 forceps, Thornton ring, or not at all. The laser then delivered a series of pulses, predetermined through a rotating series of 15 apertures, lasting 20 to 90 seconds. This has been called the "recipe." In PTK, after the initial ablation, the patient may be reexamined at the slitlamp and additional ablation carried out as needed.

In some cases of PTK, an attempt was made to compensate for the corneal flattening and resulting hyperopic shift that was seen in some patients. After the initial corneal scar was removed, usually through a wide aperture or myopic series of apertures, a secondary set of pulses was then delivered to steepen the peripheral portion of the central cornea. This has been referred to as "secondary hyperopic correction." Most scar patients received this "combined cut."

POSTOPERATIVE REGIMEN

After the ablation, Tobradex drops and 5% Homatropine methylbromide were instilled and a disposable soft contact lens (Vistakon Acuvue) was placed on the eye. On the first postoperative day, the patients were started on fluoromethalone 0.1% (FML), every 2 hours for the first week, q.i.d. for the first month, t.i.d. for the second month, and gradually tapered over the next 4 to 5 months. Tobramycin 0.3% solution (Tobrex, Alcon) was administered q.i.d. until the epithelium healed. The contact lens was also removed at this time.

PHOTOREFRACTIVE KERATECTOMY

The 28 cases described here are the phase IIB cases performed by multiple surgeons in our group. The myopia (spherical equivalent) ranged from −8.25 D to −2.5 D with a mean preoperative refraction of −5.22 D and a mean postoperative refraction at 6 months of +0.62 D. Fig. 41-6 shows the mean change in refraction after surgery in this series of eyes.

For most patients, the attempted correction was designed to achieve emmetropia. Fig. 41-7 shows attempted versus achieved corrections at 6 months or in a few cases 3 months. Seventy-four percent of patients achieved correction within 1 D of attempted, and 96% achieved the attempted amount of correction within 2 D. These data show improved predictability compared to an earlier series of 31 patients we reported from our preliminary phase II and IIA studies.[13] In that study, only 55% of our patients had achieved the desired amount of correction within 1 D because there were significant undercorrections of the myopia, believed to be related to a problem in calibration of the laser, which was subsequently corrected. The latest study showed several significant overcorrections, all of which were seen in

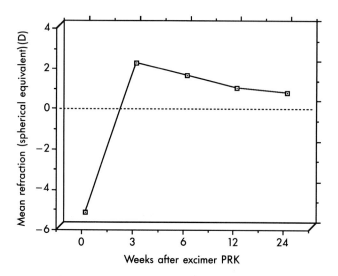

Fig. 41-6. Mean change in refraction (spherical equivalent) in 28 eyes over time.

the first several patients of this series treated with the new laser on the same day. Again, calibration of beam output was believed to be the cause of the laser running at a higher than desirable fluence. Since that time, the laser is currently calibrated by multiple techniques including ablations of standardized plastic blocks and measurement of the central depth of cut as well as direct energy measurements with a meter. We found the last technique alone inadequate.

The epithelium healed within 3 to 4 days and no recurrent erosions were seen. All patients achieved the return of their best corrected visual acuity by 3

to 6 months postoperatively. No statistically significant astigmatism was induced or reduced after PRK. There were no significant changes noted in endothelial cell counts or other intraocular effects except several cases of ocular hypertension, believed to be steroid induced, which resolved after discontinuation of the FML.

Significant postoperative pain was common in our patients. We found that the use of narcotic analgesia followed by ice packs, cycloplegics, and disposable contact lenses as well as patient counseling, provided some relief. The pain was usually ameliorated by 36 hours after surgery. Paradoxically, we found the postoperative pain much less when topical anesthesia was used compared to retrobulbar or peribulbar blocks.

Quantitative grading of corneal haze, especially at minimal levels, was difficult and numerical grades were not very meaningful. As Zabel described,[9] a fine reticulation was observed at the epithelial stromal interface and in the anterior 25 μm of the stroma at the end of the first and second weeks. A diffuse nebular haze with patchy granularity was seen in some patients, as viewed by sclerotic scatter. These changes gradually diminished in most patients over time and were frequently gone by the 6-month visit. One patient in this series had visually significant haze with corneal scarring. This patient preoperatively measured −8.50 D, had significant overcorrection (+3.0 D at 6 months), and was believed to be treated with a higher than desired fluence. The best corrected vision was 20/30 at 6 months post operatively. The patient had epithelial hyperplasia that resembled the haze seen once previ-

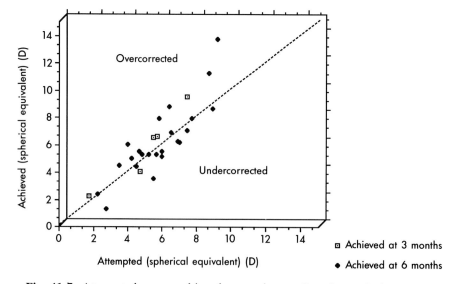

Fig. 41-7. Attempted versus achieved corrections at 3 or 6 months in 28 eyes.

ously in one of our phase II patients. In that patient, the hyperplastic epithelium was debrided and the opacity was removed without recurrence by the 6-month visit. Epithelial hyperplasia after excimer PRK has been reported by other investigators.[3]

If one compares these data to results from radial keratotomy (RK), as reported in the Prospective Evaluation of Radial Keratotomy (PERK) Study,[20] some rough comparisons can be made. At 1 year, 38% of the eyes in PERK with a baseline refraction of −4.50 to 8.00 had achieved correction between −1.00 and +1.00 D of emmetropia. In this small series of excimer PRK, 16 of 21 eyes (76%) with the same range of myopia achieved the same range. We saw no evidence of diurnal shifts of refraction or progressive myopia or hyperopia after 3 months. In contrast to RK, there was minimal glare sensitivity, no perforations and no apparent significant structural weakening of the cornea.

Our past experience shows good stability of the correction after approximately 9 months with little reversal of correction in the 1-year to 2-year interval. Analysis of larger series will be necessary to determine smaller amounts of regression.

We believe that the larger 6.0 mm ablation zone used in our patients has several advantages. Seiler reported that nearly one fourth of his patients experienced night glare when a 3.5 mm diameter beam was used and that this incidence was reduced with a 5.0 mm beam.[10,11] Night glare and halos seldom occurred in our series. Utilization of a larger-diameter optical zone may alleviate problems with centering of the area to be ablated. Uozato and Guyton have stressed the importance of centering corneal procedures over the entrance pupil rather than the corneal light reflex while the patient fixes a target coaxially placed with the surgeon's sighting eye.[19] Corneal topography data have shown that decentrations of 1.0 mm are not uncommon[7,8] and that use of a larger diameter optical zone would help mitigate these errors. The only theoretic disadvantage to a larger optical zone is that a deeper ablation is required. It is our clinical impression that the presence of clinically significant haze is not associated with the deeper ablation depths seen with the 6.0 mm diameter. Most recently, we have performed a small series of PRK on 6 highly myopic patients (−10.00 to −15.00 D) and have seen no noticeable difference in corneal haze.

Our heavy use of postoperative topical corticosteroids slowly tapered over 6 months was based on experimental work by Tuft,[18] who demonstrated in rabbits that types III and VI collagen formation, present within the ablation zone, is greatly reduced with topical corticosteroid treatment. It is not known how intense or prolonged this therapy needs to be to minimize the new collagen and related corneal haze.

PHOTOTHERAPEUTIC KERATECTOMY

The use of the excimer laser to treat pathologic conditions was first suggested by Sedarevic[9] and later reported by Steinert[15] and others.[1] We reported on a multicenter series of 33 patients with corneal scars and irregular astigmatism with a variety of pathologic conditions.[13] Approximately half of these patients in this preliminary study had improved vision, and a small but significant number avoided the need for penetrating keratoplasty.

The following series of PTK cases expands on this original series of 33 patients reported and includes additional patients contributed by Jon Frantz, M.D. (Florida Eye Center, Ft. Meyers, Florida) and Richard Eiferman, M.D. (University of Louisville).

Improvement of visual acuity alone was not the only parameter used to judge the success of excimer PTK. Alleviation of discomfort, reduction of glare, and treatment of recurrent erosions were other therapeutic goals. Table 41-1 reviews 66 cases of PTK, which were followed for at least 6 months.

Following are six illustrative case reports:

Case 1. A 52-year-old woman had diffuse corneal scarring from bacterial keratitis; a 60 μm ablation

Table 41-1. Summary of Etiology and Outcome of Phototherapeutic Keratectomy

Etiology	Number of Patients	Goal Achieved*
Postinfection scar	11	5
Herpes simplex	7	3
Herpes zoster	3	1
Post traumatic scar	17	7
Salzmann's nodular corneal dystrophy	4	3
Anterior corneal dystrophy		
Mat-dot-fingerprint	2	2
Reis-Bückler's corneal dystrophy	3	2
Lattice dystrophy	1	0
Granular dystrophy	5	2
Schneider's dystrophy	1	1
Band keratopathy	8	5
Recurrent erosions	3	3
Keratoconus apical scar	2	1
Post keratoplasty scar	1	1
TOTAL	66	36

*Goals were one or more of the following: improvement of two or more Snellen lines of acuity, reduction of glare, significantly improved comfort, or lack of recurrent erosions.

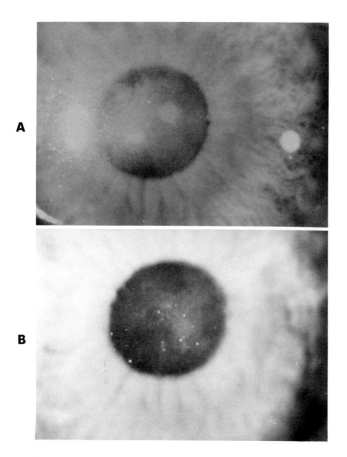

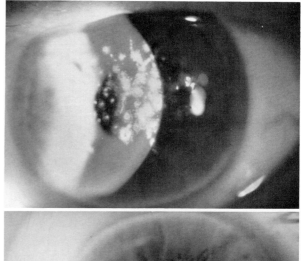

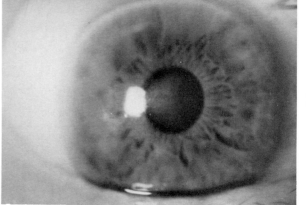

Fig. 41-8. A, Preoperative appearance of 52-year-old woman with corneal scarring from bacterial keratitis. Vision improved from 20/200 to 20/25. **B,** Six-month postoperative appearance. (From Sher NA et al: *Arch Ophthalmol* 109(4):491-498, 1991.)

Fig. 41-9. A, Preoperative appearance of 60-year-old man with granular dystrophy and anterior stromal opacities, which caused severe photophobia and glare. Visual acuity was 20/30. **B,** Postoperative appearance 6 months after surgery shows considerable reduction in deposits. Vision was unchanged, but symptoms improved.

was performed. Visual acuity improved from 20/200 to 20/20−2, and a penetrating keratoplasty was avoided (Fig. 41-8).

Case 2. A 60-year-old man had granular dystrophy, severe photophobia, and disabling glare symptoms. Fig. 41-9, *A*, reveals the typical anterior stromal opacities found in granular dystrophy. A 50 μm combined ablation was performed. After surgery, almost complete removal of the hyaline deposits was achieved. Fig. 41-9, *B*, shows the postoperative appearance at 6 months with considerable improvement in symptoms. The visual acuity did not change, but there was considerable reduction of glare.

Case 3. A 50-year-old-man had Reis-Bücklers' corneal dystrophy with recurrent erosions. A 50 μm combined ablation was performed; visual acuity improved from 20/50 to 20/25 6 months later. No further corneal erosions developed. A significant

hyperopic shift was noted, requiring contact lens fitting.

Case 4. A 43-year-old man had a 35-year history of recurrent corneal erosions from trauma. He had multiple treatments for his erosions, which included stromal micropuncture but suffered from incapacitating erosions several times a year. A 30 μm combined ablation was performed. There have been no recurrent erosions in the 18 months since surgery.

Case 5. A 79-year-old man with Avellino anterior corneal dystrophy had best corrected vision of 20/70 (Fig. 41-10, *A*). He underwent a combined 140 μm ablation. By week 10 (Fig. 41-10, *B*), there was significant reduction in the scar. However, by 6 months after PTK there was a significant recurrence of the corneal dystrophy (Fig. 41-10, *C*), which necessitated corneal transplantation.

Case 6. A 49-year-old man with an unusual bilat-

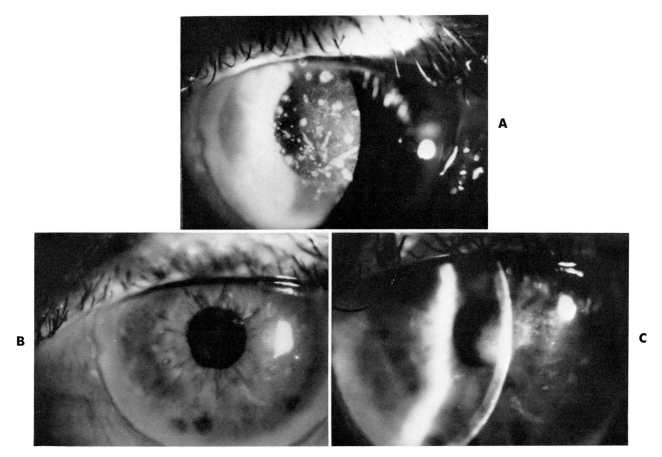

Fig. 41-10. A, Preoperative appearance of 79-year-old man with Avellino corneal dystrophy with superficial opacities. **B,** Postoperative appearance at 10 weeks after 140 μm ablation showing decrease in opacities. **C,** Six-month postoperative appearance showing recurrence of corneal scarring, which necessitated penetrating keratoplasty.

eral familial anterior dystrophy, believed to be a variant of Schnyder's crystalline dystrophy, had a best corrected vision of 20/70 in the left eye with severe glare (Fig. 41-11, *A*). The left eye was treated with a "combined" ablation of 175 μm through intact epithelium. At 3 weeks postoperatively, his best corrected vision was 20/25^{+2} with a dramatic reduction in scarring (Fig. 41-11, *B* and *C*).

Surgical technique and judgment are more critical in PTK cases than in the refractive cases. The assessment of scar depth may be difficult and can be assisted by optical pachymetry.[14] During surgery, the cornea becomes opaque from drying, and the intraoperative evaluation of the amount of residual scar becomes difficult. To accomplish this, the patient should be brought to a slitlamp after the initial ablation to determine if further treatment is required.

The limitations in success of PTK were the result of several factors. Irregular surfaces were difficult to

smooth and resulted in persistent irregular astigmatism. To achieve smoothing of the cornea, the use of modulators such as 2.5% methylcellulose was sometimes used. This was difficult to apply smoothly and was susceptible to drying and rippling from the air flow over the eye as well as flaking from interaction with the laser beam. If applied too thickly, the laser energy is absorbed by the modulator and minimal or no ablation will be carried out. There have been some recent experimental reports[4] on the use of other agents such as Tears Naturale II (Alcon). In more recent cases, we have treated through the intact epithelium, which acts as a modulator.

Excimer PTK should be considered a refractive procedure because any flattening of the cornea will produce a hyperopic shift. In almost all the above cases, the globe was fixated and the patient was treated in an identical manner to that of our refractive cases. To minimize the hyperopic shift we deliv-

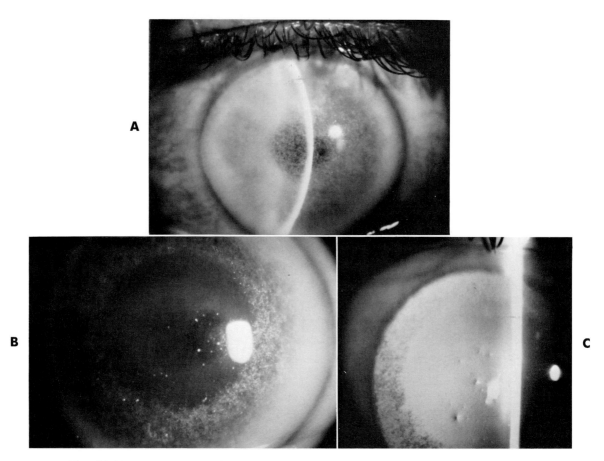

Fig. 41-11. Man 49 years of age with a bilateral familial anterior corneal dystrophy, probably a variant of Schnyder's crystalline dystrophy. **A,** Preoperative vision was 20/70. **B,** and **C,** Postoperative appearance 3 weeks after excimer phototherapeutic keratectomy. Vision improved to 20/25.

ered a secondary series of pulses to the paracentral cornea to produce steepening. This was referred to as a "combined cut." Preliminary analysis of over 40 cases of PTK using this combined cut show considerable reduction in hyperopic shifts from the hyperopia, which was expected with a standard ablation (unpublished data, N.A. Sher, A. Tucci, 1991).

At present, the ideal cases for excimer PTK include superficial scars with minimal irregular astigmatism, anterior membrane dystrophies, granular dystrophy, recurrent erosions, and band keratopathy resistant to EDTA. Poor candidates include those with scarring deeper than 150 μm, eyes with irregular astigmatism, and patients who may be unable to tolerate potential anisometropia from hyperopic shifts.

CONCLUSIONS

The Taunton Technologies (now VISX) excimer laser was used for both refractive surgery for myo-

pia and in the treatment of superficial corneal scarring. In our latest series of 28 myopic patients, 74% achieved their desired correction within 1 D and 96% within 2 D. There were no serious complications or intraocular effects. Significant corneal haze was seen in only one patient and patient satisfaction was high.

In a separate study of excimer PTK for the treatment of superficial corneal scars and irregular astigmatism, 66 patients were treated with a variety of different conditions. Overall, over half of the patients showed improvement of vision or comfort. The laser was particularly effective in the treatment of corneal dystrophies such as Reis-Bücklers', Map-dot-fingerprint, Salzmann's dystrophy and recurrent corneal erosions. It proved very useful in eyes with band keratopathy that were resistant to conventional therapy with EDTA. It was less successful in eliminating irregular astigmatism.

We have seen several recurrences of opacities in

cases of granular dystrophy as well as Avellino dystrophy. This is not unexpected because these dystrophies can reappear within penetrating grafts. It has yet to be determined if the physical disruption of Bowman's layer provides a stimulus to a more rapid recurrence of the underlying disease.

The 193 nm excimer laser gives the ophthalmologist a new tool in the treatment of superficial scarring from a variety of conditions. It also offers great promise as a refractive surgical tool and will have a significant impact on ophthalmic practice within the next decade.

ACKNOWLEDGMENT

This research was supported in part by a grant from Taunton Technologies (now VISX), Health One Corporation, The Friends of Phillips Foundation, Minneapolis, Minnesota, and the Humana Corporation, Louisville, Kentucky. Dr. Sher has received renumeration for travel expenses from VISX Co. and owns stock in VISX Co. bought on the open market. The other authors have no financial interest in VISX Co.

We appreciate the help of Kris Barnes, C.O.T., Ira Younger, M.D., S. Michael Sharp, Angela Tucci, and Susan Sutton.

REFERENCES

1. Dausch D, Schröder E: The treatment of corneal and scleral diseases with the excimer laser, *Fortschr Ophthalmol* 87:115-120, 1990.
2. Draft clinical guidance for the preparation and contents of an investigational device exemption (IDE) application for excimer laser devices used in ophthalmic surgery for myopic photorefractive keratectomy (PRK). Office of Device Evaluation, Division of Ophthalmic Devices, Food and Drug Administration, *Refract Corneal Surg* 6:265-269, 1990.
3. Goodman GL et al: Corneal healing following laser refractive keratectomy, *Arch Ophthalmol* 107:1799-1803, 1989.
4. Keates RH et al: Absorption of 308-nm excimer laser radiation by balanced salt solution, sodium hyaluronate, and human cadaver eyes, *Arch Ophthalmol* 108:1611-1613, 1990.
5. L'Esperance FA et al: Excimer laser instrumentation and technique for human corneal surgery, *Arch Ophthalmol* 107:131-139, 1989.
6. L'Esperance FA et al: Human excimer laser corneal surgery: preliminary report, *Trans Am Ophthalmol Soc* 86:208-270, 270-275, 1989.
7. McDonald MB et al: Clinical results of 193 nm excimer laser central photorefractive keratectomy for myopia; the partially sighted and sighted eye studies, *Invest Ophthalmol Vis Sci* 31(suppl):245, 1990.
8. Maguire LJ et al: Topography and ray tracing analysis of patient with excellent visual acuity 3 months after excimer laser photorefractive keratectomy for myopia, *Refract Corneal Surg* 7:122-128, 1991.
9. Sedarevic O et al: Excimer laser therapy for experimental *Candida* keratitis, *Am J Ophthalmol* 99:534-538, 1985.
10. Seiler T, Kahle G, Kriegerowski M: Excimer laser (193 nm) myopic keratomileusis in sighted and blind human eyes, *Refract Corneal Surg* 6:165-173, 1990.
11. Seiler T, Wollensak J: Myopic photorefractive keratectomy with the excimer laser: one year follow up, *Ophthalmology*.
12. Sher NA, Bowers RA, Zabel RW, et al: Clinical use of the 193-nm excimer laser in the treatment of corneal scars, *Arch Ophthalmol* 109(4):491-498, 1991.
13. Sher NA et al: Excimer laser photorefractive keratectomy in high myopia—a multicenter study, *Arch Opthalmol* 110:935-943, 1992.
14. Stark WJ et al: Optical pachometry in the measurement of anterior corneal disease: an evaluative tool for phototherapeutic keratectomy, *Arch Ophthalmol* 108:12-13, 1990.
15. Steinert RF, Puliafito CA: Excimer laser phototherapeutic keratectomy for a corneal nodule, *Refract Corneal Surg* 6:352, 1990.
16. Taylor DM et al: Human excimer laser lamellar keratectomy: a clinical study, *Ophthalmology* 96:654-664, 1989.
17. Trokel SL, Srinivasan R, Braren B: Excimer laser surgery of the cornea, *Am J Ophthalmol* 96:710-715, 1983.
18. Tuft S, Marshall J, Rothery S: Stromal remodeling following photorefractive keratectomy, *Lasers in Ophthalmology* 1:177-183, 1987.
19. Uozato H, Guyton DL: Centering corneal surgical procedures, *Am J Ophthalmol* 103:264-275, 1987.
20. Waring GO et al: Results of the Prospective Evaluation of Radial Keratotomy (PERK) Study one year after surgery, *Ophthalmology* 92:177-207, 1985.
21. Zabel RW et al: Myopic excimer laser keratectomy: a preliminary report, *Refract Corneal Surg* 6:329-334, 1990.

Technique and current status of photorefractive keratectomy with the Summit Excimed UV 200 excimer laser

DANIEL S. DURRIE

VANCE M. THOMPSON

The ExciMed UV 200 LA excimer laser (Summit Technology, Watertown Massachusetts) has been used in well-controlled clinical studies over the past few years in the pursuit of the ideal refractive surgery procedure. In this chapter, we discuss the technique of wide-area photoablation, or photorefractive keratectomy (PRK), and the current status of Summit Technology's Food and Drug Administration (FDA)-approved clinical study of their excimer laser.

LASER AND DELIVERY SYSTEM

The ExciMed UV 200 LA is an excimer laser system designed specifically for ophthalmology (Fig. 41-12). This system uses a premixed blend of argon, fluorine, and buffer gases to produce pulsed, laser radiation in the ultraviolet range of the electromagnetic spectrum at a wavelength of 193 nm.[7] In the laser, a dimer is formed when an inert gas (argon) and a halogen (fluorine) are combined with the assis-

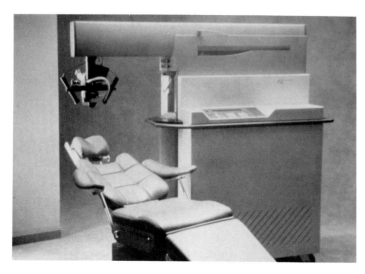

Fig. 41-12. Summit Technology's OmniMed Excimer/Holmium Refractive Laser System.

tance of an electrical discharge, thus producing an excited complex, argon fluoride (ArF).[8] When the excited ArF complex loses some of its energy and falls back to the ground state, a photon of energy, with a wavelength of 193 nm is released. Through a sophisticated series of mirrors the beam is amplified and then leaves the laser cavity through an optical rail, which consists of a series of monitors, optics, and aperturing devices that evaluates, shapes, and focuses the beam.

The beam then strikes a point on the cornea defined by the intersection of two helium-neon (HeNe) aiming beams. At this point the laser beam has the proper characteristics of size, shape, and energy density for the intended surgical procedures.

Each photon in the beam has 6.4 electron volts (eV) of energy, sufficient to easily overcome the intermolecular bond energy of 3.5 eV between molecules of the cornea. Because each photon contains a high amount of energy, the laser beam can be shaped into a parallel beam rather than needing to be focused to achieve necessary power levels as seen with YAG or argon lasers.[1]

PHOTOREFRACTIVE KERATECTOMY TECHNIQUE

At the start of each day, a beam profile and alignment test is performed with a test kit provided by Summit Technology. The only variables requiring entry into the laser computer are the desired correction and optical zone diameter. The computer then makes the necessary calculations. After this the laser is armed and tested. The internal test mode provides

verification that the proper energy levels are being attained for the desired correction.

Next, the patient, who is lying on a comfortable bed, is centered under the laser microscope utilizing the two HeNe aiming beams so that the cornea is centered on. This centration is performed on the patient's pupil, which has been constricted with pilocarpine given 30 minutes before the procedure. A drop of topical anesthetic is instilled. The nonoperative eye is typically gently patched so that the patient can concentrate on fixation with the operative eye. The patient is instructed to fixate on an annular target inside the laser delivery system. When the patient is fixated on the target and the HeNe beams are centered on the cornea and the pupillary axis, the patient is in precise focus with the laser. It is of note that after the HeNe beams are brought to a pinpoint focus on the cornea, they diverge and are seen as two spots equally spaced at the 3 and 9 o'clock positions in the midperiphery of the iris.

At this point a training session is performed to familiarize the patient with the upcoming PRK procedure. First the laser is programmed for a 3-diopter correction. One percent hydroxypropyl methylcellulose is applied on to the entire corneal surface. This layer of liquid will block any laser ablation on the patient's cornea. The patient is instructed that no corneal ablation will take place during this test but that the goal is to see how well the patient can fixate while the laser is being fired. The laser is armed and then fired. While the laser is being fired, the patient is closely observed for the ability to continuously fixate on the internal target.

The final patient training exercise is then performed on the patient's dry epithelium. The goal of this portion of the procedure is threefold: (1) to allow the patient to hear the louder, snapping noise made when the laser is hitting dry tissue, (2) to mark the epithelium over the visual axis so that adequacy of concentration can be checked, and (3) to determine the size of the optical zone and extent of corneal epithelial removal for laser keratectomy directly upon Bowman's membrane.

After the physician is satisfied with the testing phase of the procedure, an optical zone marker, 1 mm larger than the optical-zone treatment area, is centered over the epithelial mark and an indentation is made. A 64 Beaver blade or Patan spatula is then used to remove the corneal epithelium out to the border marked by the optical zone marker. The epithelium is ablated at a different rate from that of Bowman's membrane, and it is believed that epithelial removal improves the accuracy of the procedure.[6] Epithelial removal is achieved with the patient under the laser to minimize the period between débridement and laser ablation and avoid corneal stromal dehydration. Bowman's membrane is carefully cleaned of debris using a Weck-Cel or similar sponge. Next a very small amount of hydroxypropyl methylcellulose is applied to the corneal surface, and further cleaning of the Bowman's membrane is performed with the Weck-Cel sponge. The methylcellulose also acts to smooth out surface irregularities commonly present in Bowman's membrane. The cleaning of the surface should be continued until all the methylcellulose and any residual epithelium is removed. The goal is to complete the cleansing procedure in approximately 1 minute to minimize dehydration of the Bowman's membrane and stroma.

The patient is again asked to fixate on the fixation target of the laser. The HeNe beams are recentered on the cornea with use of the constricted pupil, and the patient is warned that the procedure is about to begin. After again emphasizing fixation, the laser pedal is pressed and the laser begins firing. The foot pedal is continuously pressed until the laser stops firing. Fixation is monitored very closely. Most pa-

tients fixate well, but should a rare patient lose fixation, the procedure is stopped, the patient is directed to refixate, and the procedure is completed (Fig. 41-13). Antibiotic ointment is instilled, and the eye is patched. The patient is reminded about the preoperative discussion of probable pain that evening and instructed on the use of pain medications.

Until reepithelialization is complete in 1 to 3 days, only antibiotic ointment is used on the epithelium. After reepithelialization, topical cortical steroids are utilized. In the Summit Technology–sponsored Food and Drug Administration PRK study, the steroid protocol consists of FML Forte 5 times per day for the first month and then FML 0.1% 4 times a day for the second month. For the third month FML is used 3 times a day and thereafter at the discretion of the individual physician based on the patient's refraction and degree of corneal haze.

PHOTOREFRACTIVE KERATECTOMY CLINICAL STUDIES

As of September 1, 1991, over 6500 photorefractive keratectomy procedures had been performed in the world using the Summit ExciMed UV 200 excimer laser.[3] The first report on PRK performed on sighted, human eyes was published in May, 1990, by Theo Seiler, utilizing the Summit excimer laser.[4] He concluded that the excimer laser showed good predictability in reducing myopia.[4,5]

In the United States, the study of PRK has undergone carefully controlled FDA clinical trials. Phase I of the clinical trials was performed on animal and blind, human eyes with the results supporting the idea that excimer laser could be a safe and effective technique for reducing myopia. Patients included in phase IIA of the clinical trials were either amblyopic, anisometropic, or both. The most significant finding of this phase was the lack of stability in the higher dioptric attempted powers. Even though success was initially reported of up to 15.0 diopters of myopic correction by some investigators, almost all patients with greater than 6.0 diopters of attempted correction had significant regression over time. Nevertheless, in almost all cases best corrected vision was preserved.

In phase IIB, 100 patients from five different sites in the United States were treated and have been followed up, at the time of this printing, for 15 months. The 1-year results of these 500 phase IIB patients are pending publication. It is of note that because of the regression of correction in the patients with greater than 6 diopters of myopia in phase IIA, the upper limit of correction in phase IIB was limited to 6.0 diopters of myopia.[2]

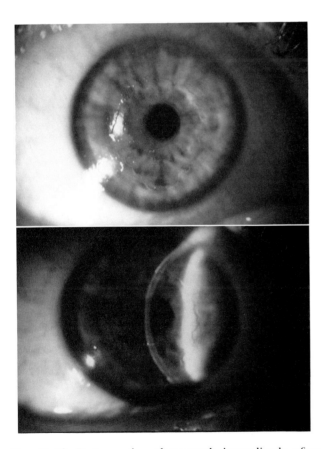

Fig. 41-13. Postoperative photograph immediately after photorefractive keratectomy.

Phase III was initiated in July 1991 and included 700 patients at 10 different sites in the United States. All were completed by January 1992. A 2-year hiatus must take place before these data can finally be turned in to the FDA. After this, it would take approximately 6 months before the FDA could complete its analysis of the data and act upon it. Thus one could predict possible approval of the excimer laser for general use by the autumn of 1994. The beauty of the FDA-controlled clinical trial is that it will provide both patients and ophthalmologists sufficient data for informed decision making about photorefractive keratectomy.

Currently, studies are being performed to expand the range of correction of PRK and also to improve its stability. Active research is being performed in the area of wound modulation in an attempt to control the rate and amount of epithelial hyperplasia and anterior stromal remodeling. Use of the two-optical-zone treatment to perform PRK is being evaluated in an attempt to make a peripheral blend zone to create a smoother, peripheral transition and, one would hope, a more stable refractive result. Using a combination of radial keratotomy and PRK is also being evaluated to possibly expand the range of both procedures. Another exciting area of research is in the field of myopic keratomileusis. By removal of the corneal cap and performance of the excimer ablation on the stromal side of the cap, the surgeon is able to leave the epithelium undisturbed and potentially achieve higher corrections with less chance of regression. With the refinements in microkeratomes, we have found that keratomileusis can be performed in a safer and more predictable fashion than was possible previously. Another area that Summit Technology is actively researching is the use of an ablatable mask. The mask consists of a substance that gradually erodes and can help shape the beam that hits the corneal surface. One can see that when the thickness of the mask is varied in different areas the beam can be shaped in multiple configurations for the correction of myopia or astigmatism. Early results with the ablatable mask have been encouraging.

SUMMARY

Photorefractive keratectomy has the potential to revolutionize the field of refractive surgery. Early results have been encouraging, and as time goes on the stability of the procedure is looking good for an eye with less than 6 diopters of myopia. Current areas of research appear to be on the right track for the eventual long-term stability and treatment of higher levels of myopia. Through the carefully FDA-controlled clinical study of excimer laser, physicians and patients will eventually be able to incorporate this exciting new technology into their practices and lives.

REFERENCES

1. Durrie DS, Thompson VM: Excimer laser and its uses in refractive surgery, *Ophthalmic Pract* 9:112-117, 1991.
2. Hunkeler JD, Durrie DS, Thompson VM, et al: *Photorefractive keratectomy with the Summit excimer laser: interim results on sighted patient eyes,* Presented at the Third International Laser Congress, November 3, 1990, Atlanta, Ga.
3. Muller D: *Summit Technology introductory lecture,* Presented at the First Annual Congress Summit International Laser Group, August 31, 1991, Geneva, Switzerland.
4. Seiler TS, Kahle G, Kriegerowski M: Excimer laser (193 nm) myopic keratomileusis in sighted and blind human eyes, *Refract Corneal Surg* 6:165-173, 1990.
5. Seiler T, Kriegerowski M: *Excimer laser keratomileusis (PRK) for myopic correction: 1 year follow-up in sighted eyes,* Presented at the Third International Laser Congress, November 3, 1990, Atlanta, Ga.
6. Seiler T, Kriegerowski M, Schnoy N: Ablation rate of human corneal epithelium and Bowman's layer with the excimer laser (193 nm), *Refract Corneal Surg* 6:99-102, 1990.
7. Summit Technology, Inc: *ExciMed® UV 200 LA laser system user's manual,* Watertown, Mass, 1991, pp 2,1-2,3.
8. Waring GO (AOS thesis): Development of a system for excimer laser corneal surgery, *Trans Am Ophthalmol Soc* 87:854-983, 1989.

Part V

EYE BANKING—MEDICAL ASPECTS

Chapter 42

Medical Standards for Eye Banks

Development

MARK J. MANNIS

WILLIAM J. REINHART

Quality assurance is a term born of two concepts. The first of these is the physician's oath, obligating him above all to do no harm. The second is a major theme of modern medical consumerism—the right of the patient to expect the very highest quality of care. The development of medical standards for eye banking was the natural and inevitable outgrowth of these two basic concepts. The major thrust of the establishment of these standards was to assure both physician and patient that corneal tissue being used for transplantation is of the highest quality and will do no harm.

HISTORY

When the American Academy of Ophthalmology and Otolaryngology formed a committee on eye banks in 1957, one of the avowed purposes was to generate standardization of procedures among eye banks throughout the country.[7] The trend toward this standardization gained the momentum through the formative years of the Eye Bank Association of America (EBAA) beginning in 1961. It was not however, until the mid-1970s that standardization became linked with the notion of regulation, and it was this link that brought to fruition established medical standards. Three forces contributed to the codification of these standards. The most important of these was the growing concern among medical directors and corneal surgeons that all eye banks function properly. The first reports of disease transmission from donor tissue to healthy recipients had begun to appear in the medical literature, an indication that transmission of infectious diseases was a real hazard

of corneal transplantation and that effective screening and processing of tissue was crucial in order to avoid potentially disastrous complications.[9,16,24,26,29] This potential for disease transmission is now well established.[8] In the absence of any regulation, there was no way to be assured that tissue was being screened or handled properly. Secondly, the eye banking community believed strongly that the most effective and pertinent quality assurance program would be one that came from within the professional ophthalmologic and eye banking community. Last, realizing the importance of standardization and self-regulation, the Eye Bank Committee of the academy strongly urged codification of medical standards by the EBAA.[10,11]

The first meeting at which medical standards were discussed at length took place at Callaway Gardens, Georgia, in April 1977.[10] Subsequently, in October 1978, the EBAA established a committee to formulate uniform medical standards. This began a series of long and arduous deliberations over the purposes, contents, and mode of implementation of the standards document.[11] The first draft of a workable document was completed after a lengthy meeting at O'Hare International Airport in Chicago in March 1979.[12] The tasks before these committees were extremely difficult. Based on only limited data about the transmissibility of a variety of diseases through corneal transplants, they were faced with making decisions about donor suitability. Practices, such as culturing of donor tissue, were not uniform at that time, and decisions had to be made as to whether such practices were mandatory or optional. Care had to be taken to be sure that decision making was not arbitrary; nonetheless, some decisions had to be made on the basis of limited or seemingly anecdotal data.

531

Even more compelling were issues such as the specificity of standards and how restrictive they should actually be. Based on limited data, these were difficult and sometimes very controversial decisions to make. In meetings of legendary length, the medical standards were hammered out point by point. The "O'Hare report" produced by this committee included the first draft of detailed medical standards for eye banks. The document that was produced encompassed (1) training and education of medical personnel within the eye bank, (2) assurance of donor quality control, (3) sterility control of the eye bank laboratory, (4) assurance of equitable distribution of tissue, and (5) a system of inspection of eye banks ensuring continued maintenance of standards. The O'Hare draft was presented at the interim board meeting of the EBAA in Colorado Springs later that year.[13] Second and third drafts were to emerge from the ensuing meetings of its medical standards committee until, in November 1980, the final document was approved at the annual meeting of the EBAA in Chicago.[14] By May 1981, the first medical standards inspection questionnaires were distributed to member eye banks for completion. These questionnaires were the first step in implementing medical standards nationwide through an inspection and certification process.

THE DOCUMENT

The complete EBAA Medical Standards Document is included in the second part of this chapter. The EBAA Medical Standards and Certification Procedure for Eye Banks has been developed to apply to any and all aspects of eye banking from the identification and screening of donors to the distribution of tissue for transplantation, research, and teaching. Included are requirements for the procurement of corneal and other ocular tissue and the laboratory processing of that tissue including its preservation, evaluation, and storage. The document outlines the responsibilities of the eye bank director, the medical director, and the technical staff along with the educational and certification requirements of the medical director and technical staff.

From its inception, the EBAA Medical Standards Document was intended as a "living document." True to this intent, included in the formulation is a method for ongoing revision of the standards in order to keep pace with the rapidly changing field of tissue transplantation. The EBAA Medical Standards Document underwent its first major revision in 1983 and has been amended to some extent every 6 months at meetings of the EBAA Medical Standards Committee. The last major revision in the

format of the EBAA Medical Standards Document was adopted in 1990. In the most recent document, details concerning eye bank procedures have been removed so that the document now is primarily concerned with eye bank medical policy. An accompanying procedures manual is presently being developed and is now available. The EBAA Procedures Manual standardizes the eye bank procedures through which EBAA-certified eye banks implement the policies of the EBAA Medical Standards Document.

EVOLUTION

The evolution of medical standards for eye banking over the past decade has focused upon ensuring quality donor tissue and eliminating the possibility of disease transmission through keratoplasty.

Corneal transplant surgeons have known that viral disease can be transmitted by donor corneal tissue since 1974 when a single case report of transmission of Creutzfeldt-Jakob disease (CJD), resulting in the death of the recipient, appeared[9] 5 years after the infectivity of CJD was recognized.[17] Since then, evidence of transmission of CJD virus by preserved dura mater homografts[4] and by pituitary-derived human growth hormone[15] have been documented. In the 1975 Gifford Lecture Dr. A.G. DeVoe recommended that corneal tissue from donors dying of neurologic disease of known or suspected viral etiology such as CJD, subacute sclerosing panencephalitis, and progressive multifocal leukoencephalopathy should not be used for transplantation and that tissue from donors dying of chronic central nervous system disorders of obscure origin should be used with extreme caution.[8]

In 1978 a 37-year-old corneal recipient died of rabies 7 weeks after receiving a cornea from a 39-year-old donor who had died of presumed Guillain-Barré syndrome.[2] Fluorescent antibody and viral isolation studies confirmed the transmission of rabies virus as the cause of death in both donor and recipient.[20] Subsequently three additional cases have been reported.[18] In all four cases the diagnosis of rabies was not suspected before the donor's death, underscoring the importance of not using transplant tissue from persons who have died of neurologic illness of unknown cause.[3]

These cases of donor transmission of a fatal viral disease to a corneal transplant recipient served as the catalyst for developing stringent medical screening of donors when the first EBAA Medical Standards Document was developed in 1980. The potential transmission of other viral diseases by corneal transplantation has been an ongoing concern of the

EBAA Medical Standards Committee meetings ever since.

The continued revision of these medical standards during the 1980s was in large part defined by the newly discovered acquired immunodeficiency syndrome (AIDS).[18] The first cases were diagnosed in 1981 in young homosexual men in the United States and by 1982 the collection of clinical conditions associated with a compromised immune system as the common denominator was named the "acquired immunodeficiency syndrome" (AIDS). In 1982 there was already clear evidence that an infectious agent associated with AIDS could be transmitted by blood transfusion and that there was a prolonged incubation period. In 1983 the U.S. Public Health Service was able to publish risk factors for AIDS and recommendations for its prevention. Exclusion criteria were developed for blood donors and were adapted for the medical screening of eye donors by the EBAA Medical Standards Committee. In 1983 and 1984 a virus now called the "human immunodeficiency virus type 1" (HIV-1) was identified as being the causative agent.

In 1985 the first laboratory test to detect the HIV-1 virus was licensed by the FDA and became the first mandated donor serologic test required by EBAA Medical Standards. Since 95% of patients who are exposed to HIV through blood transfusions become infected, blood collection agencies, the American Association of Blood Banks, and the FDA, which regulates blood banks, have been most rigorous and sophisticated in developing a donor deferral system for blood and plasma donors who have high-risk behavior. Exclusion of blood donors based solely on geographic or national origins has recently been eliminated and replaced by an expanded oral interview aimed at identifying donors who are at high risk for transmitting HIV disease.[22] The advisory notice also extends the existing donor exclusion period from 6 to 12 months for those who have received a blood transfusion or who have paid money or provided drugs or other material payment for sex.

In 1989 an estimated 1 million living persons in the United States were infected with HIV with an annual incidence of 1500 to 2000 in newborns and 40,000 in adults.[5] The majority of these HIV-infected people are young adults, an age group considered by many corneal surgeons to be the ideal donor group for corneal tissue for transplantation. Screening deceased donors for high-risk behavior cannot be as reliable as it is for living donors, and there is therefore an implicit greater reliance on serologic donor testing for HIV. Fortunately, the first

enzyme immunoassay licensed by the FDA for the detection of HIV-1 antibody has been a reliable test, with an overall analytic performance of 99.3%.[21] There is evidence that careful screening of medical examiner cases by eye bank procurement personnel for historical or physical evidence of HIV risk factors is an effective first step in eliminating a substantial proportion of HIV-infected cases as potential donors.[21] Although screening donors for possible HIV infection by history, examination, and serologic testing must remain a major concern of eye banking, it is reassuring that even with eight cases of corneal transplantation from cadaveric donors that tested positive for antibodies against HIV and an average of over 30,000 corneal transplant cases a year over the last 10 years of the HIV epidemic, there have been no known cases of either seroconversion or HIV-associated disease.[23,25]

In 1986 the EBAA was informed of the probable transmission of hepatitis B by corneal transplantation in 2 cases which were subsequently the subject of a poster presentation at the American Academy of Ophthalmology meeting in October 1988 by Hoft and associates.[19] Donor specific screening for HBV by HBsAg was the second serologic test required by EBAA Medical Standards in 1986. The major problem with the screening test for hepatitis surface antigen in the past has been false-positive results caused by hemolysis of donor blood. For blood donors, a hemolyzed blood sample can be managed by redrawing blood for testing. This is not feasible for a cadaveric eye donor in whom a suspected false positive on a hemolyzed blood sample results in the inability to distribute already processed donor corneal tissue for transplantation that is otherwise completely acceptable. New methods for obtaining and processing drawn blood and newer protocols for testing have eliminated this as a major loss of transplantable corneal tissue.

Viral hepatitis caused by non-A, non-B viruses and, in particular, parenterally transmitted non-A, non-B hepatitis now recognized as hepatitis C virus (HCV) has remained an epidemiologic problem and has been of particular concern to blood bankers.[28] Although acute HCV hepatitis is often clinically undetected unless liver function tests are monitored after transfusion, it is a serious infection, since 50% of acute HCV cases become chronic, 20% of chronic HCV carriers develop cirrhosis in a mean time of 17 years, and there is an increased risk of developing hepatocellular carcinoma in a mean time of 20 years.[1] In 1990, blood banks immediately adopted the test for screening the blood supply on hand and for all future donors.[27] The American Association of

Tissue Banks mandated the test for HCV soon thereafter. After the validity of the HCV test for cadaver donors had been evaluated by several eye banks for a 6-month period, the EBAA Medical Standards Committee also mandated that eye donors be screened for HCV, using the test in early 1991. The HCV test is less specific than commercially available tests for HBV and HIV, and at present there are not yet confirmatory tests for suspected false-positive HCV donor screening tests. In addition, it is not known whether HCV has been or can be transmitted by corneal transplantation though the epidemiology is similar to that for HBV virus, which can be transmitted by corneal transplantation. As with all issues of serologic screening, HCV testing of corneal donors continues to undergo scrutiny.

CERTIFICATION

Closely linked to the development of the Medical Standards policy is a certification process initiated in 1981 and made available to any eye bank that can comply with EBAA Medical Standards. Certification, which is currently valid for 3 years, requires a site visit by one or more members of the EBAA Medical Standards Site Visit Subcommittee. The details of the site visit and certification process are outlined in Chapter 47, p. 670.

In 1990, the Health Care Financing Agency (HCFA) of the Department of Health and Human Services (HHS) published the proposed regulations to implement the Clinical Laboratory Improvement Amendments passed by the United States Congress in 1988 (CLIA-88).[6] These regulations would require that all laboratories in the United States and its territories that examine human specimens meet performance requirements based on test complexity and risk factors related to erroneous test results in order to be certified by the HHS and would require that laboratories associated with tissue banks and tissue repositories meet federal requirements.

Eye banking falls under the CLIA-88 amendments as proposed by HCFA. As a result, it is already apparent that adjustment of the EBAA Medical Standards and the certification process for eye banks will be required. Proficiency testing programs will also have to be developed for periodic evaluation of an eye bank's performance in donor medical history and chart review, corneal evaluation by slitlamp and specular microscopy, and other laboratory functions. The EBAA will work closely with the federal government to ensure that the Medical Standards are consistent with CLIA regulations.

FUTURE OF THE EBAA MEDICAL STANDARDS

Eye banking represents the oldest organized tissue-banking effort in transplantation medicine. The establishment of medical standards and the internal regulation of the medical practices of eye banks is a landmark accomplishment. With the increasing need for transfer of tissues nationwide and internationally, the medical standards program ensures that tissues coming from a certified eye bank can be relied upon as meeting the screening and handling requirements that make it safe and efficacious. The medical standards process is in continual evolution. New disease entities and their implications for transplantation require constant revisions of the standards document. New uses for and methods of processing human corneal tissue will alter what types of tissue are acceptable for distribution and how they are handled. The establishment of medical examiner's laws have changed the way in which tissue is screened and handled.

The explosive growth of organ and tissue transplantation is moving from self-regulation through the EBAA Medical Standards toward an increasing role of the federal government in the control of transplant activities. The self-regulatory process may become the province of a team of professionals dedicated solely to the maintenance of quality assurance in eye banking. The EBAA is now established as the standard-setting agency for eye banking in the United States and will, no doubt, continue to mediate and refine the quality assurance programs developed in the last decade.

ACKNOWLEDGMENTS

The medical standards document is the product of many dedicated persons. We have purposely avoided individual names in recounting the evolution of the standards program. Special thanks are due to Arthur Boruchoff, Fred Brightbill, Margaret Kelm, and Jay Krachmer for their help in providing background information.

REFERENCES

1. Alter MJ, Sampliner RE: Hepatitis C and miles to go before we sleep, *N Engl J Med* 321:1538-1539, 1989 (Editorial).
2. Centers for Disease Control: Human-to-human transmission of rabies by a corneal transplant—Idaho, *MMWR* 28:109-111, 1979.
3. Centers for Disease Control: Human-to-human transmission of rabies via corneal transplant—Thailand, *MMWR* 30:473-474, 1981.
4. Centers for Disease Control: Update: Creutzfeldt-Jakob disease in a second patient who received a cadaveric dura mater graft, *MMWR* 38:37-43, 1989.
5. Centers for Disease Control: Estimates of HIV prevalence and projected AIDS cases: summary of a workshop, Oct. 31–Nov. 1, 1989, *MMWR* 39:110-119, 1990.

6. Centers for Disease Control: Public Health Service interagency recommendations for screening donated blood, plasma, organs, tissues, and semen for evidence of hepatitis B and hepatitis C, *MMWR*. (In press.)
7. Committee on Eye Banks: American Academy of Ophthalmology and Otolaryngology: Minutes of open meeting, New York, June 29 1961.
8. DeVoe AG: Complications of keratoplasty, the Gifford Lecture, *Am J Ophthalmol* 79:907-912, 1975.
9. Duffy P et al: Possible person-to-person transmission of Creutzfeldt-Jakob disease, *N Engl J Med* 290:692, 1974.
10. Eye Bank Association of America: Minutes, board of directors meeting, April 1977.
11. Eye Bank Association of America: Minutes, board of directors meeting, Oct 1978.
12. Eye Bank Association of America: O'Hare Report, Minutes, Medical Standards Committee, March 1979.
13. Eye Bank Association of America: Minutes, interim board meeting, May 1979.
14. Eye Bank Association of America: Minutes, board of directors meeting, Nov 1980.
15. Fradkin JE, Schonberger LB, Mills JL, et al: Creutzfeldt-Jakob disease in pituitary growth hormone recipients in the United States, *JAMA* 265:880-884, 1991.
16. Gandhi S, Lamberts DW, Perry HD: Donor to host transmission of disease via corneal transplantation, *Surv Ophthalmol* 25:306-311, 1981.
17. Gibbs CJ Jr, Gajdusek DC: Infection as the etiology of spongiform encephalopathy in Creutzfeldt-Jakob disease, *Science* 165:1023-1025, 1969.
18. Historical data abstracted from: What science knows about AIDS—a single topic issue, *Sci Am* 299:Oct issue, 1988.
19. Hoft RH, Pflugfelder SC, Ullman S, et al: Clinical evidence for hepatitis B transmission resulting from corneal transplant. Scientific Poster presentation #39, annual meeting of the American Academy of Ophthalmology, Oct 1988.
20. Hough SA, Burton RC, Wilson RW, et al: Human-to human transmission of rabies virus by a corneal transplant, *N Engl J Med* 300:603-604, 1979.
21. Hwang DG, Ward DE, Trousdale MD, Smith RE: Human immunodeficiency virus seroprevalence among potential corneal donors from medical examiner cases, *Am J Ophthalmol* 109:92-93, 1990 (Letter).
22. Marwick C: Will more donor questions make blood safer? *JAMA* 265:838-839, 1991.
23. O'Day DM: Diseases potentially transmitted through corneal transplantation, *Ophthalmology* 96:1133-1138, 1989.
24. Payne JW: New directions in eye banking, *Trans Am Ophthalmol Soc* 78:983-1026, 1980.
25. Pepose JS: Transfer of infection via corneal transplantation, *Transplant Proc* 21:3130-3132, 1989.
26. Shaw EL, Aquavella JV: Pneumococcal endophthalmitis following grafting of corneal tissue from a (cadaver) kidney donor, *Ann Ophthalmol* 9:435-440, 1977.
27. Soloway HB: The advent of hepatitis C testing, *Med Lab Observer* Nov:33-36, 1990.
28. Stevens CE, Taylor PE, Pindyck J, et al: Epidemiology of hepatitis C virus, *JAMA* 263:49-53, 1990.
29. White JH: Fungal contamination of donor eyes, *Br J Ophthalmol* 53:30-33, 1969.

EBAA Medical Standards— October 1991

These standards have the approval of the Eye Banking Committee of the American Academy of Ophthalmology.

A1.000 **Introduction and purpose**
   A1.100 Scope
B1.000 **Certification**
   B1.100 Eye bank inspection
C1.000 **Personnel**
   C1.100 Director
   C1.200 Medical director
   C1.300 Technical staff
C2.000 **Training, certification, and continuing education of technical personnel**
C3.000 **Facilities**
   C3.100 Eye bank laboratory
   C3.200 Equipment, maintenance and cleaning
   C3.300 Instruments and reagents
   C3.400 Procedures manual
   C3.500 Satellite laboratories
   C3.600 Infection control and safety
   C3.700 Waste disposal
D1.000 **Donor screening**
   D1.100 Screening of donors
      D1.110 Potentially hazardous donors
      D1.120 Contraindications
   D1.200 Documentation of donor information
   D1.300 Method of consent
   D1.400 Donor age
   D1.500 Interval between death, enucleation, excision, and preservation
   D1.600 Eye maintenance prior to enucleation
   D1.700 Living donors
E1.000 **Procurement and preservation procedures**
   E1.100 Enucleation procedure
   E1.200 In situ and laboratory removal of the corneoscleral rim
   E1.300 Use of short or intermediate term preservation medium
   E1.400 Long term preservation
   E1.500 Whole globe preservation
   E1.600 Scleral preservation
F1.000 **Tissue evaluation**
   F1.100 Gross examination
   F1.200 Slit-lamp examination
   F1.300 Specular microscopy

G1.000 **Quality assurance**
    G1.100   Quality control
    G1.200   Testing
           G1.210   Microbiologic culturing
           G1.220   HIV screening
           G1.230   Hepatitis B screening
           G1.240   Hepatitis C screening
           G1.250   HTLV-I and HTLV-II screening
           G1.260   Syphilis screening
H1.000 **Non-surgical donor tissue**
I1.000 **Storage**
J1.000 **Labeling**
K1.000 **Distribution of tissue**
    K1.100   Review of donor medical history
    K1.200   Receivers of tissue
    K1.300   Fair and equitable system
L1.000 **Documentation to accompany donor tissue**
    L1.100   Tissue report form
    L1.200   Package insert form
L2.000 **Packaging, sealing, and packing for transport**
M1.000 **Eye Bank records**
    M1.100   Length of storage
    M1.200   Confidentiality
    M1.300   Donor screening forms
    M1.400   Minimum information to be retained
    M1.500   Recipient follow-up information
N1.000 **Amendments**

A1.000 **Introduction and Purpose**

These standards have been developed to assure consistently acceptable levels of quality, proficiency and ethics in dealing with eye tissue for transplantation and to define the minimum standards of practice in the procurement, preservation, storage and distribution of eye tissue for transplantation and research, as determined by the ophthalmological medical community.

    A1.100   Scope

These standards are intended to apply to any and all aspects of eye banking, to include:

- Identification and screening of donors
- Procurement of eye and corneal tissue
- Laboratory processing of tissue, including preservation and biomicroscopic examination of tissue

- Storage of tissue
- Distribution of tissue for transplantation, research and teaching

These standards shall be reviewed at least annually and revised as necessary to incorporate current research findings and improved clinical practice.

B1.000 **Certification**

In order for an eye bank to become an accredited member of the Eye Bank Association of America, it must comply with the EBAA Bylaws and the following:

1. Demonstrate compliance with EBAA Medical Standards.
2. Pass the site visit inspection by the EBAA Medical Standards Committee.
3. Demonstrate proficiency in all aspects of eye banking by procuring, processing and distributing (within the geographic territory it defines as its service area) at least 25 surgical corneas for penetrating keratoplasty annually and provide documentation of their performance.

Eye Banks applying for EBAA membership must complete the Medical Standards Committee Questionnaire. Pending approval of the EBAA Board of Directors, the applicant may be accepted for provisional EBAA membership and will be subject to an on-site inspection within one year. A provisional member eye bank must complete the certification process within one year after obtaining provisional membership status in the EBAA. Any provisional member eye bank failing to complete the certification process after a site visit will have until the time of the next meeting to correct deficiencies and satisfy certification requirements. If, at the end of this period, the provisional member eye bank fails to meet certification standards, it may not proceed to full membership with voting rights.

Once certified, an eye bank must be inspected and recertified at least every three years to maintain certification and voting membership in the EBAA.

    B1.100   Eye Bank Inspection

The Medical Standards Committee of the EBAA shall be responsible for inspecting member Eye Banks as outlined in the written procedures of the Committee.

Certification and recertification site visits shall be scheduled following written notification of the impending inspection.

Unannounced visits may be conducted should an allegation of violation of Medical Standards be made to the Committee. Failure to permit an inspection will result in suspension or revocation of an eye bank's certification.

Demonstration of proficiency in any and all aspects of eye banking may be required during the site visit and of any or all technical personnel.

C1.000 Personnel

C1.100 Director

All policies and procedures of each eye bank shall be under the supervision of a Director appointed by the eye bank's board of Directors, Board of Regents or other governing body. The Director shall be responsible for all administrative operations including compliance with these standards.

The Director shall be the individual responsible for the day to day operation of the Eye Bank. It is this individual's responsibility to carry out policies of the Eye Bank's Board, to determine what tissues are to be collected, and to prescribe clinically acceptable means for their processing, quality control, storage and distribution.

The Director, if not a physician, shall consult with the Medical Director, as well as other medical and legal authorities, in carrying out prescribed responsibilities as necessary. These consultations shall be documented and made available for review during a site visit inspection.

The Director shall provide all staff members with adequate information to perform their duties safely and competently.

Delegation of responsibility for the clinical work of the eye bank shall be as follows:

C1.200 Medical Director

The Eye Bank must have a Medical Director.

The Medical Director must be an ophthalmologist who has completed a corneal fellowship or who has demonstrated an expertise in external eye disease, corneal surgery, research or teaching in cornea and/or external disease. If the medical director has not served a corneal fellowship, then the eye bank must have and document a consulting relationship with an ophthalmologist who has.

The Medical Director, in order to maintain his position, shall provide written documentation that he or she has attended an EBAA annual meeting or approved course at least once every three years. This written documentation must be available at the time of the eye bank's site visit inspection. The EBAA office shall be notified of a change of Medical Directors.

C1.300 Technical Staff

The Director shall appoint technical staff and ensure that staff has the appropriate qualifications and training for the performance of their job responsibilities. The Director shall ensure that there are a sufficient number of qualified eye bank technicians and supportive technical staff to promptly and proficiently perform all eye bank laboratory tests and procedures.

Each eye bank must have at least one EBAA certified technician in a supervisory role. If the medical director fulfills this role, he or she must pass an EBAA Technician Certification exam and maintain that certification. For non-certified technicians, the eye bank Executive Director or Medical Director must designate in writing those nonphysician technicians who are qualified and authorized to perform eye bank laboratory procedures.

C2.000 Training, Certification, and Continuing Education of Technical Personnel

An eye bank must provide an orientation program for each new technician and the employee's participation must be documented.

An eye bank must provide educational opportunities such as in-service training programs, attendance at meetings, seminars, and workshops for all technical personnel, including laboratory supervisors, at a frequency that is defined and reasonable for the size and needs of the technical staff.

For an eye bank technician to receive EBAA Certification, he or she must pass the EBAA Technician Certification examination. To sit for the examination, the eye bank technician must be employed by a transplant organization and be recommended by the Executive Director or a physician meeting the requirements of a medical director, as outlined in Section C1.200. A passing grade in both the written and practical portions of the exam will result in EBAA certification, provided that the appropriate fees have been paid. An EBAA certified technician must renew his or her certification at least once every three years by documenting the specified minimum number of continuing education units (CEU's) which have been approved by the EBAA Technician Subcommittee.

C3.000 Facilities

Each eye bank must have sufficient space, equipment and supplies to perform the volume of laboratory services with optimal accuracy, efficiency, sterility, timeliness and safety.

C3.100 Eye Bank Laboratory

The laboratory must be a separate area with limited access in which activities directly related to eye banking are carried out. The laboratory shall have a sink with a drain and running water. There must be adequate counter space for preparation of donor material. The room including walls, floor and sink must be kept clean at all times. Appropriate documentation of regular laboratory cleaning schedules must be maintained and kept on file for a minimum of three years.

Each eye bank laboratory must have an adequate stable electrical source and a sufficient number of grounded electrical outlets for operating laboratory equipment.

C3.200 Equipment, Maintenance and Cleaning

Each eye bank laboratory shall have a refrigerator with an external device for recording temperature variations. Temperature variations must be recorded daily and remain within the range of 2° to 6° C. These records must be kept for a minimum of three years. The refrigerator shall be maintained for the exclusive use of the eye bank and must contain clearly defined and labeled areas for all tissue stored, i.e., quarantined tissue, surgical tissue awaiting distribution, and research tissue.

In the event of a power failure, there must be provision for immediate notification and action to be taken, which may include an emergency power supply to maintain essential refrigeration.

Appropriate maintenance and certification records must be maintained on each piece of equipment. These records must show dates of inspection, performance evaluations and any maintenance procedures or repairs performed. These records must be kept at least three years.

The eye bank must include in its procedures manual, the monitoring, inspection and cleaning procedures and schedules for each piece of equipment. Documented cleaning schedules for laboratory equipment must be kept on file for a minimum of three years.

C3.300 Instruments and Reagents

Adequate instrumentation must be available to provide for sterile removal of whole eyes and corneas. Instruments must be inspected frequently enough to assure that they function properly.

All sterilized instruments, supplies and reagents, such as corneal preservation medium, must contain expiration dates that are current at all times.

C3.400 Procedures Manual

Each eye bank shall maintain its own procedures manual that details all aspects of its specific retrieval, processing, testing, storage, distribution and quality assurance practices. Each procedure must be initially approved, signed and dated by the Director. Each eye bank must maintain copies of each procedure it uses and the length of time the procedure was in use.

C3.500 Satellite Laboratories

Satellite laboratories that procure, process and distribute tissue must have a certified technician and be supervised by and have access to a qualified Medical Director or his/her delegate. Such satellite laboratories must be inspected as part of the certification process of the parent bank.

C3.600 Infection Control and Safety

Written safety procedures for the eye bank operation shall be established in compliance with the Occupational Safety and Health Act (OSHA Act) of 1970 and/or applicable state statutes, which may supersede. All eye bank personnel must operate under the current Universal Precautions for health care workers issued by the Centers for Disease Control (CDC) of HHS.[1] These written procedures must be included in the eye bank's procedure manual.

C3.700 Waste Disposal

Human tissue and waste items shall be disposed of in such a manner as to minimize any hazard to Eye Bank personnel and the environment and to comply with state and federal regulations. Dignified and proper disposal procedures shall be used to obviate recognizable human remains.

D1.000 **Donor Screening**

Each eye bank shall have a consistent policy for the physical inspection of the donor and examination and documentation of the prospective donor's available medical record or death investigation. Review of all available records on each donor shall be performed by an individual who is qualified by profession, education or training to do so, and who is familiar with the intended use of the tissue.

D1.100 Screening of Donors Must be Conducted for the Following:

D1.110 Tissue from donors with the following are potentially hazardous to eye bank personnel and requires special handling:

- Active viral hepatitis
- Acquired immunodeficiency syndrome (AIDS) or HIV seropositivity
- Active viral encephalitis or encephalitis of unknown origin
- Creutzfeldt-Jakob disease
- Rabies

D1.120 Contraindications

Tissue from donors with the following are potentially health threatening for the recipient(s) or pose a risk to the success of the surgery and shall not be offered for surgical purposes:

A. Penetrating Keratoplasty

---

[1] The Occupational Safety and Health Administration (OSHA) of the Department of Labor (DOL) relies on the CDC's published guidelines in determining compliance with its occupational exposure to HBV and HIV regulations (see DOL OSHA Instruction CPL 2-2.44B dated February 27, 1990). The CDC Guidelines may be found in *MMWR*:36(2), August 21, 1987 and *MMWR*:37(24), June 24, 1988. They are also available from the Superintendent of Documents, U.S. Government Printing Office, Washington, DC 20402, in a publication titled "Guidelines for Protecting the Safety and Health of Health Care Workers."

1. Death of unknown cause
2. Death from central nervous system diseases of unknown etiology
3. Creutzfeldt-Jakob disease
4. Subacute sclerosing panencephalitis
5. Progressive multifocal leukoencephalopathy
6. Congenital rubella
7. Reye's syndrome
8. Active viral encephalitis or encephalitis of unknown origin
9. Active septicemia (bacteremia, fungemia, viremia)
10. Active bacterial or fungal endocarditis
11. Active viral hepatitis
12. Rabies
13. Intrinsic eye disease
    a. Retinoblastoma
    b. Malignant tumors of the anterior ocular segment
    c. Active ocular or intraocular inflammation: conjunctivitis, scleritis, iritis, uveitis, vitreitis, choroiditis, retinitis
    d. Congenital or acquired disorders of the eye that would preclude a successful outcome for the intended use, e.g., a central donor corneal scar for an intended penetrating keratoplasty, keratoconus, and keratoglobus.
    e. Pterygia or other superficial disorders of the conjunctiva or corneal surface involving the central optical area of the corneal button
14. Prior intraocular or anterior segment surgery
    a. Refractive corneal procedures, e.g., radial keratotomy, lamellar inserts, etc.
    b. Laser photoablation surgery
    c. Anterior segment surgery, e.g., cataract, intraocular lens implant, glaucoma filtration
    d. Laser surgical procedures such as argon laser trabeculoplasty, retinal and panretinal photocoagulation do not necessarily preclude use for penetrating keratoplasty but should be cleared by the medical director

15. Active leukemias
16. Active disseminated lymphomas
17. Hepatitis B surface antigen positive donors (as specified in Section G1.230)
18. Recipients of human pituitary-derived growth hormone (pit-hGH) during the years from 1963 to 1985[2]
19. HIV seropositive donors (as specified in Section G1.220)
20. Acquired immunodeficiency syndrome (AIDS)
21. Children (under 13 years old) and infants of mothers with AIDS or at high risk of HIV infection
22. High risk for HIV infection based on data on AIDS cases published by the Public Health Service, Centers for Disease Control,[3] defined by HHS:
    a. Clinical or laboratory evidence of HIV infection (symptoms include: unexplained weight loss; night sweats; blue or purple spots typical of Kaposi's sarcoma on or under the skin, or on mucous membranes; swollen lymph nodes lasting more than one month; persistent white spots or unusual blemishes in the mouth; fever greater than 99° F for more than 10 days; persistent cough and shortness of breath; persistent diarrhea).
    b. Men who have had sex with another man one or more times since 1977;
    c. Past or present intravenous drug abusers;
    d. Persons immigrating since 1977 from Pattern II countries where heterosexual activity is reported as the predominant means of transmission of HIV, e.g., Haiti, Central Africa;

[2]Potential donors who received human pituitary-derived growth hormone (pit-hGH) during childhood at any time during the years from 1963 to 1985 should not be accepted as eye or corneal donors because of the potential risk of transmitting Creutzfeldt-Jakob disease (CJD). Some 7,000 U.S. children received therapeutic pit-hGH through early 1985 and there are unknown numbers of persons who may have used this drug non-therapeutically, e.g., during rigorous physical training. All known recipients and their treating endocrinologists have been notified and a fact sheet is available, HIH Publication No. 88-2793, December 1987.

[3]See CDC HIV/AIDS Surveillance, AIDS cases reported through October 1989, issued November 1989, and Department of Health and Human Services memorandum to all registered blood establishments dated October 30, 1986, from the FDA's Center for Drugs and Biologics.

e. Persons with hemophilia who have received clotting factor concentrates;

f. Sexual partners of any of the above; and

g. Men and women who have engaged in prostitution since 1977 and persons who have been their heterosexual partners within the past six months.

23. HTLV-I or HTLV-II infection

24. Active syphilis

25. Hepatitis C seropositive donors

B. Lamellar or Patch Grafts

Criteria are the same as listed for penetrating keratoplasty except that tissue with local eye disease affecting the corneal endothelium or previous ocular surgery that does not compromise the corneal stroma, e.g., aphakia, iritis, is acceptable for use.

C. Epikeratoplasty

Criteria are the same as listed for penetrating keratoplasty except that tissue with local eye disease affecting the corneal endothelium, e.g., aphakia, iritis, is acceptable for use. Death to preservation time may be extended.

D. Scleral Tissue

Criteria are the same as listed for penetrating keratoplasty except that tissue with local eye disease affecting the corneal endothelium, e.g., aphakia, iritis, is acceptable for use. Death to preservation time may be extended.

D1.200 Documentation of Donor Information

Donor screening forms and/or copies of medical charts, medical examiner or coroner review forms and gross autopsy results must be completed and retained on all donated eye tissue as part of the donor record. *See Section L1.000.*

D1.300 Method of Consent

Documentation of legal consent for enucleation or in situ excision is essential for medical-legal reasons. Consent procedures and forms must conform with state law and documentation for consent must be retained. In medical examiner's/coroner's cases, the eye bank shall adhere to the consent regulations specified by the medical examiner's or coroner's legislation in its state. In each case the consent designation and restrictions, if any, must be adhered to and cannot be altered without the witnessed resigning or redesignation of the donee.

D1.400 Donor Age

Since no definite relationship has been established between the quality of donor tissue and age, the upper and lower age limit is left to the discretion of the Medical Director.

D1.500 Interval Between Death, Enucleation, Excision and Preservation

Acceptable time intervals from death, enucleation or excision to preservation may vary according to the circumstances of death and interim means of storage of the body. It is generally recommended that corneal preservation occur as soon as possible after death. All time intervals for each donor, i.e., the time of death to the time of enucleation and preservation and/or the time to corneal excision, shall be recorded. If the donor has been refrigerated prior to enucleation or in situ corneal excision, this information shall be noted.

D1.600 Eye Maintenance Prior to Enucleation

The prospective donor's corneal integrity should be maintained. Recommended procedures for eye maintenance shall be found in the procedures manual. Each individual eye bank's procedure is left to the discretion of the Medical Director and shall be clearly documented.

D1.700 Living Donors

Eye tissue that is removed and processed for surgical use from a living donor shall have the same standards applied as for all cadaveric tissue, e.g., the same donor medical history shall be obtained, the same records, serology, etc. No extended quarantine period, outside of the usual 24-48 hours for serology results, shall be required for corneal tissue used for transplantation that is stored in short or intermediate term tissue culture medium.

E1.000 **Procurement and Preservation Procedures**

Specific procurement procedures can be found in the EBAA Procedures Manual. Variations of these procedures are at the discretion of the eye bank's Medical Director as long as they do not violate standard aseptic practice and are documented. This manual has been approved by the Medical Policy and the Technician's Subcommittees and shall be periodically reviewed and modified as necessary.

E1.100 Enucleation Procedure

Ultimate responsibility for personnel to perform enucleation rests with the Director, the Medical Director and existing state law.

E1.200 In situ and Laboratory Removal of the Corneoscleral Rim

Removal of the corneoscleral rim shall be performed using sterile technique by individuals specifically trained in in situ retrieval and/or laboratory removal of the corneoscleral segment. For in situ corneal removal, tissue should be examined with the use of a penlight prior to excision.

E1.300 Use of Short or Intermediate Term Preservation Medium

Eye Banks shall use an appropriate corneal storage medium that has been manufactured in accordance with FDA Good Manufacturing Practices. The medium shall be used and stored according to the manufacturer's recommendations for temperature, date and other factors.

E1.400 Long Term Preservation

Some eye banks employ long-term preservation of corneal tissue, such as organ culturing. While these methods are not in widespread use, an eye bank that uses long-term preservation shall carefully document the procedure in their procedures manual, and adhere to rigid aseptic technique.

E1.500 Whole Globe Preservation

Procedures for whole globe preservation may be found in the EBAA Procedures Manual. Eye banks that store whole eyes for lamellar or refractive keratoplasty shall employ aseptic practice using one of the preservation methods given in the procedures manual. The selected preservation method must be documented in the eye bank's own procedures manual.

E1.600   Scleral Preservation

Various methods of preserving sclera may be found in the EBAA Procedures Manual. Eye banks shall preserve scleral tissue aseptically, using one of these methods. The selected preservation method must be documented in the eye bank's own procedure manual.

An expiration date for use of tissue shall be indicated based on the container capability and/or other factors documented or recommended by the eye bank.

F1.000   **Tissue Evaluation**

The ultimate responsibility for determining the suitability of the tissue for transplantation rests with the transplanting surgeon.

F1.100   Gross Examination

The corneal-scleral segment shall be initially examined grossly for clarity, epithelial defects, foreign objects, contamination and scleral color, e.g., jaundice.

F1.200   Slit-lamp Examination

The cornea shall be examined for epithelial and stromal pathology and in particular endothelial disease. Enucleated whole globes should be examined in the laboratory prior to distribution and/or corneal excision. If in situ corneal excision is performed, examination of the donor eye anterior segment with a portable slit lamp is recommended, although not required. After corneal excision, the corneal-scleral rim shall be evaluated by slit lamp biomicroscopy, even if the donor eye has been examined with the slit lamp prior to excision of the corneal-scleral rim, to insure that damage to the corneal endothelium or surgical detachment of Descemet's membrane did not occur.

The minimum information that must be documented with slit lamp biomicroscopy is outlined in the EBAA Procedures Manual.

F1.300   Specular Microscopy

Specular microscopy may provide additional useful information in screening donor corneal tissue to determine suitability for transplantation.

G1.000   **Quality Assurance**

Each eye bank shall have a formally established quality assurance program. This program shall include ongoing monitoring and evaluation of activities, identification of problems, and development of plans for corrective action. These standards shall provide the basis for development of the QA program. Each eye bank shall document all aspects of its QA program and maintain records of all QA activities for a minimum of three years. These include any corrective or remedial action taken for detected deficiencies. These records shall be available for review at the time of site visit inspection.

The eye bank's quality assurance program shall include a method for the receiving surgeon to report adverse reactions from the transplantation of corneal, scleral or other ocular tissue to the source eye bank which in turn, must forward the adverse reaction information within a reasonable time to the EBAA office for review by the Medical Standards Policy Subcommittee. An Adverse Reaction file shall be available for review by the site visitor at the time of inspection and must be kept for a minimum of three years. Serious adverse reactions shall be reported immediately to the EBAA office for review by the Medical Standards Committee.

G1.100   Quality Control

The Director shall prescribe tests and procedures for measuring, assaying or monitoring properties of tissues essential to the evaluation of their safety for transplantation, e.g., hepatitis B surface antigen and human immunodeficiency virus (HIV) antibody, and to conform with federal requirements as well as individual state laws. Results of all such tests or procedures, together with evaluations based on these findings, shall become part of the permanent record of all tissues processed.

G1.200 Testing

If an eye bank performs its own microbiologic or serologic testing, it must meet applicable certification requirements established under the Clinical Laboratories Improvement Act (CLIA). Verification of satisfactory compliance with a College of American Pathologists (CAP) Proficiency Testing Program shall be available at the time of site visit inspection.

G1.210 Microbiologic Culturing

Culturing of Eye Bank donor eyes is advised despite the recognition by many that bacteriologic contamination of donor eyes does not necessarily lead to infection and that presurgical or surgical cultures may not correlate with postoperative infection if it should occur. Cultures may be performed either before and/or at the time of surgery.

A. Presurgical Cultures

Eye Banks may elect to perform corneal-scleral rim cultures at the time of corneal preservation in tissue culture medium. Positive culture reports shall be reported to the receiving surgeon or recipient eye bank.

B. Surgical Culturing

Each eye bank shall recommend culturing of the corneal-scleral rim for corneal transplantation, or a piece of sclera for scleral implantation at the time of surgery. Positive results in cases of postoperative infection shall be reported to the eye bank that processed the tissue.

G1.220 HIV Screening

A. All member eye banks must have operational an HIV screening program using an FDA approved test for all donors of surgically designated tissue. A negative screening test must be documented prior to release of tissue for transplantation.

B. If a donor has had a blood transfusion within the 48 hours preceding cessation of circulatory function, i.e., a non–heart beating donor, a pre-transfusion sample should be obtained to test for HIV. If a pre-transfusion sample is unavailable, and if the adult donor has received four or more units of whole blood or equivalent within the 48 hours preceding cessation of circulatory function, or if a child under the age of twelve years has received any transfusion of blood or non-sterilizable fraction, the donor tissue is unacceptable for transplantation and shall be considered potentially hazardous and labeled as such (see **Section G1.000**).

G1.230 Hepatitis B Screening

All member eye banks must have operational a hepatitis B screening program using an FDA approved test for hepatitis B surface antigen for all donors of surgically designated tissue. A negative screening test or neutralization or confirmatory test must be documented prior to release of tissue for transplantation.

G1.240   Hepatitis C Screening

All member eye banks must have operational a Hepatitis C screening program using an FDA approved test for all donors of surgically designated tissue. A negative screening or confirmatory test must be documented prior to release of tissue for transplantation.

G1.250   HTLV-I and HTLV-II Screening

Donor screening for HTLV-I and HTLV-II is not required. However, if donor screening for HTLV-I and HTLV-II has been performed, a negative screening test must be documented prior to release of tissue for transplantation.

G1.260   Syphilis Screening

All member eye banks must have operational a syphilis screening program using an FDA approved test for all donors of surgically designated tissue. If the screening test is positive, a negative confirmatory test must be documented before tissue is released.

H1.000   **Non-Surgical Donor Tissue**

If donor tissue is provided for purposes other than surgery, e.g., research, practice surgery, etc., and if that donor tissue is not screened for HIV, hepatitis or syphilis, a label stating that screening for HIV-antibody, hepatitis B, hepatitis C, or syphilis has not been carried out or stating "potentially haz-

ardous biological material" or some other designation acceptable under the guidelines of the CDC must be attached to the container used for the donor tissue storage and/or transport.

I1.000   **Storage**

All surgical tissue shall be stored in quarantine until results of HIV, HBsAg, HCV, and syphilis, and any other relevant donor screening tests have been recorded as non-reactive.

All tissue shall be stored aseptically at a temperature appropriate to the method of preservation used. Eye banks must precisely document their procedures for storage of corneal tissue, whether it is in the form of the whole eye or the cornea only in an appropriate medium.

J1.000   **Labelling**

Each corneal or scleral tissue shall be clearly and indelibly labeled to include at least the information below.

1. Name of source eye bank.
2. Tissue identification number. *There must be a unique identification number for each ocular tissue or fraction thereof that is distributed for surgical use.*
3. Type of tissue
4. Date and time of donor's death.
5. Date and time of corneal/scleral preservation.
6. Expiration date for scleral tissue and long-term preserved tissue.
7. A statement that the tissue is intended for single patient application only and that it is not to be considered sterile and that the FDA therefore recommends culturing or reculturing.
8. A statement that the tissue was procured from a donor who was non-reactive when tested for HIV antibody, hepatitis B surface antigen (HBsAg), hepatitis C antibody (HCV), and syphilis using a test approved by the U.S. Food and Drug Administration (FDA).

K1.000   **Distribution of Tissue**

K1.100   Review of Donor Medical History

Prior to distribution of tissue for transplantation, the Medical Director or his/her designee shall review and document the medical and laboratory information in accordance with medical standards.

K1.200   Receivers of Tissue

Tissue shall be distributed to physicians, dentists, institutions and other eye banks.

K1.300   Fair and Equitable System

Eye banks shall establish and document a system of distribution that is just, equitable and fair to all patients served by the eye bank. Documentation of distribution (time and date of requests for, offers of, and delivery of eye tissue) shall be available for inspection by this Committee. Access to tissue shall be provided without regard to recipient sex, age, religion, race, creed, color or national origin.

L1.000   Documentation to Accompany Donor Tissue

L1.100   Tissue Report Form

A copy of the tissue report form and/or donor screening form shall accompany the tissue. See **Section M1.000.**

L1.200   Package Insert Form

A "Package Insert" form that meets the EBAA requirements defined below shall accompany the tissue for transplantation. This form shall include the following:

1. Recommended storage temperature with specific emphasis on DO NOT FREEZE.
2. That the surgeon should check for integrity of the seal and immediately report to the eye bank any evidence of possible tampering.
3. That color change per the manufacturer's guidelines may indicate a change in pH, in which case the tissue should not be used and a report made immediately to the eye bank.
4. Whether pre-surgical microbiologic cultures were performed by the eye bank, including the advisement that cultures of the donor rim and sclera should be

performed at the time of surgery.

5. The form shall also advise the receiving surgeon that the tissues are delivered with no warranty as to merchantability or fitness for a particular purpose, and that the receiving surgeon is ultimately responsible for judging if the tissue is suitable for use.

This information may be included on the eye bank's donor screening form as long as it is easily noticed; otherwise a separate package insert form is advised.

L2.000   Packaging, Sealing and Packing for Transport

Each tissue shall be individually packaged and sealed with a tamper-proof shrink wrap. The tissue shall be packed in a water-proof container with wet ice, so as to maintain the temperature of the tissue at an acceptable level. Packing shall be done so that the package insert and tissue label do not become wet. Special instructions shall be included on a Package Insert. See **Section L1.200.**

M1.000   Eye Bank Records

M1.100   Length of Storage

All records shall be kept for a minimum of seven years from the date of transplantation/implantation.

M1.200   Confidentiality

All eye bank records and communications between the eye bank and its donors and recipients shall be regarded as confidential and privileged.

M1.300   Donor Screening Forms

Donor screening forms shall contain information regarding the circumstances surrounding the death of the donor and adequate medical history so that the suitability of the tissue for transplantation may be judged.

M1.400   Minimum Information to be Retained

A standard tissue report form for

retaining donor and recipient information shall be established for permanent record and shall be readily accessible for inspection by the Medical Standards Committee. The record shall include the following minimum information:

Eye Bank Identification Number unique to each tissue graft
Name of Eye Bank
Location of Eye Bank
Phone Number
Type of Preservation
Age of Donor
Cause of Death
Death Date and Time
Enucleation or In Situ Excision Date and Time
Preservation Date and Time
Slit Lamp Report
Specular Microscopy (if done)
Name of Enculeator/Evaluator/ Technician
Name of Surgeon Receiving Tissue
Recipient Identification readily identifiable and traceable to each unique graft identification number - See *Section M1.500*
Date, Time and Method of Transportation
Utilization of Non-Transplantable Tissue
Printed results of all EBAA required serologic screening tests

Microbiologic Screening Results if performed
Microbiologic reports of positive donor rim cultures from the receiving surgeon
Adverse Reactions if reported

M1.500   Recipient Follow-up Information

Each eye bank shall retain recipient information from each using surgeon on each surgically used tissue. This information shall include the following:

Patient's name
Unique identification according to the following order:
Social security number
Driver's license number
Hospital identification number
Alien identification
Passport number
Age
Date of birth
Diagnosis
Date of surgery
Location of surgery
Post-operative complications

N1.000   **Amendments**

These standards may be amended as required.

The Medical Standards Committee shall be charged with proposing amendments to these standards as new medical technology, techniques and information require. A comment period may be provided prior to the intended effective date.

Chapter 43

Donor Selection

Donor tissue

DENIS M. O'DAY

Three factors influence the selection of donor corneal tissue for penetrating keratoplasty—the potential for transmission of disease to the recipient, the health of the donor cornea, and the potential for graft rejection. The rapid growth and organization of eye banking in the last decade in the United States is a reflection of the increasing importance of these issues for the ultimate success of corneal transplantation. In this chapter, disease transmission and the quality of the donor tissue are considered.

DISEASE TRANSMISSION FROM DONOR CORNEAS

Corneal transplantation is usually a safe procedure with little associated morbidity. This coupled with the success of corneal transplantation has led to a dramatic increase in the number of donor corneas required each year. According to figures compiled by the Eye Bank Association of America (EBAA) over 40,000 corneal transplants were performed in the United States in 1990. The resulting strain on procurement resources has in turn spurred enactment of medical examiner laws in many states, as well as the development of other innovative methods for enhancing the harvesting of donor corneas. With much of the tissue made available as a result of sudden death, little may be known of the donor's medical history. It is against this background of an increasing volume of donor tissue and, at the same time, an uncertain knowledge of its pedigree that it is useful to examine the potential for disease transmission by corneal transplantation.

Transmission of donor disease to the recipient appears to be a rare event. In a review of the world literature published in 1986, Payne[37] could document only 18 such reports since 1939. In that year, Hata[21] described the development of retinoblastoma in an eye that had received a cornea from a donor with proved retinoblastoma. However, despite the small number of cases contained in the literature, the subject merits careful attention. The broad spectrum of disease these cases represent, the potential for transmission of other disease, and the difficulties in diagnosis they may pose have implications both for eye banking and criteria used for donor selection.

Diseases with the potential for transmission by corneal transplantation fall into three categories: infections, neoplastic disease, and corneal disorders.

Infections. Corneal surgeons have long worried about the possibility of transmitting an infectious disease during corneal transplantation. Reflecting this concern, as eye banks have developed in this country, elaborate procedures have evolved to screen potential donors who may be carriers of an infection.[14] However, the screening process is imperfect at best and so there is always the risk that one of these diseases will be transmitted.

Viral infections are clearly the greatest hazard in corneal transplantation because of their capacity to cause serious harm to the recipient. It is important to distinguish those viruses that appear to have a potential for transmission from those that have been actually documented to cause disease in the recipient. There is also a group of viruses for which transmission is considered to be extremely unlikely if not impossible (Table 43-1).

Viruses With Proved Transmission By Corneal Transplantation

Rabies. The rabies virus transmission as a result of corneal transplantation has been documented on four occasions.[57] All four recipients died. One of

Table 43-1. Transmissivity of Various Viral Diseases

Proved	Possible	Unlikely
Rabies	HIV (human immuno-	Varicella
Creutzfeldt-	deficiency virus)	zoster
Jakob	HSV (herpes simplex	
Hepatitis B	virus)	
	Cytomegalovirus	
	Epstein-Barr	
	Adenovirus	
	Rubella	
	Hepatitis C	

these cases occurred in the United States. Three donors were involved, one of whom had a progressive neurologic disorder. The second donor suffered from a progressive quadriplegia, whereas the third died after a 3-day history of headache, cyanosis, and confusion. All four instances of rabies transmission occurred before the risk of rabies transmission was recognized. Although there have been no further cases reported, the potential for transmission still exists, and experience with the last donor indicates that the classic feature of rabies infection may not always be present. The possibility of a slow or latent viral infection is one reason why the EBAA lists "death from central nervous system disease of unknown etiology" as an exclusion criterion.[14]

Creutzfeldt-Jakob disease. Creutzfeldt-Jakob disease is a rare but fatal progressive neurologic disorder caused by a slow virus.[17] Only one instance in which the disease was acquired by corneal transplantation has been recorded in the literature.[12,13] Nevertheless, the problem posed by Creutzfeldt-Jakob disease exemplifies the difficulty of screening for diseases caused by slow or latent viruses. Because of this risk, the EBAA prohibits the use of donor corneas from recipients of human pituitary-derived growth hormone during the years of 1963 to 1985. As more efficient harvesting of donor tissue leads to a greater volume of donor corneas, the risk of inadvertent use of corneas from patients with this or other slow virus diseases may increase.

Hepatitis B virus. The possibility of acquiring viral hepatitis through corneal transplantation has long been recognized. Hepatitis B surface antigen has been detected in the tears of patients whose serum was positive for hepatitis B surface antigen. The antigen has also been demonstrated in donor tissue.[11,40] Recently, Hoft and associates, in a poster presentation of at the American Academy of Ophthalmology meeting in October 1988, reported two

cases of hepatitis B virus infection after penetrating keratoplasty. The serum from both donors was positive for hepatitis B surface antigen. Clinical and serologic screening of donors can do much to eliminate the risk of transmitting this potentially fatal disease.

Viruses Possibly Transmitted Via Corneal Transplantation

Human immunodeficiency virus. When human immunodeficiency virus (HIV) was first isolated from the tears of infected patients, there was an immediate fear that corneal tissue from such donors presented a very real risk for the corneal transplant recipient.[16,34,39] This concern was heightened by the demonstration of HIV in donor corneal tissue itself.[43] Experience with transplantation of other organs was hardly reassuring with several patients demonstrating seroconversion after the transplantation of infected kidney tissue from HIV-infected donors.[33,45]

Pepose and associates[38] in 1987 described four patients who received corneal tissue from HIV-infected donors. In none of the recipients was there evidence of seroconversion. Three other cases reported by Schwartz and co-workers[45] also remained seronegative. There have been no reports to the Centers for Disease Control (CDC) of seroconversion after corneal transplantation. Thus, despite the theoretical risk, it is reassuring that transmission of the virus does not seem to have occurred, though late seroconversion is still possible. The most obvious reason appears to be the nature of the donor tissue. There is now strong evidence that contact with blood or semen are prerequisites for HIV transmission.[8] The cornea may enjoy a degree of protection that other vascularized tissues do not share. Although it is still possible that passenger lymphocytes infected with the virus may be present in the donor tissue, the quantity of virus is probably much below an inoculating dose. There is some evidence that other cellular components of the donor tissue such as epithelial cells, may harbor virus, but whether the virus actually invades epithelial cells or is present in wandering cells is unknown.

The failure of recipients with grafts from HIV-positive donors to show seroconversion provides no justification to lessen or abandon the present prohibition on the use of corneas from HIV-infected donors. There remains, of course, the additional concern of inadvertent use of tissue from recently infected individuals in whom an antibody response has yet to develop. There currently appears to be no way to exclude such individuals with certainty from the donor pool, though the use of clinical criteria for screening certainly will help. However, a more sensitive means of identifying HIV carriers by detecting the virus itself rather than the antibody are being developed. These should be applied to the screening process when available.

Herpes simplex virus. Herpes simplex virus (HSV) resides in a latent state in the trigeminal and other spinal ganglia after an initial infection.[35] Target tissue disease occurs when the virus is reactivated and spreads transneuronally. Recently, there is growing evidence to support the concept that the cornea in some patients may also be the site of latent infection.[42,48] Some years ago, Salisbury and associates[44] described three patients in whom a keratitis developed because of HSV infection after penetrating keraoplasty. Although the authors attributed the condition in the recipient to recurrent disease activated by surgery and steroid treatment, it is still conceivable that virus introduced by the donor cornea may have been responsible. This theory gains some support from recent animal studies demonstrating the induction of HSV infection in HSV-negative recipients by transplantation of clinically normal corneas from rabbits with latent HSV infection.[48] Clearly, there are major differences between this experimental model and human disease. Fortunately, most transplant recipients, being in the older age group, are likely to have already acquired the virus[41] and therefore are immune to further infection.

Cytomegalovirus. It is estimated that at least half the adult population is infected with cytomegalovirus (CMV) and the incidence of positive serologic responses increases with age.[22] Most persons who acquire the infection are asymptomatic, and although the virus persists in a latent state, reactivated disease is rare unless the immune system is impaired by disease or drug therapy.

Transmission of CMV by major organ transplantation is well recognized and is an important cause of illness and death in kidney, heart, liver, and bone marrow recipients.[32] In such patients, the likelihood for a seronegative patient acquiring the infection from a seropositive donor has been estimated at between 60% and 100%.[22]

The risk of transmitting CMV in corneal transplantation appears minimal. Holland and associates[22] studied the postoperative rise in CMV titer in previously seronegative patients who received corneas from seronegative or seropositive donors. In each group, 9% of the recipients demonstrated seroconversion. Presumably, the recipients of seronegative donor corneas in whom seroconversion occurred acquired the infection from another source. In no instance did the patients exhibit signs or symptoms of infection. The conclusions should be treated with some caution because the number of patients was small. However, the fact that corneal transplant patients are seldom systemically immunosuppressed and are usually otherwise healthy indicates that the risk of overt CMV disease may be slight. In the presence of a compromised immune system, CMV transmission may prove a serious risk.

Epstein-Barr virus, adenovirus, rubella virus. With each of these viruses, there is to some degree a theoretical risk of transmission. However, the lack of any clinical cases after corneal transplant surgery indicates that the risk may be extremely remote. As far as adenovirus is concerned, it seems unlikely that infected donors would survive prescreening criteria. Because of the increasing use of corneas from young donors, even though most children are immunized, the risk of rubella infection may be greater. There is a good reason to be cautious with such tissue, especially if the donor is younger than 2 years of age.

Viral Diseases in Which Transmission is Considered Extremely Unlikely

Varicella zoster. Although varicella zoster is a latent viral infection and in many ways similar to HSV, it does differ in certain important aspects, most notably the absence of virus in target tissue sites when the disease is quiescent. In contrast to HSV infection, there are no reports in the literature of patients shedding varicella zoster virus when the virus is in a latent state.

Diseases of Possible But Unproved Viral Etiology. Reye's syndrome, subacute sclerosing panencephalitis, progressive multifocal leukoencephalopathy, pseudopresumed ocular histoplasmosis (pseudo-POHS), other progressive neurologic disorders, acute leukemia, lymphoma, and Hodgkin's disease are disorders in which a viral cause is possible but unproved. Unknown slow or latent viruses may be involved. There is recent evidence to indicate that some cases of acute leukemia may be caused by a retrovirus.[18] It is also possible that the decreased efficiency of immunologic surveillance mechanisms in hematologic disorders, such as leukemias, lymphomas, and Hodgkin's disease, increases the incidence of opportunistic viral infections which may then be transmitted to the graft recipients. For these reasons, tissue from such donors should not be used in corneal transplantation. Reye's syndrome is also listed by the EBAA as one of the conditions in a donor that is a contraindication to use of the tissue. Although Reye's syndrome is linked to a viral infection—usually influenza—a viremia does not occur, and so ocular involvement with the virus is only a remote possibility.

Bacterial and Fungal Infections. Infection with bacteria or fungi acquired at the time of surgery is an uncommon but important complication of keratoplasty.[2,20,23,28] Whereas many such cases appear unrelated to primary donor sepsis, a sufficient number have now been linked to ocular or systemic infectious disease in the donor to substantiate concerns regarding the risk of transplanting tissue from individuals who at the time of death have a significant infection. Severe loss of vision or the eye is the most common outcome in cases reported in the literature,[2] but in one instance the patient died either as a result of the infection or the treatment required to eradicate it.[27] The source of the infection has been the subject of several studies.[2,20,23,28,30] Positive culture results from the donor rim is an established risk factor for the development of endophthalmitis and is associated with a twenty-twofold greater risk of infection according to one study.[28] When an infection develops postoperatively, a positive culture result from the corneal rim is reasonable evidence that the infection is donor related, though contamination of the preservation solution at the time of harvesting is still a possible explanation.

Disseminated or local sepsis in a potential donor is always a matter for concern. In two disastrous cases, both corneas taken from a patient who died of pneumonia apparently were contaminated with *Diplococcus pneumoniae* (properly *Streptococcus pneumoniae*).[47] Both eyes were lost to *S. pneumoniae* endophthalmitis, and two kidney recipients from the same donor died. Infection with *Pseudomonas aeruginosa* in two other patients was apparently acquired from corneas harvested from a donor with septicemia.[25] In one instance, corneal tissue from a patient with disseminated cryptococcal infection apparently transmitted the infection to one recipient.[3] In another, *Torulopsis glabrata* was cultured from the donor rim and from the vitreous of the recipient with endophthalmitis.[27]

It is important therefore to search for evidence of bacterial and fungal infection in potential donors. The problem of donor tissue contamination is unlikely to be resolved easily. Experience indicates that most will fail to show clinical evidence of external eye infection. Donor rim tissue cultures therefore are an important routine step that may provide the earliest evidence of an impending infection.

What is clear though is the notion that sepsis in the donor is a risk factor for the development of infection in the recipient. Although it remains impossible to quantitate this risk, the relationship is undeniable. At the current state of our knowledge, evidence of septicemia, meningitis, or a localized sepsis, specifically pneumonia, should be grounds for rejecting donor tissue.

Two different studies have examined one set of circumstances that may be associated with increased risk of donor contamination with bacteria or fungi and have arrived at very different conclusions. Sugar and Liff[49] concluded that mechanical ventilator support increases the risk of donor contamination by potentially pathogenic bacteria. However, Seedar and colleagues,[46] in a controlled study, were unable to demonstrate any relationship. Despite the finding in the latter study, it would seem prudent to consider corneas from such patients as potentially contaminated.

Neoplastic Diseases. The possibility of inadvertently implanting a malignant tumor is a recurring nightmare for most corneal surgeons, yet only one case has been reported in which this apparently unequivocally occurred. In this well-documented case, retinoblastoma was transferred from the donor to the recipient eye.[21] Although, theoretically, the greatest risk appears to be with the lymphoproliferative disorders and leukemias (the latter because of the possible viral cause), no cases of transmission have been reported. In an important study, Wagoner and co-workers[51] examined a population of patients who had received corneal tissue from donors with a variety of neoplastic diseases. They observed no evidence of disease transmission over a long period. Nevertheless, the concern is real, and it is desirable, as the EBAA recommends, to avoid use of such tissue.

Corneal Disorders. Transmission of local corneal disorders is a definite risk of corneal transplantation, yet it is remarkable that the literature contains very little comment on this matter. Presumably, formal or informal screening methods used for many years have been successful in identifying such donors, but it is probable that minor and perhaps inconsequential corneal disease is at times transferred. It is extremely unlikely in the current era of specular microscopy and careful examination of donor material that major stromal dystrophies will be missed. However, anterior and posterior membrane dystrophies and keratoconus, particularly in the early stage, may escape detection. It is also likely that corneas that are destined to develop Fuchs' dystrophy are being transplanted. Although there are no data to substantiate this, most corneal surgeons are familiar with the finding of cornea guttata in otherwise apparently healthy donor corneas, which may be the harbinger of full-blown dystrophy in many years' time. Likewise, the increased use of corneas from young donors may mean that early keratoconus is likely to be missed in the routine screening of donor corneas. However, despite these comments, it is reassuring to recognize the rarity of such an event.

HEALTH OF THE DONOR CORNEA

For the past decade there has been a major effort to upgrade the quality and safety of corneal tissue using corneal transplantation. This process has paralleled the gradual evolution of eye banking techniques from the use of fresh tissue to the use of tissue preserved for longer periods of time. As a result, there are now in place explicit standards for eye banking in the United States that address the issue of safety from the point of view of diseases potentially transmitted by corneal transplantation and the quality of the tissue with regard to its suitability as a replacement for the diseased cornea.[14] The standards are broad in scope and reflect an intense effort by the EBAA to develop standards that would be universally applicable. The process mandates a continuous review of eye banking practices with modification being implemented as new knowledge and insights develop. The standards are comprehensive and are designed to ensure that member eye banks remain in compliance with the stated goals of the EBAA. Eye banks are reviewed on a regular basis. In addition, the EBAA maintains a constant communication with member eye banks to update them on changes and new developments. These organizational approaches seem to be contributing in a large part to the relatively trouble-free history of corneal transplantation in the United States.

The EBAA has established criteria for screening of potential donors. Each member eye bank is required to have a consistent policy for the physical inspection of a donor and the examination and docu-

---

Contraindications for the use of Donor Tissue for Penetrating Keratoplasty

Systemic Disorders

- Death of unknown cause
- Death from central nervous system diseases of unknown cause
- Creutzfeldt-Jacob disease
- Subacute scleorsing panendophthalmitis
- Progressive multifocal leukoencephalopathy
- Congenital rubella
- Reye's syndrome
- Active viral encephalitis or encephalitis of unknown origin
- Active septicemia (bacteremia, fungemia, viremia)
- Active bacteria or fungal endophthalmitis
- Rabies
- Active syphilis
- Active leukemias
- Active disseminated lymphomas
- Hepatitis B surface antigen–positive donors
- Hepatitis C–seropositive donors
- Recipients of human pituitary-derived growth hormone (pit-hGH) during the years from 1963 to 1985.
- HIV-seropositive donors
- Acquired immunodeficiency syndrome (AIDS)
- Children (under 13 years old) and infants of mothers with AIDS or at high risk of HIV infection
- High risk for HIV infection
  1. Clinical or laboratory evidence of HIV infections
  2. Men who have had sex with another man one or more times since 1977
  3. Past or present intravenous drug abusers
  4. Persons immigrating since 1977 from pattern II countries where heterosexual activity is reported as the predominant means of transmission of HIV (such as Haiti, central Africa)
  5. Persons with hemophilia who have received clotting factor concentrates
  6. Sexual partners of any of the above
  7. Men or women who have engaged in prostitution since 1977 and persons who have been their heterosexual partners within the past 6 months.
- HTLV-I or HTLV-II infection

Intrinsic Eye Disease

- Retinoblastoma
- Malignant tumors of the anterior ocular segment
- Active ocular or intraocular inflammation: conjunctivitis, scleritis, iritis, uveitis, vitritis, choroiditis, retinitis congenital or acquired disorders of the eye that would preclude a successful outcome for the intended use, such as central donor corneal scar for an intended penetrating keratoplasty, keratoconus, and keratoglobus
- Pterygia or other superficial disorders of the conjunctiva or corneal surface involving the central optical area of the corneal button

Prior Intraocular or Anterior Segment Surgery

- Refractive corneal procedures, such as radial keratotomy, lamellar inserts
- Laser photoablation surgery
- Anterior segment surgery, such as cataract, intraocular lens implant, glaucoma filtration

mentation of a prospective donor's available medical records or investigation of cause of death. In accordance with this policy, potential donors are screened for diseases potentially transmissible by corneal transplantation, and a set of absolute contraindications to the use of corneal tissue has been established. These contraindications are most rigorous for penetrating keratoplasty (see box on p. 553). They also apply to tissue intended for lamellar or patch grafts or epikeratophakia except that endothelial disease is not considered a contraindication provided that the corneal stroma is not affected. The criteria for the use of scleral tissue are similar to those of penetrating keratoplasty.

In addition to these standards for screening potential donors, the EBAA has established standards for examination of the tissue. Thus the eye bank technician examines the corneoscleral segment grossly for optical clarity, the presence of epithelial defects or foreign bodies, and scleral color and by slitlamp exams for evidence of epithelial and stromal pathosis. However, the ultimate responsibility for determining the suitability of the tissue rests with the corneal surgeon, who should be knowledgeable about changes that develop in corneal tissue post mortem.

Attrition of the corneal endothelium commences immediately after death. The cell loss, though retarded somewhat by modern tissue preservation techniques, continues during transplant surgery and for as long as 5 years postoperatively.[10,31] Indeed, up to half the cells may be lost within 2 years, even with an apparently uneventful procedure.[31] It is also known that the endothelial cell count of normal corneas declines with increasing age.[4] Both these facts indicate that success of corneal transplantation would be enhanced by avoidance of the use of tissue over a certain age. Studies, however, do not support this conclusion. Increasing donor age of itself is not a risk factor for corneal graft failure.[1,9,10,15,24,19,36,50]

The status of the endothelium is, however, of crucial importance. Fortunately, specular microscopy techniques can now be applied to donor corneas so that an accurate assessment of the cell count is possible. Although a direct relationship between the cell count and the presence of corneal edema has not been established, the preoperative donor cell count provides an estimate of the margin of safety, with recognition that as many as 70% of the cells may eventually be lost, and as the cell count falls below 1000 mm^2, the likelihood of corneal edema increases progressively. Thus it would seem desirable to seek to use donor corneas with a minimum of 2000 cells/mm^2.

Given that there are no strict upper age limits on the use of donor tissue based on that criterion alone, what about the use of very young donors to obtain as healthy an endothelial layer as possible? Unfortunately other problems emerge, particularly with donors 2 years of age and younger because of a myopic shift induced by steep transplantation curvatures.[19,26] Therefore the use of young donor tissue should be limited to donors over 2 years of age.

CONCLUSION

In the past decade corneal transplantation has come to be an extraordinarily safe and effective procedure. Maturation of the eye banking system with the development and implementation of rigorous standards for the collection, preservation, and selection of donor material has made an important contribution to this record of success. The standards for donor selection outlined in this chapter are logical, scientifically sound, and readily applied. Undoubtedly, they will undergo modification as knowledge progresses, but the principles upon which they rest are unlikely to change.

ACKNOWLEDGMENTS

Portions of this chapter were adapted from and published courtesy of O'Day DM: Diseases potentially transmitted through corneal transplantation, *Ophthalmology* 96:1133-1138, 1989, and the Eye Bank Association of America: *Technician manual*, Washington, D.C., 1990.

REFERENCES

1. Abbott RL, Forster RK: Determinants of graft clarity in penetrating keratoplasty, *Arch Ophthalmol* 97:1071-1075, 1979.
2. Baer JC, Nirankari VS, Glaros DS: Streptococcal endophthalmitis from contaminated donor corneas after keratoplasty: clinical and laboratory investigations, *Arch Ophthalmol* 106:517-520, 1988.
3. Beyt BE, Waltman SR: Cryptococcal endophthalmitis after corneal transplantation, *N Engl J Med* 298:825-826, 1978.
4. Bourne WN, Kaufman HE: Specular microscopy of human corneal endothelium *in vitro*, *Am J Ophthalmol* 81:319-323, 1976.
5. Centers for Disease Control: Human-to-human transmission of rabies by a corneal transplant—Idaho, *MMWR* 28:109-111, 1979.
6. Centers for Disease Control: Human-to-human transmission of rabies via a corneal transplant—France, *MMWR* 29:25-26, 1980.
7. Centers for Disease Control: Human-to-human transmission of rabies via a corneal transplant—Thailand, *MMWR* 30:473-475, 1981.
8. Centers for Disease Control: Update: universal precautions for prevention of transmission of human immunodeficiency virus, hepatitis B virus, and other bloodborne pathogens in health-care settings, *MMWR* 37:377-388, 1988.
9. Cherry PMH, Pashby RC, Tadros ML, et al: An analysis of corneal transplantation: I-graft clarity, *Ann Ophthalmol* 11:974-976, 1979.

10. Culbertson WW, Abbott RL, Forster RK: Endothelial cell loss in penetrating keratoplasty, *Ophthalmology* 89:600-604, 1982.

11. Darrell RW, Jacob GB: Hepatitis B surface antigen in human tears, *Arch Ophthalmol* 96:674-676, 1978.

12. DeVoe AG: Complications of keratoplasty: the Gifford Lecture, *Am J Ophthalmol* 79:907-912, 1975.

13. Duffy P, Wolf J, Collins G, et al: Possible person-to-person transmission of Creutzfeldt-Jakob disease, *N Eng J Med* 290:692-693, 1974.

14. Eye Bank Association of America: *Technician manual*, 1990; available from Eye Bank Association of America, 1511 K Street NW, Suite 830, Washington, DC 20005.

15. Forster RK, Fine M: Relation to donor age to success in penetrating keratoplasty, *Arch Ophthalmol* 85:42-47, 1971.

16. Fujikawa LS, Salahuddin SZ, Palestine AG, et al: Isolation of human T-lymphotrophic virus type III from the tears of a patient with acquired immunodeficiency syndrome, *Lancet* 2:529-530, 1985.

17. Gajdusek DC: Slow infections with unconventional viruses, *Harvey Lectures* 72:283-353, 1976-1977.

18. Gallo RC: HTLV: the family of human T-lymphotrophic retroviruses and their role in leukemia and AIDS, *Med Oncol Tumor Pharmacother* 3:265-267, 1986.

19. Gloor P, Keech RV, Krachmer JH: Young donor age associated with high myopia following penetrating keratoplasty in infants, *Ophthalmology* 98(8)(suppl):156, 1991.

20. Guss RB, Koenig S, DeLaPena W, et al: Endophthalmitis after penetrating keratoplasty, *Am J Ophthalmol* 95:651-658, 1983.

21. Hata B: The development of glioma in the eye to which the cornea of a patient, who suffered from glioma, was transplanted, *Nippon Ganka Gakkai Zasshi* 43:1763-1767, 1939.

22. Holland EJ, Bennett SR, Brannian R, et al: The risk of cytomegalovirus transmission by penetrating keratoplasty, *Am J Ophthalmol* 105:357-360, 1988.

23. Insler MS, Cavanagh HD, Wilson LA: Gentamicin-resistant *Pseudomonas* endophthalmitis after penetrating keratoplasty, *Br J Ophthalmol* 69:189-191, 1985.

24. Jerkins MS, Lempert SL, Brown SI: Significance of donor age in penetrating keratoplasty, *Ann Ophthalmol* 11:974-976, 1979.

25. Khodadoust AA, Franklin RM: Transfer of bacterial infection by donor cornea in penetrating keratoplasty, *Am J Ophthalmol* 87:130-132, 1979.

26. Koenig S, Graul E, Kaufman HE: Ocular refraction after penetrating keratoplasty with infant donor corneas, *Am J Ophthalmol* 94:534-539, 1982.

27. Larsen PA, Lindstrom RL, Doughman DJ: *Torulopsis glabrata* endophthalmitis after keratoplasty with an organ-cultured cornea, *Arch Ophthalmol* 96:1019-1022, 1978.

28. Leveile AS, McMullen FD, Cavanagh HD: Endophthalmitis following penetrating keratoplasty, *Ophthalmology* 90:38-39, 1983.

29. Linn JG Jr., Stuart JC, Warnicki BA, et al: Endothelial morphology in long-term keratoconus corneal transplants, *Ophthalmology* 88:761-770, 1981.

30. Matoba A, Moore MB, Merten JL, McCulley JP: Donor-to-host transmission of streptococcal infection by corneas stored in McCarey-Kaufman medium, *Cornea* 3:105-108, 1984.

31. Matsuda M, Bourne WM: Long-term morphologic changes in the endothelium of transplanted corneas, *Arch Ophthalmol* 103:1343-1346, 1985.

32. Nankervis GA, Kumar ML: Diseases produced by cytomegalovirus, *Med Clin North Am* 62:1021-1035, 1978.

33. Neumayer HH, Fassbinder W, Kresse S, Wagner K: Human T-lymphotrophic virus III antibody screening in kidney transplant recipients and patients receiving maintenance hemodialysis, *Transplant Proc* 19:2169-2171, 1987.

34. O'Day DM: The risk posed by HTLV-III–infected corneal donor tissue, *Am J Ophthalmol* 101:246-247, 1985.

35. O'Day DM: Herpes simplex keratitis. In Duane TH, Jaeger EA, editors: *Clinical ophthalmology*, Philadelphia, 1988, Lippincott, vol 4, Chapt 19.

36. Paglen PK, Fine M, Abbott RL, Webster RG: The prognosis of keratoplasty in keratoconus, *Ophthalmology* 89:651-654, 1982.

37. Payne JW: Donor selection. In Brightbill FS, editor: *Corneal surgery: theory, technique, and tissue*, St. Louis, 1986, Mosby–Year Book.

38. Pepose JS, MacRae S, Quinn TC, Ward JW: Serologic markers after the transplantation of corneas from donors infected with human immunodeficiency virus, *Am J Ophthalmol* 103:798-801, 1987.

39. Pepose JS, MacRae S, Quinn TC, et al: The impact of the AIDS epidemic on corneal transplantation, *Am J Ophthalmol* 100:610-613, 1985.

40. Raber IM, Friedman HM: Hepatitis B surface antigen in corneal donors, *Am J Ophthalmol* 104:255-258, 1987.

41. Rawls WE, Campione-Piccardo J: Epidemiology of herpes simplex virus type 1 and type 2 infections. In Nahmias AJ, Dowdle W, Schianzi RF, editors: *The human herpesvirus, an interdisciplinary perspective*, New York, 1981, Elsevier.

42. Rong BL, Kenyon KB, Bean KM, et al: Detection of the HSV genome in human corneal buttons, *Invest Ophthalmol Vis Sci* 29(suppl):158, 1988 (ARVO Abstracts).

43. Salahuddin SZ, Palestine AG, Heck E, et al: Isolation of the human T-cell leukemia/lymphotropic virus type III from the cornea, *Am J Ophthalmol* 101:149-152, 1986.

44. Salisbury JD, Berkowitz RA, Gebbhardt BM, Kaufman HE: Herpesvirus infection of corneal allografts, *Ophthalmic Surg* 15:406-408, 1984.

45. Schwarz A, Hoffmann F, L'Age-Stehr J, et al: Human immunodeficiency virus transmission by organ donation: outcome in cornea and kidney recipients, *Transplantation* 44:21-24, 1987.

46. Seedor JA, Stulting RD, Epstein RJ, et al: Survival of corneal grafts from donors supported by mechanical ventilation, *Ophthalmology* 94:101-108, 1987.

47. Shaw EL, Aquavella JV: Pneumococcal endophthalmitis following grafting of corneal tissue from a (cadaver) kidney donor, *Ann Ophthalmol* 9:435-440, 1977.

48. Stamler JF, Bean KM, Vaslet CA, et al: Transfer of HSV nucleic acid by transplantation of latently infected corneas to non-infected rabbits, *Invest Ophthalmol Vis Sci* 29(suppl):155, 1988 (ARVO Abstracts).

49. Sugar J, Liff J: Bacterial contamination of corneal donor tissue, *Ophthalmic Surg* 11:250-252, 1980.

50. Völker-Dieben JH, Kok-van Alphen CC, Lansberger Q, Persijn GG: Different influences on corneal graft survival in 539 transplants, *Acta Ophthalmol* 60:190-202, 1982.

51. Wagoner MD, Dohlman CH, Albert DM, et al: Corneal donor material selection, *Ophthalmology* 88:139-145, 1981.

Donor age

STEVEN B. KOENIG

Donor-exclusion criteria have been established by the Eye Bank Association of America (EBAA) to reduce the threat of transmissible disease by means of the donor cornea and to increase the success rate of corneal transplantation.[12] To increase the chances of a successful graft, the donor cornea must have a healthy endothelium and a normal contour and be optically clear. Upper age limits have been adopted by many eye banks and corneal surgeons to ensure the viability of the donor endothelium. Lower age limits have been established by some surgeons to minimize the technical problems associated with transplanting immature corneal tissue and to ensure a normal corneal contour. However, the age criteria for donor corneal tissue are not well defined and vary between eye banks and corneal surgeons. Given the current demand for and limited supply of suitable corneal tissue, any age restrictions should be carefully reexamined.

LOWER AGE LIMITS

The Medical Standards of the EBAA state that the lower age limit is left to the discretion of the medical director of the eye bank.[12] A majority of eye banks and corneal surgeons surveyed by Binder accepted tissue from donors as young as 6 months of age.[3] Surgeons have traditionally preferred young donor corneas, believing that a high endothelial cell density provides greater buffer against perioperative endothelial cell loss. In addition, the pliability of the infant cornea may allow it to assume a normal curvature early in the postoperative period and provide rapid visual recovery.[33,45] However, the small diameter, thinness, and elasticity of the infant cornea are characteristics that may cause technical problems for the corneal surgeon.

INFANT TISSUE FOR PENETRATING KERATOPLASTY

The average corneal diameter of the full-term infant is less than 10 mm.[4,31] Premature infant corneas may be smaller. This small size limits the diameter of the donor corneal button and makes trephination of the donor cornea technically more difficult. Eccentric trephination may cause inclusion of scleral fibers and remnants of conjunctiva or episcleral tissue from the donor eye.

The extreme thinness and pliability of the infant cornea makes handling more difficult. The donor cornea may actually fold upon itself during transfer to the host corneal bed. The thinness and flexibility of the infant cornea may also interfere with accurate placement of corneal sutures. Inadvertently deep sutures may cause microperforations, with the potential complications of wound leak, flat anterior chamber, and endophthalmitis. Shallow suture placement

may cause the suture to cut through the tissue, loosen, and produce high postoperative astigmatism. Graft-host thickness disparity will occur if infant corneal tissue is placed in a thick or edematous recipient corneal bed. This may cause poor apposition between Descemet's membrane of the donor and host cornea, or cause overriding of the recipient cornea at the wound margin. Retraction of Descemet's membrane occurs after trephination of the infant cornea and may also interfere with proper wound apposition. Deep suture placement must be used to prevent posterior wound gape and its potential complications of peripheral graft edema and graft failure.[33]

Donzis and co-workers have documented the exceedingly steep curvature of the premature infant cornea.[11] Their longitudinal measurements of premature infant corneas demonstrate significant corneal flattening during the last few months of gestation.[11] Nevertheless, the dioptric value of the full-term infant cornea remains much steeper than the curvature of the adult cornea;[4,14,20,38] values as high as 54 diopters have been reported.[15] Although the diameter of the infant cornea stops growing after 2 years of age, the curvature probably reaches adult dimensions during the second 6 months of life.[14,15,31]

The extremely steep anterior curvature of the infant cornea may also cause technical problems when the donor button is punched from the endothelial side on a Teflon block. Standard corneal punching blocks have relatively flat radius wells, which may cause folding of the donor cornea, oversized corneal buttons, and beveled edges.[33] One may overcome this problem by trephining the donor corneal button from the anterior surface of the whole globe.[33]

The most important complication associated with the use of infant donor corneal tissue is the induction of postoperative myopia.[24,33,41,45] Vannas recognized severe myopia as a complication of penetrating keratoplasty when donor tissue was obtained from stillborn infants.[41] Wood noted a myopic shift

Table 43-2. Preoperative Clinical Data

Patient	Age	Diagnosis	Procedure	Donor age
1	28	Leukoma	PK	1 month
2	48	Fuchs' dystrophy	PK	5 days
3	69	Fuchs'/cataract	PK/ICCE	3 months
4	77	Fuchs'/cataract	PK/ICCE	3 weeks
5	63	Aphakic bullous	PK	1 month

ICCE, Intracapsular cataract extraction; *PK,* penetrating keratoplasty.

Table 43-3. Preoperative and Postoperative Refractive Errors

Patient	Manifest Refraction (Diopters): Spherical Equivalent Refractive Error		Postoperative K	Vision
	Preoperative	Postoperative		
1	−0.75	−5.00	50.25	20/25−1
2	+0.12	−16.50	59.37	20/25
3	−2.00	−3.25*	55.75	20/30
4	+1.75	−4.00*	60.75	20/30
5	+9.25	−8.00*	62.25	20/30
Mean	+1.67	−7.35	57.67	

*Aphakic eye.

in refraction after keratoplasty with infant donor corneas and related the refractive error to the steep anterior corneal curvature.[45]

Koenig and co-workers examined five adult patients who underwent penetrating keratoplasty using corneal tissue from donors 3 months of age and younger.[24] The preoperative diagnoses included corneal leukoma, Fuchs' corneal dystrophy, and aphakic bullous keratopathy (Table 43-2). Two of the three patients with Fuchs' dystrophy had coexisting cataracts and underwent combined intracapsular cataract extraction and penetrating keratoplasty.

In each case, the transplanted cornea was optically clear and the postoperative vision was 20/30 or better (Table 43-3 and Fig. 43-1). The average preoperative spherical equivalent refractive error was +1.67 diopters. After surgery, however, all patients, in-cluding three who were aphakic, demonstrated myopic refractive errors. The average postoperative refractive error was −7.35 diopters (Table 43-3). This represents a mean myopic shift in refraction of approximately 9 diopters. Postoperatively, all patients had extremely steep anterior corneal curvatures. The average keratometry reading measured 57.67 diopters compared to a normal value of 43 diopters (Fig. 43-4).[42] This finding indicates that the postoperative myopia is attributable to the high refractive power of the transplanted infant donor cornea. The postoperative corneal curvature and refractive error could not be predicted on the basis of donor age.

The postoperative myopic shift in refraction is important because it was responsible for clinically significant anisometropia in each case. The mean postoperative anisometropic error was nearly 13 diopters

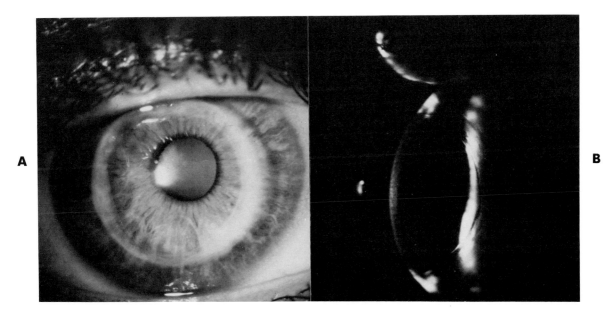

Fig. 43-1. A, Case 2. Slitlamp photograph of infant donor cornea 11 months after keratoplasty. **B,** Notice extremely steep curvature of donor cornea.

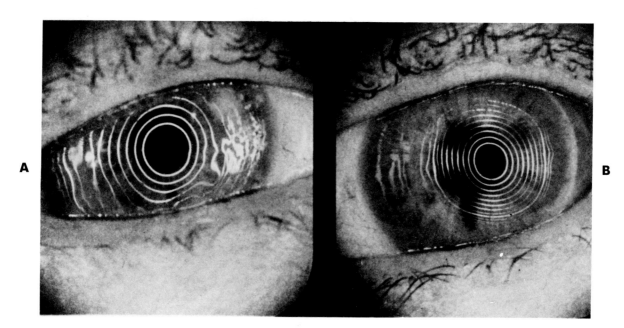

Fig. 43-2. A, Case 5. Corneoscope photograph demonstrates normal corneal curvature (43.75 D) in right eye, which received adult donor tissue. **B,** Left eye received infant donor tissue and demonstrates a steep postoperative curvature (62.25 D).

(Table 43-4). The anisometropia precluded spectacle correction in each case. However, because of the extremely steep corneal curvature, contact lens correction was unsuccessful in four of five patients. One patient (case 3) was successfully fit with a Soper E keratoconus contact lens. One patient (case 2) underwent a repeat penetrating keratoplasty with adult donor tissue in an attempt to correct the anisometropia.

This study indicates that corneal tissue from donors 3 months of age or younger may be unsuitable for penetrating keratoplasty in emmetropic adults or anisometropic patients undergoing surgery in the more myopic eye. Similar results occur after penetrating keratoplasty with tissue from donors up to 2.5 years of age.[23] Our findings also indicate that do-

nor and recipient age should be matched as closely as possible for infants undergoing penetrating keratoplasty. A relatively flat adult donor cornea could induce hyperopia and anisometropia after pediatric keratoplasty.

INFANT TISSUE FOR REFRACTIVE SURGERY

The use of infant donor corneas has been suggested as a possible form of refractive surgery to correct large ametropias in aphakic patients undergoing penetrating keratoplasty.[33] However, the inability to predict the postoperative refractive error and the difficulty with contact lens correction make this an unsuitable form of refractive keratoplasty.

Table 43-4. Postoperative anisometropia

| Patient | Manifest Refraction (Diopters): Spherical Equivalent Refractive Error | | Fellow Eye | Anisometropia |
	Preoperative	Postoperative		
1	−0.75	−5.00	Plano	5.00
2	+0.12	−16.50	+0.375	16.87
3	−2.00	−3.25*	+7.75*	11.00
4	+1.75	−4.00*	+7.62*	11.62
5	+9.25	−8.00*	+11.75*	19.75
Mean	+1.67	−7.35	+5.50	12.85

*Aphakic eye.

UPPER AGE LIMITS

The Medical Standards of the EBAA state that the upper age limit for corneal donors should be left to the discretion of the medical director of the eye bank.[12] The guidelines also indicate that endothelial abnormalities and decreased endothelial cell density occur with aging. Binder's survey of eye banks and corneal surgeons found that the majority accept tissue from donors up to 75 years old.[3] Although intended to exclude donor endothelial abnormalities, an older age limit is arbitrary and may restrict the available supply of donor corneal tissue.

SPECULAR MICROSCOPY STUDIES

The human corneal endothelium is a nonreplicating, monolayer of closely spaced hexagonal cells.[44] *In vivo* specular microscopy demonstrates a gradual and progressive decrease in endothelial cell density and increase in cell size (polymegethism) with age.[8,19,25,26,44] The rate of decline is greatest during infancy and reflects the rapid increase in the corneal diameter during the first 2 years of life.[26,31] The subsequent decline in cell density is more gradual and presumably reflects the true endothelial cell loss. This has been estimated at 0.56% per year.[31] However, there are wide variations in endothelial cell density at any given age, and cell size cannot be accurately predicted on the basis of age.[19,40,43] Furthermore, endothelial cell density may vary between different races. Matsuda and co-workers demonstrated that the endothelium of the Japanese has a greater cell density than that of an age-matched American population.[29] This may represent differences in endothelial cell density at birth or differential rates of cell loss with aging between the two groups.[30] However, it is important to recognize that age alone may not be predictive of endothelial cell density.

The aging endothelium may also demonstrate changes in cell shape (pleomorphism) with loss of the orderly hexagonal pattern.[30] Such changes may indicate a stressed endothelium with less functional reserve.[34,39] Additional aging changes include the presence of cornea guttata. Kaufman found a surprisingly high incidence of cornea guttata (15%) in older but otherwise normal corneas; all dystrophic corneas in their series were harvested from donors over 50 years of age.[22] Nevertheless, older donor corneas may have normal endothelial morphology and no guttate changes. In one series, nearly 75% of corneas from donors older than 67 years demonstrated normal endothelial morphology and density by specular microscopy.[32]

PREKERATOPLASTY AND POSTKERATOPLASTY CELL COUNTS

Since young donors may have higher endothelial cell densities, it has been assumed that young donor buttons would yield higher postoperative cell counts and better withstand the trauma of surgery.[7,9,16,37] However, studies with long-term postoperative follow-up observation demonstrate similar endothelial cell densities after keratoplasty, regardless of donor age.[1,10,27] Culbertson and co-workers have shown that preoperative donor endothelial cell count rather than donor age is a more important determinant of postoperative endothelial cell count.[10] Their study demonstrated no statistically significant correlation between donor age and postoperative endothelial cell density.[10]

DONOR AGE AND GRAFT SUCCESS

Most importantly, no studies have confirmed a relationship between the age of the donor and postoperative graft success. Forster specifically evaluated the effect of donor age upon graft clarity and found no significant difference in the number of clear grafts between a group receiving tissue from donors older than 70 years of age and donors less than 50 years.[13] Others have clearly shown that corneas from donors over 70 years of age can withstand the trauma of preservation and surgery and maintain transparency for long postoperative intervals.[13,21] The diagnosis of the recipient and the surgeon's experience are more important than donor age in determining graft clarity.[2] Age alone is therefore a poor criterion for selecting healthy donor corneal endothelium.

CELL LOSS AFTER KERATOPLASTY

Factors such as surgical trauma, postoperative inflammation, and endothelial cell migration may contribute to decreased endothelial cell density after keratoplasty. Bourne demonstrated a nearly 60% loss of endothelial cells from the central graft during the first 3 years after keratoplasty.[6] Although the rate of cell loss diminishes during the late postoperative period, specular microscopy has demonstrated average cell densities of approximately 700 cells/mm^2 in optically clear grafts with long-term follow-up study.[1] Although not clearly defined, a critical endothelial cell density is probably necessary to maintain normal corneal hydration; this value is estimated between 400 and 500 cells/mm^2.[44]

EVALUATION OF DONOR CORNEAS

The majority of eye banks rely upon biomicroscopy to assess the quality of the donor endothelium

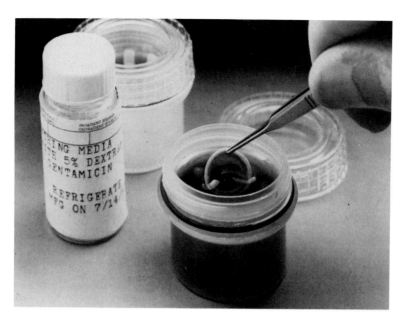

Fig. 43-3. Corneal viewing and storage chamber allows atraumatic and sterile examination of donor endothelium by specular microscopy. (Courtesy CooperVision Laboratories, Menlo Park, Calif.)

before transplantation.[17] One can obtain an indirect assessment of endothelial function by grading the amount of corneal stromal edema and folds in Descemet's membrane and identifying cornea guttata. Although specular microscopy is a more sensitive method of evaluating endothelial morphology, only 15% of eye banks and 7% of corneal surgeons recommend it as a screening tool.[3] Reluctance to adopt this technique most likely reflects concern about expense, inconvenience, and the possibility of contamination and excessive manipulation of donor corneal tissue.[32]

Specular microscopy can be performed upon whole donor globes supported in special fixation devices.[18] A more popular method is to examine the excised cornea with its scleral rim by use of modified corneal storage containers.[28] New synthetic materials allow the same chamber to be used for viewing and storage. This minimizes the risk of contamination and endothelial trauma, which may result from excessive tissue manipulation (Fig. 43-3).[5,32] The system may be modified with a high-sensitivity video camera and video recording system and can be used in the noncontact mode for rapid endothelial screening.[32,35] Endothelial evaluation is best performed early after excision of the corneoscleral specimen, since prolonged storage time may cause stromal edema and folds in Descemet's membrane, which degrade the specular image.

Although high endothelial cell density alone does not guarantee a healthy, functioning endothelium, there is a positive correlation between normal endothelial morphology and the functional reserve of the endothelium.[34,39,44] A high percentage of hexagonal cells and an absence of polymegethism imply a stable endothelial monolayer.[39] Such pathologic endothelial changes may not be associated with clinically significant stromal edema or cornea guttata and may be detected only with specular microscopy. Since endothelial morphology and cell density are not strictly age dependent, the specular microscope may allow safe extension of the donor age criterion by allowing identification of older donors with morphologically normal endothelium (Fig. 43-4).[30] Similarly, young donor tissue with abnormal endothelial morphology or unusually low cell density may be identified and rejected for transplantation (Fig. 43-4).

Specific criteria for donor endothelial cell density are uncertain and may vary with the recipient corneal pathologic condition. Patients with a primary endotheliopathy may require a healthier donor endothelium than patients undergoing keratoplasty for keratoconus or corneal scarring. Presumably, the latter have healthy peripheral host endothelium, which may contribute to the final cell density. Given the large postoperative endothelial cell loss and cell loss with aging, the donor endothelial cell density should probably be greater than 1500 cells/mm^2 to ensure sufficient density for corneal deturgescence.

In conclusion, age alone is a poor guideline for

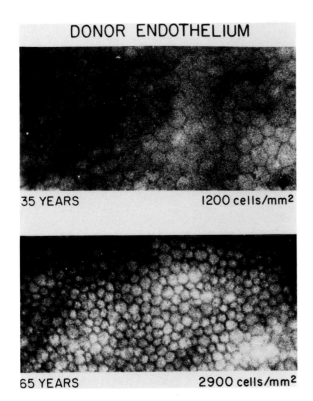

Fig. 43-4. Specular micrograph from 35-year-old donor cornea demonstrates pronounced polymegethism and cellular pleomorphism and low endothelial cell count. In contrast, cornea from 65-year-old donor shows uniform hexagonal cells and high endothelial cell density. (Courtesy Dr. Mamoru Matsuda, Osaka, Japan.)

the selection of donor corneal tissue. A donor cornea with normal endothelial cell density and morphology may be suitable for transplantation regardless of age.

REFERENCES

1. Abbott RL, Fine M, Guillet E: Long-term changes in corneal endothelium following penetrating keratoplasty, *Ophthalmology* 90:676, 1983.
2. Abbott RL, Forster RK: Determinants of graft clarity in penetrating keratoplasty, *Arch Ophthalmol* 97:1071, 1979.
3. Binder PS: Eye banking and corneal preservation. In *Symposium on Medical and Surgical Diseases of the Cornea,* Transactions of the New Orleans Academy of Ophthalmology, St. Louis, 1980, Mosby–Year Book, pp 320-354.
4. Blomdahl S: Ultrasonic measurements of the eye in the newborn infant, *Acta Ophthalmol* 57:1048, 1979.
5. Bourne WM: Examination and photography of donor corneal endothelium, *Arch Ophthalmol* 94:1799, 1976.
6. Bourne WM: Morphologic and functional evaluation of the endothelium of transplanted human corneas, *Trans Am Ophthalmol Soc* 81:403, 1983.
7. Bourne WM, Kaufman HE: The endothelium of clear corneal transplants, *Arch Ophthalmol* 94:1730, 1976.
8. Bourne WM, Kaufman HE: Specular microscopy of human corneal endothelium *in vivo, Am J Ophthalmol* 81:319, 1976.
9. Bourne WM, O'Fallan WM: Endothelial cell loss during penetrating keratoplasty, *Am J Ophthalmol* 85:760, 1978.
10. Culbertson WW, Abbott RL, Forster RW: Endothelial cell loss in penetrating keratoplasty, *Ophthalmology* 89:600, 1982.
11. Donzis PB, Insler MS, Gordon RA: Corneal curvatures in premature infants, *Am J Ophthalmol* 99:213, 1985.
12. Eye Bank Association of America, Inc: *Medical Standards,* Washington DC, 1990.
13. Forster RK, Fine M: Relation of donor age to success in penetrating keratoplasty, *Arch Ophthalmol* 85:42, 1971.
14. Gordon RA, Donzis PB: Refractive development of the human eye, *Arch Ophthalmol* 103:785, 1985.
15. Grignolo A, Rivara A: Biometry of the human eye from the sixth month of pregnancy to the tenth year of life (measurement of the axial length, retinoscopy refraction, total refraction, corneal, and lens refraction), *Acta Facultatis Medicae Universitatis Brunensis* 35:251, 1968.
16. Hiles DA, Biglan AW, Fetherolf EC: Central corneal endothelial cell counts in children, *Am Intra-Ocular Implant Soc J* 5:292, 1979.
17. Hirst LW, Stark WJ: Donor corneal endothelium: slit-lamp examination of buttons in storage medium, *Ophthalmic Surg* 9:51, 1978.
18. Hoefle FB, Maurice PM, Sibley RC: Human corneal donor material: a method of examination before keratoplasty, *Arch Ophthalmol* 84:741, 1970.
19. Hoffer KJ, Kraff MC: Normal endothelial cell count range, *Ophthalmology* 87:861, 1980.
20. Inagaki Y et al: Rearranged automated keratometer for newborn infants and patients in the supine position, *Am J Ophthalmol* 99:664, 1985.
21. Jenkins MS, Lempert SL, Brown SI: Significance of donor age in penetrating keratoplasty, *Ann Ophthalmol* 11:924, 1979.
22. Kaufman HE, Capella JA, Robbins JE: The human corneal endothelium, *Am J Ophthalmol* 61:835, 1966.
23. Koenig SB: Myopic shift in refraction following penetrating keratoplasty with pediatric donor tissue, *Am J Ophthalmol* 101:740, 1986.
24. Koenig SB, Graul E, Kaufman HE: Ocular refraction after penetrating keratoplasty with infant donor corneas, *Am J Ophthalmol* 94:534, 1982.
25. Laing RA, et al: Changes in the corneal endothelium as a function of age, *Exp Eye Res* 22:587, 1976.
26. Laule A, et al: Endothelial cell population changes of human cornea during life, *Arch Ophthalmol* 96:2031, 1978.
27. Linn JG et al: Endothelial morphology in long-term keratoconus corneal transplants, *Ophthalmology* 88:761, 1981.
28. McCarey BE, McNeill JI: Specular microscopic evaluation of donor corneal endothelium, *Ann Ophthalmol* 9:1279, 1977.
29. Matsuda M, Yee RW, Edelhauser HF: Comparison of the corneal endothelium in an American and a Japanese population, *Arch Ophthalmol* 103:68, 1985.
30. Matsuda M et al: Specular microscopic evaluation of donor corneal endothelium, *Arch Ophthalmol* 104:259, 1986.
31. Murphy C et al: Prenatal and postnatal cellularity of the human corneal endothelium, *Invest Ophthalmol Vis Sci* 25:312, 1984.
32. Nesburn AB et al: A specular microscopic viewing system for donor corneas, *Ophthalmology* 90:686, 1983.
33. Pfister RR, Breaud S: Aphakic refractive penetrating keratoplasty using newborn donor corneas, *Ophthalmology* 90:1207, 1983.

34. Rao G et al: Endothelial morphology and corneal deturgescence, *Ann Ophthalmol* 11:885, 1978.

35. Roberts CW, Koester CJ: Video with wide-field specular microscopy, *Ophthalmology* 88:146, 1981.

36. Roberts CW, Rosskothen HD, Koester CJ: Wide-field specular microscopy of excised donor corneas, *Arch Ophthalmol* 98:881, 1981.

37. Ruusuvaara P: Effects of corneal preservation, donor age, cadaver time and postoperative period on the graft endothelium, *Acta Ophthalmol* 57:868, 1979.

38. Scammon RE, Wilmer HA: Growth of the components of the human eyeball, *Arch Ophthalmol* 43:620, 1950.

39. Schultz RO et al: Corneal endothelial changes in type I and type II diabetes mellitus, *Am J Ophthalmol* 98:401, 1984.

40. Sperling S: Endothelial cell density in donor corneas, *Acta Ophthalmol* 58:278, 1980.

41. Vannas M: Remarks on the technique of corneal transplantation, *Am J Ophthalmol* 33(suppl):70, 1950.

42. Waltman SR: The cornea. In Moses RA, editor: *Adler's physiology of the eye*, St. Louis, 1981, Mosby–Year Book.

43. Waring GO III et al: Individual corneal endothelial cell size correlates poorly with age, *Invest Ophthalmol Vis Sci* 19(suppl):263, 1980.

44. Waring GO III et al: The corneal endothelium, *Ophthalmology* 89:531, 1982.

45. Wood TO, Nissenkorn L: Infant donor corneas for penetrating keratoplasty, *Ophthalmic Surg* 12:500, 1981.

Chapter 44

Tissue Removal

MARSHA A. LISITZA

The retrieval of corneal tissue, either by enucleation and subsequent corneal excision or by in situ corneal removal, is the first surgical step in the chain of events that leads to a successful corneal transplant. Enucleation of the eye is performed by eye bank staff or other trained individuals as authorized by the eye bank medical director and state laws; however, both in situ corneal removal and surgical removal of the corneoscleral rim are performed by personnel trained in the aseptic technique of medium-preserved corneas.[2] These procedures are included in the *Eye Bank Association of America (EBAA) Medical Standards Document* and *Procedures Manual.* The EBAA also offers training courses and grants certification to eye bank technicians in this area.

PREPARATION FOR TISSUE REMOVAL (ENUCLEATION AND IN SITU)

Consent. Consent laws for eye-tissue removal vary, but each eye bank must conform to its state laws. The consent may be given by the donor, by the next of kin or those in charge of the body, or by various state medical examiner laws. Regardless of the form of consent, it must be verified before tissue removal and a copy retained in the eye bank records.[2] Even if consent has been obtained, the coroner (medical examiner) can restrict tissue removal in cases under his jurisdiction and may ask the technician to collect vitreous or return the globe as part of their investigation.

Preparation of Donor. Before the arrival of the technician, the donor's head should be elevated above the chest with a head block or equivalent item. To reduce postmortem changes that affect the corneal endothelium the eyes should be cooled by either local application of ice packs or refrigeration of the donor's body. Upon arrival the technician must identify the donor's body as corresponding to the legal consent and elevate the head, if not already done. A complete review of the donor's chart or circumstances of death should be done before tissue removal so that any donors requiring precautions will be identified. EBAA Medical Standards recognize five diseases that require special handling because they are potentially hazardous to personnel (see Chapter 42). Individual eye banks may have chosen to decline such tissue or have additional restrictions. If an eye bank accepts such tissue, technicians should follow the protocol prescribed by the eye bank. After reviewing the chart the technician should perform a gross inspection of the body for evidence of intravenous drug abuse or infection sites. Since donor tissue retrieval exposes the technician to body fluids, Universal Precautions for health care workers must be observed.[1] Aseptic technique must be employed for all tissue suitable for transplant. The EBAA has developed a complete procedures manual to provide a standardized method for the aseptic procurement of human eye tissue. It describes the detailed steps for enucleation, corneal excision, and in situ corneal removal. To avoid duplication, only supplemental topics are addressed here.

BLOOD SAMPLE

Blood tests for HIV, hepatitis B and C, must be performed on all donor tissue used for transplant.[2] Individual states or programs may require additional testing. Postmortem blood (10 ml) can be obtained from various sites: existing lines, direct heart puncture, or accessible blood vessels. All blood samples should be put into a plain blood collection tube, identified, and transported in plastic bags for protection. Universal Precautions must be observed during the collection.[1] The potential for biohazard injury to the technician, either by needle stick or blood contact, is significant. Certain transfused donors must have their pretransfusion rather than their postmortem blood tested.[2] This sample is usually available in the blood bank as the "type and cross" sample. The blood bank records will contain the times and amount of transfusions, as well as the collection time of the pretransfusion sample.

ENUCLEATION

Surgical Procedure. The goal of an enucleation is to perform an aseptic eye removal without damage to the corneal endothelium. It must also allow for the natural-looking reconstruction of the donor by the funeral director. The surgical technique will affect both endothelial quality and reconstruction of the donor. Two important considerations are that *the donor cornea should not be touched or physically distorted while the whole globe is being removed and the fragile tissues surrounding the eye should not be excessively manipulated during the eye removal.*

The enucleation (Fig. 44-1) may be performed in an operating room, a hospital room, a morgue, a funeral home, or a medical examination facility. Prepare and drape the donor in accordance with the recommended procedure.[3] Insert a solid-blade eye speculum, which will provide even pressure distribution on the lid margins while containing the eyelashes. The use of an adjustable opening speculum may help prevent overextension and subsequent swelling of the eyelids. While you insert the speculum, the blades should not abrade the epithelial surface. The space for speculum insertion can be provided by elevation of the eyelid away from the globe with a cotton-tipped applicator. Perform a limbal peritomy of the conjunctiva, 360 degrees around the cornea, using forceps and blunt-tipped scissors. If excessive traction is applied to the conjunctiva, the cornea can be distorted and corneal pseudoguttae will be induced (personal observation). A blunt dissection under the conjunctiva and Tenon's fascia may be needed to facilitate access to the ocular muscles, especially on young donors. Locate each rectus muscle with a single insertion of a small muscle hook, since continual probing will damage the surrounding tissue. To accomplish this, place the muscle hook directly on the surface of the globe, either proximal or distal to the point of muscle attachment. Insert the hook deeper than the expected location of the muscle and slide it along the globe to catch the muscle. Cut the muscle distal to the hook to avoid cutting the sclera. A hemostat may be clamped onto the muscle before cutting, which leaves a muscle stump that is convenient to help elevate the globe during subsequent procedures. After the first three rectus muscles are cut, the globe will be more likely to swivel and the last rectus muscle may not be in the expected position. The two oblique muscles remain attached. They can be dealt with in one of three ways: (1) locate with the muscle hook, realizing that the insertion is much deeper than the rectus muscles, and cut, (2) clamp the medial rectus muscle with a hemostat and rotate the globe laterally to identify the muscles and cut; or (3) leave attached until after the optic nerve is severed and cut as the globe is removed.

To sever the optic nerve, elevate the globe with either a hemostat clamped to a muscle stump, or with an enucleation spoon. If not sufficiently elevated, the back of the globe might get cut, causing vitreous leakage or collapse of the globe. Although the spoon provides protection for the back of the globe, its presence may cause stretching of the eyelid margins. Insert the enucleation scissors either medially or laterally. Medially is closer to the optic nerve, however, the bridge of the nose may cause physical interference. The scissors should be inserted slightly open to surround the nerve and pushed toward the back of the orbit so that a 3 to 6 mm nerve stump will remain. With the attached hemostat or enucleation spoon, remove the globe, severing any remaining connective tissue and the oblique muscles if still attached. During the entire procedure avoid cutting the eyelashes or lid margins. Place the globe, cornea upright, in a sterile eye jar or equivalent container and secure in a metal eye cage or on a bed of gauze. Irrigate balanced salt solution and ophthalmic antibiotics over the globe, such that the gauze is moist but the eye is never submerged in fluid. Eye jars should be labeled OD or OS and with the donor name. Placed on wet ice, the jars are ready to be transported to the eye bank laboratory. Removal of the tissue *must* be documented in the donor's medical record in hospitals[5] and should be done at all other facilities.[3]

Temporary Donor Reconstruction. The goal of temporary donor reconstruction is to minimize postenucleation edema and color changes so that the funeral director can restore normal appearance. It is important to retain moisture in the surrounding tissue after the globe has been removed. The socket is filled with *moist* cotton or gauze, or some funeral directors have recommended a globe-sized marble. An

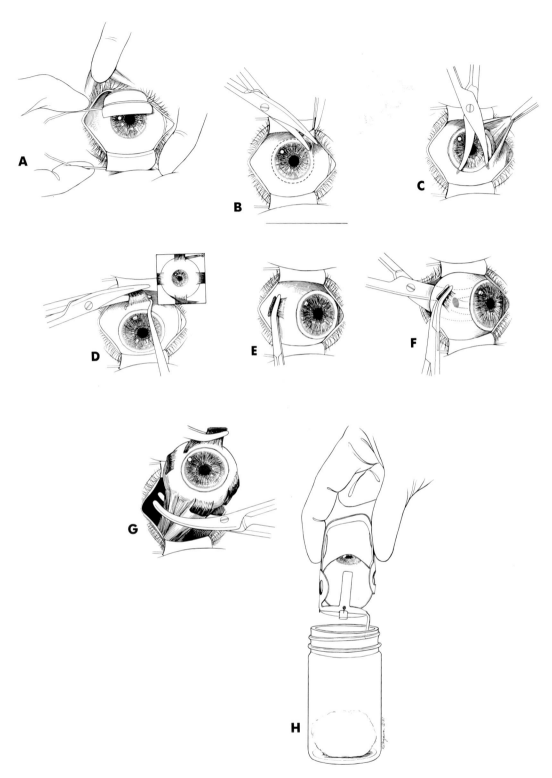

Fig. 44-1. Eye enucleation. **A,** Insert lid speculum. **B,** Grasp conjunctiva and cut around cornea. **C,** Bluntly dissect conjunctiva using scissors-spreading technique. **D,** Isolate and cut superior, medial, and inferior rectus muscles. **E,** Isolate lateral rectus muscle and *clamp*. Cut lateral rectus muscle distally to clamp. **F,** Insert enucleation scissors laterally and cut optic nerve *with ¼-inch stump*. **G,** Elevate eye and excise remaining tissues; cut inferior and superior oblique muscles. **H,** Transfer eye to cage and pin optic nerve. (Courtesy Lynn Kitagawa, Portland, Oregon.)

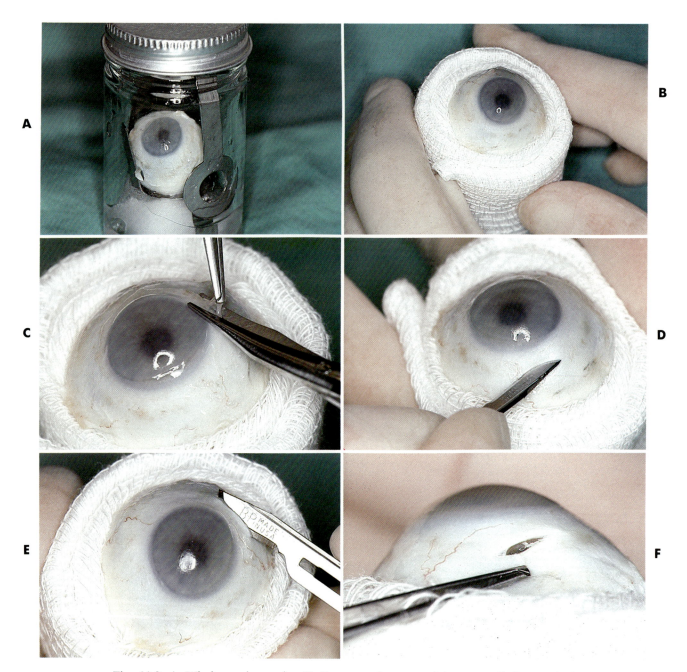

Fig. 44-2. A, Whole eye in eye jar. **B,** Eye securely wrapped in gauze. **C,** Removal of conjunctival remnants with scissors. **D,** Scraping at limbus to remove additional conjunctiva. **E,** Sclerotomy into suprachoroidal space. **F,** Sclerotomy has not penetrated into vitreous.

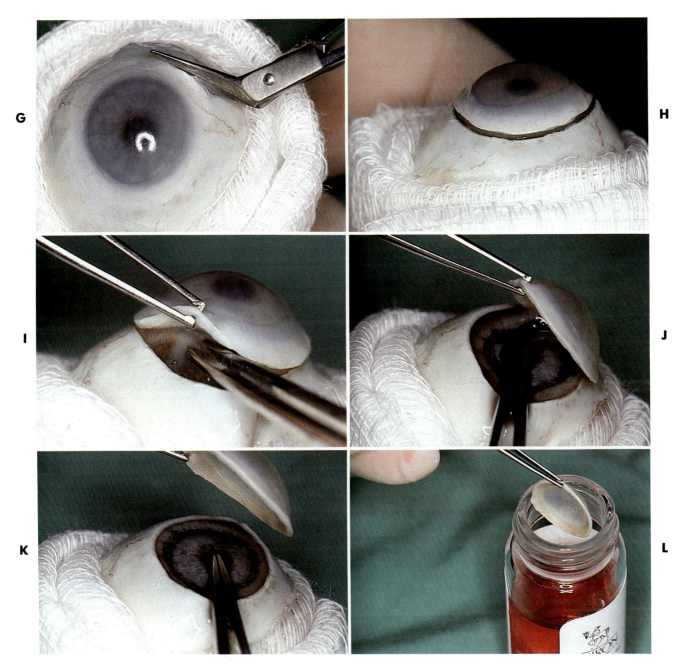

Fig. 44-2, cont'd. G, Scissors introduced into suprachoroidal space for incision. **H,** Complete 360-degree incision without entering vitreous. **I,** Enter anterior chamber by pushing ciliary body down. **J,** Push ciliary body down while without distortion lift cornea up. **K,** Completed corneal removal. **L,** Cornea placed in preservation medium. (Courtesy Patrick Saine, C.R.A., Madison, Wisc.)

eye cap may be placed over the fill; however, it is advisable to check with local funeral directors concerning their preference. Coat the lids both internally and externally with a lubricant and gently close using a cotton-tipped applicator, never forceps. Wipe off any povidone-iodine solution that remains with mild soap, rather than 70% ETOH, which will dry the skin. Skin cream may be applied to the area around the eyes for moisture retention. The head should be left elevated to retard fluid leakage and edema during any further procedures or transportation.

Postenucleation Complications. Postenucleation bleeding within the orbit is a common complication. Bleeding occurs in donors that have elevated pressure in their vascular system upon death. Most funeral directors agree that attempting to stop the bleeding with pressure packing of the socket results only in forcing the blood into the delicate tissues surrounding the eye, causing tissue discoloration and edema. Trocar buttons, chemical cautery, or vessel ligatures have been successfully utilized to stop bleeding. If they are not available, allow the blood to freely exit the socket until the pressure is released. Communication with the funeral director is essential in this situation.

Donors with an eyelid fold, infants, and some elderly donors have a small lid opening area in proportion to the globe size, which may restrict easy removal of the globe. An infant speculum, which is removed before the globe is lifted out, or softening the globe by the sterile removal of a small amount of vitreous, will provide the necessary space.

CORNEOSCLERAL RIM EXCISION

The goals of the corneoscleral rim (CS rim) excision are removal of the CS rim with minimal endothelial cell loss and reduction of bacterial flora adjacent to the excised rim. Follow the aseptic technique outlined in the EBAA Procedures Manual.[3] The use of a laminar air flow hood is highly recommended.[3] Some centers have incorporated additional rinses with sterile saline, a 3- to 5-minute immersion in ophthalmic antibiotic solutions, or a 3-minute immersion in 1% povidone-iodine to decontaminate the globe. The 1% povidone-iodine effectively reduces a broad range of bacteria, fungi, yeast, viruses, and protozoa on contact.[6] Presurgical microbial cultures, though not required, may be performed after decontamination. Positive cultures should be reported to the receiving surgeon or eye bank.[2]

The surgical removal of the CS rim (Fig. 44-2) begins with securely wrapping the posterior globe with a 4 × 4 gauze without excessive pressure. The wrapped globe is either handheld, or, if it is placed on the work surface, a hemostat secures the gauze closure. Remove any remnants of conjunctiva with either a Wescott scissors or by scraping with a no. 11 or 15 blade. This maneuver must be done circumferencially and extend at least 5 mm from the limbus. Exercise care not to distort the cornea by pulling on the conjunctiva or to scratch the epithelial surface with the blade. Using a second blade, make a sclerotomy 2 to 3 mm from the limbus without penetrating the underlying choroid. Gently introduce a Castroviejo scissors into the space and complete a 360-degree incision around the cornea, maintaining a 2 to 3 mm scleral rim. The underlying choroid is delicate, and to avoid breaking into the vitreous, complete the incision with a limited number of scissor reintroductions. The pressure exerted on the globe by the gauze wrap or the hand-holding can also increase choroid breakage. If a vitreous leak does occur, remove and reintroduce the scissors (to avoid continual cutting of the choroid) and reduce pressure on the globe. If the scissor tips enter and collapse the anterior chamber, the iris will contact and potentially damage the corneal endothelium. To avoid this, introduce the scissor tips pointing away from the limbal area and maintain the 2 to 3 mm scleral rim. If the iris contacts the endothelium, it should be documented in the excision record.

To excise the corneoscleral rim, first check for adhering tissue or an incomplete incision and then use one forceps to hold the scleral edge and a second forceps (alternatively a no. 15 blade) to detach the ciliary body by pushing down on it. An air bubble will appear in the anterior chamber if the chamber is entered correctly. Occasionally, the ciliary body is strongly attached to the cornea, and the initial entry into the anterior chamber occurs behind the iris. If this occurs, either grasp the iris with a forceps and pull it down before proceeding with the detachment, or abandon the entry spot and restart at another position. Continue to push the ciliary body circumferencially away from the corneoscleral rim until it is free. Avoid distorting the normal corneal shape with excessive traction, since stress lines of pseudoguttae may be induced in the endothelium. Do not touch the endothelium or allow long exposure to air during the maneuver. Endothelial damage and tears can occur during the removal process. Once free, the corneoscleral rim should immediately be placed in corneal storage medium. After both corneas are in their media, the bottle should be labeled according to EBAA Medical Standards and sealed with a shrink seal. The vials are stored at 4° C in a quarantined area until blood test results have been received.

IN SITU EXCISION

An in situ excision of the corneoscleral rim is performed when the legal consent dictates that only the corneas may be removed from the donor. The aseptic technique is outlined in the EBAA Procedures Manual. Because the in situ excision is performed in a variety of locations and no additional decontamination of the tissue is possible, the technician must be aware of the bacteriologic considerations outlined in Chapter 45. Ideally, the in situ procedure should be performed in a well-lit, disinfected area that has a minimum of airflow and no traffic. The initial preparation is the same as for an enucleation; however, two bottles of cornea storage medium must be present. Before removal the corneas should be examined with a penlight for foreign material. The initial irrigation of the eye will be the only opportunity to remove this material. Ophthalmic antibiotic solutions may be added during the donor preparation.[3] As in the enucleation a 360 degree peritomy of the conjunctiva is performed at the limbus. Since no later conjunctival removal is possible, any remnants must be completely removed by scraping with a blade. The sclerotomy and excision are performed as described in the corneoscleral rim procedure; however, because of the limitation of space, several additional surgical techniques may be useful. To facilitate the excision some centers utilize both left-and right-handed Castroviejo scissors or score and complete the scleral incision with a 15 mm trephine. The corneoscleral rim is removed as previously described and placed directly into the corneal storage medium. Since only the cornea has been removed, the temporary donor reconstruction requires only an eye cap. Follow the same considerations for the tissue around the eye as in an enucleation.

ACKNOWLEDGMENTS

I wish to thank Patrick Saine, C.R.A., for the ophthalmic photography and Lynn Kitagawa for use of the eye enucleation illustrations.

REFERENCES

1. Centers for Disease Control: Update: universal precautions for prevention of transmission of human immunodeficiency virus, hepatitis B virus, and other bloodborne pathogens in health care settings, *MMWR* 37:377-382, 387-88, 1988.
2. Eye Bank Association of America: *Medical standards*, Washington, DC, 1990.
3. Eye Bank Association of America: *Procedures manual*, Washington, DC, 1992.
4. Grutzmacher RD et al: Donor corneal endothelial striae, *Am J Ophthalmol* 102(4):508-515, 1986.
5. Joint Commission on Accreditation of Healthcare Organizations: *Accreditation manual for hospitals*, vol 1, Oakbrook Terrace, Ill, 1990.
6. Mindrup EA, Dubbel PA, Doughman DJ: Betadine decontamination of donor globes. (In preparation.)

Chapter 45

Tissue Evaluation

Gross and slitlamp examination of the donor eye

WILLIAM J. REINHART

Unlike many manufactured items, donor corneas supplied by an eye bank carry no warranty or guarantee. Indeed, the donor information form enclosed with the donor corneal tissue from most eye banks includes a disclaimer stating that the using ophthalmic surgeon is ultimately responsible for evaluating the donor tissue and determining its suitability for use. Even the most diligent surgeon, however, cannot determine from examination of the donor eye alone if the donor may have been septic, infected with transmissible fatal viruses such as rabies or Creutzfeldt-Jakob disease, or that antibiotics had not been added to the excised corneoscleral rim. The surgeon's review of the donor information form is useful, therefore only if all the appropriate information has been actively sought for and recorded by eye bank personnel. Obviously the using surgeon must trust the care, precision, and thoroughness of the eye bank team. It has been the goal of the medical standards committee of the Eye Bank Association of America to ensure that this trust is well placed.

The enucleator, eye bank technician, and ophthalmic surgeon assume that the thermometers, autoclave, tissue culture media, antibiotics, and so on meet certain standards. It is wise to harbor a small degree of paranoia about any system where errors of manufacture, design, or preparation technique may creep in. Protocol manuals help ensure that mistakes will not be made, but it is wise to review procedures periodically and share experience with others involved in eye banking through telephone, news letters, electronic mail, scientific meetings, and scientific publications.

PROCUREMENT

Donor corneal tissue may be obtained using the following techniques:

1. *In situ corneoscleral rim excision* with immediate transfer into storage media
2. *Whole-globe enucleation* with moist chamber storage
3. Whole-globe enucleation followed by *laboratory corneoscleral rim excision* with transfer to the following:
   a. Storage media
      (1) Short-term, such as McCarey-Kaufman medium (MK)[11]
      (2) Intermediate-term, such as K-Sol,[7] CSM,[9] Dexsol,[8] Optisol,[6,10] and ProCell[15]
   b. Organ culture[2]
   c. Cryopreservation[1]

All methods require a careful in situ examination of the donor eye and the orbit. Laboratory examination of the donor globe or excised corneoscleral rim with the aid of a written evaluation form should then precede the offer of tissue to the requesting surgeon. Careful attention to detail will improve the eye bank technician's competence and, in turn, the ophthalmic surgeon's confidence in the eye bank system.

IN SITU EXAMINATION OF EYE AND ORBIT

The enucleator should perform a careful inspection of the forearms and antecubital fossa for evidence of intravenous drug abuse especially manifested by the hyperpigmented linear lines of sclerosed veins from repeated injections. Examination of the periorbital and orbital tissues in cases involving facial trauma such as vehicular accidents, homicide, and so on may indicate how severely the eye itself may have been traumatized before death. The lids, lashes, and periorbital tissues should be carefully examined for signs of infection such as styes, skin pustules, or accumulation of mucopurulent material on the lid margins and lashes from conjunctivitis. Findings on gross examination may help explain asymmetric findings on later slitlamp laboratory examination and should be carefully recorded. Any of these findings may be important information in deciding if the tissue is suitable for transplantation. Obviously examination of the enucleated eye or excised corneoscleral rim in the laboratory cannot reveal any of these associated findings, and so the enucleator must be diligent in seeking and recording this information.

When enucleation is performed, in situ examination of the anterior segment of the eye is less important, since a careful gross and slitlamp examination will be performed in the laboratory. However, a careful in situ gross examination may allow the enucleator to supply an educated guess as to the suitability of tissue for transplantation, and a telephone call placed immediately after enucleation may permit the transplant coordinator an early opportunity for a distribution alert before laboratory confirmation of suitability, especially if there will be a long transfer time involved between enucleation and arrival of tissue at the laboratory. For in situ corneoscleral rim excisions, however, a careful gross examination is very important. Since few eye banks include a portable slitlamp in situ examination in their protocol, the technician must be adept at a careful penlight examination for two major reasons. First, if the donor eye has been subjected to anterior segment surgery, such as cataract surgery, cataract intraocular lens implant surgery, and laser surgery involving the iris, or if there are congenital anomalies of the iris or lens, or both, not involving the cornea, these findings cannot be detected on subsequent laboratory examination of the excised corneoscleral rim. In addition, an evaluation of the degree of stromal folds and stromal edema will be more precisely assessed before placement in storage media containing osmotic agents, such as dextran, which will decrease the stromal hydration of a previously swollen cornea. When the same technician is responsible for both the enucleation or corneoscleral rim in situ excision and later examination in the laboratory, the slitlamp examination will gradually improve the technician's ability to predict abnormalities from the gross examination.

GROSS EXAMINATION

In Situ. A penlight with fresh batteries is used to provide oblique illumination for the optically un-

aided eye to allow detection of the following:
1. Epithelial edema (haze), epithelial defects—exposure, trauma, foreign bodies
2. Stromal opacities
   a. Arcus senilis
   b. Central corneal stromal scars
   c. Nonulcerated anterior stromal infiltrates
   d. Microbial infiltrates
3. Estimate of stromal edema
   a. Clarity of cornea
   b. Number and severity of deep stromal folds (light, obvious, and heavy striae)
4. Keratitic precipitates
5. Abnormal corneal shape
   a. Keratoconus
   b. Microcornea or megalocornea
6. Condition of anterior chamber
   a. Formed, shallow, or flat
   b. Evidence of gross blood
   c. Abnormal anterior segment anatomy
      (1) Congenital
      (2) Acquired, such as intraocular surgery
   d. Haziness of aqueous humor

Enucleated Eye. The examination is conducted in the same manner as described for the in situ eye except that the external posterior area of the globe can also be examined for abnormalities such as previous retinal detachment surgery. In addition, evidence of poor enucleation technique as manifested by traumatic corneal epithelial abrasions, retention of excessive orbital tissue, lacerations of the globe, or sectioning of the posterior area of the globe may alert the laboratory to the possibility of a poorly trained enucleator. A globe improperly transported immersed in saline solution may help explain an excessive amount of stromal edema and may not necessarily negate use of the eye if adequate endothelial function can be determined as, for example, by specular microscopy.

SLITLAMP EXAMINATION

A careful slitlamp examination of the donor globe or excised corneoscleral rim is the sine qua non quality control of a first-class eye bank before the release of tissue to the accepting surgeon. The major skill that eludes many technicians is the ability to adequately evaluate the corneal endothelium. The improved optics of a corneal storage viewing chamber will allow even the neophyte, however, to rapidly acquire the ability to evaluate the corneal endothelial sheet, which in turn will improve his ability to detect abnormalities that may require interpretation by the medical director. The technician will then feel more confident in evaluating the endothelium in whole globes or excised corneoscleral rims stored in bottles where the optics make endothelial evaluation much more difficult even for the experienced technician or surgeon.

Whole Globe Examination

1. Remove the eye jar lid and place it upside down in a sterile area such as a laminar flow hood or an ultraviolet-lamp tissue-transfer hood if the whole eye is to be shipped in the same container. Decant any excessive fluid from the jar and then clamp the jar in place in a viewing brace attached to the slitlamp. The eye in its holding cage should be brought forward using sterile forceps, hemostat, or cotton-tipped applicators.

2. Using low magnification and either the diffuse illumination provided by a filter or a wide slit beam held at 45 degrees, examine the anterior globe. Major defects, which might be missed at higher magnification, will be more easily identified at low magnification for subsequent study. In general, after an overall view of the eye has been obtained, the exam should proceed in a systematic fashion from the corneal epithelium back to the anterior surface of the iris and lens using first a broad and then a more narrowed slit for each aspect of the examination.

3. Adjust the microscope head and the slit beam so that they are almost coaxial, creating retroillumination, which with searching, may reveal defects or opacities in the stroma that may not have been noticed with an oblique slit.

Corneal epithelium. Microcystic edema, abrasions, and retained foreign bodies should be looked for. Nonvital epithelium may have lost its adhesion to the underlying stroma and may have been rubbed off by lid action. If the epithelium is missing, it is necessary to carefully rule out stromal injury. Foreign bodies embedded in the epithelium should be carefully examined with a narrow slit beam to determine if they have penetrated into the corneal stroma. The interpalpebral area of the corneal epithelium, which may have been exposed ante and post mortem, should be carefully examined for the presence of missing epithelium (Fig. 45-1), underlying evidence of stromal opacification or inflammatory infiltrate. It is not always possible to distinguish between stromal scars, noninfectious stromal infiltrates, and microbial infiltrates. In general, stromal scars have a more slate gray appearance without adjacent stromal edema, whereas microbial infiltrates have more discrete borders, adjacent stromal edema, and a white or yellowish white appearance. If the stromal opacity involves

the central cornea, the cornea should not be offered for transplantation, whereas marginal opacities are primarily of concern if microbial infection cannot be ruled out. Unless it is obviously an inactive stromal scar, the medical director and using surgeon should make the final decision regarding acceptability for transplantation.

Corneal stroma. Major stromal opacities will already have been identified with the gross examination, low-magnification scan, and retroillumination. Higher magnification using a narrow slit beam is used to define the extent, depth, location, and appearance of stromal opacities in an attempt to characterize them as congenital or acquired inactive scars or as inflammatory infiltrates (Figs. 45-2 and 45-3). Corneal stromal folds are associated with stromal edema (Fig. 45-4). There is a complex interaction between the barrier and pump function of the corneal endothelium that determines the degree of stromal hydration.[13] At 4° C the pumping action of the endothelium ceases, and the normal cornea will swell. The anatomy of the cornea is such that most of the increased stromal hydration will be accompanied by increased thickening of the cornea toward the endothelial cell layer, throwing the elastic Descemet's membrane into folds, which in turn lead to folds in the deeper corneal stroma. Thus the number and severity of stromal folds depend on factors such as antemortem endothelial function and traumatic disruption of the barrier function of the endothelium as well as postmortem conditions such as temperature, elapsed time from death, and the integrity and hydration of the overlying corneal epithelium. An appreciation for what is normal will help the technician identify tissue with abnormal endothelial function as well as tissue that may have been improperly labeled by an outlying collection station, or allow him to suspect that the estimated time of death to examination time may be longer than indicated.

Corneal endothelium. The use of specular refraction for examination of the corneal endothelium in the whole globe is a skill acquired by practice and experience. The beginning eye bank technician can rapidly acquire experience by examining live subjects,[5] particularly those with Fuchs' endothelial dystrophy. The experience one gains in identifying the abnormal endothelial appearance of these eyes becomes invaluable when later attempting in vitro endothelial assessment in the eye bank laboratory. If the epithelial surface is dried out or irregular, placing a drop or two of antibiotic on the anterior surface of the enucleated eye will improve viewing conditions. The slitlamp is the most efficient and rapid

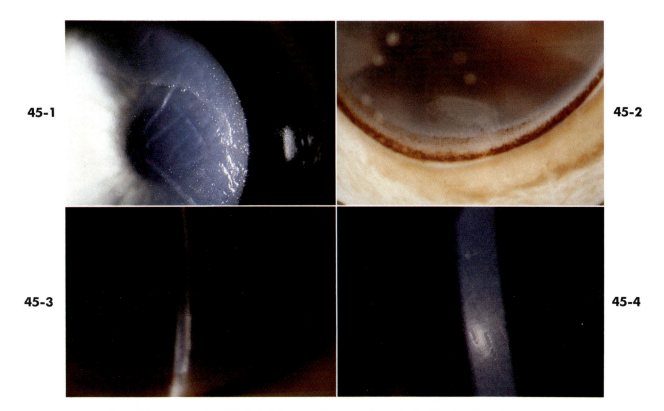

Fig. 45-1. Edges of epithelial defect as shown in broad slit illumination. Mild stromal corneal folds also visible.

Fig. 45-2. Oval anterior stromal infiltrate in excised corneoscleral rim.

Fig. 45-3. Appearance of anterior stromal infiltrate as shown in Fig. 45-2 examined with narrow slit.

Fig. 45-4. Slitlamp appearance of stressline-induced pseudoguttate excrescences.

means for the technician to determine the quality of the endothelial sheet with respect to density of cells, the degree of cell uniformity, the intactness of the endothelial sheet and Descemet's membrane, and the detection of cornea guttata, endothelial vesicles, Descemet's tears, and stress fractures in the endothelial sheet from the trauma of excision (Figs. 45-44 and 45-5).

Eye banks do not determine the refractive status of the donor cornea. Acquired disorders of corneal shape such as keratoconus in its earlier stages can be almost impossible for the eye bank technician to detect in the laboratory though central cornea stromal thinning, deep stromal striae, and stromal scars should all be sought for diligently on slitlamp examination. A donor history of contact lens wear should prompt an even more exhaustive search for such slitlamp signs of keratoconus. Of more concern is the increased prevalence of donors who may have undergone refractive corneal surgery with proce-

dures such as radial keratotomy, epikeratoplasty, keratomileusis, and excimer laser photorefractive ablation. The incisional scars of radial keratotomy, epikeratoplasty, and keratomileusis are usually visible on slitlamp examination though the change in corneal contour may be much more subtle. However, the stromal scarring from laser ablation surgery may be almost undetectable by ophthalmologists using the slitlamp to examine the eye in vivo and so it is unlikely that an eye bank technician will be able to detect all such cases in the laboratory. A donor history of refractive corneal surgery or keratoconus will remain the most reliable means for screening out eye donors with abnormally shaped corneas.

Anterior chamber. A crystalline-appearing aqueous in the anterior chamber may indicate that the eye has been frozen, and it should not be offered for use. The iris should be evaluated for evidence of prior trauma, laser surgery, or intraocular surgery.

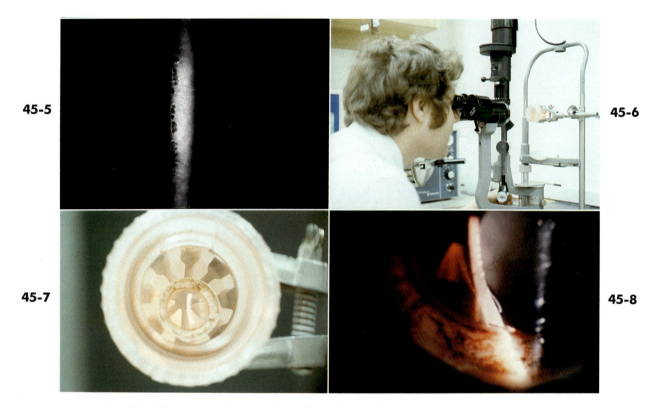

Fig. 45-5. Higher magnification view of stressline-induced pseudoguttate excrescences.
Fig. 45-6. Slitlamp examination of excised corneoscleral rim in a corneal storage viewing chamber.
Fig. 45-7. Excised corneoscleral rim in a corneal storage viewing chamber.
Fig. 45-8. Detached Descemet's membrane in excised corneoscleral rim. (Courtesy G. Rowell, Kansas City Eye Bank, Kansas City, Missouri.)

The presence or absence of the crystalline lens should be determined and an intraocular lens implant, if present, should be identified.

Excised Corneoscleral Rim. Short-term storage containers are usually provided either as glass bottles or plastic viewing chambers each holding approximately 20 ml of storage medium. Before corneoscleral rim excision and transfer, the clarity of the storage medium should be confirmed on slitlamp examination. If there is an excessive amount of ciliary body debris in the medium after transfer of the excised corneoscleral rim, the corneoscleral rim should be transferred to a new storage container. In a humid environment, condensation of moisture on the walls of the container may prevent adequate viewing if the container has been refrigerated. The glass vials may be clamped so that the cornea may be viewed through the side of the bottle or through the bottom directly with a viewing mirror. Many technicians and surgeons prefer a corneal viewing chamber because of the superior optical qualities (Figs. 45-6 and 45-7).

The slitlamp evaluation of the excised corneoscleral rim proceeds in the same fashion as described for the whole globe from epithelium back. If the same technician has performed the whole eye slitlamp examination and corneoscleral rim excision, the major effort is directed at detecting any evidence of epithelial or endothelial trauma as a result of the excision. Particular attention should be directed at detection of Descemet's membrane detachments, which may be too small to be of any significance but should be pointed out to the accepting surgeon (Fig. 45-8).

EVALUATION FORM

Finally, a laboratory pro forma should be completed, detailing the findings noted above. Details regarding time of death, time of death to refrigeration, time of enucleation, transport time, warming time in the laboratory for specular microscopy or slitlamp examination, and endothelial cell density determinations with an estimation of cell shape and variation (pleomorphism) should be recorded and forwarded with the tissue along with the name of the examining technician or medical director.

SPECULAR MICROSCOPY

Specular microscopy is very appealing to eye bank technicians, since it allows for a seemingly precise determination of endothelial cell density and allows cornea guttata to be easily identified. One must remember, however, that the area of the central corneal endothelium in a typical 8 to 8.5 mm donor button is much larger than any area that can be sampled by the specular microscope even with multiple field examinations.[4] In addition, there may be a significant amount of rewarming time needed to allow viewing of the corneal endothelial mosaic. A careful slitlamp examination remains the most important means of assessing the overall character of the endothelial sheet, and specular microscopy should be regarded as a supplementary tool. Since many eye banks have a significant turnover in part-time personnel, the publications listed in the bibliography are particularly didactic for the novice and can be recommended as permanent additions to the eye bank laboratory library.[3-5,12,14]

REFERENCES

1. Capella JA, Kaufman HE, Robbins JE: Preservation of viable corneal material, *Arch Ophthalmol* 74:669-673, 1965.
2. Doughman DJ: Prolonged donor cornea preservation in organ culture, *Trans Am Ophthalmol Soc* 78:577-628, 1980.
3. Hirst LW, Lees GP, Requard J: *Slit lamp training atlas for eye bank technicians*, Tissue Banks International, Inc., The Eye Bank Building, 815 Park Ave., Baltimore, MD 21201.
4. Hirst LW, Yamauchi K, Enger C, et al: Quantitative analysis of wide-field specular microscopy, *Invest Ophthalmol Vis Sci* 30:1972-1979, 1989.
5. Holladay JT, Bishop JE, Prager TC: Quantitative endothelial biomicroscopy, *Ophthalmic Surg* 14:33-40, 1983.
6. Kaufman HE, Beuerman RW, Steinemann TL, et al: Optisol corneal storage media, *Arch Ophthalmol* 109:864-868, 1991.
7. Kaufman HE, Varnell ED, Kaufman S, et al: K-Sol corneal preservation, *Am J Ophthalmol* 100:299-304, 1985.
8. Lass JH, Reinhart WJ, Skelnik DL, et al: An in vitro and clinical comparison of corneal storage medium with and without dextran, *Ophthalmology* 97:96-103, 1990.
9. Lindstrom RL, Doughman DJ, Skelnik DL, Mindrup EA: Minnesota system corneal preservation, *Br J Ophthalmol* 70:47-54, 1986.
10. Lindstrom RL, Skelnik DL, Lass JL, et al: Optisol—a new 4° C corneal preservation solution, *Invest Ophthalmol* 31(suppl):475, 1990.
11. McCarey BE, Kaufman HE: Improved corneal storage, *Invest Ophthalmol* 13:165-173, 1974.
12. Martonyi CL, Bahn CF, Meyer RF: Clinical slit lamp biomicroscopy and photo slit lamp biomicrography, *J Ophthalmic Photogr* 7:3-77, 1984.
13. Mishima S: Clinical investigations on the corneal endothelium, *Am J Ophthalmol* 93:1-29, 1982.
14. Requard JJ: *Evaluation of donor corneas, Eye bank technician manual*, IX-1-5, 1984, Eye Bank Association of America, 1511 K Street, Suite 830, Washington, DC 20005-1401.
15. Skelnik DL, Pearlstein CS, Mindrup EA, Lindstrom RL: Corneal preservation at 4° C with chondroitin sulfate containing medium supplemented with dextran and epidermal growth factor (EGF), *Invest Ophthalmol Vis Sci* 29(suppl):111, 1988.

Specular microscopy of donor corneas

RONALD A. LAING

The primary concern in evaluating the suitability of donor corneal tissue for use in penetrating keratoplasty is the condition of the corneal endothelium, the region of the cornea that is primarily responsible for the maintenance of normal corneal turgor and transparency. Through changes in cell morphology, the corneal endothelium reflects stresses and strains that have been placed on the cornea. Thus any morphologic changes that are seen in the endothelium are indicative of the current status of the endothelium as well as its functional reserve.

Specular microscopy is a method of evaluation that allows for, in either a clinical or eye bank setting, the direct observation of the corneal endothelium. Other tissues that may be seen with the specular microscope include the corneal epithelium, the cells of the crystalline lens, various types of ocular debris, inflammatory cells, and optically reflecting structures. The optical principles of specular microscopy[10] and the evaluation of corneal endothelium using specular microscopy;[11] have been described. Also, several reviews of the general field of ocular specular microscopy have been published.[7,12,14]

In many respects, the information obtained in specular microscopy of the corneal endothelium is similar to that received from scanning electron microscopy (SEM) but has the distinct advantage of allowing the observation to occur without inflicting any damage to the cornea. If desired, serial observations may be made to observe morphologic changes over time in the same cornea. In addition, the specular microscope allows for the observation of reflecting structures within the cells that cannot be discerned with SEM.

The importance in the determination of the viability of the corneal endothelium in the evaluation of potential penetrating keratoplasty donor corneas makes specular microscopy a valuable tool as a non-invasive, nondamaging method of endothelial cell evaluation. Recent technologic advances have brought about computerized morphometric analysis of specular micrographs, which allows for rapid quantitative analysis regarding the state of the donor corneal endothelium.

PRINCIPLES OF EYE BANK SPECULAR MICROSCOPY

The specular microscope is an optical reflection microscope that reflects a slit of light from the cornea and allows observation of this specularly reflected beam. In this context, the term "specular reflection" refers to the situation where, as with a mirror, the angle the reflected beam of light makes with the reflecting surface is equal to the angle that the incident light beam makes with the reflecting surface.

Because of its design, the specular microscope does not allow nonspecular light rays to be observed so that the image that is seen is, essentially, attributable solely to the specularly reflected light rays.

Fig. 45-9 shows a simplified optical design of the eye bank specular microscope. As is seen in this figure, a projected slit is focused onto the posterior endothelial surface by an objective lens. The light that is reflected from this surface is collected by the same objective lens and either is focused onto the film plane or may be directly observed by the examiner. An image of the posterior surface is seen at the film plane. By focusing the specular microscope at places other than the posterior corneal surface, one may observe various other reflecting surfaces. For example, by focusing the instrument on a plane within the stroma, one may detect the presence of ghost vessels, which are typically seen as linear refractile structures.

In the normal endothelial image, one sees the cells as having dark cell borders and bright cell surfaces. The reason for this appearance is illustrated in Fig. 45-10, which shows the nature of the specular reflection from various types of endothelial surfaces. Demonstrated are surfaces that are smooth, rough, wavy, and with excrescences respectively. In each

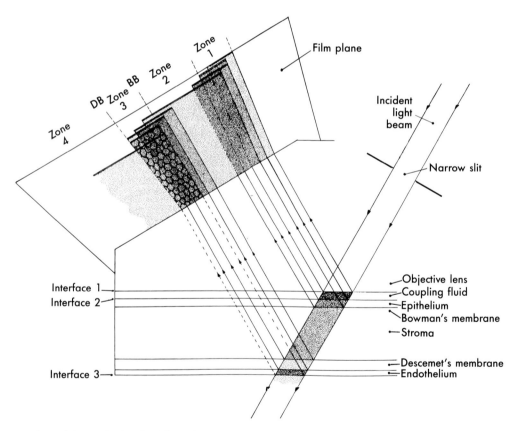

Fig. 45-9. Optical principles of the eye bank specular microscope. A slit of light is focused onto surface of interest (normally posterior endothelial surface). Specularly (mirrorlike) reflected light rays are focused onto film plane. In general, image at film plane can be viewed with a viewing ocular lens or seen on a real-time video monitor.

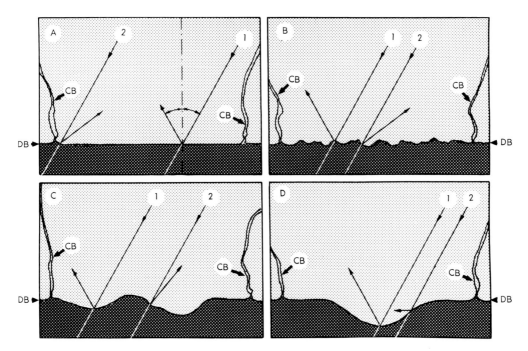

Fig. 45-10. Nature of specular reflection from various types of posterior endothelial surfaces. Surfaces shown are, **A,** smooth; **B,** rough; **C,** wavy; and **D,** a posterior endothelial surface containing an excrescence. In each figure, cell boundary is denoted by *CB;* ray denoted as *1* is collected by objective lens of specular microscope and results in a bright area on film whereas ray denoted as *2* is not collected by objective lens and result is a dark region on film plane. *DB,* Dark boundary as seen on specular micrographs.

case, the ray indicated as *1* reflects from a "flat" portion of the surface and is specularly reflected directly into the objective lens, thus causing the surface to appear as a bright structure to the observer. The rays indicated as *2* are specularly reflected from a curved part of the surface and as such are not collected by the objective lens. Therefore curved surfaces, such as the cell borders, the sides of rough areas, and the sides of an excrescence, appear dark to the observer. In specular microscopy then, the normal endothelial cell having a smooth surface appears as a bright circle surrounded by a dark border. If, instead of a smooth surface, the cell has a rough surface, the inside of the cell will have a granular appearance with the spacing between the granular dark regions being indicative of the degree of roughness of the surface. As may be seen in Fig. 45-10, *D,* isolated corneal guttae will appear as roundish dark structures with a central bright spot, which marks the apex of the excrescence.

EYE BANK SPECULAR MICROSCOPE

A typical eye bank specular microscope is shown in Fig. 45-11. This and similar instruments allow ob-

servation of the corneal endothelium, epithelium, and stroma in either whole globes or excised corneas stored in preservation media. The instrument shown allows the cornea to be tilted about its center of curvature, allowing observation of the peripheral as well as the central endothelium. Since the optics head is mounted to a rigid column, a variety of cameras may be attached to a unit without concern for the weight of the camera. In general, both direct observation and documentation of the image on film are used concomitantly.

TECHNIQUES OF EYE BANK SPECULAR MICROSCOPY

With the specular microscope, the donor cornea may be evaluated in either the enucleated globe or as an excised corneal button stored in a preservation medium. The clinical specular microscope also allows for the physician to observe the corneal endothelium of the donor cornea after transplant in the recipient's eye.

For optimal analysis of the corneal endothelium, the cornea to be examined must be at room temperature, around 25° C, to eliminate artifacts associated

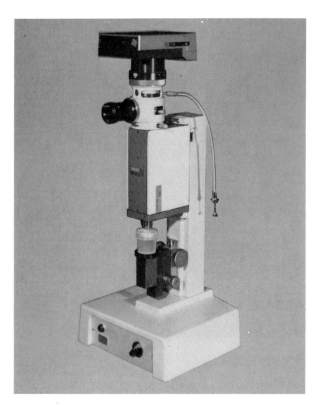

Fig. 45-11. Eye bank specular microscope. Various magnifications and modes of operation are possible when objective or ocular lens are changed. As well as high-resolution direct observation, this instrument allows for real-time viewing on a video monitor, hard-copy documentation on 35 mm, Polaroid, or other film type, and recording of image obtained on videotape. This instrument also has capability of direct input of image into a computerized morphometric analysis system. (Courtesy Bio-Optics, Inc., Arlington, Mass.)

with the appearance of the corneal endothelium at low temperature. Fig. 45-12 shows a comparison of the appearance of the corneal endothelium at both 4° C, *A,* and after warming to room temperature, *B.* As may be seen in these photographs, there is a noticeable abnormality in the appearance of the endothelium of the cornea at 4° C, yet the cells appear normal after warming to room temperature. The cycle of cooling, warming, and recooling of a donor cornea has been shown to have no adverse affects on the metabolic or morphometric status of the donor cornea.[17]

Although examination of the endothelium may be carried out with a whole globe, this necessitates the objective lens coming into contact with the donor cornea. Therefore maximal care must be taken to ensure that the instruments used are sterile. Observation of the endothelium in the whole globe is rela-

tively easy until folds begin to occur in Descemet's membrane concurrent with the advent of corneal edema, at about 6 hours post mortem. However, even after storage for 19 hours in a moist chamber at 4° C, meaningful endothelial cell observations can be made on the donor eye[13] if one looks between the folds of Descemet's membrane. By applying pressure to the globe for a period of time, one can eliminate (or at least minimize) the folds, thus allowing for endothelial cell observation.[6] Whether this practice affects the endothelium adversely is not known, and it is not recommended for use in the evaluation of potential penetrating keratpplasty donor corneas if other, less stressful, procedures are available.

For the observation of the corneal endothelium of the whole globe, the enucleated globe is placed in a special chamber that is then put on the stage of the microscope. The most convenient objective lens to use for this examination is a W10× or a W20× contact objective. With such a lens, the use of the eye bank specular microscope is similar to the use of the clinical version. The stage is moved up until the cone of the objective lens just touches the cornea. The objective lens ring is then turned until the endothelial surface is in focus. At this point, it is generally the case that the cellular outlines are not seen, though a somewhat amorphous structure is apparent. For visualization of the cell borders, the stage on which the globe sits is carefully moved laterally until the conditions necessary for specular microscopy are met; that is, the endothelial surface is perpendicular to the optical axis of the objective lens. Alternately moving the field of observation and refocusing will allow for the cellular image to be obtained. Once the cellular pattern is seen, the focus can be readjusted to sharpen the image of the cell borders and the stage can be tilted to enable peripheral regions of the cornea to be examined. The appearance of the endothelium should be noted on an eye bank donor evaluation form, and documentation of the image should be obtained. This documentation may be either a still photograph (an "instant" Polaroid or video print, or a 35 mm print) or a videotaped recording of the image. If possible, the image should also be analyzed for examination of such parameters as cell density, average cell area, and uniformity of cell shape. This analysis is accurate and easy to perform with a computerized morphometric analysis system.

If the cornea to be evaluated has been excised and placed in a specular microscope viewing chamber,[3] the procedure for examination is as follows. The most convenient objective lens to use in this case is the 13× noncontact objective lens. If necessary, the

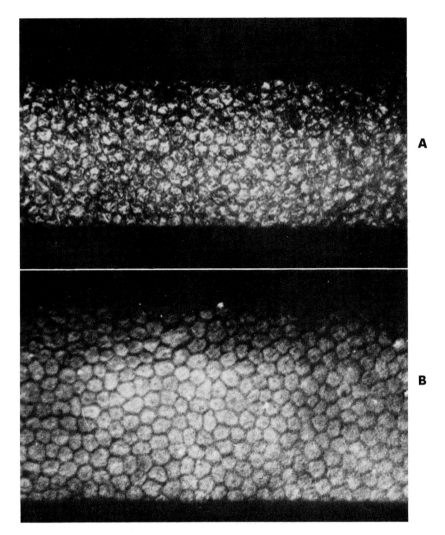

Fig. 45-12. Appearance of corneal endothelium at different temperatures. **A,** 4° C. **B,** Room temperature.

stage of the microscope should be lowered to obtain sufficient clearance for the chamber. The chamber is then placed on the stage of the microscope. The stage is then manipulated so that the cornea is aligned centrally with the objective lens and is as flat as possible relative to the objective lens. The stage can then be moved up toward the objective lens as one looks through the eyepiece of the instrument for the various structures that may be seen as the cornea moves progressively toward the lens. The first surface to come into focus will be the top of the plastic viewing chamber. As the chamber continues to be raised toward the objective lens, the next surface that will come into focus will be the bottom surface of the top of the viewing chamber. As the stage is carefully moved up, the next image that will come into focus will be the endothelial surface. It is un-

likely that the image seen at this point will resemble, at least to the inexperienced user, anything remotely familiar to the appearance of the endothelial cells in the photographs in this book. Here the cell borders may not be seen, in that the conditions necessary to see the specular image have not yet been met, that is, that the endothelial surface is flat relative to the objective lens. With practice, the nonspecular image is easy to recognize as an amorphous, low-contrast image that moves as the chamber is moved laterally. To visualize the cell borders of the endothelium, the stage upon which the viewing chamber rests is carefully moved around until the surface of the endothelium is flat with respect to the objective lens, thus assuring a specular image. By gentle tilting of the rocking mechanism of the stage, the peripheral endothelial surface may also be made to be flat relative to the lens, allowing for observation of the peripheral endothelium. Although the rocking stage of the specular microscope is designed to keep the image of the endothelium in focus when the stage is rocked, it is a good practice to continuously observe the image, either through the eyepiece or on the video monitor, so that the focus may be adjusted and the stage moved laterally to retain a sharp image of the endothelium. All observations of the appearance of the endothelium should be noted on the donor evaluation form, and a photographic record of the image should be retained, either with a still photograph or on videotape.

To facilitate the evaluation of donor corneal endothelium, computerized image processing and evaluation systems have been developed.[8] One such system that has been available and in wide use for several years is the Bambi endothelial evaluation system (Bio-Optics, Inc., Arlington, Massachusetts), which is shown in Fig. 45-13. This system allows direct video input of the endothelial image from the video specular microscope. Alternatively, images may be entered from 35 mm negatives or from prints. This system enables the user to rapidly enhance the image contrast, thus improving the amount of information available to the evaluator, and to quickly generate a print of the contrast-enhanced image. Determination of such evaluation parameters as cell density, degree of pleomorphism and polymegethism, and

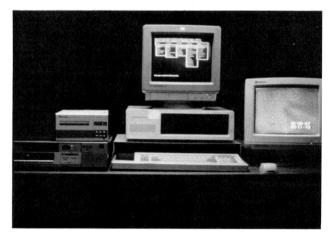

Fig. 45-13. Computer morphometric analysis system. Depicted here is a typical system, with menu-driven capabilities and ability to receive either direct image input from specular microscope or from a previously recorded image on videotape or still photograph. This system allows for a rapid, highly accurate assessment of various aspects of corneal endothelial morphometric parameters, such as cell density, cell area, and degree of polymorphism and polymegethism. (Courtesy Bio-Optics, Inc, Arlington, Mass.)

cell areas are easy and fast with such a computerized image analysis system. The data obtained in this automated evaluation may be printed out on a donor evaluation sheet, to accompany the prints of the images analyzed. If desired, the data files may be stored into a data base program, allowing the eye bank to maintain an easily accessible file of the corneas evaluated. This data base could prove valuable as a tool for determining important parameters in the evaluation of donor endothelium and the acceptable ranges of these parameters. Such a computerized analysis system speeds up the entire process of specular microscopic endothelial evaluation and provides additional information not accessible by the traditional manual methods of evaluation.

After transplantation, the donor cornea may be examined by use of a standard clinical specular microscope. Further evaluation using a computerized morphometric analysis system also may be performed at this time and provides the clinician with valuable information regarding any postoperative changes that may occur in the endothelium.

EVALUATION OF THE CORNEAL ENDOTHELIUM

The specular microscopic image of a young, normal endothelium is shown in Fig. 45-14. The cells are similar in size and shape, with no abnormally dark or bright structures being apparent and no evidence of inflammatory cells or adherent debris. The cell density is between 2000 and 3500 cells/mm^2 on the corneal surface. This is an ideal image of the endothelium of a donor cornea. In practice, the appearance of the endothelium of most donor corneas cannot be expected to be this good. In the corneas from older donors and from those whose corneas have suffered various types of previous trauma or disease, the endothelium will have a much different appearance. Other factors contributing to the change from normal in the appearance of the donor endothelium include time from death to preservation, whether the eyelids were closed after death, whether any light ice packs were applied to the lids of the donor, and trauma inflicted upon the donor, especially head and face trauma.

Ideally one would prefer that a donor cornea's endothelium has cells that are uniform in size, shape, and appearance. In practice, however, a variety of cell shapes (pleomorphism) and size (polymegethism) and abnormally bright or dark structures are encountered. (Figs. 45-15 to 45-17).

For corneas that are in the process of healing or recovering from certain types of stress, the process of coalescence can occur[9,15,16] and appears as is

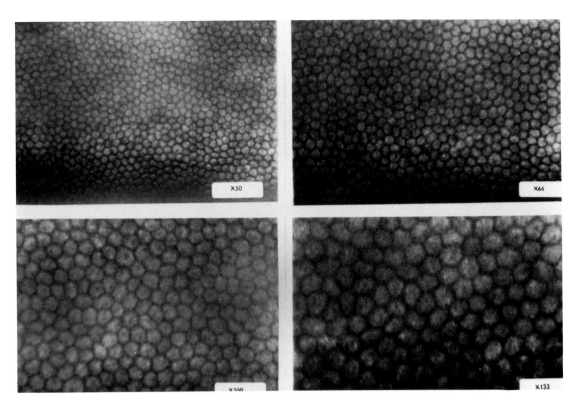

Fig. 45-14. Appearance of young, normal endothelium at room temperature. Viewed at different magnifications. Cells are hexagonal and uniform in size and appearance.

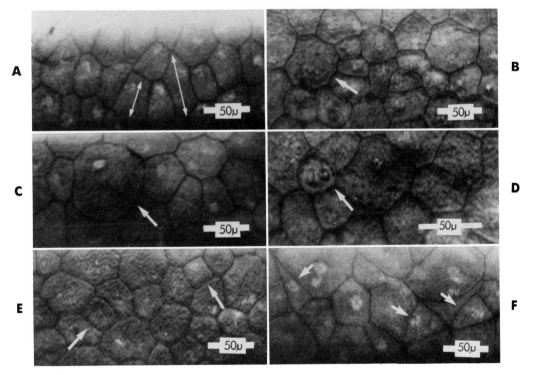

Fig. 45-15. Various abnormal endothelial cell shapes, *arrows* **A,** Stretched. **B,** Scalloped. **C,** Large, rounded. **D,** Small, rounded. **E,** Square. **F,** Triangular.

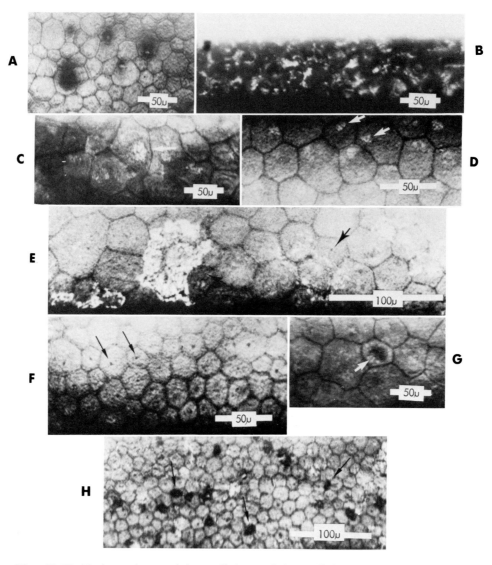

Fig. 45-16. Various abnormal intracellular and intercellular structures. **A,** Isolated smooth excrescences (cornea guttata). **B,** Multiple coalesced guttae. **C,** Pigment deposits and linear structures. **D,** Bright structures (presumably nuclei). **E,** Adherent pigment deposits. **F,** Central cilia. **G,** Large, dark structure. **H,** Inflammatory cells.

shown in Fig. 45-18. In this process, a common cell border between two cells disappears and the two cells fuse into a single cell. Although it is not presently known if this would contraindicate the use of the cornea in transplant, prudence dictates that, as long as other suitable tissue is available, corneas exhibiting such cells should not be considered for use in penetrating keratoplasty.

It has been reported that corneas with considerable polymegethism or pleomorphism have an increased incidence of postoperative decompensation[18] and have a reduced functional reserve.[19] These studies would indicate that such corneas

should not be used in transplant surgery and should be offered solely for research purposes.

As is shown in Fig. 45-19 one may observe cornea guttata on examination with the specular microscope. Cornea guttata has been reported to reduce endothelial function or functional reserve,[2,5] and for this reason, any cornea showing guttae should not be considered as acceptable for use in transplant surgery.

Bacteria and inflammatory cells are easily seen under the specular microscope. Bacteria are observed as small, bright twinkling objects whose shape and position rapidly change. Inflammatory cells have a

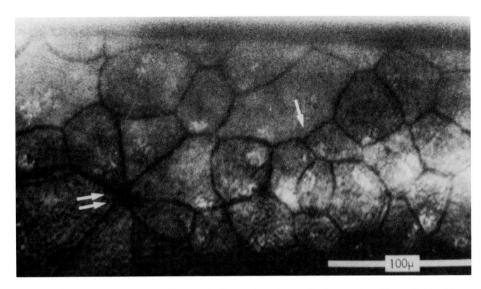

Fig. 45-17. Abnormal corneal endothelium showing a "reformation figure" *(double arrow)* believed to be indicative of endothelial repair by sloughing and cell sliding. Also seen is a cluster of "smaller" cells *(single arrow)*, probably resulting from mitosis. Large, multisided cells seen are believed to have resulted from coalescence of cells.

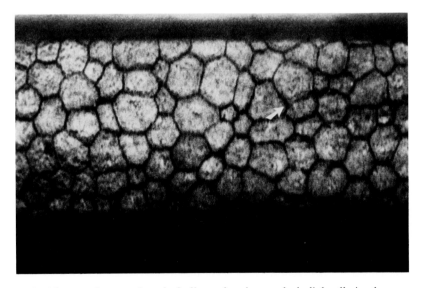

Fig. 45-18. Abnormal corneal endothelium showing endothelial cells in the process of "healing," or recovering from stress, by process of cell coalescence. *Arrow,* Cell border, which was seen to disappear over time. Endothelium exhibits pronounced polymegethism and pleomorphism.

similar appearance but are slower in their motions than the bacteria. The presence of either bacteria or inflammatory cells (Fig. 45-16, *H*) indicate probable contamination of either the storage media or the cornea and, as such, would contraindicate the use of such a cornea for transplantation.

Other abnormal appearances are indicative of disease states (Figs. 45-20 and 45-21) when seen under the specular microscope. Such corneas should naturally be considered only for use in research.

EVALUATION CRITERION

The presence of an abnormal, or "bad looking," corneal endothelium most likely indicates that the

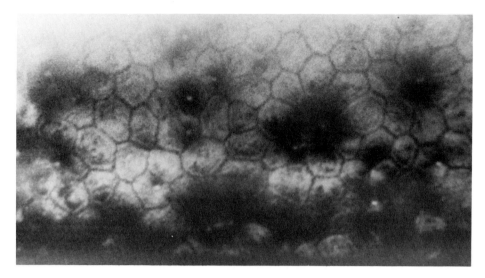

Fig. 45-19. Abnormal appearance of corneal endothelium resultant from Fuchs' dystrophy. Notice guttae, seen as irregular, dark patches.

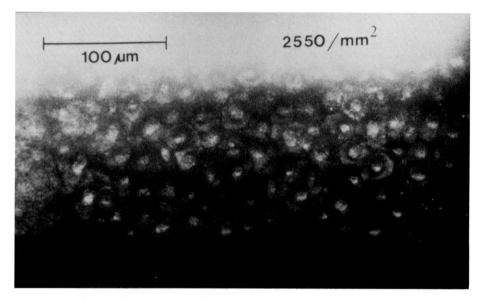

Fig. 45-20. Abnormal appearance of corneal endothelium as seen in patients with posterior polymorphous dystrophy.

cornea is functionally deficient and compromised, as has been generally presumed to be true. It would therefore seem prudent not to consider as suitable for transplant those corneas that appear either qualitatively or quantitatively abnormal. These corneas should be made available only for research.

Presently, corneas that are considered as not suitable for surgical use exhibit one or more of the following characteristics on specular microscopic examination:

1. An endothelial cell density less that 1500 cells/mm². (In general, corneas whose only flaw is a low cell density still present the risk of a continued cell loss,[4] which could ultimately lead to a density low enough for corneal decompensation.)
2. Severe polymegethism or pleomorphism of the endothelial cell pattern.
3. Presence of cornea guttata.
4. Presence of many abnormally shaped cells, such as those seen in coalescence.

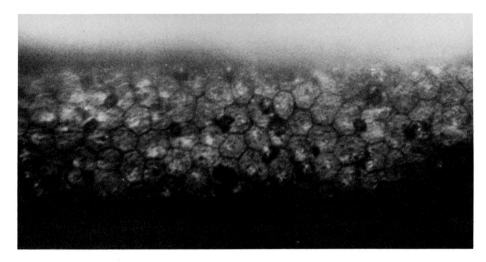

Fig. 45-21. Effects of heterochromic cyclitis on corneal endothelium as seen in a specular photomicrograph.

5. Abnormal single cell defects.
6. Extensive areas of severe edema.
7. Presence of inflammatory cells or of bacteria on the endothelium.
8. Presence of ghost vessels in the stroma.

The age of corneal donors appears to be of secondary consideration, and suitable corneas from older donors that have passed the specular microscopic criteria have provided excellent grafts.[1] An older donor whose cornea has a high endothelial cell count, low degrees of polymegethism and of pleomorphism, and a normal overall appearance is most likely functionally superior to a cornea from a younger donor if the younger cornea has a lower cell density or exhibits an abnormal appearance. Specular microscopy, especially when used with computerized morphometric analysis, proves to be extremely useful in the evaluation of the corneas from older donors, as in the range of 60 to 74 years of age, because it allows for the determination of the suitability of the tissue rather than an arbitrary dismissal of it solely on the basis of age. In general, corneas from donors over 75 years of age are rarely considered for use in penetrating keratoplasty.

SUMMARY

The specular microscope is a valuable tool for use in the evaluation of potential donor corneas before their use in penetrating keratoplasty. The routine use of the specular microscope, with slitlamp evaluation and computerized morphometric image analysis, can help to improve the quality of the tissue used in penetrating keratoplasty and reduce the number of grafts that fail secondary to faulty donor tissue.

ACKNOWLEDGMENT

I would like to thank Setsuko S. Oak and E. Gregory Marchand for their invaluable assistance in the preparation of this manuscript and for their numerous incisive comments concerning its contents and ways in which it could be improved.

REFERENCES

1. Bigar F, Schimmelpfennig B, Giesler R: Routine evaluation of endothelium in human donor corneas, *Albrecht von Graefes Arch Klin Exp Ophthalmol* 200:195-200, 1976.
2. Bigar F, Schimmelpfennig B, Hurlzeler R: Cornea guttata in donor material, *Arch Ophthalmol* 96:653-655, 1978.
3. Bourne WM: Examination and photography of donor corneal endothelium, *Arch Ophthalmol* 94:1799-1800, 1976.
4. Bourne WM: Morphologic and functional evaluation of the endothelium of transplanted human corneas, *Trans Am Ophthalmol Soc* 81:403-450, 1983.
5. Burns RR, Bourne WM, Brubaker RF: Endothelial function in patients with cornea guttata, *Invest Ophthalmol Vis Sci* 20:77-85, 1981.
6. Hoefle FB, Maurice DM, Sibley R: Human corneal donor material: a method of examination before keratoplasty, *Arch Ophthalmol* 84:741-744, 1970.
7. Laing RA: Specular microscopy of the cornea. In Zadunaisky J, Davson HH, editors: *Current topics in eye research*, vol 3, New York, 1980, Academic Press.
8. Laing RA: Image processing of corneal endothelial images. In Cavanagh D, editor: *The cornea, Transactions of the World Congress on the Cornea III*, New York, 1988, Raven Press.
9. Laing RA, Neubauer L, Leibowitz HM, Oak SS: Coalescence of endothelial cells in the traumatized cornea. II. Clinical observations, *Arch Ophthalmol* 101:1712-1715, 1983.
10. Laing RA, Sandstrom MM, Leibowitz HM: Clinical specular microscopy, I. Optical principles, *Arch Ophthalmol* 97:1714-1719, 1979.
11. Laing RA, Sandstrom MM, Leibowitz HM: Clinical specular microscopy, II. Qualitative evaluation of corneal endothelial photomicrographs, *Arch Ophthalmol* 97:1720-1725, 1979.
12. Leibowitz HM, Laing RA: Specular microscopy. In Leibowitz

HM, editor: *Corneal disorders: clinical diagnosis and management,* Philadelphia, 1984, Saunders.

13. McCarey BE, McNeill JI: Specular microscopic evaluation of donor corneal endothelium, *Ann Ophthalmol* 9:1279-1283, 1978.
14. Mayer DJ: *Clinical wide-field specular microscopy,* London, 1984, Bailliere Tindall.
15. Neubauer L, Laing RA, Leibowitz HM, Oak SS: Coalescence of endothelial cells in the traumatized cornea. I. Experimental observations in cryopreserved tissue, *Arch Ophthalmol* 101:1787-1790, 1983.
16. Neubauer L, Baratz RS, Laing RA, et al: Coalescence of endothelial cells in the traumatized cornea. III. Correlation between specular and scanning electron microscopy, *Arch Ophthalmol* 102:921-922, 1984.
17. Oak SS, Laing RA, Chiba HM, Tsubata K: Thermal cycling effects on the stored cornea, *Invest Ophthalmol Vis Sci* 30:1584-1587, 1989.
18. Rao GN, Shaw EL, Arthur EJ, Aquavella JV: Endothelial cell morphology and corneal deturgescence, *Ann Ophthalmol* 97:885-899, 1979.
19. Yee RW, Geroski DH, Matsuda M, et al: Correlation of corneal endothelial pump site density, area function and morphology in wound repair, *Invest Ophthalmol Vis Sci* 26:1191-1202, 1985.

Bacteriology

DAVID S. HULL

DONOR CONTAMINATION

The microbiologic evaluation of donor tissue is of extreme importance to prevent the transmission of host-carried infectious disease to the recipient of the donor cornea. Donor corneas have a high incidence of surface bacterial contamination, with the incidence of positive postmortem cultures reported in one study to be as high as 100%.[24,26] Gram-positive cocci are the most frequently cultured organisms; however, a significant number of gram-negative cocci are also present on the surface of postmortem eyes.[21,22,24]

DONOR HISTORY

The microbiologic evaluation of donor eyes should begin with the history of the donor where such things as facial trauma may possibly predispose to the presence of particulate matter on the surface of the globe. In addition, sepsis or the presence of infection anywhere on the surface of the body, as in burn patients, may be important historical facts. A patient who has been on a respirator may be at increased risk for ocular-surface contamination. One study has demonstrated a 61.5% positive culture rate in eye tissue recovered from donors who had been maintained on a respirator compared with a control series where 28.9% of the cultures were positive.[28]

Possible reasons for eye donors maintained on a respirator being at a high risk for ocular contamination include internal factors such as sepsis and reduced host defenses as well as external factors including corneal exposure, secretions from a tracheostomy site or suction apparatus, and open wounds. There is probably insufficient evidence to warrant rejection of these donor eyes; however, a high index of suspicion should be maintained, especially in those persons who have been on a respirator for periods exceeding 1 week.

There are conflicting reports regarding intraocular colonization of ocular tissue recovered from septic donors, with one report demonstrating intraocular contamination of donor eye tissue recovered from septic donors.[13] This is in contrast to another report, which demonstrated no correlation between bacteremia and aqueous humor contamination.[5] Until there is further clarification regarding such donor tissue, sepsis should be a contraindication to usage. One study has demonstrated that the contamination rate of eyes removed by certified morticians was twice the rate of contamination of eyes removed by medical personnel (89% versus 49%).[2] This was attributed to a modified procedure used by morticians that included a 3-minute hand scrub with commercial soap and no conjunctival irrigation with antibiotic before the enucleation. However, the same study demonstrated that washing of donor eyes in the eye bank with antibiotic reduced the contamination rate to similar levels and there was no eventual difference in the microbiologic contamination of the eyes. It was concluded that eyes recovered by morticians can safely be used for penetrating keratoplasty if washing with antibiotics is performed in the eye bank.[2]

DONOR-TO-HOST DISEASE TRANSMISSION

Although there is a high incidence of surface contamination of donor eyes, infectious keratitis or endophthalmitis occurring after penetrating keratoplasty is relatively rare.[4,21,23] One report of 200 consecutive keratoplasties showed no clinical infection even though corneoscleral rim cultures were positive for bacteria in 25 cases and for fungi in three cases.[18]

Although cases of endophthalmitis and infectious keratitis have been reported after penetrating keratoplasty, well-documented cases of donor-to-host disease transmission are fewer in number.[8,22] It is probable that the number of reported cases is less than the actual number of cases. Representative well-documented cases of donor-to-host disease transfer include a case of cryptococcal endophthalmitis. The donor blood cultures were subsequently found to be positive for *Cryptococcus neoformans*.[1] A case of Creutzfeldt-Jakob disease was transmitted to a recipient. The donor was diagnosed as having the disease at autopsy.[7] A case of *Flavobacterium* endophthalmitis after penetrating keratoplasty has been reported in a patient from whom subsequently the same organism was cultured from residual corneoscleral rim and from the culture medium in which the donor tissue had been stored.[16] Human-to-human transmission of rabies by corneal transplant has been reported.[11] Three cases of fungal endophthalmitis were reported in which the donor rim cultures yielded the same organism as that in the infected recipient eye.[4] *Streptococcus pneumoniae* endophthalmitis was reported in both recipients of corneas from a 12-year-old donor who died after acute trauma but who had been receiving cardiovascular support for 26 hours. The patient suffered a febrile illness, and an autopsy demonstrated bronchial pneumonia.[27] Two cases of *Pseudomonas aeruginosa* endophthalmitis were reported in both recipients of a donor who died of Hodgkin's disease complicated by peritonitis and possible septicemia. Blood cultures were not obtained from the donor.[14] Additional cases of *Streptococcus, Staphylococcus, Pseudomonas, Klebsiella,* and *Enterococcus* infection after keratoplasty have been reported[4,17] There has been concern about the relationship of intermediate-term corneal preservation and the incidence of endophthalmitis after keratoplasty. Girard reported five cases of endophthalmitis after using corneas preserved in McCarey-Kaufman medium.[9] Intermediate-term corneal preservation solutions contain gentamicin, which does not give adequate protection against streptococcal species.

Remember that not all cases of infection after keratoplasty are transmitted by the donor. Ocular infections can occur after a variety of ophthalmic surgical procedures. Other possible factors involved in the transmission of infection to a host include infection from the patient's own lids, a break in surgical technique, and a compromised host who is receiving steroids or antibiotics. Also the presence of a bandage contact lens as well as patient hygiene and dust and dirt in the environment may play a role. Evidence of disease transmission to a recipient many times is only circumstantial if the offending organism cannot be cultured from the donor.

EYE BANK EVALUATION AND TREATMENT OF DONOR WHOLE-EYE TISSUE

Upon receipt of eyes at the eye bank microbiologic evaluation should begin with the slitlamp examination. If dirt or other gross particulate matter is

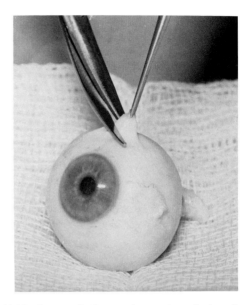

Fig. 45-22. Removal of excessive conjunctival and adnexal tissue from globe of whole eye is performed to remove possible sites where bacteria may be harbored.

found on the ocular surface, concern for contamination of the donor should be considered and such eyes should not be utilized. The presence of inflammatory corneal ulceration is also cause for nonutilization of tissue. After the slitlamp examination excision of all excess conjunctiva and adnexal tissue should be performed in order to remove possible sites where bacteria may be harbored (Fig. 45-22). Vigorous irrigation of the cornea and eye with saline or antibiotic should follow because it has been well documented that vigorous irrigation substantially reduces the surface bacterial count in postmortem eyes[10,21] (Fig. 45-23).

After vigorous saline or antibiotic irrigation the eyes should be immersed in an antibiotic solution for 5 minutes because this has been found to be superior to simple irrigation of the ocular surface with antibiotics in reducing the surface contamination[3,28] (Fig. 45-24). It has been reported that after whole donor eye irrigation with 5 ml of a commercially available ophthalmic solution containing polymyxin B, neomycin, and gramicidin, there was a 47.5% incidence of positive ocular cultures. However, if the whole eye was immersed for 10 minutes in the same solution, the incidence of positive cultures was reduced to 24.5%.[28] Increasing the concentration of thimerosal from 0.001% to 0.01% has been recommended to promote the killing of fungi. It was found that vigorous saline irrigation of eyes followed by immersion for 5 minutes in a commercially avail-

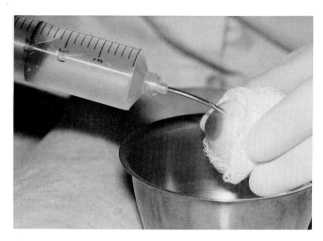

Fig. 45-23. Vigorous irrigation of cornea and limbus of eye with saline solution or antibiotic is performed in eye bank so that bacteria, mucus, dead cells, and particulate matter are physically removed from surface of cornea to reduce chance of bacterial contamination.

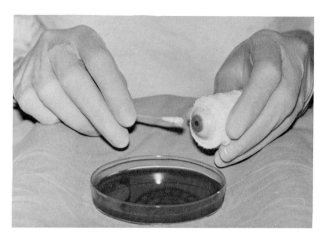

Fig. 45-25. Corneal and limbal cultures are performed and plated on blood agar and Sabouraud's medium. It is additionally recommended that eye banks advise operating surgeons to perform cultures of corneoscleral rim at time of surgery.

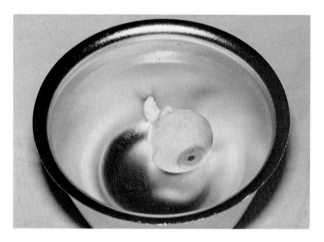

Fig. 45-24. Immersion of whole eye in an appropriate antibiotic solution for 3 to 5 minutes has been found to be of value for further reducing surface contamination with bacteria. After immersion of whole eye in antibiotic solution, a subsequent irrigation with saline solution is recommended to protect corneal endothelium from any toxic effects that could potentially arise from residual antibiotic or its preservative present on ocular surface when cornea and scleral rim are subsequently excised.

able antibiotic preparation consisting of polymyxin B sulfate, neomycin sulfate, and gramicidin in which the thimerosal concentration was increased to 0.01% resulted in a sharp reduction in bacterial and fungal growth.[10] Doughman has reported that a 3-minute immersion of the donor eye in gentamicin ophthalmic solution reduced surface flora by 78% com-

pared to a reduction of only 36% in eyes similarly soaked in a commercially available ophthalmic solution containing polymyxin B, neomycin sulfate, gramicidin, alcohol, and thimerosal.[6] The use of povidone-iodine complex for the decontamination of donor tissue has also been reported and has been found to be effective.[19,20] After immersion of the donor eye in the antibiotic solution, repeated irrigation with or immersion in saline is advised to prevent endothelial toxicity from residual antibiotic or preservative. After this second saline immersion or irrigation, corneal and limbal cultures should be performed and plated on blood agar, Sabouraud's medium, and possibly anaerobic media (Fig. 45-25). If bacterial cultures are positive (which usually results 1 to 2 days after the eyes are sent to the surgeon for transplant) identification of the organism along with antibiotic sensitivities should be reported to the recipient surgeon. Culture of the residual corneal scleral rim and corneal preservation medium in the operating room should be strongly recommended by eye banks to the operating surgeon.[25]

EYE BANK RETRIEVAL AND TREATMENT OF DONOR CORNEOSCLERAL RIM TISSUE

Donor corneas retrieved in medical examiner's cases are of unique concern because of the lack of prior medical history and the less-than-ideal conditions of sterility under which such corneas may be recovered. Preparation of donors in medical examiner's cases should include the application of povidone-iodine to the lids and skin followed by normal saline irrigation of the globe. Application of 0.1 ml

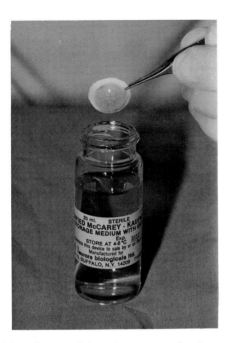

Fig. 45-26. After careful ocular preparation in an attempt to assure sterility, cornea and 2 mm scleral rim are excised and placed in corneal preservative medium with gentamicin 100 µg/ml.

of an ophthalmic antibiotic solution containing polymyxin B, neomycin, and gramicidin has been recommended.[22,25] The cornea and 2 mm of scleral rim are subsequently excised and placed in corneal storage medium with gentamicin sulfate, 100 µg/ml (Fig. 45-26). It has been reported that 76% of medical examiners cases initially showed positive ocular cultures. After preparation with a commercially available antibiotic solution containing polymyxin B, neomycin, and gramicidin, the incidence of positive cultures was reduced to 22%.[22] The question has been raised whether corneal tissue obtained in medical examiners' cases should be placed with a surgeon before the results of cultures are known. Payne believes that delay is not warranted because it may result in placement of culture-negative tissue near the limits of intermediate-term corneal preservation. Such a policy would also eliminate the utilization of potentially useful donor tissue.[22]

ORGAN-CULTURED CORNEAS

Corneal preservation by organ culture techniques presents additional problems with sterility. Techniques of organ culture and the microbiologic evaluation of tissue stored by this technique are reviewed by Doughman.[6] (See Chapter 46.)

ANTIBIOTICS IN INTERMEDIATE-TERM STORAGE MEDIUM

Corneal storage medium, as used for intermediate-term corneal storage, is available with gentamicin, 100 µg/ml. Since bacteria at 4° C are not in their replicating phase, there is concern as to whether gentamicin is effective for inhibiting bacterial growth under these conditions. It is possible that warming the tissue to room temperature just before use allows bacteria to begin to replicate, at which time gentamicin may be effective. It is also possible that gentamicin may be imbibed by the corneal stroma during storage and that it subsequently acts as a reservoir for the slow release of the antibiotic in the hours immediately after penetrating keratoplasty. *Streptococcus* and *Pseudomonas* species may be resistant to gentamicin, and therefore consideration should possibly be given to the utilization of additional antibiotics in corneal storage medium, which would provide for better gram-positive as well as gram-negative coverage.[25] Additional consideration should also be given to the utilization of antifungal agents for inclusion in intermediate-term corneal storage medium.[15] The addition of alternative antibiotics should be proved to be effective as well as nontoxic to the corneal endothelium. Previous work has identified a selected group of antibiotics related to their endothelial toxicity when they are incorporated in McCarey-Kaufman corneal storage medium.[12] Eye banks may consider recommending the use of prophylactic subconjunctival or prophylactic parenteral antibiotics for transplant surgeons. Poole and Insler have recommended the use of parenteral antibiotics in recipients of donor corneas.[25] It must be noted that there is no warranty of tissue as to merchantability or fitness for a particular purpose and that the final responsibility for judging corneal tissue rests with the surgeon receiving the tissue.

SUMMARY

The microbiologic evaluation of donor eyes should begin with a careful history of the donor followed by sterile enucleation technique. After slit-lamp examination, removal of excess adnexal and conjunctival tissue should be performed, after which vigorous saline or antibiotic irrigation should be performed. Immersion of the globe in antibiotic for 5 minutes should be followed by repeated irrigation or immersion of the globe in saline. Cornea and limbal cultures should be performed at this time, and any positive results subsequently should be reported to the surgeon receiving the tissue. Operating surgeons should be strongly encouraged to perform cultures of the residual corneoscleral rim as well as the intermediate-term preservative at the time of surgery. The use of subconjunctival and possible parenteral antibiotics at the time of surgery and postoperatively is the choice of the individual surgeon.

REFERENCES

 1. Beyt BW Jr, Waltman SR: Cryptococcal endophthalmitis after corneal transplantation, *N Engl J Med* 298:825-826, 1978.
 2. Bonner T et al: Mortician retrieval of donor globes: the Minnesota experience, *Cornea* 2:251-254, 1983.
 3. Brightbill FS, Terrones C, Gould S: Experimental studies with *Staphylococcus aureus* in M-K medium, *Invest Ophthalmol* 15:32-34, 1976.
 4. Cameron JA, Antonios SR, Cotter JB, Habash NR: Endophthalmitis from contaminated donor corneas following penetrating keratoplasty, *Arch Ophthalmol* 109:54-59, 1991.
 5. Clark WM et al: Donor eye contamination, *Am J Ophthalmol* 94:395-397, 1982.
 6. Doughman DJ: Prolonged donor cornea preservation in organ culture: long-term clinical evaluation, *Trans Am Ophthalmol Soc* 78:567-628, 1980.
 7. Duffy P et al: Possible person-to-person transmission of Creutzfeldt-Jakob disease, *N Engl J Med* 290:692-693, 1974.
 8. Gandhi SS, Lamberts DW, Perry HD: Donor to host transmission of disease via corneal transplantation, *Surv Ophthalmol* 25:306-311, 1981.
 9. Girard LJ: Bacterial endophthalmitis following the use of contaminated preserved corneal tissue, *Cornea* 1:255-257, 1982.
10. Goldman KN et al: Prevention of surface bacterial contamination of donor corneas, *Arch Ophthalmol* 96:2277-2280, 1978.
11. Houff SA et al: Human-to-human transmission of rabies virus by corneal transplant, *N Engl J Med* 300:603-604, 1979.
12. Hull DS et al: Modification of the antibiotic system in M-K medium, *Am J Ophthalmol* 83:198-205, 1977.
13. Keates RH, Mishler KE, Riedinger D: Bacterial contamination of donor eyes, *Am J Ophthalmol* 84:617-619, 1977.
14. Khodadoust AA, Franklin RM: Transfer of bacterial infection by donor cornea in penetrating keratoplasty, *Am J Ophthalmol* 87:130-132, 1979.
15. Kowalski RP et al: Antifungal synergism: a proposed dosage for corneal storage medium, *Arch Ophthalmol* 103:250-256, 1985.
16. LeFrançois M, Baum JL: *Flavobacterium* endophthalmitis following keratoplasty, *Arch Ophthalmol* 94:1907-1909, 1976.
17. Leveille AS, McMullan FD, Cavanagh HD: Endophthalmitis following penetrating keratoplasty, *Ophthalmology* 90:38-39, 1983.
18. Mascarella K, Cavanagh HD: Penetrating keratoplasty using McCarey-Kaufman preserved corneal tissue, *South Med J* 72:1268-1271, 1979.
19. Mindrup EA et al: A comparative study of the use of povidone-iodine and gentamicin in the decontamination of human donor globes, *Invest Ophthalmol Vis Sci* 26(suppl):68, 1985.
20. Nash RW, Lindquist TD, Kalina RE: An evaluation of saline irrigation and comparison of povidone-iodine and antibiotic in the surface decontamination of donor eyes, *Arch Ophthalmol* 109:869-872, 1991.
21. Pardos GJ, Gallagher MA: Microbial contamination of donor eyes, *Arch Ophthalmol* 100:1611-1613, 1982.
22. Payne JW: New directions in eye banking, *Trans Am Ophthalmol Soc* 78:983-1026, 1980.
23. Polack FM: Ocular infections after keratoplasty, *Cornea* 3:3-4, 1984.
24. Polack FM, Locatcher-Khorazo D, Gutierrez E: Bacteriologic study of "donor" eyes, *Arch Ophthalmol* 78:219-225, 1967.
25. Poole TG, Insler MS: Contamination of donor cornea by gentamicin-resistant organisms, *Am J Ophthalmol* 97:560-564, 1984.
26. Richards RD, Catzen M: Statistics of eye collections, *Ann Ophthalmol* 7:221-224, 1975.
27. Shaw EL, Aquavella JV: Pneumococcal endophthalmitis following grafting of corneal tissue from a (cadaver) kidney donor, *Ann Ophthalmol* 9:435-440, 1977.
28. Sugar J, Liff J: Bacterial contamination of corneal donor tissue, *Ophthalmic Surg* 11:250-252, 1980.

Changes in eye bank medical standards in response to the AIDS epidemic

JAY S. PEPOSE

GARY N. HOLLAND

DAVID G. BUERGER

SCOTT M. MACRAE

THE AIDS EPIDEMIC

In 1981, the first cases of the acquired immunodeficiency syndrome (AIDS) were reported from New York City and Los Angeles, manifesting as Kaposi's sarcoma, *Pneumocystis carinii* pneumonia, and other opportunistic infections in homosexual men and intravenous drug abusers with acquired cellular immune dysfunction.[26,35,52] From 1981 through 1990, the number of AIDS victims reached epidemic proportions, with an increase in heterosexual and prenatal transmission. During this period, 100,777 deaths from AIDS in the United States were reported to the Centers for Disease Control.[12] AIDS emerged as the second leading cause of death among men 25 to 44 years of age, surpassing heart disease, cancer, suicide, and homicide.[6] Human immunodeficiency virus (HIV) infection/AIDS also now ranks among the five leading causes of death among women in the United States between 25 and 44 years of age.[13]

The full-blown syndrome known as AIDS (that is, meeting the surveillance case definition by the Centers for Disease Control) reflects one end of the spectrum of HIV-1 infection, which ranges from AIDS to AIDS-related complex (ARC) to a clinically asymptomatic state. Reported cases of AIDS represent only the tip of the iceberg when compared to the much larger number of HIV-infected individuals, the majority of whom are without symptoms. The United States Public Health Service estimates

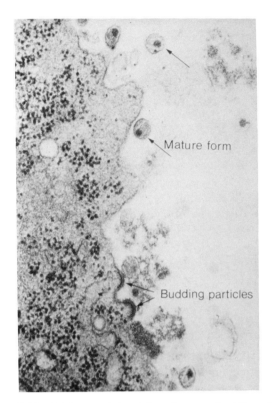

Fig. 45-27. HIV type 1 lentivirus is seen budding from surface of infected cell and also in its mature cell-free form. (Transmission electron microscopy, 100,000×.)

that between 1 and 1.5 million people in the United States currently are infected[43] with HIV type 1, the lentivirus causing AIDS[3,42] (Figs. 45-27 and 45-28). The high prevalence of infection of young people (a likely source of transplantable tissue) and the long incubation period from infection until the development of AIDS (estimated at a median of 9.8 years[2]) have had a major, lasting impact on the eye bank community.

HIV AND THE EYE

HIV type 1 has been isolated from contact lenses,[56] tears,[1,22,23] conjunctiva,[21] cornea,[8,17,28,45,46] aqueous humor,[20,23] iris,[8] vitreous,[54] and retina[8,41,44,48,53] and demonstrated in optic nerve tissue by specific viral antigen staining and the polymerase chain reaction using primers to HIV (Pepose JS and Laycock CA: unpublished studies).

The location and specific cell type harboring HIV in infected corneal tissue are less clear. Detailed histologic studies of normal corneas reveal a moderate number of passenger lymphocytes,[47] some of which bear the CD4 surface marker, which is a receptor for HIV. Studies of two culture-positive corneas from a cadaver that was repeatedly positive on enzyme-

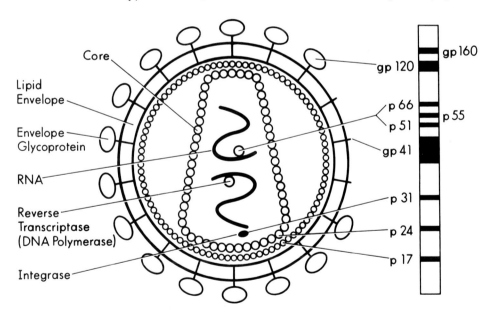

Fig. 45-28. Schema of HIV, *left*, along with its representative component bands on a typical Western blot profile, *right*. This RNA-containing lentivirus harbors a reverse transcriptase (also called DNA polymerase) and ribonuclease (p66 and p51), as well as an integrase protein (p31) that facilitates integration of proviral DNA into host-cell DNA. The nucleoid shell p24 protein and p17 protein are viral-core components derived from a larger protein precursor (p55). The viral envelope comprises a lipid bilayer containing a high molecular weight envelope glycoprotein gp120 and transmembrane envelope protein gp41, which are cleavage products of larger precursor envelope glycoprotein, gp160.

linked immunosorbent assay (ELISA) testing for HIV antibodies but was Western blot indeterminate (p24 band only) showed positive fluorescence in approximately 2% of corneal epithelial cells stained with a fluorescein-tagged antibody against the HIV p24 core antigen.[46] Virus was isolated from both central and peripheral tissue in one cornea from this cadaver and from central tissue only in the other. Qavi and colleagues[45] detected HIV transcription using in situ hybridization in cells interpreted as stromal keratocytes in a HIV culture-positive cornea. Others have implicated HIV-infected macrophages in other culture-positive ocular structures, such as retina.[35] Attempts to infect corneal stromal cells[19] and corneal epithelium in tissue culture or whole cornea in organ culture with HIV have been unsuccessful (Pepose JS, Young E, Pomerantz RJ, Hirsch MS, Skolnik PR: unpublished studies). A recent study has found evidence of HIV and human herpesvirus 6 in one of 40 corneas tested from HIV-seropositive cadavers by use of the sensitive polymerase chain reaction (PCR), as well as by isolation in tissue culture, raising the possibility of coviral interactions. Infection with human herpesvirus 6 appears to be widespread, and the virus has been demonstrated to be the etiologic agent causing exanthema subitum in children.[60] Probable transmission

of human herpesvirus 6 has been reported after liver, renal, and heart transplantation.[31,36,57]

We extracted DNA from the central 8.0 mm cornea, limbal cornea, aqueous humor, and retina from 15 HIV-seropositive cadavers and, using two sets of primers to HIV,[60] searched for evidence of HIV using polymerase chain-reaction amplification. The results of these studies are illustrated in Fig. 45-29. HIV nucleic acid was identified in 3 of 30 corneas (10%), 2 of 30 aqueous samples (7%), and 7 of 30 retinas (23%). In no case did both central and limbal cornea show HIV-specific bands; in one case only the peripheral cornea was positive and in two cases the central alone was positive. Similarly, the demonstration of HIV nucleic acid in aqueous humor did not correlate with its detection in corneal tissue from the same eye. Thus, neither the peripheral corneal rim nor the aqueous could be utilized reliably to determine whether the central transplantable cornea harbored HIV. In addition, the PCR is a method highly dependent on technical expertise and meticulous performance.[51] At this time, no PCR test for HIV detection has been licensed for screening purposes by the Food and Drug Administration (FDA).

SEROLOGIC AND HISTORICAL SCREENING OF CORNEAL DONORS

The discovery in 1984 that HIV-1 causes AIDS[5] led to the rapid development of serologic tests to screen for HIV infection. ELISA screening tests for use in detecting HIV-1 antibodies in blood or plasma was licensed by the Food and Drug Administration[40] in 1985. Acting on recommendations by the Centers for Disease Control (CDC)[9] that serum or plasma from all blood and organ donors be tested for HIV-1 using an FDA-approved screening test, the Eye Bank Association of America (EBAA) rapidly incorporated HIV-1 serologic and historical screening of all potential cornea donors into its medical standards in December 1985. Cadaveric donors with AIDS, HIV seropositivity or at high risk of HIV infection, as well as children (under 13 years of age) and infants of mothers with AIDS or at high risk of HIV infection, are excluded as sources of surgical tissue. If a potential donor has had a blood transfusion within the 48 hours preceding cessation of circulating function (that is, a non–heart beating donor), a pretransfusion sample test for HIV-1 antibodies is required. If a pretransfusion sample is unavailable and if an adult donor has received four or more units of whole blood or the equivalent within the 48 hours preceding cessation of circulating function, or if a child under 12 years of age has received any transfusion of blood or nonsterilizable fraction,

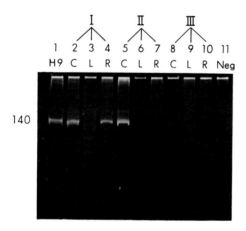

Fig. 45-29. Amplification products of the polymerase chain reaction performed with the SK (Shirley Kwok) 68/SK 69 HIV primer pair and DNA extracted from ocular tissues from two HIV-seropositive cadavers (I and II) and one seronegative cadaver (III), which were electrophoresed on a polyacrylamide gel. Sample 1 contains DNA from HIV-infected H9 cells, and sample II contains no DNA. DNA from central corneas (lanes 2, 5, 8), limbus (lanes 3, 6, 9), and retina (lanes 4, 7, 10) from the three cadavers was processed. The HIV-specific band visualized in lanes 1, 2, 4, and 5 is a 140 base-pair fragment.

the donor tissue is unacceptable for transplantation. These precautions are taken to avoid the risk of a false-negative ELISA test for AIDS antibodies as a consequence of serum dilution.

Historical screening of cornea donors is based on the identification of high-risk factors, as outlined by the CDC. Such information could be obtained from friends or family of the deceased, from a coroner's office, from hospital or physician's records, or by physical findings at autopsy, such as needle-track marks. The CDC considers the following groups to be of sufficient risk to warrant premortem ELISA testing for HIV antibody:[10] (1) persons seeking treatment for sexually transmitted diseases, (2) persons with a history of intravenous drug abuse, (3) persons who consider themselves at risk of HIV infection, (4) women of childbearing age who have used intravenous drugs, engaged in prostitution, or had sexual partners who are infected or at risk of infection, (5) persons who received blood transfusions between 1978 and 1985, (6) male and female prostitutes, (7) men who engaged in sexual activities with other men, and (8) persons in correctional systems. Such groups would therefore be the focus of postmortem historical screening. In addition, persons immigrating since 1977 from countries where heterosexual activity is reported as the predominant means of transmission of HIV-1 may be considered at risk. Corneal tissue is not to be released for transplant from any donor with an identified risk factor, regardless of the results of serologic testing. This precaution is taken because the individual at the time of death may have been in a "seronegative window" period after HIV-1 infection but before the production of antibodies against HIV at a level detectable by ELISA screening.[14,29,58] Screening programs, however, cannot replace antibody testing. In many cases, survivors may be unaware of or reluctant to reveal a donor's risk factor for HIV infection. In some cases, the donor him- or herself may not have been aware of an exposure to HIV. And in rare cases of HIV infection, no risk factors are identified.

Currently licensed ELISA test kits for the detection of antibodies against HIV-1 predominantly utilize HIV-1 target antigens derived from disruption of whole virus cultured in human-derived cell lines; some kits are supplemented with partially purified viral proteins.[40] Tests utilizing recombinant proteins have been developed but have not yet been licensed by the FDA for screening purposes. To perform the licensed ELISA assays for the detection of HIV antibodies, one adds the cadaveric test serum, various diluents, and an enzyme conjugated with anti–human gamma globulin (IgG) to HIV antigens that are fixed to a solid support in microwell plates. If an HIV antigen–HIV antibody–antihuman IgG antibody complex is formed, a colorimetric reaction occurs. The test results are defined either by comparison of the optical density of the specimen to a cutoff value or as the ratio of the optical densities of the sample to a control specimen.[50]

Since licensure of the first ELISA test kits in 1985, the manufacturers have systematically improved the sensitivity, specificity, and reproducibility of their assays, which are now greater than 99% sensitive in testing premortem serum.[11] By contrast, in testing cadaveric sera, three licensed HIV-antibody ELISA kits showed between 94.3% and 97.1% sensitivity and 99.2% to 99.6% specificity, as compared to the autopsy diagnosis of AIDS.[37] Positive results were obtained on sera from AIDS cadavers even when the time of blood draw was delayed for 35 hours after death and the time of serum preparation was delayed up to 176 days. Although relatively effective compared to other screening tests, both the sensitivity and the specificity of these ELISA assays on cadaveric sera are somewhat lower than in premortem serum testing. These tests have been carefully optimized for performance on premortem samples, as opposed to cadaveric sera. Whereas the U.S. Public Health Service has emphasized that a person should be considered to have serologic evidence of HIV infection only after an HIV-1 antibody ELISA is repeatedly reactive and another confirmatory test such as the Western blot test has validated the results,[10] corneal tissue is not deemed suitable for transplantation when an ELISA screening test is positive two out of three times, regardless of the results of confirmatory testing.

The incidence of HIV infection may vary considerably, depending on the demographic characteristics of the donor population, the urban or rural nature of the population, and the part of the country being considered. Of 262 potential corneal donors from Baltimore and Los Angeles without known-risk of HIV infection, 3 to 5 (1.1% to 1.9%) were ELISA seropositive.[37] In tests on 199 potential corneal donors in Dallas, 6 (3%) were ELISA-positive for HIV antibodies, of which 5 were confirmed on the Western blot test and 1 had an identifiable risk factor.[28] Other groups have reported cadaver seropositivity of between 0.3% and 2.4%; many seropositive cadavers were over 50 or under 25 years of age, and most had no identifiable risk factor for HIV infection.[4,14,15,29,58] Of 1517 eye donors screened in Houston, 13 (0.85%) initially tested positive on ELISA, but less than half (5, or 0.33%) were repeatedly reactive.[58] In Los Angeles, 1680 of 4451 potential corneal donors (37.7%) were excluded before serologic testing on the basis of historical risk factors or physical signs such as needle tracks.[29]

Although ELISA testing of cadaveric sera is a relatively, though not absolutely, effective method of screening for antibodies, ELISA testing of aqueous humor is not a reliable method of screening corneal donors for HIV antibodies.[37] Similarly, ELISA testing of postmortem vitreous humor specimens from ELISA-test seropositive cadavers may frequently give negative results for HIV antibodies.[34]

We have recently evaluated the use of an FDA-licensed ELISA test for HIV-1 *antigens* as a supplemental method to accompany HIV antibody screening,[7] in an effort to identify cadavers that are HIV infected and HIV antigen positive but are not positive for HIV antibodies at the time of death.[16,27,30,32,55,59] In tests on 18 AIDS and 96 high-risk cadavers, no serum samples were identified as HIV-antigen positive that were not also positive for antibodies to HIV-1 by ELISA and Western blot. The specificity of the HIV *antigen* assay in testing cadaveric sera was low; false positively correlated with hemolysis and with increasing death to puncture time. This test has therefore not been recommended as a supplementary assay to accompany HIV antibody ELISA screening of potential corneal donors. A much larger study of approximately one million blood donors in Europe and the United States by the American Red Cross, the American Association of Blood Banks, and the Council of Community Blood Centers has similarly failed to uncover any confirmed HIV antigen-positive samples in the absence of antibody.[16] The ELISA test for HIV antigen therefore has not been adopted for screening blood or plasma donors.

LACK OF DOCUMENTED HIV-1 TRANSMISSION BY CORNEAL TRANSPLANTATION

Concern over the potential for HIV transmission by corneal transplantation is heightened by the fact that other viral diseases, such as hepatitis B, rabies, and Creutzfeldt-Jakob disease, have been acquired through that route. Up to now, however, no cases of HIV transmission or seroconversion after corneal transplantation have been reported. Ten corneas from HIV-seropositive cadavers (including two from a recently reported case in Virginia) have been inadvertently transplanted to individuals without known risk factors for AIDS.[38,49] Six years have passed without seroconversion or clinical signs of HIV infection in these recipients. Two of the corneal do-

nors were multiple organ donors.[49] The four recipients of kidneys and other organs and tissues from these cadavers did seroconvert shortly after transplantation, in contrast to the recipients of corneas from these same cadavers. It is likely that the inoculum of HIV in corneal tissue is quite low and may often be below the threshold required to initiate infection. In contrast, HIV has been transmitted after transplantation of liver, pancreas, bone marrow, skin, heart, kidney, and multiple organs.[18,25]

Current historical and serologic screening procedures should minimize the likelihood of corneal transplantation from an HIV-infected donor. These test methods remain a relatively, though not absolutely, effective means of screening. One mathematical projection[24] of the average risk of inadvertently transplanting a cornea from an HIV-infected donor, because of the latency period of seroconversion and the false-negative rate of the ELISA test, was 0.03%. With over 40,000 corneal transplants performed annually in the United States alone, this conservative estimate allows one to predict that 6 corneas will be transplanted from HIV-infected donors each year, if one assumes a prevalence of HIV infection in the donor population of 0.005. Given these data, the lack of evidence up to now of HIV-1 transmission after penetrating keratoplasty is of some comfort but emphasizes the need for continued screening programs and for the development of more sensitive screening assays optimized for testing cadaveric donors. The EBAA should be commended for rapidly implementing important changes in its medical standards in response to the AIDS epidemic in order to reduce the likelihood of transmitting this fatal disease by corneal transplantation.

ACKNOWLEDGMENT

This study was supported in part by Public Health Service Grant EY 08143-01 from the National Eye Institute (JSP).

REFERENCES

1. Ablashi DV et al: Presence of HTLV-III in tears and cells from the eyes of AIDS patients, *J Exp Pathol* 3:693-703, 1987.
2. Bacchetti P, Moss AR: Incubation period of AIDS in San Francisco, *Nature* 338:251-253, 1989.
3. Barré-Sinoussi F et al: Isolation of a T-lymphotropic retrovirus from a patient at risk for acquired immunodeficiency syndrome, *Science* 220:868-871, 1983.
4. Bialasiewicz AA, Jahn GJ: Screening for potentially pathogenic agents in cornea donors, *Am J Ophthalmol* 102:104-105, 1987.
5. Broder S, Gallo RC: A pathogenic retrovirus (HTLV-III) linked to AIDS, *N Engl J Med* 311:1292-1297, 1984.
6. Buehler JW et al: Impact of the human immunodeficiency virus epidemic on mortality trends in young men, United States, *Am J Public Health* 80:1080-1086, 1990.

7. Buerger DG, Pepose JS: New developments in serologic screening of cornea donors for HIV and hepatitis B, *Invest Ophthalmol Vis Sci* 32(suppl):766, 1991.

8. Cantrill HL et al: Recovery of human immunodeficiency virus from ocular tissues in patients with acquired immune deficiency syndrome, *Ophthalmology* 95:1458-1462, 1988.

9. Centers for Disease Control: Update: acquired immunodeficiency syndrome (AIDS) United States, *MMWR* 32:465-468, 1983.

10. Centers for Disease Control: Public health service guidelines for counseling and antibody testing to prevent HIV infection and AIDS, *MMWR* 36:509-515, 1987.

11. Centers for Disease Control: Update: serologic testing for antibody to human immunodeficiency virus, *MMWR* 36:833-845, 1988.

12. Centers for Disease Control: Mortality attributable to HIV/ AIDS - United States, 1981-90, *MMWR* 40:41-44, 1991.

13. Chu SY, Buehler JW, Berkelman RL: Impact of the human immunodeficiency virus epidemic on mortality in women of reproductive age, United States, *JAMA* 264:225-229, 1990.

14. Conway MD, Insler MS: The identification and incidence of human immunodeficiency virus antibodies and hepatitis B virus antigens in corneal donors, *Ophthalmology* 95:1463-1467, 1988.

15. Danneffel MB, Sugar A: Incidence of HIV antibody—positive eye/cornea donors in hospital versus medical examiner cases, *Cornea* 9:271-272, 1990.

16. Dodd RY, Barker LF: Early markers of HIV-1 infection in plasma donors, *JAMA* 202:92-93, 1989.

17. Doro S et al: Confirmation of HTLV-III virus in cornea, *Am J Ophthalmol* 102:390-391, 1986.

18. Dummer JS et al: Infection with human immunodeficiency virus in the Pittsburgh transplant population, *Transplantation* 47:134-139, 1989.

19. Dutt K et al: Replication of HIV in human fetal retinal cultures and established pigment epithelial cell lines, *Invest Ophthalmol Vis Sci* 30:1535-1541, 1989.

20. Farrell PL et al: Response of human immunodeficiency virus—associated uveitis to zidovudine, *Am J Ophthalmol* 106:7-10, 1988.

21. Fujikawa LS et al: Human T-cell leukemia/lymphotropic virus type III in the conjunctival epithelium of a patient with AIDS, *Am J Ophthalmol* 100:507-509, 1985.

22. Fujikawa LS et al: Isolation of human T lymphotropic virus type III from the tears of a patient with the acquired immunodeficiency syndrome, *Lancet* 2:529-530, 1985.

23. Fujikawa LS et al: HTLV-III in the tears of AIDS patients, *Ophthalmology* 93:1479-1481, 1986.

24. Goode SM et al: Adequacy of the ELISA test for screening corneal transplant donors, *Am J Ophthalmol* 106:463-466, 1980.

25. Gottesdiener KM: Transplanted infections: donor-to-host transmission with the allograft, *Ann Intern Med* 110:1016-1017, 1989.

26. Gottlieb MS et al: *Pneumocystis carinii* pneumonia and mucosal candidiasis in previously healthy homosexual men: evidence of a new acquired cellular immunodeficiency, *N Engl J Med* 305:1425-1431, 1981.

27. Goudsmit J et al: Antigenemia and antibody titers to core and envelop antigens in AIDS, AIDS-related complex, and subclinical human immunodeficiency virus infection, *J Infect Dis* 155(3):558-560, 1987.

28. Heck E et al: ELISA HIV testing and viral culture in the screening of corneal tissue for transplant from medical examiner cases, *Cornea* 8:77-80, 1989.

29. Hwang DG et al: Human immunodeficiency virus seroprevalence among potential corneal donors from medical examiner cases, *Am J Ophthalmol* 109:92-93, 1990.

30. Imagawa DT et al: Human immunodeficiency virus type 1 infection in homosexual men who remain seronegative for prolonged periods, *N Engl J Med* 320:1458-1462, 1989.

31. Irving WL et al: Antibody to both human herpesvirus 6 and cytomegalovirus, *Lancet* 2:630-635, 1988.

32. Kessler HA et al: Diagnosis of human immunodeficiency virus infection in seronegative homosexuals presenting with an acute viral syndrome, *JAMA* 258:1196-1199, 1987.

33. Kestelyn P, de Perre PV, Sprecher-Goldberger S: Isolation of the human T-cell leukemia/lymphotropic virus type III from aqueous humor in two patients with perivasculitis of the retinal vessels, *Int Ophthalmol* 9:247-251, 1986.

34. Klatt EC, Shibats D, Strigle SM: Postmortem enzyme immunoassay for human immunodeficiency virus, *Arch Pathol Lab Med* 113:485-487, 1989.

35. Masur H et al: An outbreak of community-acquired *Pneumocystis carinii* pneumonia: initial manifestation of cellular immune dysfunction, *N Engl J Med* 305:1431-1438, 1981.

36. Okuno T et al: Human herpesvirus 6 infection in renal transplantation, *Transplant* 49:519-522, 1990.

37. Pepose JS et al: Screening cornea donor for antibodies against human immunodeficiency virus: efficacy of ELISA testing of cadaveric sera and aqueous humor, *Ophthalmology* 94:95-100, 1987.

38. Pepose JS et al: Serologic markers after the transplantation of corneas from donors infected with human immunodeficiency virus, *Am J Ophthalmol* 103:798-801, 1987.

39. Pepose JS et al: Co-factors associated with cytomegalovirus infection of the retina. In Usui M, Ohno S, Aoki K, editors: *Ocular immunology today*, Amsterdam, 1990, Elsevier Scientific Publishers.

40. Petricciani JC: Licensed tests for antibody to human T-lymphotropic virus type III: sensitivity and specificity, *Ann Intern Med* 103:726-729, 1985.

41. Pomerantz RJ et al: Infection of the retina by human immunodeficiency virus type 1, *N Engl J Med* 317:1643-1647, 1987.

42. Popovic M et al: Detection, isolation and continuous production of cytopathic retroviruses (HTLV-III) from patients with AIDS and pre-AIDS, *Science* 224:497-500, 1984.

43. Public Health Service: Coolfront report: a PHS plan for prevention and control of AIDS and the AIDS virus, *Public Health Rep* 101:341-348, 1986.

44. Qavi HB et al: Demonstration of HIV-1 and HHV-6 in AIDS-associated retinitis, *Curr Eye Res* 8:379-387, 1989.

45. Qavi HB et al: The incidence of HIV-1 and HHV-6 in corneal buttons, *Curr Eye Res* 10(suppl):97-103, 1991.

46. Salahuddin SZ et al: Isolation of the human T-cell leukemia/ lymphotropic virus type III from the cornea, *Am J Ophthalmol* 101:149-152, 1986.

47. Scheiffarth OF et al: T-lymphocytes of the normal human cornea, *Br J Ophthalmol* 71:384-386, 1987.

48. Schmitt-Graff A et al: Evidence for cytomegalovirus and human immunodeficiency infection of the retina in AIDS, *Virchows Arch Pathol Anat* 416:249-253, 1990.

49. Schwarz A et al: Human immunodeficiency virus transmission by organ donation: outcome for cornea and kidney recipients, *Transplantation* 44:21-24, 1987.

50. Schwartz JS, Dans PE, Kinosian BP: Human immunodeficiency virus test evaluation, performance and use: proposals to make good tests better, *JAMA* 259:2574-2579, 1988.

51. Sheppard HW et al: A multicenter proficiency trial of gene amplification (PCR) for the detection of HIV-1, *J Acquired Immune Deficiency Syndrome* 4:277-283, 1991.

52. Siegal IP et al: Severe acquired immunodeficiency in male homosexuals, manifested by chronic perianal, ulcerative herpes simplex lesions, *N Engl J Med* 305:1439-1444, 1981.

53. Skolnik PR et al: Dual infection of retina with human immunodeficiency virus type 1 and cytomegalovirus, *Am J Ophthalmol* 107:361-372, 1989.

54. Srinivasan A et al: Isolation of HIV-1 from vitreous humor, *Am J Ophthalmol* 108:197-198, 1989.

55. Stramer SL et al: Markers of HIV infection prior to IgG antibody seropositivity, *JAMA* 262:64-69, 1989.

56. Tervo T et al: Recovery of HTLV-III from contact lenses, *Lancet* 1:379-380, 1986.

57. Ward KN, Gray JJ, Efstathio S: Brief report: primary human herpesvirus 6 infection in a patient following transplantation from a seropositive donee, *J Med Virol* 28:69-72, 1989.

58. Wilhelmus KR, Farge EJ: HIV antibody screening of corneal donor, *Ophthalmologica* 195:57-60, 1987.

59. Wolinsky SM et al: Human immunodeficiency virus type 1 (HIV-1) infection a median of 18 months before a diagnostic Western blot: evidence from a cohort of homosexual men, *Ann Intern Med* 111:961-972, 1989.

60. Yamanishi K et al: Identification of human herpesvirus-6 as a causal agent for exanthem subitum, *Lancet* 1:1065-1067, 1988.

Chapter 46

Tissue Storage and Tissue Typing

Short term—state of the art

BERND H. SCHIMMELPFENNIG

The donor tissue of the first documented corneal graft in humans was retrieved and judged by the surgeon himself.[59] Today his successors would be overwhelmed in a similar situation. A functioning eye bank laboratory is now on duty to procure and evaluate suitable donor corneas for busy surgeons who want to perform their procedures on a regular schedule. The method by which the donor material is being stored in an eye bank is mainly determined by the supply and demand for donor tissue. The most desirable situation in order to maintain a satisfactory supply of donor material exists if cadavers are routinely dissected in a department of pathology close to the local eye bank. The enucleating physician can then either select donor eyes on the basis of the known preceding disease or make his final decision after the report of autopsy has been released. The Zurich Eye Bank is operating under such conditions.

CADAVER TIME (TIME FROM DEATH TO ENUCLEATION)

Depending on the ambient temperature the corneal endothelial cells facing a stagnant aqueous humor show progressive cytolysis, which ultimately results in cell death.[2,4,34,50,54] The exact point in time from which cell changes lead to irreversible failure is unknown. On the other hand, knowledge about that "point of no return" is of great importance, since any extension of the cadaver time enables eye banks to reduce the number of unsuitably discarded eyes and to increase the supply. From clinical reports the accepted cadaver time ranges from 4 to 48 hours.[28,35,39,41] Usually, the cadaver time includes

two periods: (1) For some time after death the cadaver is exposed to room temperature. During this period the cessation of aqueous humor formation causes increasing nutritional problems for the endothelium. A prolonged duration of this state may be critical for endothelial viability and survival. (2) Cadaver storage between 4° and 8° C. The low temperature slows down endothelial pump mechanisms[22] and metabolic stress is avoided. Under these circumstances donor endothelium has a better chance to survive. In a laboratory study, the viability of donor corneas after different cadaver times (including the period of time at room temperature, 4 ± 2 hours) was investigated.[48] The isolated corneas were perfused at 34.5° C (Fig. 46-1) with modified Ringer's solution,[16] and the decrease of swelling as well as reversibility of ultrastructural changes were recorded. It could be demonstrated that even after 41 hours of cadaver time donor corneas revealed functioning endothelium. At present, the average cadaver time of donor eyes at the Zurich Eye Bank is 11 hours, 24 minutes (range, 1 to 49 hours).

EVALUATION OF DONOR MATERIAL

After enucleation donor eyes are immediately immersed in precooled isotonic saline containing gentamicin 200 μg/ml and polymyxin 50 μg/ml (Fig. 46-2). Within 10 minutes they are brought to the eye bank laboratory. Screening for corneal opacities, scars, and injuries is done with the slitlamp (Fig. 46-3). The donor endothelium is examined under an in vitro specular microscope (Fig. 46-4). The presence of cornea guttata changes (Fig. 46-5), which exclude a cornea from surgical use, can be identified only by means of this technique.[9,46]

Specular micrographic cell evaluations, such as measurements of numerical cell-density and cell-size

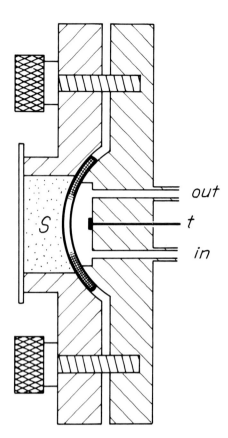

Fig. 46-1. Perfusion chamber for isolated human corneas, allowing specular microscopic recording of corneal function (thickness measurements) during perfusion with test substances. *In,* Inlet tube; *out,* outlet tube, *t,* temperature regulation, *s,* silicon oil cover (removable) of epithelium to prevent evaporation.

variations, have been abandoned for three reasons:

1. The limited sample size (between 40 and 80 cells), which is often additionally impaired by stromal edema, does not allow an accurate quantitative judgment of the endothelium (Figs. 46-6 and 46-7).
2. It has been shown in vitro that age-related decrease of endothelial cell density is far less than originally suggested[29,45] (Fig. 46-8). Thus old age is no reason to reject donor material.[25, 19]
3. Any negative influence of variation in cell size and shape on the quality of donor cell population is not yet established.

After specular microscopic examination the globe is vigorously rinsed with gentamicin- and polymyxin-containing saline. The excision of the cornea with a 3 to 4 mm scleral rim is best done with the globe sucked onto a Plexiglas plate (Fig. 46-9). Bacterial swabs are not taken. After excision the donor button

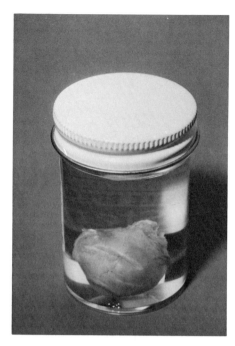

Fig. 46-2. Donor eye immersed in precooled isotonic saline solution (containing gentamicin, 200 μg/ml, and polymyxin, 50 μg/ml) after enucleation.

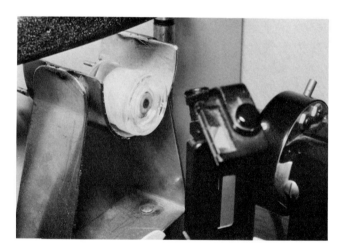

Fig. 46-3. Slitlamp evaluation of a donor eye.

is stored in a modified tissue-culture medium 199 (TC 199) at 4° C (Fig. 46-10). The corneoscleral rim, which remains after surgical trephination, is kept in its storage solution for 1 week at 4° C to have it available for investigational bacterial cultures.

SHORT-TERM STORAGE

Corneal donor tissue can be stored for short-term purposes (3 to 4 days) by means of two techniques:

1. Keeping the whole globe in a saturated moist chamber at 4° C (Fig. 46-11).

2. Immersion of the excised cornea in a defined culture medium at 4° C (Fig. 46-10).

The prevailing storage practice today is the excision of the cornea from the enucleated donor eye[6] in order to avoid its prolonged exposure to the small volume of stagnant and probably changing aqueous humor.[8] The most convenient replacement for the aqueous is a tissue-culture medium that is commercially available. The storage solution serves four purposes:

1. It provides a chemically defined and stable environment at 4° C.
2. It enables some basic metabolic activities of the stored tissue.[15]
3. With antibiotic additives it keeps the tissue under sterile conditions and may, to a certain extent, sterilize the corneas.
4. Added colloidosmotically active substances counterbalance the stromal swelling pressure thereby preventing excessive swelling.

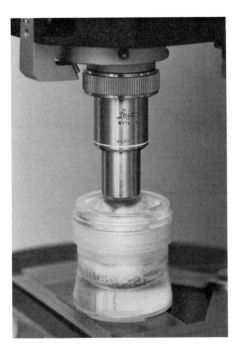

Fig. 46-4. Specular microscopic evaluation of donor endothelium under saline immersion.

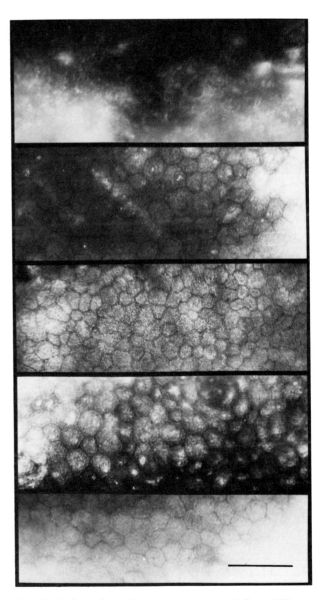

Fig. 46-6. Specular photomicrographs of five different suitable donor endothelia. (Cadaver time, 16 hours; magnification bar, 75 μm.)

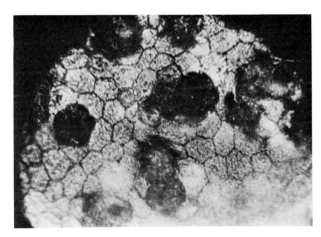

Fig. 46-5. Cornea guttata (*dark areas*, or corneal guttae) in donor endothelium.

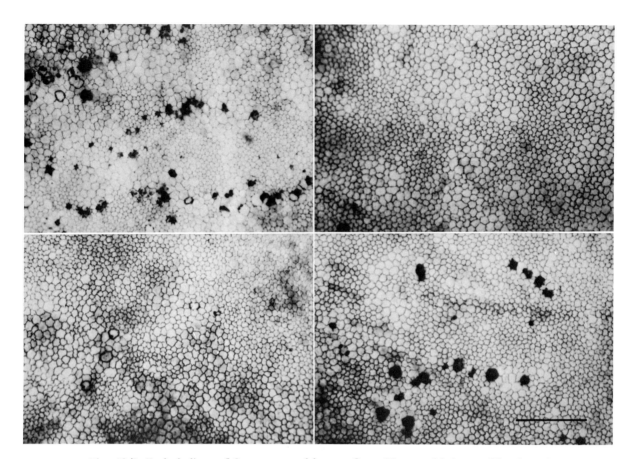

Fig. 46-7. Endothelium of 8 mm corneal button from 65-year-old donor. The four 1 mm areas were photographed 2 to 3 mm off center after Alizarin red staining. Area distribution of different cell sizes would have made precise cell-density measurements difficult. (Magnification bar, 250 μm.)

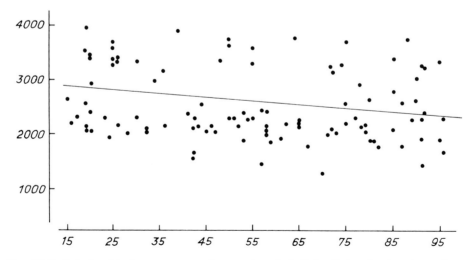

Fig. 46-8. Relationship between central corneal endothelial cell density (y axis) and age (x axis) in 105 human eyes. Weak linear correlation between increasing age and decreasing cell density ($y = 2937 - 6.89x$, $r^2 = 0.036$, correlation coefficient $r = 0.19$, cell loss per year = 0.22%). Data obtained from counts on Alizarin red–stained corneas. Sampled area per individual cornea, 3 mm × 1 mm.

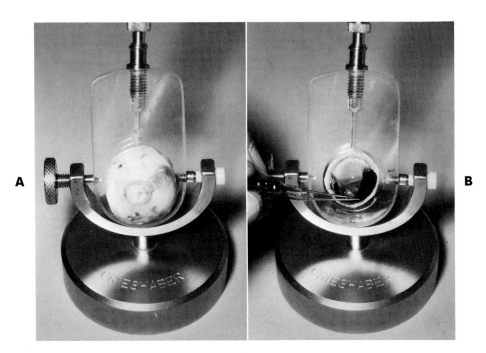

Fig. 46-9. Excision of corneoscleral donor button. **A,** Donor eye is sucked to a Plexiglas plate. **B,** Its contents are being removed without damaging distortion of remaining donor button.

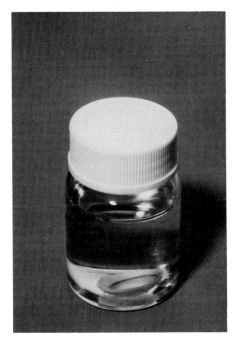

Fig. 46-10. Twenty-five milliliter (class I, lead-free glass) vial for short-term storage of corneoscleral buttons (endothelial side up).

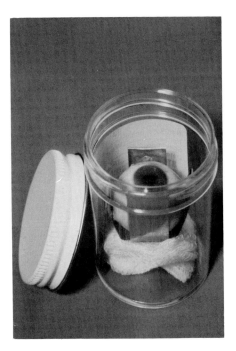

Fig. 46-11. Common vial for moist chamber storage of donor eyes.

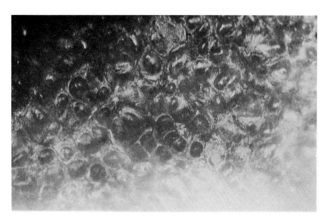

Fig. 46-12. Specular microscopic appearance of donor endothelium 4 days after storage at 4° C in modified TC-medium 199. Indistinct cell borders and darkening of cells suggestive of edematous changes make qualitative and quantitative evaluation after storage difficult.

TC-MEDIUM 199 AND ITS ADDITIVES

Dextran. Sachs[40] was the first to add Dextran to a bathing solution for donor globes to prevent excessive stromal swelling. Later, McCarey and Kaufman[32] were able to demonstrate functional and ultrastructural integrity of excised rabbit corneas, which had been stored in Morgan and co-workers[37] well-established TC (tissue culture medium) 199 at 4° C up to 14 days. The medium contained 5% dextran (molecular weight, 40,000) and penicillin. Favorable clinical reports confirmed the efficacy of dextran in preventing excess stromal swelling.[1,5,52]

This ability, however, has its limitations. It has been shown that dextran enters the cornea.[10,24] The average stromal thickness after 4 days of storage in dextran-containing medium ranges from 0.65 to 0.75 mm. Together with endothelial changes (Fig. 46-12) it does not allow routine specular microscopic investigations of the endothelium after short-term storage.

pH Buffering. Early commercial short-term storage solutions had very unstable pH values (own observation). This was not surprising in view of the fact that tissue culture media contain a substantial amount of bicarbonate, which has to be balanced with carbon dioxide gas. Its controlled supply in sealed storage vials, however, is difficult to maintain. The introduction of a synthetic pH-stabilizing substance that could be used in tissue culture systems was of great importance. The compatibility of HEPES® (N'-2-hydroxyethylpiperazine-N-ethanesulfonic acid) with human corneal donor tissue was tested in long-term perfusion experiments.[43] It is now added to the storage medium at a concentration of 15 to 20 mM/L and stabilizes the pH at 7.3.[58] In the presence of HEPES, pH indicators, such as phenolsulfonphthalein (phenol red), can be omitted.

Antibiotics. The outer surface of a cadaver eye is heavily contaminated.[13,17,26,38,48] Bacterial growth increases further with advancing cadaver time. A corneoscleral button, even after removal of the conjunctiva, is considered to be infectious. Thus any measure should be taken to sterilize the tissue.[12,18] Vigorous rinsing under tap water or with a syringe can mechanically remove quite a few microorganisms. The storage medium itself should provide a sterile environment with at least bacteriostatic properties.[14] Penicillin, which at high concentrations still is an efficient broad-spectrum antibiotic, has the disadvantage of early decay. During short-term storage an antibiotic is needed, which combines stability with bactericidal activity. In addition, it should not be toxic for corneal tissue and should have sufficient efficacy against common pathogenic microorganisms. A study on bacterial contamination of donor eyes from the local university department of pathology revealed gentamicin and polymyxin to be most effective against pathogenic bacteria such as *Pseudomonas aeruginosa* and staphylococci.[48] Gentamicin at a concentration of 100 μg/ml was able to decontaminate 85% of 122 donor eyes (Fig. 46-13) under short-

	122 donor-eyes	122 donor-corneas
contaminated	100 (82%)	18 (15%)
not contaminated	22 (18%)	104 (85%)

Fig. 46-13. Extent of bacterial contamination of donor eyes obtained at autopsy in comparison to that of same corneas after storage in gentamicin-containing culture medium at 4° C.

	S. aureus	Klebsiella pneumoniae	E. coli	Proteus	P. aeruginosa	Enterococci	mean value of sensitivity
Gentamicin	100	72	100	100	75	70	86
Chloramphenicol	100	52	53	100	8	53	61
Polymyxin	72	100	87	0	100	0	60
Neomycin	82	65	67	72	5	67	60
Tetracycline	79	75	100	14	23	27	53
Kanamycin	75	40	40	26	25	50	43
Cephalotin	85	33	34	86	0	15	42
Erythromycin	73	45	53	57	7	13	41
Ampicillin	22	18	0	72	0	100	35
Penicillin	25	25	8	43	7	0	18

Fig. 46-14. Sensitivity (%) of potentially pathogenic bacteria cultured from donor eyes obtained at autopsy.

term storage conditions. Since there were gentamicin-resistant strains in this series and polymyxin was 100% effective against them (Fig. 46-14), both antibiotics are now being used. Baum and co-workers[3] reported similar results with the use of gentamicin under low temperature conditions. The modified storage medium now contains gentamicin 200 μg/ml and polymyxin 50 μg/ml. In the eye department in the University of Zurich 750 perforating corneal grafts have been performed, so far, without a single postoperative endophthalmitis.

DONOR TISSUE VIABILITY

The most important question about the use of stored donor material concerns the viability of its endothelium.* A suitable definition, which includes biologic as well as surgical aspects, would describe viable endothelium as a sufficient number of endothelial cells with intact pump sites and proper adhesion to Descemet's membrane. Before a graft finally resides in the recipient's eye, its viability had been stressed on several occasions (Fig. 46-15). The sud-

*References 11, 21, 23, 27, 28, 34, 50, 51, 53, 54.

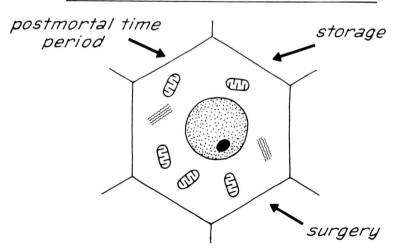

Fig. 46-15. Schema of factors affecting viability of donor endothelium.

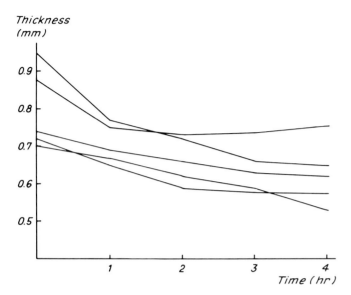

Fig. 46-16. Decrease of corneal thickness during perfusion with modified Ringer's solution at 34° C. Corneas had previously been stored in a moist chamber for 4 days.

den stop of aqueous humor formation after death and the depletion of nutrients and oxygen at room temperature causes the first damage to the cells.[50] However, I believe that as long as the cell membrane is intact and the exposure to room temperature has not exceeded 4 or 5 hours, the cells can resume their metabolic activity even after 40 hours of storage at 4° C.[44]

Moist Chamber Storage. Storage of excised donor corneas in modified culture media has decreased the

use of donor material from refrigerated moist chamber eyes.[6,30] Despite the advantages of having the excised cornea ready for trephination in a large volume of defined culture medium, the latter method should not be discounted. At present, our knowledge about postmortem changes in the aqueous in human cadaver eyes is very limited. One should also consider that the total volume of aqueous includes the vitreous space. Thus the nutritional basis for the cadaver endothelium may be larger than expected. As opposed to an isolated cornea, the intact donor eye enables the surgeon to modify shape and excision technique of the graft.

If the cadaver time does not exceed 4 or 5 hours an enucleated eye can be kept at least 3 days in a saturated moist chamber of 4° C without loosing its endothelial pump activity. This can be demonstrated during perfusion of isolated human corneas that had previously been stored under moist chamber conditions (Fig. 46-16). The individual cells can be visualized with the specular microscope (Fig. 46-17). Although the majority of studies indicate more serious ultrastructural changes in moist-chamber corneas,* the areas of endothelial cell loss compare closely with those corneas stored in modified culture medium at 4° C (Fig. 46-18).

Short-Term Tissue Culture Storage (TC 199) at 4° C. The viability of corneas that have been stored in dextran-containing culture media at 4° C is difficult to determine. From ultrastructural observations

---

*References 7, 20, 31, 33, 36, 42, 53, 55.

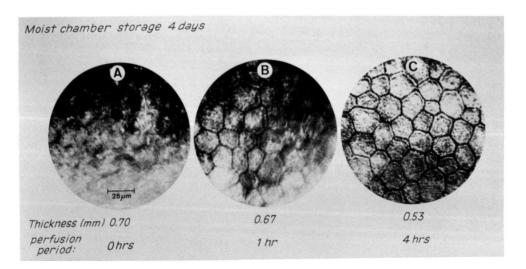

Fig. 46-17. Specular microscopic observations on endothelial changes during perfusion of moist chamber–stored donor corneas. There is improving visualization of cell pattern because of functioning endothelial pump and decreasing stromal thickness.

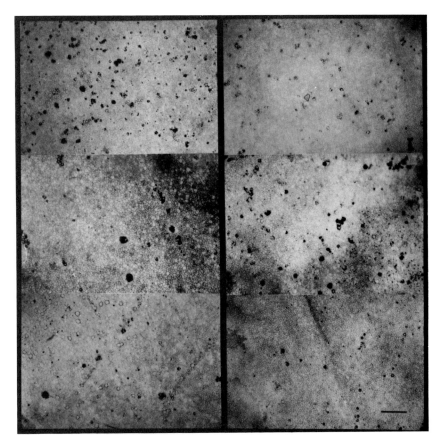

Fig. 46-18. Comparison of cell loss in Alizarin red–stained endothelia from three pairs of corneas (cadaver time, 12, 13, and 15 hours). *Left row from top to bottom,* 3 days after storage in modified TC-medium 199 at 4° C. *Right row,* Moist chamber storage 3 days at 4° C. Areas of cell loss are dark because of staining of denuded Descemet's membrane. (Magnification bar, 250 μm.)

one can conclude that endothelial cells at that temperature are dying cells.[27,56,57] After several days they inevitably reveal signs of autolysis (Fig. 46-19) if compared to partner cells that have been cultured at 37° C (Fig. 46-20). From clinical experience a certain in vivo reversibility of those changes can be suggested, since those corneas can do well as a graft 7 days after short-term storage.[5] However, before any conclusions can be drawn about viability, some additional aspects should be considered:

1. Dextran enters the cornea[10,24] and thereby changes its swelling properties. Thinning curves obtained during perfusion are difficult to interpret.

2. We do not know if the reversibility of storage-induced cell changes concern all cells uniformly. There may be a substantial number of cells in a donor endothelium that have reached conditions beyond safe recovery.

3. During storage, cells are lost at variable degrees

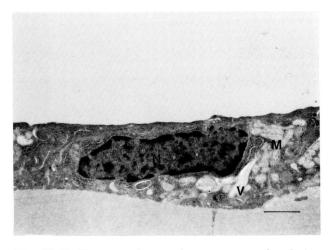

Fig. 46-19. Electron microscopic appearance of endothelium 7 days after storage in modified TC-Medium 199 at 4° C. (Cadaver time, 8 hours.) *N,* Nucleus with clumping of its chromatin; *M,* swollen or lysed mitochondria; *V,* cytoplasmic vacuoles. (Magnification bar, 2.5 μm.)

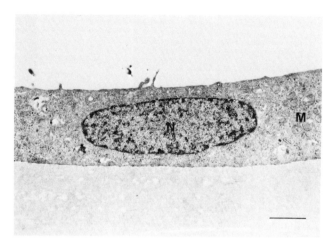

Fig. 46-20. Ultrastructure of partner cornea (see Fig. 46-19) after 7 days of organ culture at 37° C. *N,* Regularly dispersed nuclear chromatin; *M,* mitochondria. (Magnification bar, 2.5 µm.)

(Fig. 46-21). At present, we can neither exactly determine the cell loss,[30,56] nor indicate the tolerable range.[49]

4. Cell adhesion to Descemet's membrane decreases with increasing storage time at 4° C, which could be the most important limiting factor for extension of the storage time. It can be demonstrated experimentally that cell loss induced by surgical manipulations of the graft runs parallel with increasing storage time[47] (Figs. 46-22 and 46-23).

5. The corneal donor epithelium seems to survive well during the storage period. Thus, in high-risk corneal grafts, short-term donor material yields better results than medium-term (Dexsol) donor corneas (own observation).

After these considerations it seems reasonable to use TC 199–stored donor corneas before a maximum storage period of 4 days. A death-to-enucleation time of 3 to 6 hours allows for 4 days, whereas one of 7 to 12 hours allows for only 2 days. In our series of 740 penetrating keratoplasties we had only 5 primary graft failures with an average death-to-operation time of 46 hours (range, 1 hour to 7 days). Donor corneas can be grafted successfully after longer storage periods with use of newer intermediate-term media, reviewed in the next section.

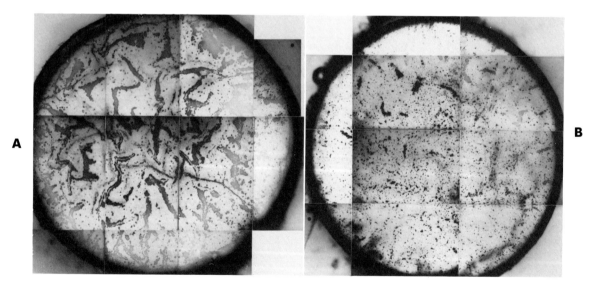

Fig. 46-21. A, Endothelial cell loss 7 days after storage in modified TC-Medium 199 at 4° C. Entire endothelial surface of 8 mm corneal button has been stained with Alizarin red. Dark areas indicate cell loss (approximately 40%). **B,** Another 8 mm donor button, stored under the same circumstances as in **A.** Multiple small areas of cell loss (approximately 15%).

Fig. 46-22. Demonstration of decreased endothelial cell adhesion after short-term storage. **A,** Fresh 8 mm donor button that had experimentally been grafted to a living rabbit eye. Alizarin red staining immediately after removal of the sutured graft. Dark areas indicate cell loss (approximately 20%). **B,** In comparison, endothelium of an 8 mm donor button 7 days after short-term storage and subsequent grafting shows pronounced endothelial cell loss (approximately 65%).

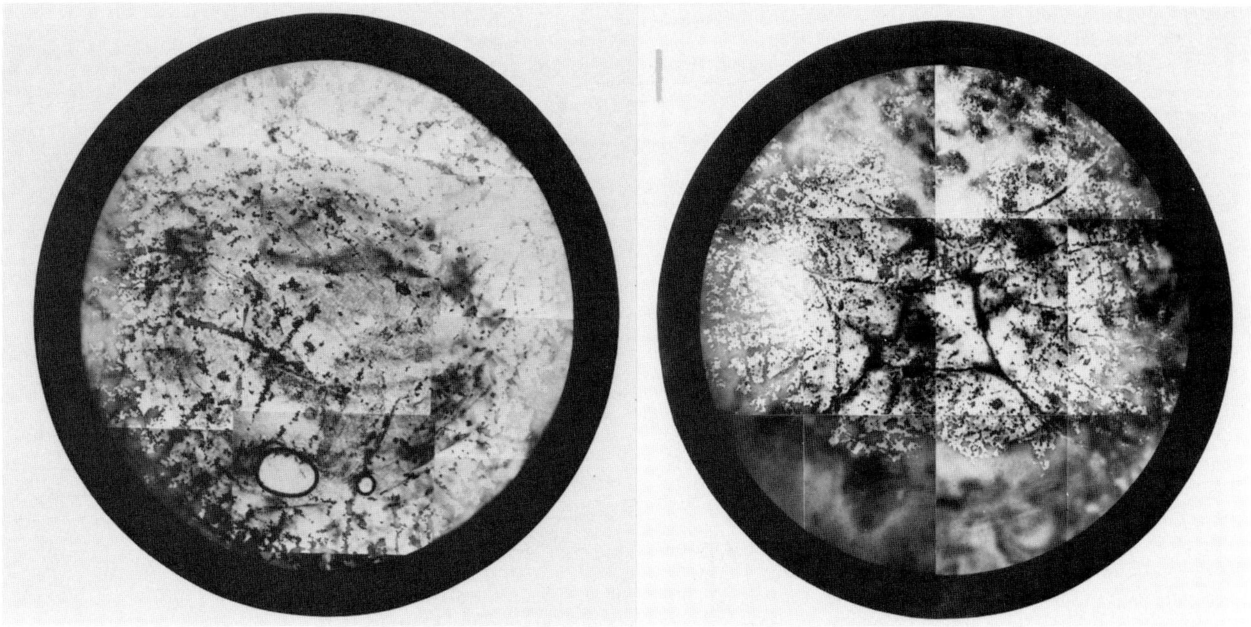

ACKNOWLEDGMENTS

This work was supported by the A. Bruppacher Eye Bank Foundation, Zürich, Switzerland.

I am grateful to Drs. E. Korach and T. Haubensak, both in Zürich, for reviewing the manuscript.

REFERENCES

1. Aquavella JV, Van Horn DL, Haggerty CJ: Corneal preservation using M-K medium, *Am J Ophthalmol* 80:791, 1975.
2. Basu PK, Hasany S: Autolysis of the cornea of stored human donor eyes, *Can J Ophthalmol* 9:229, 1974.
3. Baum JL, Barza M, Kane A: Efficacy of penicillin G, cefazolin, and gentamicin in M-K medium at 4° C, *Arch Ophthalmol* 96:1262, 1978.
4. Beveridge B: Eye banking. In Casey TA, editor: *Corneal grafting,* New York, 1972, Appleton-Century-Crofts.
5. Bigar F, Kaufman HE, McCarey BE, Binder PS: Improved corneal storage for penetrating keratoplasties in man, *Am J Ophthalmol* 79:115, 1975.
6. Binder PS: Eye banking and corneal preservation. In *Symposium on medical and surgical diseases of the cornea,* Transactions of the New Orleans Academy of Ophthalmology, St. Louis, 1980, Mosby–Year Book.
7. Binder PS, Wickham MG: M-K medium and post mortem cytologic damage, *Invest Ophthalmol Vis Sci* 17:159, 1978.
8. Bito LZ, Salvador EV: Intraocular fluid dynamics. II. Post mortem changes in solute concentration, *Exp Eye Res* 10:273, 1970.

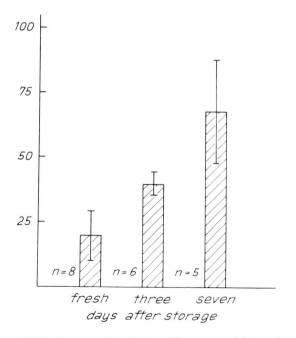

Fig. 46-23. Extent of cell loss (% on *y* axis) in three groups: *left,* fresh corneas; *middle,* 3 days' storage; *right,* 7 days' storage of 8 mm corneal buttons after experimental grafting to living rabbit eye. (For details see reference 47.)

9. Bourne WM: Examination and photography of donor corneal endothelium, *Arch Ophthalmol* 94:1799, 1976.

10. Breslin CW, Kaufman HE, Centifanto YM: Dextran flux in M-K medium-stored human corneas, *Invest Ophthalmol Vis Sci* 16:752, 1977.

11. Breslin CW, Sherrard ES, Marshall J, Rice NSC: Evaluation of the McCarey-Kaufman technique of corneal storage, *Arch Ophthalmol* 94:1545, 1976.

12. Brightbill FS, Terrones C, Gould S: Experimental studies with *Staphylococcus aureus* in M-K media, *Invest Ophthalmol* 15:32, 1976.

13. Buxton JN, Brownstein S: Bacterial cultures from donor corneas, *Arch Ophthalmol* 84:148, 1970.

14. Christensen J, Kastl PR, Caldwell DR: Bacterial contamination of donor corneas stored in McCarey-Kaufman medium, *Ophthalmic Surg* 13:231, 1982.

15. De Roeth A Jr: Metabolism of the stored cornea, *Arch Ophthalmol* 65:659, 1957.

16. Dikstein S, Maurice DM: The metabolic bases to the fluid pump in the cornea, *Br J Ophthalmol* 221:29, 1972.

17. Doctor V, Hughes I: Prophylactic use of Neosporin for donor eyes, *Am J Ophthalmol* 46:351, 1958.

18. Escapini H Jr, Olson RJ, Kaufman HE: Donor cornea contamination with McCarey-Kaufman medium preservation, *Am J Ophthalmol* 88:59, 1979.

19. Forster RK, Fine MF: Relation of donor age to success in penetrating keratoplasty, *Arch Ophthalmol* 85:42, 1971.

20. Friedland BR, Forster RK: Comparison of corneal storage in McCarey-Kaufman medium, moist chamber, or standard eye-bank conditions, *Invest Ophthalmol* 15:143, 1976.

21. Hanna C: Ultrastructural changes and RNA and protein synthesis in cells of human eye bank corneas. In Capella JA, Edelhauser HF, Van Horn DI, editors: *Corneal preservation: clinical and laboratory evaluation of current methods*, Springfield, Ill, 1973, Charles C Thomas, Publisher.

22. Harris JE, Byrnes P: Reversal of induced hydration of human corneas stored in a moist chamber at refrigeration temperatures for various periods of time. In Capella, JA, Edelhauser HF, Van Horn DL, editors: *Corneal preservation; clinical and laboratory evaluation of current methods*, Springfield, Ill, 1973, Charles C Thomas, Publisher.

23. Hull DS, Green K, Bowman K: Corneal water and electrolyte content following storage in moist chamber and M-K medium, *Invest Ophthalmol* 15:778, 1976.

24. Hull DS, Green K, Bowman K: Dextran uptake into, and loss from, corneas stored in intermediate-term preservative, *Invest Ophthalmol* 15:663, 1976.

25. Jenkins MS, Lemper SL, and Brown SI: Significance of donor age in penetrating keratoplasty, *Am Ophthalmol* 11:974, 1979.

26. Keates RH, Mishler KE, Riedinger D: Bacterial contamination of donor eyes, *Am J Ophthalmol* 84:617, 1977.

27. Kobayashi S: Electron microscopy of stored corneal grafts, *Acta Soc Ophthalmol Jap* 68:952, 1964.

28. Kuming BS, Rycroft RV: A study of post mortem viability of corneal endothelial cells. In Rycroft PW, editor: *Corneoplastic surgery*, Proceedings of the Second International Plastic Conference, Oxford, 1969, Pergamon Press.

29. Laing RA, Sandstrom MM, Berrospi AR, and Leibowitz HM: Changes in the corneal endothelium as a function of age, *Exp Eye Res* 22:587, 1976.

30. McCarey BE: Corneal storage and handling. In Zimmerman TJ, Kaufman HE, editors: *Current concepts in ophthalmology*, St. Louis, 1977, Mosby–Year Book.

31. McCarey BE: In vitro specular microscope perfusion of M-K and moist chamber-stored human corneas, *Invest Ophthalmol Vis Sci* 16:743, 1977.

32. McCarey BE, Kaufman HE: Improved corneal storage, *Invest Ophthalmol* 13:165, 1974.

33. McCarey BE, Sakimoto T, Bigar F: Ultrastructure of M-K and refrigerated moist chamber-stored corneas, *Invest Ophthalmol* 13:859, 1974.

34. McKinnon JR, Walters GD: Cadaver storage time: an important factor in donor cornea survival, *Arch Ophthalmol* 94:217, 1976.

35. McLean JM: Symposium: corneal transplantation: II. Technique, *Am J Ophthalmol* 31:1370, 1948.

36. Meyer RF, McCarey BE, Valenti J, et al: Scanning electron microscopy of postoperative M-K and moist chamber-stored corneas, *Invest Ophthalmol* 15:260, 1976.

37. Morgan JF, Morton HJ, Parker RC: Nutrition of animal cells in tissue culture: initial studies on synthetic medium, *Proc Soc Exp Biol Med* 73:1, 1950.

38. Polack FM, Locatcher-Khorazo D, Gutiérrez E: Bacteriologic study of "donor" eyes: evaluation of antibacterial treatments prior to corneal grafting, *Arch Ophthalmol* 78:219, 1967.

39. Poyales A: Queratoplastia parcial penetrante, *Arch Soc Oftalmol Hispano-Am* 11:746, 1951.

40. Sachs A: A new medium for the storage of donor eyes for corneal grafts, *Br J Ophthalmol* 41:558, 1957.

41. Saleeby SS: Keratoplasty: results using donor tissue beyond 48 hours, *Arch Ophthalmol* 87:538, 1972.

42. Schaeffer EM: Ultrastructural changes in moist chamber corneas, *Invest Ophthalmol* 2:272, 1963.

43. Schimmelpfennig B: Long-term perfusion of human corneas, *Invest Ophthalmol Vis Sci* 18:107, 1979.

44. Schimmelpfennig B: Evaluation of endothelial viability in human donor corneas, *Arch Ophthalmol* 100:472, 1982.

45. Schimmelpfennig B: Human corneal endothelium—*in vitro observations on growth and age related changes*, doctoral thesis, Zürich, 1987, University of Zürich.

46. Schimmelpfennig B, Bigar F, Witmer R, Gieseler R: Endothelial changes in human donor corneas, *Albrecht von Graefes Arch Klin Exp Ophthalmol* 200:201, 1976.

47. Schimmelpfennig B, Cosgrove J: Decreasing adhesion of human donor endothelium during storage at 4° C, *Invest Ophthalmol Vis Sci* 24(suppl):125, 1983.

48. Schimmelpfennig B, Hürzeler R: Bacterial flora of stored human donor corneas after antibiotic treatment, *Albrecht von Graefes Arch Klin Exp Ophthalmol* 202:181, 1977.

49. Shaw EL, Rao GN, Arthur EJ, Aquavella JV: The functional reserve of the corneal endothelium, *Trans Am Acad Ophthalmol Otolaryngol* 85:640, 1978.

50. Sherrard ES: The quality of donor corneas for penetrating keratoplasty. In Jones BR, chairman: Corneal graft failure, *Ciba Found Symp* 15:43-56, Amsterdam, 1973, Associated Scientific Publishers.

51. Sherrard ES: The corneal endothelium in vitro: its survival during banking at 4° C, *Trans Ophthalmol Soc UK* 94:80, 1974.

52. Stark WJ, Maumenee AE, Kenyon KR: Intermediate-term corneal storage for penetrating keratoplasty, *Am J Ophthalmol* 79:795, 1975.

53. Van Horn DL, Hanna C, Schultz RO: Corneal preservation. II. Ultrastructural and viability changes, *Arch Ophthalmol* 84:655, 1970.

54. Van Horn DL, Schultz RO: Ultrastructural changes in the endothelium of human corneas stored under eye bank conditions. In Capella JA, Edelhauser HF, Van Horn DL, editors: *Corneal preservation: clinical and laboratory evaluation of current methods*, Springfield, Ill, 1973, Charles C Thomas, Publisher.

55. Van Horn DL, Schultz RO: Comparison of serum vs. eye bank storage of cat corneas, *Arch Ophthalmol* 92:142, 1974.

56. Van Horn DL, Schultz RO: Corneal preservation: recent advances, *Surv Ophthalmol* 21:301, 1977.
57. Van Horn DL, Schultz RO, DeBruin J: Endothelial survival in corneal tissue stored in M-K medium, *Am J Ophthalmol* 80:642, 1975.
58. Waltman SR, Palmberg PF: Human penetrating keratoplasty using modified M-K medium, *Ophthalmic Surg* 9:48, 1978.
59. Zirm E: History of corneal grafting, *Albrecht von Graefes Arch Ophthalmol* 64:580, 1906.

Intermediate-term storage media (K-Sol, Dexsol, Optisol)

THOMAS L. STEINEMANN
HERBERT E. KAUFMAN
RICHARD L. LINDSTROM
ROGER W. BEUERMAN
EMILY D. VARNELL

The purpose of developing an intermediate-term corneal storage medium is to permit greater flexibility in the use of donor tissue and to prevent waste of tissue that can occur when surgery is postponed or rescheduled. Improvement in corneal preservation for up to 2 weeks allows flexible surgical scheduling, allows the surgeon to select the most desirable tissue without waste, and provides adequate time for performing various cultures. It is important that the use of such a medium involves no complex technical procedures—only standard eye bank procedures, a container, the medium, and 4° C refrigerator storage.

The addition of chondroitin sulfate has been a key development in the genesis of intermediate-term storage media. Chondroitin sulfate has been used in storage media in Japan for more than 20 years. Early studies by Mizukawa and Manabe[21] reported the successful preservation of whole globes immersed in a solution of chondroitin sulfate at 4° C for up to 3 days, but the medium was not used to bathe and preserve the endothelium. The exact mechanism by which chondroitin sulfate exerts its effect is unknown, but it may act as an antioxidant[33] and free-radical scavenger[7] to protect cell membranes. Also chondroitin sulfate may act as a cation-exchange resin to regulate cation fluxes across cell membranes through the formation of chelation complexes.[6]

Chondroitin sulfate is a constituent of all four intermediate-term storage media that have been or are being used in the United States: K-Sol, CSM, Dexsol, and Optisol. K-Sol was manufactured by Cilco, Inc., Belleview, Washington. It is no longer commercially available. CSM was produced by Aurora Biologicals, Williamsville, New York, which was brought out by Chiron Intraoptics, Irvine, California. At this writing, Chiron is producing CSM for investigational use only and manufacturing Dexsol and Optisol for commercial use in the preservation of donor corneal tissue.

K-SOL

In 1983 Kaufman and co-workers[11] described a storage medium (K-Sol) and method intended for simple refrigerated corneal storage up to 2 weeks. The results of this preliminary study were later corroborated by a clinical report of 17 patients who underwent corneal transplantation in 1985.[12] The mean corneal storage time was 8 days (range 2 to 16 days), and there was one primary graft failure. K-Sol contains tissue culture medium 199 (TC 199), 2.5% chondroitin sulfate, HEPES buffer, and gentamicin sulfate (100 µg/ml) (Table 46-1). Low-molecular-weight chondroitin sulfate polymers were removed during preparation to prevent small pieces of chondroitin sulfate from entering corneal tissue, thereby increasing osmotic pressure and causing excessive swelling of the donor tissue when it is placed in the eye. The larger polymers were believed to be less likely to permeate the tissue and more likely to remain in the preserving solution. The storage technique used with K-Sol was identical to that used with McCarey-Kaufman (MK) medium[19] in terms of eye bank handling.

Yau and Kaufman[34] studied rabbit corneas transplanted after 12 days of storage in K-Sol and found no significant differences from controls in terms of postoperative corneal thickness and endothelial cell loss. Stein and co-workers[30] compared endothelial disruption by scanning electron microscopy in canine and human corneas stored in K-Sol and MK medium for 14 days. Endothelial morphology was better maintained after storage in K-Sol at 4° C for 2 weeks. However, a clinical study by Bourne[4] reported large endothelial cell losses with increased time in the K-Sol storage. In this report 37 patients were transplanted with tissue that had been stored an average of 6 days (range 1 to 13 days). There were 2 primary graft failures. Based on these findings, Bourne recommended using tissue as early as possible and limiting corneal storage in K-Sol to 10 days.

In 1988 *Propionibacterium acnes*, a gram-positive anaerobic bacterium, was cultured from five donor corneal rims and from two lots of unopened K-Sol.[26] Despite the excellent record of corneal preservation, no previous reports of contamination, and the absence of clinical infection in any of the five trans-

Table 46-1. Constituents of Five Corneal Storage Media

Constituent	MK	K-Sol	CSM	Dexsol	Optisol
Base medium	TC 199	TC 199	MEM	MEM	Hybrid of TC 199 and MEM
Chondroitin sulfate	None	2.5%	1.35%	1.35%	2.5%
Dextran*	5%	None	None	1%	1%
HEPES buffer	Yes	Yes	Yes	Yes	Yes
Gentamicin sulfate	Yes	Yes	Yes	Yes	Yes
Nonessential amino acids	None	None	Yes	0.1 mM	0.1 mM
Sodium bicarbonate	No	Yes		Yes	Yes
Sodium pyruvate	None	None		1 mM	1 mM
Additional antioxidants	No	No		Yes	Yes
Other	No	No		No	Yes†

*Dextran (molecular weight 40,000 daltons).
†Ascorbic acid; vitamin B_{12}; adenosine triphosphate precursors.
CSM, Chondroitin sulfate–based medium; *MEM*, minimal essential medium; *TC 199*, tissue culture medium 199.

planted patients, all unopened lots of K-Sol medium were recalled by the manufacturer, and commercial production of this medium was halted. Because gentamicin has poor activity against anaerobes, staphylococcal, and streptococcal species,[25] current research is focusing on the safety and efficacy of additional antibiotic enrichment of storage media. Preliminary studies indicate that vancomycin may provide an additional spectrum of coverage in the prophylaxis of infection during corneal storage without toxicity to the donor tissue.[5,20,22,31]

CSM

Since 1983 Lindstrom, Doughman, and colleagues at the University of Minnesota Lions Eye Bank have performed laboratory and clinical studies on the use of a chondroitin sulfate–based medium (CSM) for organ culture.[15,16,18] CSM contains minimal essential medium (MEM), 1.35% chondroitin sulfate, 0.025 M HEPES buffer, gentamicin sulfate (100 μg/ml), mercaptoethanol, and nonessential amino acids (Table 46-1). A major qualitative difference in the chondroitin sulfate used in CSM, compared with K-Sol, is the retention of a low-molecular-weight (less than 10,000-dalton) fraction of chondroitin sulfate in CSM. In vitro studies have shown increased growth rates of human endothelial cells when the low-molecular-weight fractions are retained.[27] The formulation is intended to provide a single preparation for intermediate-term corneal storage at both 4° and 34° C.

Early laboratory studies demonstrated the maintenance of a normal-appearing endothelial mosaic in cat corneas stored for 3 weeks and human corneas stored for 1 week in CSM at 4° C.[15] Human corneas were also used to compare the preservative efficacy of CSM with that of K-Sol. No statistically significant differences in corneal thickness or central endothelial cell counts were found after 7 or 10 days of storage at 4° C. However, CSM-stored corneas displayed superior endothelial cell morphology at 14 and 22 days of storage as judged by vital staining with trypan blue and alizarine red.[18] Saggau and Bourne compared endothelial morphology by scanning electron microscopy and found no significant differences between corneas stored in CSM or K-Sol at 4° C for 14 days.[23]

Lass and co-workers studied the metabolic activity of paired K-Sol– and CSM-stored feline corneas using magnetic resonance spectroscopy.[10] After 2 weeks of storage at 4° C, there was no significant difference in the phosphatic metabolites such as adenosine triphosphate (ATP) in corneas with intact epithelium. In corneas denuded of epithelium, however, there were significantly higher levels of phosphatic metabolites in the CSM-stored corneas.

A clinical study by Lass and co-workers[13] compared the efficacy of CSM and K-Sol in a prospective, paired, and randomized fashion. Fifty-one pairs of corneas were stored up to 4 days at 4° C before transplantation. No significant differences between the groups were found in terms of endothelial cell density at 3, 6, and 12 months postoperatively. However, within the two groups, the K-Sol–stored corneas showed a significant decline in mean cell density and increase in mean cell area by 3 months, compared to preoperative levels. A similarly significant decline in cell density and increase in cell area was seen again between 6 and 12 months postoperatively in the K-Sol group but not in the CSM group. In the CSM-group a significant decline in mean cell density and increase in mean cell area was observed between the preoperative and 12-month postoperative assessments. The mean cell losses for tissue stored in both media at 3 and 6 months (7% for CSM, 11% for K-Sol) were comparable to the 6% cell loss reported for K-Sol–stored grafts at 2 months.[4] The mean cell losses at 1 year (27% for K-Sol and 17% for CSM) were comparable with the cell loss reported for tissue stored in MK medium for less than 50 hours.[1-3,32]

Saggau and Bourne also compared the preservative efficacy of K-Sol– and CSM-stored corneas for 2 weeks at 4° C by scanning electron microscopy of the endothelium.[24] A total of 22 pairs of corneas were evaluated in three groups. In group 1 (10 pairs) the tissue stored in K-Sol showed better endothelial preservation. In groups 2 and 3 (6 corneal pairs each), preservation in CSM was equal or possibly superior to preservation in K-Sol based on the percentage of intact endothelial cells. At the end of 2 weeks of storage, three CSM-stored corneas in group 1 had no remaining endothelial cells. Four K-Sol–stored corneas (two each in groups 2 and 3) also showed complete destruction of the endothelium. The authors ascribed these differences to the variability of composition of different lots of storage medium from the same manufacturer.

In summary, laboratory and clinical evidence indicates that storage in CSM at 4° C is safe and effective for 7 to 10 days. There is no conclusive proof, however, that CSM is superior to K-Sol for intermediate-term corneal storage or that it improves the endothelial survival time observed with short-term storage in MK medium.

DEXSOL

One disadvantage of CSM is related to the retention of low molecular weight chondroitin sulfate. Although these small polymers have a beneficial effect on corneal endothelial growth and metabolism,[27] their presence also results in increased corneal thickness intraoperatively and 1 day postoperatively.[13] This makes preoperative specular microscopy and intraoperative handling of tissue more difficult.

Dextran is an osmotically active agent that reduces corneal swelling during storage by preventing water in the medium from entering the corneal stroma. The use of dextran to maintain thinner donor tissue was studied extensively in MK medium,[3,29,32] but neither K-Sol nor CSM contained this molecule. The next intermediate-term storage medium to appear, Dexsol, was developed in 1988 when 1% dextran (with a 40,000-dalton molecular weight) was added to CSM[14,28] (Table 46-1).

Few laboratory and clinical studies have been performed using Dexsol. Lass and co-workers[14] studied the safety and efficacy of tissue stored in Dexsol at 4°

C. First, an in vitro bioassay of corneal endothelium was performed in cell culture. In this technique, cells are maintained in a proliferative state, actively undergoing mitosis. Decreased incorporation of ^{3}H-thymidine by endothelial DNA is a reflection of cytotoxicity in the culture system. No significant differences were noted between cells in CSM and cells in CSM plus dextran (Dexsol). This indicates that supplementation of CSM with 1% dextran may have no deleterious metabolic effects on the endothelium.

Lass and co-workers[14] also described a prospective randomized double-masked clinical trial comparing corneal thickness and endothelial survival in 21 pairs of corneas stored in at 4° C in CSM or CSM plus dextran for 5 days or less. Intraoperative corneal thickness was significantly less in the corneas stored in the dextran-containing medium. However, corneal thickness measurements obtained from 1 week to 4 months postoperatively were not significantly different between the groups. This clinical study also included a morphometric analysis of endothelial survival measured before storage and at 2 and 4 months postoperatively. No significant differences in endothelial cell density were noted between the groups at 2 and 4 months postoperatively. There were significant declines (13% to 16%) in mean endothelial cell density within each group at 4 months postoperatively, compared to preoperative densities. This degree of cell loss is comparable to that previously described in CSM- and K-Sol–stored corneas at 6 months.[13] No significant differences in endothelial cell area or coefficient of variation (a measure of polymegethism) were noted between the groups. Lass and colleagues currently recommend limiting storage time in Dexsol at 4° C to 1 week.

OPTISOL

Optisol was introduced in 1989 as an investigational medium for intermediate-term corneal storage.[8] It is a hybrid of K-Sol and Dexsol with additional constituents (Table 46-1). The base medium combines TC 199 (used in K-Sol) and MEM (used in Dexsol). The main difference between Optisol and Dexsol is that Optisol contains a higher concentration of chondroitin sulfate (2.5% versus 1.35%), ATP precursors, iron, cholesterol, L-hydroxyproline, and numerous vitamins (cobalamin, ascorbic acid, alpha-tocopherol, D-biotin, calciferol, niacin, pyridoxine, and *p*-aminobenzoic acid.[17] ATP precursors such as adenosine, inosine, and adenine are important components in this medium, since ATP is depleted during 4° C storage.

Lindstrom and co-workers[17] have described several preclinical studies examining the safety of Opti-

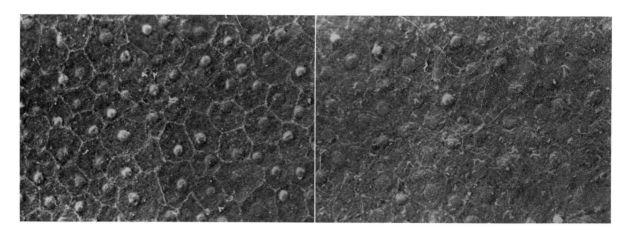

Fig. 46-24. Paired corneas were stored in Optisol, *left,* or Dexsol, *right,* for 14 days at 4° C. Endothelial cell borders in Optisol-stored tissue are distinct, and nuclei are well centered and clearly demarcated. In the Dexsol-stored tissue, endothelial cell borders and nuclei are less clear, and surface debris is visible. (500×.) (From Kaufman HE, Beuerman RW, Steinemann TL, et al: Optisol corneal storage medium, *Arch Ophthalmol* 109:864-868, 1991.)

sol. First, a human endothelial cell culture is assayed for the incorporation of ^{3}H-thymidine. Cells incubated in Optisol showed significantly greater ^{3}H-thymidine incorporation than those in Dexsol. Further studies revealed that adenosine was the single component responsible for this increased mitotic activity. Whether comparable mitotic activity occurs after 4° C storage and, indeed, in situ after penetrating keratoplasty remains to be seen.

Another study in this report[17] examined human corneas stored up to 12 days in Dexsol or in Optisol containing varying concentrations of chondroitin sulfate (up to 2.5%). The thinnest corneas were those stored in Optisol with 2.5% chondroitin sulfate. Paired human corneas were also examined by scanning electron microscopy after storage in Dexsol or Optisol. Endothelial cell borders and cell shape were better maintained in the Optisol storage group at 1, 3, 5, and 7 days. At 14 days, both groups displayed poor intracellular contact and indistinct cell borders. Transmission electron microscopy of endothelial cells from Optisol-stored tissue for 5 days showed less tissue sloughing, fewer pinocytotic vesicles, and fewer cytoplasmic vacuoles, compared to Dexsol-stored tissue. Also, the endothelial basilar surface showed a smoother appearance in the Optisol-stored corneas.

A report by Kaufman and associates[9] examined the scanning electron microscopic appearance of paired human corneal endothelial tissue after storage in Optisol or Dexsol at 4° C for 2 weeks (Fig. 46-24). A grading system based on cell shape, cell borders, cell swelling, and apical holes was used. The Optisol-stored corneas showed significantly fewer abnormalities in all categories. Corneas stored in Optisol for 2 weeks at 4° C were also significantly thinner than those stored in Dexsol under the same conditions.

Finally, the results of an open-label, uncontrolled clinical study of 51 patients enrolled at 6 centers was reported by Lindstrom and co-workers.[17] Patients were transplanted with tissue stored in Optisol for 20 to 154 hours (mean, 86 hours). One primary graft failure occurred. Endothelial cell counts were estimated by an analysis of specular photographs preoperatively and again in 3 and 6 months (on 35 and 33 patients respectively). Mean endothelial cell density decreased by 5.3% at 3 months and 11.4% at 6 months. This degree of cell loss is comparable to that observed in CSM- and K-Sol–stored corneas at 6 months postoperatively.[13]

Preliminary data indicate that corneal tissue can be safely and effectively maintained in Optisol storage medium. The upper limits of storage time remain to be determined, however. Future studies are necessary to assess whether the formulation of Optisol will actually improve endothelial survival in a long-term follow-up study compared to short-term storage methods such as whole-globe moist-chamber storage or storage of donor corneas in MK medium.

A prospective randomized, double-masked clinical trial using paired corneas would be helpful in answering these important questions.

ACKNOWLEDGMENT

This work was supported in part by U.S. Public Health Service grants EY-02580 and EY-02377 from the National Eye Institute, National Institutes of Health, Bethesda, Maryland.

REFERENCES

1. Bourne WM: One-year observation of transplanted human corneal endothelium, *Ophthalmology* 87:673-679, 1980.
2. Bourne WM: Chronic endothelial cell loss in transplanted corneas, *Cornea* 2:289-294, 1983.
3. Bourne WM: Morphologic and functional evaluation of the endothelium of transplanted human corneas, *Trans Am Ophthalmol Soc* 81:403-450, 1983.
4. Bourne WM: Endothelial cell survival on transplanted human corneas preserved at 4° C in 2.5% chondroitin sulfate for one to 13 days, *Am J Ophthalmol* 102:382-386, 1986.
5. García-Ferrer FJ, Pepose JS, Murray PR, et al: Antimicrobial efficacy and corneal endothelial toxicity of DexSol corneal storage medium supplemented with vancomycin, *Ophthalmology* 98:863-869, 1991.
6. Höök M, Kjellén L, Johansson S: Cell-surface glycosaminoglycans, *Annu Rev Biochem* 53:847-869, 1984.
7. Hull DS, Strickland EC, Green K: Photodynamically induced alteration of cornea endothelial cell function, *Invest Ophthalmol Vis Sci* 18:1226-1231, 1979.
8. Kaufman HE, Beuerman RW, Steinemann TL, Varnell ED: *Optisol corneal storage medium,* Eye Bank Association of America, 28th scientific session, October 28, 1989.
9. Kaufman HE, Beuerman RW, Steinemann TL, et al: Optisol corneal storage medium, *Arch Ophthalmol* 109:864-868, 1991.
10. Lass JH, Greiner JV, McBride M, et al: Effects of intermediate-term storage on corneal metabolism: K-Sol versus CSM. In Cavanagh HD, editor: *The cornea,* Transactions of the World Congress on the Cornea III, New York, 1988, Raven Press, pp 73-79.
11. Kaufman HE, Varnell ED, Kaufman S: Chondroitin sulfate in a new cornea preservation medium, *Am J Ophthalmol* 98:112-114, 1984.
12. Kaufman HE, Varnell ED, Kaufman S, et al: K-Sol corneal preservation, *Am J Ophthalmol* 100:299-304, 1985.
13. Lass JH, Reinhart WJ, Bruner WE, et al: Comparison of corneal storage in K-Sol and chondroitin sulfate corneal storage medium in human corneal transplantation, *Ophthalmology* 96:688-697, 1989.
14. Lass JH, Reinhart WJ, Skelnik DL, et al: An in vitro and clinical comparison of corneal storage with chondroitin sulfate corneal storage medium with and without dextran, *Ophthalmology* 97:96-103, 1990.
15. Lindstrom RL, Doughman DJ, Skelnik DL, et al: Minnesota system corneal preservation, *Br J Ophthalmol* 70:47-54, 1986.
16. Lindstrom RL, Doughman DJ, Skelnik DL, et al: Corneal preservation at 4° C with chondroitin sulfate—containing medium, *Trans Am Ophthalmol Soc* 55:332-349, 1987.
17. Lindstrom RL, Kaufman HE, Skelnik D, et al: *Optisol: a new corneal storage medium.* [Submitted, 1991.]
18. Lindstrom RL, Skelnik DL: Corneal preservation at 4° C with chondroitin sulfate—containing medium. In Cavanagh HD, editor: *The cornea,* Transactions of the World Congress on the Cornea III, New York, 1988, Raven Press, pp 81-89.
19. McCarey BE, Kaufman HE: Improved corneal storage, *Invest Ophthalmol Vis Sci* 13:165-173, 1984.
20. Matoba AY, O'Brien TP, Robinson NM, et al: *Antimicrobial efficacy of vancomycin in tissue culture media supplementation,* Ocular Microbiology and Immunology Group, 23rd annual meeting, October 28, 1989.
21. Mizukawa T, Manabe R: Recent advances in keratoplasty with special reference to the advantage of liquid preservation, *Folia Ophthalmol Jpn* 19:1310-1318, 1968.
22. Roth BP, Lindquist TD: *Safety and efficacy of vancomycin in corneal storage media,* Eye Bank Association of America, 29th scientific session, October 27, 1990.
23. Saggau DD, Bourne WM: A comparison of CSM and K-Sol by scanning electron microscopy of preserved endothelium, *Invest Ophthalmol Vis Sci* 28(suppl):166, 1987.
24. Saggau DD, Bourne WM: A comparison of two preservation media (CSM and K-Sol) by scanning electron microscopy of preserved corneal endothelium, *Arch Ophthalmol* 107:429-432, 1989.
25. Sande MA, Mandell GL: The aminoglycosides. In Gilman AG, Goodman LS, Gilman A, editors: *The pharmacologic basis of therapeutics,* ed 6, New York, 1980, MacMillan, pp 1162-1180.
26. Seick EA, Enzenauer RW, Cornell FM, Butler C: Contamination of K-Sol corneal storage medium with *Propionibacterium acnes, Arch Ophthalmol* 107:1023-1024, 1989.
27. Skelnik DL, Novak AF, Gregerson DS, et al: An in vitro assessment of corneal storage media CSM, MK and K-Sol using human corneal endothelial cells, *Invest Ophthalmol Vis Sci* 27(suppl):126, 1986.
28. Skelnik DL, Pearlstein CS, Mindrup EA, et al: Corneal preservation at 4° C with chondroitin sulfate—containing medium supplemented with dextran and epidermal growth factor (EGF), *Invest Ophthalmol Vis Sci* 29(suppl):111, 1988.
29. Stainer GA, Brightbill FS, Calkins B: A comparison of corneal storage in moist chamber and McCarey-Kaufman medium in human keratoplasty, *Ophthalmology* 88:46-49, 1981.
30. Stein RM, Bourne WM, Campbell RJ: Chondroitin sulfate for corneal preservation at 4° C, *Arch Ophthalmol* 104:1358-1361, 1986.
31. Steinemann TL, Kaufman HE, Beuerman RW, et al: *Vancomycin enriched corneal storage medium.* [Submitted, 1991.]
32. Sugar A, Meyer RF, Heidemann D, et al: Specular microscopic follow-up of corneal grafts for pseudophakic bullous keratopathy, *Ophthalmology* 92:325-329, 1985.
33. Trawkin AG, Gundorowa RA, Bordjugowa GG, et al: Erforschung des Zustandes der Zellmembran und der Mechanismen der Hornhautautolyse bei der Konservierung, II. Rolle der Antioxydationsmittel in der selbstregelnden Oxydation struktureller Lipoide von Zellmembranen der Hornhaut bei ihrer Konservierung, *Klin Monatsbl Augenheilkd* 169:500-504, 1976.
34. Yau C-W, Kaufman HE: A medium term corneal preserving medium (K-Sol), *Arch Ophthalmol* 104:598-601, 1986.

Long-term organ culture corneal storage: Minnesota system

DONALD J. DOUGHMAN
RICHARD L. LINDSTROM
DEBRA L. SKELNICK
ELIZABETH A. MINDRUP
J. DANIEL NELSON

Since Stocker's classic treatise on this subject,[43] the importance of the endothelial cell in maintaining normal corneal transparency has been firmly established. The success of penetrating keratoplasty in humans depends in part on transplanting an adequate amount of functioning donor endothelium. Therefore any method used to store the donor cornea from death of the donor to transplantation in the recipient must maintain endothelial viability.

We have been investigating organ culture of the cornea at the University of Minnesota since 1972 and have developed it as a method of long-term corneal storage.[8,9] The purpose of this chapter is to give a historical perspective of the development of the organ culture technique at the University of Minnesota, to review our recent developments in modifying the media, to review our most recent clinical results, and to briefly mention present investigations for future developments of this technique.

HISTORICAL BACKGROUND

1972-1982. Our work in organ culture began when one of us (D.J.D.) arrived in Minnesota in 1972 and joined work that had been started by one of the residents, George E. Miller, M.D., with William Summerlin, M.D. Dr. Summerlin had reported increased survival of skin allografts after organ culture of skin of mice[45] and humans.[44] Based upon Summerlin's work, we began experiments to see if corneal antigenicity could be modified by passage through organ culture. In 1973, the first report from this laboratory on organ culture of the cornea showed that by light microscopy, human and animal corneas could be preserved for at least 1 month in organ culture.[46] This stimulated research in utilization of organ culture as a method of long-term donor cornea preservation.

In 1972 refrigeration (4° C) of the whole globe was the traditional method of donor storage. However, progressive loss of endothelial cells at this low temperature compelled most surgeons to use donor

corneal tissue stored in this manner as soon as possible. Cryopreservation had been reported by Kaufman and Capella to preserve donor endothelium for as long as 1 year and had been used successfully in corneal transplantation.[6,7,20-22] However, its complex technology and high incidence of primary donor graft failure limited its use to only a few eye bank centers.[22,40]

In 1974 McCarey and Kaufman introduced their MK medium.[32] With this method, the corneoscleral segment is immersed in TC (tissue culture) medium 199 and stored at 4° C. Dextran is added (5% final concentration as an osmotic agent used to thin the cornea), and an antibiotic is added to control bacterial contamination. Animal studies[5,31,48] demonstrated the possibility of 14-day storage in rabbits. Further laboratory studies confirmed the viability of human endothelium[19,32,48] stored in MK medium for at least 4 days. However, studies in our laboratory as well as in others[16,18,38,48] showed no difference between MK-medium corneas and fresh corneas with regard to preservation of endothelium, and as time has passed, most surgeons have been reluctant to use MK-medium tissue beyond 72 hours of storage.

The technique of organ culture has evolved through many stages in our laboratory. These changes have occurred because of laboratory findings or clinical needs. We began by using a "batch" system, that is, placing corneas in 20 ml petri dishes and changing the medium three times per week. This has evolved to a closed system in which the medium is not changed. This latter method is described in more detail below.

Laboratory Evaluation. We have reported maintenance of human endothelial ultrastructural integrity for up to 120 days.[8-11,24] Epithelial ultrastructure has also been maintained for at least 35 days in organ culture, though there is a moderate intercellular and intracellular edema with loss of superficial epithelium including Langerhans' cells.[24,49] After storage for longer than 40 days, epithelial overgrowth onto the endothelial surface may be seen.[8] This occurs when there is endothelial cell damage, a confirmation of the work of Yanoff.[53] Accumulation of glycogen often occurs in the epithelial, stromal, and endothelial cells after 11 days of organ culture.[10,11,24,49] Although some degeneration of stromal cells toward the center of the stroma is seen, most stromal cells appear ultrastructurally intact up to 35 days in organ culture.[24,49]

One of our early findings was that corneas in organ culture demonstrated a complete layer of ultrastructurally intact endothelial cells by transmission

This investigation was supported in part by National Eye Institute Grant EY-01211, in part by Research for the Prevention of Blindness and the Minnesota Lions Eye Bank.

electron microscopy (TEM) and scanning electron microscopy (SEM), whereas fellow corneas in moist chamber storage of 4° C had areas of endothelial cell lysis and disruption.[10,11] This indicated that a process of endothelial cell repair occurred during organ culture incubation. We confirmed this finding in an endothelial wound-healing experiment in which we induced a 4 mm freeze-thaw endothelial wound and then placed the cornea in organ culture from 1 to 21 days. By SEM, we detected a layer of large endothelial cells completely covering the defect by 7 days.[13] The presumed healing process was enlargement and spreading rather than mitoses. TEM confirmed the presence of ultrastructurally intact endothelial cells with normal intracytoplasmic organelles. Chamber-diffusion studies indicated functional integrity of the regenerated endothelium and showed that anatomic and functional endothelial regeneration in vitro in corneas from donors as old as 85 years of age occurred in this model.[13]

Glucose metabolism was also studied in corneas stored up to 35 days in organ culture.[24] Changing the medium twice a week resulted in glucose concentrations falling from 110 to 30 mg/dl and lactate concentrations rising from 7 to 84 mg/dl between changes. The pH changed from 7.22 to 7.28, which indicated adequate buffering capacity of the medium, even with the elevated lactate concentration. By day 12, glucose uptake and lactate release decreased by approximately 50%. Glucose uptake stabilized at this level, but lactate release continued to fall. By day 25, it was 20% of its original rate. Transmission electron microscopic studies revealed normal endothelial, stromal, and epithelial cells that contained glycogen granules. These data demonstrated maintenance of an adequate but reduced rate of glucose metabolism during organ culture. In another study, the activity of corneal cytoplasmic and lysosomal enzymes from human fetal corneas were measured and showed maintenance of normal enzyme activity after 8 days of organ culture.[52] After 22 days of organ culture there was a sharp increase in lysosomal enzyme activity, suggestive of in vitro protein synthesis.

In an attempt to find the ideal storage temperature for organ-cultured corneas, endothelial ultrastructure at 37° C, 4° C, and room temperature (25° to 27° C) in organ culture medium was compared.[25] The temperature of 4° C was associated with ultrastructural damage as early as 48 hours using organ culture medium alone, organ culture medium with 5% dextran, or MK medium. However, human corneas could be left at ambient room temperature in organ-culture medium as long as 12 days in a closed system where the medium was not changed. Therefore there appeared to be no rigid restrictions on temperature maintenance during transportation of corneas. Successful transplants were performed by other surgeons, as well as ourselves, using organ-cultured corneas where ambient temperature prevailed for up to 48 hours during shipping. This study was also the first indication that a closed system of organ culture was feasible.

Since the stimulus for our beginning work in organ culture was the possibility that immune modification might occur, we studied the effect of organ culture and corneal immune rejections using experimental xenograft and allograft models. Utilizing intralamellar corneal xenografts, 3- to 4-week organ-cultured chicken and guinea pig corneas transplanted to rabbits had significant delayed rejection times compared with control corneas.[12,46] In addition, 22% of the 4-week organ-cultured chick xenografts did not reject. However, organ-cultured human-to-rabbit xenograft rejection was not delayed. This indicated species specificity. Histologically, organ-cultured nonrejected xenografts and organ-cultured xenografts with delayed rejection times were hypocellular with a decrease or absence of donor epithelium. This indicated that prolonged survival of xenografts after organ culture may represent reduced antigenicity secondary to donor hypocellularity. With regard to allograft rejection, all rabbit studies were done using "second-set" or prior sensitization of the recipient with skin grafts from the donor to enhance immune rejection.[33] The results of these studies showed no significant delay or modification of rejection in the rabbit model.[13] Finally, in collaboration with Hall and Smolin from the Proctor Foundation, we found that 3-week organ-cultured bovine corneas lacked a strong antigenic protein present in control bovine corneas.[17] Although this is caused in part by the loss of epithelium during organ culture, the antigen was absent from the stroma as well, an indication of loss of soluble antigens known to accelerate heterograft rejection.

In summary, extensive investigations in our laboratory using a system of 37° C organ-cultured human corneas stored for at least 5 weeks demonstrated preserved endothelial cell function and metabolism. Although there is some evidence that modification of experimental xenograft reactions occurs, we were unable to demonstrate this in the allograft model in rabbits.

Clinical Studies. After reassuring ourselves that human endothelial cell function was maintained during organ culture, we performed our first organ-cultured corneal transplant in January 1974. We reported our first clinical study in 1975 on 41 cases with at least 6-month follow-up observation and 22 cases followed less than 6 months using donor corneas, with an average storage time of 13 days in organ culture.[12] Sixty-seven percent of the long-term cases were clear, and 34% had failed. The length of storage time could not be associated with graft failure or immune rejection. Wound separation at the time of suture removal was a major complication.

Our second clinical report was a long-term study of 114 penetrating keratoplasties in 106 patients using organ-cultured corneas.[13] These corneas had been stored for an average of 16.5 days in 37° C organ culture incubation before transplantation and were performed by one of us (D.J.D.) (Table 46-2). A total of 80.7% of the grafts remained clear after a minimum of 6 months follow-up time. Compared with other published methods using 4° C refrigeration in MK medium, there appeared to be no significant difference between the success rate or cause of graft failure between these methods. Except for an increased incidence of wound separation using organ-cultured corneas, the postoperative complications were similar to that reported by other storage methods. There was no apparent modification of immune graft rejection. There was one case of endophthalmitis attributable to *Torulopsis glabrata* in this study.[23] In addition, two other cases of fungal endophthalmitis have occurred, the most recent in March 1982. This emphasizes the major concern we have using organ culture, that is, microbial contamination of the medium and transplanting infected corneas to the recipient.

Although our initial specular microscopic evaluation of organ-cultured corneas showed no apparent

Table 46-2. Organ Culture Transplants: Donor Cornea Data, 1979

Parameter	Total 114	Successful 92	Failed 22
Duration of organ culture (days)	16.5 ± 6.5	16.5 ± 5.8	16.6 ± 8.9
Donor age (years)	35.3 ± 17.7	35.4 ± 17.1	32.4 ± 20.9
Postmortem time (hours)	3.8 ± 3.8	3.5 ± 3.8	4.9 ± 4.1
Postenucleation time (hours)	6.4 ± 5.0	6.2 ± 4.5	7.4 ± 6.6
Follow-up period (months)	31.0 ± 19.0	28.8 ± 18.8	40.5 ± 17.6

difference between endothelial cell counts utilizing organ-cultured, MK-medium, or fresh corneas,[2] subsequent studies by Bourne and co-workers in collaboration with our laboratory showed that corneas stored in organ culture compared to their fellow corneas stored in MK medium showed a 20% reduction in cell counts 3 months after surgery.[4] Since endothelial cell counts before and after organ culture showed no loss of endothelial cells, it appeared that the endothelial cells from organ-cultured corneas did not survive the surgical procedure as well as those from MK-medium corneas. We presumed that the major reason for this vulnerability was intracellular and intercellular edema that occurred as a consequence of organ culture.

1983-1985. If organ culture was ever to be adopted as a universal method of donor cornea storage, four major problems had to be overcome. First, we needed a way to thin the donor cornea. Corneal tissue becomes thick and opaque as a result of its storage in organ culture. Second, microbial contamination, particularly fungal, is a significant hazard as mentioned above. Third, this method is technically complicated and expensive. Fourth, significant endothelial cell loss occurred after surgery using organ-cultured corneas as opposed to MK medium—stored corneas.

In 1979, the work of Sperling from Denmark came to our attention (personal communication), indicating that corneas could be organ cultured in a closed system, that is, with no medium changes, for a minimum of 30 days. The addition of 5% dextran to this medium seemed to limit corneal swelling. In the fall of 1980, two of us (D.J.D. and R.L.L.) traveled to Denmark to observe surgery and examine patients who had received organ-cultured transplants. We also spent time in their laboratory observing preparation of the donor corneas. Although the corneas in the early postoperative period appeared to have stromal haze, the postoperative endothelial cell counts and the success rates appeared to be similar to the open system in which media were changed two or three times per week. After further investigations of the endothelial cell we adopted a long-term closed system of organ culture.[27-29] Dextran, however, was omitted when endothelial toxicity was shown. The cornea was suspended in a bottle containing 100 ml of organ-culture medium (Fig. 46-25). With this method we were able to reduce the complexity of the system and limit access to the medium thereby reducing the opportunity for microbial contamination.

Microbial Studies. From the beginning we had always used terminal quarantine procedures to check

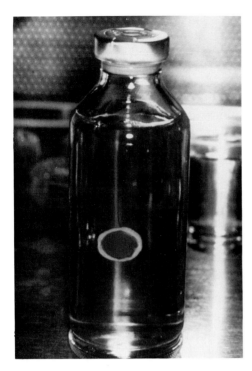

Fig. 46-25. Closed bottle containing organ-culture medium and donor corneas suspended on a bent spiral needle.

the sterility of the cornea at the time of transplantation. The first routine included the following: 48 hours before transplantation a final change of medium was performed. As a sterility check, samples of the medium from that final change were streaked on blood agar and Sabaraud's medium. The petri dish with the donor cornea was kept closed until opened by the surgeon in the operating room at the time of surgery. If the microbial medium grew organisms or if the medium and petri dish containing the cornea became turbid or changed in pH as evidenced by a change in the phenol red indicator, the cornea was discarded.[12] In January 1976, in order to thin the corneas before transplantation, this routine was modified by placing the donor corneas in MK media containing penicillin, streptomycin, and amphotericin at the final medium change 48 hours before surgical treatment.[13] Incubation was continued at room temperature or 37° C for an additional 48 hours and sterility check procedures were carried out as prescribed above. After our first case of fungal endophthalmitis in 1976[23] we changed the sterility check to a closed system for at least 7 days before surgery. In addition, in the open medium change before the terminal storage, antibiotics and amphotericin B were removed to avoid antibiotic carryover. Samples from

the last open medium change and the terminal closed media were inoculated into diagnostic media for bacteria, fungi, and yeast checks by the University Hospital Diagnostic Microbiological Laboratory according to a sterility check protocol already established for parental solutions and serums. If no contamination was found, the corneas were shifted in MK medium 18 hours before surgery and stored at 4° C in order to thin them preoperatively. However, two more cases of fungal endophthalmitis occurred after use of organ-cultured corneas in September 1982 and March 1983.

In determining the cause of fungal contamination in organ culture, we published a study showing that corneas from donors on respirators at the time of death, corneas with long postmortem times, corneas with positive postwash cultures, and corneas shifted into MK medium 48 hours before surgery were identified as risk factors for fungal-contamination organ culture.[36] It was apparent from this study that if terminal sterility quarantines were going to be utilized, any inhibitory effect from antibiotics in the media had to be overcome. In all three cases of endophthalmitis the corneas were transplanted with sterility checks that lasted less than 7 days. We now know it may take at least 2 weeks for fungus to become apparent in the sterility check routine, especially if antibiotics and antimycotics have been utilized. In addition, corneas shifted into MK medium before surgery opened the system for contamination. Based upon this information, we changed our sterility routine to that noted on Table 46-3. Utilizing this terminal sterility method in over 400 corneal transplants, no cases of endophthalmitis occurred.

Although our new method of terminal quarantine solved the sterility problem, eliminating MK medium at the end of the quarantine meant transplanting thick, swollen, opaque corneas. In December 1982 one of us (R.L.L.) visited the Eye Bank in Sri Lanka, which supplies tissue to many parts of Asia and Africa. Eyes sent to Japan were being shipped in a medium containing chondroitin sulfate that was used to keep the corneas thin and clear.[35] We later found that corneas kept in a 1.35% solution of chondroitin sulfate remained thin during organ-culture incubation.[23] In addition, we have found that with chondroitin sulfate in the media, endothelial cell counts are no longer reduced after surgical trauma compared to those from MK media.[27] This indicates that chondroitin sulfate in some way protects the organ-cultured endothelial cell from loss after surgery (Table 46-4). This finding has been confirmed by Bourne and co-workers[3] (Table 46-5).

Clinical Studies. To compare our most recent

clinical results with those obtained before 1982, we did a retrospective review of 101 consecutive corneal transplants (performed by three of us, D.J.D., R.L.L., J.D.N.) using organ-cultured cornea between January 1, 1982, and June 1983. Table 46-6 gives donor corneal data. The average organ culture duration was 25.1 days with no differences noted be-

tween the storage time of successful versus failed transplants. Eighty percent of the corneal transplants remained clear and 20% failed. No difference between the successful and failed corneal transplants was found when donor age, postmortem time, or postenucleation time were compared. Tables 46-2 and 46-6 show that although both the donor age and

Table 46-3. Flow of Corneas in Minnesota System

Day 1	Cornea in medium with gentamicin
Day 3	Change of medium with gentamicin
Day 6	Cornea into closed system medium with gentamicin†
Day 13*	Sample from closed system medium for microbiologic assay
Day 26-35	Transplant if sterile

*The 7-day interval allows time for the inhibitory effect of gentamicin to disappear.
†Gentamicin is now used to reduce the incidence of bacterial contamination that may occur early in the culture period. Its antimicrobial effect is gone by day 10, and therefore there is no carry-over.

Table 46-4. Chondroitin Sulfate Clinical Studies at the University of Minnesota
Postoperative endothelial cell loss in 23 paired corneas at 1.5% CDS

Media	% Cell Loss
Organ Culture with CDS	7.93 ± 12.19
Organ Culture without CDS	28.71 ± 13.36

CDS, Chondroitin sulfate.

Table 46-5. Chondroitin Sulfate Clinical Studies—Mayo Clinic Results
Postoperative endothelial cell loss in 22 paired corneas in organ culture ±1.5% CDS versus McCarey-Kaufman medium

Medium	% Cell Loss
Organ culture with CDS	11% ± 11%
McCarey-Kaufman	9% ± 16%

CDS, Chondroitin sulfate.

Table 46-6. Organ Culture Transplants: Donor Cornea Data, 1983

	Total 101	Successful 81	Failed 20
Duration of organ culture (days)	25.1 ± 7.4	25.5 ± 6.7	23.2 ± 9.6
Donor age (years)	42.1 ± 17.8	41.4 ± 17.9	46.4 ± 17.1
Postmortem time (hours)	3.9 ± 3.2	3.2 ± 2.7	4.5 ± 4.6
Postenucleation time (hours)	5.0 ± 5.3	5.1 ± 5.6	4.6 ± 4.1
Follow-up period (months)	18.6 ± 9.6	19.8 ± 9.1	13.6 ± 10.3

Table 46-7. Causes of Failed Keratoplasties in Organ-Cultured Corneas

Type	1979 Number (%)	1983 Number (%)
Immune rejection	8 (36.4)	2 (10)
Uncontrolled glaucoma	6 (27.3)	3 (15)
Epithelial defect	3 (13.6)	10 (50)
Wound separation	2 (9.0)	0 (0)
Retinal detachment	1 (4.5)	0 (0)
Epithelial downgrowth	1 (4.5)	0 (0)
Unknown	1 (4.5)	5 (25)
TOTAL	22 (19%)	20 (20%)

Table 46-8. Postoperative Complications with Organ-Cultured Corneas

Type	1979 Number (%)	1983 Number (%)
Immune rejection	33/114 (30)	8/10 (8)
Wound separation	11 (10)	2 (2)
Epithelial defect	10 (9)	24 (24)
Endophthalmitis	1 (1)	2 (2)

the duration of organ culture have increased over this 4-year period the number of successful and failed transplants has not changed. There were major differences in postoperative complications and causes of failed penetrating keratoplasty between the two series. Table 46-7 shows that the incidence of immune rejection, uncontrolled glaucoma, and wound separation was greatly reduced in the 1983 series compared with the 1979 series. However, the incidence of epithelial defects with attributable graft failure had greatly increased (Tables 46-7 and 46-8). We believe that the pathogenesis of epithelial defects in organ-cultured corneas was related to intracellular and intercellular epithelial edema during storage. We now coat the cornea at the time of surgery with sodium hyaluronate and have reduced the incidence of epithelial defects to less than 10%.

1985-1988. During this period we continued to preserve corneas in organ culture with the addition of chondroitin sulfate (Table 46-9) using the terminal quarantine method as described in Table 46-3. We reported another series of 82 cases done in 1986 using chondroitin-containing media with results similar to those in our earlier series.[14] It is interesting to note that in this series none had failed at 1 year from immune rejection, again suggestive that modification of allograft rejection occurs during the culture process. However, this was a retrospective study and therefore not proof that such modification did occur.

During this period our laboratory, as well as others, was developing corneal storage media with chondroitin sulfate for intermediate storage at 4° C.[3,26,42,47,50] At the same time, commercial development of the media occurred for 4° C use. Because of the success of this method, 34° C organ culture storage was used with less frequency so that by the end of 1988, 34° C organ culture was only occasionally used for clinical purposes.[30]

Table 46-9. Organ Culture Media

Medium	Value
Minimum essential medium (Eagle's) (with 25 mM HEPES buffer and Earle's salts)	
Defined fetal bovine serum	10%
Chondroitin sulfate	1.35%
L-Glutamine	2.0 mM
Sodium pyruvate	1.0 mM
Nonessential amino acids	0.1 mM
2-Mercaptoethanol (antioxidant)	0.44 mM
Gentamicin sulfate	100 mg/ml, or 100 mg/L

1988-Present. In our eye bank, as well as in most of the eye banks in the United States and Canada, the shift to intermediate storage at 4° C has been attributable to the fact that 7 days of storage is adequate for the need of most eye banks. Tissue is usually used on an elective basis, and the risks of infection inherent with 34° C culture are reduced. The availability of commercially prepared media adds to the desirability of using this method. In addition, the supply of donor corneas continues to increase in the United States, so that enough tissue can be banked to meet the demand within the storage limits of 4° C chondroitin-containing media.

In Europe, 34° C organ culture has become an important method of donor corneal storage.[38] It has been used since the early 1980s by eye banks in Denmark[15,41] and the Netherlands.[51] Recently, a series of organ culture–preserved corneas was reported from France citing a 92% success rate at 1 year.[37] Organ-cultured corneas have been successfully used for transplantation in acute corneal ulceration.[15] Since 1986, when organ culture was introduced to the United Kingdom, the number of corneas supplied from the Corneal Transplant Service and eye bank in Bristol has risen from 59 to over 1500 in 1989, with over 100 hospitals using these corneas.[1] Organ culture provides significant advantages, especially when linked to an organization such as the United Kingdom Corneal Transplant Service. It allows for elective surgery and for evaluation of tissue for tissue typing. Therefore, in countries that have a shortage of donor tissue and have the technologic resources, organ-culture donor corneal preservation is an acceptable option for donor storage.

THE MINNESOTA SYSTEM OF ORGAN CULTURE

Whole globes are received in the Eye Bank where microbial decontamination and corneal excision are done under a laminar flow hood using sterile technique (Fig. 46-26). The technician carefully trims all conjunctiva and excessive tissue from the globe using sterile instruments and then immerses the globe in 1.0% povidone-iodine for 3 minutes, a technique we have found very effective in decontaminating the globes of bacteria and fungi.[34] The globes are then rinsed for 1 minute in normal saline and flushed with saline. A swab taken from the limbus is then cultured in tryptic soy broth until positive, or for 2 weeks, if negative. Corneal excision is performed by an incision being made 2 to 3 mm from the limbus into the suprachoroidal space. The anterior chamber is maintained during this removal process. The cor-

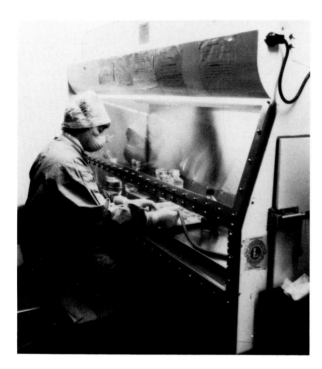

Fig. 46-26. Technician changing organ-culture medium under laminar flow hood.

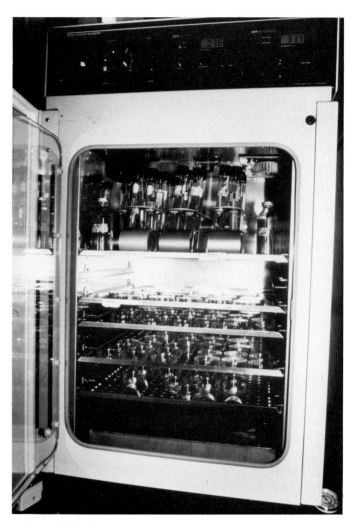

Fig. 46-27. Incubator containing organ-cultured corneas.

neoscleral segment is placed endothelial side up in a petri dish with 15 ml of medium. The constituents of the organ-culture medium are listed in Table 46-6. The corneas are then examined with an inverted-phase microscope for epithelial, stromal, and endothelial pathosis. The corneas are maintained in these petri dishes for 2 to 3 days for one or two medium changes and stored at 34° C in 5% CO_2 in water-jacketed incubators (Fig. 46-27). After two medium changes, the corneas are suspended in 130 ml of medium by a spinal needle hook inserted through the scleral rim and then stored at 34° C (Fig. 46-25). One makes the cornea hook is made by placing a 25-gage disposable spinal needle through the inner lip of the rubber stopper and bending it at the beveled end. The cap is a rubber stopper that is crimped with an aluminum seal, ensuring a secure tamper-proof closure. The cap also permits removal of 7 to 10 ml of medium 7 days later to be sent to the University Microbiological Laboratory for a sterility check (Table 46-3). The bottle containing the cornea, as well as the plates and the medium, are examined daily for evidence of contamination. If after 10 days no growth is observed in any of the microbiologic media, and the media in the closed bottles containing the corneas are clear without pH change, the system is considered sterile, and the corneas may be transplanted.

THE FUTURE

Organ culture has proved its value in situations where there is a shortage of donor tissue in the face of high demand and where the technical demands of 34° C organ culture that allow its safe use for eye banking can be met. It is likely that more areas of the developing world will turn to this method if enough donor tissue becomes available.

The ability to quarantine donor corneas for prolonged periods during organ culture allows for detection and perhaps elimination of infectious agents. A temperature of 34° C allows antibiotics to act on most bacteria and many fungi with the potential to sterilize donor material. Additionally, prolonged storage of donor corneas at metabolic temperatures may permit future manipulation of factors such as epithelial and endothelial enhancement by growth factors, modification of immune rejection and wound healing, or other, yet-to-be-discovered bioengineering techniques.

In summary, 34° C organ culture has become an accepted technique of long-term donor corneal storage in America and Europe with the potential to provide improved donor corneal quality in the future.

REFERENCES

1. Armitage WJ, Moss SJ, Easty DL, et al: Substantially improved supply of corneal tissue in the U.K. brought about by organ culture, *Invest Ophthalmol Vis Sci* 32(suppl):1924, 1991.
2. Bourne WM, Doughman DJ, Lindstrom RL: Organ-cultured corneal endothelium *in vivo, Arch Ophthalmol* 95:1818, 1977.
3. Bourne WM, Lindstrom RL, Doughman DJ: Endothelial cell survival on transplanted human corneas preserved by organ culture with 1.5% chondroitin sulfate, *Invest Ophthalmol Vis Sci* 26(3)(suppl):239, 1985.
4. Bourne WM, Doughman DJ, Lindstrom RL, et al: Increased endothelial cell loss after transplantation of corneas preserved by a modified organ-culture technique, *Ophthalmology* 91:285, 1984.
5. Breslin CW: Evaluation of the McCarey-Kaufman technique of corneal storage, *Arch Ophthalmol* 94:1545, 1976.
6. Capella JA, Kaufman HE: Corneal cryo-preservation and its clinical application. In Casey TA, editor: *Corneal grafting*, New York, 1972, Appleton-Century-Crofts.
7. Capella JA, Kaufman HE, Robbins JE: Preservation of viable corneal tissue, *Arch Ophthalmol* 74:669, 1965.
8. Doughman DJ et al: Endothelium of the human organ cultured cornea: an electron microscopic study, *Trans Am Ophthalmol Soc* 71:304, 1973.
9. Doughman DJ et al: The ultrastructure of human organ-cultured corneas: 1. Endothelium, *Arch Ophthalmol* 92:516, 1974.
10. Doughman DJ et al: Human corneal endothelial layer repair during organ culture, *Arch Ophthalmol* 94:1791, 1976.
11. Doughman DJ et al: The fate of experimental organ-cultured corneal xenografts, *Transplantation* 22:132, 1976.
12. Doughman DJ, Harris JE, Schmitt MK: Penetrating keratoplasty using 37° C organ-cultured cornea, *Trans Am Acad Ophthalmol Otolaryngol* 81:778, 1976.
13. Doughman DJ: Prolonged donor cornea preservation in organ culture: longterm clinical evaluation, *Trans Am Ophthalmol Soc* 81:567, 1980.
14. Doughman DJ, Falk S, Mindrup B, et al: Minnesota Corneal Storage System: 34° C organ culture. In Cavanagh HD, editor: *The cornea*, Transactions of the World Congress on the Cornea III, New York, 1988, Raven Press.
15. Ehlers N, Andersen J: Treatment of central corneal ulcers by *à chaud* transplantation of organ culture preserved donor tissue, *Acta Ophthalmol* 65:516-520, 1987.
16. Friedland BR, Forster RK: Comparison of corneal storage in McCarey-Kaufman medium, moist chamber or standard eye-bank conditions, *Invest Ophthalmol* 15:143, 1976.
17. Hall JM et al: Changes in the antigenic composition of cultured bovine corneas, *Invest Ophthalmol* 14:295, 1975.
18. Holtmann HW, Stein HJ: Zur Kurzzeitlagerung menschlicher Hornhaute im Medium NCTC 135, *Klin Monatsbl Augenheilkd* 173:838, 1978.
19. Holtmann HW, Stein HJ, Dardenne MU: Experiments on corneal preservation (short-time storage), *Ophthalmic Res* 8:124, 1976.
20. Kaufman HE: Corneal cryopreservation and its clinical application, *Transplant Proc* 8(2, suppl 1):149, 1976.
21. Kaufman HE, Capella JA: Preserved corneal tissue for transplantation, *J Cryosurg* 1:125, 1968.
22. Kaufman HE, Escapini H, Capella JA, et al: Living preserved corneal tissue for penetrating keratoplasty, *Arch Ophthalmol* 76:471, 1966.
23. Larsen PA, Lindstrom RL, Doughman DJ: *Torulopsis glabrata* endophthalmitis after keratoplasty with an organ-cultured cornea, *Arch Ophthalmol* 96:1019, 1978.
24. Lindstrom RL et al: A metabolic and electron microscopic study of human organ-cultured cornea, *Am J Ophthalmol* 82:72, 1976.
25. Lindstrom RL et al: Organ culture and corneal storage at ambient room temperature, *Arch Ophthalmol* 22:132, 1977.
26. Lindstrom RL et al: Organ culture corneal preservation with chondroitin sulfate, *Invest Ophthalmol Vis Sci* 25(suppl):266, 1984.
27. Lindstrom RL et al: Minnesota system cornea preservation, *Invest Ophthalmol Vis Sci* 26(suppl):239, 1985.
28. Lindstrom RL et al: Minnesota system cornea preservation, *Dev Ophthalmol* 11:37, 1985.
29. Lindstrom RL et al: Minnesota system cornea preservation, *Br J Ophthalmol* 70:47-54, 1986.
30. Lindstrom RL et al: Corneal preservation at 4° C with chondroitin sulfate containing medium, *Trans Am Ophthalmol Soc* 85:332-349, 1987.
31. McCarey BE, Kaufman HE: Improved corneal storage, *Invest Ophthalmol* 13:165, 1974.
32. McCarey BE, Kaufman HE: In vitro specular microscope perfusion of M-K and moist chamber—stored human corneas, *Invest Ophthalmol Vis Sci* 16:743, 1977.
33. Maumenee AE: The influence of donor recipient sensitization on corneal grafts, *Am J Ophthalmol* 34:141, 1951.
34. Mindrup EA et al: A comparative study of the use of povidone-iodine and gentamicin in the decontamination of human donor globes, *Invest Ophthalmol Vis Sci* 26(3, suppl):68, 1985.
35. Mizukawa T, Manabe R: Recent advances in keratoplasty: with special references to the advantage of liquid preservation, *Nippon Ganka Kiyo* 19:1310, 1968.
36. Nelson JD et al: Fungal contamination in organ culture, *Arch Ophthalmol* 101:280, 1983.
37. Piquot X, Delbosc B, Hervé P, Royer J: Preservation of human corneas in organ culture: results of a feasibility clinical protocol, *Bull Soc Ophthalmol Fr* 90:429-432, 1990.
38. Schimmelpfennig B, Witmer R: Hornhautkonservierung bei +37° C in kontinuierlichen Gewebekulturmedium, *Ophthalmologica* 175:275, 1977.
39. Skelnik DL et al: Culturing and application of HCE cells in human corneal endothelial enhancement, *Invest Ophthalmol Vis Sci* 26(3, suppl):147, 1985.
40. Slappey TE: Corneal preservation, *Transplant Proc* (2 suppl 1):223, 1976.
41. Sperling S, Olsen T, Ehlers N: Fresh and cultured corneal grafts compared by post-operative thickness and endothelial cell density, *Acta Ophthalmol* 59:566-575, 1981.
42. Stein RM, Bourne WM, Campbell RJ: Comparison of 1.5% chondroitin sulfate and 5% dextran for corneal storage, *Invest Ophthalmol Vis Sci* 26(3)(suppl):238, 1985.
43. Stocker FW: The endothelium of the cornea and its clinical implications, *Trans Am Ophthalmol Soc* 51:669, 1953.
44. Summerlin WT: Allogeneic transplantation of organ cultures of adult human skin, *Clin Immunol Immunopathol* 1:372, 1973.
45. Summerlin WT et al: Acceptance of phenotypically differing cultured skin in man and mice, *Transplant Proc* 5:707, 1973.
46. Summerlin WT et al: Transplantation of organ cultured cornea: an in vitro and in vivo study, *Fed Proc* 32:362, 1973.

47. Tamaki K et al: Two new cornea preserving media: histology of stored corneas, *Invest Ophthalmol Vis Sci* 26(3)(suppl):238, 1985.

48. Van Horn DL, Doughman DJ, Harris JE, et al: Ultrastructure of human organ-cultured cornea: II. Stroma and epithelium, *Arch Ophthalmol* 93:275, 1975.

49. Van Horn DL, Schultz RO, DeBruin J: Endothelial survival in corneal tissue stored in M-K medium, *Am J Ophthalmol* 80:642, 1975.

50. Varnell ED, Kaufman HE, Beuerman RW: K-Sol: a new preserving medium for 14 day storage of donor corneas, *Invest Ophthalmol Vis Sci* 26(3, suppl):238, 1985.

51. Völker-Dieben HJ, D'Amaro J, Kok-van Alphen CC, Pels E: The survival of organ-cultured donor corneas. In Brightbill FS, editor: *Corneal surgery: theory, technique, and tissue*, St. Louis, 1986, Mosby–Year Book.

52. Whitley CB: *Studies of heritable and induced lysosomopathies*, doctoral thesis, 1977. University of Minnesota, Minneapolis.

53. Yanoff M: In vitro biology of corneal epithelium and endothelium, *Trans Am Ophthalmol Soc* 73:571, 1975.

Organ culture in the Netherlands

PRESERVATION AND ENDOTHELIAL EVALUATION

LIESBETH PELS
YVONNE SCHUCHARD

When it became clear that corneas of deceased persons could successfully be used for penetrating keratoplasty, methods were developed for storage of the donor tissue.

The McCarey-Kaufman (MK) medium,[14,15] introduced in 1974 enabled a preservation of 2 to 3 days at a temperature of 4° C. This period, however, is still rather short when tissue typing of the donor tissue[36] is necessary. A medium-term storage method using tissue culture medium (TC medium, Minimum Essential Medium, MEM) and a storage temperature of 31° to 37° C was developed.[6,7,24,32] Sperling[19] added Dextran T500 to the medium to keep the cornea thin, whereas Doughman and co-workers[6,7] dehydrated the corneas shortly before the operation in the dextran-containing MK medium at 4° C. The advantage of Sperling's method is that the cornea is kept thin during the whole period. Although a direct toxic effect of high-molecular-weight dextran on corneal endothelium could not be demonstrated, the finding of increasing amounts of dextran in all layers of the cornea during storage contraindicates a long storage period in a medium containing dextran.[35]

The vitality of the donor endothelium is of ultimate importance for the success of penetrating keratoplasty. Sperling[23,26] described a method for the evaluation of the corneal endothelium by light microscopy after staining with trypan blue. With this method it was possible to define criteria for the quality of the endothelium.[17] In this chapter the methods and results of an organ-culture storage procedure modified after Doughman and co-workers[6,7,32] and Sperling[24] are described.

Materials and Methods

Donor eyes. The human donor eyes were donated to the Eurotransplant Foundation (Leiden, the Netherlands) for transplantation. They were sent to the Cornea Bank for tissue evaluation and preservation. Contraindications for acceptance of corneal tissue before enucleation and contraindications for tissue offered for surgical purposes were according to the EBAA medical standards.

Eyes were transported in a moist chamber on ice. The time between death of the donor and enucleation varied from 0.1 to 29 hours (average, 7 hours). The mean age of the donor was more than 60 years

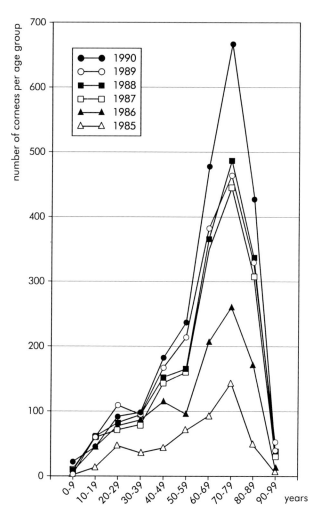

Fig. 46-28. Distribution of donor eyes to Eurotransplant Foundation from 1985 to 1990 by age groups.

and was slowly increasing during the latter years. The distribution of the donors over the different age groups is given in Fig. 46-28. Donor corneas that could not be used for transplantation (see tissue evaluation criteria below and on p. 624) were used for organ-culture experiments.

Decontamination of donor eyes. The method of Sperling and Sørensen[28] was used for decontamination of the donor eyes. In short, after rinsing of the eyes with tap water for 1 minute, the eyes were subsequently immersed in the following sterile solutions: 0.5% polyvinylpyrrolidone-iodine (povidone-iodine) for 2 minutes, 0.1% sodium thiosulfate in phosphate-buffered saline (PBS) for 1 minute and finally rinsed in PBS.

Preparation of corneoscleral button. The time between death and preparation varied from 0.3 to 51 hours (mean, 15 hours). Corneas were trephined (diameter, 14 mm) including a scleral rim of 1 to 2 mm. The incision was completed by a pair of scissors. The ciliary body and the iris were carefully removed from the scleral rim with a knife and a pair of forceps. During this procedure the cornea was kept in a vertical position enabling air to enter the anterior chamber, which kept the cornea in shape.

Tissue evaluation

1. *Macroscopy.* The cornea was first macroscopically examined for clarity, epithelial integrity, foreign objects, opacities, and scleral color (such as jaundice).

2. *Slitlamp examination.* Corneas were discarded for transplantation during slitlamp examination because of presence of a macula or a nebula, senile changes of the endothelium including cornea guttata and Fuchs' dystrophy, or previous eye operations except for strabismus.

3. *Examination of the corneal endothelium by light microscopy.* The methods and criteria for the evaluation of corneal endothelium are discussed in detail elsewhere.[17] In short, the presence of dead cells before and after preservation was studied using 0.3% trypan blue in PBS, and the cell borders were visualized by provoked swelling in 1.8% sucrose[12,22] or PBS. The whole surface of the endothelium was scanned with a light microscope at a magnification of 125. The number of cells was estimated with the help of a calibrated graticule in the ocular for routine purposes. In case of experiments the cell density was determined with the help of micrographs as described.[17] The following criteria for acceptance were adopted:

   a. Minimally 2000 cells/mm² before and after preservation.

   b. Before preservation the presence, number, and location of cells stained by trypan blue are recorded. If there are stained cells left or present after preservation, the corneas are discarded.

   c. A regular cell mosaic (no polymegethism, no pleomorphism).

   d. Swelling of the intercellular borders after exposure to PBS in case of preserved corneas, or a hypotonic 1.8% sucrose solution in case of fresh corneas and corneas preserved in media containing dehydrating agents like dextran or chondroitin sulfate.

   e. Folds caused by the swelling during preservation covered with endothelium.

   f. Clear-cut cell borders and a smooth appearance.

   g. A maximum cell loss of 20%. Cell loss is calculated according to the formula:

$$\frac{N_{\text{pre}} - N_{\text{post}}}{N_{\text{pre}}} \times 100\% = \text{Cell loss}$$

in which N_{pre} is the number of endothelial cells before preservation and N_{post} those after preservation.

Organ culture. After a first evaluation of the endothelium the corneoscleral button was suspended in a sterilized 100 ml glass infusion bottle by a suture tied to the scleral rim. It was incubated in 60 ml of culture medium at 31° C. During experiments, when the preservation time exceeded 7 weeks, the medium was renewed. About 3 to 5 days before the scheduled date of operation the endothelium of the cornea was reevaluated. If it passed the criteria, the cornea was transferred to a 60 ml glass bottle completely filled with transport medium to reduce the corneal swelling and incubated 24 to 48 hours at 31° C. Subsequently the cornea was transported in the same bottle at room temperature. The time in transport medium varied from less than 1 hour to maximally 7 days.[18] The culture medium contained the following ingredients:

1. Minimum essential medium with Earle's salts (Eagle's) with L-glutamine and 20 mM HEPES buffer (powder, Flow, Meckenheim, Germany)

2. Sodium bicarbonate (2 gm/L)

3. Fetal bovine serum, 2% (Flow)

4. Antibiotics: penicillin, 100 IU/ml (Gist-Brocades, Weybridge Surrey, U.K.) and streptomycin, 0.05 mg/ml (Gist-Brocades).

The transport medium was identical to the culture medium but contained in addition 5% Dextran T500 (Pharmacia, Uppsala, Sweden), unless stated otherwise. Shortly before use nystatin was added (50 IU/ml). The media were aseptically prepared by membrane filtration (pore size, 0.22 μm) and stored at −20° C until use.

Corneal thickness. The thickness of the corneoscleral button was estimated by use of the micrometer screw of the microscope. First the epithelial side of the corneas was focused and then the endothelial side. The difference between the micrometer readings is correlated with the thickness of the cornea. The mean thickness was calculated from five consecutive measurements in the center of the cornea. The readings found were not corrected for errors induced by different refractive indices of the tissue.

Microbiologic control. All organ-culture procedures were performed in a horizontal laminar flow hood according to a strict protocol. During preservation the culture bottles were daily checked for contamination by looking at the clearness and the color of the medium. After overnight incubation of the cornea in the transport medium (the thinning period) at 31° C a sample of this medium was taken with a syringe through the stopper of the closed vial. This medium sample was controlled for microbial contamination by incubation on blood agar plates at 21° and 37° C and TSB broth at 37° C. The plates and broth were daily inspected for 10 days. Without microbial growth the cornea was dispatched after 1 day and transplanted after 2 days.

Electron microscopy. Corneas, unsuitable for transplantation and used in experiments, were prepared for transmission electron microscopy as described before.[18,35] The sections were inspected in a Philips 201 electron microscope.

Results

Tissue evaluation

1 and 2: *Gross examination and slitlamp examination.* About 17% of all corneas donated were discarded according to the described criteria. With increasing age of the donor this percentage increased from 0% (age group, 0 to 9 years) to 23% (age group, 80 to 89 years), see Fig. 46-29.

3. *Primary evaluation of the corneal endothelium.* After staining with trypan blue and sucrose-induced swelling of the intercellular spaces of the endothelium on the fresh corneoscleral buttons four classes were discerned:

a. Endothelium with trypan blue–stained nuclei in the center of the cornea (Fig. 46-30, *A*). Stained nuclei may be present in rows. In such case the trypan blue–stained nuclei are probably the result of folds in the cornea generated during storage or preparation. Stained nuclei may also be found scattered in small to large groups throughout the endothelium. Small groups are often present when the postmortem time is rather long. Larger groups are more probably the result of mechanical damage.

b. Endothelium with no trypan blue–stained

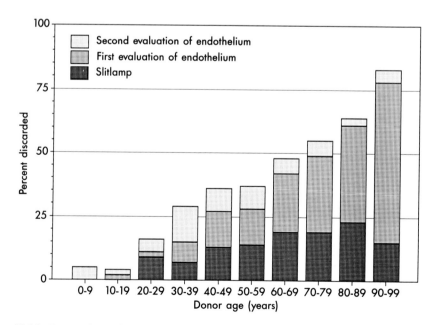

Fig. 46-29. Percentage of discarded donor eyes by age after (1) evaluation by slitlamp, (2) trypan blue and sucrose-induced swelling (first evaluation), (3) organ-culture preservation (second evaluation).

A   B   C   D

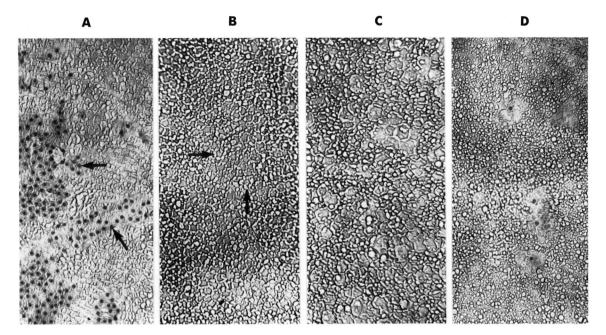

Fig. 46-30. Bright-field light micrographs of endothelium of fresh human corneas after staining with 0.3% trypan blue and swelling of the intercellular borders with 1.8% sucrose. Final magnification, 135.5×. **A,** Endothelium with trypan blue–stained nuclei, class I *(arrows)*. **B,** Regular endothelial cell mosaic visualized by the swollen intercellular space *(arrows)* and absence of trypan blue–stained nuclei in the center, class II. **C,** Irregular endothelial cell mosaic, class III. **D,** Endothelium with an abnormal swelling pattern, class IV.

cells in the center of the cornea, a regular cell mosaic, and nicely swollen intercellular spaces (Fig. 46-30, *B*).

c. Endothelium with nicely swollen intercellular spaces and irregular cell mosaic (polymegethism, pleomorphism) was observed in elderly donors. The irregular cell mosaic was not correlated with a low cell density (Fig. 46-30, *C*).

d. Endothelium with abnormal or badly swollen intercellular spaces (Fig. 46-30, *D*). Trypan blue–stained nuclei may also be present.

A correlation between age of the donor and endothelial cell count did not exist. However, with increasing age the lowest cell counts decreased within the age groups from 3300 (age group of less than 10 years) through 2900 (age, 10 to 20 years) and 2500 (20 to 30 years) to 2300 (30 to 40 years). After the primary evaluation 30% of all corneas did not meet the quality criteria. The discard rate was correlated with the age of the donor (Fig. 46-29) and increased from 0% (age group, 0 to 9 years) to 63% (age group, >90 years).

4. *Second evaluation of corneal endothelium.* Corneas belonging to evaluation class I passed in 50% of the cases the second evaluation. The preservation period was considered as a kind of stress test. Despite that the endothelium of corneas belonging to evaluation class II did not show any morphologic defects before organ culture, the endothelium did not always tolerate the preservation; endothelial defects, an increased endothelial cell loss (>20%) in 4% to 5% of the cases, or complete endothelial cell death in less than 0.5% of the cases, was observed. The same happened to corneas belonging to class III. Remarkable in this case is that the endothelium of young donors showing polymegethism lost more cells than the endothelium of the elder donors in this same class. The endothelium of corneas belonging to class IV died within 1 to 2 weeks of organ culture in 80% of the cases.

In general 6% of all corneas were discarded at the end of the first preservation phase. This was independent of the age of the donor (Fig. 46-29). The overall percentage of transplanted corneas varied from 46% to 60% during the different years.

Table 46-10. Corneal Thickness During Organ Culture

Preservation Period (Days)	Corneal Thickness (mm)			Number of Corneas
	Mean ±SD	Minimum	Maximum	
<4	0.73 ± 0.09	0.65	0.85	6
4-8	0.90 ± 0.13	0.62	1.16	47
9-15	0.94 ± 0.14	0.58	1.41	66
16-30	1.00 ± 0.16	0.72	1.29	55
>30	0.96 ± 0.14	0.72	1.18	30

SD, Standard deviation.

Organ culture. During the first 2 weeks the thickness of the corneas increased from 0.56 ±0.07 mm (mean ±SD) to more than 1 mm (Table 46-10). The individual variation between swelling rate and final thickness in the culture medium was substantial. The corneas of younger donors (age, <45 years) swelled significantly more than the corneas of the older ones (Mann-Whitney U-test, p <0.01). The swelling resulted in numerous folds. After culture periods of up to 40 days the endothelial monolayer appeared to be intact even over the folds, trypan blue–stained nuclei were very rare, and the endothelial cells reacted equally as well to a hypotonic 1.8% sucrose solution as the cells on the fresh cornea did. Artificial swelling of the intercellular borders could also be induced with PBS after more than 3 to 5 days in culture. This latter method was preferred. With increasing preservation time the incidence of deformation of the endothelial cell layer increased. The on-

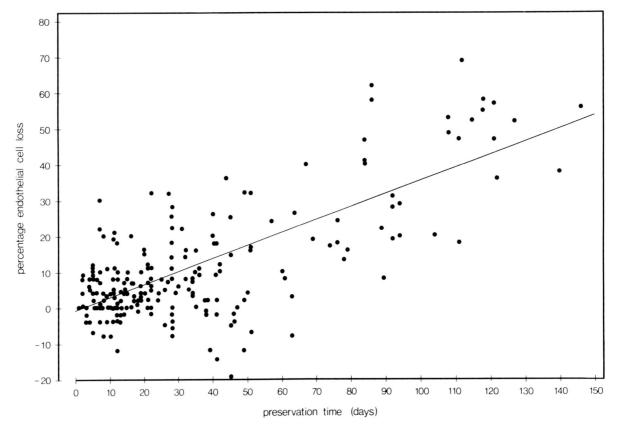

Fig. 46-31. Relative loss of endothelial cells during organ culture in modified MEM (minimum essential medium). Number of cells present before organ culture (n_{pre}) is compared to number of cells present after organ culture (n_{post}). Percentage of endothelial cell loss is calculated according to formula: $\dfrac{n_{\text{pre}} - n_{\text{post}}}{n_{\text{pre}}} \times 100\%$. Line represents significant (p <0.001) correlation between relative cell loss and preservation time. A negative cell loss does not indicate multiplication of endothelial cells but must be ascribed to errors made by estimation of the number of endothelial cells per square millimeter.

set of these phenomena varied among individual corneas. During organ culture the number of endothelial cells gradually decreased, but up to 35 days the cell loss was not significantly correlated with the preservation time (data not shown). However, with increasing preservation time the correlation was highly significant ($p < 0.001$) (Fig. 46-31).

As shown by electron microscopy the cellular junctions of the endothelium remained intact up to 122 days of organ culture, but the apical intercellular space was occasionally swollen (Fig. 46-32). With increasing preservation time more cells exhibited degenerative changes, such as electron-lucent vacuoles (Fig. 46-32, *B*). After culture the corneal endothelium had an increased incidence of Golgi fields and endoplasmic reticulum and an increased size of mitochondria (Fig. 46-32). The epithelial layer decreased from a value of six to seven layers in the fresh cornea to that of one to three layers after 1 week of organ culture. The intercellular space of the epithelium was swollen, and the tight junctions between the cells were almost all detached (Fig. 46-33). Bowman's membrane, however, was always covered with a thin, irregular, layer of epithelial cells during at least 50 days of organ culture.

In the stroma ultrastructurally normal keratocytes were found between the stromal lamellae. Most likely because of the swelling of the stroma during organ culture, the collagen fibers were not so tightly packed as those in fresh corneal stroma.

Deswelling of cornea. For determination of the rate of thinning and the ultimate thickness of the corneas after organ culture three groups of five swollen corneas were incubated in organ-culture medium with 4%, 6%, and 8% Dextran T500 for 30 hours. As shown in Fig. 46-34 the thickness of the corneas de-

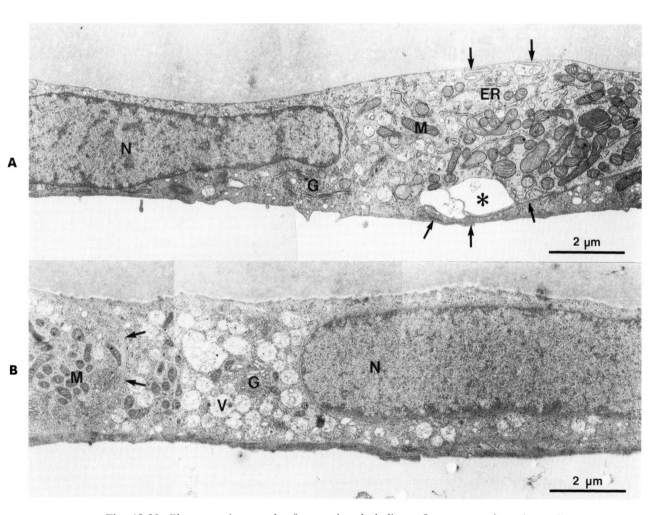

Fig. 46-32. Electron micrograph of corneal endothelium after organ culture in modified MEM for 35 days, **A,** and 122 days, **B.** *Arrows,* Cellular junctions; *asterisk,* swollen intercellular space; *N,* nucleus; *M,* mitochondria; *G,* Golgi fields; *ER,* endoplasmic reticulum; *V,* electron-lucent vacuoles.

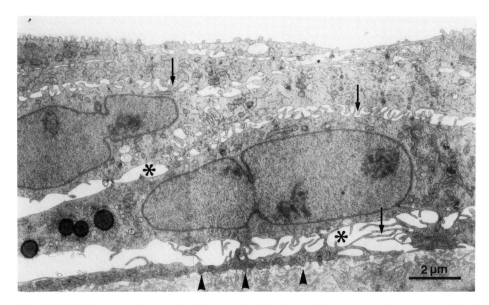

Fig. 46-33. Electron micrograph of corneal epithelium after organ culture in modified MEM for 35 days. Notice presence of only two or three cell layers on Bowman's membrane, broken tight junctions *(arrows),* swollen intercellular space *(asterisk),* and intact hemidesmosomes *(arrowheads).*

creased from about 1 mm to a range of 0.41 to 0.55 mm within 12 hours. The thinning rate appeared to be independent of the dextran concentration. However, the ultimate thickness appeared to be dependent on the dextran concentration. Based on these results the culture medium with 5% dextran was preferred to dehydrate the cornea before transplantation. After 24 hours of incubation in dextran-containing medium, vacuoles with dextran were electron microscopically found in the endothelium, but these vacuoles were still rare.

Microbiologic control. Despite the decontamination procedure 0.5% to 2% of the corneas turned out to be contaminated during the first week of organ culture, with *Pseudomonas* species and *Staphylococcus epidermidis* being the most frequent contaminants. The transport medium was checked 1 and 2 days respectively before transportation and transplantation of the cornea. In two out of more than 1000 cases microbial growth on the blood agar plates and TSB broth was observed, and the operations were canceled.

Discussion

Endothelial evaluation. The quality of the corneal endothelium is one of the important factors in the success of penetrating keratoplasty. The evaluation of donor endothelium is a help to ensure this quality.

Because the adult human corneal endothelium has a limited regenerative capacity,[33] the number of donor endothelial cells is an important factor. Minimally 2000 cells/mm^2 are considered to be necessary. After the loss from the surgical procedure[2,3,27] sufficient cells will be present to maintain a clear graft. A simple correlation between donor age and endothelial cell density does not exist.[16,25,29] By counting the endothelial cells before keratoplasty one can deliver corneas with minimally 2000 cells/mm^2 without restriction of donors because of age. About 15% of the donor corneas had an irregular endothelial cell pattern, whereas the endothelial cell density was above the minimal level. This irregular pattern (polymegethism) was predominantly found in the endothelium of elderly donors. Stefansson and co-workers[29] found a positive correlation between donor age and variation in cell size. Therefore this irregular cell pattern must be considered as a senile change, contraindicating transplantation. In some cases polymegethism was also observed in the endothelium of younger donors (less than 40 years). In two cases the donors turned out to have been contact lens wearers. It is known that contact lens wear can be associated with changes in the corneal endothelium.[11,31] Functional abnormalities of this endothelium however were not yet demonstrated.[4]

Cell number and cell pattern are not fully satisfying as criteria to guarantee the quality of the donor endothelium. The cells must be healthy and func-

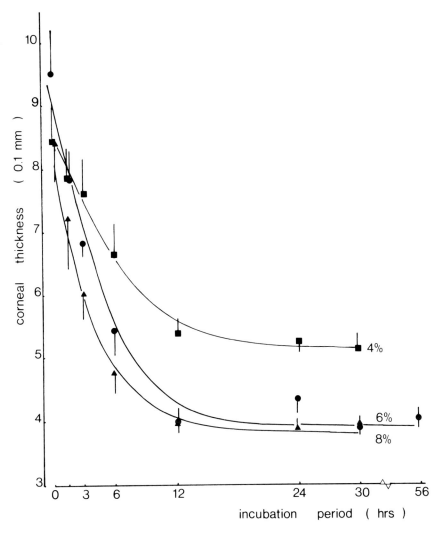

Fig. 46-34. Corneal thickness during incubation in MEM supplemented with 8% *(squares)*, 6% *(triangles)*, and 4% *(circles)* Dextran T500 at 31° C after organ-culture preservation. *Bars,* Standard deviation.

tioning as well. So, in addition, the endothelium was evaluated after being stained with trypan blue and incubation with a hypotonic solution.[10] Trypan blue stains the nuclei of dead cells and appears to be harmless for vital endothelium.[30] Exposure of the endothelium to a hypotonic solution leads to swelling of the intercellular space if the endothelial cells are able to counterbalance water inflow.[18] Counterbalancing of the osmotic equilibrium presupposes intactness of the metabolically dependent barrier function of the endothelium. The swelling also enables the visualization of the endothelium by normal light microscopy. It was possible to scan the whole endothelial surface including folds. Ultrastructurally no defects were found in the endothelial cells because

of the incubation with 1.8% sucrose and staining with trypan blue.[18,35] Unfortunately up to now there is no functional test that can be used before transplantation. Cell number and cell pattern and the morphology of the cells have to suffice.

During organ culture in modified MEM at 31° C the number of endothelial cells decreased slowly. The mean endothelial cell loss became significant after 5 weeks.[18] The variation in cell loss between the individual corneas was substantial and may be attributable to normal variation in cell behavior. However, during organ culture the endothelium is provocatively tested by exposure to the abnormal environment of tissue culture. The differences in cell loss may also reflect differences in the vitality of the endothelium, since the organ culture is a kind of stress test. The percentage of corneas that did not tolerate the organ culture, however, was small, and they were detected by the second endothelial evaluation. With other storage methods (CSM and K-Sol) it was also observed that normal corneas (7 out of 44) did not tolerate prolonged storage.[21] Some of the corneas had numerous dead cells in the center of their endothelium before preservation because of storage or mechanical damage. These endothelia suffered a tremendous cell loss during subsequent organ culture. Dead cells, however, were seldom found after culture because necrotic cells were eliminated. The monolayer was restored by the sliding and stretching of adjacent cells.[7,18] Minor damages were repaired in the same way, but afterwards cell loss and reformation were not significant. Most of the corneas with endothelium that reacted abnormally to the hypotonic sucrose solution at the first evaluation (80%) died quickly during organ culture. Whether these endothelia could have been successfully used for penetrating keratoplasty is uncertain. These endothelia were considered less vital than others because they showed an enhanced cell loss during organ culture. By evaluation of the endothelium before and after organ culture about 30% of the corneas donated were excluded. This was in addition to the about 17% of the corneas discarded during slitlamp examination.

Organ culture. Corneal graft survival significantly improved by the use of HLA class I matched corneal grafts in high-risk cases (vascularized corneas, regrafts).[9,18,36] The storage of corneoscleral buttons in MK medium at 4° C[14,15] offers limited time (2 to 3 days) for HLA typing and matching procedures, scheduling of the operation, and transportation and exchange of corneas between different centers. As the need for a longer storage period arose, the introduction of an organ-culture preservation method enabled a medium-term storage period.[7,14,17,32]

The endothelium and keratocytes looked ultrastructurally vital during 35 days of organ culture, thus concurring with the results of Doughman and co-workers.[7] Data concerning the endothelial cell loss during organ culture are not available from other groups, and so comparisons cannot be made. Whether the differences between each organ-culture procedure (2% or 10% fetal calf serum; HEPES or carbonate buffer; volume of culture medium; incubation temperature) are essential for the survival of the endothelial cells and the cornea in general is discussed below. It is generally agreed that 10% fetal calf serum (FCS) is necessary for cell growth in culture. Because the organ culture of corneas is only a storage method, a lesser amount of FCS might suffice. As described, the epithelium was reduced during incubation with 2% FCS in the medium. Because this layer is constantly growing, it may need a higher amount of FCS for optimal growth.

The epithelial layer bears the larger part of the HLA class I antigens, and reduction of this layer may improve the survival of the corneal allograft[34] without damaging the basal membrane and Bowman's membrane. In addition, dendritic cells bearing HLA class II antigens could no longer be detected in the epithelium and corneal stroma after 1 week of organ culture.[19] It was shown that the immunogenicity of heterotopic corneal grafts in mice is directly dependent on the number of dendritic cells in the cornea bearing histocompatibility complex class II antigens.[20] Whether the reduction of the presence of HLA class II antigens by organ culture affects corneal graft survival is not yet known.

In the Dutch system a HEPES buffer was used. With HEPES buffer similar results were obtained as with carbonate-buffered media (unpublished observations). The primary advantage of HEPES however is that closed bottles and dry incubation (no humidified atmosphere and 5% CO_2 in air) can be used, diminishing the chance of microbial contamination. Sixty milliliters of organ-culture medium was sufficient for the survival of the endothelial cells for about 5 weeks. During that period the pH of the medium decreased from 7.3 to 7.0. The endothelium has a high pH tolerance,[10] and so the small pH decrease appears to be no problem. However, after 40 to 60 days the significantly increased cell loss might be caused by a further decrease of the pH caused by more waste products.[18] A larger volume or renewal of the medium may postpone or prevent this phenomenon. Different incubation temperatures are used in the literature;[5,7,13,30] 37°, 34°, 32°, 31° C, and room temperature. Therefore the temperature appears to be not very important, provided that it is not too high or too low.

During the first phase of preservation 0.5% to 2% of the corneas turned out to be contaminated. During the second phase, however, this amount was only 0.2%. This indicates to our opinion that the use of closed bottles, a dry incubator, no renewal of the medium, and a strict protocol helped to keep the contamination rate low without significant effect on the survival of the corneas during 35 days. The decontamination procedure,[28] however, is not yet sufficient to kill all microbes present.

A disadvantage of the organ-culture procedure described here is the swelling of the corneal stroma. Elsewhere, swollen corneas were successfully transplanted,[6] or corneas were kept thin during organ culture by the addition of high-molecular-weight dextran.[24] Although a direct toxic effect of dextran could not be demonstrated,[18,35] the long-term use of dextran before keratoplasty was contraindicated. Doughman and co-workers[5] deswelled the corneas in MK medium at 4° C. In the Dutch procedure culture medium supplemented with Dextran T500 was used to dehydrate the corneas at 31° C. It was found that the deswelling rate was independent of the dextran concentration. The corneas reached their minimal thickness within 12 hours. The ultimate thickness depended on the dextran concentration. A 5% solution was preferred for surgical reasons. The use of culture medium supplemented with 5% Dextran T500 during a week at room temperature did not have morphologically demonstrable effects on the endothelium, enabling a week for transportation.

Conclusions. Organ culture of corneas enables a preservation period up to 35 days without remarkable loss of endothelial cells and ultrastructural defects. Evaluation of the corneal endothelium offers the opportunity to exclude corneas with partly damaged endothelium, senile changes, or latent anomalies. It offers also the opportunity to select good corneas from less favorable donor groups (high age, relatively long postmortem time), increasing the donor supply. By a combination of organ culture and endothelial evaluation corneas with a well-defined endothelial quality can be delivered; thus the chance of primary failures is reduced and an optimal scheduling of the keratoplasty is allowed for the convenience of patient, surgeon, hospital, and tissue-typing laboratory.

REFERENCES

1. Batchelor JR, Casey TA, Werb A, et al: HLA matching and corneal grafting, *Lancet* 1:551-554, 1976.
2. Bigar F: Specular microscopy of the corneal endothelium, *Dev Ophthalmol* 6:1-94, 1982.
3. Bourne WM: Chronic endothelial cell loss in transplanted corneas, *Cornea* 2:289-294, 1983.
4. Carlson KH, Bourne WM, Brubaker RF: Effect of long-term contact lens wear on corneal endothelial cell morphology and function, *Invest Ophthalmol Vis Sci* 29:185-193, 1988.
5. Doughman DH, Harris JE, Mindrup E, Lindstrom RL: Prolonged donor cornea preservation in organ-culture: long-term evaluation, *Cornea* 1:7-29, 1982.
6. Doughman DJ, Harris JE, Schmidt KM: Penetrating keratoplasty using 37° C organ-cultured cornea, *Trans Am Acad Ophthalmol Otolaryngol* 81:778-793, 1976.
7. Doughman DJ, Van Horn D, Harris JE, et al: The ultrastructure of human organ-cultured cornea. I. Endothelium, *Arch Ophthalmol* 92:516-523, 1974.
8. Ehlers N, Kissmeyer-Nielsen F: Corneal transplantation and HLA-histocompatibility: a preliminary communication, *Acta Ophthalmol* 57:738-741, 1979.
9. Foulks GN, Sanfilippo F: Beneficial effects of histocompatibility in high risk corneal transplantation, *Am J Ophthalmol* 94:622-629, 1982.
10. Gonnering R, Edelhauser HF, Van Horn DL, Durant W: The pH tolerance of rabbit and human corneal endothelium, *Invest Ophthalmol Vis Sci* 18:373-390, 1979.
11. Holden BA, Sweeney DF, Vannas AA, et al: Effects of long-term extended contact lens wear on the human cornea, *Invest Ophthalmol Vis Sci* 26:1489-1501, 1985.
12. Kirk AH, Hassard DTR: Supravital staining for the corneal endothelium and evidence for a membrane on its surface, *Can J Ophthalmol* 4:404-415, 1969.
13. Lindstrom RL, Doughman DJ, Van Horn DL, et al: Organ-culture corneal storage at ambient room temperature, *Arch Ophthalmol* 95:869-878, 1977.
14. McCarey BE, Kaufman HE: Improved corneal storage, *Invest Ophthalmol Vis Sci* 13:165-173, 1974.
15. McCarey BE, Meyer RF, Kaufman HE: Improved corneal storage for penetrating keratoplasty in humans, *Ann Ophthalmol* 9:1488-1495, 1977.
16. Olsen T: Noncontact specular microscopy of human corneal endothelium, *Acta Ophthalmol* 57:986-997, 1979.
17. Pels E, Schuchard Y: Organ-culture of human corneas, *Doc Ophthalmol* 56:147-153, 1983.
18. Pels E, Schuchard Y: The effects of high molecular weight dextran on the preservation of human corneas, *Cornea* 3:219-227, 1984-1985.
19. Pels E, Van der Gaag R: HLA-A, B, C and HLA-DR antigens and dendritic cells in fresh and organ culture preserved corneas, *Cornea* 3:231-239, 1984-1985.
20. Rubsamen PE, McCulley J, Bergstresser PR, Streilein JW: On the immunogenicity of mouse corneal allografts infiltrated with Langerhans cells, *Invest Ophthalmol Vis Sci* 25:513-518, 1984.
21. Saggau DD, Bourne WM: A comparison of two preservation media (CSM and K-Sol) by scanning electron microscopy of preserved corneal endothelium, *Arch Ophthalmol* 107:429-432, 1989.
22. Schröder HD, Sperling S: Polysaccharide coating of human corneal endothelium, *Acta Ophthalmol* 55:819-826, 1977.
23. Sperling S: Early morphological changes in organ cultured human corneal endothelium, *Acta Ophthalmol* 56:785-791, 1978.
24. Sperling S: Human corneal endothelium in organ culture: the influence of temperature and medium of incubation, *Acta Ophthalmol* 57:269-276, 1979.
25. Sperling S: Endothelial cell density in donor corneas, *Acta Ophthalmol* 58:278-282, 1980.
26. Sperling S: Cryopreservation of human cadaver corneas regenerated at 31° C in a modified tissue culture medium, *Acta Ophthalmol* 59:142-148, 1981.
27. Sperling S, Olsen T, Ehlers N: Fresh and cultured corneal grafts compared by post-operative thickness and endothelial cell density, *Acta Ophthalmol* 59:566-575, 1981.
28. Sperling S, Sørensen IG: Decontamination of cadaver corneas, *Acta Ophthalmol* 59:123-133, 1981.
29. Stefansson A, Müller O, Sundmacher R: Non-contact specular microscopy of the normal corneal endothelium: a statistical evaluation of morphometric parameters, *Graefes Arch Clin Exp Ophthalmol* 218:200-205, 1982.
30. Stocker FW, King EH, Lucas DO, Georgiade NA: Clinical test for evaluating donor corneas, *Arch Ophthalmol* 84:2-7, 1970.
31. Stocker EG, Schoessler JP: Corneal endothelial polymegathism induced by PMMA contact lens wear, *Invest Ophthalmol Vis Sci* 26:857-863, 1985.

32. Summerlin WT, Miller GE, Harris JE, Good RA: The organ-cultured cornea: an in vitro study, *Invest Ophthalmol Vis Sci* 12:176-180, 1973.

33. Treffers WF: *Corneal endothelial wound healing*, Nijmegen, 1982, Janssen Printers.

34. Tuberville AW, Foster CS, Wood TO: The effect of donor cornea epithelium removal on the incidence of allograft rejection, *Ophthalmology* 90:1351-1356, 1983.

35. Van der Want JJL, Pels E, Schuchard Y, et al: Electron microscopy of cultured human corneas: osmotic hydration and the use of a dextran fraction (Dextran T500) in organ culture, *Arch Ophthalmol* 101:1920-1926, 1983.

36. Völker-Dieben HJ, Kok-van Alphen CC, Lansbergen Q, Persijn GC: The effect of prospective HLA-A and B matching on corneal graft survival, *Acta Ophthalmol* 60:203-212, 1982.

THE SURVIVAL OF ORGAN-CULTURED DONOR CORNEAS

H.J. VÖLKER-DIEBEN

J. D'AMARO

C.C. KOK–van ALPHEN†

LIESBETH PELS

The success of corneal grafts depends chiefly on whether the donor corneas have sufficient numbers of viable endothelial cells.

Since the introduction of keratoplasty, methods have been sought for optimal preservation of donor material. Clinically good results have been reported in penetrating keratoplasties with donor corneas preserved by several different methods. A simple and well-tried method is the storage of the intact globe in a moist chamber at 4° C.[22] In general, a storage period of 48 hours is acceptable for this method. Storage of corneoscleral buttons in McCarey-Kaufman (MK) medium at 4° C[15] has doubled the storage time to 96 hours. Thereafter pronounced marked endothelial damage can be observed.[31] Within this limited period, we experienced medical problems regarding the optimal preoperative preparation of senior patients often with anticoagulant, cardiac or antihypertensive therapies. Moreover, organizational problems interfered with the selection of high-risk patients who were in need of tissue typed and HLA A and B matched grafts. Since the beneficial effect of HLA-matched donor corneas for high-risk patients has been reported by several authors,[32,34,36] we were interested in extending the storage time. Although cryopreservation allows a storage time of at least 1 year, the complex technology limits its use to a few centers.[5,9]

The intermediate-term storage method described by Doughman and co-workers[7] presented us with a possible solution to our storage problems. Therefore we developed a new preservation method based on the organ culture techniques described by Doughman and Sperling.[25]

This chapter presents the results of 238 penetrating keratoplasties performed between 1982 and 1984 using organ-cultured donor corneal tissue. A comparison is made with the results of 239 penetrating keratoplasties performed between 1980 and 1982 using MK medium–stored donor corneal tissue. The analysis of 52 organ cultured and 46 MK-stored donor corneas transplanted in 1982 in a randomized manner revealed the clearly beneficial effect of organ culture. Consequently, we believed that the continued use of MK-stored corneas was not in the best interest of our patients and that it would have been unethical to continue to use that procedure. In the period 1985-1990 we performed an additional 626 penetrating keratoplasties using organ-cultured donor corneal tissue. The effect of the length of organ-culture time and the effect of HLA-A, B, and DR matching in a total number of 864 cases are analyzed.

Materials and Methods. Apart from the first 16 corneas, which were organ cultured by Sperling and co-workers in Arhus, Denmark, and sent to Holland by train, the remaining donor material was prepared as follows.

Donor corneas. The corneoscleral buttons were provided by the Eurotransplant Foundation (Leiden, the Netherlands) and preserved in MK medium. The storage time in this MK medium varied from 6 to 68 hours (mean, 25 hours). The time between death and the start of the organ culture varied from 13 to 75 hours (mean, 35 hours).

Organ culture. Corneoscleral buttons were suspended in sterilized 100 ml glass infusion bottles by a suture tied to the scleral rim and were incubated in 30 ml of culture medium at 31° C.[25]

The medium consisted of minimal essential medium (MEM) with Earle's salts (Eagle's) with L-glutamine and 20 mM HEPES buffer, MEM (Flow) 2% and fetal calf serum (Flow), and penicillin, 100 IU/ml (Gist-Brocades), streptomycin, 0.05 mg/ml (Gist-Brocades) and nystatin, 50 IU/ml (Labaz).

In order to reduce the swelling of the corneas before use, they were incubated at 31° C for 24 hours in 30 ml glass vials completely filled with culture medium supplemented with 5% Dextran T500 (Pharmacia). Those closed vials may be used to transport at room temperature. The transportation time can be up to 4 days.

Evaluation of Corneal Endothelium. The endothelium was stained in 0.3% trypan blue in 0.9% NaCl for 1 minute. After staining, the cornea was

---

†Deceased 1987.

rinsed with phosphate-buffered saline. The endothelial cell borders were visualized by provoked swelling in 1.8% sucrose.[15] Random micrographs were obtained by use of a total linear magnification of 135.5 with a Zeiss microscope, Standard 14, equipped with a test frame of 2 × 2 cm, and the density of cells was determined. Total cell counts and standard error were obtained. A standard error of about 10% was often observed.[26] After photography the corneas were placed in culture medium. At the end of the culture period the endothelium was reevaluated. The length of the culture period depended on the date of the transplantation.

The following criteria were adopted as indicators of the structural and functional integrity of the corneal endothelium:[17]

1. Descemet's folds must be covered with endothelium.
2. Minimally 2000 endothelial cells/mm.[2]
3. A regular cell mosaic.[24]
4. The intercellular borders must swell.
5. The cell loss may not exceed a maximum of 20% during a 30-day preservation period.
6. The cells must show clean-cut cell borders and have a smooth appearance like the cells of fresh corneas.

Description of Cases. All 1103 (238 + 626 organ-cultured and 239 MK medium–stored donor tissue) penetrating keratoplasties were performed between 1980 and 1990 by a single surgeon (H.J.V.D.).

The technique of penetrating keratoplasty remained constant throughout the study and has been previously described.[35] Disparate-sized grafts, 0.5 mm larger than the trephination opening, were used in aphakic and pseudophakic eyes. In all cases, the postoperative treatment consisted of dexamethasone 1% eyedrops, 3 times daily combined with antibiotic eyedrops, for at least 1 year. No systemic steroid or immunosuppressive therapy was given to the patients. High-risk cases, that is, patients with moderately or severely vascularized corneas with or without previous corneal grafts, received HLA A and B matched grafts with a maximum of two mismatches. All HLA typings of the patients and donors were performed in the National Reference Center in Leiden (Department of Immunohaematology, University Hospital). Tissue typing was performed with a standard microlymphocytotoxicity assay.[33]

HLA-DR matching was not performed prospectively, since no significant effect on corneal graft survival was observed in a previous studies.[38,40-42]

All patients and graft donors were whites of Dutch

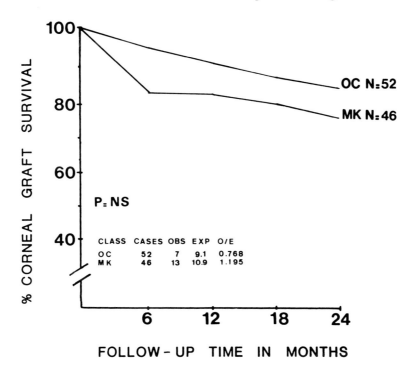

Fig. 46-35. Influence of two storage methods on corneal graft survival; corneas cultured at 31° C (*OC*, organ culture) or stored at 4° C (*MK*, McCarey-Kaufman) in the year 1982. Beneficial effect of use of organ-cultured donor corneas (*OC*) is
$$\left[1 - \left(\frac{0.768}{1.195}\right)\right] \times 10^2 = 35.7\%.$$

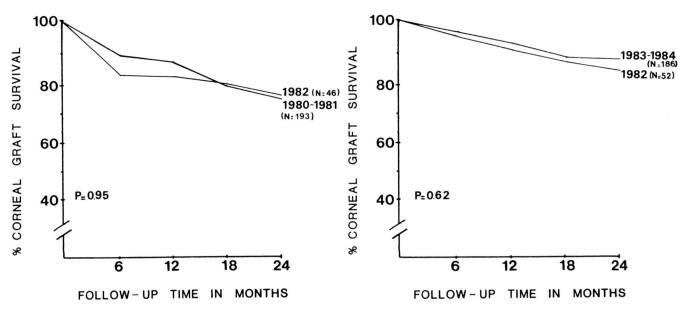

Fig. 46-36. Effect of McCarey-Kaufman stored donor corneas *(MK)* on graft survival in two different time periods.

Fig. 46-37. Effect of organ-cultured donor corneas *(OC)* on graft survival in two different time periods.

origin. All survival times were calculated using the actuarial life table method. The significance of the difference between the various classes were tested with a χ^2 statistic derived from the Logrank test.[18] The numbers to the right of the follow-up curves (Figs. 46-35 to 46-44) indicate the numbers of the patients at risk at the start of the study. The criteria for the survival of corneal allografts are those described by Jones[13] with the clarity of the cornea as the major criterion. Two-dimensional χ^2 tests were used to find the significance of the differences in the distributions of various parameters in the organ-cultured and MK-medium study groups.

Results. In 1982, organ-cultured (OC) and MK-stored donor corneas were used in a randomized manner. No selection for whatever reason was made. The survivals of the 52 corneal grafts performed with OC donor tissue and the 46 corneal grafts with MK-stored material were 96.1% and 84.3% at 6 months, 92.1% and 84.3% at 12 months, and 86.0% and 78.5% respectively at 24 months (Fig. 46-35). Although the differences between the two classes were not statistically significant, a beneficial effect of

$$35.7\% \left(\left[1 - \left(\frac{0.768}{1.195} \right) \right] \times 10^2 \right), \text{ according to}$$

Peto[19] was observed with the OC donor corneas.

There were no significant differences in the survival of 193 grafts with MK-stored tissue performed in the years 1980 and 1981 as compared to the graft survival of 46 similarly stored grafts that were per-

formed in 1982 (Fig. 46-36). The survival of 52 corneal grafts performed with OC donor tissue in 1982 and of 186 grafts with the same preservation technique performed in 1983 and 1984 were not significantly different (Fig. 46-37). The homogeneity in the above results justified the pooling of those data and the computing of survival curves for the 239 corneal grafts performed with MK-stored tissue in the years 1980, 1981, and 1982 versus the survival of 238 corneal grafts performed with OC corneas in the years 1982, 1983, and 1984. The OC donor corneas had a graft survival of 97.3%, 94.1%, and 87.9% at 6, 12, and 24 months versus 89.4%, 86.06%, and 76.51% for the time intervals for the MK-stored donor corneas ($p = 0.0029$) (Fig. 46-38).

The distribution of recipient ages and sex, donor age, diagnoses at transplant, numbers of aphakic and pseudophakic patients, the number of repeated grafts, and the number of HLA A and B−matched grafts demonstrated no significant heterogeneity in the two study groups.[39] However a significantly larger number of vascularized recipient corneas were observed among the patients who received MK-stored donor material ($p = 0.017$) than among those who received OC corneas (Table 46-11). In the MK-stored corneas there were significantly more large-diameter grafts than in the OC grafts ($p = 0.002$) (Table 46-12).

To rule out the effect of these potentially confounding factors the survival curves were recom-

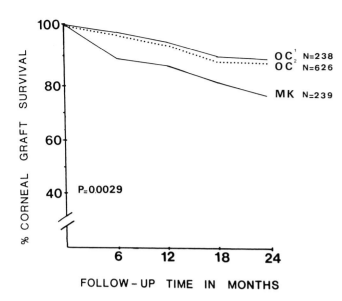

Fig. 46-38. Survival of grafts performed with McCarey-Kaufman–stored donor corneas (MK) versus organ-cultured donor corneas (OC). The OC corneas are divided into two time periods. OC^1 represents period 1982-1984 and OC^2 1985-1990.

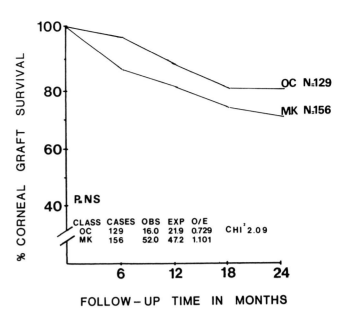

Fig. 46-39. Influence of two storage methods on corneal grgraft survival; corneas cultured at 31° C *(OC)* or stored at 4° C *(MK)* in moderately or severely vascularized recipient corneas only.

Table 46-11. Comparison of Degree of Vascularization of Recipient Corneas in Patients Who Received Organ-Cultured Versus MK Medium–Stored Donor Corneas.

Degree of Vascularization of Recipient Cornea	Organ-Cultured Donor Corneas	MK Medium–Stored Donor Corneas
Nonvascularized	24 ⎱ 109	28 ⎱ 83
Slightly	85 ⎰	55 ⎰
Moderately	39 ⎱ 129	52 ⎱ 156
Severely	90 ⎰	104 ⎰

$\chi^2(1) = 5.63 \qquad p = 0.017$

Table 46-12. Comparison of Diameter of Grafts in Patients Who Received Organ-Cultured Versus MK Medium–Stored Donor Corneas

Graft Size	Organ-Cultured Donor Corneas	MK Medium–Stored Donor Corneas
Small diameter, 7.1	147 ⎱ 129	77 ⎱ 197
Medium diameter, 7.2 to 7.9	72 ⎰	120 ⎰
Large diameter, 8.0	19	42

$\chi^2(1) = 9.98 \qquad p = 0.002$

puted after stratifying the data for the degree of vascularization (none and slightly versus moderately and severely). In these two groups, the survivals of OC corneas was always better than that of the MK-stored corneas. In recipients with moderately or severely vascularized corneas the differences were not statistically significant but nevertheless interesting.

In the none or slightly vascularized recipient beds, the survival of the OC and MK donor corneas were both excellent with that of the OC corneas slightly better than the MK corneas (100% survival at 6 and 12 months, 95.3% at 24 months for the OC and 98.5%, 96.9%, and 88.7% at 6, 12, and 24 months for the MK-stored corneas in the non- or slightly vascularized recipient corneal beds). In moderately or severely vascularized corneas, survivals of 95.0%, 88.9% and 80.9% at 6, 12, and 24 months were observed for the OC corneas and 87.0%, 82.4%, and 72.1% survival at the same time intervals for the MK-stored corneas (Fig. 46-39). The use of OC donor corneas yielded a beneficial effect of 38% as compared to the use of MK-stored corneas.

We had previously demonstrated that the survivals of small versus medium-sized grafts were not significantly different, whereas large grafts (diameter ≥8.0 mm) are less favorable.[37] The survival of small or medium-sized OC corneas (diameter ≤7.9 mm) was better than that of similarly sized MK corneas

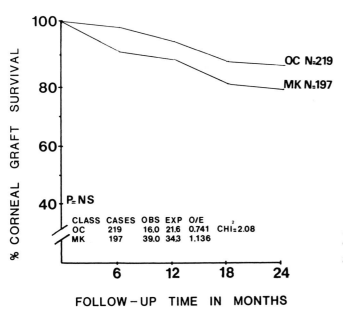

Fig. 46-40. Influence of two storage methods on corneal graft survival; corneas cultured at 31° C *(OC)* or stored at 4° C *(MK)* in small or medium-sized grafts (0 ≤ 7.9) only.

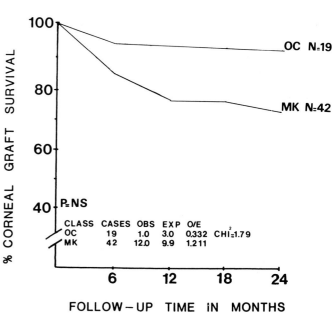

Fig. 46-41. Influence of two storage methods on corneal graft survival; corneas cultured at 31° C *(OC)* or stored at 4° C *(MK)* in large grafts (0 ≥ 8.0) only.

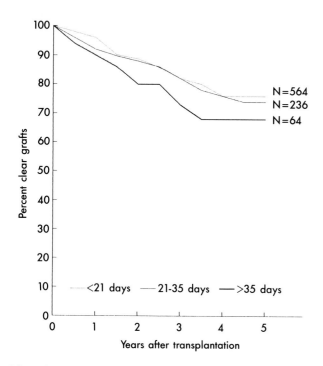

Fig. 46-42. Influence of length of organ-culture time of donor cornea on graft survival.

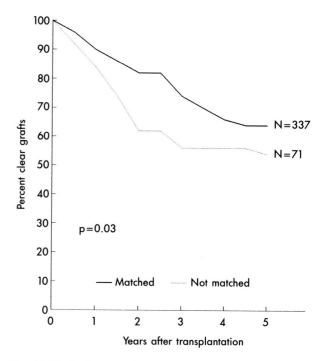

Fig. 46-43. Influence of HLA-A and HLA-B matching in keratoplasties performed with organ-cultured donor corneas in moderately or severely vascularized corneal beds.

(98.0%, 94.2%, and 87.0% survival at 6, 12, and 24 months for the OC corneas and 92.6%, 89.5%, and 80.1% for the MK corneas at the same time intervals). Although the differences are not statistically significant, the use of OC corneas yielded a beneficial effect of 34.8% (Fig. 46-40). The survival of large organ-cultured grafts (diameter ≥8.0 mm) was 94.6% at 6, 12, and 24 months and 85.1%, 77.4%, and 74.6% at the same time intervals for MK-stored corneas (Fig. 46-41). Once again, the results were not statistically significant, but the beneficial effect of the use of OC corneas was 72.6% with only one failure occurring in OC grafts.

The effect of the duration of organ culture on graft survival is analyzed in the total number of 864 grafts and set out in Fig. 46-42. There were no statistically significant differences in the survival of corneas cultured up to 21 days versus up to 35 days or longer than 35 days. However, transplants performed with donor corneas that had been cultured for longer than 35 days had the poorest survival times.

The beneficial effect of HLA A and B matching previously reported by us was most evident in vascularized recipient beds.[40-42] HLA A and B matching also appears to influence graft survival in keratoplasties performed with organ-cultured material in moderately or severely vascularized corneal beds (90.1%, 82.3%, 74.1%, 66.0%, and 64.1% survival at 1, 2, 3, 4, and 5 years for the HLA A and B–matched grafts versus 84.2%, 62.1%, 55.9%, 55.9%, and 54.1% for the group not matched) (Fig. 46-43).

Discussion. The aim of this study was to investigate the survival of organ-cultured (OC) donor corneas used for penetrating keratoplasties. The first analysis of 52 OC corneas and 46 MK-stored corneas demonstrated a beneficial effect of the use of OC corneas (Fig. 46-35). The second comparison of the survival of 238 OC corneas and 239 MK-stored corneas demonstrated a statistically significant ($p = 0.0029$) improved survival of OC corneas (Fig. 46-38).

The survival of 626 penetrating keratoplasties using OC corneas in the period 1985 to 1990 demonstrated similar results when compared to the results observed in the period 1982 to 1984 (Fig. 46-38).

These observations are not in concordance with those of Bourne,[4] who reported a statistically significant increased endothelial cell loss, naturally leading to more opaque grafts, in OC corneas already 2 months after keratoplasty when compared to MK-stored donor corneas. Bourne's observation indicates that more graft failures should be expected in OC corneas in a long-term survival analysis. However,

their procedure for organ culture was different from ours, especially at the end of the culture period when Bourne placed the cultured corneas again in MK medium for 2 days before transplantation was performed. In a long-term clinical evaluation of organ-cultured corneas Doughman[8] reported graft survival of 80.7% at 6 months, which was comparable to the survival of grafts obtained from moist chamber–stored globes as reported by Salabee,[23] Stark and co-workers,[28] and Abbott and Forster.[1] They observed survivals of 83%, 78%, and 69% respectively. Aquavella et al.,[2] McCarey et al.,[16] Bigar et al.,[3] and Stark et al.[29] reported similar results for corneal grafts performed with MK-stored corneas. Our observation of 97.3% survival at 6 months compares favorably with these reports. Further comparison of our and their results is not possible since none of the authors just mentioned analyzed their results using the actuarial life table method. The actuarial life table method as used in the evaluation of renal transplants and used by us since 1982 in the evaluation of corneal transplants is the only valid method for such data.

The partition of recipients into different prognostic groups according to Polack's criteria[20] may result in substantial levels of classification bias. Consequently we prefer to define the prognostic groups according to the degree of vascularization of the recipient bed: none, slightly (one-fourth peripheral vessel ingrowth only), moderately (more than one-fourth vessel ingrowth), and severely (vessel ingrowth in all four quarters and in the central part of the cornea). Previous graft failures attributable to immune rejections almost always coincide with vascular ingrowth.

The highly significant influence of the degree of vessel ingrowth is demonstrated in Fig. 46-44, which presents the results of our complete series of corneal grafts performed since 1977 (at $p < 0.0000$). Because of the possible confounding effect of the smaller number of vascularized corneal beds in the group of OC corneas (Table 46-11) we stratified our cases with regard to that factor. In both subgroups, (nonvascularized or slightly, and moderately or severely) the survival of OC corneas was better than the survival of MK corneas (Fig. 46-5). This type of stratified analysis has not been previously performed, and so it is not possible to make any comparisons. Stainer and Brightbill[29] compared moist chamber storage with MK medium storage. Their patients were divided in five prognostic groups according to Polack's criteria, and the survival was reported in percentages of clear grafts with follow-up periods varying from 4 to 35 months. Doughman

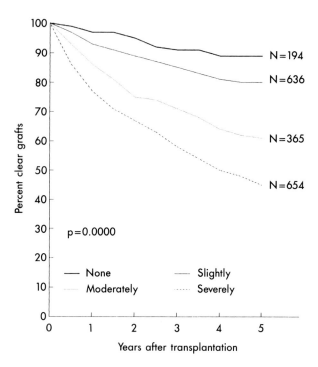

Fig. 46-44. Influence of degree of vascularization of recipient cornea on graft survival (total *n* = 1649).

and co-workers[8] classified 114 grafts into three prognostic groups, but they discussed only the survival of the total group of 114 OC grafts and not of the 3 separate groups. Clear grafts were followed for an average of 28.8 months, and the 22 failed grafts for an average of 40.4 months.

In Table 46-12 a second possible confounding factor is reported. In the group of MK-stored corneas a large number of large-diameter grafts were used. However, division of the patient material according to the graft size, that is, grafts with a diameter up to 7.9 mm and those of 8 mm and more was made (Figs. 46-40 and 46-41). In both study groups, the survival of OC corneas was superior to that of MK-stored corneas. Although the differences were not statistically significant, a clear beneficial effect was observed. The relation between large-diameter grafts and an increased number of immune reactions was reported by Chandler and Kaufman.[6] In their study, only moist chamber–stored donor material was used for penetrating keratoplasties. Our report represents the only one on the relationship between donor graft size and the survival of organ-cultured donor corneas.

Since we have eliminated the confounding factors

by analyzing the survival of OC corneas and MK-stored corneas in these four subgroups, we consider the superior graft survival of OC corneas as the result of improved donor material and maintenance of viable endothelial cells by means of the organ-culture method.

Corneas cultured for more than 35 days seem to survive less favorably after transplantation than cultured for shorter periods. Pels and Schuchard[17] reported a positive correlation between the percentage of dead endothelial cells and the time since donor death. Although cell densities of almost 3000 cells/mm^2 are reported after 30 days of culturing, a 3 to 4 weeks culture time might represent a more certain maximum culture period.

Doughman and co-workers[7] reported that in experimental grafts no modification in immune responsiveness occurred until at least 3 weeks after organ culture. However van der Gaag and co-workers[30] observed a disappearance of HLA-DR antigens on corneoscleral buttons after a 1-week culture time, whereas HLA A, B, and C antigens were still detectable. In our total group of 408 OC grafts in vascularized recipient corneal beds, the influence of HLA A and B matching was still present (Fig. 46-43), confirming the reports of Doughman and van der Gaag. Since HLA-DR matching was not prospectively performed, no comments can be made in regard to the disappearance of HLA-DR antigens on corneoscleral buttons after a 1-week culture time. However, the influence of HLA-DR matching on corneal graft survival may be expected only with large grafts where the dendritic cells are detectable only in the peripheral third of the cornea.[21]

Conclusions

The survival of grafts performed with organ-cultured donor corneas is at least as good or better than that of MK medium–stored donor material. This conclusion applies not only in recipient subgroups divided according to the degree of corneal vascularization, but also in subgroups with different corneal graft sizes.

The prolonged preservation time of the organ-culture method helps us to resolve the medical and organizational problems related to the preoperative patient care. That procedure is especially true for high-risk patients who should preferably receive HLA A and B matched corneal grafts.

Since our results demonstrate the lack of a statistically significant but clearly beneficial effect of the use of organ-cultured corneas in comparison to MK medium–stored corneas used in a randomized manner, we believe that it would be unethical to continue to use MK-stored corneas, which may expose our patients to an increased risk of graft failure.

Retrospective analysis of different procedures (that is, storage methods) may yield useful results if attention is paid to stratification of the data so that the possible effect of confounding factors may be ruled out.

REFERENCES

1. Abbott RL, Forster RK: Determinants of graft clarity in penetrating keratoplasty, *Arch Ophthalmol* 97:1071, 1979.
2. Aquavella JV, Van Horn DL, Haggerty CJ: Corneal preservation using M-K media, *Am J Ophthalmol* 80:791-799, 1975.
3. Bigar F et al: Improved corneal storage for penetrating keratoplasties in man, *Am J Ophthalmol* 79:115-120, 1975.
4. Bourne WM et al: Increased endothelial cell loss after transplantation of corneas preserved by a modified organ culture technique, *Ophthalmology* 91(3):285-289, 1984.
5. Capella JA, Kaufman HE, Robbins JE: Preservation of viable corneal tissue, *Arch Ophthalmol* 74:669-673, 1965.
6. Chandler JW, Kaufman HE: Graft reactions after keratoplasty for keratoconus, *Am J Ophthalmol* 77:543, 1974.
7. Doughman DJ, Harris JE, Schmitt MK: Penetrating keratoplasty using 37° C organ cultured corneas, *Trans Am Acad Ophthalmol Otolaryngol* 81:778-793, 1976.
8. Doughman DJ et al: Prolonged donor cornea preservation in organ culture: long-term clinical evaluation, *Cornea* 1:7-20, 1982.
9. Eastcott HHG et al: Preservation of corneal grafts by freezing, *Lancet* 1:237-239, 1954.
10. Ehlers N, Kissmeyer-Nielsen F: Influence of histocompatibility on the fate of the corneal transplant. In Corneal graft failure, *Ciba Found Symp* 15:307-322, Amsterdam, 1973, Elsevier.
11. Foulks GN, Sanfilippo FP: Histocompatibility testing for keratoplasty in high risk patients, *Ophthalmology* 90:239-244, 1983.
12. Gibbs DC et al: The influence of tissue typing compatibility on the success rate of full-thickness corneal grafts, *Trans Ophthalmol Soc UK* 94:101-126, 1974.
13. Jones BR: In Corneal graft failure, *Ciba Found Symp* 15:344, Amsterdam, 1973, Elsevier.
14. Kirk AH, Hassard DTR: Supravital staining of the corneal endothelium and evidence for a membrane on its surface, *Can J Ophthalmol* 4:405-415, 1969.
15. McCarey BE, Kaufman HE: Improved corneal storage, *Invest Ophthalmol* 13:165-173, 1974.
16. McCarey BE, Meyer RF, Kaufman HE: Improved corneal storage for penetrating keratoplasties in humans, *Ann Ophthalmol* 8:1488-1495, 1976.
17. Pels E, Schuchard J: Organ culture preservation of human corneas, *Doc Ophthalmol* 56:147-153, 1983.
    Pels E, van der Gaag R: (See reference 30.)
18. Peto R et al: Design and analysis of randomized clinical trials requiring prolonged observation of each patient. I. Introduction and design, *Br J Cancer* 34:585, 1976.
19. Peto J: *The calculation and interpretation of survival curves*, Oxford, 1984, Oxford University Press.
20. Polack FM: Influence of host corneal disease in the prognosis of keratoplasty. In *Corneal transplantation*, New York, 1972, Grune & Stratton.
21. Rodrigues MM et al: Langerhans cells in the normal conjunctiva and peripheral cornea of selected species, *Invest Ophthalmol Vis Sci* 21(5):759, 1981.

22. Rycroft BW: *Corneal grafts*, London, 1955, Butterworth.
23. Saleeby SS: Keratoplasty: results using donor tissue beyond 48 hours, *Arch Ophthalmol* 87:538, 1972.
24. Sperling S: Early morphological changes in organ cultured human corneal endothelium, *Acta Ophthalmol* 56:785-792, 1978.
25. Sperling S: Human corneal endothelium in organ culture: the influence of temperature and medium of incubation, *Acta Ophthalmol* 57:269-276, 1979.
26. Sperling S, Gundersen HJG: The precision of unbiased estimates of numerical density of endothelial cells in donor corneas, *Acta Ophthalmol* 56:793-802, 1978.
27. Stainer GA, Brightbill FS, Calkins B: A comparison of corneal storage in moist chamber and McCarey-Kaufman medium in human keratoplasty, *Ophthalmology* 88(1):46-49, 1981.
28. Stark WJ et al: The results of one or two penetrating keratoplasties using 10-0 monofilament nylon suture, *Ophthalmic Surg* 3:11-25, 1972.
29. Stark WJ, Maumenee AE, Kenyon KR: Intermediate-term corneal storage for penetrating keratoplasty, *Am J Ophthalmol* 79:795-802, 1975.
30. Pels E, van der Gaag R: HLA-A,B, C and HLA-DR antigens and dendritic cells in fresh and in organ culture preserved corneas, *Cornea* 3(4):231-239, 1984-1985.
31. Van Horn DL, Schultz RO, DeBruin J: Endothelial survival in corneal tissue stored in M-K medium, *Am J Ophthalmol* 80:642-647, 1975.
32. Vannas S et al: HLA-compatible donor for prevention of allograft reaction, *Albrecht von Graefes Arch Klin Ophthalmol* 198:217-222, 1976.
33. Van Rood JJ: Microlymphocytotoxicity method. In Ray J, editor: *NIAID Manual of tissue typing techniques*, Maryland, 1979, National Institutes of Health (NIH), 80-545.
34. Völker-Dieben HJ et al: First experiences with HLA-matched corneal grafts in high risk cases, *Doc Ophthalmol* 44:39-48, 1977.
35. Völker-Dieben HJ et al: Different influences on corneal graft survival in 539 transplants, *Acta Ophthalmol* 60:190-202, 1982.
36. Völker-Dieben HJ et al: The effect of prospective HLA-A and B matching on corneal graft survival, *Acta Ophthalmol* 60:203-212, 1982.
37. Völker-Dieben HJ: *The effect of immunological and nonimmunological factors on corneal graft survival*, The Hague, 1984, Dr. W. Junk bv Publisher, p 88.
38. Völker-Dieben HJ: The interactions of HLA-DR, donor graft size and corneal vascularisation of the recipient on graft survival. Chapter 7 in *The effect of immunological and non-immunological factors on corneal graft survival*, The Hague, 1984, Dr. W. Junk bv Publisher.
39. Völker-Dieben HJ et al: The survival of organ-cultured donor corneas. In Brightbill FS, editor: *Corneal surgery*, St. Louis, 1986, Mosby—Year Book.
40. Völker-Dieben HJ et al: Hierarchy of prognostic factors for corneal allograft survival, *Aust NZ J Ophthalmol* 15:11-18, 1987.
41. Völker-Dieben HJ et al: Corneal transplantation: a single center experience 1976-1988. In Terasaki P, editor: *Clinical transplants 1988*, Los Angelos, 1989, UCLA, Tissue Typing Lab, p 249.
42. Völker-Dieben HJ et al: Interaction between prognostic factors for corneal allograft survival, *Transplantation Proc* 21(1):3135-3138, 1989.

Tissue typing

PRESENT STATE OF THE ART AND RESULTS

DANIEL J. MAYER

The human cornea is one of the most successfully transplanted tissues in clinical practice, yet it still remains one of the least studied in experimental transplantation systems. Despite the recent impetus in the understanding of the immunology of organ transplantation, the complex interaction involved in the afferent and efferent loops of the recognition and rejection responses of the host against foreign tissue is still a matter of speculation. However, the old belief that the cornea is nonantigenic and that the loading dose of this tissue in transplantation is insufficient to stimulate the host's immune response is both outmoded and wrong.[8,22]

It is known that foreign substances usually evoke specific immune responses of both a cellular and a humoral nature when introduced into an organism. In 1948 Sir Peter Medawar demonstrated the homology between leukocytes and tissue antigens in rabbits and that allograft rejection is based on a specific reaction to these histocompatibility antigens of the donor.[29] Similar leukoagglutinins have been demonstrated after blood transfusions and pregnancies.[30,34,47] Techniques have been developed to specify these tissue antigens. The earlier macroleukoagglutination techniques have been replaced by the microlymphocytotoxicity complement–dependent assays that were initially introduced by Terasaki and McClelland in 1964.[42,46] These tissue-typing techniques have become more standardized, more rapid, more reliable, and more reproducible in laboratories throughout the United States, Europe, and the rest of the world.

HLA Loci. The cellular antigens have been named the "human leukocyte antigens" (HLA) and represent the major histocompatibility complex (MHC) in man, accounting for the main target in the rejection process. These antigens, which are present on the surface of virtually all nucleated cells, are the products of a closely linked cluster of genes on a single chromosome (six). Each HLA locus has multiple alleles that code for different tissue antigens, with the four major loci designated HLA A, B, C, and DR. There are now over 80 specificities in the major histocompatibility complex, and there have been 10 international histocompatibility workshops and conferences to determine and define new antigen types.[53]

Structure of HLA A, B, C, and DR. There are two main structural classes of antigens—class I, or HLA

A, B, C, and class II, or HLA DR, DQ, or DP. HLA-A,B,C is a polypeptide and has a heavy chain of molecular weight 44,000 daltons that possesses a single asparagine-linked oligosaccharide unit, which carries the allotypic determinant.[33] These products are transmembrane glycoproteins associated with a smaller peptide, a nonpolymorphic beta$_2$-microglobulin, and are located on the surface of virtually all nucleated cells.[9]

In contrast to the HLA A, B, and C, the HLA-DR antigen is a class II antigen that comprises two polypeptide chains of molecular weight 34,000 and 28,000 daltons—the transmembrane alpha and beta chains. The main structural polymorphism and therefore the alloantigenic determinant resides in the beta chain.[33] There are now at least three loci encoding class II antigens, officially designated HLA DP, DQ, or DR and in all cases the products include an alpha and beta glycoprotein.[38] It is believed that the HLA-DR antigen is of major concern in transplantation immunology.[2]

Localization of Human Leukocyte Antigens in Cornea. Immunohistologic techniques using monoclonal antibodies directed against the monomorphic determinants of class I and class II molecules succeeded in mapping out the location of these antigens in the human cornea. The corneal epithelium stains for class I antigen with an increase in staining pattern located nearer the limbus than centrally.[11,52] The stromal keratocytes also express class I antigens. It has recently been confirmed that the corneal endothelium can express these antigens not only in vitro but also in vivo induced after the stimulation with interferon.[16,54]

Class II antigens are found on a limited number of cells in man—the cell surface of B-lymphocytes, macrophages, glomerular endothelium, and mesangium and on intertubular structures of the kidney and dendritic cells.[9,38] They have been found in the corneal epithelium in the form of Langerhans' cells.[20,27,43] These cells seem to be more prominent in the limbal and conjunctival area but can be induced to migrate to the central corneal area with inflammation.

Class II antigens have recently been found in the corneal stroma in the form of dendritic cells, which also appear in the kidney and many other organs.[27,43] These cells help process foreign antigen to stimulate the host's immune system and are themselves highly immunogenic.[38] Recent reports of rejected corneal discs revealed class II antigens on the corneal endothelium. Rabbits can be induced to express this antigen on the corneal endothelium after ovalbumin-induced primary uveitis.[10] Using a rat model of corneal transplantation we were able to induce class II antigen on corneal epithelium, keratocytes, and endothelium in corneal grafts. Whether this was attributable to the inflammatory response, to the release of lymphokines or interferon, or to the rejection response itself remains unclear.[28]

HLA and Rejection. How are these antigens related to the corneal rejection response? The polymorphism in the A, B, and DR antigens of the recipient and the donor are the most important stimuli for graft destruction. Recent evidence indicates that helper T-cells may be critical for the induction of an effective rejection response. It seems that both the cytotoxic T-cell (directed mainly at class I antigens) and helper T-cells (stimulated mainly by class II antigens for such delayed hypersensitivity reactions) contribute to the rejection of MHC-incompatible allografts.[24,25] The efficacy of how the response is provoked or how it arises depends on the expression or accessibility of these antigens within the graft.[31,35]

Microlymphocytotoxicity Test. The process of determining the specificities of the human leukocyte antigens is called "tissue typing" and is performed using the microlymphocytotoxicity complement–dependent test, which has not changed dramatically since introduced by Terasaki and McClelland in 1964.[42,46] Briefly the patient's lymphocytes are separated by density-gradient centrifugation. T-lymphocytes express class I antigen on their cell surface, whereas B-lymphocytes express both class I and II antigens. For HLA class I (A, B, C) typing, the patient's T-lymphocytes (or B-cells for class II) are tested against a large panel of known antisera, which define each of the HLA class I alleles. Briefly, 1 μl of cells (2 × 10^2) are mixed with 1 μl of antiserum in a microtest tray under liquid paraffin (to prevent evaporation). After a 30-minute incubation, 5 μl of rabbit serum is added as a source of complement. The trays are then incubated further for 1 hour (class I) or 2 hours (class II) followed by staining with eosin and fixation with formalin. Each well is then examined, and the percentage of cell lysis is assessed. From this analysis the tissue type is determined. More recently the use of immunomagnetic beads have been introduced to enable cell purification. These procedures are now quite routine in many laboratories throughout the United States and the world. Certainly any hospital where kidney or heart transplantation is performed utilizes these tests.

Crossmatching. We now know that class I and class II antigens can induce an antibody response.[29,39,44] Their role in the success of kidney grafts has been known for many years. The phenomenon of hyperacute rejection of kidney grafts

whereby antigen-antibody complexes form and are deposited in the vasculature of the kidney during surgery is also well known.[23] Invariably the kidney dies. For this reason all kidney transplantation centers and those engaged in other organ transplantation require a crossmatch between the patient's serum and the donor's lymphocytes to see if there has been any prior sensitization to these antigens.

The technique is not difficult and is less costly than HLA A, B, or DR tissue typing. The patient's serum is tested against a panel of typed lymphocytes in a microlymphocytotoxicity test as previously described. The patient's serum can be frozen, stored, and tested against a potential donor's lymphocytes to determine if there had been any prior sensitization before renal transplantation.

The role of these performed antibodies in corneal graft rejection is not clear.[32,36] Because the donor cornea is not vascularized, hyperacute rejection cannot take place, but it may act as a marker for cellular sensitization. Stark reported initially good results using negatively crossmatched corneal grafts. He noted a 78% survival rate in 86 high-risk cases.[40,41] Although this study provides evidence that these performed antibodies may be involved in the rejection response, there were no positive crossmatch controls to determine if there was an increased incidence of rejection in these cases.

High-Risk Cases. One must establish what constitutes a high-risk case, thereby justifying the use of tissue-matched material. Those patients with either previous graft rejection and failure or corneal vascularization in more than two quadrants represent a high risk for corneal transplantation.[22]

Results of Cases. The following report reviews the results of 450 cases performed at Queen Victoria Hospital (East Grinstead, England) over a 14-year period using tissue-typed and tissue-matched corneal grafts.[6,7,17-19,28] Our risk factors were as follows: At low risk are those patients with avascular corneas in first-time grafts, usually patients with keratoconus, the classic stromal dystrophies, and Fuchs' dystrophy as well. At medium risk are those patients with minimal to moderate vessels and no, one, or two previous grafts, usually patients with herpes simplex keratitis, bacterial keratitis, and failures from the first group. At high risk are those cases with the two worst features in common— severe vascularization and at least two previous grafts failing from rejection—usually patients with chemical burns or regrafted herpes simplex keratitis.

In the present study there were 142 low-risk, 156 medium-risk, and 152 high-risk cases. The low-risk cases seemed to do well whether matched or not, because they were 88%, 94%, 91%, and 100% clear at 1 and 2 years respectively for no, one, two, and three antigen matches. In the medium-risk cases, the survival rates were 76%, 78%, 90%, and 100% clarity at 1 and 2 years for no, one, two, and three antigen matches respectively. When those patients sharing no or one antigen were grouped against those sharing two or three antigens, the results were 76% versus 92% clarity at 1 and 2 years—significant at the *p* <0.1 level.

The high-risk cases showed survivals of 65%, 75%, 74%, and 92% for no, one, two, and three matches respectively. At 2 years the survival rate dropped to 57%, 51%, 74%, and 69%. When we examined the no match and one match versus two and three matches, the difference became 72% versus 76% at 1 year and 50% versus 76% survival at 2 years (*p* <0.1). Other researchers have confirmed our findings.[3,12-15,45] Recently Boisjoly and co-workers[4,5] in Canada in a prospective study of 438 recipients of known HLA type showed that recipients with zero or one mismatched antigen at the HLA-A or HLA-B locus had lower rejection rates than recipients with two mismatched antigens. Her group took into account corneal vascularization and donor size. Having two mismatched antigens of either the HLA-A or the HLA-B locus increased the likelihood of endothelial allograft reactions approximately twofold. Two mismatches resulted in 60% 36-month allograft survival versus 81% survival in grafts with zero or one mismatch (*p* <0.0002). They had an unexpected finding of a strong association between allograft reactions and HLA-A or HLA-B incompatibility in unvascularized recipients of small grafts. Such results need to be confirmed by other investigators. Their analysis of HLA-DR matching was not statistically significant but 4 of 18 recipients with perfect HLA-A and HLA-B matches suffered a rejection episode; none of these had a perfect HLA-DR match. On the other hand, 15 of 18 recipients with a total of four mismatched antigens at the HLA-A and HLA-B loci did not suffer from an allograft reaction. They all had good HLA-DR matches or 1 mismatched antigen. Beekhuis also had a 3-year survival rate of 76.3% in high-risk transplantation using HLA-A and B matching. They were unable to achieve statistical significance with HLA-DR matching.[1] Völker-Dieben, Kok-van Alphen, and Foulks have published similar results.[14,48-51] More and more centers in the United States and Europe have been using tissue-typed grafts.[21]

It may be difficult to draw conclusions from a series of grafts with so many variables because even a four-antigen HLA-A,B match is not an autograft. For this reason further study of the class II system, the HLA-DR antigens, seems warranted.[37] Many kidney transplant centers use HLA-DR matching as a criterion for the recipient. In corneal transplantation a small series of cases provided evidence that HLA-DRw6–positive patients had a worse prognosis if they were not matched.[48] We have begun a prospective study of HLA-DR tissue-matched transplants using criteria similar to those in our previous series of HLA-A,B–matched grafts. Using only small numbers at this time we may be able to improve graft survival to 75% at 1 year in 85% of the patients with previous graft rejections.[28]

Tissue Matching for Eye Banks. It behooves the eye bank to know the indications for corneal transplants performed in the community and to speak to the ophthalmologists in the area to see if there are several high-risk cases being performed. If that is so, the corneal surgeon and the eyebank must have access to a tissue-typing laboratory that can store recipient serum for later tissue matching and crossmatching.

Certain logistical problems must be considered before one begins tissue matching. A large volume of donor corneal tissue is ideal, particularly from younger age groups. In older donors dying of cancer who have received chemotherapy there may be a depletion of white cells, which makes it difficult to obtain a tissue type. Cadaver time is also an important factor because as the time lengthens there is less of a likelihood that the peripheral blood lymphocytes will be viable enough for obtainment of the tissue type. Technicians need training in the techniques of obtaining blood from cadavers. We have seen many instances whereby the donor cornea has been excellent and used as a donor but donor blood could not be obtained or it clotted in the test tube. Finally once a reasonable match has been obtained, a recipient must be called, the case scheduled in the operating room, and the surgery completed within the usual times for available corneal storage media.

Excellent sources of donor material that are fresh, relatively young, usually without severe systemic disease, and already tissue typed are the donors that are used for kidney transplantation. Unfortunately many of the eyes from these donors are not obtained principally because of lack of communication between kidney transplant teams and eye banks. All too often permission is not obtained for removal of the eyes for fear of jeopardizing obtaining consent for the kidneys. If some of theses obstacles were overcome, more donor tissue could be obtained.

There have been recent trends in this country to correct this.

REFERENCES

1. Beekhuis WH et al: Corneal graft survival in HLA-A and HLA-B– matched transplantation in high-risk cases with retrospective review of HLA-DR compatibility, *Cornea* 10:9, 1991.
2. Bodmer J, Bodmer W: Histocompatibility 1984, *Immunol Today* 5:251, 1984.
3. Boisjoly HM et al: Results of HLA-A/B and DR matching in corneal grafting, *Invest Ophthalmol Vis Sci* 26(suppl):78, 1985 (ARVO abstracts).
4. Boisjoly HM et al: Effect of factors unrelated to tissue matching on corneal endothelial rejection, *Am J Ophthalmol* 107:647, 1989.
5. Boisjoly HM et al: HLA-A,-B, and -DR matching in corneal transplantation, *Ophthalmology* 93:1290, 1986.
6. Callahan D et al: Rejection of orthopic corneal transplant in the rat, *ARVO Abstracts,* p 195, 1987.
7. Casey TA, Mayer DJ: *The influence of HLA compatibility in corneal graft rejection,* Presented at the International Ophthalmological Congress, San Francisco, 1982.
8. Casey TA, Mayer DJ: *Corneal grafting: principles and practice,* Philadelphia, 1984, Saunders.
9. Daar AS et al: The detailed distribution of IILA-A,B,C antigens in normal human organs, *Transplantation* 38:287, 1984.
10. Donnelly JJ, Li W, Rockey JH, Prendergast RA: Class II (Ia) alloantigens induced on corneal endothelium in vivo, *Invest Ophthalmol Vis Sci* 26(suppl):316, 1985 (ARVO abstracts).
11. Dreizen NG et al: Laser densitometric analysis of class I HLA antigens in corneal epithelium, *Invest Ophthalmol Vis Sci* 26(suppl):78, 1985 (ARVO abstracts).
12. Ehlers N, Kissmeyer-Nielsen F: Influence of histocompatibility on the fate of the corneal transplant. In Porter R, Knight J, editors: Corneal graft failure, *Ciba Found Symp* 15:307-322, Amsterdam, 1973, Elsevier.
13. Ehlers N, Kissmeyer-Nielsen F: Corneal transplantation and HLA histocompatibility: a preliminary communication, *Acta Ophthalmol* 57:738, 1979.
14. Foulks GN, Sanfilippo F: Beneficial effects of histocompatibility in high-risk corneal transplantation, *Am J Ophthalmol* 94:622, 1982.
15. Fronterre A, Trimarchi F, Bo G: HLA antigens and selection of donors in corneal transplantation, *Curr Ther Res* 27:749, 1980.
16. Fujikawa LS et al: Expression of HLA-A/B/C and DR locus antigens on epithelial, stromal, and endothelial cells of the human cornea, *Cornea,* 1:213, 1982.
17. Gibbs DC, Batchelor JR, Casey TA: The influence of HLA compatibility on the fate of corneal grafts. In Porter R, Knight J, editors: Corneal graft failure, *Ciba Found Symp* 15:293, Amsterdam, 1973, Elsevier.
18. Gibbs DC et al: The influence of tissue type compatibility on the fate of full-thickness corneal grafts, *Trans Ophthalmol Soc UK* 94:101, 1974.
19. Gibbs DC et al: HLA matching and corneal graft rejection, *Doc Ophthalmol Proc Series* 20:139, 1980.
20. Gillette TE, Chandler JW, Greiner JV: Langerhans cells of the ocular surface, *Ophthalmology* 89:700, 1982.
21. Hoffman F et al: Importance of HLA-DR matching for corneal transplantation in high risk cases, *Cornea* 5:139, 1986.
22. Khodadoust AA: The allograft rejection reaction: the leading cause of late failure of clinical corneal grafts. In Porter R, Knight J, editors: Corneal graft failure, *Ciba Found Symp* 15:151, Amsterdam, 1973, Elsevier.
23. Kissmeyer-Nielsen F et al: Hyperacute rejection of kidney allografts associated with pre-existing humoral antibodies against donor cells, *Lancet* 2:662, 1966.
24. Loveland BE, McKenzie IFC: Which T cells cause graft rejection? *Transplantation* 33:217, 1982.
25. Mason DW et al: Functions of rat T-lymphocyte subsets isolated by means of monoclonal antibodies, *Immunol Rev* 74:57, 1984.
26. Mayer DJ: Induction of class I and class II major histocompatibility complex antigens in a rat model of corneal transplantation, Acta XXV Concilium Ophthalmologicum, Rome, May 4-10, 1986, p 125, 1987.
27. Mayer DJ et al: Localization of HLA-A,B,C, and HLA-DR antigens in the human cornea: practical significance for grafting technique and HLA typing, *Transplant Proc* 15:126, 1983.
28. Mayer DJ et al: Reducing the risk of corneal graft rejection: a comparison of different methods, *Cornea* 6:241, 1987.
29. Medawar P: Immunity to homologous grafted skin. II. The fate of skin homografts transplanted to the brain, to subcutaneous tissue, and anterior chamber of the eye, *Br J Exp Pathol* 29:58, 1948.
30. Miescher P, Fauconnet M: Mise en évidence de différents groupes leucocytaires chez l'homme, *Schweiz Med Wochenschr* 84:597, 1954.
31. Milton AD, Fabre JW: Massive induction of donor type class I and class II major histocompatibility complex antigens in rejecting cardiac allografts in the rat, *J Exp Med* 161:98, 1985.
32. Nelken E, Nelken D: Serological studies in keratoplasty, *Br J Ophthalmol* 49:159, 1965.
33. Owen MJ, Crumpton MJ: Biochemistry of major human histocompatibility antigen, *Immunol Today* 1:117, Dec 1980.
34. Payne R, Rolfs MR: Fetomaternal leukocyte incompatibility, *J Clin Invest* 37:1756, 1958.
35. Peeler JS, Niederkorn JY, Matoba AY: Cellular immune response to murine heterotopic corneal allografts: induction of cytotoxic T-lymphocytes but not delayed type hypersensitivity, *Invest Ophthalmol Vis Sci* 26(suppl):75, 1985 (ARVO abstracts).
36. Polack FM: Clinical and pathological aspects of the corneal graft reaction, *Trans Am Acad Ophthalmol Otolaryngol* 77:418, 1973.
37. Ray-Keil L, Gillette TE, Chandler JW: Murine heterotopic corneal transplantation: reduction in rejection rates by pretreatment of donor corneas with ultraviolet light, *Invest Ophthalmol Vis Sci* 26(suppl):78, 1985 (ARVO abstracts).
38. Shackelford DA et al: HLA-DR antigens: structure, separation of subpopulations, gene cloning and function, *Immunol Rev* 66:133, 1982.
39. Stark WJ et al: Sensitization to human lymphocyte antigens by corneal transplantation, *Invest Ophthalmol Vis Sci* 12:639, 1973.
40. Stark WJ et al: Histocompatibility (HLA) antigens and keratoplasty, *Am J Ophthalmol* 86:595, 1978.
41. Stark WJ et al: Transplantation antigens and keratoplasty, *Austral J Ophthalmol* 11:333, 1983.
42. Terasaki PI, McClelland JD: Microdroplet assay of human serum cytotoxins, *Nature* 204:998, 1964.
43. Treseler PA, Foulks GN, Sanfilippo F: The expression of HLA antigens by cells in the human cornea, *Am J Ophthalmol* 98:763, 1984.
44. Treseler PA, Foulks GN, Sanfilippo F: Contribution of major histocompatibility complex (MHC) antigens and individual corneal cell populations to the immunogenicity of corneal allografts, *Invest Ophthalmol Vis Sci* 26(suppl):316, 1985 (ARVO abstracts).

45. Vannas S et al: HLA-compatible donor cornea for the prevention of allograft rejection, *Albrecht von Graefes Arch Klin Exp Ophthalmol* 198:217, 1976.

46. van Rood JJ: Microlymphocytotoxicity method. In Ray J editor: *NIAID manual of tissue typing techniques*, National Institute of Health (NIH) 80:104, 1980.

47. van Rood JJ, Ernisse JG, van Leeuwen A: Leukocyte antibodies in sera from pregnant women, *Nature* 181:1735, 1958.

48. Völker-Dieben HJM: *The effect of immunological and non-immunological factors on corneal graft survival*, The Hague, 1984, Dr. W. Junk bv Publisher.

49. Völker-Dieben HJM, Kok-van Alphen CC, Kruit PJ: Advances and disappointments, indications and restriction regarding HLA-matched corneal grafts in high risk cases, *Doc Ophthalmol* 46:219, 1979.

50. Völker-Dieben HJM et al: First experiences with HLA-matched corneal grafts in high risk cases, *Doc Ophthalmol* 44:39, 1977.

51. Völker-Dieben HJM et al: The effect of prospective HLA-A and HLA-B matching on corneal graft survival, *Acta Ophthalmol* 60:203, 1982.

52. Whitsett CF, Stulting RD: The distribution of HLA antigens on human corneal tissue, *Invest Ophthalmol Vis Sci* 25:519, 1984.

53. World Health Organization HLA Nomenclature Committee meeting summary: Nomenclature for factors of the HLA system 1980: In Terasaki P, editor: *Histocompatibility testing 1980*, Los Angeles, 1980, UCLA Tissue Typing Lab.

54. Young F, Stark WJ, Prendergast RA: Modulation of cell surface antigen expression in cultured human corneal cells, *Invest Ophthalmol Vis Sci* 26(suppl):316, 1985 (ARVO abstracts).

THE ROLE OF CORNEAL ANTIGENS IN GRAFT SUCCESS OR FAILURE
GARY N. FOULKS
FRED SANFILIPPO

The human cornea is an immunogenic tissue. It is well recognized that a cornea transplanted from a donor to a recipient is capable of evoking an immune response that can result in graft rejection and failure. The nature of antigen expression by the cornea that is responsible for such events has only recently been explored, however. Localization of the antigens of the human major histocompatibility complex (HLA) to certain corneal cells has been reported,[19,38,51,58] as has the presence of other important transplantation antigens such as the ABH antigens.[12,16,26,46] The presence of passenger cells of hematopoietic origin within the corneal tissue also may significantly contribute to the immunogenicity of grafted corneal tissue, but information about the types and numbers of such cells is incomplete.[35] Furthermore, the expression of intercellular adhesion molecules pertinent to the processing and trafficking of leukocytes that participate in the immune response has only recently been characterized.[15,29,36] Similarity of structural antigenic markers between corneal cells and analogous noncorneal cells with immunogenic potential may provide additional infor-

mation about the immunologic basis of corneal allograft rejection.

Antigen Expression in Human Cornea
Methods of analysis. The search for antigen markers in the cornea has taken many technical turns, and thus interpretation of the reported results and comparison of data hinge on recognition of the method of analysis used and its limitations. Extremely sensitive improvements in immunoperoxidase techniques[31] and the use of monoclonal as well as polyclonal antibodies have enhanced the detection of antigen markers and allowed critical evaluation of previously reported data. An excellent example is the data regarding expression of ABO blood group antigens by the cornea.

ABO antigens. Nelken and associates found A and B blood group antigens in preparations of whole, minced cornea in 1956.[39] Using immunofluorescence techniques available in 1972, Herold detected ABO antigens only in the epithelium of corneas obtained at autopsy.[26] Later studies of specific red blood cell adherence indicated the possible presence of ABO antigens in corneal epithelium and endothelium but not in stroma.[12] Peroxidase-antiperoxidase methods localized these same blood group antigens to the corneal endothelium.[46] Using the very sensitive avidin-biotin-complex immunoperoxidase technique and monoclonal antibodies directed against human ABO blood group antigens, we found these antigens expressed by normal human corneal epithelial cells but absent from other layers including stroma and endothelium[52] (Fig. 46-45). Our studies also indicate that the strength of expression of blood group antigen A on corneal epithelial cells may increase with age and proceeds with maturation from H precursors similar to that observed with erythrocytes.[8,24,49,57] Since ABH antigens have been shown to act as important human histocompatibility antigens,[9,25,34,37,44] the expression of these antigens on epithelial cells of the cornea could implicate them in corneal allograft rejection but not necessarily in destruction of the endothelium.

HLA antigens—class I. Cultured corneal epithelial and stromal cells express class I HLA antigens as originally described by Newsome and co-workers[40] and as confirmed by Whitsett and Stulting.[58] Cultured endothelial cells as reported by Fujikawa[19] and confirmed by Whitsett and Stulting[58] also express class I HLA antigens. Testing in vivo for expression of such antigens has given mixed results, however.[19,58] Fujikawa and co-workers using immunofluorescent and immunoperoxidase techniques could not detect class I HLA antigens on endothelial whole flat mounts.[19] Similar results are reported by

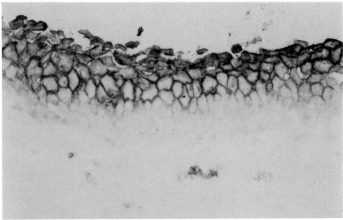

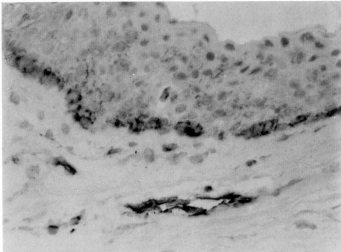

Fig. 46-45. Immunoperoxidase labeling of blood group A antigen expression of human corneas. **A,** Staining is predominantly of superficial epithelium (525×). **B,** Staining is predominantly of basal epithelium (325×). Both corneas also show staining of limbal vascular endothelium. (From Treseler PA, Foulks GN, Sanfilippo F: *Am J Ophthalmol* 98(6):763-772, 1984. Published with permission from The American Journal of Ophthalmology. Copyright by The Ophthalmic Publishing Company.)

Williams and co-workers.[59] With an indirect immunofluorescence and immunoperoxidase technique Whitsett and Stulting demonstrated class I HLA antigens only on cornea from donors less than 2 years of age but not on older donors.[58] Using the sensitive ABC immunoperoxidase technique and a panel of monoclonal antibodies reactive with various monomorphic and polymorphic HLA antigen determinants, we readily demonstrated class I HLA antigens on corneal epithelial, stromal, and endothelial cells regardless of donor age[52] (Figs. 46-46 and 46-47). Interestingly, in our studies the intensity of antigen

expression increased greatly from the central to the limbal epithelium where staining generally matched or exceeded that of vascular endothelial cells at the limbus. We noticed no appreciable variation of intensity of staining with age.

HLA antigens—class II. Class II HLA antigens have been localized in normal corneas to dendritic and cuboidal cells scattered through the central and peripheral epithelium and stroma of the cornea but not to keratocytes or endothelial cells (Figs. 46-48 and 46-49).[19,21,38,45,51,58] This is consistent with the findings in cultured corneal fibroblasts and endothelial preparations that also fail to express class II antigens.[19,40]

Induction of expression of class II antigens has been seen in endothelial cells in culture when exposed to gamma-interferon and during episodes of graft rejection and uveitis.[11,18,60] This process may be analogous to that seen in epidermis and gut epithelium.[4,10,41,42]

The class II HLA antigen expression present in normal corneal tissue probably represents the presence of Langerhans cells.[21,45,52,59] Their presence probably contributes to the immunogenicity of the corneal tissue and indicates that passenger cells may be an important part of the process of graft rejection.[59]

Intercellular adhesion molecules. Constitutive expression of the intercellular adhesion molecule-1 (ICAM-1), which serves as the cellular ligand that binds the lymphocyte function—associated antigen-1 (LFA-1) present on all leukocytes, has been confirmed for corneal endothelial cells.[15,29] Since this ligand appears to regulate binding of leukocytes both to vascular and to corneal endothelium,[13] it is reasonable to surmise a role in the clinical inflammatory conditions attended by focal adherence of leukocytes to the corneal endothelium. Also, since ICAM-1 appears to modulate leukocyte trafficking in the inflamed dermis,[14] it may exert a similar modulation for corneal inflammation. Since the expression of ICAM-1 is responsive to cytokine stimulation in a manner similar to that of HLA-DR and with the observation that coexpression of ICAM-1 and HLA-DR is critical to HLA class II antigen—restricted, cell-specific T-cell activation, ICAM-1 probably plays an important role in T-cell immunity[48] and may be important in antigen recognition and processing.

Hematopoietically derived cell antigens. Using the panel of monoclonal antibodies directed against hematopoietically derived cells listed in Table 46-13 in combination with the ABC immunoperoxidase technique, we were able to demonstrate reactivity of cells

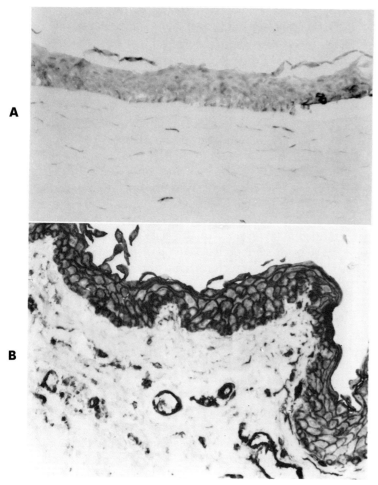

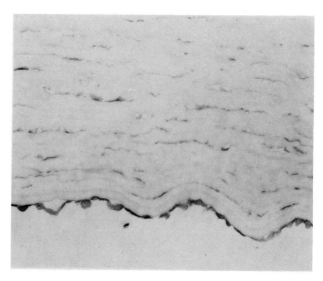

Fig. 46-47. Immunoperoxidase staining of adult human corneal endothelium using monoclonal antibody (W6/32) against human class I HLA antigens. (325×.) (From Treseler PA, Foulks GN, Sanfilippo F: *Am J Ophthalmol* 98:763, 1984.)

Fig. 46-46. Immunoperoxidase staining of central, **A,** and peripheral, **B,** corneal epithelium and stroma from human cornea using monoclonal antibody (anti-HLA) against human class I HLA antigens. (325×.) (From Treseler PA, Foulks GN, Sanfilippo F: *Am J Ophthalmol* 98:763, 1984.)

scattered throughout the cornea but with more prominent reaction at the limbus[52] (Fig. 46-50). Isolated cells staining with CD45, which identifies virtually all hematopoietically derived cells except mature erythrocytes, were sometimes dendritic but often lacked cytoplasmic processes. These probably represent Langerhans cells, which have also been identified by their HLA-DR antigen expression. Williams and co-workers have reported similar localization of passenger cells in human corneas and have documented increased numbers of such cells in diseased corneas carrying an anticipated high risk of graft rejection.[59]

Cell-specific antigens. Table 46-14 summarizes the expression of a variety of antigens as detected by the ABC immunoperoxidase technique.[52] The expression of a vascular endothelial cell marker by the corneal endothelium (Fig. 46-51) as well as endothelium of the limbal vasculature may indicate antigenic similarity as does reactivity with antisera specific for human myosin. Absence of staining of the corneal endothelium with anti–factor VIII related antigen, however, shows that they are not strictly comparable. This dissimilarity of corneal endothelium and vascular endothelium holds as well for antigens recognized by a monoclonal antibody that is raised against corneal endothelium in Balb/c mice (designated 2B4.14.1) and strongly reacts with corneal endothelium but is nonreactive with vascular endothelial cells. The corneal endothelium apparently shares antigenic expression, however, with several other tissues recognized by mAb 2B4.14.1, including renal tubules, glandular epithelia, mesothelial surfaces, and Tamm-Horsfall urinary glycoprotein.[29,30] Antibodies reactive with human keratin consistently stain corneal epithelial cells, whereas antisera specific for human myosin and myoglobin stain some epithelial cells mildly to moderately and most endothelial cells intensely. Antiserum against human fibronectin stains stromal cells as well as basal lamina of both corneal endothelial and limbal vascular endothelial cells.

Clinical Studies of Histocompatibility. Data regarding possible benefit of histocompatibility testing

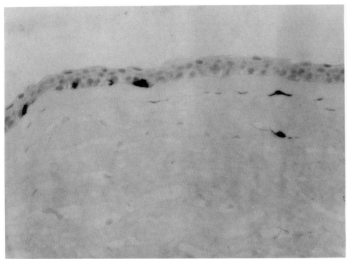

Fig. 46-48. Immunoperoxidase staining of central corneal epithelium and stroma from human cornea using monoclonal antibody (1.19.15) against class II HLA antigens. (325×.) (From Treseler PA, Foulks GN, Sanfilippo F: *Am J Ophthalmol* 98:763, 1984.)

Fig. 46-49. Immunoperoxidase staining of adult corneal endothelium using monoclonal antibody (1.19.15) against class II HLA antigens. (325×.) (From Treseler PA, Foulks GN, Sanfilippo F: *Am J Ophthalmol* 98:763, 1984.)

Table 46-13. Antibodies Used to Localize Hematopoietic Cell Antigen Expression

Specificity	Antibody
CD45	T29/33
CD2	T11
CD7	3A1
CD5	Leu 1
CD4	Leu 3a
CD8	Leu 2a
CD3	Leu 4
CD57	Leu 7
CD20	B1
CD14	Leu M3

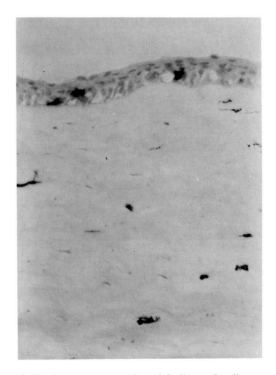

Table 46-14. Expression of Cell-Specific Antigens in Human Cornea

	Antibody Specificity			
Location	Vascular Endothelium	Factor VIII	Keratin	Myosin
Epithelium	1+	—	4+	1-2+
Stroma	—	—	—	—
Endothelium	2-4+	—	—	2-4+
Limbal vessel	2-4+	2-4+	—	3-4+

1+, Slight but significantly above background.
4+, Maximal staining intensity.

Fig. 46-50. Immunoperoxidase labeling of cells expressing CD45 (leukocyte common antigen) in the human cornea. Positive cells are present in the epithelium and stroma. (525×.) (From Treseler PA, Foulks GN, Sanfilippo F: *Am J Ophthalmol* 98:763, 1984.)

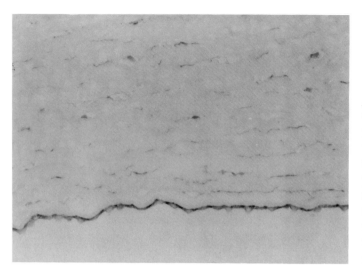

Fig. 46-51. Immunoperoxidase staining of cells expressing HuEE12 antigen (human vascular endothelium) in the human cornea. Staining is predominantly of corneal endothelium. (525×.) (From Treseler PA, Foulks GN, Sanfilippo F: *Am J Ophthalmol* 98:763, 1984.)

for human corneal transplantation are conflicting.* Early studies indicated no probable direct benefit of tissue matching for either ABO or HLA antigen systems.[1,2] Later retrospective studies in Europe and prospective studies in Europe and the United States addressing patients at high risk of allograft rejection by virtue of corneal vascularization and prior graft rejection strongly indicated an improved graft survival in patients well matched at the class I HLA antigen loci.† Most recent analysis of our data in a prospective, double-masked observational trial shows that patients well matched for the class I HLA antigens have a better chance of avoiding allograft rejection. After a 3-year follow-up study well-matched patients (two or more shared class I HLA antigens) experienced rejection episodes in 18% of patients, whereas poorly matched patients had a 39% incidence of allograft reaction.[47] Interestingly, a small subset of these high-risk patients receiving ABO-incompatible donors had a much worse result with respect to graft rejection, but it is difficult to interpret such data because of the small number of patients with ABO incompatibility.

Implications for Corneal Graft Rejection. The patterns of antigen expression described for the human cornea may help us to understand some of the clinical observations that have been made of corneal allograft rejection. Presence of class I HLA antigens on corneal epithelium indicates a possible source of immunogenic and target antigens in that densely populated layer and may explain the clinical observation that removal of epithelium at the time of keratoplasty may decrease the incidence of graft rejection.[53] Our finding that such class I HLA antigen expression is greater in the periphery provides supplemental information to explain the improved survival of smaller corneal grafts, which was previously attributed solely to the exclusion from such grafts of peripheral dendritic cells with reduction of HLA-DR antigen load.[38] Identification of class I HLA antigens on all three layers of the cornea (epithelium, stroma, and endothelium) would be consistent with the recognized rejection of individual layers of the cornea.[32] The presence of class I HLA antigens on the endothelium could also represent target antigens involved in graft rejection and would help to explain the reports of improved allograft survival in patients well matched at the class I HLA locus.*

The expression of class II HLA antigens by scattered dendritic cells in the epithelium with increased frequency in the limbal periphery is well established.[21,45,59] This distribution along with identification of similar cells in the stroma[51,58] has been used to explain the better survival of smaller corneal grafts as previously mentioned[38,56] and indicates that even in the absence of epithelium human corneal grafts contain passenger cells that may provide allogenic stimulation with ultimate graft rejection.[53] Improvement of graft survival by depletion of such cells through physical or chemical treatment adds further evidence to the immunomodulating capability of such cells.[5,7,43]

Our finding in a small number of high-risk patients that ABO incompatibility of the donor and recipient may mean greater chance of graft rejection is compatible with the expression of ABH antigens on the corneal epithelium and the information available about the immunogenicity of such antigens in other transplantation systems.[9,25,34,40,44] The expression of non-MHC antigens on the corneal endothelium provides evidence of other potential targets of allograft rejection that may contribute to the immunogenicity of the cornea upon transplantation.[29,30]

The antigenic similarities of corneal endothelium and vascular endothelium raise interesting questions. The functional similarities of the two cell types include the ability to secrete basal laminae and provide an active fluid pump.[22] Since the vascular endothelium has been shown to participate in al-

---

*References 1, 2, 3, 17, 20, 23, 33, 50, 54, 56.
†References 3, 17, 20, 23, 33, 50, 54, 56.

*References 3, 17, 20, 23, 33, 47, 50, 54, 56.

lograft rejection in vascularized organs and to possess certain immune processing capabilities, it is conceivable that the corneal endothelium may under certain conditions perform in an analogous manner.[6,22,27,28,55]

The presence on the corneal endothelium of intercellular adhesion molecules that are relevant to the trafficking of leukocytes in vascularized tissue would support such a role in mediation of allograft rejection of the cornea.

ACKNOWLEDGMENT

Jim Burchette and Julie Fuller provided excellent technical assistance.

This work is supported in part by NIH grant EY-03819 and a grant from the North Carolina Lions Association for the Blind.

REFERENCES

1. Allansmith MR, Drell DW, Kajiyama G, Fine M: ABO blood groups and corneal transplantation, *Am J Ophthalmol* 79:493-501, 1975.
2. Allansmith MR, Fine M, Payne R: Histocompatibility typing and corneal transplantation, *Trans Am Acad Ophthalmol Otolaryngol* 78:445-460, 1974.
3. Batchelor JR, Casey TA, Gibbs DC, et al: HLA matching and corneal grafting, *Lancet* 1:551-554, 1976.
4. Barclay AN, Mason DW: Induction of Ia antigen in rat epidermal cells and gut epithelium by immunological stimuli, *J Exp Med* 156:1665, 1982.
5. Braude LS, Chandler JW: Corneal allograft rejection: the role of the major histocompatibility complex, *Surv Ophthalmol* 27:290-305, 1983.
6. Burger DR, Ford D, Vetto RM, Hamblin A, et al: Endothelial cell presentation of antigen to human T cells, *Hum Immunol* 3:209-230, 1981.
7. Chandler JW, Ray-Keil L, Gillette TE: Experimental corneal allograft rejection: description of a murine model and a new hypothesis of immunopathogenesis, *Curr Eye Res* 2:387-397, 1983.
8. Cohen F, Warezak W, Zuelzer WW: Interrelationship of erythrocyte blood group substances A, B, and H studied with immunofluorescence, *Vox Sang* 16:105-118, 1969.
9. Dausset J, Rapaport FT: Blood group determinants of human histocompatibility. In Rapaport FT, Dausset J, editors: *Human transplantation*, New York, 1968, Grune & Stratton.
10. De Wall RMW, Bogman MJJ, Maass CN, et al: Variable expression of Ia antigens on the vascular endothelium of mouse skin allografts, *Nature* 303:426, 1983.
11. Donnelly JJ, Li W, Rochey SH, Prendergast RA: Class II alloantigens induced on corneal endothelium in vivo and in vitro, *Invest Ophthalmol Vis Sci* 26(suppl):316 1985 (ARVO abstracts).
12. Dua HS, Shidham VB: Application of specific red cell adherence test to the human cornea and conjunctiva, *Am J Ophthalmol* 88:1067-1071, 1979.
13. Dustin ML et al: Induction by IL1 and interferon-gamma: tissue distribution, biochemistry, and function of a natural adherence molecule (ICAM-1), *J Immunol* 137:245, 1986.
14. Dustin ML, Singer KH, Tuck DT, Springer TA: Adhesion of T lymphoblasts to epidermal keratinocytes is regulated by interferon-gamma and is mediated by intercellular adhesion molecule-1 (ICAM-1), *J Exp Med* 167:1323, 1988.
15. Elner VM et al: Intercellular adhesion molecule-1 in human corneal endothelium, *Am J Pathol* 138:525, 1991.
16. Foster CS, Allansmith MR: Lack of blood group antigen A on human corneal endothelium, *Am J Ophthalmol* 87:165-170, 1979.
17. Foulks GN, Sanfilippo F: Beneficial effects of histocompatibility in high-risk corneal transplantation, *Am J Ophthalmol* 94:622-629, 1982.
18. Fujikawa LS, Chan CC, McAllister C, et al: Activation of endothelial cells in experimental autoimmune uveitis, *Invest Ophthalmol Vis Sci* 26(suppl):97, 1985 (ARVO abstracts).
19. Fujikawa LS, Colvin RB, Bhan AK, et al: Expression of HLA-A/B/C and -DR locus antigens on epithelial, stromal, and endothelial cells of the human cornea, *Cornea* 1:213-222, 1982.
20. Gibbs DC, Batchelor JR, Werb A, et al: The influence of tissue-type compatibility on the fate of full-thickness corneal drafts, *Trans Ophthalmol Soc UK* 94:101-126, 1974.
21. Gillette TE, Chandler JW, Greiner JV: Langerhans cells of the ocular surface, *Ophthalmology* 89:700-710, 1982.
22. Gospodarowicz D, Vlodavsky I, Greenburg G, et al: Studies on atherogenesis and corneal transplantation using cultured vascular and corneal endothelia, *Recent Prog Horm Res* 35:375-443, 1979.
23. Gronterre A, Trimarchi F, Bo G: HLA antigens and selection of donors in corneal transplants, *Curr Ther Res* 27:749-756, 1980.
24. Grundbacher FJ: Changes in the human A antigen of erythrocytes with the individual's age, *Nature* 204:192-194, 1964.
25. Havener WH, Stine GT, Weiss LL: Corneal donor selection by blood type, *Arch Ophthalmol* 60:443-447, 1958.
26. Herold W: Zum Nachweis der Blutgruppenantigene A und B in der menschlichen Hornhaut mittels der Immunofluoreszenztechnik, *Klin Monatbl Augenheilkd* 161:658-662, 1972.
27. Hirschberg H, Bergh OJ, Thorsby E: Antigen-presenting properties of human vascular endothelial cells, *J Exp Med* 152:249s-255s, 1980.
28. Hirschberg H, Evenson SA, Henriksen T, Thorsby E: The human mixed lymphocyte-endothelium culture interaction, *Transplantation* 19:495-504, 1975.
29. Howell DN, Burchette J, Foulks GN, Sanfilippo F: Antigen expression by human corneal endothelium, *Invest Ophthalmol Vis Sci* 32(suppl):1178, 1991.
30. Howell DN, Burchette JL Jr, Paolini JF, Geier SS, et al: Characterization of a novel human corneal endothelial antigen, *Invest Ophthalmol Vis Sci* 32:2473-2482, 1991.
31. Hsu S, Raine L, Fanger H: Use of avidin-biotin-peroxidase complex (ABC) in immunoperoxidase techniques: a comparison between ABC and unlabeled antibody (PAP) procedures, *J Histochem Cytochem* 29:577-580, 1981.
32. Khodadoust AA, Silverstein AM: Transplantation and rejection of individual cell layers of the cornea, *Invest Ophthalmol* 8:180-195, 1969.
33. Kissmeyer-Nielsen F, Ehlers N: Corneal transplantation and matching for HLA-A and HLA-B. In Ferrone S, Curtoni E, Gorini S, editors: *HLA antigens in clinical medicine and biology*, New York, 1979, Garland Publishers.
34. Kissmeyer-Nielsen F, Thorsby E: Transplantation antigens, *Transplant Rev* 4:72-85, 1970.
35. Lafferty KJ, Prowse SJ, Simeonovic CJ: Immunobiology of tissue transplantation: a return to the passenger leukocyte concept, *Annu Rev Immunol* 1:143-173, 1983.
36. Lauweryns B, van den Oord JJ, Volpes R, et al: Distribution

of very late activation integrins in the human cornea, *Invest Ophthalmol Vis Sci* 32:2079, 1991.

37. Mailath L, Stenszky V, Alberth B, Aszodi L: Die Rolle der Blutgruppenkompatibilität bei Keratoplastik, *Klin Monatsbl Augenheilkd* 160:550-553, 1972.

38. Mayer DJ, Daar AS, Casey TA, Fabre JW: Localization of HLA-A,B,C and HLA-DR antigens in the human cornea: practical significance for grafting technique and HLA typing, *Transplant Proc* 15:126-129, 1983.

39. Nelken E, Michaelson IC, Nelken D, Gurevitch J: ABO antigens in the human cornea, *Nature* 177:840, 1956.

40. Newsome DA, Takasugi M, Kenyon KR, et al: Human corneal cells in vitro: morphology and histocompatibility (HL-A) antigens of pure cell populations, *Invest Ophthalmol Vis Sci* 13:23, 1974.

41. Pober JS, Collins T, Gimbrone MA, et al: Lymphocytes recognize human vascular endothelial and dermal fibroblast Ia antigens induced by recombinant immune interferon, *Nature* 305:726, 1983.

42. Pober JS, Gimbrone MA, Cotran RS, et al: Ia expression by vascular endothelium is inducible by activated T cells and by human interferon, *J Exp Med* 157:1339, 1983.

43. Ray-Keil L, Gillette TE, Chandler JW: Murine heterotopic corneal transplantation: reduction on rejection rates by pretreatment of donor corneas with ultraviolet light, *Invest Ophthalmol Vis Sci* 26(suppl):78, 1985 (ARVO abstracts).

44. Richter, S.: Untersuchungen über Isoantikörper bei Keratoplastik, *Albrecht von Graefes Arch Klin Exp Ophthalmol* 168:131-135, 1965.

45. Rodrigues MM, Rowden G, Hackett J, Bakos I: Langerhans cells in normal conjunctiva and peripheral cornea of selected species, *Invest Ophthalmol Vis Sci* 21:759-765, 1981.

46. Salisbury JD, Gebhardt BM: Blood group antigens on human corneal cells demonstrated by immunoperoxidase staining, *Am J Ophthalmol* 91:46-50, 1981.

47. Sanfilippo F, MacQueen M, Vaughn W, et al: Histocompatibility testing in high risk corneal transplantation, *Invest Ophthalmol Vis Sci* 25(suppl):27, 1984 (ARVO abstracts).

48. Siu G, Hedrick SM, Brian AA: Isolation of the murine intercellular adhesion molecule 1 (ICAM-1) gene: ICAM-1 enhances antigen-specific T-cell activation, *J Immunol* 143:3813, 1989.

49. Solomon JM: Comparison of fetal and adult ABH antigens by the quantitative hemagglutination technic, *Transfusion* 3:185-191, 1963.

50. Stark WJ, Taylor HR, Bias WB, Maumenee AE: Histocompatibility (HLA) antigens and keratoplasty, *Am J Ophthalmol* 85:595-604, 1978.

51. Treseler PA, Foulks GN, Sanfilippo F: The expression of HLA antigens by cells in the human cornea, *Am J Ophthalmol* 98:763-772, 1984.

52. Treseler PA, Foulks GN, Sanfilippo F: The expression of HLA antigens by cells in the human cornea, *Am J Ophthalmol* 98(6):763-772, 1984.

53. Tuberville AW, Foster CS, Wood TO: The effect of donor cornea epithelium removal on the incidence of allograft rejection reactions, *Ophthalmology* 90:1351, 1983.

54. Vannas S, Karjalainen K, Ruusuvaara P, Tiilikainen A: HLA-compatible donor cornea for prevention of allograft reaction, *Albrecht von Graefes Arch Klin Exp Ophthalmol* 198:217-222, 1976.

55. Vetto RM, Burger DR: Endothelial cell stimulation of allogenic lymphocytes, *Transplantation* 14:652-654, 1972.

56. Völker-Dieben HJM, Kok-van Alphen CC, Kruit PJ: Advances and disappointments, indications and restrictions regarding HLA-matched corneal grafts in high-risk cases, *Doc Ophthalmol* 49:219-226, 1979.

57. Watkins WM, Morgan WTJ: Possible genetical pathways for the biosynthesis of blood group mucopolysaccharides, *Vox Sang* 4:97-119, 1959.

58. Whitsett CF, Stulting RD: The distribution of HLA antigens on human corneal tissue, *Invest Ophthalmol Vis Sci* 25:519-524, 1984.

59. Williams KA, Ash JK, Coster DJ: Histocompatibility antigen and passenger cell content of normal and diseased human cornea, *Transplantation* 39:265-269, 1985.

60. Young E, Stark WJ, Prendergast RA: Modulation of cell surface antigen expressions on cultured human corneal cells, *Invest Ophthalmol Vis Sci* 26(suppl):316, 1985 (ARVO abstracts).

DONOR EPITHELIUM AND REJECTION
THOMAS E. GILLETTE

Although the rejection rates of corneal transplants may be as low as 2.3% in selected cases,[40] rejection rates of 20% to 35% are more common,[15] and rejection rates as high as 40% to 65% have been reported in poor-prognosis recipients with inflamed eyes or vascularized corneas, or both.[61] Clearly, then, the concept of the cornea as an immunologically privileged transplant site is relative, and new concepts are required to understand the immunobiology of corneal graft rejection. Changes in the general concepts of allograft immunobiology have opened the door to the possibilities of donor tissue pretreatment to reduce immunogenicity in lieu of more traditional approaches to suppression of the host's immune system.[52] These approaches may be applicable to donor corneal tissue and more specifically the donor corneal epithelium, which represents the largest share of nucleated cells and thus the largest share of transplant antigens.

Allograft Immunobiology. Once Medawar had established the immunologic basis of the allograft reaction, tissue antigen was seen to be the major barrier to the allografting of tissues and organs.[54] This postulate was based on the unquestioned assumption that antigen recognition causes lymphocyte activation; that is, antigen recognition and lymphocyte activation are considered part of the same process. The concept was an important impetus for work elucidating the major histocompatibility complex (MHC) but has not solved the allograft problem.

Two-signal theory. Antigen recognition alone may not be sufficient for lymphocyte activation, however.[3,44] In a study of the graft-versus-host (GVH) reaction in chicken embryos, Lafferty unexpectedly

Supported in part by NIH grant EY-03951.

found that the reaction was species specific. Adult chicken lymphoid cells introduced into immunologically immature embryos survived, proliferated, and caused a graft-versus-host reaction. Pigeon spleen and sheep lymph node cells, however, though surviving in the embryonic host, did not cause a GVH reaction. The failure of the xenogeneic cells to cause a GVH reaction indicated that antigen contact was not a sufficient requirement for transplantation reactions.[45]

A similar conclusion came from studies of T-cell activation in vitro.[51,69] Cells killed by a variety of procedures did not stimulate incompatible T-cells, though the dead cells could be shown to express transplantation antigen. Furthermore, not all viable cells had the capacity to stimulate allogeneic T-cells in vitro. Antigen-bearing nonlymphoid cells such as fibroblasts, erythrocytes, or platelets did not stimulate normal allogeneic lymphocytes in vitro.[37]

In an attempt to explain these phenomena, Lafferty and Cunningham[44] took up the Bretscher-Cohn suggestion that two signals were required for lymphocyte activation[11] and developed a two-signal model for the initial step in T-cell activation (Fig. 46-52). Their model postulates a stimulator cell (S+) requirement for the presentation of antigen to the potentially responsive T-cell. Antigen binding by the T-cell provides one signal, whereas an inductive molecule (CoS, cosignal) is postulated to provide the second signal. Once the responsive T-cell is activated, factors that greatly amplify the overall level of proliferation in the T-cell population may be released. Provision of signal one alone (antigen recognition/binding) does not cause T-cell activation and may be tolerogenic.[5,21]

There is now clear evidence in support of the two-signal model for T-cell activation by mitogen[48] and by alloantigen.[96] The species specificity of alloreactivity is expressed at the level of the second signal (CoS). Using cloned tumor lines as the source of allogeneic stimulation, Talmage and co-workers have demonstrated the existence of stimulating (S+) and nonstimulating (S−) tumor lines, both expressing identical histocompatibility antigens; metabolic inactivation of the S+ population with ultraviolet irradiation destroys its capacity to activate a cytotoxic T-cell response. Neither the antigen on the S− cells nor CoS activity alone are sufficient for cytotoxic T-cell activation.[85]

Role of class I and class II MHC antigens. Bach et al. developed an alternative two-signal model for allogeneic T-cell activation in which recognition of the Ia epitope on the allogeneic cell activated the helper T-cell subset, which then provided the second signal for cytotoxic T-cell activation.[3] There is now evidence, however, that recognition of class II antigen is not required for cytotoxic T-cell activation, the clearest being the demonstration of cytotoxic T-cell activation when stimulator and responder strains differ only in the K region of MHC.[56] Rather, two-signal activation is seen to be important for both cytotoxic and helper T-cells and is closely correlated with but not restricted to class II (Ia antigen–bearing) cells. Class I and class II antigens are believed to activate cytotoxic and helper T-cells respectively,[12] with cells of either subclass mediating graft rejection by the synergistic effects of lymphokine release and an associated inflammatory process[2] (Fig. 46-62).

The Ia+ cell is probably the cell responsible for stimulation of both class I and class II MHC reactive T-cells in vivo, however, with the most likely candidate being the Ia-rich dendritic cell.[50] This same cell, of *host* origin, may then provide the CoS activity (second signal) necessary for allograft rejection in the face of restricted class I or minor antigen differences.[72] The two-signal model would allow prediction of an extended survival for grafts allogeneic at minor loci only, in H-2–*incompatible* hosts, avoiding an H-2–compatible S+ cell population. Silvers and co-workers have demonstrated this effect in mice.[71]

The two-signal model would also predict tissue-specific rejection phenomena based on lymphoreticular (S+ cellular) content. Lafferty and Simeonovic have seen this effect in mice, and clinical experience supports this concept.[46]

Passenger cell concept. The concept of passenger leukocytes originated in a review of the "homograft

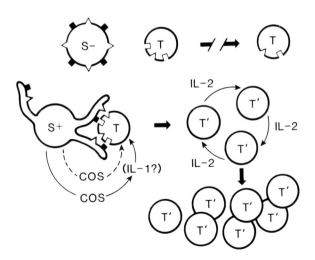

Fig. 46-52. Two-signal theory of allogeneic T-cell stimulation. S+ stimulator cell carrying transplantation antigen (signal 1) and providing CoS (signal 2). *T*, T cells.

reaction" published by Snell in 1957.[74] Snell suggested that donor leukocytes in grafts might play a particularly significant role in the induction of transplantation immunity. This was based on reports that allografted tissues taken from donors pretreated with radiation, immunosuppressive drugs, or steroids showed a reduced ability to immunize hosts to challenge allografts.[79] Implicit in Snell's reasoning was the assumption that donor pretreatment with leukocidal agents reduced graft immunogenicity by depleting the allogeneic leukocytes present in the allograft.

Supporting this concept were the observations that (1) immunization of a recipient animal with donor spleen or lymph node cells would sensitize the animal to a tumor allograft, whereas antigen extracts of the tumor were only weakly immunogenic;[39] (2) parental strain spleen cells injected into syngeneic kidneys recently grafted to F_1 hybrid rats resulted in graft destruction;[25] (3) skin isografts from murine bone marrow chimeras induced, in syngeneic hosts, a state of allograft immunity indistinguishable from that induced by skin allografts taken from normal donors;[75] (4) perfusion of embryonic heart with leukocytes before grafting to chicken embryos resulted in the activation of a violent allograft reaction.[45]

The passenger cell concept has evolved and in a sense now embraces the two-signal theory. Passenger "immunocytes" are now believed to represent Ia+ dendritic cells, the CoS provider of the two-signal theory.

Critics of the theory point to two experimental observations seemingly in conflict with the theory. Streilein and co-workers found that if donor and host differ only at the K region of the H_2 complex, heterotopic corneal allografts are rejected acutely.[80] This was interpreted to mean that class II bearing cells (Langerhans cells) were unimportant in the initiation of that rejection. Although it is arguable whether donor Langerhans cells (LC) were present to participate, in this model (matched at the I locus) it is not important. As Silvers and co-workers have shown,[72] recipient dendritic cells (LC) may have presented the allogeneic class I antigen of the donor, thus providing the S+ cell required in the two-signal theory.

Steinmuller[76] and Stuart[81] have been unable to demonstrate prolongation of mean survival time for chimeric skin grafts bearing bone marrow–derived (BMD) cells syngeneic to recipient mice. (In contrast, Woodward and colleagues[95] have shown mean survival time prolongation in this model.) Although these data also appear to refute the passenger cell theory, Silvers' data[72] must again be noted. Al-

lografts syngeneic for class II antigens can be rejected across class I differences by presentation of those class I antigens on recipient "S+" dendritic cells. An alternative explanation envisions Ia antigen induction on non-bone marrow derived (NBMD) cells of the skin graft. Other reports indicating induced expression of Ia on NBMD cells[19,20,42,47] lend credence to this possibility.

Most still believe that passenger leukocytes (dendritic cells) may be significant immunogens in organ allografts. Donor pretreatment does prolong the survival of heart and kidney allografts in laboratory animals,[34,58] and two reports indicate that rat kidney allografts taken from bone marrow chimeras survive longer than controls in untreated hosts.[35,76] The passenger cell concept may be a valuable framework then to examine the problem of corneal allograft rejection.

Corneal Allograft Rejection. As mentioned previously, the older concept of corneal immunologic privilege is clearly relative. Rejection rates are substantial in vascularized hosts.[61] New approaches are needed then to understand the mechanisms operative in corneal graft rejection. Recent data from our laboratory and others lend validity to the use of the two-signal theory and the passenger cell concept as theoretical frameworks by which to better understand corneal allograft rejection.

Histocompatibility antigens. Critical to the employment of these concepts are the presence of histocompatibility antigens within corneal tissue. An initial study of this question found class I (HLA-A,B,C) antigens on corneal epithelial and stromal cells in culture.[57] Certain recent studies were unable to detect class I antigens on stromal keratocytes,[29,53] whereas others have[87,92] (Table 46-15). All investigators have found class I antigens on corneal epithelial cells, probably indicating high antigenic density. Variance in stromal keratocyte results may indicate decreased antigenic density requiring very sensitive immunohistology for detection.[87]

Class II (HLA-DR/Ia) bearing cells have been noted in corneal epithelium by several authors,[29,43,53,87,90,92] whereas scattered stromal class II–positive cells have been occasionally seen.[29,53,87]

HLA matching. Both of the concepts just discussed would allow prediction of improved graft survival with greater matching of donor and recipient HLA antigens. This predicted improvement has been substantiated in kidney transplantation.[59]

Data relating to corneal transplantation are less clear. Stark has shown improved graft survival in crossmatch negative pairs[77] and several retrospective studies have indicated that increased matching at the

Table 46-15. Histocompatibility Antigens on Corneal Cells

	Epithelium	Stroma	Endothelium
Newsome et al., 1974 (57)	Class I (in culture)	Class I (in culture)	—
Fujikawa et al., 1982 (29)	Class I Scattered peripheral class II	— Scattered peripheral class II	Class I in culture only
Mayer et al., 1983 (53)	Class I Scattered peripheral class II	— Scattered peripheral class II	—
Whitsett et al., 1984 (91)	Class I Scattered peripheral class II	Class I	Class I below 2 years of age
Treseler et al., 1984 (87)	Class I Scattered central and peripheral class II	Class I Scattered central and peripheral class II	Class I

HLA-A and B loci may improve graft survival.[4,27,28,41,89] Others have failed to confirm these findings, however.[1,22] HLA matching appears to be most efficacious in high-risk patients.[4,6,29,38] Long-term results relating to matching at the DR locus are not available as yet, but preliminary results look promising.[9] The key importance of DR matching in kidney allograft survival[55] indicates that this issue may need further attention.

Corneal epithelial Langerhans cells. Recent evidence has been collected by several investigators defining a distinct population of dendritic cells (Langerhans cells) of mesenchymal origin residing in the epidermal surfaces of many mammalian species.[7,78] These cells carry class II histocompatibility antigen believed to be of central importance in the afferent arm of allograft rejection; that is, Langerhans cells represent the S+ phenotype in Lafferty's two-signal hypothesis for allograft rejection and can represent a significant portion of the passenger cell load in allografts of epidermal tissue (including cornea).

Historically, atypical or dendritic cells resident within conjunctival and corneal epithelium have been noted since the earliest microscopic examinations of the ocular surface.[23] No fewer than 10 investigators have noted unusual dendritic or polygonal cells in corneal epithelium by various optical and electron microscopic techniques since their earliest description by Engelmann in 1867.[26]

In recent years these cells have been assigned various names and functions including peculiar branched wiry bodies,[8] polymorph elements,[68] basal layer branched cells,[91] secretory cells,[86] polygonal cells,[83] and dendritic cells.[70]

The first investigator to suggest a similarity of these cells to the Langerhans cells of the skin was apparently Ribbert in 1878.[64] The suggestion was repeated in 1934 by Egorow[24] and again in 1957 by

Pau and Conrads,[60] but these suggestions were made within the context of then current misconceptions concerning the origin and function of Langerhans cells.

An immunofluorescence study of guinea pig corneas in 1979 indicated that this frequently seen and misinterpreted cell may be the equivalent of the epidermal Langerhans cell.[43] Gillette and Chandler reported the presence of Langerhans cells in murine and human corneal epithelium in 1981,[31] and further confirmations have been reported.[14,32,33,65]

In a review of ocular-surface Langerhans cells Gillette and co-workers arbitrarily divided the ocular surface into four concentric zones (Fig. 46-53). The center third of the cornea constitutes the central cornea. The peripheral ring of one-sixth corneal diameter is defined to constitute the peripheral cornea. This zone is in turn overlapped by the "limbal ring." Examination of normal donor globes revealed the following LC densities (cells/mm^2): conjunctiva, 200 to 400; limbus, 150 to 350; peripheral cornea, 75 to 150; pericentral cornea, 25 to 50 (Fig. 46-53). LC identification was confirmed by ATPase enzyme histochemistry, immunofluorescence for HLA-donor antigen, and electron microscopy[33] (Figs. 46-54 and 46-55).

The striking finding of this study was the number of cells within the boundary of the average 7 to 8 mm donor button for keratoplasty. Topographic distribution of corneal LC would seem to require the inclusion of corneal LC (S+ cell?, passenger leukocyte?) in the average human corneal transplant, and larger grafts could be expected to include more of these cells. It is tempting to suggest that the well-known decrease in prognosis for larger corneal grafts[10,17] is partially accounted for by inclusion of larger numbers of class II cells at the time of surgery.

Rubsamen and co-workers[66] and Williams and co-

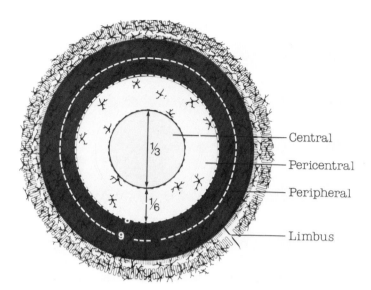

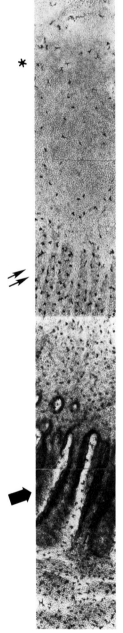

Fig. 46-53. Normal human distribution of ocular-surface Langerhans cells, *LC. Above,* Diagram of ocular surface with four concentric zones of corneal surface arbitrarily defined. Notice that LC populations lie within customary 7.0 to 8.5 mm donor button dimensions. *Below,* Surface densities of Langerhans cells in ocular surface epithelium (cells/mm^2) in several species:

Region	Species			
	Human	*Guinea Pig*	*Mouse*	*Rat*
Conjunctiva	200-400	200-300	100-150	200-400
Limbus	150-350	200-300	150-200	200-400
Peripheral cornea	75-150	25-50	50-100	25-50
Pericentral cornea	25-50	None	25-50	None
Central cornea	*	None	None	None

*Density varied from nearly zero in young healthy corneas to greater than 400 cells/mm^2 in diseased corneas.

Fig. 46-54. Langerhans cell distribution in normal human donor epithelium. *Large arrow,* Palisades of Vogt; *double arrows,* epithelial fingers of peripheral cornea; *asterisk,* pericentral cornea. (Epithelial flat mount; originally 40×; ATPase.)

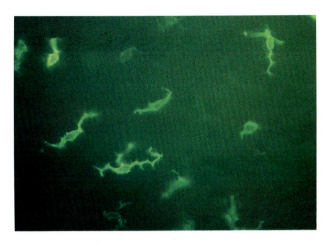

Fig. 46-55. Langerhans cells by the fluorescent antibody technique. (3 weeks, 25×.)

Table 46-16. Pretreatment of Donor Tissue in Heterotopic Corneal Allograft Model

Graft Pretreatment	Donor/Recipient	Rejection
None	BALB/c/C57B1/6	32/39 (82%)
In vitro culture in hyperbaric O_2	BALB/c/C57B1/6	12/56 (21%)
EDTA	BALB/c/C57B1/6	18/23 (78%)
EDTA with epithelium off	BALB/c/C57B1/6	1/25 (4%)
None	BALB/c/C57B1/6	27/42 (64%)
Ultraviolet bulb, 75 mJ/cm^2	BALB/c/C57B1/6	5/20 (25%)
NMS with complement	C_3H/He/C57B1/6	15/24 (63%)
Anti-Ia antiserum with complement	C_3H/He/C57B1/6	6/23 (26%)

NMS, Normal mouse serum.

workers[93] speculate that class II+ cells in the cornea are potent immunogens and that the larger the number of these cells present in the cornea, the more likely an immune graft reaction would occur.

Gebhart has recently shown data indicating that class II+ cells in the cornea may be sufficient to elicit local immune reactions but may not be present in numbers sufficient to generate systemic immunity in the recipient.[30]

Experimental corneal allograft. To investigate the question of histocompatibility antigens and corneal graft rejection, Chandler and associates have developed a murine heterotopic corneal transplant model.[16] Whole corneas from genetically defined donors are inserted into subcutaneous pockets of genetically defined recipients and examined 21 days later. The model allows for pretransplant maneuvers designed to perturbate, remove, or otherwise inhibit the S+/passenger cell population discussed above (if one assumes its presence in murine corneal epithelium).

Four maneuvers have been reported:

1. In vitro culture in hyperbaric oxygen[15]
2. EDTA removal of donor epithelium[62]
3. Exposure to anti-Ia antiserum plus complement[62]
4. Ultraviolet irradiation of the epithelial surface[63]

Each of these maneuvers was predicated on previous successes in other allograft models,[13,49,73,84] and each has been relatively successful in reduction of corneal allograft rejection in this model (Table 46-16).

Low-dose ultraviolet-B pretreatment of donor corneal *endothelium* has also been shown to be effective in a rabbit model, but toxic side effects were also observed.[6]

There are many explanations for the success of these maneuvers, but one unifying explanation stands out: perturbation of S+/passenger cells, that is, corneal epithelial Langerhans cells. Indeed, parallel evidence has been published by Rubsamen and co-workers using another murine heterotopic corneal allograft model. In their model, corneal tissue trimmed of LC-bearing limbal epithelium was not immunogenic at the H-2 locus whereas LC-infiltrated corneal epithelium was.[66] Further work will be required to prove the hypothesis, that is, perturbation followed by S+/LC reconstitution.

What emerges is the possibility of clinical presurgical treatment of human corneal grafts. Both hyperbaric oxygen and ultraviolet light are potentially clinically practical, and other pretreatments are available including cyclosporin A.[67] Indeed, presurgical removal of donor epithelium has been historically advocated and has been looked at prospectively and retrospectively.[88]

Donor epithelial removal. Tuberville, Foster, and Wood studied 152 patients retrospectively and found an incidence of 24.7% rejection reactions in patients with epithelium transplanted compared to 7.2% in the epithelium-removed group ($p = 0.008$). In a prospective study of 55 patients, there was a rejection incidence of 30% in the epithelium-on group versus 8% with the epithelium removed ($p = 0.04$).[88]

These data again support the concept of an S+ cell population in corneal epithelium, presumably corneal epithelial LC. Critics will question, however, the persisting levels, albeit low, of rejection. Three possible explanations are at hand:

1. Incomplete removal of epithelium (and DR+LC)—mechanical removal of corneal epithelium is imprecise and may leave adherent basally sited DR+ LC.[36]

2. HLA-DR–compatible graft/host[72] allowing for *recipient* LC presentation of allogeneic class I antigens of donor corneal stroma and endothelium.

3. Possible presence of DR+ (S+) cells in donor corneal stroma.[53,87]

Summary. Over the last two decades, clinical corneal transplantation has been based on the idea that transplantation antigen alone is the major barrier to successful grafting. As a consequence, tissue typing and host immunosuppression have been seen as the only rational means of attaining allograft acceptance by an immunocompetent host.

A new theory of allogeneic reactivity sees antigen as only a *potential* barrier to allotransplantation. The theory places overriding emphasis on the way antigen is presented to the recipient's immune system and postulates that transplantation antigen, whether it be class I or class II major histocompatibility complex antigen, will be highly immunogenic only when presented to recipient T-cells on the surface of donor stimulator cells (S+).

We and others have identified an Ia+ cell population in corneal epithelium putatively identical to epidermal Langerhans cells. As such they are potentially stimulatory in the perspective of the two-signal theory of allograft rejection, serving a pivotal role in the afferent arm of corneal allograft rejection. By virtue of their restricted localization within corneal epithelium, they are potentially targets for selective maneuvers to remove or inactivate them. Strategies have been developed, and additional strategies may be developed in the future. With the potential to inactivate the afferent arm of corneal graft rejection, we may be able to place less emphasis on the treatment of the efferent arm—our current therapeutic mainstay.

REFERENCES

1. Allansmith MR, Fine M, Payne R: Histocompatibility typing and corneal transplantation, *Trans Am Acad Ophthalmol Otolaryngol* 78:444, 1974.
2. Andrus L, Prowse SJ, Lafferty KJ: Interleukin 2 production by both Ly2+ and Ly2– T-cell subsets, *Scand J Immunol* 13:297-301, 1981.
3. Bach FH, Bach ML, Sondel PM: Differential function of major histocompatibility complex antigens in T-lymphocyte activation, *Nature* 259:273-281, 1976.
4. Batchelor JR et al: HLA matching and corneal grafting, *Lancet* 2:551-554, 1976.
5. Batchelor JR et al: Failure of long surviving, passively enhanced kidney allografts to provoke T-dependent alloimmunity, *J Exp Med* 150:445-464, 1979.
6. Beckhuis WH et al: Corneal graft survival in HLA-A- and HLA-B-matched transplantations in high risk cases with retrospective review of HLA-DR compatibility, *Cornea* 10(1):9-12, 1991.
7. Bergstresser PR, Fletcher CR, Streilein JW: Surface densities of Langerhans cells in relation to rodent epidermal sites with special immunologic properties, *J Invest Dermatol* 74:77-80, 1980.
8. Billingham RE, Medawar PB: A note on the specificity of the corneal epithelium, *J Anat* 84:50, 1950.
9. Boisjoly HM et al: Results of HLA A/B and DR matching in corneal grafting, *Invest Ophthalmol Vis Sci* 26(3, suppl):78, 1985.
10. Boisjoly HM et al: Histompatibility among other risk factors of corneal transplant rejection, *Invest Ophthalmol Vis Sci* 29(suppl):113, 1988.
11. Bretscher P, Cohn M: A theory of self-nonself discrimination, *Science* 169:1042, 1970.
12. Cantor H, Boyse EA: Functional subclasses of T-lymphocytes bearing different Ly antigens, *J Exp Med* 141:1390-1399, 1975.
13. Chandler JW: Immunologic protection of corneal allografts: prolonged survival of allografts pretreated with homologous antibody against transplantation antigens, *Invest Ophthalmol Vis Sci* 15(3):213-216, 1976.
14. Chandler JW, Cummings M, Gillette TE: Presence of Langerhans cells in the central corneas of normal human infants, *Invest Ophthalmol Vis Sci* 26:113, 1985.
15. Chandler JW, Kaufman HE: Graft reactions after keratoplasty for keratoconus, *Am J Ophthalmol* 77:543-547, 1974.
16. Chandler JW, Ray-Keil L, Gillette TE: Experimental corneal allograft rejection: description of murine model and a new hypothesis of immunopathogenesis, *Curr Eye Res* 2(6):387-397, 1982-1983.
17. Cherry PMH et al: An analysis of corneal transplantation: I. Graft clarity, *Ann Ophthalmol* 11:461-469, 1979.
18. Dana MR et al: Low-dose ultraviolet-B irradiation of donor corneal endothelium and graft survival, *Invest Ophthalmol Vis Sci* 31(11):2261-2268, 1990.
19. Daynes RA, Emam M, Krueger GG, Roberts LK: Expression of Ia antigen on epidermal keratinocytes after the grafting of normal skin to nude mice, *J Immunol* 130:1536, 1983.
20. de Waal RMW et al: Variable expression of Ia antigens on the vascular endothelium of mouse skin allografts, *Nature* 303:426, 1983.
21. Donohoe JA et al: Cultured thyroid allografts induce a state of partial tolerance in adult recipient mice, *Transplantation* 35:62-67, 1983.
22. Ducrey NM, Gauser MP, Frei PC: Corneal transplantation: ABO bloodgroups and HLA compatibility, *Ann Ophthalmol* 12(7):880-884, 1980.
23. Duke-Elder S, editor: *System of ophthalmology*, vol 2: *The anatomy of the visual system*, London, 1961, Henry Kimpton, pp 98-99.
24. Egorow I: Nervenelemente der Cornea im Meerschweinchenauge, *Albrecht von Graefes Arch Ophthalmol* 131:531-553, 1934.
25. Elkins WL, Guttmann RD: Pathogenesis of a local graft versus host reaction: immunogenicity of circulating host leukocytes, *Science* 159:1250-1251, 1968.
26. Engelman TW: Über die Hornhaut des Auges, Leipzig, 1867. Cited by Virchow H: *Graefe-Saemisch Handbuch der gesammten Augenheilkunde*, ed 2, Leipzig, 1910, Engelmann, vol 1, pp 30-31.
27. Fonterre A, Trimarchi F, Bo G: HLA antigens and selection

of donors in corneal transplants, *Curr Ther Res* 27:749, 1980.

28. Foulks GN, Sanfilippo F: Beneficial effects of histocompatibility in high-risk corneal transplantation, *Am J Ophthalmol* 94:622-629, 1982.

29. Fujikawa LS et al: Expression of HLA-A/B/C and -DR locus antigens on epithelial, stromal, and endothelial cells of the human cornea, *Cornea* 1:213-222, 1982.

30. Gebhart, BM: The role of Class II Antigen-Expressing cells in corneal allograft immunity, *Invest Ophthal Vis Sci* 31(11):2254-2260, 1990.

31. Gillette TE, Chandler JW: Immunofluorescence and histochemistry of corneal epithelial flat mounts: use of EDTA, *Curr Eye Res* 1:249-253, 1981.

32. Gillette TE, Chandler JW: Langerhans cells of the ocular surface, *Invest Ophthalmol Vis Sci* 20(suppl):98, 1981.

33. Gillette TE, Chandler JW: Langerhans cells of the ocular surface, *Ophthalmology* 89(6):700-710, 1982.

34. Guttmann RD, Lindquist RR: Renal transplantation in the inbred rat. XI. Reduction of allograft immunogenicity by cytotoxic drug pretreatment of donors, *Transplantation* 8:490-495, 1969.

35. Guttmann RD, Lindquist RR, Ockner SA: Renal transplantation in the inbred rat. IX. Haemopoietic origin of an immunologic stimulus of rejection, *Transplantation* 8:472-484, 1969.

36. Haik BG, Zimmy ML: Scanning election microscopy of corneal wound healing in the rabbit, *Invest Ophthalmol Vis Sci* 16:787-796, 1977.

37. Hardy DA, Ling NR: Effects of some cellular antigens on lymphocytes and the nature of the mixed lymphocyte reaction, *Nature* 221:545-548, 1969.

38. Hoffmann F, von Keyserlingk HJ, Wiederholt M: Importance of HLA-DR matching for corneal transplantation in high risk cases, *Cornea* 5:139-143, 1986.

39. Kaliss N, Kandutsch AA: Acceptance of tumor homografts by mice injected with antiserum. I. Activity of serum fractions, *Proc Soc Exp Biol Med* 91:118-121, 1956.

40. Khodadoust AA: The allograft rejection reaction: the leading cause of late failure of clinical corneal grafts. In Corneal graft failure, *Ciba Found Symp* 15:151-163, Amsterdam, 1973, Elsevier.

41. Kissmeyer-Nielson F, Ehlers N: Corneal transplantation and matching for HLA-A and HLA-B. In Ferone S, Curtoni E, Gorini S, editors: *HLA antigens in clinical medicine and biology,* New York, 1979, Garland STPM.

42. Klareskog L, Forsum U, Peterson PA: Hormonal regulation of the expression of Ia antigens on mammary gland epithelium, *Eur J Immunol* 10:598, 1980.

43. Klareskog L et al: Expression of Ia antigen like molecules on cells in the corneal epithelium, *Invest Ophthalmol Vis Sci* 18:310-313, 1979.

44. Lafferty KJ, Cunningham AJ: A new analysis of allogeneic interactions, *Aust J Exp Biol Med Sci* 53:27, 1985.

45. Lafferty KJ, Jones MAS: Reactions of the graft versus host (GVH) type, *Aust J Exp Biol Med Sci* 12:198, 1969.

46. Lafferty KJ, Simeonovic CJ: Immunology of graft rejection, *Transplant Proc* 16(4):927-930, 1984.

47. Lampert IA, Suitters AJ, Chisholm PM: Expression of Ia antigen on epidermal keratinocytes in graft-versus-host disease, *Nature* 293:149, 1981.

48. Larsson EL, Iscove N, Continho A: Two distinct factors are required for induction of T cell growth, *Nature* 283:644, 1980.

49. Lau H, Reemtsma K, Hardy MA: Prolongation of rat islet allograft survival by direct ultraviolet irradiation of the graft, *Science* 223:607-608, 1984.

50. Lechler RI, Batchelor JR: Restoration of immunogenicity to passenger cell–depleted kidney allografts by the addition of donor strain dendritic cells, *J Exp Med* 115:13-41, 1982.

51. Lindahl-Kiessling K, Satwenberg J: Inability of UV-irradiated lymphocytes to stimulate allogeneic cells in mixed lymphocyte culture, *Int Arch Allergy* 41:670-678, 1971.

52. Maugh TH: Transplants (II): altering the donor organ, *Science* 210:177-179, 1980.

53. Mayer DJ et al: Localization of HLA-A,B,C and HLA-DR antigens in the human cornea: practical significance for grafting technique and HLA typing, *Transplant Proc* 15(1):126-129, 1983.

54. Medawar PB: The immunology of transplantation, *Harvey Lect* 52:144-176, 1956-1957.

55. Moen T et al: Importance of HLA-DR matching in cadaveric renal transplantation, *N Engl J Med* 303:850, 1980.

56. Nairn R, Yamaga K, Nathenson SG: Biochemistry of the gene products from murine MHC mutants, *Annu Rev Genet* 14:241-277, 1980.

57. Newsome DA et al: Human corneal cells in vitro: morphology and histocompatibility (HL-A) antigens of pure cell populations, *Invest Ophthalmol Vis Sci* 13(1):23, 1974.

58. Nowygrod R et al: Donor pretreatment in cardiac allografts, *Transplant Proc* 11(2):1462-1464, 1979.

59. Opelz G, Michey MR, Terasaki PI: Calculations on long term graft and patient survival in human kidney transplantation, *Transplant Proc* 9:27-30, 1977.

60. Pau H, Conrads H: Die Bedeutung der Langerhansschen Zellen für die Nerven des Hornhautepithels, *Albrecht von Graefes Arch Ophthalmol* 158:427-433, 1957.

61. Polack FM: Clinical and pathological aspects of the corneal graft reaction, *Trans Am Acad Ophthalmol* 77:418, 1973.

62. Ray-Keil L, Chandler JW: Rejection of murine heterotopic corneal transplants, *Transplantation* 39(5):473, 1985.

63. Ray-Keil L, Gillette TE, Chandler JW: Murine heterotopic corneal transplantation: reduction in rejection rates by pretreatment of donor corneas with ultraviolet light, *Invest Ophthalmol Vis Sci* 26(3, suppl):78, 1985.

64. Ribbert H: Beiträge zur Anatomie der Hautdecken bei Säugetieren, *Arch Naturgesch* 44:321, 1878.

65. Rodrigues MM et al: Langenhans cells in the normal conjunctiva and peripheral cornea of selected species, *Invest Ophthalmol Vis Sci* 21:759, 1981.

66. Rubsamen PE et al: On the Ia immunogenicity of mouse corneal allografts infiltrated with Langerhans cells, *Invest Ophthalmol Vis Sci* 25:513-518, 1984.

67. Ricker J et al: Improvement of kidney transplant survival after graft pretreatment with cyclosporin A, *Transplantation* 34(6):356-359, 1982.

68. Scharenberg K: The cells and nerves of the human cornea: a study with silver carbonate, *Am J Ophthalmol* 40:368-379, 1955.

69. Schellekans PTA, Eijsvoogel VP: Lymphocyte transformation in vitro. III. Mechanism of stimulation in the mixed lymphocyte culture, *Clin Exp Immunol* 7:229-239, 1970.

70. Segawa K: Electron microscopic studies on the human corneal epithelium: dendritic cells, *Arch Ophthalmol* 72:650, 1964.

71. Silvers WK, Fleming HL, Naji A, Barker CF: The influence of removing passenger cells on the fate of skin and parathyroid allografts: evidence for major histocompatibility complex restriction in transplantation immunity, *Diabetes* 31(8):60-62, 1982.

72. Silvers WK et al: Major histocompatibility complex restriction and transplantation immunity: a possible solution to the allograft problem, *Transplantation* 37(1):28-32, 1984.

73. Simeonovic CJ et al: Modulation of tissue immunogenicity by organ culture, *Transplantation* 30(3):174-179, 1980.

74. Snell GD: The homograft reaction, *Annu Rev Microbiol* 11:439, 1957.

75. Steinmuller D: Immunization with skin isografts taken from tolerant mice, *Science* 158:127-129, 1967.

76. Steinmuller D: Passenger leukocytes and the immunogenicity of skin allografts: a critical reevaluation, *Transplant Proc* 13(1):1094-1098, 1981.

77. Stark WJ et al: Histocompatibility (HLA) antigens and keratoplasty, *Am J Ophthalmol* 86(5):595-604, 1978.

78. Stingl G, Tanaki K, Katz S: Origin and function of epidermal Langerhans cells, *Immunol Rev* 53:149, 1980.

79. Stoerk HC: Cortisone and immunity to homoiogeneous tissue—loss of "individually differentials" from tissues of cortisone treated rats, *Ann NY Acad Sci* 56:742-747, 1953.

80. Streilein JW, Towes GB, Bergstresser PR: Corneal allografts fail to express Ia antigens, *Nature* 282:326-327, 1979.

81. Stuart PM, Beck-Maier B, Melvold RW: Provocation of skin graft rejection across murine class II differences by non-bone-marrow-derived cells, *Transplantation* 37(4):393-396, 1984.

82. Stuart FP et al: Role of passenger leukocytes in the rejection of renal allografts, *Transplant Proc* 3:461-464, 1971.

83. Sugiura S: The "polygonal cell" of the corneal epithelium. In Langham ME, editor: *The cornea macromolecular organization of a connective tissue*, Baltimore, 1969, The Johns Hopkins Press.

84. Talmage DW, Dart GA: Effect of oxygen pressure during culture on survival of mouse thyroid allografts, *Science* 200:1066-1067, 1978.

85. Talmage DW et al: Activation of cytotoxic T cells by nonstimulating tumor cells and spleen cell factor(s), *Proc Natl Acad Sci USA* 74:4610, 1977.

86. Teng CC: Fine structure of the human cornea: epithelium and stroma, *Am J Ophthalmol* 54:969-1002, 1962.

87. Treseler PA, Foulks GN, Sanfilippo F: The expression of HLA antigens by cells in the human cornea, *Am J Ophthalmol* 98:763-772, 1984.

88. Tuberville AW, Foster CS, Wood TO: The effect of donor cornea epithelium removal on the incidence of allograft rejection reactions, *Ophthalmology* 90(11):1351-1356, 1983.

89. Vannas S et al: HLA compatible donor cornea for prevention of allograft rejection, *Albrecht von Graefes Arch Klin Exp Ophthalmol* 198:217, 1976.

90. Van Trappen L et al: Lymphocytes and Langerhans cells in the normal human cornea, *Invest Ophthalmol Vis Sci* 26:220-225, 1985.

91. Whitear M: An electron microscope study of the cornea in mice, with special reference to the innervation, *J Anat* 94:387-409, 1960.

92. Whitsett CF, Stulting RD: The distribution of HLA antigens on human corneal tissue, *Invest Ophthalmol Vis Sci* 25(5):519-524, 1984.

93. Williams KA, Ash JK, Coster DJ: Histocompatibility antigen and passenger cell content of normal and diseased human cornea, *Transplantation* 39:265, 1986.

94. Williams KA et al: The role of resident accessory cells in corneal allograft rejection in the rabbit, *Transplantation* 42:667, 1986.

95. Woodward JG, Shigekawa BL, Frelinger JA: Bone marrow derived cells are responsible for stimulating I region incompatible skin graft rejection, *Transplantation* 33:254, 1982.

96. Woolnough JA, Misko IS, Lafferty KJ: Cytotoxic and proliferative lymphocyte responses to allogeneic and xenogeneic antigens in vitro, *Aust J Exp Biol Med Sci* 57:467-477, 1979.

INDICATIONS FOR HLA TISSUE TYPING IN CORNEAL TRANSPLANTATION

MICHAEL E. HETTINGER

Host acceptance of donor tissue, decreasing the incidence or severity of allograft reactions, and decreasing the time required to reverse a rejection episode are events that will enhance allograft survival from immunologic failure. Various means of increasing host acceptance of homologous donor corneal tissue have been studied. This chapter is concerned with investigations that questioned whether or not host sensitization to donor tissue could be reduced or prevented by HLA (human leukocyte antigen) tissue matching of donor and recipient and which recipients benefited from this matching.

The major histocompatibility complex in man is the HLA system found on chromosome 6.[15] Gorer and co-workers[16] and Little[19] documented that rejection of transplanted tissue was controlled by histocompatibility antigens on the cell surface, and these antigens are influenced by several genetic loci. The genetic loci of the HLA system can be found in Fig. 46-56. Medawar[20] and others documented that a specific set of immune responses by the recipient to the histocompatibility antigens on the donor were responsible for transplantation rejection reactions. Nearly all nucleated cells have human leukocyte antigens, glycoproteins, within their plasma membranes,[8] and corneal tissue is no exception.[22] HLA-A, B, and C antigens have been identified on human corneal epithelium, keratocytes, and endothelium, with epithelium and keratocytes having greater amounts than endothelium.[6] In normal corneas, HLA-DR antigens have only been detected on Langerhans' cells in the peripheral cornea;[6] however, detection of HLA-DR antigens on corneal endothelial cells, on cells in the stroma, and on basal epithelial cells have been reported in rejected corneas.[26] During corneal allograft rejection, lymphocytes causing cell lysis have been found in epithelium, stroma, and endothelium.[27,28] Other antigen groups also play a role in allograft rejection and are referred to as the minor histocompatibility system, which includes the ABO system, Lewis antigens, sex antigens, and possibly the monocytes and endothelial system.[8] These antigens are not believed to be membrane-bound glycoproteins; however, they are capable of inducing a cell-mediated graft reaction in vivo.[5] Much of the early clinical investigation regarding HLA matching was performed in association with renal transplantation.

Since allograft rejections have been reported to be the greatest cause of delayed corneal graft failure,[9,18] corneal surgeons seeking to limit or elimi-

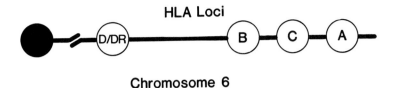

HLA Loci

Chromosome 6

Fig. 46-56. Genetic loci on chromosome 6.

nate immunologic rejection have investigated this by matching the HLA system between donor and recipient.[1,3,7,13,33,37]

Defining Patient Risk. Some surgeons tend to define patient risk to immunologic rejection by placing patients into low-risk and high-risk groups,[4,13,33] whereas others[7] define risk by adding medium[13,33] risk to the above two categories. For simplicity, two categories are employed in this chapter—those recipients at low risk and those at increased risk. In patients with normal lid anatomy and function, normal intraocular pressure, adequate tear function, healthy ocular surface, and normal corneal sensation and those without recurring uveitis, there presently exists two known conditions—vascularized corneas and previous sensitization to HLA antigens—that predispose the recipient to an allograft rejection. Age may be an additional factor to be considered. Alldredge and Krachmer[2] substantiated the clinical impression that younger patients have a higher rate of allograft rejections, lending indirect support to the hypothesis that younger patients have a more active immune system. Additional studies are needed for verification.

Patients at Increased Risk. Recipients at increased risk are often defined as those having two or more quadrants of stromal vascularization into the area to be grafted (Figs. 46-57 and 46-58) or a history of prior HLA sensitization (Figs. 46-59 and 46-60). Hoffman and co-workers[17] also include the recipient's graft-bed diameter of 7.5 mm or greater and the presence of blood or fibrin in the anterior chamber on the first postoperative day as factors that increase the risk of an immune reaction. Tuberville and co-workers[36] found no significant correlation between graft size and allograft rejection in low-risk patients.

HLA sensitization of recipient. Prior HLA sensitization to HLA antigens results in the host developing lymphocytotoxic antibodies to the neoantigens. The exact role of humoral immunity in corneal allograft rejections is uncertain,[34] yet lymphocytotoxic antibodies may play a role in allograft rejections.[6] These antibodies have been detected after corneal transplantation,[35] renal transplantation,[21] skin transplantation,[38] blood and platelet transfusion,[23,39] and pregnancy.[11] Lymphocytotoxic antibodies can be detected preoperatively with an in vitro test, a lympho-

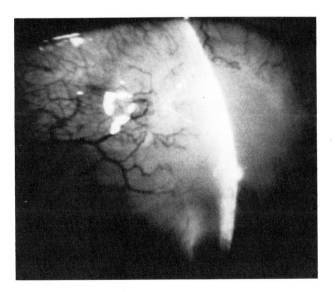

Fig. 46-57. Corneal opacification and deep stromal vascularization in all quadrants after alkali injury.

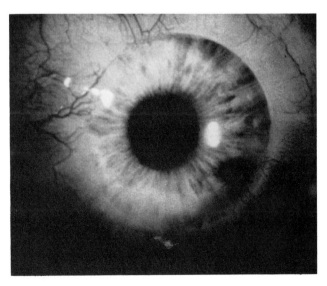

Fig. 46-58. Same eye as in Fig. 46-57 2 years after HLA-matched penetrating keratoplasty.

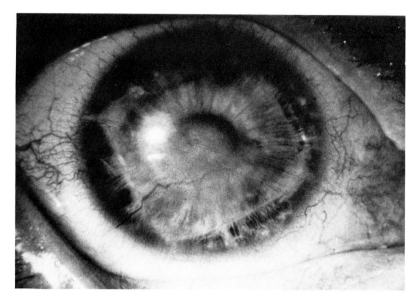

Fig. 46-59. Square allograft having failed after severe allograft rejection.

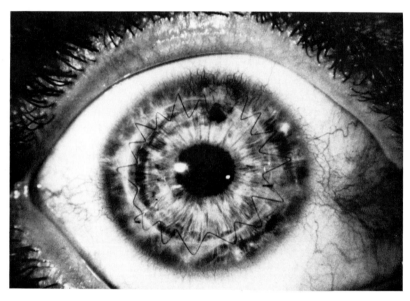

Fig. 46-60. Regraft of eye in Fig. 46-59.

cyte crossmatch, in which donor and recipient lymphocytes are mixed. A negative crossmatch is indicative of no preformed antibody to donor antigens, whereas a positive crossmatch means circulating antibodies to one or more of the donor antigens. Investigators,[4,13] have demonstrated a lower rate of rejection in patients at increased risk by having a negative lymphocyte crossmatch and HLA matching, yet in a retrospective study Stark and co-workers[33] were unable to show a positive correlation between the num-

ber of HLA antigens shared and graft outcome. They did substantiate a beneficial effect from lymphocyte crossmatching in patients at increased risk. A prospective, controlled, single-masked study of HLA-A and B matching with a negative lymphocyte crossmatch demonstrated a long-term benefit of reducing the number of episodes of allograft rejection and subsequent failure in recipients with two or more antigen matches.[31] A prospective controlled randomized, unmasked study demonstrated significant graft survival at 2 years and 5 years in HLA-A and B matched corneas.[25]

Stromal vascularization. In unmatched transplants, Khodadoust[18] found a 65% rate of rejection with heavy vascularization of the cornea, a 28% rate of rejection with moderate vascularization, and 13.3% rate of rejection in mildly vascularized ones. A positive correlation between increased rate of rejection has been substantiated by others.[10,14] Since lymphatics have been found in vascularized corneas,[30] the anatomic architecture necessary for the afferent arc and efferent arc of the immune response in allograft rejection is present. Opremcak and co-workers[24] conducted in vitro experiments resulting in natural killer cells against human corneal endothelium. Natural killing is a lymphocyte-mediated activity detectable without previous sensitization, whereas humoral immunity and cell-mediated immunity require prior sensitization. This response has not been documented in vivo; however, if it were to occur, the requirement for an afferent arc of the immune system for endothelial rejection would be negated.

Low-Risk Patients. Patients at low risk are defined as those having an avascular cornea and no history of prior sensitization to HLA antigens. Corneal allograft rejection rates in initial avascular grafts have been reported to be as high as 35% in one report;[9] however, most investigators have found the rate to be around 10%.[12,13,29,32] These observations do not corroborate the hypothesis that the avascular cornea is an immunologically privileged tissue; however, it appears to be relatively privileged when compared to vascular transplantable tissue (kidney, heart, lung, and liver).[6] The high success rate without an attempt at matching donor and recipient in initial avascular corneas (90%) makes it difficult to demonstrate statistical significance in HLA-matched donor and recipient. Casey and Mayer[7] were unable to demonstrate a beneficial effect of HLA matching A and B loci in their low-risk patients, defined as first-time grafts and avascular corneas. Boisjoly and co-workers[4] recently reported that matching the DR loci in addition to the A and B loci along with a negative lymphocyte crossmatch may play an important role in decreasing the incidence of allograft rejection in low-risk patients. Do all corneal transplant recipients benefit from HLA matching? HLA matching of low-risk patients may be beneficial when studied after 5 to 10 years of follow-up study. Until there is better evidence, most surgeons do not believe that low-risk patients benefit from HLA matching.

Acceptable Match. It should be noted that in addition to recipient blood, HLA matching requires donor blood, and lymphocyte crossmatching requires either donor blood, a lymph node, or a specimen from the spleen. Since it is extremely difficult to match each antigen between donor and recipient, one must define an acceptable match. In some studies, matches were made on the basis of the fewest mismatched antigens. Corneal surgeons often want to know what an acceptable match is for a specific patient at increased risk. No conclusive answer is available; however, an acceptable match is usually defined as a negative lymphocyte crossmatch and a donor containing 50% or more of the HLA-A and B manifested by the recipient.

Summary. Lymphocyte crossmatching and matching of the major histocompatibility complex have been studied in cases at increased risk of allograft rejection and subsequent graft failure. The majority of the reports indicate a beneficial effect. Results of the collaborative corneal transplant study (CCTS) which is a 5-year multicenter study will, one would hope, provide more information on HLA-matching in high-risk patients. Furthermore, the benefit of topical cyclosporin A in high-risk cases, though promising, is also being investigated in a prospective, randomized, double-masked, multicenter clinical trial. Because of the added expense to perform HLA testing and lymphocyte crossmatching and until the results of the CCTS and the topical cyclosporin A study are made available, I am not performing the test in high-risk patients unless there is a multiple organ donor in which the HLA tests are available at no additional cost to the patient or health care system. The results of the above studies could significantly influence whether HLA-A, B, and DR matching and lymphocyte crossmatching will be employed in high-risk cases.

REFERENCES

1. Allansmith MR, Fine M, Payne R: Histocompatibility typing and corneal transplantation, *Trans Am Acad Ophthalmol Otolaryngol* 78:445, 1974.
2. Alldredge OC, Krachmer JH: Clinical types of corneal transplant rejection, *Arch Ophthalmol* 99:599, 1981.
3. Batchelor JR et al: HLA matching and corneal grafting, *Lancet* 1:551, 1976.
4. Boisjoly HM et al: HLA-A, B and DR matching in corneal transplantation, *Ophthalmology* 93:1290, 1986.
5. Bouchard CS, Belin MW: The use of topical cyclosporin in high-risk corneal transplants, *Ophthalmology* 97:691, 1990 (Letters to the Editor).
6. Braude LS, Chandler JW: Corneal allograft rejection: the role of the major histocompatibility complex, *Surv Ophthalmol* 27:290, 1983.
7. Casey TA, Mayer DJ: *The influence of HLA compatibility on corneal graft rejection*, Presented to the International Ophthalmic Congress, San Francisco, 1982.
8. Casey TA, Mayer DJ: *Corneal grafting*, London, 1984, Saunders.

9. Chandler JW, Kaufman HE: Graft reactions after keratoplasty for keratoconus, *Am J Ophthalmol* 77:543, 1974.

10. Cherry PMH et al: An analysis of corneal transplantion. I. Graft clarity, *Ann Ophthalmol* 11:461, 1979.

11. Dausset J: Leuco-agglutinins and blood transfusion, *Vox Sang* 4:190, 1954.

12. Donshik PC, Cavanagh HD, Boruchoff SA, Dohlman CH: Effect of bilateral and unilateral grafts on the incidence of rejections in keratoconus, *Am J Ophthalmol* 87:82, 1979.

13. Foulks GN, Sanfilippo F: Beneficial effects of histocompatibility in high-risk corneal transplantation, *Am J Ophthalmol* 94:622, 1982.

14. Gibbs DC et al: The influence of tissue-type compatibility on the fate of full thickness corneal grafts, *Trans Ophthalmol Soc UK* 94:101, 1974.

15. Goldman JN, Goldman MB: What the clinician should know about the major histocompatibility complex, *JAMA* 246:873, 1981.

16. Gorer PA, Lyman S, Snell GD: Studies on the genetic and antigenic basis of tumor transplantation: linkage between a histocompatibility gene and 'fused' in mice, *Proc R Soc, London,* sB 135:499, 1948.

17. Hoffman F, Pahlitzsch T: Predisposing factors in corneal graft rejection, *Cornea* 8:215, 1989.

18. Khodadoust AA: The allograft rejection reaction: the leading cause of late failure of clinical corneal grafts. In Porter R, Knight J, editors: *Corneal graft failure, Ciba Found Symp* 15:151, Amsterdam, 1973, Elsevier.

19. Little CC: The genetics of tumor transplantation. In Snell GD, editor: *Biology of laboratory mouse,* Philadelphia, 1941, Blakiston, p 279.

20. Medawar PB: The immunology of transplantation, *Harvey Lect* 52:144, 1957.

21. Morris PJ, Williams GM, Hume DM: Serotyping for homotransplantation, *Transplantation* 6:392, 1968.

22. Newsome DA et al: Human corneal grafts in vitro: morphology and histocompatibility (HL-A) antigens of pure cell populations, *Invest Ophthalmol* 13:23, 1974.

23. Opelz G, Terasaki PI: Histocompatibility matching utilizing responsiveness as a new dimension, *Transplant Proc* 4:433, 1972.

24. Opremcak EM, Whisler RL, Dangel ME: Natural killer cells against human corneal endothelium, *Am J Ophthalmol* 99:524, 1985.

25. Ozdemir O: A prospective study of histocompatibility testing for keratoplasty in high risk patients, *Br J Ophthalmol* 70:183, 1986.

26. Pepose JS et al: Detection of HLA class I and II antigens in rejected human corneal allografts, *Ophthalmology* 92:1480, 1985.

27. Polack FM: Scanning electron microscopy of corneal graft rejection: epithelium rejection, endothelial rejection and formation of posterior graft membranes, *Invest Ophthalmol* 11:1, 1972.

28. Polack FM: Clinical and pathological aspects of the corneal graft reaction, *Trans Am Acad Ophthalmol Otolaryngol* 77:418, 1973.

29. Polack FM: *Corneal graft rejection: clinico-pathological correlation, in corneal graft failure,* Amsterdam, 1973, Associated Scientific Publishers.

30. Polack FM: *Corneal transplantation,* New York, 1977, Grune & Stratton.

31. Sanfilippo F et al: Reduced graft rejection with good HLA-A and B matching in high-risk corneal transplantation, *N Engl J Med* 315:29, 1986.

32. Stark WJ, Paton D, Maumenee AE, Michelson PE: The results of 102 penetrating keratoplasties using 10-0 monofilament nylon suture, *Ophthalmol Surg* 3:11, 1972.

33. Stark WJ, Taylor HR, Bias WB, Maumenee AE: Histocompatibility (HLA) antigens and keratoplasty, *Am J Ophthalmol* 86:595, 1978.

34. Stark WJ, Taylor HR, Bias WB, Maumenee AE: Keratoplasty: the role of histocompatibility (HLA) antigens. In Steinberg GM, Gery I, Nussenblatt RB, editors: *Immunology of the eye,* Workshop: I, Spec. Suppl. to Immunology Abstracts, pp 221-232, 1980.

35. Stark WJ et al: Sensitization to human lymphocyte antigens by corneal transplantation, *Invest Ophthalmol* 12:639, 1973.

36. Tuberville AW, Foster CS, Wood TO: The effect of donor corneal epithelium removal on the incidence of allograft rejection reactions, *Ophthalmology* 90:1351, 1983.

37. Vannas S, Karjalainen K, Ruusuvaara P, Tiilikainen A: HLA-compatible donor cornea for prevention of allograft rejection, *Albrecht von Graefes Arch Klin Exp Ophthalmol* 198:217, 1976.

38. Walford RL, Carter PK, Anderson RE: Leukocyte antibodies following skin homografting in the human, *Transplant Bull* 29:16, 1962.

39. Yankee RA, Grumet FC, Rogentine GN: Platelet transfusion therapy: the selection of compatible platelet donors for refractory patients by lymphocyte HLA typing, *N Engl J Med* 281:1208, 1969.

Part VI

EYE BANKING—ADMINISTRATIVE ASPECTS

Chapter 47

The Eye Bank

Starting an eye bank

DONNA OILAND

Starting a new eye bank is more difficult than it was 40 or 50 years ago when the need for such programs first appeared.

The first eye banks consisted of a telephone, a refrigerator, and containers to ship eye tissue. Individual surgeons had their own criteria for suitable donor material, and the numbers of sets of criteria depended on the number of surgeons doing transplants. Record keeping was poor or nonexistent, and most of the staff was part-time or volunteer.

Modern eye banks have developed into professional operations with highly trained staff members and certified technicians, 24-hour-a-day service, and growing public and professional recognition. Like any institution, an eye bank must be systematically organized. It must run smoothly technically, clerically, and financially and must have strong public relations and professional education programs.

Once it has been determined there is a need for a local eye bank facility, one of the first options should be to consider associating with an established eye bank program as a satellite laboratory. If there is a well-run, fully EBAA (Eye Bank Association of America) certified eye bank within the same geographic region, not only is becoming affiliated with that program cost effective but also many functions of your eye bank would already be up and running. Some of the advantages would be to have policies, procedures, forms, public relations materials and campaigns, financial support, and professional education programs already in place.

If it is evident that associating with an established eye bank program is not politically or geographically feasible and there is support from the local medical association and community, an eye bank program should be started.

The first step is to seek assistance from the Eye Bank Association of America in Washington, D.C., and obtain copies of the eye bank operations procedures manuals developed by that organization. The manuals address administration, public relations, tissue procurement, as well as other technical aspects of running an eye bank program. Since federal regulations require hospitals to develop policies and procedures to help routinely identify potential donors in their facility, most hospitals will already have a working relationship with other organ/tissue procurement agencies. It would be also prudent for those working to start a new program to enlist the support of appropriate organ/tissue procurement agencies.

BOARD OF DIRECTORS

When you are starting an eye bank, a strong active board of directors is essential. Board members must be committed to the cause of eye donation and corneal transplantation and be willing to work to develop a strong eye bank program.

This group of people will formulate a budget, help develop job descriptions for staff members, hire an executive director, be responsible for major fund raising, and develop public and professional relations campaigns. It is useful to choose board members carefully. There are obvious advantages to including influential community leaders, people in key positions in hospitals, members of the local media, and people who have a special desire to promote the program such as corneal transplant recipients or donor family members. Persons with political influence and business contacts will also strengthen your board. Legal counsel is also an asset.

Once the board has been established its first job is to form a clearly stated purpose and objective so that direction can be given to the foundation's work. It is helpful to state the purpose of the eye bank in public relations material and a display in the eye bank facility. This gives the staff, volunteers, and general public an understanding of the goals of your program and will help give direction to decisions that must be made.

SERVICE AND OBJECTIVES FOR AN EYE BANK PROGRAM

The local eye bank shall:

1. Procure, process, and distribute tissue of the highest quality for transplantation.
2. Provide and process eye tissue for research or teaching as needed.
3. Provide families of potential donors and donor families the mechanism to donate a decedent's eyes.
4. Provide support to donor families and thank them for their donation.
5. Cooperate with other organ and tissue procurement agencies by providing professional education programs and donor referrals.
6. Promote public relations activities and enhance public awareness of organ and tissue donation.

FINANCIAL SUPPORT

To operate any business including public service programs, one must have financial support to pay salaries, to purchase equipment and supplies, to support laboratory functions such as virology testing, and to develop public relations and professional education material. The board of directors should help raise funds not only to start the program, but also to help sustain it. Some of the support may come from local service organizations, the United Way Fund, and philanthropic foundations interested in community service. Local surgeons and hospitals may be approached to donate supplies or equipment to help get the lab up and running.

Some newly formed as well as established eye bank programs may choose to hire a development officer to be responsible for fund raising. After the eye bank is established, part of the budget will be derived from processing fees charged for tissue supplied for transplant and research. It has become apparent, however, from established eye banks that processing fees alone are not adequate to supply the entire budget, and supplemental support must continue to come from other sources.

Items for Budget Consideration

1. *Salaries*
   Director's salary
   Secretarial salary
   Technicians' salaries
   Fringe benefits
2. *Equipment*
   Laminar flow hood
   Specular microscope
   Slitlamp (biomicroscope)
   Computer or computers and software
   Refrigerator
   Instruments
   Furniture
   Autoclave (optional)
3. *Supplies*
   Storage media
   Jars and cages
   Antibiotics
   Donor preparation solutions
   Hats, masks, gloves, gowns
   Shipping containers, etc.
4. *Services*
   Laboratory testing fees (virology and microbiology)
   Printing (labels, forms, stationary, professional educational materials)
   Telephone
   Transportation of tissue
   Facilities costs (if not provided)
   Pager rental
   Postage
   Central services for sterilization
5. *Travel*
   Allowance for staff to attend professional or educational meetings
   Mileage allowance for personal car use

EXECUTIVE DIRECTOR

Hiring an executive director is a critical step when you are laying the foundation for a program that will grow and develop into a strong eye bank. Because there are a limited number of eye banks and other organ donation programs, it is difficult to find a person with special eye bank or organ-donation experience. One of the ways to find a person with specific donation experience would be to obtain mailing lists from national organizations (American Association of Tissue Banks, AATB; Eye Bank Association of America, EBAA; North American Transplant Coordinators Organization, NATCO) and publicize your opening for a new director. If it is not possible to recruit a person with organ or tissue donation experience, a person with a background in medicine, counseling, or public relations may help but is not essential. Whoever is hired should be a strong leader and dedicated to developing a growing eye bank program.

Some of the qualities necessary for a good executive director include the ability to present oneself in public, to have compassion and a high level of energy, be resourceful, have the ability to be committed to a cause, and be organized yet flexible. An executive director must be intelligent, a positive thinker, and above all enthusiastic!

No matter how much experience the new executive director might have, additional training is necessary in all aspects of eye banking. Since the executive director will oversee the hiring of other personnel in the establishment of clerical and technical activities, this person should be familiar with every aspect of the eye bank program.

In the beginning, at least, the new director may have to act as the administrator, secretary, technician, public relations person and professional education consultant. Since the new executive director will always be responsible for the day-to-day aspects of the eye bank, it is helpful that this person also be a certified technician. The Eye Bank Association of America offers training and certification courses for eye bank technicians, and member eye banks periodically also offer courses on how to approach potential donor families for consent and how to present inservices and so on.

EBAA meetings are held several times a year on both a regional and national level, and the interaction with other eye banks will be very beneficial, especially to someone new in the field.

One of the most valuable experiences for a prospective executive director is the opportunity to spend several days in one or more established eye banks. The knowledge gained by observing the day-to-day operations of an eye bank will be invaluable. This time will also give the prospective or new employee the opportunity to get ideas for developing forms, lists of vendors for supplies, public relations ideas, professional education materials, and suggestions for implementing hospital procedures. If the new executive director is still excited about eye banking after spending time with other eye banks, you may have found the right person for the job. Even for executive directors with years of experience, visits to other eye banks can give them fresh ideas and renewed energy.

MEDICAL DIRECTOR

An ophthalmologist who has a special interest in corneal and external diseases of the eye and performs corneal transplant surgery should be appointed as medical director of the new eye bank program. The medical director must be appointed and accept this position with the understanding of the vital role that this person will play in orchestrating an eye bank laboratory that meets all requirements of the EBAA Medical Standards.

The medical director of a new eye bank will be actively involved in establishing laboratory policies and procedures for procurement, screening, grading, and distribution of donor eye tissue. Since the medical director is responsible for the day-to-day operation of the technical aspects of the program, this person must be accessible to answer technician's questions, review medical histories, examine corneas by slitlamp, periodically review donor charts, and participate in staff meetings. The office of the medical director should be located in or close to the eye bank or be very accessible.

The board of directors of a new eye bank may also want to develop a medical advisory board consisting of community ophthalmologists interested in the eye bank to help establish procedures and policies and to help resolve medical issues that might arise. Often the medical director is chosen from this board and acts as its chairman.

The medical advisory board will be instrumental in gaining the support of the local medical community and in making contacts in local hospitals to establish procedures for identifying and facilitating donations.

LOCATION

A hospital location for an eye bank is a logical answer to the question of where the facility might be housed. The proximity to potential donors and other support services such as a central supply, a pharmacy, and virology and microbiology laboratories will be beneficial to the day-to-day operation of the eye bank. If the eye bank is in a hospital where a large amount of eye surgery is done, the convenience of having the facility close to the operating room is an additional bonus. With the growing competition between hospitals, a new eye bank program might find a hospital willing to provide space and some support services free of charge in exchange for the added visibility the program will offer to that institution. If it is determined that the eye bank will not be housed in a hospital, it will be helpful to have it located close to a medical facility, the medical director, and the laboratory support services.

When determining where the eye bank is to be housed, you must consider the requirements laid out in the EBAA Medical Standards. The space where the laboratory is located must be dedicated solely to the eye bank's technical activities and have access limited to eye bank personnel. There must be running water and an adequate amount of counter space for the technical staff to perform the processing of tissue, evaluation and preparation of supplies, and equipment for use. Special consideration must be given to where a flow hood will be located, and room for an appropriate (see EBAA Medical Standards) refrigerator for tissue storage must be available. There must also be room for a slitlamp and adequate storage space for supplies. Most eye banks find storing empty shipping containers one of the real challenges when it comes to space consideration. Other obvious space considerations have to be for the storage of donor records and the necessary furnishings and equipment to operate a smoothly functioning eye bank program.

CONCLUSION

When a new eye bank is started, the very first step should be to contact the Eye Bank Association of America in Washington, D.C., for support and experience from people who have worked in the field. I have been acquainted with people who have worked for years to establish a new eye bank before they were ready to procure and process tissue. There is so much ground work to be done before specific procedures, forms, and communications systems can be developed and implemented. Before donor tissue can be processed, the laboratory must be equipped and functional. Staff members and volunteers working with an eye bank program must be committed to the cause of providing renewed sight through corneal transplantation. The frustrations are many and the hours are long, but the rewards of working in an area that positively touches so many lives makes the effort eminently worthwhile.

Modern local eye banking

MARY BETH DANNEFFEL

Eye banking has achieved significant growth and development in the nearly 50 years since the first eye bank was founded in New York in 1944.[4] Overseeing and guiding this development has been the Eye Bank Association of America (EBAA), which celebrated its thirtieth birthday in 1991. The EBAA's 1990 eye banking statistics reported that 107 eye banks in North America received a total of 86,076 eye donations and provided 40,631 corneas for keratoplasty.[3] Although not all eye banks are certified members of the EBAA, most are. Certification, which requires site visit inspection and adherence to

EBAA medical standards, remains voluntary in the early 1990s; this is expected to change in the near future. This section is a brief summary of events leading to proposed federal regulation of eye and tissue banking, followed by an overview of what a modern local eye bank is and what services it provides.

THE REGULATORY CLIMATE

Congress passed the National Organ Transplant Act in 1984, which led to the establishment of the Office of Organ Transplantation within the Health Resources and Services Administration, Department of Health and Human Services. This legislation, Public Law 98-507, also created the OPTN, or the Organ Procurement and Transplant Network. Rules were subsequently promulgated for the certification of organ procurement organizations by the Health Care Financing Administration (HCFA). Under the 1984 National Organ Transplant Act the definition of organs specifically and carefully omitted inclusion of tissues. As a result, eye and tissue banks escaped federal regulation in the mid-1980s. However, the Eye Bank Association of America and its member banks took a proactive role. Recognizing that federal regulation was inevitable and necessary in order to be publicly accountable for high-quality standards and provision of safe tissue for corneal transplantation, the EBAA House of Delegates and Board of Directors voted to recommend to the United States Federal Government that eye and tissue banks be included under the Clinical Laboratories Improvement Act of 1988 (CLIA). At the same time, the EBAA Medical Standards Policy Committee adopted a revised medical standards document, which contained more stringent standards and subsequently strengthened its certification process. A formal procedures manual was written in 1991 to operationalize the EBAA Medical Standards. This procedures manual further standardized and defined eye bank procedures performed by EBAA-certified member banks.

In May 1991, the first case of transmission of HIV to multiple recipients of organs and tissues was reported from a donor in Virginia. Over 50 recipients of organs and tissues, including corneas, were involved. Several organ and tissue recipients died from AIDS-related problems. Notably, the corneal recipients remain seronegative. Nevertheless, this raised public outcry for regulation of tissue banks. In particular, the FDA, which had already begun to regulate certain tissues, such as corneal lenticules for epikeratophakia, dura, and human heart valves, escalated its involvement. As of mid-1992, it had not been determined which federal agency would be assigned regulatory oversight for eye banking. Federal regulation became a *fait accompli*, with only a remaining decision of exactly when and through what mechanism.

As the EBAA and member eye banks were developing a strategy and taking a proactive role regarding federal regulation, eye banks also faced external pressure from organ procurement organizations (OPOs). HCFA begun promulgating regulations and developing standards to certify OPOs in the late 1980s. These standards called for a minimum number of donors per year and geographic service areas with assignment of territories to designated OPOs. Organ procurement organizations became increasingly concerned about meeting these standards to remain certified. Despite required request laws that had been enacted in almost every state, a decline in the number of organ donors was experienced in the latter 1980s. Increased national attention was focused on OPO effectiveness in identifying organ donors and providing cost-effective retrieval of organs. The Association of Organ Procurement Organizations, or AOPO, called for single telephone referral numbers controlled by local OPOs. This was countered by the EBAA, which maintained that in some areas of the country a common donor 800 number might be very effective but would not work in other areas, given the local dynamics between the OPO and the eye and tissue banks within the community. However, this external pressure exerted by OPOs led to a need for increased professionalism and assertiveness of eye banks. Collaborative and cooperative efforts with OPOs to coordinate services became extremely important.

THE EYE BANK OF THE 1990s

To ensure survival and success, the eye bank of the 1990s has become far more sophisticated than ever before. A modern local eye bank is one that provides a full range of services with a paid professional staff, facilities, equipment, and operations to meet the stringent EBAA Medical Standards. Formal quality assurance programs and a requirement to have at least one EBAA-certified technician in a supervisory role became a requirement.[1] Eye banks were also required to have procedures manuals.

A full-service eye bank implies that an eye bank provides many of the following functions: hospital development and professional education to ensure the appropriate identification of suitable donors and referral to the local eye bank or donor hotline; professional staff available to approach families to offer the option for donation; the appropriate screening of donors to include evaluation of donor medical history and evaluation of donor risk for HIV, hepatitis, and other infectious diseases including inspection of the body and documentation of autopsy results, if applicable; the timely retrieval and processing of the eye tissue according to EBAA and local standards and procedures; the laboratory evaluation by slitlamp and specular biomicroscopy; and ensuring fair and equitable distribution of tissue to surgeons and their patients on the eye bank's waiting list. Many local eye banks have formed liaisons with their local OPO and tissue banks leading to shared responsibilities, including a donor hotline in many instances. Not all eye banks provide all these services directly; these services may be shared with the tissue bank and OPO. Public relations is another aspect that eye banks have devoted considerable amount of attention to.

Eye banks have had to critically examine their structure, management, and operations in order to remain competitive and meet increasingly stringent standards. Looking ahead into the 1990s and beyond into the next century, it is doubtful that many new eye banks will be formed in the United States. Rather, it is likely that the total number of United States eye banks will decline just as the number of OPOs decreased after federal regulation when consolidation of organ procurement organizations occurred.

EYE BANK STRUCTURE AND FUNCTION

Depending on the circumstances within a particular community, eye banks may be part of a university medical school, usually within the ophthalmology department, or they may be independent nonprofit organizations totally separate from any other institution or a department within a hospital, or they may be incorporated in a tissue bank or organ procurement agency. Regardless, an eye bank must have a medical director who is an ophthalmologist specializing in corneal surgery as stipulated in EBAA Medical Standards.[2] The eye bank medical director must be actively involved in overseeing the functioning of the eye bank laboratory. He or she should be readily available for consultation and be frequently on site. The medical director should also attend periodic staff meetings, review technical policy and procedures, and attend national EBAA meetings.

Most eye banks also have a board of directors, or, if they are within a university, a board of directors may be replaced by regents, board of governors, or other policy setting body. Eye banks also have an executive director, president or chief executive officer, manager, or other administrative director. Eye bank executive directors have responsibility for implementing policies set by the board of directors or other governing authority and report progress in providing service and number of tissues provided for transplantation. The executive director is also responsible for setting an annual budget, formulating goals and objectives for the organization, and deciding what equipment and instrumentation to purchase. This person assumes day-to-day responsibility for recruitment and hiring of technical and other staff for the eye bank, technical staff training, adherence to medical standards in conjunction with the medical director, marketing and public relations, development of hospitals, professional and public education, and collaborative efforts with organ procurement agencies and tissue banks in the community.

Many eye banks have implemented computerized data base management systems. These systems are designed to store donor and recipient records, produce statistical reports, and automatically generate invoices for tissue-processing fees. Computer programs have also been written to run a tissue distribution system.

Regardless of whether an eye bank owns the most advanced equipment and has a state-of-the-art laboratory, it is the technical staff that is the most critical component of modern eye bank function and service it provides. It is the technical staff that carries out the daily critical functions of coordinating donor referrals, screening and retrieval of tissue, followed by preservation of tissue in the laboratory. The eye bank technician evaluates corneal tissue by slitlamp and specular biomicroscopy and distributes tissue to waiting recipients and surgeons. Technical staff are also involved in quality assurance and monitoring activities as well as in providing important professional education and public education. The technical staff form the pivotal crux of an eye bank's operation. If they are not carefully selected, trained, developed, and supervised, the most modern-appearing eye bank laboratory cannot function efficiently and according to EBAA Medical Standards. The Eye Bank Association of America provides technician training and certification. Technicians must be recertified every 3 years. However, the local eye bank must assume the day-to-day responsibility of ensuring a technician's competence in this growing specialty.

CONCLUSION

A modern eye bank must be prepared to meet the challenges of the 1990s and beyond into the next century. It must be flexible to accommodate and survive change yet firm in meeting increasingly stringent standards and federal regulation. Quality of tissue and service must be the main focus, not merely the quantity of tissue provided. Eye banks must have well-formulated quality assurance programs and monitoring activities in place. The public has the right to expect safe tissue for corneal transplantation that will not pose a health risk by transmitting an infectious disease to a recipient. An eye bank is not modern merely by its high-technology laboratory, with the most sophisticated and latest equipment, such as laminar airflow hoods, automated endothelial cell counting apparatus, and computerized data base management systems. These items are simply tools that must be operated by highly qualified and well-trained staff. Competent and capable technical staff assisted by the right tools enable eye banks to meet the need for high-quality corneal tissue for transplantation.

Eye banking has undergone tremendous change in the latter half of the twentieth century. From its early altruistic beginnings as a largely volunteer organization supported by lay members of the community such as the Lions and the Oddfellows, eye banking has strived to become integrated with other healthcare organizations and the transplant medical community as a whole. Its evolution will be further influenced by federal regulation as eye banking struggles for survival and maintenance of its own unique identity as it undergoes transition into the twenty-first century.

REFERENCES

1. EBAA Medical Standards, Oct 1990, sections C1.300 and G1.000.
2. EBAA Medical Standards, Oct 1990, section C1.200
3. Eye Bank Association of America: 1990 eye banking statistics, Washington, D.C., April 26, 1991.
4. McLean JM: Symposium: corneal transplantation. II. Technique, *Am J Ophthalmol* 31:1310-1374, 1948.

Certification of eye banks

ELLEN HECK

Certification, or the process of certifying, attests to the quality or worth, documents that one has met specified requirements, and vouches for or guarantees.[7] It is the normal extension of the development of medical standards and the desire to provide quality service and protect the patient from undue risk.

HISTORY

After the adoption in 1980 of Medical Standards by the Eye Bank Association of America (EBAA), the first steps in determining the level of practice of eye banks in relationship to these standards began with survey questionnaires. Through these questionnaires and the publication of its standards, it began to be possible for eye banks to compare their practices not just with a neighboring or collaborating eye bank, but also with virtually all eye banks nationwide. In 1982, the eye bank site visit inspections were instituted. Beginning with 12 bank inspections, 29 EBAA member banks were reviewed in the first year for adherence to the first published document for the EBAA Medical Standards for eye banking. Of the first 12 inspections, nine banks were certified and three were denied certification. At that time, the certification of eye banks became an established practice of EBAA, and all new eye bank members were inspected as part of their application for membership. In addition, all certified eye banks were and are reinspected every 3 years. During the June 1991 review, 35 banks were inspected, and, of them, 32 were certified and 3 were denied certification.

THE PROCESS

The process of certification inspection has been evolutionary, developing and changing as the Medical Standards document has been revised and as the level of eye bank practice has progressed. In June 1988, the EBAA Medical Standards Committee also revised the minimum criteria for education, experience, and training for eye bank inspectors. These minimum criteria were an additional aid in assuring a uniformity of inspections that would attest to the validity of peer view certification. The criteria are as follows:

1. Corneal surgeon with 2 years of active involvement in eye banking or EBAA experience.
2. An EBAA-certified eye bank technician with minimum of 5 years in eye banking.
3. An individual with a bachelor of science (B.S.) degree, a physician assistant (P.A.) or registered nurse (R.N.) or other medical professional licensure, and at least 3 years' experience in eye banking.

Preference in site visitor selection is given to the eye bank professionals who best meet or exceed minimum criteria and who have demonstrated an interest in serving EBAA in this capacity by providing a curriculum vitae and support letters to the committee and association chairs. To achieve broad representation and balance on the committee, member rotation occurs, with senior members relieved of service after 3 years for a period of at least 1 year and new members added to fill these vacancies.

The site visit inspection is arranged through notification by the EBAA office to both the committee and the eye bank for which a certification or recertification inspection is due. The committee chair assigns a member or members of the committee to perform the visit, and the inspector and the eye bank arrange the timing for the inspection. This process of date or time arrangement has been an advantage of voluntary peer review not enjoyed in certification processes such as the FDA (Food and Drug Administration) or the JCAHCO (Joint Commission on Accreditation of Health Care Organizations). Site visitors are provided an inspection document that addresses questions directly related to Medical Standards. Each question is referenced by number to the Medical Standard to which it applies. The inspection document is computer graded in a weighted program that assigns greater value to questions that are considered critical criteria for eye bank operation. The result of the computer analysis, the inspectors' summary, and the full committee's review are used to determine an eye bank's level of compliance with the EBAA Medical Standards and thereby its certification status.

During each meeting of the EBAA Certification Committee, a portion of the committee's time is devoted to understanding and improving the inspection process. Time is spent reviewing the inspection criteria, the documentation processes, and any revisions of Medical Standards that become additions to the site visit process. Members receive a guideline for conducting a site visit. This guideline addresses policy and procedures manuals and required sections, such as donor history, tissue evaluation, and records. It also references documentation, operations, maintenance and cleaning, instrumentation, technical performance, facilities and labeling. Combined with a checklist, a chart review documentation sheet, and the computer-graded survey sheets, the site inspector has the basic materials for the performance of a certification or recertification inspection. Even so, no inspector conducts a site visit without first accompanying an experienced inspector on a visit.

THE CONTENT

Just as the association attempts to prepare the certification committee inspectors for a site visit, so too does it provide assistance to eye banks in understanding and adherence to EBAA Medical Standards and to attainment of certification. Although the basis for certification is contained in the Medical Standards document, the EBAA provides a guide, *Building Blocks for a Site Visit*, a reference with examples of standard practices in eye banking that meet minimum standards. In this document, areas of quality assurances, donor screening, policies and procedures, labeling, and package inserts are addressed. The EBAA produced this document to accompany the June 1990 revisions of its Medical Standards and to assist with the policy and procedures requirements of the standards document. As these standards are revised, additional materials will be available from the EBAA for eye banks to consider in their operating practices.

At present, the areas of standards which are most emphasized in the inspection process are those that relate to recipient safety and to the documentation necessary to determine recipient safety.

These areas include donor screening, physical assessment, and serologic testing; medical history, chart review, interview and preliminary or gross autopsy results, and serology. Review for and screening and detection of all absolute contraindications to donation, such as Creutzfeldt-Jakob disease and rabies, which have demonstrated transmissibility to corneal recipients,[1,5] and AIDS (acquired immunodeficiency syndrome) or hepatitis,[2,3,6] which have perhaps a more limited potential for transmissibility, must be the desired outcome of any quality assurance, standards, or certification program for patient safety. So too are the identification and removal of risk from primary or secondary infective processes, bacterium or sepsis, or the potential hazards encountered with high-risk behavioral patterns like intravenous drug abuse.[4] These critical areas of concern are also affected by the criteria of labeling, identification, and tracking and by storage and conditions of maintenance and distribution, which assure that tissue can be promptly and properly identified, quarantined, recalled, or researched in regard to its outcome. Integrally related to all these categories are areas of instrumentation and sterility, quality assurance, security, technical proficiency, and tissue assessment, all of which play a role in the safe and efficient operation of an eye bank. All are important components of the overall content of the review process.

RESULTS

Once visited, the eye bank review information, computer survey, inspectors' summary report, and committee review are compiled, and the category of certification is determined, or certification is denied. The certification categories are defined as follows:

Category I. No deficiencies or only very limited deficiencies with none in the areas defined as critical or absolute criteria. Corrective action plan to be provided within 30 days and corrective action completed and documented with verification received by the certification committee with 90 days.

Category II. Limited deficiencies with not more than one deficiency within the areas defined as critical. Corrective action plan to be received within 60 days and corrective actions to be completed and documented with verification received by the certification committee within 6 months.

Category III. Deficiencies that are more frequent and may include up to two deficiencies within the areas defined as critical. Corrective action plan to be received within 60 days and corrective actions to be completed and documented with verification received by the certification committee within 6 months and the possible requirement for revisit within 18 months.

Certification Denied. Frequent or numerous deficiencies that because of number, inclusion of two or more deficiencies from the critical areas, or failure to appropriately correct and maintain previously cited deficiencies results in the need for reinspection within 1 year, corrective action plan within 6 months, progress reports within 9 months, and revisit in 12 months.

These categories are based, as previously mentioned, on areas of critical criteria. Using the 1990 EBAA Medical Standards, one can identify these criteria as follows:

1. *Medical Standards C3.400.* A policy and procedures manual with sufficient documentation to demonstrate adherence to requirements D1.200, E1.000, F1.000, G1.100, and K1.000.
2. *Medical Standards C2.100.* An actively involved medical director who is an ophthalmologist.
3. *Medical Standards C1.300.* EBAA certified technician.
4. *Medical Standards C1.200.* Demonstration of satisfactory corneoscleral rim removal by a member of each technician category who performs such procedures.
5. *Medical Standards F1.200.* Slitlamping of all potentially transplantable tissue.
6. *Medical Standards C2.100.* Functional limited-access laboratory.
7. *Medical Standards C2.100.* Appropriate functional equipment, such as a refrigerator with recording temperature monitor.
8. *Medical Standards E1.200.* Sterilization and supply maintenance with appropriate documentation and indicators.
9. *Medical Standards G1.210.* FDA-approved negative or nonreactive testing for required serologic types with documentation before tissue release.
10. *Medical Standards J1.000.* Unique identification number for all tissue with label content to

identify bank, serology, and donor data sufficient to trace tissue.

11. *Medical Standards G1.1000.* Documented report, before release of tissue, of autopsy or inquest, if performed.

Eye banks that receive certification in category I or II will not normally require a revisit for 3 years. Certification in category III may require that an eye bank be revisited within 18 months. This revisit is intended to ensure that actual implementation of corrective actions is understood and applied equally and correctly by all affected members of the eye bank's staff. When certification is denied, an eye bank seeking to attain certification should be prepared for revisit within 12 months. Most of the items of correction should be accomplished and documentation of compliance supplied to the committee well in advance of any revisit inspection. Technical proficiency will be reassessed at the time of revisit.

CONCLUSIONS

Eye bank certification is an educational process by which the eye banks and the Eye Bank Association of America continually evaluate the standards of eye banking practice. Scientific and technical advancements, disease prevalence, and levels of professional achievement are constantly changing; so too are the practices and procedures of eye banking and the criteria by which they are measured. Certification is a guideline of achievement but not the boundary of attainment. It will always be extended as eye banks improve the standards by which they provide service to the patients, physicians, and donor families.

ACKNOWLEDGMENT

My thanks to Elizabeth Cummings and Betty McMasters for research and manuscript preparation assistance.

REFERENCES

1. Centers for Disease Control: Human-to-human transmission of rabies by a corneal transplant—Idaho, *MMWR* 28:109-111, 1979.
2. Heck E, Petty C, Palestine A, et al: ELISA HIV testing and viral culture in the screening of corneal tissue for transplant from medical examiner cases, *Cornea* 8(2):77-80, 1989.
3. Hoft RH, Pflugfelder SC, Ullman S, et al: *Clinical evidence for hepatitis B transmission resulting from corneal transplant,* scientific poster presentation 39, annual meeting of The American Academy of Ophthalmology, Oct 1988.
4. The HIV/AIDS epidemic: the first 10 years, *Morbidity and Mortality Weekly Report* 40:357-375, 1991.
5. Pepose JS: Transfer of infection via corneal transplantation, *Transplant Proc* 21:3130-3132, 1989.
6. Salahuddin SZ, Palestine AG, Heck E, et al: Isolation of the human T-cell leukemia/lymphotropic virus type III from the cornea, *Am J Ophthalmol* 101:149, 1986.
7. *Webster's new world dictionary of the American language,* second college ed, New York, 1980, Simon & Schuster.

Chapter 48

The Eye Bank Association of America

History and development

EMILE J. FARGE

It would seem that a very loose federation of eye banks would serve a very useful purpose, not only in the exchange of ideas and development of better methods, but also in forming an exchange for the better distribution of available eyes.

Frederick C. Cordes
(*Am J Ophthalmol* 41:142, 1956)

BEFORE THE BEGINNING

The first of all eye banks, the Eye Bank for Sight Restoration in the State of New York, began in 1944 and received its certificate of incorporation on February 21, 1945. Its medical director was Dr. R. Townley Paton; its executive director was Mrs. Aida Breckinridge. Reporting in the *American Journal of Ophthalmology*[5] in 1946, Dr. Derrick Vail remarked that ". . .after a year of difficulties and achievement in spite of these, the eye bank has become firmly established and is fulfilling its most important function, . . . the collection and distribution of eyes, the corneas of which are to be used as material for the transplantation operation."[8]

Advances in transplantation came quickly after the first eye bank's birth with banks in Buffalo, Toronto, Chicago, and New Orleans established in rapid order. These, however, operated as almost unofficial branches of the New York bank, where the majority of the tissue was procured. A national board of directors guided the operation.

By 1950, when the first international symposium on corneal surgery was held in New York, 1200 eyes had been received and supplied to surgeons through the Eye Bank for Sight Restoration.

Five years later 37 representatives from eye banks in Boston, Buffalo, Chicago, Memphis, New Orleans, New York City, Rochester, Washington, D.C., Iowa City and Winston-Salem (N.C.), urged a thorough assessment of eye banking needs.[4] As a result, in 1956, under the leadership of Derrick Vail and Frederick C. Cordes, two contributing editors to the *American Journal of Ophthalmology*,[1,7] a committee was appointed to investigate eye banking, ways in which activities might be controlled and standardized, and a possible search for a unification of the approximately 20 eye banks in existence. The American Academy of Ophthalmology and Otolaryngology (AAOO), the American Medical Association (AMA), the American Ophthalmological Society, and the Association for Research in Ophthalmology were represented on the committee, which was active for two years and produced several recommendations. These included:

1. An eye bank organization, composed of all acceptable eye banks, should be formed.
2. A central clearinghouse should be formed to aid in the distribution of eye tissues.
3. Ethical means should be formulated for fundraising, publicity, and seeking of donors.
4. Medical aspects must be governed by ophthalmologists, and investigation must accompany the growth of eye banking primarily in appropriate ways of obtaining, transporting, and preserving corneal material

By this time, Dr. Paton reported,[6] the national eye bank and its branches had distributed 3800 eyes in its 10-year history.

The joint committee proved unwieldy; its members had to take suggestions back to each of four organizations, wait for deliberation, and report back to the committee. Leadership, therefore, was given instead to the American Academy of Ophthalmology and Otolaryngology. AAOO formed a permanent committee on eye banks in October 1960 to investigate the establishment of an association of affiliated eye banks in the United States. With the concurrence of ophthalmologists and lay directors of many eye banks throughout the country, the organization began at the academy meeting later that year.

EARLY YEARS OF THE EBAA: 1961 TO 1965

Ten eye banks were represented at an organizational meeting[3] on October 7, 1961. They were:

Buffalo Eye-Bank
Colorado Eye-Bank
The Eye-Bank for Sight Restoration, Inc., New York
Eye Foundation of Delaware Valley (Pa., N.J., Del.)
Iowa Eye Bank
Lions of District 22-C of Washington, D.C.
North Carolina Eye-Bank
Hawaii Eye-Bank
Southern Eye-Bank
Rochester Eye-Bank

The original name "Eye-Bank Association of America" (EBAA) was adopted unanimously. The hyphen, which was part of the EBAA name for many years, was intended to separate eye banking from the concept that a "bank" was a depository of monetary funds.

The EBAA adopted the following purposes:
1. To establish uniform standards and procedures
2. To exchange information from member eye-banks
3. To establish central and regional clearing-houses
4. To promote legislation of interest to eye-banks
5. To establish eye-banks where needed
6. To promote eye research
7. To promote cooperation between lay and professional groups operating in the eye-bank field
8. To serve as a center of information in all matters pertaining to eye-bank organization and operation

Membership in the EBAA required that member eye banks be legally incorporated; be affiliated with a hospital or medical center; and have a medical-surgical director, a responsible board of directors, and an executive secretary with an office and 24-hour telephone service. Such eye banks must also be recommended by their local medical association and employ medically approved methods for collecting eyes.

Within a year an interim board meeting was held,

appropriate committees were appointed, and the officers and directors were urged to keep in touch with each other on a frequent basis.

At the first annual meeting of the EBAA in Las Vegas in 1962 the constitution was adopted, a statistical research project was approved, and the securing of a national permanent headquarters was given high priority.

From the first, the question of fees and charges was to plague the fledgling organization. The first discussion hinged on reimbursement of costs incurred by one eye bank (such as the large New York eye bank) for collecting, handling, and distributing an eye to another eye bank. It was decided that the eye banks would reimburse each other, but these charges must not be passed on to the patient receiving the graft. Beyond the questions of financing and reimbursement, a model law that could be adopted by any or all of the states was presented and approved. Such a law would enable a living person to "will" his eyes to an eye bank or for the next of kin to donate the eyes by means of a simple legal document.

Subsequent meetings focused on the need for a central office and secretary, continuous liaison with the American Academy of Ophthalmology and Otolaryngology, and a need for standards and procedures. Dr. Herbert Kaufman, of the Gainesville, Florida, eye bank, prepared an enucleation procedure to be distributed to all member eye banks. A procedure for admitting new members was established by a committee headed by Dr. Robert Fitzgerald of the Illinois eye bank, which recommended that the primary officials must sign an application for membership and must be approved by the medical society in their country of origin and by the member eye banks nearby. Leonard Heise, also of Illinois, represented the EBAA with Lions International, seeking the help of the Lions in the formation and maintenance of member eye banks throughout the country.

Under EBAA urging, members established close alliances with local funeral directors and participated in a network of "ham" radio enthusiasts.

In 1965, EBAA headquarters were established in the North Carolina Eye Bank Building in Winston-Salem. By unanimous motion of the board, the eye bank was instructed to move its files and few belongings to Winston-Salem. Thus, on November 11, 1965, the 4-year-old organization had a board of directors, 18 members in 13 states, and a new home—a single office that was part of an eye bank of one of its members and its home for approximately 15 years.

THE NORTH CAROLINA YEARS: 1965 TO 1980

Board meetings that lasted a full 2 days and house of delegates' meetings that lasted an entire day were to mark the next decade of EBAA practices. From its Winston-Salem home it convened these meetings generally with the American Academy of Ophthalmology or one of its regional meetings. Much of the infrastructure on which the eye banking of the 1980s and 1990s was to be built was established during this time.

In 1968 the board discussed the need for accreditation of eye banks, saying that teams of qualified eye bankers and ophthalmologists should visit member eye banks. No deadline or protocol was established, and so this practice was left in abeyance.

Also in 1968 service charges by eye banks were brought up by Dr. Alfred Sadler, who pointed out that blood banks had been charging service fees for several decades without this being construed as an unethical practice or a charge for the tissue itself.

Dr. William Clark, a New Orleans ophthalmologist, was executive director of the EBAA from 1968 to 1970. It was a time of turbulence and high expectation. With the national headquarters in Winston-Salem and Dr. Clark working out of New Orleans, progress was made. About 10 new members were admitted, but the continuous call for a "full-time executive" to lead the organization sometimes drowned out the progress that was in fact taking place.

The Rochester Eye Bank announced in 1969 that Blue Cross was beginning to reimburse its patients for costs of services incurred in producing corneas for surgery. That same year, graduating morticians at the University of Iowa took the first course in eye enucleation, taught by Dr. Alson Braley.

Fifty-seven eye banks held membership in the EBAA at that time. A sliding scale of dues between $150 and $1,000, based on the number of eyes produced was established briefly, but the flat membership of $300 per member per year was later reinstated.

Helen Bunce was retained as executive secretary of the EBAA after Dr. Clark's resignation as executive director. In 1971, cryopreservation was adopted by many eye banks, and freezing units were being recommended by Dr. Herbert Kaufman of Gainesville, Florida.

At this time the Medical Eye Bank of Maryland announced that it had exported over 500 corneas to surgeons outside the state of Maryland. Under the strong executive directorship of Frederick L. Griffith, the eye bank based at Baltimore had begun to gather over 1000 whole-globe eyes per year. Under

ophthalmologist Richard Richards of the Wilmer Institute at Baltimore, the EBAA's annual scientific session was beginning to make a name for itself with outstanding corneal meetings.

In 1972 standing committees were finally established. The eye network run by "ham" radio operators reported that 6200 eyes had been distributed throughout its 12-year history. At the 1973 Dallas meeting attended by 43 member eye banks and 33 nonmember eye banks, the issue of charging a service fee for eyes first arose. Philips B. Jankus of the Southern Eye Bank, New Orleans, presented a resolution stating that fees or handling costs would be interpreted by the public as the sale of eyes.

By the mid-1970s eye banking had changed. Some eye banks, especially in Baltimore and New York, were gathering many eyes; eye banks in Rochester, Baltimore, and Houston were regularly passing on service charges. President Jack McTigue, M.D., of Washington, D.C., pointed out that kidney banks were charging over $2,000 per organ and perhaps it was time for the EBAA to recognize that a service charge connected with tissue was no longer a difficulty. Finally, in 1976, Attorney Paul Byrnes stated the following: "I find nothing in the Constitution and Bylaws that would prohibit an eye bank from making a charge for servicing, processing, and transporting of tissue." He recommended that this should be done on a local option basis.

In 1977 at his last meeting as president, Dr. McTigue announced that the American Academy of Ophthalmology had recognized the EBAA as its eye-banking arm for accreditation and had stated strongly that the EBAA must set up and implement standards. The academy stated that the EBAA should set its own policy regarding fees, saying that charging fees was in no way in conflict with AAO regulations.

The years 1978 and 1979 were times of growth in all tissue banking. Eye banking was no exception. More eye banks began to charge a service fee, hire specific personnel to serve as donor procurement and enucleation technicians, and generally increase the lay or nonophthalmologic personnel connected with the eye banks. The Medical Standards Committee of the EBAA, guided principally by Drs. Jay Krachmer of Iowa City, Frederick Brightbill of Madison, James Aquavella of Rochester, and Donald Doughman of Minneapolis, drafted medical standards to be implemented according to the instructions of the AAO.

After several years and several drafts the board of directors unanimously adopted the medical standards of the EBAA for the first time on June 6,

1980. The original purpose of a union of eye banks—the standardizing of medical and ethical practices—had come about 24 years after Dr. Cordes's original recommendation.

THE TEXAS YEARS: 1981 TO 1985

To declare medical standards was one thing; to implement them certainly was another. Accordingly, the Search Committee of the EBAA sought an executive director to lead the organization through its next few highly critical years. Past President W.H. "Mac" Goldfinch, Jr., chairman of the EBAA Search Committee, explained that it must be a person who knew something of eye banking, fund raising, and administration. Dr. Emile J. Farge, executive director of the Lions Eye Bank at Houston, was named to the post and moved EBAA headquarters to Houston.

President James Jerva of Syracuse was completely supportive of the new administration. The committee structure was enlarged, and Jerva appointed two key committee chairmanships: Dr. Jay Krachmer continuing as chairman of the Medical Standards Committee and Dr. Frederick Brightbill as chairman of the Technicians' Committee. Both of these chairmen were encouraged to gather around them persons committed to the task of technician training and medical standards implementation.

The first technicians' training course was taught under the leadership of Mary Ann Gallagher later that year. Thirteen students became the most senior approved eye-bank technicians under this new program.

The Medical Standards Committee formulated a questionnaire asking eye banks about their current medical practices in the procurement, enucleation, storage, and distribution of eye tissue, recommending that the initial certification be granted by registered mail, with the questionnaire having been filled out correctly by the medical director and executive director of each eye bank, signed in front of a notary, and posted to the EBAA's Committee on Medical Standards based at Chairman Jay Krachmer's office in Iowa City.

At this same meeting the board approved a $160,000 fund-raising task to be undertaken by Farge to expand to meet the needs of an organization that now, for the first time, was to certify both medical standards at eye banks and technicians. A challenge gift 1 month later by the Moody Foundation of Galveston, Texas, in the amount of $40,000, predicated upon the EBAA's ability to raise the additional $120,000, formed the financial keystone of this new operation.

Concurrently, membership in EBAA was growing from 80 members in 1981 to 86 at the end of 1982 and 94 at the end of 1984. The budget was growing accordingly, from $10,114 in 1980 to $251,000 in 1984.

Frederick Brightbill became president in 1982, strongly stressing the need for donor procurement. Government relations, continuing donor procurement, and national public relations efforts were priorities of his successor, A. Howard Snyder, of Dallas.

During Snyder's presidency the board voted to allow Emile Farge to hire Thomas J. Moore as associate director for public relations, allowing the EBAA to intensify its work. Four manuals were written and edited during his year as president, including the *Eye Bank Administrative Manual, Eye Bank Technical Manual, Eye Bank Public Relations Manual,* and *Eye Bank Tissue Procurement.*

At this meeting Y.T. Abernathy, chairman of the Constitution and Bylaws Committee, engineered a change in the EBAA's constitution to allow heightened constitutional status for the executive employees of EBAA, the ability to allow any North American eye bank to become a full member of EBAA and to allow South American eye banks to become associate members, and to clarify finally that charging a service fee for tissue was in no way an abridgment of EBAA ethical standards. All were approved unanimously by the board and house of delegates.

The international theme was to be taken up by the 1984 president, Busharat Ahmad of Marquette, Michigan. That year the EBAA cosponsored with the International Eye Foundation the Fifth World Congress of Ophthalmology held in Cairo, Egypt. During this year the EBAA and Pan American Association of Ophthalmology also sponsored the first training course for Latin American eye bankers. Executive director trainees were received at the Houston offices from Argentina, Colombia, Ecuador, Panama, Paraguay, Peru, and Puerto Rico. Additionally, President Ahmad announced the formation of the International Association of Eye Banks, a project in which he pledged to be active even after his presidential year.

EBAA headquarters moved to Washington, D.C., in 1984, hiring a full-time director for the first time. Having begun with Rosario Guglielmo running the office from his own home and Dr. Holt running it from his office, the EBAA had become a 15-year "roommate" with the North Carolina Eye and Tissue Bank and had spent 4 years in an office across the street from the Lions Eye Bank of Houston. Now it was to be its own independent self, leaving it free from the criticism that any local eye bank was profiting unduly.

When Dr. Farge chose not to go to Washington, Associate Director Thomas J. Moore was hired to lead the EBAA, now as president rather than as executive director.

During its time in Houston, the number of member eye banks had grown from 72 to 94 and tissue procurement had grown from 18,000 per year to 42,000 total eyes and corneas donated each year. Seven new medical examiner laws were passed, and assets increased from $10,000 to $100,000. After loading the furniture, literature, computers, files, and other equipment, the moving company announced that the EBAA's possessions weighed 7½ tons. The 50-month tenure in Texas had seen the 40 pounds of files brought from North Carolina blossom from a seedling to a viable plant.

THE WASHINGTON YEARS: 1985 TO PRESENT

Opening its doors in Washington, D.C., on March 7, 1985, the EBAA faced several structural as well as geographic changes. The voluntary office of president became known as chairman of the board with a 2-year term to allow for a greater continuity and ability to work with the staff. The chairman's position was first held by Bill Temples of North Carolina, followed by Jay Krachmer, M.D., of Iowa; Richard Fuller of Ann Arbor (1988-1990, who during his tenure accepted a position with Tissue Bank International); Mark Mannis, M.D., of Sacramento (1990-1992); and Ellen Heck of Dallas (1992-1994).

Faced with the opportunity to be at the nerve center of decision-making for health care matters meant the retaining of a full-time public relations associate to assist the president as well as a full-time secretary. The EBAA also needed legislative and legal counsel on a retainer basis.

This need for expanded services brought about total independence from any local eye bank and brought increased operating expenses and restructured dues. In place of the $500 annual dues assessed during the previous 5 years, a review committee recommended a basic dues of $700, which would increase incrementally based upon an eye bank's production of corneas for transplant. Thus some eye banks would pay $700 per year, whereas others had dues over $10,000. These larger banks, it was believed, could better afford to pay the higher fee and received a greater benefit from having a strong organization.

There were some initial disagreements on the size of the dues; many eye banks were paying tenfold or more of what they had previously paid. The 11 eye banks that were members of the Tissue Bank International group of eye banks temporarily left EBAA, rejoining as a global member 2½ years later.

An endowment fund and an annual fund to establish research awards for breaking new ground in areas crucial to eye banking, such as sterile procedure, corneal preservation, corneal evaluation, and quality control in eye banking, was established. A national campaign ("The Goal is in SIGHT") was undertaken raising $700,000 over an 18-month period.

On the legislative side, the EBAA's government affairs counsel worked to maintain a legislative identity for eye banks separate from that of organ banks or tissue banks. In this regard, EBAA approached the Health Care Finance Administration to have the regulation of eye banks included under the purview of the Clinical Laboratories Improvement Act (CLIA) as modified in 1988. Efforts have been undertaken for over a year and a half and are still in process as of this writing.

When President Thomas Moore accepted an invitation to return to Houston to resume work with eye banking in that state, Patricia Aiken-O'Neill, formerly of the Washington office of the American Academy of Ophthalmology, was chosen to be the third paid executive and second president of the EBAA. She took office on March 1, 1990.

The memorable events of the first 5 years in Washington of the EBAA might be summarized thus:

1. The EBAA took a more active national role in legislation through its national and state government affairs program. The membership became more supportive of the need for working with the government to help protect the public's trust in the eye donation process.

2. Eye banking began greater participation with national leaders in organ and tissue procurement by greater involvement of EBAA members with the North American Transplant Coordinators Organization, the American Association of Tissue Banks, the Association of Organ Procurement Organizations, and the American Council on Transplantation.

3. The EBAA's expanded services, particularly in the medical standards and administrative areas, helped to strengthen the growing trends for professionalism and public accountability within eye banking.

4. The EBAA achieved much greater financial stability through the membership's dedication to building operating reserve and endowment funds.

L

REFERENCES

1. Cordes FC: Federation of eye-banks, *Am J Ophthalmol* 41:140-142, 1956 (Editorial).
2. Cordes FC: The Eye Bank Committee *Am J Ophthalmol* 43:310-311, 1957 (Editorial).
3. Holt LB: *History of the Eye-Bank Association of America: 1944-1965* (pamphlet), Eye Bank Association of America, 1001 Connecticut Avenue, Suite 601, Washington, DC 20036.
4. King JH Jr: Eye-bank programs, *Am J Ophthalmol* 54:5, 1962.
5. Paton RT: Corneal transplants, *Am J Ophthalmol* 33(3, part II):1, 1950.
6. Paton RT: Eye-bank programs, *Am J Ophthalmol* 41:419-424, 1956.
7. Post LT: Eye banks, *Am J Ophthalmol* 30:920-922, 1947 (Editorial).
8. Vail D: The Eye-Bank for Sight Restoration, Inc., *Am J Ophthalmol* 29:46-48, 1946 (Editorial).

Purposes and programs

THOMAS J. MOORE
PATRICIA AIKEN-O'NEILL

The Eye Bank Association of America (EBAA) is a voluntary health organization composed of non-profit eye banks united "to restore sight through the promotion and advancement of eye banking." As of June 1991, the EBAA had 98 member eye banks from 43 states, the District of Columbia, Puerto Rico, and Canada, with satellites and local offices in more than 125 locations.

MEMBERSHIP

Membership in the association is available to those eye banks from United States that meet the following criteria: (1) They must be exempt under 501(c)(3) or 5(c)(6) of the Internal Revenue Code; (2) they must comply with the purpose and Code of Ethics of the EBAA; and (3) they must be recommended for membership by their local or regional medical society. Eye banks in North America, outside the United States, also are eligible for membership if they are in compliance with the above requirements. Associate memberships are available for eye banks from Central America and South America if they meet the above requirements and are affiliated with a university hospital, an eye hospital, or a general hospital with a well-established eye department.

MEDICAL STANDARDS

The EBAA's commitment to quality control is one of its most important functions. Its roots are found in the EBAA's Medical Standards, a document that originally was developed in June 1980 and has been updated regularly since then.

In the late 1970s the need for those standards became paramount for several reasons. Eye banking was growing rapidly, and an increasing number of eye banks with varied practices were being formed. The number of corneal transplants being performed was growing quickly, causing a greater demand for donor tissue. Several cases of transmitted disease from donor corneas were being reported, and concern was increasing that state and federal agencies would be evaluating the quality of eye-banking practices. The American Academy of Ophthalmology looked to the EBAA to develop medical standards covering the operations of eye banks. All these factors related to the need to improve the effectiveness and efficiency of eye banks.

The EBAA's Medical Standards is the only set of eye-banking standards that has been endorsed by the American Academy of Ophthalmology. The EBAA has consistently reviewed and refined its standards and procedures to a level that results in the maximum availability of tissue for either transplantation or for research and education. As a consequence, corneal transplantation serves as a model for the greater transplantation arena, with an over 90% success rate in transplantation and few adverse reactions.

As federal and state organizations begin the certification of eye and tissue banks, the value of the EBAA's Medical Standards has grown. Several states have accepted these standards as the requirements for state certification. Medical Standards undergo stringent annual review and revision.

The EBAA in 1991 and 1992 undertook a major initiative and developed a thorough operations manual to outline technical procedures and necessary monitoring of eye banks through quality assurance and quality control. This process will maintain eye banking's commitment to ensuring patient safety.

SITE VISITS

The creation of the Medical Standards provided the EBAA with a solid foundation for conducting site-visit evaluations to determine that its members were adhering to proper eye-banking procedures. The chairman of the EBAA Medical Standards Site Visit Subcommittee appoints a team of inspectors to inspect an eye bank due for inspection. One or two inspectors may visit, depending on the size of the laboratory. Inspectors are drawn from the EBAA Site Visit Subcommittee and are either eye bank administrators, technicians, or medical doctors, who are ophthalmologists with a specialty in cornea. Appointment as an inspector is based on a review of a candidate's curriculum vitae, experience and willingness to serve. At present, pay to an inspector is limited to reimbursement of expenses incurred.

Before the visit, eye banks are sent a preinspection checklist of certification requirements that, when completed, provides the Site Visit Subcommittee with an approximate understanding of the eye bank's readiness to be inspected. After the site visit, the inspector submits a completed Inspection Questionnaire form to the chairman of the Medical Standards Site Visit Committee. This form is processed through a standardized computerized program to provide an analysis of the eye bank's laboratory proficiency. In addition, the inspector prepares a written report to present at the next committee meeting (held biannually).

The tabulated computer results and narrative report are used with the inspector's verbal assessment to help the committee determine the bank's certification status. This method works very effectively as a check-and-balance mechanism.

The medical director or executive director of the inspected eye bank laboratory also completes an evaluation report after the site visit and submits the report to the chairman of the Medical Standards Committee. The chairman's responsibility is to review this report and, if the report raises any questions of fairness and objectivity, to determine whether an appeal to the Standards Committee is appropriate. After an appeal to the Medical Standards Committee, the inspected laboratory retains the option to petition the EBAA's Arbitration Committee.

TECHNICAL TRAINING

The development of the Medical Standards also made possible the EBAA's technician training program, which began in 1981. The training program combines a standardized didactic course, practical or "laboratory" experience, and completion of a comprehensive examination. In addition, technicians are required to pass a review of their technical skills by their medical director. This need for local involvement reflects the EBAA's belief that the examination and certification process should be a cooperative effort.

The EBAA entered into a contractual agreement with the Joint Commission of Allied Health Professionals in Ophthalmology (JCAHPO) in 1991 to administer technician examinations. This change is ex-

pected to confer an enhanced professional standing and image to eye bank technicians within the greater transplantation community.

In 1984, the Technician's Recertification Program was established for those technicians who had been certified 3 years previously. Recertification credit now can be earned through courses sponsored by the EBAA or courses taught by other organizations that meet the content guidelines established by the EBAA's Technicians' Committee.

EBAA MANUALS

In 1984, the EBAA published four manuals covering the key elements of eye banking: administration, technical skills, donor procurement, and public relations. In 1987 the Legislative Affairs Manual was published, and in 1990 the Public Education Resource Manual was published. These manuals, which feature articles from experts in eye banking, have been accepted by those within the transplant community as a premier set of reference books. The comprehensive manuals are updated periodically as new developments and trends arise.

SCIENTIFIC SESSIONS, MEETINGS, AND PROFESSIONAL TRAINING

The commitment to training extends beyond the four eye banking manuals. Since 1963, the EBAA traditionally has held a scientific session during the annual meeting of the American Academy of Ophthalmology. This half-day session features presentations by leaders in corneal surgery and research and in eye banking. Many of the new research and clinical developments, such as improved preservation techniques and new surgical innovations, are presented. The EBAA publishes the abstracts of these presentations. The EBAA also is committed to sponsoring larger scientific programs, such as the First International Cornea and Eye Banking Symposium in 1985 and this publication.

The EBAA also conducts an annual meeting, an educational conference, and various regional meetings each year. The annual meeting is held in late spring or early summer. It includes presentations on all areas of eye banking, and a business meeting of the board of directors and house of delegates (the legislative arm of the EBAA composed of representatives from each eye bank). The educational seminar is held either directly before or after the AAO's annual meeting and includes the scientific session and a 2-day program on a variety of topics. The EBAA's meetings are open to all interested parties.

INTERACTION WITH OTHER ORGANIZATIONS

The EBAA long has recognized that cooperation, both internal and external, is one of the keys to its success. The EBAA's network of supporting organizations has been instrumental in the promotion and growth of the eye banking. The AAO's Committee on Eye Banks has given the EBAA a strong liaison to the academy. This group has been instrumental in the formation of the EBAA's Medical Standards, as well as in helping to coordinate centralized eye-banking policy and legislative efforts. The EBAA also works closely with specialty groups in ophthalmology, such as the American Society of Cataract and Refractive Surgery, to gain a better understanding of the issues affecting ophthalmology and eye banking.

The EBAA has strong working relationships with many critical research organizations, including the National Diabetes Research Interchange, the Juvenile Diabetes Foundation, and Project ORBIS. The EBAA's members have been one of the main suppliers of tissues to the Retinitis Pigmentosa Fighting Blindness Foundation and the Foundation for Glaucoma Research. For 20 years, the EBAA has been a member of the National Health Council, and EBAA eye bankers have held membership in the Ocular Council of the American Association of Tissue Banks (AATB) since its inception in 1977. EBAA members also belong to other transplant organizations, such as the North American Transplant Coordination Organization (NATCO), to help enhance relationship with other professionals in organ and tissue procurement.

The EBAA's move to Washington in March 1985 has enhanced the opportunity for interorganizational involvement. The EBAA was actively involved in the American Council on Transplantation (ACT) during its existence from 1984-1991. An EBAA representative sat on its board of directors, and in 1984, EBAA President Busharat Ahmad, M.D., served as the first chairman of the ACT's Public Education Forum. This type of national cooperation is possible only through the united effort of eye banks because membership in many national organizations often is limited only to other national groups.

The EBAA has worked closely with two kindred organizations, the Association of Nurses Endorsing Transplantation (ANET) and the National Ambassadors for Corneal Transplants (NACT), which have promoted the involvement of nurses and corneal recipients, respectively, in the eye donation process. These groups are successfully allowing eye banks to increase their abilities to serve their communities and are providing strong support services to their constituents.

INTERNATIONAL PROGRAMS

Improving eye banking internationally is an important goal of the association. In 1984, the EBAA held a training program in which representatives from seven Central American and South American countries were trained to become executive directors. Each of the trainees were carefully selected by ophthalmologists from their local areas. The course, which had the support of the International Eye Foundation and the Pan-American Association of Ophthalmology, included a 2-week workshop at the EBAA's headquarters followed by 3 weeks in residence at one of the EBAA's member eye banks. The course was extremely successful and was the forerunner for commitments to assist others around the world in establishing eye banks. The course initiated the creation of the Pan-American Association of Eye Banks, which now has grown from seven eye banks in six countries before the course to 27 eye banks in 16 countries as of June 1, 1991.

The EBAA and its members have a long history of cooperation with civic groups. Over 50 of the 98 members are sponsored by a civic group. The involvement of these organizations has been critical in many phases of the growth of eye banking. The support of the Lions Clubs to sight restoration is particularly noteworthy.

COMMITTEES

A major reason why eye banks become EBAA members is to have a strong cooperative relationship with other eye banks. Internal cooperation among EBAA members is best evidenced by the strong network of EBAA committees. These committees not only are vital in handling important issues (such as tissue procurement and medical standards) as they arise, but they also have initiated many of the EBAA's key programs. For example, the long-range planning committee has been critical in providing the membership with the foresight needed to prepare for future developments. The committees interact with other eye banks and the national staff to fulfill their programs.

One of the assets of the committee structure is that small task forces can be formed to handle specific assignments that need prompt action. A good example of this advantage is the Vision Planning Task Force, which in 1985 outlined a national communications program to build a stronger public image for the association and its members. The Tissue Distribution Task Force's work in the 1990s will form an important basis for major policy considerations.

EBAA RESEARCH GRANTS PROGRAM

In 1987 the EBAA established a Research Grants Program to provide support for proposals specifically concerned with issues directly related to eye banking or corneal transplantation. Preference is given to pilot projects, well-defined short-term protocols, and initial studies directed toward new research initiatives. Physicians, basic scientists, biomedical and social scientists, eye bank technicians, ophthalmology residents and fellows, and other health professionals are eligible to apply for funding.

The program has awarded more than $87,000 since its inception, thanks in large part to the generous support of ophthalmic companies, in particular, Allergan Medical Optics (Santa Ana, California) and Chiron Ophthalmics (Irvine, California). Results from the research have been detailed in major ophthalmic publications and presented at many national meetings.

OTHER ACTIVITIES

By joining forces in the EBAA, eye banks benefit from the "sum being greater than the individual parts." The EBAA has been able to negotiate with equipment vendors on a group basis to help member eye banks save money in ordering needed instruments and office equipment. These types of services have begun to meet identified needs of the EBAA's membership.

Another important EBAA program is national communication coordinated by the national office. Eye-banking statistics are complied annually from information supplied by member eye banks concerning their activity in procuring and distributing corneas and whole-eye tissue. The EBAA prepares a summary report that is distributed to its members, national organizations, and the news media. These reports have helped to generate news coverage and have been extremely well received for their detail and reporting format.

The EBAA also publishes *Foresight*, a quarterly newsletter featuring stories on the national efforts in eye banking. The newsletter, which now has a circulation of more than 5000, is available free of charge to anyone interested. The association also provides its member eye banks with monthly reports including updates on legislation and other key issues affecting day-to-day eye-bank operations.

Beginning in 1984, the EBAA, as one part of its overall fund-raising program, began the R. Townley Paton, M.D., Society for corneal surgeons and researchers in honor of the founder of eye banking in the United States. Through their annual support, the society's members are financial partners in the EBAA's mission and future. The EBAA sponsors an annual educational program and luncheon for the society.

The EBAA's Code of Ethics followed by its members stipulate that member eye banks conduct their operations in a dignified manner. The EBAA's Medical Standards and Code of Ethics both indicate the association's strong commitment to a unified, consistent, and ethical approach in eye banking to serve an eye bank's many users: transplant recipients, donors, the news media, physicians, procurement coordinators, nurses, funeral industry representatives, and so on.

The future for eye banking and the EBAA looks extremely promising. The first 30 years of the association have laid the groundwork for the EBAA to assume a prominent position in the transplant and ophthalmologic communities. The association, with the input of the membership is designing the necessary programs to ensure that the EBAA has a strong public image in the years ahead. The national staff, together with the strong volunteers within the association, are ready and able to meet the challenges facing the eye banking community in the future.

Chapter 49

Tissue Procurement

Retrieval Without a Medical Examiner Law

MARGARET C. KELM

In a state without a medical examiner law, tissue procurement involves effort by a broad range of persons, coordinated by the staff of the eye bank. It involves dedication, education, and ongoing encouragement to make it work, but it can succeed.

The Wisconsin Eye Bank has such a program. In view of its history, its volunteer support and its growing success is instructive. Established in 1969, for 8 years the Wisconsin Eye Bank remained quiet, not much more than an office receiving occasional donations of tissue from ophthalmologists, then the only legal tissue enucleators. In 1977, when state law changed to allow funeral directors, nursing staff, and any person working under the direction of a physician to enucleate eyes, a tremendous source of volunteer enucleators was available. It became the job of the Wisconsin Eye Bank to tap that potential, coordinate its effort, and truly establish an active service for those waiting for corneal transplantation.

The Eye Bank, which serves a population of 2,445,885 people and 82 hospitals, offered its first course for volunteer enucleators in 1978. That same year, a full-time technician was employed. There was growth in the number of eyes received through 1985 but with passage of the Required Request Law in Wisconsin in July of 1986, the numbers soared:

1980	643	**1986**	2236
1981	506	**1987**	2589
1982	728	**1988**	2199
1983	1029	**1989**	1975
1984	1040	**1990**	1925
1985	1080	**1991**	1928

The education and hospital support already in place eased the effort required for the sudden increase. Hospitals developed policies for required request quickly; the first 2 years' numbers under the new law are impressive. After looking at our medical criteria in 1988 and deciding not to accept eyes from septic patients, the numbers decreased. Subsequent concern that families were not being approached because of an erroneous belief that a patient was septic led to reversal of that decision, effective January 1991.

In 1991 there were more than 672 certified eye enucleators in the area, including 430 nurses, 115 funeral directors, 29 coroners and medical examiners, 22 emergency medical technicians, and 76 social workers, technicians, and others.

The Wisconsin Eye Bank accepts eyes from donors of all ages (Table 49-1).

COMPONENTS OF SUCCESS

Through combined efforts of the Lions organization, hospital staffs, coroners and medical examiners, and clergy and by making the most of promotional efforts, the Eye Bank serves its constituency.

Lions. The Wisconsin Lions organization is a strong supporter of eye banking. When increasing numbers of enucleators made tissue more readily available to the eye bank, the Lions were there, an organization ready to be tapped for manpower and financial support to get eye banking moving at the local level.

To handle the geographic spread of the Wisconsin Eye Bank, it was necessary to have local substations established to coordinate the handling and transportation of tissue. The Lions maintain this "establishment" role, purchasing enucleation kits for area hospitals and covering the cost for enucleation and pro-

Table 49-1. Donor Eyes, Wisconsin Eye Bank, 1990

Age of Donor	Number of Eyes Received
0-9	32
10-19	36
20-29	49
30-39	51
40-49	128
50-59	193
60-69	461
70-79	499
80-89	364
90-99	108
100+	4

curement training for volunteers from their communities. They also provide a structure to establish the rudiments of an eye bank substation quickly. When tissue becomes available in their communities, the Lions arrange for its transportation to the office in Madison for processing. With distances approaching 400 miles from the outer limits of the Eye Bank's territory to Madison, transportation takes varied forms. Arrangements are made with airlines to fly the tissue in; United States National Guard units are on call to help with transportation. Bus lines serve much of the state. Where these options are not satisfactory, Lions members drive the tissue in for processing.

Lion members are also excellent resources for local community awareness campaigns. During National Eye Bank Awareness month in March, Lions clubs across the state distribute pamphlets throughout their communities, speak before service clubs, make personal contacts with local media, arrange for mayoral proclamation signings, and, in some cases, meet with clergy groups, encouraging their involvement and endorsement of eye bank efforts from the pulpit. The Lions give a community pride to the eye bank effort.

Hospitals. With the training of nurses as enucleators, hospitals became an important part of the statewide eye bank team. Staff education was essential. Education in eye banking, its importance, and how to obtain consent for corneal donation from next of kin as well as the basics of removing and preparing eyes for use by the eye bank were essential.

Eye bank staff members work to gain hospital support and then offer the training necessary to make it work. Administrative support is as necessary as that of the floor nurse—each must be aware of the effort and be willing to make the time and space available to make it work.

In-service time must be available to eye bank staff who can teach the rudiments of procurement and the importance of the eye bank's work. Hospital personnel need to be made aware that for every eye donated, there will be a team ready to use that tissue for transplantation or research. One in-service session is not enough; continual retraining is necessary to bring new people into the voluntary effort and to let "veterans" know that their efforts are appreciated.

Taking the time to handle eye bank work in a hospital is an extra commitment that the eye bank asks staff to take on, and continual reaffirmation of appreciation is part of the success of this program.

Procurement seminars are offered by the Wisconsin Eye Bank twice a year, training key people from participating hospitals to effectively ask for eyes from the next of kin. For many dedicated, sincere volunteers this is a very difficult task, and it is the job of the eye bank to be certain that they have the training needed to do the job. These specially trained staff then return to their hospitals and pass on what they have learned. Top to bottom, the training passes down. Top to bottom, the support must be there for the program.

Finally, hospitals must offer coordination of eye removal. Facilities must be made available for the enucleation. Procedures must be established to make the enucleator's part of the system work.

Coroners and Medical Examiners. Coroners and medical examiners are, of necessity, with every family where a member has met an early death. Tragically, many of these deaths involve young people, and the cooperation of coroners and medical examiners makes the receipt of good, young tissue more likely.

If a good working relationship has been developed between these persons and the eye bank, that tissue can be forthcoming. Some medical examiners and coroners will make the approach to the family themselves. Others will ask clergy or hospital staff who are also involved in the case to talk to the family. But because they are there and if they have been impressed with the importance of the work, they can be invaluable resources to the eye bank. They are a prime reason that the Wisconsin group has such a strong donation of young tissue.

Clergy. Similarly, there is no overemphasizing the importance of clergy as consent seekers. Like the coroner or medical examiner, clergy are often in touch with a family immediately upon the death of a family member or, in the case of a lingering illness, even before the death. They are highly appropriate people to approach the family for organ donations, and they should not be overlooked as solid eye bank volunteers. In Wisconsin, they are offered special training in procurement.

These, then, are the major groups directly involved in support of the Wisconsin Eye Bank: Lions clubs, hospitals, medical examiners, coroners, and clergy. Through education and public relations efforts of the eye bank they are continually kept involved in its work.

Education. The Wisconsin Eye Bank believes that it owes its volunteers the best possible education for the important job that they are being asked to do.

Starting with the first group of enucleators trained in 1978, enucleation programs have been arranged to give a total picture of the eye bank to those involved. Two courses, funded by the Wisconsin Lions Foundation, are planned each year with 25 to 45 participants. Lectures are presented by the executive director, laboratory director, medical and surgical directors, an operating room nurse, legal advisors, a funeral director, and corneal transplant recipients. From viewing a videotape of an eye enucleation to performing one on a rabbit, new enucleators are thoroughly familiar with the technical aspects of the service after the 2-day session.

But the training goes beyond that. Believing that it is necessary for people to understand an organization before they will become good supporters of it, eye bank staff also emphasize the total eye bank program, acquainting the enucleator with all aspects of eye banking. In 1982, procurement training became an important part of the Wisconsin Eye Bank educational effort. Twice a year, Margaret Verble and Judy Worth, nationally recognized instructional consultants, bring an organ procurement seminar to Wisconsin (see p. 694). The 2-day invitational conference is geared to procurement leaders from hospitals around the state. An in-depth examination is made of procurement—the psychologic and social aspects as well as the role playing in a donation conversation.

Because the number who can attend a given conference is limited, participants are expected to return to their communities and pass on what they have learned. The success of this effort is obvious; in the first year after the seminars were initiated, donations increased more than 30%.

Paralleling the procurement training offered hospital personnel is clergy training. Father Michael Lynch, a chaplain at Wausau Hospital Center in Wausau, Wisconsin, coordinates the annual training for a group of clergy from throughout the state. The seminar involves information on the meaning of brain death, organ donation programs, religious doctrine, and discussions by donor families and recipients.

Brochures on how to ask for eye donations and materials to give families to back up the donation conversation are available to all who make these contacts, further increasing their confidence in this difficult task. A total commitment to education, from in-service training to enucleation and procurement programs, is basic to the success of the Wisconsin program. The volunteers who do the eye bank's work across that state are the first contact that most potential donor families have with the bank. It only makes sense to help them do that job well.

Public Relations. Finally, nearly everything that an eye bank does involves public relations. Dealing with these vital organizations that keep the eye bank going, attracting and keeping the persons who make the local programs run, and making the general public aware of the purpose of eye banking and therefore more likely to become donors are all public relations functions and are business as usual for the successful eye bank.

In Wisconsin, this effort means thousands of miles of travel each year to work with hospitals to reinforce the ongoing efforts. It means attending annual Lions meetings and conventions of medical examiners and coroners; these groups, which do so much, must be constantly told that their efforts make a difference.

In meeting with local groups and attracting local media coverage, first-hand stories from cornea-transplant recipients and families of donors are dramatic and remembered. Their stories bring the overall picture of eye donation into sharp focus for those who hear them.

But the good will of those recipients and donor families must also be sought. Recipients, in general, are enthusiastic supporters, but follow-up observation and personal concern shown by eye bank staff allow that enthusiasm to surface. Donor families are always thanked by letter in Wisconsin, letting them know that the eyes they gave were used. Frequently they respond with their enthusiasm for the decision to donate tissue. Frequently they are willing to tell others of the enthusiasm, either through public appearances of interviews for local media or eye bank publication.

Publications. Publications, including a newsletter and annual report, are further reminders to those involved that the Wisconsin Eye Bank cares about them and that it is making good use of their services. In Wisconsin, the annual report emphasizes the human side of corneal donation; the newsletter highlights individual substations and reminds the reader of the ongoing efforts to make the program stronger through education and involvement of individuals and organizations around the service area and through staff efforts.

Every letter, every phone call made by an eye bank to a "constituent" is a public relations gesture. When your success or failure depends on your relations with those who voluntarily do your work, you must proceed carefully!

SUMMARY

Wisconsin is proof that it is possible to have a successful eye-banking program without a medical examiner law. But it is necessary for you to evaluate carefully the needs of your service area, seeing how you can meet those needs, and carefully to develop a strategy to carry through. It involves work with organizations, with hospitals, and with others who can make your job easier, and it involves letting all those persons who make your success possible know that they are important to you. There are many components to such a program. You, the eye bank, are the force for bringing them all together.

Corneal retrieval by legislative consent (medical examiner statutes)

RICHARD L. FULLER

The need for corneal tissue has exceeded availability since eye banks became organized entities in the 1940s.[4]

The development of new procedures and indications for transplantation will probably continue this trend.[7] In 1990, patient waiting lists were determined to be approximately 6787,[11] thus eye banks supplied about 85% of the corneas needed in the United States.[3] Many areas, especially states that have legislative consent statutes, also known as medical examiner coroner laws, have eliminated their waiting lists.

During the 1940-1970 period, most eye donations were received through hospital programs. In 1968, the Uniform Anatomical Gift Act addressed the subject in detail and thus helped to facilitate donations. It was recognized, however, that medical examiner and coroner cadavers were a potential source of additional corneas. The development of this idea encompassed the fact that the surgical technique to excise only the cornea was much less invasive than the routine autopsy procedure performed by the medi-

cal examiner/coroner. This fundamental, along with the clear need and limited recovery time for viability, formed the basis for early discussions regarding possible legislation.

The first medical examiner/coroner statute, spearheaded by Russell S. Fisher, M.D., Chief Medical Examiner of Maryland, was passed in 1975. This statute recognized the uniqueness of the cornea as a transplantable tissue and medical examiner/coroner cadavers as a significant source of corneas.[1] In 1987, the National Association of Medical Examiners (NAME) officially recognized the potential value of human organs and tissues for transplantation and further that "medical examiner/coroner cases constitute the single most important source for healthy organ and tissue donation."[8]

Medical examiner/coroner statutes are written in a variety of formats; however, 12 states have modeled their statutes on the Maryland statute of 1975. The model and most effective form is legislative or implied consent and may also be known as presumed consent.[1]

LEGISLATIVE CONSENT

Corneas may be released to an eye bank when:
- The decedent is under medical examiner/coroner jurisdiction.
- An autopsy is required.
- Release will not interfere with subsequent investigation.
- There will be no mutilation of the decedent.
- There is no known objection by next of kin.

Other less effective formats include:
- Diligent or reasonable search; an effort must be made to contact next of kin within a specified time before release of the cornea.
- Consent only; release only upon consent of next of kin.

States That Have Enacted Legislative Consent Statutes[1,9]

Implied Consent	Diligent Search	Consent Only
1. Alabama	1. Arizona	1. Colorado
2. California	2. Hawaii	2. Illinois
3. Connecticut	3. Louisiana	3. Nebraska
4. Delaware	4. Massachusetts	4. New York
5. Florida	5. Mississippi	5. North Carolina
6. Georgia	6. Tennessee	6. Virginia
7. Kentucky	7. Washington	
8. Maryland		
9. Michigan		
10. Ohio		
11. Texas		
12. West Virginia		
13. (Puerto Rico)		

Foreign Countries That Have Legislative Consent Statutes[1]

Austria	Finland	Japan	Spain
Belgium	France	Morocco	Sweden
Czechoslovakia	Greece	Norway	Switzerland
Denmark	Israel	Poland	
Egypt	Italy	Singapore	

Cornea retrieval by legislative consent has been challenged in the courts; however, the constitutionality of these statutes has been upheld. Cases of note include *Tillman* v. *Michigan Eye Bank et al.*, 1984-1985; *Georgia Lions Eye Bank, Inc.*, *et al.* v. *Lavant*, 1985-1986; and *Powel* v. *Florida et al.*, 1986. In the Georgia case, appeal was made to the United States Supreme Court, which refused to hear the case, in essence upholding the decision of the lower court.

Some have questioned the medical suitability of corneas retrieved from medical examiner/coroner cadavers, particularly since the recognition of the HIV risk. The Centers for Disease Control estimated a range of 0.4% to 0.6% HIV seroprevalence among the United States population in 1988.[6] A retrospective study in Los Angeles, California, reviewed 4451 consecutive potential donors from Los Angeles County Medical Examiner cases to determine HIV seroprevalence. Of the 2771 potential donors who were screened for HIV antibody, 0.97% were repeatedly reactive for HIV. This study concluded that the risk of transplanting a cornea from HIV-infected but antibody-negative donors is 0.01%.[5]

A retrospective study on HIV-incidence antibody-positive eye/cornea donors in hospital versus medical examiner cases in Michigan concluded that the difference was neither clinically nor statistically significant.[2]

Careful screening of medical examiner/coroner cases utilizing the Eye Bank Association of America, Inc., Medical Standards should be followed. These cases presently have a low rate of HIV seropositivity and can be considered an important and safe source of surgical quality corneas, especially since no instance of HIV seroconversion has yet been reported.[2]

Cornea retrieval from medical examiner/coroner cadavers enabled eye banks to provide 15,527 corneas in 1990, representing 18% of the 86,076 cornea or eye donations in that year.[3]

Since the implementation of retrieval programs by legislative consent, much discussion has ensued regarding the pros and cons of this approach. On the positive side, it has been clearly demonstrated that eye banks utilizing legislative consent–driven programs recover a significant number of surgically suitable corneas. In fact, among the largest providers of surgical corneas in the United States are those eye banks utilizing legislative-consent programs. Further, these programs enable the recovery of corneas from younger and primarily trauma type of cadavers. In addition, the ratio of surgically usable corneas compared to non–medical examiner/coroner cases is significantly higher. In the TBI (Tissue Banks International) network 85% of the corneas obtained from medical examiner/coroner cadavers are surgically suitable, compared to 35% of all other procurement programs.[12] Significant to surgeons utilizing the TBI Tissue Distribution and Information Center (TDIC) is the fact that availability of corneas made possible through TBI's utilization of legislative-consent programs enables them to routinely schedule surgery. This not only benefits the patient, but also saves dollars for hospitals and better utilizes facility time as well as surgeon time. Utilization of legislative consent programs provides an opportunity for local eye banks to maximize the potential donor resources in their area and to recognize economies of scale with regard to their operational costs to procure corneas.

On the negative side, some argue that legislative consent is simply not in the best interest of the potential donor family. This issue is purely an individual matter and must be so resolved. Some also feel that adequate medical history may not be available to adequately screen the case. Because the concept of legislative consent is relatively new, it may not be well understood by the majority of the population thus creating the possibility of misunderstanding and perhaps litigation. Further, from the perspective of the eye bank, these programs are less than "secure" in that the statutes specify that the medical examiner/coroner "may" release the corneas under specified conditions because he has no mandate to do so.

The TBI experience has been positive in using retrieval by legislative consent because of the development of positive working relationships with medical examiners and coroners. Successful retrieval programs in medical examiner/coroner facilities require constant attention from appropriate eye bank staff and in particular an appreciation for and respect of the primary legislative mandate to which the medical examiner/coroner must adhere. The TBI network, composed of 12 eye banks and 26 locations, provided 8149 surgical corneas for penetrating keratoplasty in 1990, of which 77% represented corneas from medical examiner/coroner cadavers. One of TBI's basic objectives has traditionally been to eliminate patient waiting lists for corneal transplantation. A strong commitment within the TBI network to this objective has enabled the network eye banks to provide corneas on a schedules basis, with better than a 95% performance rate, to their surgeons and patients. This has virtually eliminated network waiting lists.

Corneal retrieval programs, by legislative consent, are an important part of the total eye banking enterprise. Statistics have clearly indicated that the significant number of corneas obtained from this source are necessary to close the gap between needed and available corneas. Further, studies have clearly indicated that corneas from this source are safe for surgical use. Although arguments can be made on both sides of the legislative consent issue, the courts have determined that these statutes are in the public interest.

It must be remembered, in all discussions, that the basic reason eye banks were established was to develop an organized way to retrieve adequate numbers of corneas to meet patient needs. We have been quite successful in the development of a safe, efficient, and effective eye banking system; however, we have yet fully to meet the need for surgical corneas in a timely manner. Careful weighing of the evidence clearly indicates that retrieval of corneas by legislative consent is an acceptable means toward the end of meeting the need and should be developed to its fullest potential.

REFERENCES

1. Bernstein TD: *The role of the medical examiner coroner in eye banking*, TBI pamphlet, Baltimore, Jan 1991, Tissue Banks International (TBI).
2. Danneffel MB, Sugar A: Incidence of HIV antibody-positive eye/cornea donors in hospital versus medical examiner cases, *Cornea* 9(3):271-272, 1990.
3. Eye Bank Association of America: *Eye banking activity, 1990*, Washington, DC, May 1991, the Association; telephone 1-(202)-775-4999.
4. Farge EJ: Eye banking, 1944 to the present, *Surv Ophthalmol* 33:260-263, 1989.
5. Hwang DG, Ward DE, Trousdale MD, Smith RN: Human immunodeficiency virus seroprevalence among potential corneal donors from medical examiner cases, *Am J Ophthalmol* 109(1):92-93, 1990 (Letters).
6. Karon JM, Dondero TJ Jr, Curran JW: The projected incidence of AIDS and estimated prevalence of HIV infection in the United States, *J Acquir Immune Defic Syndr* 1:542, 1988.
7. Lee PP, Stark WJ, Yang JC: Cornea donation laws in the United States, *Arch Ophthalmol* 107:1585-1589, Nov 1989.
8. National Association of Medical Examiners: Proposed National Association of Medical Examiners policy and guidelines on human organ and tissue procurement, St. Louis, Sept 1987.
9. National Health Publishing, State Statutes, 1987-1989.
10. O'Day DM: Diseases potentially transmitted through corneal transplantation, *Ophthalmology* 96:1133, 1989.
11. Prottas JM: *Study of unmet demand and corneal distribution in North America*, Report for EBAA/TBI, March 1991.
12. TBI (Tissue Banks International): *TBI statistical report*, 1990, Baltimore, Feb 1991; telephone 1-(410)-752-3800.

Evolution of required request and routine referral laws

MARY JAYNE STEVENS

In describing the laws that require health care workers to request donation of organs and tissues, the terms "required request" and "routine referral" are used interchangeably and are basically the same. "Required request" laws require hospitals to request from families permission for organ or tissue donation. "Routine inquiry" laws require hospitals to ask patients if they have signed a donor card and to record that information in their medical record, or to inform the families of deceased patients of their option to consent to or deny donation. There is little difference in the way these two terms are used. These laws require a conscious act on the part of families.

HISTORICAL PERSPECTIVES

In 1968, the Uniform Anatomical Gift Act (UAGA), which made organ and tissue donation legal in the United States, was passed by Congress. Adopted by all 50 states, this act allowed individuals to determine what will be done with their organs after their death. The mechanism used to declare the individual's choice was the organ donor card. This system of organ procurement was best characterized as encouraged altruism. However, with few cards actually signed and often not even found after an accident, this system rarely resulted in actual donations.

The concept of "required request/routine inquiry" was originally proposed by Arthur Caplan. This proposal would create a policy that would require hospitals to ask surviving family members whether they would like to donate a deceased one's organs. Required request would restrict volunteerism but only on the part of hospitals and health care providers, not individual prospective donors or their families.[2] A study by Prottas found that 75% of families grant permission when asked.[7] Therefore required request would potentially create more than double the number of organs available for transplantation.

In 1984, Congress passed the Organ Transplant Act, which created the Task Force on Organ Procurement and Transplantation. Members of the task force included physicians and representatives of organ-procurement agencies, as well as agents from the fields of law, theology, ethics, finance, the general public, and health insurance agencies.

In 1986, the task force delivered its report and recommendations,[6] one of which was that "all hospitals should adopt the required request policy."

This policy could help meet the need for organs and be ethically acceptable. It was preferable to other policies of presumed consent because it supports active generosity, even though family members respond to an inquiry or request for a gift rather that offering it on their own initiative. It also focused on the family rather than the individual, on hospitals rather than professionals, and on explicit rather than presumed consent. Presumed consent laws take for granted that the deceased and the next of kin have no known objections to organ or tissue removal. Today 18 states have presumed consent for corneas in medical examiner laws. Many European countries use presumed consent for all organs.

New York and Oregon were the first states to pass required request laws in 1985. These two laws are very similar—each required that, in the absence of prior notification, hospital personnel or their designees request consent for anatomic gifts from potential donors or their families. Each request and its outcome must be recorded in the medical record and on the death certificate. California's law, passed after the New York and Oregon legislation was signed into law, has no requirement for recording the outcome of the request. Instead, California hospitals are directed to inform families of the option to consent for donation, rather than to request consent.

Most of the state laws follow one of these two models. Twenty-six states and the District of Columbia have the required request laws modeled after New York and Oregon, whereas 23 require hospitals to inform families about donation, more like California's law. South Dakota is the only state that has not passed any type of state legislation and relies only on the federal legislation (Table 49-2).

FEDERAL LEGISLATION

The Omnibus Budget Reconciliation Act of 1986 (Public Law No. 99-509) implemented the recommendations of the Task Force on Organ Procurement and Transplantation by adding Section 1138 to the Social Security Act.[5] The goal of this 1986 legislation was to increase the percentage of actual donors from the pool of potential donors. Using a hospital's eligibility to participate in Medicaid or Medicare as a constraint, Section 1138 requires all Medicaid or Medicare hospitals to institutionalize a required request policy. Hospitals must establish written protocols for identifying potential organ do-

Table 49-2. States With Required Request/Routine Inquiry Laws*

1985	1986	1987	1988	1989	1990	1991
California	Alabama	Arkansas	Alaska	Idaho	Utah	South Carolina
New	Arizona	Colorado	Hawaii		Vermont	
York	Connecticut	Iowa	Virginia		Wyoming	
Oregon	Delaware	Minnesota				
	Florida	Mississippi				
	Georgia	Montana				
	Illinoiis	Nebraska				
	Indiana	Nevada				
	Kansas	New Jersey				
	Kentucky	New Mexico				
	Louisiana	North Carolina				
	Maine	North Dakota				
	Maryland	Oklahoma				
	Massachusetts	Texas				
	Michigan	Washington, D.C.				
	Missouri					
	New Hampshire					
	Ohio					
	Pennsylvania					
	Rhode Island					
	Tennessee					
	Washington					
	West Virginia					
	Wisconsin					

*South Dakota has not passed any required request/routine inquiry laws.

nors and for notifying an organ-procurement agency of the potential donor.

In 1987, the National Conference of Commissioners on Uniform State Laws drafted a revised version of the UAGA, which was then introduced to all states for individual action. The 1987 revisions incorporated many aspects of required request and routine referral laws. They mandated that hospitals discuss with family members of dying patients the option of donation if there was no indication of the patient's decision in the medical record and if the patient was medically suitable as a donor candidate. This revised UAGA, with its routine inquiry and required request provisions, would hopefully increase opportunities for requesting consent for anatomic gifts. It also required emergency personnel to search for information (such as a donor card or driver's license donor notification) that a person who is dead or near death is a possible donor.

EFFECTS OF LEGISLATION

After utilizing the new routine inquiry legislation for 12 months the Lions Eye Bank of Oregon obtained 2312 donated eyes, sustaining a 135% increase in donor eye procurement over the yearly average for 1984-1985.[1] However, they stated that the >70-years-of-age category represented 45% of the donations obtained in 1986.[1]

In a telephone conversation with the technical director of the Lions Eye Bank of Oregon, it was indicated that the increase in eye donations continued until 1988, when a plateau was reached, and that in 1990 there was a decrease in donations. By July 1991, the Lions Eye Bank of Oregon was "back on track," ahead of previous years, with the increase attributed to a concentrated statewide professional education program.

Procurement agencies in Los Angeles and San Francisco reported findings similar to Oregon's, with donations increasing until 1987 and then leveling off and dropping slightly. This decrease was attributed to a decline in the number of deaths and suitable donor candidates.

Evaluating the success of required request laws has been difficult. Many states have seen significant increases in referrals and actual donations. Some states have stronger laws with varying degrees of hospital monitoring, health department involvement in regulation and implementation, and determination of whether hospitals are required to request donations or only to inform families of the option.

Caplan and Welvang[3] surveyed 10 states that had a required request law to see how the laws were being implemented. Eight of the ten states surveyed reported an increase of 20% or more in the number of eye, skin graft, and bone donations since state legislation was implemented. Five (Oregon, Arizona, Ohio, Missouri, and Minnesota) of the 10 states reported a greater than 100% increase in the number of eye donors, despite stricter medical standards for eye donation and suitability for transplant.[3]

Many states have well-written laws, but lack community understanding and enforcement. The problem of ignoring the law, combined with attitudes of resentment, present a major difficulty in many parts of the country. Doctors and nurses in many hospitals resent required request laws in general, particularly the idea that government would require them to ask families about donation. Nurses are usually the ones asked to comply with the laws and actually obtain consent from families. Nurses are generally overworked and not well-trained in organ and tissue donation requests. The situation is improving, however, since several professional training programs are now available.

In conclusion, all required request laws mandate hospitals to develop a means to ensure that all families of potential donors are offered the option of donation. The families have a right to make this decision about organ and tissue donation, and the hospital and staff do not have the right to deny their choice by not offering this option.

Legislation directing organ and tissue donation may be passed and revised regularly, but without the support of health care professionals (physicians, nurses, administrators, and other medical staff), there will continue to be a barrier in the organ and tissue donation process. The Task Force on Organ Transplantation categorized physicians of dying patients as "gatekeepers" in "raising the issue of donation with families." Fox and Swazey[4] write: "The final gatekeeper in organ exchange is the physician. Acting on behalf of the transplant team, the patient, and possible donors and their relatives, as well as for himself, he makes the ultimate judgment. He acts as mediator and interpreter in the complex social system called into play by the transplantation situation . . . the physician is not free to abnegate his responsibility nor may he exercise it arbitrarily or coercively. . . .In certain respects, the physician is under pressure to decide in favor of organ transplantation. He is propelled toward it by his own professional and personal motivation to do everything possible to save the life of a dying patient."

Hospitals and health care providers must be educated in how to make requests. Medical and nursing schools should include education programs on organ and tissue donation and transplantation in their curricula. Efforts to educate the public, including children, as well as addressing organ and tissue donation and transplantation in secondary schools and collegiate health text books must be encouraged. Required request will be successful only through the combined efforts of many individuals and a willingness to participate in finding solutions to the donor shortage.

REFERENCES

1. Burris TE et al: Impact of routine inquiry legislation in Oregon on eye donations, *Cornea* 6(3):226-230, 1987.
2. Caplan AL: Organ procurement: it's not in the cards, *Hastings Cent Rep* 14(5):9-12, 1984.
3. Caplan AL, Welvang P: Are required request laws working? Altruism and procurement of organs and tissues, *Clin Transplantation* 3:170-176, 1989.
4. Fox RC, Swazey JP: Gift exchange and gatekeeping. In *The courage to fail: a social view of organ transplants and dialysis,* Chicago, 1978, The University of Chicago Press, p 5.
5. *Omnibus Budget Reconciliation Act of 1986. An act to provide for reconciliation pursuant to Section 2 of the Concurrent Resolution on the Budget for Fiscal Year 1987,* U.S. General Purchasing Office, 1986.
6. *Organ transplantation issues and recommendations,* Report of Task Force on Organ Transplantation, U.S. Department of Health and Human Services, 1986.
7. Prottas J: Structure and effectiveness of the American organ procurement system, *Inquiry* 22:365-376, 1985.

The role of coroners, clergy, nurses, and morticians

LOWELL H. MAYS

Thousands of people lose their sight each year from corneal damage caused by disease, injury, or infection. Yet, despite all the cornea transplants performed each year, an equal number of additional transplants could be done if enough transplantable corneas were available. It appears that our society is becoming considerably more willing to entertain the possibility of corneal tissue donation than was the case some years ago. Much has been done to increase public awareness of cornea donations through publicity campaigns, literature, and person-to-person contact after the death of a relative or friend. In some instances people have been encouraged to consider donation while they are healthy so that the eventual procurement of tissue is simply done as a matter of fact and routine. In most instances, however, tissue is procured after the death of a person who has not offered tissue for donation. Hence, the roles of those who deal with persons at the time of death are well worth review.

Often, the person to make the request for dona-

tion is the person who has access. Unfortunately, those who have access may in some cases, presume that another member of the health care team has thought of the question and maybe has already posed it to the patient or family. In such cases, the professional with access should be encouraged to raise the question even if it is redundant.

ROLE OF THE CORONER

The role of the coroner is one that dates back to the foundation of English law. The coroner was one appointed by the Crown and, as such, represented the highest form of government in a given area for cases of ultimate concern. The coroner, although having responsibility under state law as the designated person who must arrest the sheriff if there is ever need, is the officer who is charged with the management of the forensic investigation for the causes of death. The services rendered by the coroner in such investigation of those deaths that require legal intervention is an essential serve of local government. Certainly no statutory responsibility is put on the coroner in most instances for the procurement of tissue, but many coroner's offices have developed public relations programs that involve conducting training seminars at schools, speaking at conferences, and cooperating with local eye banks by informing the next of kin about donation procedures. As a matter of routine procedure, the coroner's office at Dane County, Wisconsin, has a regularly stated protocol to ask each member of the coroner's staff to make sure that the family has been given an opportunity for the donation of corneal tissue.

In the case of sudden or unattended death, the coroner has the responsibility of assessing the utility of any tissue for transplantation, teaching, or research. Furthermore, the coroner is often the person who instigates the request to guarantee that the tissue is kept moist. Most coroners are organized in such a way as to have contact with donation-receiving agencies and often, through the eye banks, initiate the arrangements for enucleation.

The coroner may also be the guarantor of confidant signatures and that the signatures are *bona fide* when consent is obtained. In some instances, when written consent is impossible because of time and distance, the coroner arranges verbal consent. Coroner's in those instances, will arrange for a two-person verification of the verbal consent and then will apply their own statements attesting to such consent.

In some cases, the uniform anatomical gift acts need to be interpreted to families. Many states allow a person, by signing a statement on the back of his motor vehicle operator's license, to indicate that he is willing to donate tissue. That, by itself, is a *bona fide* contract if it is legally witnessed and should be respected. In some instances, the information that a deceased person wishes to donate corneas may be new to a family, and there may appear to be some reluctance to subscribe to the deceased's personal wishes. The coroner's office, at that time, may be a helpful authoritative influence in understanding and interpreting the law.

The coroner's office also may assist in arranging for the transport of the tissue through police agencies or other resources to the eye bank should the distance be significant.

ROLE OF THE CLERGY

Historically, the clergy have been invited to be present by families when death is near and have been requested to minister to families in the face of sudden and traumatic death.

One of the clergy's responsibilities is to be helpful in destroying myths about the donation of tissue. Some persons have the impression that any form of tissue transplantation or resection after death is a form of mutilation and in some way may desecrate the body. Almost all religious groups have strong feelings indicating that whenever cadaveric tissue may be of assistance for the enhancement of the life of the living, such transplants should be made. Jewish and Christian groups may vary somewhat, but even Orthodox Jews find that corneal donation is mandated if such activity would bring sight to someone whose life is yet to be enjoyed. The Roman Catholic Church has no restrictions on corneal donation, and Protestant perspectives only encourage such donations.

The clergy are often perceived by the dying and by those who have suffered the death of a loved one as an authority figure of positive assistance. When the clergy announce the invitation to consider donating corneal tissue, very often that announcement is perceived as a sense of permission giving. This is a valid role for spiritual leaders to fulfill.

In most instances, the clergy have rapport with the family that superseded that between the family and other professionals. When someone is suffering from end-stage disease, the family clergyperson will be frequently calling on the sick and on the family, offering support and encouragement. Such rapport is not limited, however, to times of tragedy, but rather also at times of celebration and joy. Because of that kind of balance, the clergy often have access that other professionals do not. Frequently, observers have heard families say in response to a member of the clergy's invitation to consider donation of corneal tissue, "If you think it's a good idea, pastor, we certainly will respect that." For years conservative Jews have lived with a "nonmutilation" mentality concerning the body of the dead. For a Jewish spiritual leader to make the invitation to consider donation, the invitation is frequently understood as "permission." Christians have grown up with an anthropomorphic understanding of immortality and that the dead shall be raised. Much of that thinking, though never intended to offer a literalness that the bodies will come forth from the "grave in their natural state," has given some people the metaphorical impression that you should not therefore mutilate or transplant tissue for fear that the resurrection could be altered. The clergy have the perceived authority to help people reinterpret and understand that more adequately.

The clergy also have a teaching office. If the clergy are adequately fulfilling their pastoral responsibilities, they will find ways of talking about tissue donation in teaching opportunities. Children should learn that one of the privileges human beings can offer to others is that they may, in the face of their own suffering, give life and hope to other people. Such instruction should be amplified at other times through formal opportunities. Often in pastoral conversations with families while a loved one is seriously ill, such educational transactions can occur.

Statements from within religious traditions, particularly from sacred literature, bring to mind significant altruism in behalf of one's loved ones and friends. Statements like "greater love hath no one than that they would lay down their life for their friends" are replete throughout the Bible. Religious assemblies offer a person a chance to remember such injunctions and to respond. Sometimes that response is not only in praise and thanksgiving, but also in an offering. It would be quite appropriate in religious assemblies during the offertory to ask people to take out their vehicle operator's licenses and to sign the donation form indicating that they would be willing to donate corneas and then to have it witnessed by the person next to them in the pew. This, in a very practical manner would not only yield many potentially transplantable corneas, but would also give the immediate moral approval to tissue donation.

ROLE OF THE NURSE

Nurses have a qualitative relationship not only with the patient, but also with the patient's family and, as a result, are in an excellent position to raise the issue of corneal donation. It should be said, however, that such an issue should not be raised only at the time of death but should be a part of the normal care plan that is being executed in behalf of a patient. At the time of death, however, it needs to be restated, and the nurse is in an excellent position to do so.

Outpatient care is also a setting for the nurse to be sensitive to the need for tissue donation. The nurse can include new tissue donation as a regular subject of concern with patients who are undergoing outpatient chemotherapy, those who have chronic illnesses, and, of course, those who have end-stage disease. Nurse practitioners working with adolescents would be well also to remember that patient education should include a posturing toward tissue donation so that as a person matures tissue donation would be a natural thing to consider. Furthermore, adolescents present a very high rate for those who are potential trauma victims, and unfortunately, at this point, most tissue does come from traumatic death.

Emergency services' nurses are in a particularly appropriate place for the procurement of tissue. The question of consent for tissue donation should be a matter of routine protocol for an emergency service death. The nurse, of course, would be responsible for maintaining the moist condition of the corneas and, in some cases, nurses have been trained as enucleators.

ROLE OF MORTICIANS

In many cases morticians have been trained as enucleators. After consent is verified, morticians in more remote areas (particularly in rural settings) are often the only persons who have contact with the corpse and therefore are logically appropriate people for enucleator training.

Furthermore, in recent years the mortician has developed a rather active role in prearranged funeral planning. Every mortician is interested in developing a file for whom they have prearrangement permission and with whom they have developed a relationship. A logical question that the mortician can raise at the time of the prearrangement is the question of corneal donation. If the mortician raises the issue when a person is planning a funeral, that person may then have plenty of time to check it out with religious advisers, family members, and others who may be viewed as supportive and interested people by that person.

DEATH NOTIFICATION

Police agencies are generally charged with the responsibility of notifying the next of kin of a death at the request of the coroner's offices. Statutory requirements are common in most states whereby the coroner is responsible for the notification of next of kin, but such notification may be deferred to a policy agency who have people on patrol in various geographic areas.

For the past 20 years many police agencies have hired police chaplains. Norfolk, Virginia, for example, has 20 police chaplains. Uniformed personnel in squad cars are assigned to police chaplain activity, and there is one on patrol at all times. That person is radio equipped, having one in the squad car and one as a walkie-talkie, and is often dispatched to a residence to deliver a death notification. In Dane County, Wisconsin, the sheriff's department has field chaplains who notify the next of kin in the case of all sudden and traumatic deaths. These persons have a unique access to the appropriate persons, and it is only logical for them to raise the question of the possibility of tissue donation. Historically, the Wisconsin Eye Bank has received significant tissue donations from the requests made by police chaplains and coroners. Eye banks are wise to assess what structure is used within each local jurisdiction concerning death notification, and such persons should be challenged with one or more responsibility.

HOW TO MAKE A REQUEST FOR DONATION

There are many ways to couch a request for a tissue donation. The only important thing is that the request is made and made carefully. After the notification has been made and the next of kin have had an opportunity to deal with their immediate emotions, one needs to state to the survivors that at times such as this one would presume that there are hundreds of questions these survivors may have and matters the next of kin has to take care of. Strangely enough, there are really only a few. One then says that only three things need to be obtained from them: the names of persons who need to be contacted before a release is made public to the news media concerning a sudden or traumatic death, the name of a funeral home the family feels comfortable in choosing, and permission to use the corneas of the deceased. One can say, "It is our policy always to ask this question. I have chosen to make it the final question because it is the most important question. I have full awareness that this may be a hard question at this time, but I am sure you would want the opportunity. Most families are grateful that the question is brought up." I then say, "The corneas of the deceased's eyes are in good condition and would be usable for transplantation to give sight to another human being, and it is my responsibility to ask you whether you would be willing to consent to the donation of those corneas." I then explain what the cornea is and tell them that in no way will the removal of the cornea cause them to change any plans they have for the funeral or disposition of the body. I explain that if perhaps there has been a traumatic death a person's body may not be viewable but it will not be because of corneal donation. I explain that there are numerous people who are waiting by a phone at this very hour for a call that will guarantee them an opportunity to get to the hospital on a moment's notice and that transplantation can be arranged within hours. I explain that as long as the corneas are removed within a reasonable length of time after death they are usable and sight can be given to someone within the next day. I then ask if they would be willing "to donate these corneas so that someone else can see very soon."

Time should be allowed for them to think about their decision. I generally choose to leave the area for a few moments to allow them some privacy so that they do not feel coerced. I then return to the scene and ask if they have any questions. In no way do I want to pressure them, but I do want to encourage them. Then, upon their consent, I read a standard donation agreement form to them so that they understand what is being asked. I ask them to sign the form and date it, and then I, along with another family member, will witness it. In most cases consent is given and tissue is procured.

These disciplines are traditional professions that do interface in the lives of people at important points. It appears only responsible for us from many disciplines to depend upon one another to enhance better sight for humans.

Family counseling

MARGARET S. VERBLE
JUDY K. WORTH

RATIONALE

Between 1988 and 1989 the number of corneas transplanted in the United States increased by more than 1500, reflecting an intensified effort by eye banks and other tissue-procurement agencies to procure corneal tissue for transplantation. Despite the obvious success of such efforts, the demand for corneas continues to exceed the supply of transplantable tissue. Indeed, according to current estimates, more than 6700 Americans have been evaluated as medically acceptable for corneal transplants and are currently enrolled on official waiting lists. Furthermore, this figure represents only a fraction of those Americans who could benefit from corneal transplant surgery if suitable donor tissue were available.[2,8]

Obviously, all efforts to increase the supply of transplantable tissue must begin with public education and donor registration. However, these alternatives alone will not produce sufficient tissue to meet current and projected demands. Recent polls indicate that 94% to 98% of the American public have heard or read about organ and tissue transplants. However, only 48% to 53% of those who have heard about transplants describe themselves as very likely or somewhat likely to want their own organs donated after death. Additionally, between 25% and 36% of the persons who describe themselves as very likely or somewhat likely to want their own organs donated have taken no action to ensure that such a donation takes place after their deaths.[5,11] And although 20% to 25% of those willing to donate indicate that they have signed and carry organ-donor cards, data from drivers' license bureaus indicate that the percentage of licensed drivers who have signed donor cards averages only 7% nationally.[4,11] Furthermore, anecdotal data from transplant coordinators and emergency room personnel indicate that few actual donors are carrying donor cards at the time of death and that such information is unlikely to be discovered anyway because it remains in the hands of law enforcement personnel or is overlooked by emergency room personnel who do not routinely check for organ-donor information. Finally, various studies indicate that persons who sign donor cards are not representative of the general population.[11]

More recent efforts to increase the supply of corneal tissue have resulted in the passage of medical examiner laws in 20 states and two municipalities.[1] Significant increases in the numbers of corneas obtained for transplantation have been reported in states where such legislation has been passed. Nevertheless, national concern over the potential transmission of acquired immunodeficiency syndrome (AIDS) and other communicable diseases attributable to tissue obtained from medical examiner cases and litigation in Florida, Georgia, and Ohio have dampened the enthusiasm of many eye bank representatives and corneal surgeons for more aggressive legislation of this type.

In an effort to procure more tissue, many eye banks have initiated comprehensive programs to identify and approach family members of potential donors for permission to remove corneas for transplantation or research. Such programs, including those for procuring kidneys and other organs, are reported to have an average success rate of 70% to 75%[7,9,10] Furthermore, eye banks that have initiated such programs, using liaison nurses, eye bank personnel, or other persons as procurement counselors, have reported overall increases of up to 262% in the number of corneas procured for transplantation and research.[6] Finally, follow-up studies of family responses to the request for organ donation indicate that for many family members the decision to donate corneas, kidneys, and other tissues can have a beneficial impact on the family's grief. For such persons the donation request confronts them with the reality of death in a way that helps them begin the process of grieving and gives them back some control at a time when they are otherwise powerless. Furthermore, the decision to donate may be the only good thing that happens to them in an otherwise incomprehensible and tragic series of events.

INTERVIEWING THE FAMILY

Having conversations with families about donation that are successful both in terms of obtaining permission and providing comfort and support is an art. In many cases, the interviewer is someone with whom the family already has rapport, such as a nurse who has helped care for the potential donor. However, donation conversations conducted by eye bank employees, social service personnel, chaplains, and funeral directors can also be successful. Whoever conducts the interview conversation, it is essential that concern for the family and the potential donor be communicated as more important than concern with obtaining corneas.

Most donation conversations take place while the family is still at the hospital. If the conversation is with a caregiver, that person should separate his role as caregiver from his role as interviewer. This can be done simply and effectively by a change in clothing. Slipping a jacket or sweater over whites or removing a lab coat signals to the family that the caregiver has assumed a slightly different role. Separating roles in a concrete way is important psychologically both to the family and to the interviewer. Such a separation helps reassure the family that interest in donation does not conflict with interest in providing care and reduces the likelihood that the donation conversation will be met with overt hostility. The eye bank employee who talks with the family should be dressed professionally in dark colors.

WAITING ROOM CONVERSATION

The initial conversation with the family is often in the waiting room or the emergency room lobby.

This conversation, serving as an introduction to the donation interview, should communicate four facts: the interviewer's name and title, the involvement (or lack thereof) of the interviewer in the potential donor's care, the interviewer's sympathy about the potential donor's condition, and that this conversation is what normally takes place at this time. The interviewer then asks the family to accompany her to a more private place to talk.

During this initial conversation the interviewer should place herself on the same physical plane as the next of kin. If the next of kin is seated, the interviewer should squat briefly in front of him or her or sit in an adjacent chair. Standing over the next of kin tends to put that person in an inferior position and can lead to an interaction in which she feels intimidated or coerced. The rule of same plane positioning should be followed throughout the conversation.

The interviewer should try to limit the number of family members she talks to. Legally, of course, the next of kin, as established by statute from state to state, must be included. If the next of kin is functioning reasonably well he or she may be the only person included in the interview conversation. If that person is in obvious need of support, the interviewer may want to designate another relative to join the conversation. Grown children of a surviving spouse are often helpful to both the parent and the interviewer during the conversation. As a general rule, the interviewer should include any member of the family upon whom the next of kin is obviously relying and all relatives of the same degree of kin. However, extended family members, in-laws, and children should not be included in the conversation. One "no" will outweigh several "yeses," and donation is not a topic about which everyone should have an equal say.

ESTABLISHING THE CLIMATE

The donation interview should ideally take place in comfortable, private surroundings. If a conference room is not available in the hospital, a secluded part of the cafeteria or a patio will suffice. Privacy is important because it affords fewer distractions and because family members will be very vulnerable during the conversation. Chapels should be avoided in most cases both because family members are often mad at God at this time and because they may feel a chapel setting plays unfairly upon their emotions.

Upon arriving in the conference room or setting, the interviewer should establish a climate of hospitality by offering coffee, soft drinks, ashtrays, or other helpful services. The interviewer's solicitousness, even more than his words, will convey that he knows this is a difficult time for the family and the discussion about amenities allows for small talk that gives both interviewer and family members the opportunity to take a measure of one another. Additionally, many experienced interviewers think that whether the family accepts hospitality is an important first signal about their willingness to donate. There is no doubt hospitality lowers the risk of hostility.

During the conversation, the interviewer should talk at a slower than normal rate. The perceptions of people in grief are slowed down, and in grief people do not have their normal capacity to decode. Normally paced words often sound harsh and grating to people in grief. If family members are shocked and have not had time to get into grief, they are often excitable and slower paced wording calms them down.

The interviewer also should relax his muscles during the conversation. Muscle tension, like yawning, is highly suggestive, and if the interviewer is relaxed, the family is more likely to feel at ease. On the other hand, a tense interviewer is more likely to spark anger in family members because they will catch his tension. The interviewer should sit at a slight back tilt rather than leaning forward, which is the natural inclination. Leaning forward during the conversation is likely to be perceived as threatening by family members, increases muscle tension, and at the very least makes the interviewer look impatient.

The extent and duration of the interviewer's eye contact should match the next-of-kin's pattern of gaze. Direct eye contact falls off dramatically during grief and, at all times, is less highly valued by many poor people and ethnic minorities than by health professionals. Direct gaze is perceived as aggressive by people who, for any reason, choose less direct eye contact. In most cases, the interviewer should use lowered gaze, with occasional glances upwards, throughout the conversation.

After attending to the family's comfort, the interviewer should check the next-of-kin's understanding of the potential donor's condition. The family, without exception, should be informed of the loved one's condition before the conversation takes place; however, that does not guarantee that the next of kin understands the situation. And the conversation cannot proceed until the next of kin understands his or her loved one is already dead or cannot survive much longer. If the potential donor has not yet been pronounced, understanding may have to be reached in this conversation even when the family has been told several times before that the loved one has no chance of survival. This understanding usually can

be reached by a sequence of questions: Has the doctor talked with you? What did the doctor say? What does that mean to you? In particularly difficult cases, a fourth question, What makes you think he can live? is helpful in determining exactly what the stumbling block to understanding is and addressing that specifically. It is not necessary that this conversation take place after pronouncement. The necessary prerequisites are that the family has been informed by the doctor that the potential donor cannot survive and they accept that. The research on the timing of these conversations shows that if information on death is given initially in an earlier conversation and then reinforced in this conversation, consent rates are higher than if there is only one conversation as to whether death has been pronounced.[3]

A reiteration of the medical facts of the death in language appropriate to the family's educational level reinforces understanding even in people who accept death. Additionally, such information is useful to families later on in their grief work as they go over and over the circumstances of the death in their heads. If the interviewer is not an attending nurse or physician, he should obtain the appropriate medical facts before the conversation. With practice, interviewers who are not health professionals can explain the causes of death in understandable terms as well as or better than health professionals can. However, a non–health professional who doesn't feel confident in this part of the conversation can bring a health professional with him to conduct this part of the interview.

In this and in all parts of the conversation, the interviewer should avoid medical terms and understand that metaphoric language will be the most useful in which to communicate. For instance, corneas can be likened to contact lenses, watch crystals, fish scales, or fogged windshields.

INTRODUCING THE SUBJECT

Once family understanding of the death has been established and reinforced, the subject of donation should be introduced. There are four standard introductions currently used. The make-meaning approach emphasizes that there is a way to make something meaningful come out of an otherwise senseless situation. This approach is appreciated most by families who are facing a sudden, tragic, and untimely death. The other-people-in-need approach is not effective at all in cases of sudden tragic death and may even be offensive. It works best for families who are resigned to the death of their loved one and are ready to look beyond that to a greater good. The there's-a-way-for-her-to-live-on approach is recommended for pediatric deaths, and although it often makes the interviewer uncomfortable, parents of pediatric potential donors seem to find it comforting. The our-hospital-likes-to-offer-the-opportunity approach is generic enough to work well with everybody just as the I'm-here-to-talk-to-you-about-another-decision approach does. The decision approach has the added advantages of being value free and of putting this decision in a context of other decisions the family will be making.

The most common mistake made in this conversation occurs at this point. Most interviewers, after introducing the subject, want to ask the family a question, like, "Have you all ever discussed donation?" or "Do you know if he wanted to be a donor?" *Don't ask those questions or any other at this point.* Many families will assume that because they never discussed donation with their loved one he didn't want to donate. However, the research on donation indicates that most people who want to donate don't discuss it with their families. Other families will interpret a question at this point as, "If you want to donate, tell me now," and try to give you an immediate answer. But a yes answer is useless at this point because it is not an informed consent.

EXTENDING THE SUBJECT

So, after introducing the subject, instead of asking a question, say, "I'd like to give you some information. You'll need to decide what you want to do." Then provide information necessary for informed consent and address the concerns most associated with donation. For informed consent, the family will need to know what the cornea is and specifically how it and the rest of the eye can be used to benefit other people; that they have a choice not to donate and whatever choice they make is fine; what the procedure is like and the effect it will have (or not have) on the funeral; that donation will not cost them anything; and that tissue not used for transplant can be used for research into eye disease. Other information that addresses common concerns is that the tissue would most likely be used locally, that the body would be treated with respect, that nothing would be done until after the death has been declared, and that their decision, whatever it is, will be held in confidence.

The slow, measured delivery of this information gives the family the information they need to make the decision and buys them time to think at a time they are likely to be disoriented and unable to make instant decisions. Most families will interrupt at the point when they have collected their thoughts enough to respond. However, don't be afraid of rep-

etition. Because families are hearing less well at this point in the conversation than at any other time, they are not likely to notice any repetition of information and prolonged silence or a direct request for a decision before they are ready to respond is more likely than not to generate a refusal.

ASKING QUESTIONS

When the family interrupts the information monolog, respond to whatever they say with a question. It is rare for a family member in this situation to be able to make a statement or ask a question that reflects a true concern. In short, people don't say what they mean in this part of the conversation. For instance, they may say, What would people think? and really mean, What will my mother-in-law think? or What will people see when they look into the casket? or What do I really think about this? So, if the interviewer responds to, What would people think? with, Most people think this is a generous thing to do, then the real question hasn't been answered and communication has been short circuited. The interviewer's task here is to ask questions that get the family members to extend and clarify her concern, probe for deeper concerns, invite confirmation, and offer solutions or new information as necessary.

ADDRESSING FEARS

As the conversation progresses by questioning and giving new information, real fears may arise and need to be addressed in a way that is both honest and comforting. For example, the family may be concerned about what the body will look like at an open-casket funeral. At base, they are worried about empty sockets. In addressing this fear, the interviewer needs to give correct information in a way that avoids evoking visual images that may overwhelm rational thought. For example, "empty sockets," "disfigurement," "bruising," "sunken eyeballs" are terms that should be avoided. A better choice of words is: In most instances, it is impossible to tell from looking that the eyes have been donated. The spaces are filled and the lids are closed over an eye cap that retains the shape of the face. Whatever you decide, the funeral director will place an eye cap under the lid to insure the look of the face during the visitation.

RESPONDING TO THE DECISION

The majority of families say yes to donation. Once verbal agreement is reached, the interviewer should leave the room briefly to obtain the release form and, if one has not already been completed, a medical history form. This interlude allows the family a few moments of private time to consolidate their decision. The medical history form may have been, depending on the circumstances of the death, completed already. If not, go over the form with the family before they sign the consent form. When presenting either form to the family, give them an overview of what the form says and its purpose. Even well-educated family members are unlikely to be able to read with comprehension at this time in their lives. So explaining the forms item by item is recommended.

In many cases, it is possible to donate more than eyes only. In fact, in some places in the country 45 different body parts can be donated. The proliferation of transplantable organs and issues in recent years has complicated the donation conversation. There is no doubt that families find a shopping-list recitation of body parts offensive and the timing of the mention of various possibilities for donation is sensitive. The best approach seems to be to introduce the subject of donation with solid organs, particularly the heart and kidneys, when suitable, and leave the discussion of eyes and tissues to later in the conversation when the consent form is discussed. In non–heart beating donations, it's best to introduce the subject with eye donation and leave a detailed discussion of other tissues until the consent form is discussed.

The consent form should be constructed so that the next of kin initials each and every donation the family wishes to make. Fill-in-the-blank forms do not afford either the family or the procurement agency the protection of truly informed consent. Therefore, as the form is explained to the family members, any organs or tissues not mentioned earlier in the conversation can be covered at this time.

During the explanation of the form, the family should be afforded time to ask questions and any information necessary for informed consent but not covered earlier in the conversation should be given. It is psychologically comforting for the family if all members present sign, and after the signatures are obtained, the interviewer should ask once again for questions. This final request for questions is important because signing often acts as a catharsis, and after signing, many family members will ask questions they have refrained from asking previously.

In cases where the family declines donation a questioning strategy is recommended. The purpose of the strategy is to elicit from the family either a firm, well-articulated no or a change of mind. An unexplored or weak no can be damaging to families. These are people who will return to a society that in the abstract is overwhelmingly prodonation. Within

a month after their no they are likely to see one or more medium personalities talk about how donation is the gift of life or sight and imply or directly state that good, generous people don't let their loved one's body parts go to waste. It is not uncommon for families who have declined donation to experience considerable guilt later on about their decision. The way to prevent this guilt is to gently pursue any no that is less than absolutely firm with follow-up questions.

These questions should be along the lines of, So you don't think donation would be the right decision for your family? and Could you tell me a little more about your feelings about this? These soft questions do several things simultaneously: they help the family articulate their real feelings; they uncover misinformation and declines based on reasons unrelated to donations, such as anger at the hospital admitting personnel; they give families who really don't want to donate a substantial rationale for their decision that can be affirmed by the interviewer and recalled later to assuage guilt.

The most difficult situation for the interviewer is when the family members disagree among themselves. Generally, interviewers want to run away (Why don't you just discuss this among yourselves and call me went you decide) or stay and control the family (We can't have this kind of argument here. This is a hospital and there are sick people here.) Either response is inappropriate. When family members disagree, stay with them and stay out of the conversation unless asked for information. These people have probably been disagreeing with each other for years and have a pattern of conflict resolution that they will unconsciously stick to no matter what you do. After they have said everything they have to say to one another and a lull appears in the conversation, the interviewer can successfully reframe the disagreement by saying, for example, "Mr. and Mrs. Smith, you knew Ricky better than anyone. You knew what kind of child he was and what kind of adult he would have grown into. From your knowledge of your child, can you say what he would have wanted if he were here and could make this decision for himself?" Another successful reframing technique is to say, "Mr. and Mrs. Smith, this is one of the last decisions you will ever make regarding your child. I hope you can make it together." To make either of these reframing statements work, the interviewer has to wait silently for a lull, make the statement, and then retreat into silence. If agreement cannot be reached, the donation should be turned down.

Conversations that conclude with donation are

closed when the interviewer asks the family if they are interested in receiving a letter from the bank about the use of the donation. Most families will request such a letter, and the interviewer will need to explain that only general information will be given. The need for confidentiality can be clarified by telling the family that many people who receive transplants feel guilty someone had to die for them to be helped and that confidentiality protects both the recipient and the donor family's privacy. As in conversations when permission is denied, the interviewer returns the family to the waiting room, thanks them, offers reassurance and sympathy, and tells them how to get in touch if they have questions. Leaving a brochure that explains the information necessary for informed consent is also a good idea.

TELEPHONE INTERVIEWS

Many candidates for corneal donation have no hospital admission at the time of death. In such cases, it may be necessary to approach the next of kin by telephone. This is a less desirable approach because it is more impersonal, but it can be done in a way that increases the likelihood of donation and communicates respect for the family's grief. Indeed, eye banks using telephone requests to families report success rates comparable to those in face-to-face conversations.[12]

Except for the arrangements made for witnessing the consent, the procedure for making the request by telephone is much like the face-to-face conversation. The telephone conversation is different in the following respects: If the death has taken place at a distance from the family and if it is unexpected, often family members grasp at the hope that the body has been misidentified. So, if the interviewer has access to the body, it should be examined for wounds, birthmarks, and identifying characteristics, such as height, hair color, and scars, and the family should be told early in the conversation that the interviewer has seen the body. People are less likely to interrupt on the phone than in person, and so after the subject has been extended thoroughly, the family may not interrupt with a question or statement. If that happens, the interviewer should simply say, "I've just given you a lot of information, Mrs. Smith. What questions do you have?" As many people tend to break down if sympathy is directly expressed early in the conversation, it is best to leave a direct expression of sympathy to the end. In concluding, the interviewer should ask the family member to get a pen and paper and write down her telephone number and name.

CONCLUSION

Procurement counseling is an effective method of obtaining corneas for transplantation and research. It increases the number of corneas available for transplantation and research and, unlike other methods of procuring tissue, can aid the donor family in dealing with their grief.

REFERENCES

1. Cummings E: Personal communication, Feb 27, 1991.
2. Cummings E: Personal communication, Feb 20, 1991.
3. Garrison RN et al: There is an answer to the organ donor shortage, *Surg Gynecol Obstet.* (In press).
4. Kelm M: Personal communication, Feb 28, 1991.
5. Miles MS et al: Public attitudes toward organ donation, *Dialysis and Transplantation* 17(2):74-76, 1988.
6. Polgar G: Personal communication, Lions Eye Bank of Delaware Valley, 1987.
7. Prottas JM: Structure and effectiveness of the American organ procurement system, *Inquiry* 22:365-376, 1985.
8. Prottas JM: A study of unmet demand and corneal distribution in North America, March 1991, unpublished manuscript, a survey conducted for the Eye Bank Association of America.
9. Prottas JM, Batten HL: Health professionals and hospital administrators in organ procurement: attitudes, reservations, and their resolutions, *Am J Public Health* 78:642-645, 1988.
10. Prottas JM, Batten HL: Neurosurgeons and the supply of human organs, *Health Affairs* 8(1):119-131, 1989.
11. Staff of the United Network for Organ Sharing: A comparison of surveys of the U.S. public's attitude toward organ transplants/organ donation, Richmond, Va, Nov 1989, unpublished manuscript.
12. Suss K, Pennock C: Personal communication, Arizona Lions Eye Bank, Feb 22, 1991.

Enucleation training courses

MICHAEL M. MARQUETTE

A survey of the 106 member eye banks of the Eye Bank Association of America was conducted during the spring of 1991.[1] This survey was an attempt to obtain the most current information about each eye bank's status in regard to conducting eye enucleation training courses. Of the 106 member eye banks, 50% responded to the survey. The 53 eye banks responding to the survey will equal 100% in this report. Variances in responses are attributable to eye bank size, geographic area, procedural policies, and statutory limitations governing enucleators.

TRAINING COURSES CONDUCTED BY EYE BANKS

Of the respondents, 57% conduct training courses. About one fourth of these eye banks charge for their course; the average course charge is $40 and lasts an average of 9 hours.

State agencies accredit half of the training courses.

The other training courses are accredited by mortuary schools, funeral service professional organizations, and medical schools. About two thirds of the training courses are accredited.

Eighty-four percent of the eye banks offer refresher training courses, whereas one fourth have actual recertification requirements. Most recertification requirements include a minimum number of enucleations per year or years or attending a refresher training course periodically, which may be the regular training course again. In the interest of quality assurance, recertification requirements should be a standard for those offering enucleation training.

Many of the training courses are offered either biannually or annually. The others are offered on an as-needed basis or every 2 to 3 years. They are held at either the eye bank or a university hospital or, less frequently, at a mortuary school, private hospital, or other location.

It may be that some eye banks utilize only eye bank technicians and have no need for formal training courses. For example, some areas require only an eye bank technician to provide enucleation services, whereas other areas can use only licensed funeral service professionals to perform enucleations because of statutory limitations.

There are many factors that influence an eye bank's decision to provide a formal enucleation training course. However, offering such a course enhances procurement capabilities by increasing the geographical area served and thereby the number of donations and corneas for transplantation.

WHO RECEIVES TRAINING FOR ENUCLEATION

Those who receive enucleation training fall into eight groups. The predominate group receiving training is funeral service professionals, followed in decreasing order by eye bank technicians, registered nurses and licensed practical nurses, pathology dieners, optometrists, ophthalmic technicians, medical examiners, and others (emergency medical technicians, medical doctors, surgery technicians, medical school students, laboratory technicians, operating room technicians, medical technicians, and so on). Although funeral service professionals are the dominant group receiving training, eye banks utilize individuals from all categories of enucleators or from only one. The percentage of enucleations performed by each group varies greatly from eye bank to eye bank. Some rely exclusively on one group, which may be attributable to their individual statutes.

CONTENT OF THE TRAINING COURSES

An important portion of a training course is the cadaver subject used both for demonstration of the procedure and for each student's practice surgery. For the instructor's demonstration model, the human cadaver is used most frequently, followed by rabbits or rabbit heads. Other cadaver subjects include pig (hog) head, monkeys, enucleated human eyes, models, and audio-visuals. Practice surgery models are, in descending order of use, the rabbit or rabbit head, the human cadaver, the enucleated human eye, and the pig (hog) head.

The contents of most training courses include anatomy and physiology; approaching families and counseling; aseptic technique, blood samples, and testing; legal issues and consents; cornea diseases, transplantation, and donor criteria; and enucleation, restoration, and transportation. It is essential that courses emphasize universal precautions. Some courses have a donor family and a cornea recipient as speakers.

In addition to the topics covered in the course, training manuals include sample documents, donor

---

Suggested audio-visuals for eye bank use

1. Counce, William: *Restoration of the organ and tissue donor.* (Videotape available through the Lions Eye Bank of Oregon, 1010 N.W. 22nd Ave., N120, Portland, OR 97210, (503) 229-7523.
2. *Enucleation* (slides), Alabama Eye and Tissue Bank, 700 South 18th St., Suite 308, Birmingham, AL 35233, (205) 939-3937.
3. *Enucleation* (videotape), Central New York Eye Bank, 750 East Adams St., Syracuse, NY 13210, (315) 471-6060.
4. *Enucleation* (videotape), Cleveland Eye Bank, 1909 East 101st St., Suite 10, Cleveland, OH 44106, (216) 791-9700.
5. *Enucleation* (videotape), Lions Eye Bank of Oregon (for address see 1 above).
6. *Enucleation* (videotape), Medical Eye Bank of Maryland—Tissue Banks International, 815 Park Ave., Baltimore, MD 21201, (301) 752-2020.
7. Sawyer, Don: *Restoring the Enucleated Eye* (slides with tape), The Dodge Chemical Company, Box 193, Cambridge, MA 02140, (800) 443-6343.
8. Tesh, John: *So Small a Space* (videotape), Eye Bank Association of America, Washington, D.C., (202) 775-4999.

criteria, chart review, and ethics and confidentiality. Additionally manuals should include Eye Bank Association of America Medical Standards, a list of important phone numbers, a checklist, and the proper responses to donor calls.

There are limited audio-visuals available for training courses. Many eye banks rely on one another for supplying audio-visuals because of the expense in producing one's own. See Box, p. 700, for a partial list of available videotapes.

Although many eye banks use a variety of media (videotapes, slides, films, charts, models), training courses lack satisfactory materials to enhance their training capabilities.

In response to this dearth, the Eye Bank Association of America (EBAA) produced and distributed a set of 15 by 20-inch black-and-white posters addressing enucleation and restoration procedures (1987). They provide a quick and easy reference for enucleators. The EBAA is currently producing a comprehensive slide and video show addressing donor criteria, aseptic technique, preenucleation considerations, enucleation, postenucleation considerations, restoration, and restorative problems. Corneal excision of the whole eye donor, in situ excision, and cornea donor restoration may be added to the audio-visuals in the future.

CONCLUSION

The complete status of training courses in North America was unfortunately unobtainable without the complete participation of all member eye banks. A map of training-course locations could be constructed with full participation.

There are many factors that influence an eye bank's decision regarding formal training courses for enucleators. Every eye bank should give serious consideration to offering a training course, training and certifying individuals in every community, expanding donations to every corner of North America, and providing eye bank growth and, most importantly, cornea tissue for transplantation. Enucleators may be paid or be volunteers, with trainable groups limited to the eye bank's statutory requirements.

The EBAA may want to consider adopting a minimum requirement for recertification as it does for eye bank technicians. This requirement should be tailored to fit the circumstances of enucleators; that is, those in rural communities may have infrequent opportunity to perform enucleations.

Although the training courses and training course manuals vary, they have common topics. Perhaps a minimum standard for training courses and training manuals should be adopted. The upcoming EBAA slide show and videotapes may provide a standard for training courses, recertification, and refresher training. This may be the training tool eye banks have been waiting for.

REFERENCES

1. Marquette, MM: *Eye enucleation training course survey of Eye Bank Association of America member eye banks,* April 1991, Lions Eye Bank of Oregon, Portland, Oregon.

SUGGESTED READING

Brightbill, S: *Corneal surgery: theory, technique, and tissue,* St Louis, 1986, Mosby–Year Book, pp 698-701.
Sawyer, D: Don Sawyer on embalming: eye enucleations, *The Dodge Magazine,* Sept 1976.
Whitaker, L: Helping someone in the dark, *The Dodge Magazine,* pp 6-7, 11, 25, 29, Nov 1988.

Chapter 50

Tissue Distribution

Whole globes and corneas for surgery, research, and teaching

EMILE J. FARGE

When donated globes or corneas arrive in the eye bank laboratory, quick action must follow to use this gift to its fullest potential. For the sake of completeness, we consider here the three general headings as distribution of eye tissue for (1) surgery, (2) teaching, and (3) research.

SURGICAL USE OF EYES

Originally, eye banks were developed to provide corneas for patients to restore their sight. The use of donated corneas for surgical penetrating keratoplasty accounts for less than half of the corneas donated. In 1990 there were 86,076 whole eyes and corneas donated to American eye banks that are members of the Eye Bank Association of America (EBAA). About 40,631 of these eyes were distributed to surgeons for transplants.[2]

Corneas are distributed either as whole globes or as corneoscleral discs. In the former condition the eye bank will, after verifying the absence of contraindications for use in transplantation, examine the various strata of the cornea and determine its optical quality. Then the eye bank sends the entire globe in a moist chamber with antibiotic or sterile saline or both to the operating room where the surgeon removes and transplants the appropriate part of the cornea taken from the globe.

Today, however, in North and South America corneoscleral rim storage in various media has all but entirely replaced whole globe use. The eye bank technician removes the cornea and 1 to 3 mm of adjacent sclera from the globe, assays its optical integrity, places it in a holding medium fortified with appropriate antibiotics, and ships the cornea to the operating room for transplantation. The first holding medium that was used exclusively for 10 years was McCarey-Kaufman[4] medium. It continues to be the medium of choice in many parts of the world and is used to some degree universally. The addition of chondroitin sulfate in 1984[3] appears to have added to the length of time that the endothelium could be preserved post mortem, and still more recently the use of both dextran and chondroitin sulfate, together with amino acids and antioxidants, appears to enhance corneal endothelium even more.[1]

Beyond this, an entire globe can be placed in the freezer and kept there until a surgeon requires it for a lamellar keratoplasty.

In the 1980s, another use for corneas, namely, epikeratophakia, was introduced. This procedure allows use of tissue from donors up to 80 years of age. Corneas are placed in a holding medium and sent to a laboratory where they can be freeze-dried, lathed according to prescription by the surgeon requesting the tissue, and sent to the surgeon in this freeze-dried state (devoid of epithelium or endothelium). They are rehydrated and sutured onto the corneal surface of eyes with high myopia, keratoconus, and aphakia.

Other surgical uses for donated eye tissue include use of sclera in dental packing by some oral surgeons as an aid to healing of the gums, scleral patches and scleral buckles used in accordance with certain retinal surgical procedures, orbital repair during an in vivo enucleation of a diseased eye, some eyelid plastic repairs, and most recently for reinforcement in glaucoma seton surgery.

NEED FOR CORNEAS FOR KERATOPLASTY

The need for corneas for penetrating keratoplasty and other corneal procedures has escalated tremendously. Whereas 7900 corneal transplants were performed by doctors associated with the EBAA in 1979, over 24,000 such grafts were undertaken in 1984 and 40,631 in 1990. This tremendous increase in the numbers of keratoplasties at present has shown no sign of slowing down.

Corneal disease and corneal dystrophies are being diagnosed more rapidly than ever. At one time corneal blindness was considered an unpleasant condition to be tolerated rather than reversed. With an increase in surgeons who are technically capable of performing keratoplasty, the rise of technology in the form of excellent inert suturing material, and the use of operating microscopes, the success of corneal transplants has increased and more transplants are being performed. Every year more than 3000 persons in the United States alone wait for available corneal tissue for transplantation.

It is well known that corneal disease thrives between the Tropic of Cancer and the Tropic of Capricorn, the zone of which the equator is the center. Pterygia, corneal dystrophies, and, in countries with poor public health, trachoma continue to account for a large percentage of corneal disease worldwide. Because of this, eye banks are being developed in these parts of the world.

In 1985, the Pan-American Association of Ophthalmology created an eye banking arm to serve its membership. The Pan American Association of Eye Banks (APABO) grew to 35 member eye banks in Latin America in its first 6 years. Almost all of these had been begun in the 1980s. Originally based in Houston, Texas, APABO opened a South American office in Bogotá in December 1988 and a Brazilian office in Rio de Janeiro in 1991. A coordinating and teaching association, APABO has training courses for certifying technicians and workshops and literature for teaching administration of eye banks with emphasis on public education, passing of appropriate anatomic gift legislation, and working with ministries of health.

Last year more than 1000 corneas were exported by United States eye banks to Latin American countries; this number is expected to increase dramatically as surgeons in Latin countries perform more keratoplasties. The same can hold true for the Middle East and some European countries.

The greatest need for corneas exists in India, where an estimated one million blind persons could have their sight restored with a corneal transplant. Although there are about 30 fledgling eye banks in India, modern eye banking and quality control are nonexistent. This situation will have to be addressed in the near future.

USE OF DONATED EYE TISSUE FOR TEACHING PURPOSES

For the most part, whole globes donated by families after the death of their loved ones are useful for educational purposes when they are unsuitable for penetrating or lamellar keratoplasty. Basic science courses in medical school, the histopathology laboratory during residency training, and practice surgery by residents and ophthalmologists make educational use of whole donated eyes. The whole eye can serve as study material for medical students, residents in ophthalmology, and ophthalmic personnel. Sections of the eye are made and stained after fixation in formalin for microscopic study of normal and abnormal tissues.

The final teaching use, surgical practice, is of increasing importance in today's sophisticated medical education. Whereas beef or porcine eyes may be useful for learning suturing and excision of diseased parts, the human eye has unique characteristics, and it alone is the optimal teaching instrument for those learning to perform surgery on the human eye.

INVESTIGATIVE USES OF DONATED EYES

Eye banks that collect tissue for research are quick to point out that donated eyes whose corneas are used in surgery have helped two persons to improve their quality of life. Meanwhile eyes donated and used in research projects can potentially help thousands of persons through research outcomes.

Increasingly, researchers seek corneas and lenses. The understanding of disease entities such as keratoconus and other dystrophies have been brought about directly by the use of human anterior segments for investigation. Vitreous humor is also studied biochemically.

Cataract research requires lenses because continued efforts are being made to defer by a decade or more the age at which most cataracts sufferers begin to be inconvenienced by their disease. One of the stated goals of the National Eye Institute is to seek ways to defer the onset of cataracts in the lives of those most prone to cataract problems.

Eye banks also provide posterior segments for research on the retina and pigment epithelium. Such studies include (1) the distribution of various neurotransmitters using autoradiography, immunocytochemistry, and cytologic techniques performed on early postmortem tissue; (2) studies on the comparison of various carbohydrates in metabolism of rods and cones throughout the human retina; (3) the transport of vitamin A in the retina and pigment epithelium; (4) the protective mechanisms provided by xanthine pigments in the macula; (5) the biosynthe-

SUMMARY OF USES FOR EYES DONATED TO AN EYE BANK

1. Uses for Surgery
   1.1 Penetrating keratoplasty (PKP)
   1.2 Lamellar keratoplasty (LKP)
   1.3 Cryopreservation for later PKP
   1.4 Frozen whole globe for later LKP
   1.5 Glycerin preservation for later LKP; or patch graft
   1.6 Freeze-dried for epikeratophakia
   1.7 Dental surgery for gums
   1.8 Scleral patches
   1.9 Orbital or lid repair
2. Uses for teaching
   2.1 Anatomic studies
   2.2 Histology and histopathology
   2.3 Surgical practice
3. Uses for investigation
   3.1 Corneas
       3.1.1 For corneal anatomy and physiologic functioning
       3.1.2 Studies of corneal dystrophies and diseases
       3.1.3 Endothelial viability studies
   3.2 Lenses
       3.2.1 Cataract studies
       3.2.2 Normal versus opacified lens chemistry
   3.3 Vitreous
   3.4 Posterior segments
       3.4.1 Studies of neurotransmitters in retina
       3.4.2 Comparison of carbohydrates in metabolism of rods and cones throughout retina
       3.4.3 Transplant of vitamin A in retina and pigment epithelium
       3.4.4 Protective mechanisms provided by xanthine pigments in macula
       3.4.5 Studies of interphotoreceptor matrix
       3.4.6 Studies of distribution of melatonin in retina and pigment epithelium
       3.4.7 Studies of differences between cones of fovea and other cones
       3.4.8 Studies of differences in endocytotic mechanisms of rod and cone photoreceptors
       3.4.9 Studies of pigment epithelium from human eyes maintained in organ culture
       3.4.10 Studies using normal human retinas subjected to various metabolic agents to demonstrate vulnerability of specific cell types

sis and secretion of components of the interphotoreceptor matrix; (6) the regional distribution of melatonin in the retina and pigment epithelium; (7) comparisons in the cytologic differences between foveal cones and peripheral cones; (8) the differences in the endocytotic mechanisms of rod and cone photoreceptors; and (9) the pigment epithelium from human retina subjected to various metabolic agents to show the vulnerability of specific retinal cell types.

Two organizations have successfully garnered the help of eye banks during the 1980s: The National Disease Research Interchange and the Retinitis Pigmentosa Foundation. The NDRI (2401 Walnut Street Suite 408, Philadelphia, PA 19103, [215] 557-7361) is endeavoring to intervene in the process of diabetes or to defer its effects. Through research, both basic and clinical, they are attempting to discover how to delay the onset of or to prevent the retinopathy so often associated with diabetes. Eyes of deceased diabetic patients, as well as normal eyes from eye banks, are vital to assist in their project. Usually they can pay the pharmaceutical and enucleation fees in modest amounts to reimburse eye banks.

Likewise, the Retinitis Pigmentosa Foundation (National Headquarters, 1401 Mt. Royal Ave., 4th Floor, Baltimore, MD 21217) has done an excellent job of making their appeal nationwide for donated eyes of persons with retinitis pigmentosa or other forms of retinal degeneration. In one or two laboratories, they can have the fresh retina, less than 1 hour post mortem, employed in a research protocol, a promptness requiring a tremendous cooperation between the research laboratory and the eye bank. The Retinitis Pigmentosa Foundation has a special office for donated eyes; their telephone number is (800) 638-2300.

REFERENCES

1. Chiron Intraoptics, Inc: *Advance in 4° corneal preservation media*, Irvine, California, 1990 (commercial blurb).
2. Eye Bank Association of America: *Annual activity report*, 1001 Connecticut Avenue, Suite 601, Washington, DC 20036, April 1991.
3. Kaufman HE et al: K-Sol corneal preservation, *Am J Ophthalmol* 100:299-304, 1985.
4. McCarey BE, Kaufman HE: Improved corneal storage, *Invest Ophthalmol* 13:165, 1974.

Distribution: the Tissue Banks International system

FREDERICK N. GRIFFITH
KENNETH D. STERNER

The ultimate goal for an eye bank is the delivery of a viable, disease-free donor cornea into the hands of a competent corneal surgeon to use in the life-transforming procedure of a penetrating keratoplasty. Over the years, various distribution systems have evolved toward reaching that goal, and they are summarized in the following pages.

EYE EMERGENCY NET

The first systemized networking between eye banks for the specific purpose of distributing tissue was started in the 1950s by a dedicated group of amateur radio operators (hams). In routine contact with their local eye banks, these operators would broadcast emergency needs for corneal tissue, then stored only as who whole globes, during their transmissions to other ham users. Other operators in the net receiving these broadcasts would immediately contact their local eye bank to relay the emergency tissue request. When tissue became available, the source eye bank would contact the requesting eye bank for further details. Although this method of sharing tissue and making needs known to other eye banks was indeed timely, it became burdensome as the number of eye banks increased because numerous redundant contacts were made to fill one particular need. Additionally the system was easily abused when nonemergency requests were placed on the net.

As eye banks improved their means of communication by telephone and other methods and with the use of corneal storage media instead of moist chamber storage, the need for the net disappeared. Many patients, however, owe their sight to this wonderful group of volunteers.

EYE NET

The Eye Bank Association of America in 1983 began providing member eye banks with access to a computer system based at Emory University and later at the University of Iowa to assist in the distribution of tissue to other participating eye banks through an electronic bulletin board. Users of this system notified other users that either surgical or research tissue was (1) needed at their eye bank, or (2) available from their eye bank.

If a user wanted to learn more about a particular piece of tissue, the system provided the telephone number of the source eye bank. On the other hand, if a user needed to know if there was a need for a piece of tissue with a particular description, the system generated similar contact information. The system also provided for the sending of messages to other users by electronic mail.

An advantage of this system was its centralized, single source of tissue and information. However, there was no centralized control of matching the most appropriate tissue to available patients. There was also limited prioritization of tissue needs, though an attempt was made always to fill emergency needs first by grouping them in a separate category.

The format of this system was arranged to standardize information about available tissue and patients needing grafts. However, although current technology was being used, the information accessible through the system regarding donor medical history, tissue descriptions, and recipient data has been lacking.

THE TISSUE DISTRIBUTION AND INFORMATION CENTER OF TISSUE BANKS INTERNATIONAL

Tissue Banks International (TBI) is a nonprofit network of 12 eye banks across the United States. Beginning as a single eye bank in 1962 in Baltimore processing 250 corneas, TBI processed over 8000 transplantable corneas in 1990. In every city with a TBI-affiliated eye bank, patient waiting lists have been virtually eliminated with corneal graft surgeries performed on a scheduled basis.

Recognizing the need for centralized coordination of the distribution of a growing number of available transplantable corneas being processed by its network of eye banks, TBI created its Tissue Distribution and Information Center in February 1985. TDIC's toll-free tissue request line, 1-(800) 858-2020, was made available to surgeons and eye banks across the United States in order to access the tissue resources of TBI. In practice, tissue generated at an eye bank is used for local patients before it is made available to any neighboring eye banks or regions on a scheduled basis. Having eliminated the waiting lists in the local areas served by TBI eye banks by the distribution of tissue on an elective surgery schedule, a large number of corneas is routinely available for shipment to surgeons outside these areas.

Since its inception, TDIC has been responsible for distributing more than 27,000 corneas for transplantation worldwide. In 1991 TDIC distributed 8100 corneas around the world. With the potential availability of 1000 corneas being available from a new eye bank in Prague, Czechoslovakia, more than

10,000 corneas may be handled by TDIC in 1992.

Distribution Procedure. Surgeons in need of tissue for any surgical use may contact TDIC and request tissue for specific patients. Among the required pieces of information provided about the request are the following:

Patient name
Social Security number and address
Patient age
Patient diagnosis
Hospital
Surgery date

These data are combined with those regarding a surgeon's general preference for tissue, that is, maximum donor age, storage time before surgery, donor death–to–storage interval and delivery instructions (direct or through an eye bank) in TDIC's computer system in Baltimore. In addition, each surgeon is identified as either a local surgeon or a surgeon in a particular region as designated by HCFA (Health Care Finance Administration) (Fig. 50-1). The relationships between eye banks and their geographic regions are programmed into the computer. When corneal tissue becomes available, the data regarding the tissue are entered into the system and integrated with the data concerning the many requests and the surgeons already entered. The TDIC system then provides a list of those patients, prioritized by eye bank, region, and date of surgery most appropriate to receive the particular cornea.

An advantage of this system for participating eye banks is the centralized control of its tissue distribution function, allowing the eye bank to concentrate its efforts and resources on developing donor tissue sources rather than inventing means to distribute tissue. TDIC coordinates the entire process up to the actual packaging and shipment of the tissue by processing all tissue requests, prioritizing them, contacting surgeons with available tissue, and determining the optimal shipping arrangements in order to meet a surgery schedule. This information is communicated to the surgeon's local eye bank, if requested, and to the source eye bank in a timely manner. Additionally, any inquiries regarding a request's status, tissue availability, or delivery arrangements are handled by this central office.

From a surgeon's perspective, being able to reduce a patient's anxiety about his or her upcoming surgery by actually scheduling the transplant rather than having the patient wait expectantly for an undetermined time can be extremely valuable to the patient's well-being. Also, through using the centralized TDIC system as their primary source of tissue, surgeons are getting access not only to the tissue resources of the 12 TBI eye banks, but also to another 17 non-TBI eye banks that routinely request assistance in distributing their "surplus" corneas.

Currently, enhancements are being made to the TDIC system to provide on-line data entry of available tissue into the central system to reduce the time between tissue recovery and distribution and to centralize the billing of appropriate tissue-processing fees to hospitals and surgery centers.

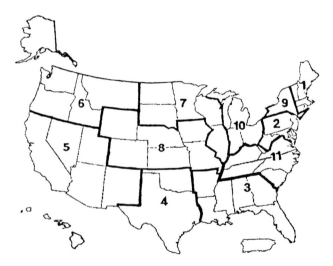

Fig. 50-1. Tissue distribution regions for the United States.

Chapter 51

Medical-Legal Aspects of Eye Banking

An overview of the law of corneal transplants[1]

DOUGLAS W. BOND
I. NELSON ROSE

Law always trails society. Whether the changes are technologic, ethical, or political, it is the nature of law to follow, not lead.

The law is slowly catching up with advancements in the field of organ transplantation, but even as it changes, the law creates new traps for the careless. An eye bank, physician, or technician can be liable for removing tissue without legal permission, for disfiguring the dead, for mishandling the tissue, and for infecting the recipient.[2] Even if found not liable, the cost of litigation can be devastating. The material presented here is intended to serve as a general overview of the laws relating to transplants and to help diminish the probability of litigation. It is important to note that the laws of each state differ in many respects and constantly change; consultation with local legal counsel is essential.

THE UNIFORM ANATOMICAL GIFT ACT

In England the rights and duties and methods of disposal of the dead were historically governed by the Christian churches and their ecclesiastical courts until the adoption of the English Burial Acts in the 1850s. Although American courts are not bound by church law, many of the ideas promulgated by the early ecclesiastical decisions influenced early American courts in deciding who had control over the remains of the dead.[3]

In the United States common law courts made the family, not the church, the entity responsible for the body's disposition.[4] In essence, a person who died no longer "owned" his body; he could will his land and even his slaves, but he had no control over his own corpse. Because of the family's role and unsettled issues at common law, doctors could not confidently remove organs based on the decedent's consent alone.

This common law is still the law of the United States, unless changed by acts of a legislature. Each state may change the common law as it deems necessary to promote the interests of its people. States enacted statutes to deal with new legal questions created by rapid advances in biotechnology and medical science for new uses of body organs. However, the result was a confusing mixture of old common law dating back to the seventeenth century and new conflicting state statutes that were inadequate in both content and coverage.[5]

To bring consistency to the law and to encourage the making of anatomical gifts, the National Conference of Commissioners on Uniform State Laws developed the Uniform Anatomical Gift Act[6] (hereinafter "the Act") in 1968. The Act has no legal effect until it is enacted into law by an individual state. In fact, virtually every state legislature made significant changes in adopting the model statute.

The Act has been adopted in some form by all 50 states and the District of Columbia. However, the Act had left some important questions unanswered. So, in 1987, the National Conference approved an amended version[7] (hereinafter "the 1987 revision"). A minority of states subsequently adopted, in whole or in part, the 1987 revision.[8] Because of the changes made by various states to the original Act, local counsel must be retained for advice as to the particular local state law when developing policies for eye banking and transplantation.

The original 1968 Act remains the basic structural

model used by the majority of states.[9] The 1968 Act allows any person of sound mind who is at least 18 years of age to make an anatomical gift.[10] The gift can be made by will, which would become effective on the death of the donor without waiting for probate,[11] or by an authorized document.[12] The document, usually a card the donor can carry, must be signed by the donor in the presence of two witnesses who must also sign in the donor's presence.[13] If consent is given by a relative, there must be a signed document, telegram, or recorded conversation.[14] Under the 1987 revision, the requirement of two witnesses signing the document has been deleted to simplify the making of a gift.[15]

If no gift were made during the decedent's lifetime and the decedent had not previously made his wishes known, the 1968 Act sets forth a prioritized list of relatives who may consent to donation: spouse, adult children, parents, adult siblings, guardian or other person authorized by law to dispose of the body.[16] The procurer can rely on the consent of a relative unless it is known that the decedent or another relative of the same or a higher priority class would object.[17]

The donor may specify a particular donee. Only those individuals and organizations listed in the 1968 Act can receive anatomical gifts. These include physicians, hospitals, schools, organ banks, and transplant recipients. The gift must be used for one of the stated purposes: research, education, advancement of science, therapy, or transplantation.[18] The donee is not required to accept the gift. If the gift of a body part is accepted, the part must be removed without unnecessary mutilation and the body returned to the next of kin.[19]

To avoid the possibility of a conflict of interest, the attending physician determines the time of death but is precluded from participation in removal or transplant.[20]

Under the 1968 Act, "A person who acts in good faith in accord with the terms of this Act or with the anatomical gift laws of another state (or foreign country) is not liable for damages in any civil action or subject to prosecution in any criminal proceeding for his act."[21] However, at least one court has construed this legal protection narrowly, to extend neither immunity to treatment of the donor before death, nor immunity to treatment of the live transplant donee.[22]

The 1987 revision has several new provisions that attempt to increase the supply of organs for transplantation. A new section[23] in the 1987 revised Act authorizes a coroner, medical examiner, or public health official to remove a part from a body in their custody for transplantation, provided that several conditions are met. The removal is not permitted where the coroner has knowledge of an objection to the removal of a part. The official must make a "reasonable effort," taking into account the useful life of the part, to locate and examine the decedent's medical records and contact the next of kin to determine if there are any objections.

Another significant addition in the 1987 revised Act is the routine inquiry and required request provision.[24] This provision requires hospitals to ask patients being admitted to the hospital if they are an organ donor. If a dying patient's file does not indicate a refusal to make a gift, the hospital must discuss making an anatomical gift with the family using reasonable discretion and sensitivity.

NATIONAL ORGAN TRANSPLANT ACT OF 1984

On October 19, 1984, Congress enacted the National Organ Transplant Act (hereinafter "the NOTA").[25] The NOTA established the National Organ Procurement and Transplantation Network to maintain a central registry for linking organ donors with potential recipients. The NOTA banned the purchase or sale of human organs if the transfer affects interstate commerce. The Task Force on Organ Transplantation was created to provide a study of organ procurement in the United States.

Recommendations by the task force led to Congress amending the Social Security Act to require hospitals participating in Medicare or Medicaid to have written procedures to make families of potential donors aware of the option of organ donation.[26]

PROCUREMENT OF CORNEAL TISSUE

The 1968 Uniform Anatomical Gift Act failed to address the question of who may remove corneal tissue, leaving the issue up to the individual states. Until recently, only licensed physicians and morticians could handle dead bodies. The need for prompt action has given rise to laws that enable others to perform cadaver enucleations. For example, in the state of Hawaii, it was often difficult to obtain a physician to perform the procedure when the donor had died on one of the outer islands. As a result, a law was passed in 1981 allowing "a technician who has successfully completed a course of training acceptable to the Board of Medical Examiners" to enucleate donor eyes under Hawaii's Anatomical Gift Act.[27]

A majority of states have enacted similar enabling statutes. Often, the trained technician must be an embalmer or funeral director who has undergone additional training.[28]

Some states afford additional legal protection for enucleators who act in compliance with these statutes.[29] However, careful adherence to the exact requirements of state law is essential. Additionally, the enucleator must competently perform according to good medical standards for enucleation and handling of corneal tissue to avoid liability for negligence.[30]

Several states have enacted provisions requiring that all organs be tested for acquired immunodeficiency syndrome before being transplanted. If the test is positive, the organ must be destroyed.[31]

Under the 1987 revision, the list of individuals authorized to remove a part has been expanded to include certified enucleators for eyes and technicians.[32] The type of certification necessary for these individuals is also indicated in the 1987 revised Act.

MEDICAL EXAMINER STATUTES

Although the 1968 Uniform Anatomical Gift Act made a variety of advances in the law of organ donation, it failed to procure sufficient organs to meet the demand. Under the 1968 Act no organs could be removed for transplant unless there was explicit authorization by the donor or relative. In practice, even when donor cards were signed and available, doctors would not retrieve the organs without first obtaining the additional consent of a family member.[33]

To overcome the problem of lack of consent where a healthy organ was available for transplant, many states enacted legislation in addition to the 1968 Act. Several states have enacted "presumed consent" laws. These statutes allow a coroner or medical examiner to authorize the removal of corneas without giving notice or obtaining consent from the next of kin. The law presumes the dying person would consent to the removal if given the opportunity; the burden of objecting rests on the decedent before death or on the family. Because there is no requirement of notice, families are often unaware that the cornea has been removed.[34]

Jurisdictions adopting presumed consent laws allow corneal tissue removal only under certain conditions. The body must be under the jurisdiction of the medical examiner. Removal must not interfere with the autopsy or other investigation or alter the deceased's postmortem facial appearance. Most importantly, no objection by the deceased or the next of kin is known by the coroner. However, this last condition does not require the coroner to inquire into the preference of the deceased or his next of kin.[35]

Statutes that presume consent or require no notice are of questionable constitutionality. Although several state courts have upheld statutes that presume consent and do not require notice as constitutional,[36] the Sixth Circuit Court of Appeals recently held that a coroner can be liable for the unauthorized removal of corneas from a body.[37]

The Sixth Circuit case involved an Ohio statute[38] that permitted the coroner to have a technician remove corneas from a body without consent provided that there was no knowledge of an objection. The policy and custom of the coroner's office was not to obtain the next of kin's consent or to inspect the medical records or hospital documents before removing corneas.[39]

Other jurisdictions have enacted statutes allowing the removal of organs only after "reasonable efforts" have been made to obtain consent by the next of kin. These statutes often require a "good faith" effort by either the coroner, hospital, or eye bank to notify the appropriate parties and obtain their consent. Only after these efforts have failed may the coroner authorize the removal of the organ. These laws often include an additional provision requiring hospitals to ask the next of kin for organs when the wishes of the deceased are unknown.[40] The 1987 revised Act has taken this approach in an effort to increase the supply of suitable organs for transplant.[41]

Some medical examiner statutes exempt individuals from donation if it is known that the decedent would have objected because of religious concerns. For example, the Tennessee medical examiners' statute states that it does not apply where the decedent is a Christian Scientist.[42]

It is important to consult local counsel to determine the particular statute your jurisdiction has adopted and possible litigation that may have resulted from it.

THEORIES OF LIABILITY

The American legal system provides monetary damages as a remedy for harm. This is true in many cases even where there was no intentional act.

In the case of unauthorized autopsy, harm is not measured by the amount of actual damages to the corpse. Instead, compensation is based upon the mental suffering of the surviving relatives.[43]

An autopsy performed after securing family consent is limited to the scope of such consent;[44] retention of body parts when unnecessary to determine cause of death has been held to be outside the scope of an autopsy.[45] Even the medical examiner's right to conduct an autopsy is limited to circumstances specifically authorized by state law.[66] Therefore liability for mutilation of a corpse under the common law[47] is extended to physicians who exceed the scope of legal authority.[48] It is not difficult to imagine a scenario in which the decedent's family discover by their own examination that an unauthorized enucleation has taken place and thus suffer extreme emotional pain. And the "good faith" immunity from liability under the Uniform Anatomical Gift Act applies only to actions taken in accord with its terms.[49] A state may also make such conduct a crime as well as a civil wrong.[50]

As in the case with all medical procedures, the law of negligence applies with respect to transplantation of a cornea into a recipient. Negligence is the failure to conform to a standard of good medical practice — what is customary and usual in the profession.[51] This standard is higher in the case of a physician who possesses an additional degree of skill and knowledge; for example, an ophthalmologist may be found negligent in a case where a family practice physician would not.[52] The breach of this standard must be the cause of the actual damage to the person suing.[53] A jury of laypersons usually decides these issues based upon expert testimony and the benefit of hindsight.

In the case of *Ravenis v. Detroit General Hospital*,[54] such negligence was found where a hospital failed to establish a procedure that would give the person determining suitability of tissue adequate access to the donor's medical history. Expert testimony at trial revealed that the donor was unsuitable, based on information that was not supplied to the resident performing the enucleation or to the surgeon performing the transplant. As a result, the jury exonerated the physicians while finding the hospital liable for negligence. Had a complete history been provided, it follows that the physician determining suitability would have been liable for failing to eliminate an inappropriate donor.

Besides negligence, physician liability can be based on failure to obtain informed consent.[55] The modern rule is that the patient must be informed of all risks that are material to the patient's decision whether to undergo a procedure.[56] A material risk is one to which a reasonable person would be "likely to attach significance."[57] In determining materiality, one must consider the probability and severity of risk. The careful physician will not substitute his own judgment for that of the patient; disclosure is essential even though the patient may choose to decline recommended treatment as a result. Risks of not having the procedure, of course, must also be disclosed.

The lack of informed consent must be the cause of the injury. In determining causation, some courts look to whether a reasonable patient in the same position would have withheld consent had the risk been disclosed;[58] others look to what the particular patient would have done if the risk were known.[59]

The relationship of informed consent to negligence can best be illustrated by the following example. A patient develops an infection after a penetrating keratoplasty. If the physician negligently used corneal tissue from a donor who died of infection, the patient could recover under a theory of negligence. If the physician did not act negligently but failed to disclose the risk of infection (assuming the failure to disclose was material and the legal cause of harm), the physician may be liable under the theory of informed consent. If both situations occur, the physician's liability would be predicated upon both legal causes of action.

Liability without negligence is also possible under a theory of strict liability. This applies whenever a product is sold in a defective condition and is unreasonably dangerous to the consumer.[60] As a product, the storage medium could be subject to this standard of liability without fault. Strict liability has also been extended by some courts to serum hepatitis transmitted by a blood transfusion.[61] However, several courts have concluded that a physician treating or diagnosing a patient is selling his services and not selling a product.[62] Many states have enacted statutes that characterize blood transfusions and organ transplants as services not sales, thus avoiding application of strict liability.[63]

Medical professionals cannot completely avoid the possibility of litigation under these or other theories. Nevertheless, there are some affirmative steps that can be taken to reduce the risk. Everyone involved in the procedure must have the requisite skill and knowledge and must perform in a competent manner within the boundaries of good medical practice. The diagnosis must be explained to the patient, as well as the treatment to be performed, the risks involved in submitting to as well as declining the treatment, and any alternatives to the proposed procedure. No warranty should be made as to the outcome. Additionally, the physician must comply with the technical requirements of all federal, state, and local laws. Finally, malpractice insurance is essential because there is no guarantee that even the most careful surgeon or eye bank will avoid a lawsuit.

REFERENCES

1. This chapter is based in part on "An overview of the law of corneal transplants," by I. Nelson Rose and Christine J. Wilson in the prior edition of this book, Brightbill FS, editor:

Corneal surgery: theory, technique, and tissue, St. Louis, 1986, Mosby–Year Book.

2. Trenkner R: "Tort Liability of Physician or Hospital in Connection with Organ or Tissue Transplant Procedures," 76 A.L.R. 3d 890 (1989).

3. Note, "The Role of the Family in Cadaveric Organ Procurement," 65 Ind. L.J. 167. (Winter 1989).

4. *Id.,* at 171.

5. Uniform Anatomical Gift Act (prefatory note), 8A U.L.A. 15 (1983).

6. 8A U.L.A. 15 (1983). This is the original version of the Act and the one adopted by most states. The most recent amended version was issued in 1987 and contains several significant changes. 8A U.L.A. 2 (Supp. 1991).

7. 8A U.L.A. 2 (Supp. 1991). The amended version is intended to simplify the manner of making an anatomical gift and require the intentions of a donor be followed.

8. Thirteen jurisdictions have adopted the revised Uniform Anatomical Gift Act of 1987: Arkansas, California, Connecticut, Hawaii, Idaho, Montana, Nevada, North Dakota, Rhode Island, Utah, Vermont, Virginia, Wisconsin. See 8A U.L.A. 2 (Supp. 1991) (table).

9. The general provisions of the 1968 Act will be discussed with differences in the 1987 Act being pointed out when relevant.

10. Uniform Anatomical Gift Act (1968), section 2(a).

11. Uniform Anatomical Gift Act (1968), section 4(a). "[I]f the will is not probated or is declared invalid for testamentary purposes, the gift, to the extent that it has been acted upon in good faith, is nevertheless valid and effective." *Id.*

12. Uniform Anatomical Gift Act (1968), section 4(b).

13. *Id.*

14. *Id.,* section 4(e)

15. Revised Uniform Anatomical Gift Act (1987), section 2(b).

16. Uniform Anatomical Gift Act (1968), section 2(b). The 1987 revised Uniform Anatomical Gift Act Section 3(a), adds "a grandparent of the decedent" after brother or sister.

17. Uniform Anatomical Gift Act (1968), section 2(c). The 1987 revised Uniform Anatomical Gift Act clarifies that if a person of a prior class is available but does not make a gift, section 3(e) authorizes a gift by a person of a lower class. Of course, a medical examiner's office will be liable if it performs an enucleation over a known objection. *Kirker v. Orange County,* 519 So.2d 682, 684 (Fla. App. 1988).

18. Uniform Anatomical Gift Act (1968), section 3. The 1987 revised Uniform Anatomical Gift Act, section 6(a) combines sections 3(1) and 3(3) of the 1968 Act to reverse the sequence of purposes for which anatomical gifts may be made, thereby emphasizing transplantation as the primary purpose.

19. Uniform Anatomical Gift Act (1968), section 7.

20. *Id.,* section 7(b). The comment to this subsection indicates that the language of the provision does not prevent the donor's attending physician from communicating with the transplant team or other relevant donees.

21. *Id.,* section 7(c). The 1987 revised Uniform Anatomical Gift Act is more explicit and includes "hospital, physician, surgeon, [coroner], [medical examiner], [local public health officer], enucleator, technician, or other person,. . ." "Acts in good faith" has been expanded to read "Attempts to act in good faith." Section 11(c).

22. *Williams v. Hoffman,* 66 Wis.2d 145, 223 N.W.2d 844 (1974).

23. Revised Uniform Anatomical Gift Act (1987), section 4.

24. *Id.,* section 5.

25. National Organ Transplant Act, Pub. L. No. 98-507, 98 Stat. 2339 (codified at 42 U.S.C. sections 273-74) (1984).

26. 42 U.S.C. section 1320b-8 (Supp. IV 1986).

27. Hawaii Rev. Stat. section 327-7(e) (Supp. 1984). One of the authors of this chapter, Prof. I. Nelson Rose, authored this amendment to the statute while serving as legal advisor to the Hawaii Lions Eye Bank and Makana Foundation. Hawaii later adopted the 1987 revisions, eliminating the need for this special amendment.

28. *See, e.g.,* Ind. Code Ann. section 29-2-16-4(d) (West 1990) (embalmer or funeral director who has completed a course in eye enucleation and was certified as competent to enucleate eyes by an accredited school of medicine).

29. *See, e.g.,* Del. Code Ann. tit. 16, section 2713(d); "shall be free from civil and criminal liability with respect to the eye enucleation;" New Jersey N.J. Stat. Ann. section 26:6-58.1(d); "shall not have any liability, civil or criminal, for the eye enucleation."

30. Some statutes clearly exempt negligence and malpractice from the definition of good faith. *See* Fla. Stat. Ann. section 732.917(3); S .C. Code Ann. section 44-43-380(c).

31. *See, e.g.,* section 23-06.2-11.1.; R.I. Gen. Laws section 23-18.6-12 (1956); Del. Code Ann. tit. 16, section 2801(b).

32. Revised Uniform Anatomical Gift Act (1987) Section 1.

33. Revised Uniform Anatomical Gift Act (prefatory note) (1987).

34. "The Role of the Family in Cadaveric Organ Procurement," *supra* note 3, at 180.

35. Note, " 'She's Got Bette Davis['s] Eyes' ": Assessing the Non-consensual Removal of Cadaver Organs Under The Takings And Due Process Clauses," 90 Colum. L. Rev. 528, 528-574 (1990).

36. Three state courts have upheld these statutes against constitutional challenges. *State v. Powell,* 497 So.2d 1188 (Fla. 1986), cert. denied, 481 U.S. 1059 (1987); *Tillman v. Detroit Receiving Hosp.,* 138 Mich. App. 683, 360 N.W. 2d 275 (1984) (no violation of right to privacy); *Georgia Lions Eye Bank v. Lavant,* 255 Ga. 60, 335 S.E.2d 127 (1985) (no deprivation of property without due process).

37. *Brotherton v. Cleveland,* 923 F.2d 477 (6th Cir. 1991).

38. Ohio Rev. Code section 2108.60.

39. *Id.,* 923 F.2d at 478 (6th Cir. 1991).

40. "She's Got Bette Davis['s] Eyes", *supra* note 35, at 536-537.

41. Revised Uniform Anatomical Gift Act (1987), section 4 allows removal by coroner or public health official provided that specific conditions are met. Section 5 requires hospitals to make routine inquiry with patients regarding organ donation.

42. Tenn. Code Ann. section 68-30-201(3) (1990).

43. *See Sworski v. Simons,* 208 Minn. 201, 293 N.W. 309 (1940); *Lott v. State,* 32 Misc.2d 296, 225 N.Y.S.2d 434 (1962).

44. *See, e.g., Terill v. Harbin,* 376 S.W.2d 945 (Tex. Civ. Appl. 1964).

45. *Hendriksen v. Roosevelt Hosp.,* 297 F. Supp. 1142 (S.D.N.Y. 1969).

46. *See, e.g., Scarpaci v. Milwaukee County,* 96 Wis.2d 663, 292 N.W.2d 816 (1980).

47. Restatement (Second) of Torts section 868 (1977).

48. *See, e.g., Koerber v. Patek,* 123 Wis. 453, 102 N.W. 40 (1905); *Palmquist v. Standard Accident Ins. Co.,* 3 F.Supp. 358 (S.D. Cal. 1933).

49. *See supra* note 21 and accompanying text.

50. *See, e.g.,* Cal. Health & Safety Code section 7114 (Deerings 1991), which provides that any person who performs, permits, or assists with an unauthorized autopsy is guilty of a misdemeanor. This section does not apply to the coroner or any other officer authorized by law.

51. W. Keeton, Prosser and Keeton on the Law of Torts, section 32 at 189 (5th ed. 1984).

52. *Cf., id.,* section 32 at 185.
53. *Id.,* section 30 at 165.
54. 63 Mich.App. 79, 234 N.W.2d 411 (1975).
55. For a detailed discussion of this topic, see Rozovsky, F.A.: *Consent to Treatment: A Practical Guide,* Little, Brown & Co., Boston (1984).
56. *See Canterbury v. Spence,* 464 F.2d 772 (D.C. Cir. 1972).
57. *Id.,* at 787 (quoting Waltz and Scheuneman, "Informed Consent to Therapy," 64 Nw. U.L. Rev. 628, 640 (1970)).
58. *See, e.g., Macey v. James,* 139 Vt. 270, 427 A.2d 803 (1981); *Cobbs v. Grant,* 8 Cal.3d 229, 104 Cal. Rptr 505, 502 P.2d 1 (1972).
59. *See, e.g., MacPherson v. Ellis,* 305 N.C. 266, 287 S.E.2d 892 (1982).
60. Restatement (Second) of Torts section 402 A (1965).
61. *Cunningham v. MacNeal Memorial Hosp.,* 47 Ill.2d 443, 266 N.E.2d 897 (1970).
62. *E.g., Hoven v. Kelble,* 79 Wis.2d 444, 256 N.W.2d 379 (1977); *Carmichael v. Reitz,* 17 Cal. App.3d 958, 95 Cal. Rptr. 381 (1971).
63. *See, e.g.,* Ala. Code section 7-2-314(4) (1990); Ga. Code Ann. section 105-1105(a) (1991); Ky. Rev. Stat. section 139.125 (1991); N.D. Cent. Code section 41-02-33(3) (d) (1989).

Eye bank–related litigation

GEORGE N. MEROS, Jr.
MARY W. CHAISSON

Corneal transplantation is an exceptionally successful tool in restoring sight to the functionally blind. In 1990 alone, 40,631 corneal transplants were performed in the United States.[1] The benefits of such successful procedures are immense. Restoration of sight to the functionally blind not only greatly improves our quality of life, but also alleviates economic burdens imposed upon state governments, which must provide for the special needs of blind citizens.

However, despite passage of the Uniform Anatomical Gift Act in all 50 states, demand for suitable corneas continued to far outstrip supply. A majority of states responded to this critical shortage of corneal tissue by enacting additional legislation. The states' efforts can be subdivided into three separate categories—presumed consent laws enacted by at least 13 states,[2] laws making consent largely irrelevant, enacted by at least two states and Puerto Rico,[3] and laws requiring efforts to obtain consent, enacted by at least 14 states.[4]

The presumed consent laws authorize the immediate removal of a decedent's corneas if the body is under the jurisdiction of a medical examiner, an autopsy is otherwise required by law, and no objection of the next of kin is known to the medical examiner. The laws impose no obligation on the medical examiner to make any attempt to obtain consent. The

laws also provide immunity from civil or criminal liability to those involved in the removal, transfer, and storage of the corneal tissue.

Because presumed consent laws operate in the realm of emotional tragedy and permit corneal removal without imposing an affirmative duty to obtain consent from the next of kin, these laws sparked heated litigation in several states. Although such statutes were upheld against constitutional challenges in Florida,[5] Georgia,[6] and Michigan,[7] the United States Court of Appeals for the Sixth Circuit recently struck down Ohio's version of a presumed consent law in *Brotherton v. Cleveland.*[8] The decisions in all these cases involved the nature of the rights involved in a decedent's remains and constitutional implications of those rights.

COMMON LAW AND CONSTITUTIONAL THEORIES INVOLVED

In the earliest days of English common law, the ecclesiastical courts were solely responsible for matters pertaining to dead bodies. There were no property rights in dead bodies because a person's remains were not characterized as property.[9] This created a vacuum in the United States, since there were no ecclesiastical courts to handle these matters.

In this century American common law created a legal right in the next of kin to control and direct the disposition of a loved one's remains. Early decisions characterized the right as a property right in the corpse itself.[10] Later decisions questioned that characterization, choosing instead to describe the right as a "quasi-property" right.[11] More recent decisions, however, have made clear that the right to direct the disposition of a body is not a property right at all but is a personal right in the next of kin against the emotional distress caused by the mutilation of a family member's remains.[12] A recognized expert in tort law aptly stated: "It seems reasonably obvious that such 'property' is something evolved out of thin air to meet the occasion, and that it is in reality the personal feelings of the survivors which are being protected, under a fiction likely to deceive no one but a lawyer."[13]

Two rights secured by the federal constitution and the constitutions of most states figure prominently in the applicable cases. The first is the right of privacy. Courts have interpreted the due process clause of the Fourteenth Amendment to the United States Constition[14] as affording a right of privacy in certain fundamentally personal, intimate matters, such as the decision to have an abortion or the decision to have children.[15] Government cannot intrude into these matters without a compelling reason for doing so. The second right is known as procedural due process. Before state action can materially affect a person's property, the due process clause requires that such person be given a meaningful opportunity to be heard and to object to that action.[16]

APPLICABLE CASE LAW

Michigan's presumed consent law was challenged on right-to-privacy grounds in *Tillman v. Detroit Receiving Hosp.;*[17] In affirming the trial court's rejection of this argument, the Michigan Court of Appeals stated the following:

Only rights that can be deemed "fundamental" or "implicit in the concept of ordered liberty" are included in the guaranty of the right of personal privacy. Plaintiff claims that as next of kin she has an inherent, fundamental right to bury her decedent's body without mutilation. While there is no property right in the next of kin to a dead body, Michigan jurisprudence recognizes a common law cause of action on behalf of the person or persons entitled to the possession, control, or burial of a dead body for the tort of interference with the right of burial of a deceased person without mutilation.

We do not find this common law right to be of constitutional dimension. The privacy right encompasses the right to make decisions concerning the integrity of one's body. This right is, however, a personal one. It ends with the death of the person to whom it is of value. It may not be claimed by his estate or his next of kin.[18]

Florida's statute was upheld against similar constitutional challenge in *State v. Powell.*[19] The Supreme Court of Florida concluded that the statute "reasonably achieves the permissible legislative objective of providing sight to many of Florida's blind citizens."[20] The court found no property right in the remains of a decedent beyond that of possession for the purpose of ultimate disposition. This limited right did not warrant constitutional protection. Although interference with the next-of-kin's right to disposal of a loved one's remains could form the basis for a tort action, such actions "may be restricted when necessary to obtain a permissible legislative objective."[21] The Supreme Court of Georgia arrived at much the same conclusion when Georgia's presumed consent law was challenged on constitutional grounds in *Georgia Lions Eye Bank, Inc. v. Lavant.*[22]

Although the law seems relatively settled in favor of the constitutionality of implied consent laws, newly emerging concerns may signal a move toward the recognition of a property interest in dead bodies that would trigger constitutional protections. The decision in *Brotherton v. Cleveland,*[23] mentioned previously, is a case in point. There the court reversed the lower court's dismissal of a widow's civil rights claim[24] for the wrongful removal of her deceased husband's corneas, finding that she had a protected property interest in her husband's corneas and that the corneal removal had been caused by established state procedures. However, the court premised its conclusion that the widow had a legitimate claim of entitlement to her deceased husband's corneas on its interpretation of Ohio's Uniform Anatomical Gift Act rather than on any inherent property interest in a dead body arising out of the common law.

Also, at least one commentator has predicted that the "[r]apid advances in the medical sciences beginning in the 1950s, and in genetic engineering since the 1970s, [that] have dramatically increased the uses for and value of bodily tissues" will lead to the recognition of property rights in the human body and its parts.[25]

Currently, the law remains favorable for the continued harvesting of healthy corneal tissue for transplantation. Emerging concerns indicate, however, that such harvesting should be handled with sensitivity, lest additional challenges provoke the courts to revisit the issue. When the next of kin of the decedent are readily available and time permits, one should consider seeking to obtain consent, even though there is no strict duty to do so. The wisdom of this approach is apparent when one considers that "before legislation authorized medical examiners in California to remove corneas without the consent of the next of kin, the majority of the families asked by the Los Angeles medical examiner's office responded positively"[26] and that there have been no constitutional challenges in the 14 states whose statutes require at least some effort to obtain consent before removal of corneal tissue.

REFERENCES

1. Telephone interview with Gail Crummer, Executive Director of the North Florida Lions Eye Bank, Inc., Gainesville, Florida (July 8, 1991).
2. Cal. Gov't Code §§ 27491.46-.47 (West 1988); Conn. Gen. Stat. Ann. § 19a-281 (West 1986); Del. Code Ann. tit. 29, § 4712 (Supp. 1988); Fla. Stat. Ann. § 732,9185 (West Supp. 1989); Ga. Code Ann. § 31-23-6 (1985); Ky. Rev. Stat. Ann. § 311.187 (Michie Supp. 1988); Md. Est. & Trusts Code Ann. § 4-509.1 (Supp. 1989); Mich. Comp. Laws Ann. § 333.10202 (1989); N.C. Gen. Stat. § 130A-391 (1989); Ohio Rev. Code Ann. § 2108.60 (Baldwin 1987); Tenn. Code Ann. § 68-30-204 (Supp. 1989); Tex. Health & Safety Code Ann. § 693,012 (Vernon pamphlet 1990); W. Va. Code § 16-19-3a (1985). *See also* Note, "*She's Got Bette Davis['s] Eyes": Assessing the Nonconsensual Removal of Cadaver Organs Under the Takings and Due Process Clauses,*" 90 Column. L. Rev. 528, 535 n.35 (1990).
3. Cal. Gov't Code § 27491.45(a) (West 1988); Haw. Rev. Stat Ann. § 841-14 (1988); Laws of P.R. Ann. tit. 18, § 731g (1989). *See* Note *supra,* note 2, at 536 n.38.
4. Ariz. Rev. Stat. Ann. §§ 36-851 to-852 (1986 & Supp. 1989); Ark. Stat. Ann. § 20-17-604 (Supp. 1989); Cal. Health & Safety Code § 7151.5 (West Supp. 1990); Colo. Rev. Stat. §

30-10-620 (1986); Haw. Rev. Stat. Ann. § 327-4 (1988); Idaho Code § 39-3405 (Supp. 1989); Ill. Ann. Stat. ch. 110 1/2, ¶¶ 351-354 (Smith-Hurd Supp. 1989); La. Rev. Stat. Ann. §§ 17:2354.1-.3, 33:1565 (West 1982, 1988 & Supp. 1989); Mass. Ann. Laws ch. 113, § 14 (La. Co-op. Supp. 1989); Miss. Code Ann. § 41-61-71 (Supp. 1989); Mont. Code Ann. § 72-17-215 (1989); N.D. Cent. Code § 23-06.2-04 (Supp. 1989); R.I. Gen. Laws § 23-18.6-4 (1989); Wash. Rev. Code Ann. § 68.50.280 (Supp. 1989). *See Note supra*, note 2, at 537 n.39.

5. *State v. Powell*, 497 So. 2d 1188 (Fla. 1986).
6. *Georgia Lions Eye Bank, Inc. v. Lavant*, 255 Ga. 60, 335 S.E.2d 127 (1985).
7. *Tillman v. Detroit Receiving Hosp.*, 138 Mich. App. 683, 360 N.W.2d 275 (Mich. Ct. App. 1984).
8. 923 F.2d 477 (6th Cir. 1991).
9. *Georgia Lions Eye Bank*, 255 Ga. at 61, 335 S.E.2d at 128.
10. *See, e.g., Dunahoo v. Bess*, 146 Fla. 182, 200 So. 541 (Fla. 1941).
11. *See, e.g., Lawyer v. Kernodle*, 721 F.2d 632 (8th Cir. 1983) (applying Missouri law); *Barela v. Frank A. Hubbell Co.*, 67 N.M. 319, 355 P.2d 133 (1960); *Sinai Temple v. Kaplan*, 54 Cal. App. 3d 1103, 127 Cal. Rptr. 80 (Ct. App. 1976); *Finn v. City of New York*, 70 Misc. 2d 947, 335 N.Y.S.2d 516 (Civ. Ct. 1972), *rev'd on other grounds*, 76 Misc. 2d 388, 350 N.Y.S.2d 552 (Sup. Ct. 1973).
12. *See, e.g., Dougherty v. Mercantile-Safe Deposit & Trust Co.*, 282 Md. App. 617, 387 A.2d 244 (Ct. Spec. App. 1978); *Jackson v. Rupp*, 228 So. 2d 916 (Fla. 4th DCA 1969), *aff'd*, 238 So. 2d 86 (Fla. 1970).
13. W. Prosser, *The Law of Torts*, 43-44 (2d ed. 1955).
14. U.S. Const. amend. XIV, § 1.
15. *See, e.g., Carey v. Population Servs. International*, 431 U.S. 678 (1977) (procreation); *Roe v. Wade*, 410 U.S. 113 (1973) (abortion).
16. *See, e.g., Perry v. Sinderman*, 408 U.S. 593 (1972).
17. 138 Mich. App. 683, 360 N.W.2d 275 (Ct. App. 1984).
18. *Id.* at 686-687, 360 N.W.2d at 277 (citations omitted). *Accord State v. Powell*, 497 So. 2d 1188, 1193 (Fla. 1986) (freedom of choice concerning personal matters exists in existing, ongoing relationships among living persons).
19. 497 So. 2d 1188 (Fla. 1986).
20. *Id.* at 1191.
21. *Id.* at 1192.
22. 255 Ga. at 61, 335 S.E.2d at 128.
23. 923 F.2d 477 (6th Cir. 1991).
24. 42 U.S.C. §1983 (1988).
25. Note, *"She's Got Bette Davis['s] Eyes": Assessing the Nonconsensual Removal of Cadaver Organs Under the Takings and Due Process Clauses*, 90 Colum. L. Rev. 521, 530 (1990) (cited in *Brotherton v. Cleveland*, 923 F.2d 477, 481 (6th Cir. 1991)). *See also Moore v. Regents of University of Cal.*, 202 Cal. App. 3d 1230, 249 Cal. Rptr. 494 (Ct. App. 1988), *rev'd in part*, 51 Cal. 3d 120, 793 P.2d 479, 271 Cal. Rptr. 146 (1990).
26. *State v. Powell*, 497 So. 2d 1188, 1191 (Fla. 1986).

Ethical considerations

PETER Y. WINDT

CHARACTER OF THE ISSUES

Identifying the Issues. People have diverse expectations regarding discussions of ethics in medicine. Some expect misbehavior to be identified, proposals made for remedying it, and exhortations to everyone to be good. In such discussion it is presumed that we all are clear enough about what ethics requires and that the primary problem is to ensure that we all meet those requirements. Others find this presumption premature and expect a discussion of ethical issues to explore situations in which it is not obvious what duty requires or precisely what the outcome should be of a decision made in good conscience. What follows is a discussion of the second sort. The good intentions of health care professionals will be assumed, and the issues to be examined will involve difficulties in determining precisely what ethical decency requires of us.

Ethical issues of this sort arise primarily out of conflicts among the values to which we subscribe. We may, for example, undertake a project the goals of which are ethically praiseworthy and then discover that some of the actions we must perform as a means to achieve those goals are suspect. Our problem then is to determine whether the positive value of the ends to be achieved outweighs the badness or wrongness we perceive in the means or whether the negative character of the means is so severe that we are ethically constrained to limit our pursuit of the ends in order to avoid the harms or wrongs involved in those means.

So it is with the activities under consideration here. The goals of transplantation, research, and medical education rank highly. They are important and deserve support. On the other hand, if these goals are to be served effectively, substantial amounts of tissue must be obtained. In the area of tissue procurement we encounter the possibility that ethically suspect means may be employed in the service of these ethically appropriate ends. For example, there is a possibility that tissue procurement policies that assure a sufficient quantity of tissue may do some harm or wrong to the (cadaver) donor. A second issue springs from the possibility that some harm or wrong may be done to surviving kin because of the manner in which tissue is obtained. A third issue arises when we consider the role of information transmission and management in tissue procurement. And, finally, serious questions may be raised about the effect that tissue-procurement policies may have on the attitudes of our society toward the *use* of persons in our pursuit of the goals of medicine. Before considering each of these issues in more detail, let us consider what would count as a solution to or resolution of the kind of problem they involve.

Coping with Ethical Issues. It is important to distinguish between *cleverness* and *ethical wisdom.* Cleverness, in this context, involves finding some alternative strategy for realizing the desirable ends without having to employ the dubious means. It is then a way of resolving an issue by making the conflict of values disappear. If, for example, we could devise a procedure for tissue procurement that involved harvesting of tissue only in accord with the wishes of completely enlightened donors and with the support of equally enlightened next of kin but that effectively met the demand for tissue, most of the issues listed earlier would evaporate. Cleverness, where we can achieve it, is the ideal way to cope with an ethical issue.

If we cannot discover a clever resolution to an issue involving conflicting values, we must make some hard choices. Doing so wisely involves *identifying* the values in conflict and managing to *assign degrees of importance or ethical weight* to each, in the light of which it may be decided what is to be sacrificed for the sake of what gains. Theoretically, this process might result in the determination that one value, no matter how slightly it is served, always takes precedence over another, no matter how extensively that one is abused. But typically we find ourselves embroiled in more complex estimations of *how much* of one value may or must be sacrificed to promote *how much* of another one. Cases in which it must be decided how much pain a patient may legitimately be required to endure in order to prolong life for a limited time amply illustrate the structure (and the sometimes excruciating difficulty) of this sort of hard choice.

Ethical wisdom is the capacity to make these hard choices with sensitivity and accuracy (and, I should add, within the available time). Although it may be reflected in policy, ethical wisdom seldom emerges as a set of rules or principles. Instead, it appears as a skill or capacity acquired through experience and finely attuned to the unique aspects of individual cases. What follows then will not be a prescription of principles that the ethically wise person would follow when confronted with perplexities about tissue procurement but is an account of some of the factors that such a person would take into consideration.

Aspects of Ethical Concern. Ethical attitudes and behavior toward other persons require that we show concern for them in at least two significantly different ways. First, we must have concern for the *condition* of other persons. That is, we must consider the effects of our actions and decisions on the lives, health, capacities, and happiness of others. Such

concern restrains us from making another person's condition worse in any of these respects and often requires us to strive for improvements in the condition of others. It is precisely this concern for others that is the source of ethical approbation of the uses to which donated tissue is put in transplantation, research, or medical education.

But ethical regard for others also requires concern for their *agency.* That is, we are required to respect the autonomy, rights, and responsibilities of other persons. Such respect prohibits interference with the making of decisions and the pursuit of chosen interest by others. Respect for agency requires that we do not preempt the responsibilities of others or their authority to make choices. More subtly, respect for the agency of others requires that we take into account their own wishes and preferences when we make decisions that will affect them. And it is this kind of concern for others that is the principal source of ethical reservations about the way in which tissue is procured.

In fact, a multitude of ethical issues arise from the conflict of these two kinds of ethical concern for persons; for it is a painfully familiar fact that in exercising our agency we often fail to promote optimal conditions for ourselves or others, and thus unrestricted respect for our agency is not compatible with single-minded concern for optimizing our condition. The proper role of informed consent, for example, is problematic because we recognize that persons are sometimes inclined to make choices that are not in their best interests, and so unrestricted respect for their agency must result in a worsening of their condition, but, on the other hand, unswerving dedication to maintenance or improvement of their condition must result in abuse of their agency.

It is not plausible to appeal to simple, extreme solutions to resolve such conflicts of value. That is, we cannot simply adopt a policy of always preferring respect for agency to concern for personal condition, or vice versa. It is clear that a substantial improvement in a personal condition will justify some slight failure to respect someone's agency, but it is also clear that a serious failure to respect agency cannot be justified in terms of a tiny improvement in a personal condition. Perplexity arises when we find something approximating a balance between the values in conflict. Accordingly, we do not find people aligned in two major camps with respect to what is ethically appropriate in tissue procurement. Rather, they are arrayed along a continuum, according to the relative importance they attribute to concern for personal condition and respect for agency. It has been observed that citizens of the United States tend to place more importance on agency than Europeans do where tissue procurement is involved. It may well be that health care professionals, whose orientation is primarily to the maintenance of optimum personal condition, place more importance on concern for condition than do lawyers, who have strong professional commitments to protecting the agency of their clients. In legislation, too, we find diversity. The Uniform Anatomical Gift Act, for example, emphasizes the importance of respect for agency in its concern for compliance with the wishes of prospective donors and next of kin. But several states (such as Florida, Maryland, Michigan, and Texas) have adopted medical examiner's laws that, to the extent that they approximate a policy of presumed consent, place a somewhat higher premium on the preservation or restoration of sight, or other considerations of human condition, and a somewhat lower premium on respect for the agency of some donors.

ANALYSIS OF ISSUES

Effects on Social Attitudes. One objection to procurement policies that favor satisfying the need for tissue over strict respect for agency is that such policies, if accepted and implemented, will contribute to a shift in our attitudes, so that we will become, in other circumstances, more ready to abuse agency for the sake of promoting better human conditions. Of course, anyone who believes that such procurement policies strike the right balance between concern for condition and respect for agency could respond with a counterargument of similar kind. Policies that place more emphasis on respect for agency, they might reply, would contribute to a tendency to ignore the needs of others for the sake of a self-centered independence that has outlived whatever usefulness it may have had in frontier societies. Thus we can see that whatever force these arguments have springs from one's estimate of the appropriateness of the procurement policy itself. If we believe a policy strikes the right balance between human condition and agency, our response to the claim that the policy will engender attitudes that are in alignment with that balance will be simply, "Good!" If we believe the procurement policy strikes an inappropriate balance, we will, of course, be alarmed at any tendency it may have to induce attitudes that favor that (inappropriate) balance more generally. The real issue then is not the effects that a policy will have on social attitudes but the ethical appropriateness of the policy itself.

In any case, claims about the effects a procurement policy will have on public attitudes are purely

speculative. We have not yet produced data that provide a foundation for predicting such effects, and without this foundation the contribution of such considerations to the selection of an ethically appropriate procurement policy is at best slight.

Management of Information. In discussing the procurement and use of tissue with prospective donors, surviving kin, and the general public, there is a strong temptation to be selective, to provide the information that will promote cooperation, and to suppress information that might induce reluctance or anxiety about tissue donation. Mention of benefits to donees and assurances that harvesting is done respectfully and is not disfiguring do not really provide a clear grasp of the nature of the procedures involved. (Taxidermy, after all, is not disfiguring either!) Is this a matter for concern?

If our ethical thought is condition oriented, we will tend to see the function of education to be the provision of a background against which enlightened (that is, condition-optimizing) choices will be made. From this perspective, of course, it can seem only perverse to offer information that might introduce confusion of anxiety or might encourage an *un*enlightened choice. With this orientation it will seem entirely appropriate to select and present information that supports the *right* choice. Doing so, after all, does not involve being untruthful.

But if our ethical thought is agency oriented, we will see this sort of *guidance* of choice as interference with the authentic decision-making of those who are "selectively informed." From this point of view the appropriate information to provide is the information that the informee might find pertinent to choice. The primary concern is not that the *best* choice be made (although, of course, we hope for that) but that the person to whom the information is provided make a choice that is genuinely his or hers. The question then is not whether *all* information should be forced upon our audience, but whether the information presented should have a directive function, or simply be responsive to the concerns of those to whom it is provided.

Interaction with Surviving Kin. Concern often is expressed that approaching surviving kin about the procurement of tissue from a loved one who has just died or is about to die will add to their grief, anxiety, and stress. This, of course, is concern for the condition of the kin, and this concern appears to be in conflict with concern for the condition of potential beneficiaries of tissue donation. It has been suggested that the best resolution of this conflict lies in a policy of presumed consent, wherein tissue is harvested unless the next of kin raise an objection. A radical version of such a policy would leave it up to the surviving kin to raise the issue, whereas a more moderate version would have one explain to survivors that tissue harvesting is routine, leaving it to them to decide whether to object. With either version, the aim is to maximize procurement of tissue, while minimizing stress for survivors.

But, of course, such solutions are unappealing from the point of view of respect for agency. If it is a right or responsibility of surviving kin to manage the disposition of a cadaver, a presumption of consent to donation, even if they are notified of that presumption, undermines an unhindered choice responsive to their own concerns and interests, or to the concerns and interests they are obliged to represent. Whether surviving kin do have such a right or responsibility cannot be settled without consideration of the ethical status of the deceased potential donor.

Ethical Status of the Dead. Is it possible to do harm or wrong to a deceased person? After all, life and health are already gone, as are capacities and functions. And since the capacity for experience is lost, no suffering or unhappiness can be incurred. Perhaps mutilation or disfigurement could be counted as harms, though they seem relatively insignificant given the inevitable deterioration the body will undergo. From a condition-oriented viewpoint, then, the idea of causing significant harm to the dead is implausible, if not absurd.

But once again things appear differently from an agency-oriented point of view. The important considerations are these: (1) It is possible to abuse a person's agency without that person ever learning of the abuse. (Withholding information from someone that a certain choice is available to him or her is an example of such an abuse.) (2) Persons can and often do have interests, concerns, and wishes regarding events that will occur only after their deaths. (Wills commonly express such interests.) These factors persuade many people that posthumous abuses of agency are quite possible. Suppose, for example, that I make a gift to a medical school, stipulating that it be used to endow an appointment in ophthalmology department in perpetuity, and suppose that an administrator in that school manages to suppress all evidence of my stipulation and diverts the funds to another use. My agency would have been abused even if I never learned of the suppression of my stipulation. But would the abuse of my agency be reduced in any way; would the interference with the success of my enterprise be any less a wrong to me, if I had happened to die after making the gift but before the administrator suppressed my stipulation? A number of people don't believe so.

If one accepts that abuses of agency are wrongs that may be committed against a deceased person, then to harvest tissue against the wishes (expressed or not) of the deceased donor will appear to be such a wrong. It would, of course, be equally wrong to refuse to harvest acceptable tissue against the wishes of a donor. And from this viewpoint policies involving presumed consent to donate abuse the agency of the donor precisely as they abuse the agency of surviving kin. Even if the presumption happens to coincide with the wishes the donor had, the opportunity for choice has been preempted.

It should be noted too that from the agency orientation the role of surviving kin is likely to be perceived, not as exercising a *right* to decide what they would like to have done with the body, but as carrying out a *responsibility* to represent the interests of the deceased in the matter. From this point of view, then, the wishes of the deceased would take precedence over those of the surviving kin, should the two conflict.

CONCLUDING REMARKS

Advocates of expedited tissue-procurement policies are apt to respond to the preceding analyses along these lines: "After all, the real issue is this—if we don't secure available tissue, some person will remain sightless whose sight might otherwise have been restored. Is it really plausible to maintain that it is more important to respect the agency of a dead person than to restore the sight of a living one?"

They are correct, of course, that this is the crux of the issues that have been discussed. But many people *do* find it plausible and even ethically appropriate to respect the agency of the dead or the living at the cost of failing to harvest some available tissue. In fact, the harvest of potentially life-saving organs is foregone for precisely these reasons. It should be noted that if these reasons are as implausible as the response implies, consistency requires us to suppose that political expediency is the only acceptable justification for failing to harvest tissue *against the clearly expressed wishes* of a deceased potential donor.

The forgoing discussion is not meant to advocate a position, but only to analyze, clarify, and focus on the hard choices. What it is meant to show is that one's position about the proper approach to tissue procurement will be fundamentally a function of one's views about the ethical status of the dead and about the relative importance of concern for the condition of persons and respect for the agency of persons.

SUGGESTED READINGS

Caplan AL: Ethical and policy issues in the procurement of cadaver organs for transplantation, *N Engl J Med* 311:981, 1984.

Dukeminier J Jr, Sanders D: Organ transplantation: a proposal for routine salvaging of cadaver organs, *N Engl J Med* 279:413, 1968.

Feinberg J: The mistreatment of dead bodies, *Hastings Cent Rep* 15:31, Feb 1985.

Kass LR: Thinking about the body, *Hastings Cent Rep* 15:20, Feb 1985.

Manninen DL, Evans RW: Public attitudes and behavior regarding organ donation, *JAMA* 253:3111, 1985.

May WF: Religious justification for donating body parts, *Hastings Cent Rep* 15:38, Feb 1985.

Nagel T: *Mortal questions,* New York, 1979, Cambridge University Press, pp 1-10.

Chapter 52

Cooperative Activities in Tissue and Organ Transplantation

An overview

GARY E. FRIEDLAENDER

Few advances in medicine have captured public attention to the degree witnessed with tissue and organ transplantation. Indeed, the concept of replacing injured or diseased body parts with allografts or xenografts has inspired ancient lore, has been a subject of visual artists for centuries, and, more recently, has caused scientists to search for methods to support these aspirations.[4] It is now feasible, and with predictable success, to transplant a wide variety of allogeneic tissues and organs including kidney, heart, heart-lung, liver, pancreas, cornea, skin, bone, cartilage, fibrous tissue (tendon, ligament, fascia, dura), nerve, reproductive cells, and blood! The efficacy of transplantation, in many specific cases, will continue to improve, and additional tissues and organs will be added to the list of practical opportunities in the future. Similarly, the numbers of tissues and organs transplanted each year will also expand

Table 52-1. Transplants in the United States

	1984	1990
Kidney	6730	9560
Heart	1673	2085
Heart-lung	17	50
Liver	308	2656
Pancreas/islet cells	87	549
Cornea	23,500	40,631
Bone	1000s	350,000
Skin	1000s	5500

Source: American Association of Tissue Banks, Arlington, Va.

(Table 52-1), provided that the necessary increase in resources to support these procedures also materialize.

THE MANDATE

Despite these enormous scientific advances, there remain considerable unmet needs.[1,11,12] Thousands of patients wait for transplantable tissues and organs and never have the opportunity to benefit from this technology. This usually reflects the unavailability of allografts, sometimes lack of sufficient financial support or adequate facilities and occasionally insufficient numbers of properly trained health care professionals. Because of these unmet needs in the face of limited resources, it behooves us to maximize opportunities for the largest possible number of appropriate patients. Herein lies both the rationale and compelling reasons for developing, implementing, and nurturing cooperative programs supportive of tissue and organ transplantation. There is a range of similarities and differences between each type of tissue and organ transplant that collectively necessitates collaborative approaches but simultaneously presents obstacles and distractions from these cooperative efforts. Appreciation of these issues should improve our ability to address our national agenda designed to provide the highest quality care to all in need and in a timely fashion.

THE BACKGROUND

The Science and the Personnel. The methodologies required for each transplantable allograft have evolved at their own pace, often relying upon advances in core knowledge of immunology, physiology, cellular and molecular biology, infectious diseases, cryopreservation, and surgical technique. Physicians and scientists have tended to focus on narrow areas of interest, often because of past training, resulting in expertise limited to one type of transplantable allograft. Funding idiosyncrasies at both the research and clinical care level have also influenced program progress in specific areas. In addition, each tissue and organ has had its own patient constituency. Organs, especially heart and liver, have been associated with considerable and well-deserved public attention and drama as well as commensurate awareness. Other transplant programs, particularly tissues like cornea and bone, have more quietly attended to the needs of large numbers of patients in whom the quality of life rather than lifesaving opportunities were the issue.

Consequently, much of the organization, policy, and progress associated with individual tissue and organ transplantation has occurred in a fragmented fashion. An element of competition and further fragmentation of efforts has resulted from limited available funding and inadequate numbers of appropriate allograft donors. Ironically the efficiencies and effectiveness of creating a cohesive mosaic program offer at least partial solutions to (rather than cause for) these vexing problems and limitations. There has clearly been substantial progress toward the necessary cooperative efforts required in strengthening the effectiveness, safety, and availability of tissues and organs for transplantation. There remain compelling reasons for continuing this trend, with issues ranging from science to public confidence playing major rolls.

The System. The sequence of events leading to the availability of transplantable tissues and organs begins with donor identification, selection, and referral to an appropriate facility and then requires mechanisms for graft retrieval and methods for preservation and storage, followed by a system for timely and equitable distribution for implantation. Over the past few years, these programs have encountered increased public scrutiny related to the prevention of disease transmission and the need for regulation. In addition, there has been an evolution in public and professional awareness of transplantation-related issues and, subsequently, legislation in support of these activities.

Tissue and organ transplantation represent altruistic gifts provided from the public to the public. This is the common basis for all transplant programs regardless of which allograft is being sought. The numerous issues reflected in the process of obtaining allografts must be the mutual and cooperative agenda of all groups interested in transplantation, whether organ or tissue oriented.

Donor recruitment and selection requires attention to public and professional education, consent, and medical criteria for suitability. Although selection criteria vary somewhat among the various types of tissues and organs, much of the process is similar, and virtually all aspects of education and consent reflect common themes.

Public Education. The public must be educated with respect to the need for and usefulness of tissue and organ donation.[9] Gallup polls commissioned by the American Council on Transplantation and other interested groups during the 1980s reported that most (more than 93%) of Americans have heard about transplantation, and at least 3 out of 4 persons indicated willingness to authorize donation of tissues and organs from their next of kin at the time of death. However, far fewer of those surveyed stated that they would consider donating their own tissues and organs.

There are many possible explanations for this discrepancy. First, many people are reluctant to think about their own death. Second, although it is clear that most of the public has *knowledge* of transplantation as a general concept, *understanding* lags behind. This lack of understanding and the resultant misperceptions regarding tissue donation and transplantation significantly detract from the public's participation in the transplant program. It is the *collective* obligation of transplant programs to improve understanding and minimize misperception. The public must come to realize that numerous tissues and organs can be recovered and transplanted with substantial success, that only minor physical changes result from these donations, that traditional funeral arrangements can proceed unimpeded, that no financial responsibilities associated with donation will be incurred by the donor (or family), and that mechanisms exist for easy and convenient implementation of a person's desire to donate. Perhaps most important, it must remain clear that willingness to donate tissues and organs will not compromise a person's health care in any way and that in fact the medical professionals responsible for screening potential donors and recovering tissues and organs are different from those participating directly and vigorously in one's treatment. Misperceptions also abound with respect to the concept of brain death specifically and the definition of death in general.

It is quite easy to see that substantially more effort must be devoted to public education and that this should ideally occur during times of good health, with information being provided by health care professionals, clergy, public advocate groups, teachers, and other family members, all of whom have a sufficiently broad perspective to represent the common needs of the entire transplant program.

Professional Education. The next major link in the transplant chain of events involves referral of potential donors to organ-procurement organizations and tissue banks. This referral requires that health care professionals, whether they are associated with emergency medical teams in the field, emergency rooms, or inpatient activities, be fully informed and educated about the need for transplants and the mechanisms for referring potential donors.

As with the public, there appear to be many obstacles and misperceptions that require attention. Health care professions may harbor feelings of failure when their patients do not survive; some are ignorant of the need for transplantable resources or lack knowledge concerning appropriate referral patterns.[10] The health care system still is not consistent in approaching brain death. It was not until 1980 that the Uniform Determination of Death Act was provided by the National Conference of Commissioners on Uniform State Laws, and now most states have adopted legislation recognizing the concept of brain death. Professionals often do not appreciate the content, objectives, and protections provided by the Uniform Anatomical Gift Act of 1968 and that of 1987. As with members of the public, health care professionals must recognize the substantial need for tissues and organs for transplantation and the fact that criteria for donor suitability vary with respect to the specific tissues and organs of interest. For example, there are rather narrow age restrictions for donation of vascularized solid organs but more liberal age guidelines for most tissues. Accordingly, the size of the potential donor pool also varies depending on the nature of transplantable resources to be recovered. Given the limited supply of potentially suitable donors, it becomes extremely important that the constraints and concerns of each focused interest be understood and accommodated. Solid organs, for example, must be removed after little if any ischemia time. These organs must then be quickly transported to recipients, since long-term preservation methods are not available. On the other hand, tissues can be acquired post mortem, though the length of tolerable elapsed time after death varies between cornea, bone, and skin.

In view of these factors, the rationale for a cooperative and coordinated approach among medical specialities to maximize opportunities for each donor becomes quite clear.

Consent. Authorization to remove tissues or organs for transplantation or research has been based traditionally on voluntary consent. In this circumstance the donor may indicate ante mortem a desire to be a donor, usually by signing a Uniform Donor Card or verbally conveying this desire to next of kin. Alternatively, the next of kin may authorize donation post mortem by specifically indicating permission in writing or by telephone, provided that it is properly witnessed. This approach is also called "opting-in." Donation does not occur unless the person or next of kin specifically decides to participate in the program and provides authorization.

Alternative mechanisms to consent include an "opting-out" principle, or presumed consent. This mechanism is based on the presumption that everyone is automatically a donor, though modifications to this approach have been proposed ranging from no opportunity to object to a system that allows a potential donor to be excluded if any objections are raised by the person or next of kin. The system would, in theory, increase the number of donations, but some would argue that it infringes upon a person's choice in favor of perceived societal needs. How vigorously would the transplant system have to search for objections to donation? Some states currently have statutes that allow for removal of corneas on the presumption that donation may occur unless objections are raised. Similarly, some states have mechanisms that empower the coroner or medical examiner to authorize donation if the next of kin cannot be identified.

Between the totally voluntary and presumed-consent approaches is a variation termed "required request." In this case, the hospital through health care professionals is required to ask the question! Individuals are free to say yes or no. The Uniform Anatomical Gift Act of 1987 and legislation subsequently enacted in nearly every state requires the health care system to request of potentially appropriate persons upon admission to the hospital whether they are willing to authorize donation should a circumstance arise that is compatible with tissue or organ recovery. Passage of this legislation grew out of a common need and reflects a coordinated approach by the transplant community. Although the effectiveness of this approach to consent is not yet clear, the trend appears favorable, especially for tissues.[8]

Disease Transmission. A major objective of tissue selection criteria and subsequent screening tools has been the elimination of potentially harmful transmissible diseases.[2] In the early stages of developing criteria for tissue and, later, organ donation the primary concerns were bacterial contamination and the presence of venereal diseases or hepatitis B. In recent years both public and professional attention has been sharply focused on the human immunodeficiency virus (HIV) and hepatitis C.

Blood transfusions and solid-organ transplantation have proved to be infrequent but tragic vectors of HIV.[13] Bone from two donors in 1985 has transmitted the virus and resulted in fatal cases of AIDS.[6] Awareness of this virus and the development of serologic tests for antibodies to HIV have greatly reduced the risk associated with transplantation to the point that the incidence associated with bone allografts has been estimated to fall between 1 in 40,000 (reflecting the risk with blood transfusions) to 1 in more than 1 million.[5] Despite the reduced risks, concern for transmission of this fatal disease-producing virus has prompted emphasis on thorough screening in the standards for donor selection of the American Association of Tissue Banks and similar professional organizations.[2] As of April 1, 1991, a 180-day quarantine of donated tissues from live donors has been imposed, reflecting the window period during which antibody formation may not be detectable.[13] New methodology targeting the viral antigens is now being evaluated and is expected to reduce this period and, consequently, the risk of disease transmission even further.

Analogous improvements have been made with the detection of hepatitis, including hepatitis C virus (HCV). Again, the need for these approaches and the development and application of these technologies transcends narrow-interest groups and progress reflects the collaborative efforts of many scientists and physicians throughout the range of allograft expertise.

Federal Regulation. Issues of safety and efficacy have always been matters of both public interest and regulatory scrutiny. The Food and Drug Administration has recently instituted activities that could lead to the regulation of human heart valves used for allotransplantation.[7] This narrow action may well widen its focus to some or many aspects of tissue and organ banking and underscores the public concern for the development and implementation of standards that assure the highest quality with the least risk. These aspirations are shared by the professional components of the many transplant programs. Vigorous controversy, however, has not concentrated upon the desired ends as much as the proper mechanism for assuring these goals. The major approaches being considered are voluntary inspection and accreditation based on peer-derived standards of activity compared to federal or state regulation. In either case, the transplant community will benefit

from a strong, coordinated approach that recognizes both the commonality and the uniqueness of the various transplant programs.

Network. Perhaps the most effective means to structure cooperative efforts in tissue transplantation approaches would be the development of a national network based on standards and an inspection-accreditation program reflecting these guidelines. The National Organ Transplant Act of 1984 created the Organ Procurement and Transplant Network and led to the authorization of federal funding to support this function. A parallel and compatible network for tissues would both assure equitable access to these scarce resources and serve to collect data needed to monitor use, efficacy, complications, and unmet need. Both the American Association of Tissue Banks and the Southeastern Organ Procurement Foundation have been exploring mechanisms for developing this type of collaborative approach.

THE SOLUTION

Cooperative approaches to tissue and organ transplantation are not only desirable, they are also crucial to fulfilling our collective obligation to society. Allografts offer enormous opportunities for life-sustaining and quality-of-life–enhancing treatment alternatives. These programs require the altruistic participation of the public based upon extensive education; the establishment of legislative, financial, scientific, moral, and ethical frameworks conducive to these efforts and to future progress and the training of health care professionals knowledgeable in these complex systems. A mosaic program must be constructed in which each piece recognizes and respects the uniqueness and special requirements of the others, yet fit together to form a cohesive pattern that emphasizes the overwhelming common nature of the mission.

REFERENCES

1. American Association of Tissue Banks, Arlington, Virginia.
2. American Association of Tissue Banks: *Standards for tissue banking,* Arlington, Va, 1987, AATB.
3. American Association of Tissue Banks: 190-day quarantine for HCV and HIV for living donors effective April 1, 1991, *AATB Newsletter* 13(4):1, 1990.
4. Bick EM: *Source book of orthopaedics,* ed 2, New York, 1968, Hafner.
5. Buck BE, Resnick L, Shah SM, Malinin TT: Human immunodeficiency virus cultured from bone: implications for transplantation, *Clin Orthop* 251:249-253, 1990.
6. Centers for Disease Control, Atlanta, Georgia.
7. Food and Drug Administration: Cardiovascular devices; effective date of requirement for premarket approval; replacement heart valve allograft, *Fed Reg* 56(123):29177-29179, 1991.

8. Gabor AO, Hall G, Britt: An assessment of the impact of required request legislation on the availability of cadaveric organs for transplantation, *Transplant Proc* 22:318-319, 1990.

9. Nathan HM, Jarell BE, Broznik B, et al: Estimation and characterization of the potential renal organ donor pool in Pennsylvania, *Transplantation* 51:142-149, 1991.

10. Spital A, Kitter DS: Barriers to organ donation among house staff physicians, *Transplant Proc* 22:2414-2416, 1990.

11. Swerdlow JL: *Matching needs, saving lives,* Washington, DC, 1989, The Annenberg Washington Program.

12. United Network for Organ Sharing, Richmond, Virginia.

13. Ward JW, Holmberg SD, Allen JR, et al: Transmission of human immunodeficiency virus (HIV) by blood transfusions screened as negative for HIV antibody, *N Engl J Med* 318:473-477, 1988.

The government, OPOs, and eye banks

PATRICIA AIKEN-O'NEILL

The relationship between organ-procurement organizations (OPOs) and eye banks, as well as tissue banks, has been inconsistent. Their success and mutual accord have depended on a convergence of multiple factors involving federal requirements and congressional expectations for OPOs tempered by the local political climate. A brief overview of the history that underlies these two communities may contribute to an understanding of their current relationship as well as provide a harbinger of the future.

HISTORY

Locally based organ-procurement organizations proliferated before the National Organ Transplant Act (NOTA) of 1984[8] and their subsequent formal acknowledgment by the federal government. OPOs were originally established in response to the growing practice and institutionalization of organ transplantation, particularly kidney transplantation in the 1960s and 1970s. The NOTA established the Task Force on Organ Transplantation to examine the status of the organ-procurement and transplantation system.

There was no system; over 100 OPOs operated with varying degrees of efficiency and effectiveness. A significant number were hospital based, most usually attached in an ancillary fashion to their department of surgery and solely beholden to that hospital; the remainder functioned as independent operational entities. Some communities housed several competing OPOs, which the task force concluded damaged the procurement process as a whole. The task force recommended sweeping changes to result in a systematic approach to procurement and distribution, which the existing network lacked.[11]

Congress accepted the recommendations of the task force by legislating them under the Omnibus Budget Reconciliation Act of 1986. The requirements were incorporated into the Social Security Act (Section 1138). The act provided for performance standards for OPOs and other specific criteria; oversight and development of a national system was assigned to the Organ Procurement and Transplantation Network (OPTN), previously established under NOTA. Medicare and Medicaid reimbursement was made contingent on designation by the Department of Health and Human Services as a qualified OPO; hospitals, in turn, were required to notify the OPO of possible donors. In order to reduce the waste and inefficiency found by the task force, the act also required that only one OPO would qualify to operate in a defined service area.[9]

HISTORY: EYE BANKS

A short recap of the factors that contributed to the state of eye banking at the time that the National Organ Transplant Act was enacted will provide some understanding of the factors that continue to influence the relationship between the organ and eye and tissue communities.

Corneal transplantation preceded transplantation of other tissues and organs by several decades. Indeed, Dr. R. Townley Paton founded the first eye bank in New York City in 1944. The past two decades have witnessed a phenomenal growth in eye banking, contributing to more than 250,000 documented corneal transplants handled by United States eye banks. The obvious conclusion is that the eye banking community can point to a demonstrated history of success in an area that is still relatively new for organs and other tissues.

Moreover, the federal government recognized the stability of tissue transplantation in the preamble to its final OPO regulations. The Health Care Financing Administration (HCFA) commented:

We have avoided specific regulation with respect to tissues because we believe that at this time it would impose an unreasonable burden on an OPO to serve as the contact point for all organ and tissue donation. The number of tissue donations far exceed vascular organ donations. We understand there are other important differences between tissue procurement and organ procurement, including different staffing requirements and medical techniques. Further, many states already have tissue donation requirements that require the hospital to notify the tissue bank as well as the OPO. These arrangements appear to be working effectively. This in no way subordinates the importance of tissue procurement but reflects what we believe is congressional intent for this provision to focus on the procurement and transplantation of vascular organs.[6]

To reinforce this view, HCFA also required that qualified OPOs participate with the tissue community in "retrieval, processing, preservation, storage, and distribution of tissues," as a condition of participation in Medicare.[4]

JOINT STATEMENT OF COOPERATION

Despite this recognition, the federal government's regulation of organ transplantation in the mid-1980s appeared to have created a presumption of "anointed leadership" among the organ community.

That the approval of the government should entitle the OPOs that qualified under federal standards to in turn control the entire procurement and distribution system within the transplantation community was perhaps understandable given the short-sighted attitude of those involved in organ transplantation. It could be argued that tissue transplantation had evaded federal focus and control. In addition, the organ community experienced increasingly strict requirements by the federal government, such as the statutory change to the Organ Transplant Act. The 1988 amendments (P.L. 100-607) in the infamous "50 donor rule" required OPOs to have a defined service area to "reasonably expect to procure 50 donors each year."[10] With the subtle deletion of the word "potential" the change would have had a drastic impact on the status of existing OPOs and would eventually be rescinded by Congress in the Transplantation Amendments Act of 1990. Nevertheless, OPOs remain "under the gun," and the 86,076 eyes procured (40,631 distributed for transplant) by the nation's eye banks in 1990 would substantively increase OPO numbers and paint a rosy statistical portrait of the current status of transplantation in the 1990s.[5]

Not only would the numbers increase with the infusion of eye tissue (and other tissues) in their statistics, but also one must pose the question: Might more organs be procured if one plugged in all the calls that an eye bank receives, and since it is the OPO that is mandated to be called for organs, would it not follow that the OPO receive all tissue calls, as well?

The nation's OPOs attempted to do just that. In a 1990 position paper on the recertification of OPOs submitted to HCFA by the national OPO association, the Association of Organ Procurement Organizations (AOPO), the organ community requested the Secretary of Health and Human Services "to require the potential donors of any transplantable human tissues to be directly notified to the designated OPO

for that service area."[3] The EBAA quickly responded. Identifying the AOPO position statement as "unilateral, monopolistic and violative of the very spirit of cooperation which it proposes for the transplant community," the EBAA stressed that it would "undermine tissue procurement by the inflexibility of its proposal." Additionally, the EBAA charged that it would strip from the province of eye banks a proved and historically successful operation.[2] The EBAA contacted the legislative and the regulatory branches of government to defend its position. HCFA, among others in the government, assured the EBAA that AOPO must first put its own house in order before it could manage others. Nevertheless, this presaged the future intentions of the organ community and put the eye bank community on notice. It also undermined any potential benefit to be gained through a cooperative agreement on the need for donation among the organ, tissue, and eye organizations. The three communities—Eye Bank Association of America, EBAA; American Association of Tissue Banks, AATB; and Association of Organ Procurement Organizations, AOPO—had finalized a joint statement on the need for donation at the time AOPO released its position paper. In the works for a year, the statement reviewed steps necessary to effectuate a coordinated service approach to procurement and agency management and had suggested models for consideration to implement a program and to stimulate local cooperation.[7] The timing was unfortunate, and the statement was lost to internecine politics.

CURRENT CLIMATE: COOPERATION OR CONFRONTATION?

In its response to the AOPO's position paper, the EBAA called for "cooperation and collaboration among the transplant community."[2] Currently, the organizations are hesitantly working together on some transplantwide initiatives proposed by the Division of Transplantation in the Department of Health and Human Services. However, fundamental disagreement remains on substantive issues such as a single line number for donor calls from hospitals, OPO charges for referral fees, and government regulation of tissue.

Even so, a fair number of eye banks and OPOs in local communities have established cooperative relationships (p. 725). Other communities engage in an uneasy truce. Contributing factors to either success or failure seem to be the personalities of the parties involved in the agreement, their flexibility, local politics, and the degree of control to be exercised by the OPO. With the establishment of a national headquarters office in Washington, D.C., in 1991 and the retention of professional staff, AOPO is positioning itself to establish more studied, consistent, and incremental policies. This could well contribute to an increased ability to work together to truly serve the community.

In a 1990 presentation to the Food, Drug, and Law Institute (FDLI), Patricia Aiken-O'Neill, Esq., EBAA president and chief executive officer, commented on the relationship between the government, OPOs, and eye banks:

No matter what the federal government may require of us, I do not think that we should expect it to be the vehicle that glues us together. We would be asking the government to do for us what not all of us have been able to do ourselves, and that is to get together. We do have a vehicle—the benefit to our recipients—and it is an incentive that can and does work when it is the driving focus. It should be up to us to put our house in order.[1]

REFERENCES

1. Aiken-O'Neill, P: EBAA perspective on OPOs, tissue banks and eye banks working together, Presented to Food, Drug, and Law Institute, Washington, D.C., July 10, 1990, pp 13-14.
2. Aiken-O'Neill, P: EBAA position response to AOPO, Washington, D.C., August 10, 1990, Eye Bank Association of America.
3. Association of Organ Procurement Organizations (AOPO): Position and recommendations for improving the National Organ Procurement System, Washington, D.C., June 1990, p 25.
4. Code of Federal Regulations: 42 C.F.R. 485.304(1) Condition: Organ procurement organization qualifications—general (1989).
5. Eye Bank Association of America: *1990 eye banking statistics,* Washington D.C., 1991, EBAA.
6. Medicare-Medicaid programs: organ procurement organization and organ procurement protocols; final rule, *Federal Register* (53 F.R. 6530), Washington, D.C., March 1, 1988.
7. Joint statement on meeting the communities needs for organ, tissue and eye donation, final draft, May 22, 1990, American Association of Tissue Banks (AATB), Association of Organ Procurement Organization (AOPO), and Eye Bank Association of America (EBAA).
8. *National Organ Transplant Act of 1984,* P.L. 98-504.
9. *Omnibus Budget Reconciliation Act of 1986,* P.L. 99-509.
10. Organ Transplant Amendments Act of 1988, P.L. 100-607, Health Omnibus Programs Extension of 1988, 402(c) 102 Stat. 3114 (1988).
11. Task Force on Organ Transplantation (established by the National Organ Transplant Act of 1984): *Organ transplantation: issues and recommendations,* Washington, D.C. (April 1986).

Shared services for procuring tissues and organs

CAROLINE BUNKER ROSDAHL

THE MINNESOTA EXPERIENCE

Is it possible for three independent and unrelated agencies to cooperate in the procurement of organs and tissues? Can cooperation exist without competition? Would results be potentiated by cooperation? Are shared services cost effective? This chapter describes the "Minnesota experience" in an attempt to answer these questions.

WHO ARE WE?

Minnesota Organ and Tissue Procurement Agencies. Three totally unrelated agencies exist in Minnesota for the purpose of organ and tissue procurement, processing, and distribution. They are:

Minnesota Lions Eye Bank at the University of Minnesota

American Red Cross (St. Paul Chapter)—Transplantation Services

LifeSource—Upper Midwest Organ Procurement Organization, Inc.

The *Minnesota Lions Eye Bank* "coordinates the procurement, processing and distribution of eye tissue" for Minnesota and North Dakota. Transplantation Services of the *American Red Cross* "operates a multi-regional tissue bank which collects, tests, processes and distributes bone, skin, heart valves and connective tissue" (as well as other tissues). *LifeSource* "is the federally licensed organ procurement organization for Minnesota, North Dakota and South Dakota."*

Goals and Objectives. How can three such different agencies work together? Each has a different structure. Yet, when we compare the mission statements, the similarities become obvious.

Minnesota Lions Eye Bank. The Minnesota Lions Eye Bank was organized in 1960 at the University of Minnesota. It is sponsored by the Lions of Multiple 5M and is one of the larger eye banks in the United States. The eye bank identifies its mission as follows: "to procure human eyes, process the tissue, and distribute the tissue to corneal surgeons, researchers and educators. . . . [The Eye Bank] is committed to providing public and professional education regarding tissue and organ donation. . . . In order to give the gift of sight, the Eye Bank works with health professionals, donor families, hospitals, enucleators, and transporters."†

American Red Cross. The American Red Cross (ARC) states that "in accomplishing the mission, the American Red Cross will . . . develop and maintain public support for tissue donation . . . educate medical professionals who will identify potential tissue donors and facilitate tissue collection . . . counsel family members . . . support hospitals . . . collect, process, store and distribute human tissues . . . [and]

---

*A FAMILY DECISION: organ and tissue donation" (Minnesota version).
†Minnesota Lions Eye Bank: *Mission and objectives,* revised 1991.

conduct research and development activities."*

LifeSource. LifeSource was formed in 1987 in response to federal regulation of organ procurement and distribution. Their brochure states: "Our mission is to promote organ donation and to facilitate the procurement and utilization of organs in transplantation. LifeSource coordinators are responsible for organ donor management, working closely with donor families, hospital staffs, and the transplant teams . . . [and] also help build community and health care professional awareness of the need for . . . donation through ongoing educational activities."†

SHARED PROCUREMENT SERVICES

800 Telephone Number Referral and Information Services. The three agencies share the cost of a 24-hour telephone information and referral service that is managed by the American Red Cross. A person anywhere in the United States need only dial 1-(800)-24SHARE to receive assistance or information about *any type of donation*. The call is sorted to determine which agency should handle the request. If the caller has a potential organ donor, he or she is referred to LifeSource. If the call relates to a potential skin or bone donor, the referral is made to the Red Cross. And, if the call relates to a person who will donate eyes only, the eye bank responds. In addition, the 800 telephone service does the initial health history screening of tissue donors and obtains telephone consents. The American Red Cross staff also responds to many questions from the general public and mails printed information in response to requests.

Joint Procurement Efforts. The agencies *work together* to procure organs and tissues. In Minnesota, American Red Cross (ARC) tissue technicians are also trained enucleators. When an ARC technician removes skin, bone, or other tissue from an eye donor, that technician also enucleates the eyes for the eye bank. The eye bank pays a set fee for each ARC enucleation, preventing duplication of effort. The accompanying table illustrates eye bank activity directly generated by calls to the 800 number, as well as the numbers of eyes directly enucleated by ARC for the Minnesota Lions Eye Bank (Fig. 52-1).

It should be noted that nearly all corneas removed from skin and bone donors are *transplantable*. The reason is that the ARC has narrow age criteria for

tissue, as compared to those for transplantable corneal tissue. The ARC obtains a donor history before selecting a person as a tissue donor, which also rules out most factors that would render corneal tissue unsuitable for transplant.

If a person is an *organ and eye donor*, the LifeSource coordinator does the health history screening, obtains the consent, and sends the blood for testing. LifeSource also notifies the 800 telephone coordinator, and so the enucleation can be done soon after the completion of the organ donation.

Blood Testing. Blood testing for the Minnesota Lions Eye Bank is performed by the St. Paul Chapter of the American Red Cross. This is true whether the eyes are removed by the American Red Cross, by an eye bank enucleator, or by a volunteer funeral director in Minnesota or North Dakota. In the case of a tissue donor, the American Red Cross would test the blood for its own purposes. Therefore blood testing need only be done once; it is not repeated for the eye donation. The fact that the American Red Cross maintains a laboratory for its other donor programs allows the Minnesota Lions Eye Bank to save the cost and administrative factors involved in setting up a separate laboratory. (The American Red Cross does much of the blood testing for LifeSource organ donors as well.)

SHARED PUBLIC RELATIONS ACTIVITIES

Minnesota Hospital Development Council. A committee consisting of the managing administrators of the three agencies meets monthly. In this way, common concerns can be discussed, and the group can plan future events. Each agency shares its schedule of hospital development activities. The other agencies may choose whether to participate in these activities. Each agency also shares procurement information, and so the agencies can determine total numbers and types of donations by hospital.

The Minnesota Hospital Development Council has developed several sample forms for hospitals, such as the generic "death checklist" (Fig. 52-2). This checklist is available to hospitals to assist them in meeting accreditation requirements and those of "required request" legislation. Hospitals can adopt the form or tailor it to meet their specific needs. In addition, the procurement agencies have developed for hospital use a generic donor consent form with the logos of all three organizations.

Advisory Committee. A combined Minnesota Funeral Director Advisory Committee meets on call to discuss common concerns. (The Minnesota Lions Eye Bank has a parallel committee which deals with specific eye bank concerns.)

*American Red Cross Tissue Services: *Line of services—mission statement,* Jan 1991.
†LifeSource brochure: *Making the promise a reality,* revised 1990.

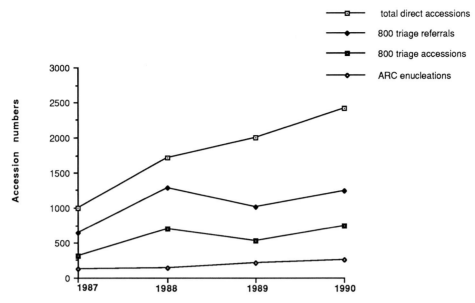

Fig. 52-1. Minnesota Lions Eye Bank (MLEB) activity generated by the shared 800 telephone triage service. The 800 area-code telephone line contributes greatly to eye donor referrals and accession of eyes by the Minnesota Lions Eye Bank, as indicated by the *two center lines* on this graph. *Top line* delineates total number of eyes received by the eye bank (not imports). Total number of accessions increased sharply from 996 globes in 1987 to 2421 globes in 1990. Of the 1990 total, 746 (nearly 31%) were procured as a direct result of the 800 referral service. This graph also illustrates gradual increase in eyes procured for the eye bank by the American Red Cross. This number, *bottom line,* increased from 125 in 1987 to 256 in 1990 (more than 10.5% of total eyes received by the eye bank). A very high percentage of the ARC-enucleated eyes yielded transplantable corneas. (NOTE: 1988 was the first full year of Minnesota's Required Request legislation.)

Seminars and Professional In-service Education Activities. In-service education has been provided by each agency for the staff of the other two agencies. This provides them with a basic knowledge of all the agencies, so that they can present seminars and answer questions.

The council discusses development activities and decides who will participate in each event. For example, if a 2- or 3- hour workshop is scheduled at a large emergency hospital, all three agencies may choose to present information. If the request comes from an agency that is likely to generate eye donors only (such as a nursing home with an older population), the eye bank would most likely conduct the program alone.

In any event, no matter which agency presents the seminar, *information about the other two agencies is also presented.* The amount of detail depends on the audience involved. The committee has jointly developed guidelines for hospital development activities in an effort to maximize effort. (See Box, p. 729.)

Audiovisual Sharing. The Minnesota Lions Eye Bank, the American Red Cross, and LifeSource have slide presentations for seminars and other public relations activities. Slides and scripts have been shared, and, so each agency has information about the others. Thus information can be presented about all the agencies. Eye bank information is included in public presentations whether eye bank staff is there.

The agencies have also developed a seven-page handout entitled *Fact Sheet on Organ and Tissue Transplants.* This is cooperatively updated yearly and distributed to interested agencies and individuals. It contains a brief history of transplantation, as well as specific information on each type of transplant performed in our region.

Public Information Activities. Public information and public relations activities are coordinated between the agencies.

Brochures. Several brochures have been developed by the Minnesota Hospital Development Committee for use by all the agencies. The one pictured here

HOSPITAL NAME
RECORD OF DEATH CHECKLIST

Patient Identification Plate

Date: _____ Time of Death: _____

Unit / Service Area: _____ Diagnosis/Cause of Death: _____

Pronounced By: _____ Primary Physician: _____

Funeral Home: _____ Autopsy: ☐ Yes ☐ No

Coroner's Case: ☐ Yes ☐ No If Coroner's Case, Jurisdiction Released By: _____

*In Consultation with Organ/Tissue Procurement Coordinator, **(291-4654 or 1-800-247-4273)**, the decedent is not a

suitable organ and/or tissue donor because: _____

_____ Signature: _____

Next of Kin: _____ Relationship: _____

Driver's License / Donor Card Located: ☐ Yes ☐ No This information may assist the next of kin
in their decision regarding donation.

Family Offered Option of Donation (next of kin): ☐ Yes ☐ No

Family Wishes to Donate: ☐ Yes ☐ No If yes, complete written consent and
notify procurement coordinator / local
enucleator.

A copy of the Consent Form accompanied the decedent: ☐ Yes ☐ No

Name / Title of Staff Who Talked With Family: _____

Belongings (List): _____

_____

Taken By (Name/Relationship): _____

Signature: _____

This Section to be Completed After Procurements

Procurement: ☐ Bone ☐ Connective Tissues ☐ Eyes ☐ Heart ☐ Kidneys ☐ Liver
☐ Lungs ☐ Pancreas ☐ Skin ☐ Other: _____

Procured by: _____ Hospital Staff Signature: _____

* You are encouraged to call the Procurement Coordinator as soon as possible to assist both in the assessment of
the potential donor and answer any questions you may have.

(4/12/91)

Fig. 52-2. Generic Death Checklist developed by the cooperating procurement agencies.

Shared Services Agreement for Minnesota Hospital Development Activities
American Red Cross/LifeSource/Minnesota Lions Eye Bank
HOSPITAL EDUCATION ATTENDANCE/CANCELLATION GUIDELINES*

- All educational activities require preregistration.
- Flyers will contain a right-to-cancel notice.
- The procurement agency reserves the right to cancel if attendance numbers are not met.
- The hospital contact person will fax the sign-up sheet before the session.
- The number of enrollees required are stated for each situation in each of these categories:
    1. Unit meetings, hospital-wide seminars, specialty-group seminars.
    2. Twin City metropolitan area, Greater Minnesota area, regional area (flying distance or long driving distance).
- Educational alternatives if a session is cancelled:
    1. Refer to the other procurement agencies.
    2. Provide other educational materials (videotapes, slides with script, and so on).
    3. Evaluate the option of providing objectives, posting tests, and evaluating for hospital-based continuing education offering.
    4. If an alternative is chosen, procurement agency requests information related to date and time of presentation, attendance, and evaluation summary.

The *coordinating agency* is the agency who received the initial request for education.
Responsibilities of the coordinating agency are to:
1. Invite other procurement agencies to participate.
2. Provide contact person's name.
3. Coordinate the date, time and location.
4. Follow attendance and cancellation requirements.
5. Finalize outline, case scenarios, post test, and so on with other agencies.
6. Finalize and assign specific content and time constraints for each presenter.
7. Provide educational packets, continuing education units, and other needed materials, including information about all three agencies.
8. Provide a written summary of evaluations to each presenter.

---

*This exhibit represents a *summary* of the actual document. The original document was developed jointly by the Minnesota Hospital Development Council of the three procurement agencies in Minnesota (adopted, 1990).

(Fig. 52-3) is a "check stuffer," which is printed on both sides of a no. 10 envelope-sized card. This is distributed to factories, department stores, electric companies, and the like for inclusion with bills or paychecks. It is also an inexpensive piece to use for displays, fairs, and other public information settings.

The *Family Decision* brochure, published by the Michigan Eye Bank and Transplantation Center, has been purchased and is distributed by all the agencies. All three logos appear on it, along with the 800 telephone number.

Cooperative display. A large display is used by the agencies at public events, such as community health fairs, and at health-related events, such as the Association of Critical Care Nurses' conference (Fig. 52-4). This display encourages donation and highlights the activities of the agencies. Recipients are pictured and the 800 telephone number is emphasized.

The Minnesota Hospital Development Council is currently designing a new display. This display encourages all types of donation; each agency will purchase one. In addition, the graphics can be changed easily, so that each agency can use the basic display for its materials, taking advantage of the same frame, carrying case, and lighting system. The cost of the display is reduced to each agency because of the multiple purchase.

US West Communication Workers' Project. A special US West Communication Workers' project is an example of a cooperative community service event. This union has chosen organ and tissue donation for special fund raising, in conjunction with the United Way campaign, for 2 consecutive years. With the money collected, they have established a fund to assist recipient families with costs that are not covered by third-party payors (such as travel and lodging).

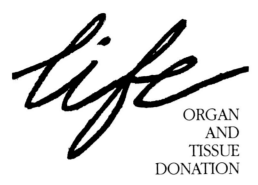

YOUR CHANCE TO GIVE

ORGAN
AND
TISSUE
DONATION

Today, organ and tissue transplantation holds the promise of life for thousands of patients with life-threatening conditions and diseases. However, the need for tissues and organs surpasses the number donated each year.

You can help! Most people think organ/tissue donation is a good idea, but few have taken appropriate steps to be sure their wishes are carried out. It is important for everyone to make the decision for themselves; but equally important, you should share your decision with your family. If your family knows your wishes, it will be easier to make a decision when the time comes.

PLEASE TALK WITH
YOUR FAMILY ABOUT
ORGAN/TISSUE
DONATION

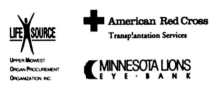

Fig. 52-3. This "check stuffer" is an attractive informational piece that has been prepared by the cooperating agencies. It helps to get the message of donation across to the general public and reinforces the fact that the three procurement agencies are working together for the common good.

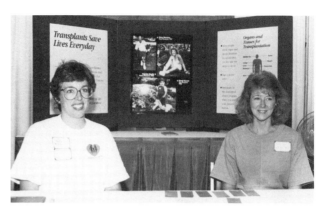

Fig. 52-4. Shown at 1991 Minnesota State Fair, this cooperative display is used to highlight option of donation and to increase awareness of local procurement agencies. It is staffed here by Kathy McCann, *left*, whose daughter, Colleen, received a human heart valve replacement in 1988, at 9 weeks of age. Colleen was born without a pulmonary valve and is now a healthy child. *On right*, Julie Bergsten, Hospital Development Representative, American Red Cross. Display is also used for health-related conferences, community health fairs, and events such as National Organ and Tissue Donor Awareness Week. (Courtesy C.B. Rosdahl, Minneapolis.)

The involvement of the procurement agencies includes informational talks to campaign workers, written information for distribution to members, and serving as an information resource.

SPECIAL PROJECTS

Drivers' Education Project. LifeSource is working with the Minneapolis Junior League on development of a teaching unit for drivers' education. This unit will present information about donation to high school students. Minneapolis is the site designated for pilot-testing, with the long-term goal being development and implementation of a statewide curriculum. The Minneapolis Junior League and LifeSource are contributing funding and personnel for this project, while the Minnesota Lions Eye Bank and the American Red Cross are providing technical assistance.

Minnesota State Fair: a Shared Effort. The Minnesota Hospital Development Council determines appropriate public relations activities for combined displays and rotates responsibility for coordination. One of these combined activities is the Minnesota State Fair, which is one of the largest in the country, attracting nearly 1.5 million people yearly. In 1991, a refrigerator magnet was developed to give away at the booth. (See Box, p. 731.)

(Text of the fluorescent-pink refrigerator magnets distributed at the Minnesota State Fair by the three cooperating transplant agencies)

MAKE A
MIRACLE
HAPPEN!

Be an Organ and
Tissue Donor
And tell your family!

For more information
1-800-24SHARE

You have been selected to participate in

A Special Workshop
by Margaret Verble and Judy Worth

SPONSORED BY

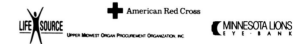

A CONVERSATION FOR A LIFETIME...
offering the option of organ and tissue donation

Fig. 52-5. Front of invitation designed and printed by Minnesota Hospital Development Council to publicize cooperative Verble-Worth donation workshop.

Revision of Minnesota's Anatomical Gift Act.[*]A great deal of effort was spent in revising Minnesota's Anatomical Gift Act in 1991. The agencies, combined with other community groups, such as the Minnesota Junior League, the Kidney Foundation, and "Second Chance for Life," helped to facilitate important changes in this law. Some of these changes are as follows:

- The applicant (for a driver's license) *may indicate a desire* to make an anatomical gift. (The option "not to donate" has been removed from the form.)
- If the applicant does not indicate a desire to make an anatomical gift when the application is made, [he or she] must be offered a donor document.
- The application form must also be accompanied by a pamphlet describing Minnesota laws regarding anatomical gifts and the need for and benefits of anatomical gifts.
- If the donor is a minor, the donor document or application must be signed by the minor donor and *one of the minor donor's parents*. . . . (Previously this section required the signature of both parents.)
- The department shall maintain a computer record of donors. Revocation, suspension, expiration, or cancellation of the license does not invalidate the anatomical gift.
- "Decedent" means a deceased individual and includes a stillborn infant or an embryo or fetus that has died of *natural causes* in utero.

- Any member of the following classes of persons, in the order of priority listed, may make an anatomical gift:
  1. Spouse
  2. Adult son or daughter
  3. Either parent
  4. Adult brother or sister
  5. *Grandparent* (a new category in Minnesota)
  6. Guardian of the person . . . at the time of death

A failure to make a decision as to an anatomical gift . . . *is not an objection* to the making of [a] . . . gift.

Special Donation Workshop. In July 1991, the agencies cosponsored a workshop entitled "A Conversation for a Lifetime: Offering the Option of Organ and Tissue Donation." Nationally known consultants Margaret Verble and Judy Worth were brought to Minneapolis to conduct the 2-day workshop. Since there was a limit of 24 participants, each agency was allowed to invite eight persons. The invitation list was finalized by the Minnesota Hospital Development Council to maximize available spaces. Because the costs were shared among the agencies, the participants paid only a minimum registration fee (Fig. 52-5).

NATIONAL ORGAN AND TISSUE DONOR AWARENESS WEEK

The activities of the National Organ and Tissue Donor Awareness Week (NOTDAW) were the result of planning and coordination by the Minnesota Hos-

---

[*]Adapted from Minnesota Statutes, sections 525.921 to 27, as amended in 1991 (Uniform Anatomical Gift Act, 1987). The Driver's License law is M S, sections 171.06 to 171.07 (1990).

pital Development Council and hard work by agency staff members.

Public Information Activities
- Governor Carlson of Minnesota signed a proclamation.
- Public information spot announcements (50+) were purchased on radio and television.
- Many local newspapers, radio, and television stations covered the week's events.
- A special memo was sent to 1500 Minnesota state agencies regarding the special week, encouraging family discussion and including the 800 telephone number.
- Information about donation was printed on Dayton's department store bills (750,000).
- Information was printed on Cub Grocery store bags (1.2 million), as well as several billboards in the Twin Cities area (sponsored by the Minneapolis Junior League).
- Information was printed on milk cartons (sponsored by Meyer's Dairy).

Professional In-service Education Activities
- Informational packets were sent to more than 100 hospitals throughout Minnesota, North Dakota, and South Dakota. The materials included brochures from each agency, public and professional education posters, "transplant trivia" table tents, organ and tissue donation fact sheets, and a press release for the local newspaper. Most of the hospitals used the table tents in their cafeterias and placed the posters and other information in prominent places.
- Large displays were set up in at least 17 hospitals, particularly the larger transplantation facilities.
- Special lectures and seminars were presented during the week by procurement agency staff.

NOTDAW Special Events
- A "kickoff breakfast" (by invitation only) was held for approximately 100 representatives of donor families, recipients, government officials, clergy, and hospital staff. The governor's proclamation was read, and speakers discussed transplantation from the perspective of the donor family and the recipient. The invitation list included a recipient representing each of the organs and tissues that are transplanted, including corneas.
- Tree planting ceremonies were held in the following locations:
  St. Paul, Minnesota (capitol approach area)
  Bismarck, North Dakota (arboretum trail, state capitol)
  Fargo, North Dakota (Hector Airport Arboretum)
  Duluth, Minnesota (Lake Superior Zoo)
  Rochester, Minnesota (Gift of Life Transplant House)
  Sioux Falls, South Dakota (Sertoma Children's Park)

The trees were donated and ceremonies were held simultaneously at all locations. Participants tied red ribbons on the trees as a memorial to donors and in recognition of the recipients and their new and improved life. A reception was held after each ceremony (Fig. 52-6).

Costs of NOTDAW. More than $4000 was contributed by outside companies and agencies for NOTDAW. This was used primarily to pay for media announcements. Items such as the grocery bags were distributed. Local media coverage included special stories related to transplantation and coverage of the tree-planting ceremonies. Agency staff,

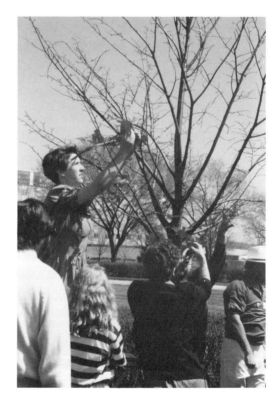

Fig. 52-6. Green-spire linden tree, donated by Minnesota Nursery Association, was planted on grounds of Minnesota State Capitol in St. Paul. Six simultaneous tree-planting ceremonies were sponsored by cooperating organizations in Minnesota, North Dakota, and South Dakota. The trees serve as living memorials to "those who have given and as a symbol of the life-renewing potential of transplantation." Shown here is Jane Habicht tying a red ribbon on the tree in memory of her father, Jim, who was an organ donor. Her sister, Jenny, is watching (striped sweater). (From American Red Cross, St. Paul Chapter.)

donor families, and recipients were featured on talk shows and in news stories.

Results of NOTDAW Activities. It is difficult to measure the long-term effects of such an effort. However, the American Red Cross reported an increase in calls to the 800 telephone number requesting information during NOTDAW week (from an average of 5 calls for each day to approximately 40 calls daily). In addition, a total of 1300 donor cards were distributed during NOTDAW week from telephone requests alone. Because of the cooperation of the three agencies and the outside financial contributions, the expense to each agency for the week-long events was not excessive.

Many human interest stories could be told about the events of NOTDAW. Perhaps one of the most touching was a meeting between a heart recipient and the wife of the donor. They did not know each other before the event, but in a mutually requested and professionally facilitated introduction, they were able to meet and share tears and the joy of life.

OVERALL COST-EFFECTIVENESS OF COOPERATION

The three agencies share in the cost of the telephone line, the triage service, the hospital development activities, and the costs of printed materials and other public relations activities. The costs to each agency is less than if each were to independently prepare and manage the activities. In addition, much greater coverage is possible. There is no way that one of the individual agencies could devote the resources of time or money to carry out this level of activity.

SUMMARY

We return to the questions presented at the beginning of this chapter: "Is it possible for three independent and unrelated agencies to cooperate in the procurement of organs and tissues? Can cooperation exist without competition? Would results be potentiated by cooperation? Are shared services cost-effective?" The answer to each of these questions is a resounding *yes!* This chapter has been presented as a model; other areas of the country can extrapolate from this point to build and individualized local program.

I believe that shared services can increase the efficiency and effectiveness of donor transplant services. We can work toward the common good to benefit our agencies and the health care system, as well as donor families and recipients. The bottom line is to *make a difference* in someone's life.

ACKNOWLEDGMENT

This document was reviewed by:

Donald J. Doughman, M.D., Medical Director, Minnesota Lions Eye Bank

Carol R. Engel, Procurement Director, Minnesota Lions Eye Bank

Betty Jane Walen, Volunteer Coordinator/Administrative Assistant, Minnesota Lions Eye Bank

Susan Gunderson, Executive Director, LifeSource–Upper Midwest Organ Procurement Organization

Gayl Rogers Chrysler, Director, Transplant Donor Services, St. Paul Chapter, American Red Cross

Chapter 53

International Supply of Corneal Tissue

FREDERICK N. GRIFFITH

CHARLES T. VALMADRID

Based on the internationally accepted definition of blindness as having vision of less than 3/60 with best possible correction, there are between 27 and 35 million blind in the world, according to recent estimates made by the World Health Organization (WHO).[58] Of this number, over 10 million are caused by corneal blindness from trachoma, xerophthalmia, onchocerciasis, ocular trauma, and other causes of corneal ulceration.[59] Only after prevention and disease management as a means to overcome corneal blindness, corneal transplantation has remained a major initiative in restoring sight.

Eye banks and corneal tissue–processing facilities have been well established in many parts of the world. Progress in eye banking methodology and awareness has followed the advances in surgical techniques, instrumentation, and research involved in corneal grafting. This is especially true of many developed countries where waiting lists for transplantation have been practically eliminated. For many developing countries and the remainder in the developed world, problems ranging from the lack of political will to sociocultural barriers and limited resources continue to limit corneal tissue supply.[50]

This chapter is an attempt to describe the current status of eye-banking facilities in international settings, largely based on our personal communications with some leading international ophthalmologists, corneal surgeons, and directors or representatives of eye banking organizations. The term "eye bank" or "eye banking facility" as used here refers to any facility or organization involved in the supply of corneal tissue for the primary purpose of grafting. Such facility performs activities that include procuring, processing, storing, importing, or distributing corneal tissues. In this chapter, the following terms describing international eye banking facilities are used: "passive," denoting an organization that merely imports or distributes corneas; "active," one that is involved in obtaining, processing, storing, and distributing corneas; "private," one that serves the needs of an individual surgeon or surgeons of just one institution; and "public," one that supplies corneas to local, regional, or international surgeons or organizations. Thus an eye bank can be passive-private, passive-public, active-private, or active-public.

INTERNATIONAL EYE BANKING: CURRENT STATUS

Facilities for supply of corneal tissues have emerged in different countries (see Box) since 1935 when Vladimir Filatov reported the enucleation, preservation at 4° to 6° C, and use of cadaver eyes for corneal grafting in Odessa in the Ukraine.[20,32] In 1945, the first American eye bank was opened in New York.[35] Today, approximately 100 eye banks are in place in the United States.[17] The rapid proliferation of eye banks and increasing interest by ophthalmologists in doing corneal grafting are indicated by some 86,000 corneas recovered and approximately 36,000 transplants done in North America alone in 1990.[18]

Many eye banks have likewise been established in several countries. Active-private eye banking facilities (Table 53-1) have served many ophthalmic surgeons and institutions, including some leading eye

Table 53-1. Active-Private Eye-Banking Facilities

Name of Eye Banking Facility	Tissue Source and Number	Tissue Storage: Medium Used	Tissue Importation Number	Number Used for Transplant	Number Used for Research
Eye Bank of Haukeland Hospital (Norway)	County hospital: 183	+ : Minimum essential medium	+ : 1-2		10-15
Eye Department, Ulleval Hospital (Norway)	Public Hospital: 50			50	
Eye Clinic, Freie Universität Berlin	Public hospital: 50 Coroner: 5	+ : Dexsol		50	

YEAR OF ESTABLISHMENT OF SOME EYE BANKS AROUND THE WORLD

1935   Modern eye banking conceived by Filatov in Odessa in the Ukraine
1945   Eye Bank for Sight Restoration, Inc. (New York, USA)
1955   Eye Bank of Canada, Ontario Division (Toronto, Canada)
1958   Sri Lanka International Eye Bank (Colombo, Sri Lanka)
1959   Corneo Plastic Unit and Eye Bank, The Queen Victoria Hospital (East Grinstead, UK)
1960   Pirogov Scientific Institute for Emergency Medicine Tissue Bank (Sofia, Bulgaria)
1962   Medical Eye Bank of Maryland—Tissue Banks International (Baltimore, USA)
1963   Osaka Eye Bank (Osaka, Japan)
1964   Hong Kong Eye Bank and Research Foundation (Hong Kong)
1965   Eye Bank, Moorfields Eye Hospital (London, UK)
1967   Kangnam St. Mary's Hospital Eye Bank (Seoul, Korea)
1968   Penyantun Mata Tunanetra (Eye Bank) DKI Jakarta (Jakarta, Indonesia)
1970   Banco de Ojos Piloto, Instituto Nacional Oftalmología, Ministry of Health (Lima, Peru)
        University Eye Clinic Steglitz (Berlin, Germany)
1974   Eye Bank Foundation of South Africa (Cape Town, South Africa)
1980   Cornea Bank Rotterdam (Rotterdam, the Netherlands)
1981   Lions Model Eye Bank (Madras, India)
1983   Lions Eye Bank of South Australia (Bedford Park, South Australia)
1984   El-Maghraby Eye Hospital Eye Bank (Jidda, Saudi Arabia)
1986   Eye Bank, Bristol Eye Hospital (Bristol, UK)
        Lions Eye Bank of Western Australia (Nedlands, Western Australia)
        Eye Bank of Shanghai Medical University (Shanghai, People's Republic of China)
1988   Eye Bank of Intersectoral Research and Technology Complex "Eye Microsurgery" (Moscow, Russia)
        Keratec Eye Bank (London, UK)
        David Lucas Eye Bank (Manchester, UK)
1989   Eye Bank of Haukeland Hospital (Bergen, Norway)
        Lions Eye Bank of New South Wales (Potts Point, Australia)
        'Ain Shams University Eye Bank (Cairo, Egypt)
        Cairo University Eye Bank (Cairo, Egypt)
        Ramayamma International Eye Bank (Hyderabad, India)
1990   Beijing Tongren Eye Bank (Beijing, China)
        Chittagong Eye Infirmary and Training Complex Eye Bank (Chittagong, Bangladesh)
        American University Eye Bank (Beirut, Lebanon)
1991   São Paulo Hospital Eye Bank (São Paulo, Brazil)
        Lions Eye Bank—Melbourne (Melbourne, Australia)
        Queensland Eye Bank (Queensland, Australia)
        Eye Bank of Prague, Czechoslovakia (Prague, Czechoslovakia)
Soon   Singapore National Eye Bank (Singapore)
to
open

Table 53-2.   Active-Public Eye Banks in Different Countries

Name of Eye Bank	Tissue Source and Number[a]	Tissue Storage: No. and Medium used[b]	Number of Imported Tissues[c]	Distribution Local[d]	Regional[e]	International[f]	Distribution Surgery[g]	Research[h]	Training[i]
Africa									
Eye Bank Foundation of South Africa	PrH 47, Cor 1436	+:1246: M-K		+	+	+	1200	46	
America									
Eye Bank of Canada (Ontario Division)	PuH 1600, Cor, MD	+: : DX		+	+				
Banco de Ojos Pioloto, INO (Peru)	National Morgue 180	+: : M-K		+			20		
São Paulo Hospital EB (Brazil)	PPH 360, Cor 120, Mrt, MD	+:	+	+			360*		120*
Banco de Córneas del Leonismo Chileño	PuH 200, Cor	+: 200: TC 199		+			200		
Asia									
Beijing Tongren Eye Bank (China)	PuH 210	+: 200: K-S, M-K		+			126	6	5
Eye Bank of Shanghai Medical University (China)	PuH 100	+: 20: Medium 1640		+	+		80	20	10
Osaka Eye Bank (Japan)	PuH 115, Cor 2, MD 20	+: 8: EP II	+: 2	+	+		12		
Kangnam St. Mary's Hospital Eye Bank (Korea)	PuH 170	+: : MC		+			130	20	20
Penyantun Eye Bank (Indonesia)		+: 19:	+:140		+		145		
Chittagong Eye Infirmary and Training Complex Eye Bank (Bangladesh)	PuH 24	+: : MC		+	+				
Ramayamma International Eye Bank (India)	PuH96*, Cor, destitute homes 24*	+: 15: MC & DX	+				96*		24*
Lions Model Eye Bank (Madras, India)	Voluntary donors 308	+: : MC		+			268	20	20

Eye Bank	Sources[a]	Import[c]	Storage[b]	[d]	[e]	[f]	[g]	[h]	[i]
Sri Lanka International Eye Bank	PPH 4800, Cor, Mrt	+:	: M-K, Optisol	+	+	+	2750		350
El-Maghraby Eye Hospital Eye Bank (Saudi)	PuH 32	+: 11:	M-K, Optisol	+:418	+	+	387	42	18
Europe									
Keratec Eye Bank (UK)	PPH 250, Cor 50 MD 5	+: 300:	QC	+: 10	+	+	150	50	10
Pigorov Scientific Institute for Emergency Medicine Tissue Bank (Bulgaria)	PuH 196			+			196		
Cornea Bank Rotterdam	PuH 100, Cor	+:	: MEM	+	+				
Oceania									
Lions Eye Bank—Melbourne	PPH 336*, Mrt 48*	+:384*:	M-K	+					
Lions Eye Bank of South Australia	PuH 286, Cor 40, Mrt 20	+ :	M-K	+	+				
Lions Eye Bank of Western Australia	PuH 164, Cor 22	+: 160:	M-K & Dx			+	121	20	
Russian Federation Eye Bank of Intersectional Research and Technology Complex "Eye Microsurgery" (Moscow)	PuH and Cor: 1718	+: 280:	Dx & Rmcs	+		970	528	220	

The unit of all numbers given is "per year," based on 1991 figures of the eye banks.

"*", An estimate, based on the figure during the month of June, July, *or* August of 1991.

"+", Activity done by the eye bank.

" " (blank), No response given by the person who answered the questionnaire.

[a] Sources of eye tissues include *Cor*, coroners, medical examiners, pathologists; *MD*, individual physicians; *Mrt*, morticians/funeral homes; *PPH*, both public and private hospitals; *PrH*, private hospitals; *PuH*, public hospitals; and others, as cited.

[b] Storage of eye tissues. Methods used include *MC* (moist chamber) and *M-K* (McCarey-Kaufman) medium for short-term storage; *K-S* (K-Sol) and *DX* (Dexsol) for intermediate-term storage; *MEM* (minimum essential medium) and *OC* (organ culture) medium for long-term storage; *Rmcs* (Russian media for corneal storage); and others, as cited.

[c] Importing of processed corneal tissues from local, regional, or international eye banks.

[d] Distribution of corneal tissues to local (within the province or state) surgeons, hospitals, or eye banks.

[e] Distribution of corneal tissues to regional (outside the province or state but within the country) surgeons, hospitals, or eye banks.

[f] Distribution of corneal tissues to foreign (international) surgeons, hospitals, or eye banks.

[g] Number of corneas distributed to surgeons, hospitals, or eye banks for corneal transplantation.

[h] Number of corneas distributed for research purposes.

[i] Number of corneas distributed for training or teaching purposes.

centers in the world. Active-public eye banks have been in place in the United Kingdom, the Netherlands, Bulgaria, the Russian Federation, Egypt, South Africa, Saudi Arabia, India, Sri Lanka, Bangladesh, Indonesia, Australia, China, Korea, Japan, Canada, Peru, Chile, and Brazil (Tables 53-2).

In recent years, some eye banking organizations in the United States have taken an active role in promoting an international network of eye banks. With support from the Saudi Eye Foundation, Tissue Banks International (TBI—formerly Medical Eye Bank of Maryland), a recognized leader among all eye banking facilities,[32] established the International Federation of Eye Banks (IFEB). This was in response to the critical need for quality eye banks and corneas in less developed and developed countries. IFEB helps establish eye banks and monitors the quality of facilities and eye tissue for its member eye banks. It also serves as an information network for them. Through the support of its board, IFEB has reached an inimitable level of understanding, sophistication, and commitment by identifying countries where the need for eye banking is apparent, the determination to generate political will and cultural acceptance is genuine for a sustainable impact, and an infrastructure exists with the potential for recovering, processing, and storing quality tissue along with training and teaching local ophthalmologists in surgical skills.[49] This has led to the establishment of active-public eye banks in Cairo, Jidda, Riyadh, and Hyderabad; the networking with eye banks in Bristol and Shanghai; and the preparations for the future opening of eye banks in Prague, Barcelona, Casablanca, Colombo, Chittagong, Damascus, and Mexico City. For a number of Latin American countries, initiatives have come from the Eye Bank Association of America (EBAA) and the Asociación Pan-Americana de Bancos de Ojos (APABO, Pan-American Association of Eye Banks) in training eye banks directors and technicians, increasing public awareness of tissue donation, and guiding and uniting, through the Sister Eye Bank Program, North and South American eye banks.[19]

Following is a description of the current status of eye banking in different regions and countries around the world, excluding the United States.

Africa. In northern Africa, two eye banks have recently opened in Egypt with the assistance of the International Federation of Eye Banks (IFEB). A total of about 1200 corneas per year are distributed from the Cairo-based 'Ain Shams University and Cairo University Eye Banks.[15] These will help restore sight to some 10,000 Egyptians with corneal blindness in Cairo alone.[21] Their success is mainly attributed to the implementation of the Presumed Consent Law, which allows the removal of eye tissue in medicolegal cases without the permission of next of kin. It also relies on the support of the IFEB, Saudi Eye Foundation, the Ministry of Health, and religious leaders in Egypt. Plans are now underway to open up an eye bank in Casablanca, Morocco.

Currently, there is no known eye bank actively operating in western[14,56] and middle Africa. In eastern Africa, corneas for keratoplasties done in Ethiopia, Malawi, and Zimbabwe in the past came directly from mortuaries and were not preserved.[43] Some tissues used in Malawi came from the Eye Bank Foundation in Cape Town, South Africa.[8] In the late 1970s, one eye bank was known to exist in Kenya, but it was not very active.[43]

In 1974, the Eye Bank Foundation of South Africa (formerly the Cape Bank Foundation) was established in Cape Town, with the assistance of one of the authors (Griffith). At present, it is processing about 1400 corneal tissues per year for supply to the whole of South Africa and its neighboring states, such as the autonomous republics of Transkei and Ciskei,[40] as well as to surgeons in Namibia, Mauritania, Zambia, Israel, and Taiwan.[41]

America. The Eye Bank of Canada (EBC) was established in 1955 and was the source of tissue for the first keratoplasty in the country. There are at least five active-public eye banks in Canada,[10] among which the EBC (Ontario Division) handles the most tissue. For ophthalmologists in centers away from the EBC, tissues from local sources are frequently used.[7]

Six years after the creation of the APABO by the Pan-American Association of Ophthalmology, there are now a total of 37 member eye banks in Latin America (Table 52-3). APABO has also been instrumental in the passage of the Presumed Consent Law in Costa Rica, Panama, Puerto Rico, Colombia, and Peru.[19] Total number of tissues collected have increased, although importation, largely from Fresno, Houston, Phoenix, and Miami, continues. Training of local eye surgeons is facilitated by ophthalmologists affiliated with Project ORBIS.* APABO continues to provide training for Latin American eye bank technicians.

In Peru, there are seven active-public eye banks, four of which are in Lima and one each in Trujillo, Arequipa and Piura.[51] Chile has one public eye bank, but each hospital collects its own corneas for

---

*Latin *orbis* 'circle (of the world), disk, hollow of the eye'.

Table 52-3. Latin American Member Eye Banks of the Asociación Pan Americana de Bancos de Ojos (APABO, Pan-American Association of Eye Banks)

Location		Name of Eye Bank
Argentina	Buenos Aires	Banco de Ojos de la Fundación Oftalmológica Argentina Malbrán
		Banco de Ojos Club de Leones
Brazil	Curitiba	Banco de Olhos de Curitiba
	Santa Catarina	Banco de Olhos de Joinvile
	Manaus	Banco de Olhos de Manaus
	Rio de Janeiro	Banco de Olhos Cruz Vermelda Brasileira
		Banco de Olhos del Hospital Bonsucesso
Chile	Santiago	Banco de Córneas del Leonismo Chileno
	Valparaíso	Banco de Córneas/Tejidos del Club de Leones
Colombia	Barranquilla	Banco de Ojos del Caribe
	Bogotá	Banco de Córneas Fundación Oftalmológica Nacional
		Banco de Ojos Fundación Santa Fe
		Banco de Ojos Hospital Militar Central
		Banco de Ojos Hospital San Juan de Dios
		Banco de Ojos Instituto Barraquer de América
	Bucaramanga	Banco de Ojos Fundación Oftalmológica de Santander
	Cali	Banco de Ojos del Occidente Colombiano
	Medellín	Banco de Ojos Cruz Roja de Antioquía
Costa Rica	San José	Asociación Filantrópica de Leones de Costa Rica
Cuba	La Habana	Banco de Ojos Hospital Hermanos Ameijeiras
Dominican Republic	Santo Domingo	Banco de Córneas de la República Dominicana
Ecuador	Quito	Banco de Ojos Nacional
	Guayaquil	Banco de Ojos de la Fundación Oftalmológica Ecuatoriana
El Salvador	San Salvador	Banco de Ojos de El Salvador
Guatemala	Guatemala City	Banco de Ojos Hospital Dr. Rodolfo Robles Valverde
Honduras	Tegucigalpa	Banco de Córneas
Mexico	Guanajuato	Banco de Ojos de León, AC
		Banco de Ojos del Hospital General Regional
	Coyoacán	Banco de Ojos Hospital Asociación Para Evitar la Ceguera en México
	Nuevo León	Banco de Córneas de Monterrey
	Puebla	Centro de Córneas de la Cruz Roja Mexicana
Nicaragua	Managua	Banco de Córneas de Managua
Panama	Panama City	Banco de Ojos del Club de Leones de Panamá
Paraguay	Asunción	Fundación Banco de Ojos
Peru	Lima	Banco de Ojos del Instituto Nacional Oftalmología
		Banco de Corneas del Hospital María Auxiliadora
Venezuela	Caracas	Banco de Ojos del Hospital Miguel Pérez Carreño

its own needs.[2] Brazil reportedly has 70 eye banking facilities, though six are considered as the major ones, two of which are in São Paulo, and one each in Macedo, Curitiba, Rio, and Belo Horizonte.[5] To achieve better cooperation among the eye banks in Colombia, the Asociación Colombiana de Bancos de Ojos was founded in 1989.[19] McCarey-Kaufman medium,[29] a modified tissue culture (TC) 199 medium for short-term storage, is now manufactured in Colombia.

Asia. Eye banks exist in major centers in China: two in Beijing and one each in Shanghai, Hangzhou, and Guangzhou and in Henan province. All facilities combined benefit about 100 to 200 patients for corneal transplant.[11] However, eye banking remains underdeveloped, largely because of the absence of a presumed consent law, as well as laws that protect physicians and coroners against lawsuits filed by donors' relatives. As a consequence, only a small proportion of ophthalmologists, about 50 out of 10,000, are trained to do corneal grafting in China.[36,37] Meanwhile, creation of a nationwide network to coordinate research work and share technology has been considered.[36] In Hong Kong, the Eye Bank and Research Foundation continues to import 15 corneal tissues per month from Sri Lanka. However, this passive eye bank is slowly transforming into an active bank by recruiting staff to counsel families of potential donors in the hospital.[57]

Japan has about 45 eye banks, approximately one

in each of the 46 prefectures.[34] The government-approved Nippon Eye Bank Association regulates eye banking activities. A total of 1400 corneas per year are collected from all eye banks, the majority of which, though classified as active-public,[30] only process one to two corneas per year.[34] Despite its advanced technologic status, Japan has encountered difficulties in organ procurement. Its legal department opposes any presumed consent law, and pathologists and coroners have yet to become committed to an important role in recovering cadaver eyes for purposes of keratoplasty.[34] Only a few eye departments, mainly those specializing in the external diseases of the eye, are active in obtaining corneal tissue. Approximately 15,000 Japanese need to undergo corneal grafting.[30]

South Korea has four major eye banks in Seoul. All eye banks serve about 300 patients for grafting in 1 year.[28] The oldest active eye bank is the Central Eye Bank of the Catholic University Medical College's St. Mary's Hospital. Other eye banks have opened in the past, but their activities were limited by religious beliefs and customs that oppose organ donation after death.[27] For the past 3 years, Korean Catholic churches have campaigned favorably for eye donation. This has led to more than 4000 registered donors and about 400 actual donations.[28]

Likewise, the picture in Southeast Asia is far from ideal. Malaysia has two eye banks, both passive-private, which account for 80 to 100 corneas per year, against the estimated 5000 needing corneal transplantation per year.[47] The removal of eyes is not only culturally considered as mutilation of the body, but also as an act that renders the spirit of the dead blind.[46] In Indonesia, the Penyantun Mata Tunanetra (Eye Bank) DKI Jakarta is the only eye bank in the country. An active-public facility, it processes 15 and imports 140 corneas per year in response to nearly 168,000 individuals with corneal blindness.[24] Singapore currently has one passive eye bank, which receives approximately six imported corneas per month from Sri Lanka. A total of 70 patients currently need keratoplasty. Procuring tissues is likewise difficult among Singaporean Chinese, who believe that sight is necessary in the afterlife, and among Malays, who hold sacred the body, which must be kept intact even after death.[53] An eye donation campaign has continued as Singapore attempts to become self-sufficient with the establishment of the proposed Singapore National Eye Bank in 1992.

Perhaps the view of many East and Southeast Asians is well expressed in the statements made by the Minister of Health of Malaysia during an address on eye donation:

Communities, religions and beliefs hold sacred the human body both in life and after death. Although it is said that dust should be returned to dust, most beliefs are that the body should not be desecrated or mutilated after death but that it should be returned whole to its Maker, whatever the individual perception of the Maker may be. Belief is particularly strong where the human eyes are concerned. There is no departed soul more hopeless in the view of many of the traditionally minded people in certain sections of our community, as one without eyes. A lost soul without eyes in their reckoning comes about when a person who has died has his eyes removed. This in turn is founded on the belief that although our ancestors may be dead and gone, they have also their benign share in shaping the destiny of those they have left behind them. And if a particular ancestor has lost his sight, then how can he guide the present generation along in its path towards prosperity? Belief in the supernatural and ties to ancestor worship can therefore also take a materialistic turn.[46]

As of 1989, there had been over 120 eye banks formally established in the whole of India, about 20 of which were collecting 50 or more eye tissues per year.[25]

The most successful ones include the Red Cross Eye Bank in Dholka, Gujarat (an IFEB member) and the eye bank at Harkish Andas Hospital in Bombay, with each harvesting 500 to 700 corneas per year.[25] In 1989, IFEB helped establish the Ramayamma International Eye Bank in Hyderabad.[38] In that year, the Eye Bank Association of India was established to improve the quality of eye bank services, provide training for technicians, and maximally coordinate all eye banks in the country. Developing a uniform set of standards for all Indian eye banks is now a priority.[39] Although relatively small, these are determined efforts aimed at decreasing corneal blindness, which is now estimated to be at least 2 million.[31]

In Bangladesh, eye banking facilities are in a developing stage, with the assistance of IFEB. One active-public eye bank, the Chittagong Eye Infirmary and Training Complex Eye Bank, processes about 24 corneas per year. A few thousand patients per year can be served by all facilities in the country.[23]

In western Asia, two active-public eye banks, the El-Maghraby Eye Bank in Jidda, Saudi Arabia, and the King Khalid Eye Hospital Eye Bank in Riyadh, Saudi Arabia, have opened. With about 36 to 40 eye tissues processed in 1 year, eye tissue donation in both banks has been relatively scarce.[16] Thus the need is supplemented by importing eyes from Egypt, Sri Lanka, and the United States. In the Arab world, more public educational programs to educate the people about eye donation and the possibility of sight restoration, along with the passage of a presumed consent law, are needed. This also applies to other countries, including Jordan, where there is a known eye banking facility. Because of certain religious beliefs, Israel continues to import their corneas for keratoplasty.[15]

Europe. There is a strong eye banking system in northern Europe. In Norway, all 200 corneal grafts done every year are performed in one of the three major University Eye Clinics, Haukeland in Bergen, and Ulleval and Rikshospitalet in Oslo.[6] About 50 and 183 corneas per year are obtained from Ulleval.[60] and Haukeland, respectively. Since all donor tissues are solely for the use of their own departments, these facilities many qualify as private eye banks. Nonetheless, their scope of service extends to all corneally blind Norwegians in a population of 4 million. In Denmark, the Århus Kommunehospital provides tissue-typing services[6] to some European eye banks, as well as quality corneal tissues using the organ culture technique. This method,[12] which was extensively researched by Doughman and associates in Minnesota in the early 1970s,[50] allows a longer preservation time for human corneas from a few days to 30 days. Similar techniques have also been in use in the United Kingdom (U.K.) and several of Western European countries,[26] such as the Netherlands (see Chapter 46), Austria, and Germany.

In the U.K., there have been significant changes in corneal tissue supply since 1983 when corneal tissue started to be nationally distributed through the U.K. Transplant Service.[3] Coupled with the adoption of the organ culture preservation method, tissue wastage has significantly decreased and access increased.[26] Currently, there are 10 eye banking facilities in the U.K., six of which are active-public banks.[42] These include the East Grinstead, Moorfields, and Keratec eye banks in London and the eye banks in Bristol, Manchester,[13] and Norwich.[3] About 2500 eye tissues are processed in 1 year in Bristol alone.[13]

In the Netherlands, there are three eye banks, the Amsterdam Cornea Bank in North Holland and the Cornea Bank Rotterdam and Eurotransplant–Leyden in South Holland. Organ culture is used in these banks, but the McCarey-Kaufman medium is still used in Rotterdam.[4] Corneas from these eye banks make up the Eurotransplant pool, hence allowing greater tissue access and less wastage. Despite these advances, administrative procedures sometimes limit organizational efficiency.[4] Further, it is believed that a presumed consent law and strong grief-counseling programs can dramatically increase tissue donation rates.[4]

The situation for the rest of western and southern Europe still remains far from ideal.[56] Although Spain has six active eye banking facilities, none of these are public. An active-private eye bank, Banco de Ojos para la Ceguera of the Clínica Barraquer in Barcelona has served patients throughout Europe since its founding in 1966.[22] A major active-public bank is anticipated to open in the same city, with the support of local health authorities and the IFEB.[22]

A major international effort, aimed at promoting eye banking in Europe, has been realized with the organization of the European Association of Eye Banks in 1989.

There is currently no eye bank functioning in Hungary. All grafts are done using fresh donor material.[1] In Bulgaria, the Tissue Bank of the Pirogov Scientific Institute for Emergency Medicine (SIEM) of the Bulgarian Ministry of Health is the only place specialized for obtaining, processing, and distributing various tissues, including corneas for grafting. Thus, the practice of many ophthalmologists is to personally obtain fresh globes from the hospitals' mortuaries.[54] Currently processing 196 corneas per year, it distributes tissue, on demand, to Sofia, Varna, Blagoevgrad, and Stara Zagora.[54] In November 1991, a modern public eye bank was opened in Prague, Czechoslovakia, with the assistance of IFEB and the endorsement of the Czechoslovakian Transplant Council. With a presumed consent law that is in place, it is hoped that this facility will become a model eye bank in Eastern Europe.

Oceania. The status of eye banking in Australia, with five eye banks in Melbourne, Sydney, South Australia, West Australia, and Queensland, is quite ideal. This is especially so in South Australia, where waiting lists for corneal grafting have been eliminated.[55] For other states and territories, further expansion, with provision of tissue on request without a waiting list, may improve the situation.[52] Better national cooperation and mutual support and assistance, including interstate exchanges of tissue-typed corneas between eye banks,[9] will benefit not only Australia, but also the rest of the Asia-Pacific region.

The Russian Federation. One of the eye banks in the Russian Federation is the Eye Bank of Intersectoral Research and Technology Complex (ITRC) "Eye Microsurgery." Established in 1988, it is processing approximately 1700 corneas per year, roughly 970 of which are utilized for grafting purposes. Both fresh and stored corneas are used.[33]

THE FUTURE OF INTERNATIONAL EYE BANKING

As different countries are in different settings and stages of eye banking development, needs and problems necessarily vary. Common to most eye banks around the world is the relative shortage of corneal tissue supply, which is largely determined by four important variables: sociocultural acceptance of tissue donation, political will to frame and take advantage of appropriate laws, load of corneal blindness in the population, and the amount of resources available for program planning, implementation, and evaluation.

For countries with adequate resources and trained surgeons in the developed world, eye banking status can be greatly improved by enhancing social acceptance of tissue donation and developing strong policies to move forward.[49] This means passing appropriate laws, designing effective public awareness programs, investing in suitable eye banking technology, and so on. On the other hand, for less developed countries that have uniformly limited resources, surgical efforts, if needed, must be aimed at addressing other more common causes of blindness, such as cataracts, where sight can be restored with easier, simpler procedures. However, for some developing countries where there are pockets, especially in large urban centers, of technical and financial resources, where other causes of blindness are adequately addressed, and where the political will can allow a sustainable eye banking technology,[49] a good eye banking program has its rightful place, provided that local ophthalmologic expertise is commonly available and appropriate quality standards are aimed for.

With a better understanding of the current status and problems of facilities for corneal tissue supply, plus the growing national and international initiatives, the prospect of a successful surgical solution to corneal blindness, regionally and globally, seems nearer than ever!

ACKNOWLEDGMENTS

We wish to thank Sir John Wilson and Drs. A. Edward Maumenee, Alfred Sommer, Kenneth Kenyon, David Easty, and Akira Nakajima for sharing with one of us (CTV) their knowledge, ideas, and perspectives on international eye banking. We are equally grateful to all eye bank directors interviewed and to all respondents to the questionnaire, including those whose reply we received after our September 10, 1991, deadline. We also acknowledge Professor A.F. Deutman, Dr. Arthur Lim Siew Ming and Ms. Charity Wai, and Dr. Emile J. Farge and Mrs. Lourdes Fernandez for providing us with the addresses of some international ophthalmologists and experts in this field.

REFERENCES

1. Alberth, Bela: Letter to author, Aug 1991.
2. Arentsen, Juan S: Questionnaire reply to author, Aug 5, 1991.
3. Armitage WJ, Moss SJ, Easty, DL: Supply of corneal tissue in the United Kingdom, *Br J Ophthalmol* 74:685-687, 1990.
4. Beekhuis, W Houdijn: Questionnaire reply to author, Aug 25, 1991.
5. Belfort, Rubens, Sr: Questionnaire reply to author, Aug 2, 1991.
6. Bertelsen, Torstein: Questionnaire reply to author, Aug 19, 1991.
7. Chipman ML, Willett P, Basu PK, Wolf A: Donor eyes: a comparison of characteristics and outcomes for eye bank and local tissue, *Cornea* 8(1):62-66, 1989.
8. Chirambo, Moses: Letter to author, Aug 8, 1991.
9. Crewe, Julie M: Questionnaire reply to author, Aug 2, 1991.
10. Dixon, William S: Questionnaire reply to author, July 23, 1991.
11. Dong Dong-sheng: Questionnaire reply to author, July 30, 1991.
12. Doughman DJ, Harris JE, Schmitt MK: Penetrating keratoplasty using 37° C organ cultured cornea, *Ophthalmology* 81:778-793, 1976.
13. Easty, David: Telephone interview with author, July 30, 1991.
14. Egbert, Peter R: Letter to author, July 26, 1991.
15. El-Maghraby, Akef: Personal interview with author, Baltimore, July 28, 1991.
16. El-Maghraby, Akef: Questionnaire reply to author, July 20, 1991.
17. Eye Bank Association of America: *Membership Directory, 1989-1990*, Washington, DC.
18. Eye Bank Association of America: *Activity Report, 1990*, Washington, DC.
19. Farge, Emilio J: Questionnaire reply to author, Aug 1991.
20. Filatov VP: Transplantation of the cornea, *Arch Ophthalmol* 13:321-347, 1935.
21. Griffith FN: The promise of international eye banking, *Int Ophthalmol* 14(3):205-210, 1990.
22. Henríquez, Antonio S: Letter and questionnaire reply to author, July 26, 1991.
23. Husain, Rabiul: Letter and questionnaire reply to author, Aug 28, 1991.
24. Istiantoro: Questionnaire reply to author, Djakarta, Aug 26, 1991.
25. Kalevar V: Eye banking in India, *Ind J Ophthalmol* 37(3):110-111, 1989.
26. Kenyon, Kenneth: Telephone interview with author, July 22, 1991.
27. Kim, JH: Corneal transplantation in Korea, *JAMA Korea*, pp 5-6, July 1988.
28. Kim Jae-Ho: Questionnaire reply to author, Aug 8, 1991.
29. McCarey BE, Kaufman HE: Improved corneal storage, *Invest Ophthalmol* 13:165, 1974.
30. Manabe, Reizo: Letter and questionnaire to author, July 29, 1991.
31. Mathew, Vimi: Letter and questionnaire reply to author, Aug 29, 1991.
32. Maumenee, A Edward: Personal interview with author, Baltimore, July 17, 1991.
33. Moroz, Zinaida I: Letter and questionnaire reply to author, Aug 9, 1991.
34. Nakajima, Akira: Telephone interview with author, July 24, 1991.
35. Payne, JW: New directions in eye banking, *Trans Am Ophthalmol Soc* 78:983-1026, 1980.
36. Qiu Xiaozhi: Telephone interview with author, July 29, 1991.
37. Qiu Xiaozhi: Questionnaire reply to the author, July 31, 1991.

38. Rao, Gullapalli N: Telephone interview with author, July 25, 1991.
39. Rao, Gullapalli N: Letter and questionnaire reply to author, Aug 30, 1991.
40. Roome, Shirley D: Letter and questionnaire reply to author, July 30, 1991.
41. Roome, Shirley D: Telephone interview with author, Aug 30, 1991.
42. Rostron, CK: Questionnaire reply to author, Aug 11, 1991.
43. Schwab, Larry: Letter to author, Aug 2, 1991.
44. Seiler, Theo: Questionnaire reply to author, Aug 6, 1991.
45. Silva, Hudson FG: Paper presented to the Pan-Ophthalmologica 1991, Sept 6-8, 1991.
46. Singh, Keshmahinder: Letter to author, Aug 5, 1991.
47. Singh, Keshmahinder: Letter and questionnaire reply to author, Aug 13, 1991.
48. Sommer, Alfred: Letter to Frederick N. Griffith, July 10, 1991.
49. Sommer, Alfred: Personal interview with author, Baltimore, July 15, 1991.
50. Summerlin WT, Miller GE, Harris JE, Good RA: The organ-cultured cornea: an in-vitro study, *Invest Ophthalmol Vis Sci* 12:176-180, 1973.
51. Takayama, Daniel A: Questionnaire reply to author, Aug 12, 1991.
52. Taylor, Hugh R: Letter and questionnaire reply to author, Aug 16, 1991.
53. Tseng, Peter SF: Questionnaire reply to author, July 30, 1991.
54. Vassileva, Petja: Letter and questionnaire reply to author, Sept 9, 1991.
55. Wedding, Trevor R: Questionnaire reply to author, Aug 6, 1991.
56. Wilson, Sir John: Telephone interview with author, July 24, 1991.
57. Woo Chipang, Victor: Questionnaire reply to author, Aug 30, 1991.
58. World Health Organization: Available data on blindness (update 1987), Geneva, WHO/PBL/87.14, pp 1-23, 1987 (unpublished).
59. World Health Organization: Report of the Interregional Meeting on control of cornea blindness within primary health care systems, Geneva, WHO/PBL/89.16, pp 1-22, 1989 (unpublished).
60. Ytteborg, Jan: Questionnaire reply to author, Aug 21, 1991.

Index

C